W9-BBY-111

SAUNDERS

Q&A REVIEW *for the*
NCLEX-RN®
EXAMINATION

"ലോക നമ്മുടെ വേദനകൾ ഏറ്റെടുക്കുകയും രോഗങ്ങൾ വഹിക്കുകയും ചെയ്തു."

SAUNDERS

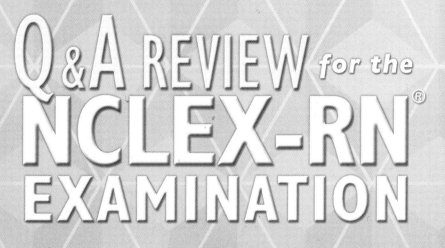

Q&A REVIEW *for the* NCLEX-RN® EXAMINATION

THIRD EDITION

LINDA ANNE SILVESTRI, MSN, RN
Instructor of Nursing
Salve Regina University
Newport, Rhode Island

President
Nursing Reviews, Inc.
and
Professional Nursing Seminars, Inc.
Charlestown, Rhode Island

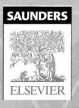

SAUNDERS

ELSEVIER

ELSEVIER
SAUNDERS

11830 Westline Industrial Drive
St. Louis, Missouri 63146

SAUNDERS Q&A REVIEW FOR THE NCLEX-RN® EXAMINATION   ISBN-13: 978-0-7216-0352-0

Copyright © 2006, Elsevier Inc. All rights reserved.   ISBN-10: 0-7216-0352-1

NCLEX-RN® is a registered trademark and service mark of the National Council of State Boards of Nursing, Inc.

No part of this publication may be reproduced or transmitted in any form or by any means, electronic or mechanical, including photocopying, recording, or any information storage and retrieval system, without permission in writing from the publisher. Permissions may be sought directly from Elsevier's Health Sciences Rights Department in Philadelphia, PA, USA: phone: (+1) 215 238 7869, fax: (+1) 215 238 2239, e-mail: healthpermissions@elsevier.com. You may also complete your request on-line via the Elsevier homepage (http://www.elsevier.com), by selecting 'Customer Support' and then 'Obtaining Permissions'.

Notice

Pharmacology is an ever-changing field. Standard safety precautions must be followed, but as new research and clinical experience broaden our knowledge, changes in treatment and drug therapy may become necessary or appropriate. Readers are advised to check the most current product information provided by the manufacturer of each drug to be administered to verify the recommended dose, the method and duration of administration, and contraindications. It is the responsibility of the licensed prescriber, relying on experience and knowledge of the patient, to determine dosages and the best treatment for each individual patient. Neither the publisher nor the author assumes any liability for any injury and/or damage to persons or property arising from this publication.

Director, Review and Testing: Loren S. Wilson
Managing Editor: Nancy O'Brien
Associate Developmental Editor: Charlene R.M. Ketchum
Production Services Manager: Jeff Patterson
Project Manager: Jeanne Genz
Designer: Jyotika Shroff

Printed in the United States of America
Last digit is the print number: 9   8   7   6   5   4   3   2   1

ISBN-13: 978-0-7216-0352-0

Working together to grow
libraries in developing countries

www.elsevier.com | www.bookaid.org | www.sabre.org

ELSEVIER   BOOK AID International   Sabre Foundation

J. Mathew

To my father,
ARNOLD LAWRENCE
My memories of his love, support,
and words of encouragement will remain
in my heart forever!

and

To my nursing students, past, present,
and future; their inspiration has
brought many professional rewards
to my life!

About the Author

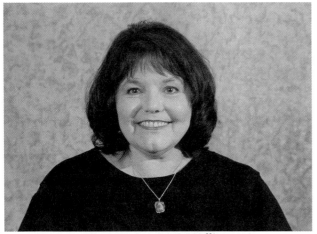

Photo by Laurent W. Valliere

ABOUT THE AUTHOR

Linda Anne Silvestri received her diploma in nursing at Cooley Dickinson Hospital School of Nursing in Northampton, Massachusetts. Afterward, she worked at Baystate Medical Center in Springfield, Massachusetts, in acute medical-surgical units, the intensive care unit, the emergency department, pediatric units, and other acute care units. She later received an associate degree from Holyoke Community College in Holyoke, Massachusetts, and then received her BSN from American International College in Springfield, Massachusetts.

A native of Springfield, Massachusetts, Linda began her teaching career as an instructor of medical-surgical nursing and leadership-management nursing at Baystate Medical Center School of Nursing in 1981. In 1985, she earned her MSN from Anna Maria College in Paxton, Massachusetts, with a dual major in Nursing Management and Patient Education. Linda is a member of Sigma Theta Tau.

Linda relocated to Rhode Island in 1989 and began teaching advanced medical-surgical nursing and psychiatric nursing to RN and LPN students at the Community College of Rhode Island. While teaching at the Community College of Rhode Island, a group of students approached Linda, asking her to help them prepare for the NCLEX examination. Based on her experience as a nursing educator and as an NCLEX item writer, she developed a comprehensive review course to prepare nursing graduates for the NCLEX examination. In 1994, Linda began teaching medical-surgical nursing at Salve Regina University in Newport, Rhode Island. She also prepares nursing students at Salve Regina University for the NCLEX-RN examination.

In 1991, Linda established Professional Nursing Seminars, Inc., and in 2000, she established Nursing Reviews, Inc. Both companies are dedicated to conducting NCLEX-RN and NCLEX-PN review courses and assisting nursing graduates to achieve their goals of becoming Registered Nurses and/or Licensed Practical/Vocational Nurses.

Today, Linda Silvestri's companies conduct NCLEX review courses throughout New England. She is the successful author of numerous NCLEX-RN and NCLEX-PN review products, including *Saunders Comprehensive Review for the NCLEX-RN Examination, Saunders Q&A Review for the NCLEX-RN Examination, Saunders Strategies for Success for the NCLEX-RN Examination, Saunders Computerized Review for the NCLEX-RN Examination, Saunders Instructor's Resource Package for NCLEX-RN, Saunders Comprehensive Review for the NCLEX-PN Examination, Saunders Q&A Review for the NCLEX-PN Examination, Saunders Review Cards for the NCLEX-PN Examination,* and *Saunders Instructor's Resource Package for NCLEX-PN.* Linda has also authored several online products, including the online specialty tests titled *Adult Health, Mental Health, Maternal-Newborn, Pediatrics, and Pharmacology,* and the *Saunders Online Review Course for the NCLEX-RN Examination.*

Contributors

Rebecca S. Blaszczak, RN
Graduate, Department of Nursing
Salve Regina University
Newport, Rhode Island

Laurent W. Valliere, BS
Vice President
Professional Nursing Seminars, Inc.
Charlestown, Rhode Island

The author and publisher would also like to acknowledge the following individuals for contributions to the previous editions of this book:

Marianne P. Barba, MS, RN
Care New England
Coventry, Rhode Island

Nancy Blasdell, MSN, RN
Doctoral Student
University of Rhode Island
Kingston, Rhode Island

Barbara Bono-Snell, MS, RN, CS
Psychiatric Clinical Nurse Specialist
St. Joseph's Certified Home Health Care Agency
Liverpool, New York

Netta Moncur Bowen, MSN, RN
Nursing Faculty
Seminole Community College
Sanford, Florida

Carolyn Pierce Buckelew, RNCS, NC, CHyp
Nursing Instructor
Charles E. Gregory School of Nursing
Raritan Bay Medical Center
Perth Amboy, New Jersey

Janis M. Byers, MSN, RNC
Nursing Faculty
Sewickley Valley Hospital School of Nursing
Sewickley, Pennsylvania

Penny S. Cass, PhD, RN
Dean, Division of Nursing
Indiana University Kokomo
Kokomo, Indiana

Deborah H. Chatham, RN, MS, CS
Assistant Professor of Nursing
William Carey College
Gulfport, Mississippi

Tom Christenbery, MSN, RN
Assistant Professor of Nursing
Tennessee State University
Nashville, Tennessee

Anita M. Creamer, RN, MS, CS
Associate Professor of Nursing
Community College of Rhode Island
Warwick, Rhode Island

Barbara A. Dagastine, EdMSN, RN
Associate Professor of Nursing
Hudson Valley Community College
Troy, New York

Jean DeCoffe, MSN, RN
Assistant Professor of Nursing
Curry College
Milton, Massachusetts

DeAnna Jan Emory, MS, RN
Assistant Professor of Nursing
Bacone College
Muskogee, Oklahoma

Mary E. Farrell, MS, RN, CCRN
Associate Professor of Nursing
Salem State College
Salem, Massachusetts

Patsy H. Fasnacht, MSN, RN, CCRN
Nursing Instructor
Lancaster Institute for Health Education
Lancaster, Pennsylvania

Dona Ferguson, MSN, RN, C
Assistant Professor of Nursing and
Chair, Nursing and Allied Health
Atlantic Community College
Mays Landing, New Jersey

Thomas E. Folcarelli, MSN, RN
Associate Professor of Nursing
Community College of Rhode Island
Newport, Rhode Island

Florence Hayes Gibson, MSN, CNS
Associate Professor of Nursing
Northeast Louisiana University
Monroe, Louisiana

Alma V. Harkey, RNC, MSN, ACCE
Instructor of Nursing
Southeast Missouri State University
Cape Girardeau, Missouri

Joyce Ellen Heil, BSN, CCRN
Assistant Instructor of Nursing
St. Margaret School of Nursing
Pittsburgh, Pennsylvania

Barbara Hicks, DSN, RN
Instructor of Nursing
Central Alabama Community College
Coosa Valley School of Nursing
Sylacauga, Alabama

Mary Ann Hogan, RN, CS, MSN
Clinical Assistant Professor
University of Massachusetts
Amherst, Massachusetts

Noreen M. Houck, MS, RN
Assistant Director
Crouse Hospital School of Nursing
Syracuse, New York

Amy Lawyer Hudson, RN, MSN
Nursing Faculty
Phillips Community College
University of Arkansas
Helene, Arkansas

Frances E. Johnson, MS, RNC
Assistant Professor of Nursing
Andrews University
Berrien Springs, Michigan

Deborah Klaas, RN, PhD
Assistant Professor of Nursing
Northern Arizona University
Flagstaff, Arizona

June Peterson Larson, RN, MS
Associate Professor of Nursing
University of South Dakota
Vermillion, South Dakota

Suzanne K. Marnocha, RN, MSN, CCRN
Assistant Professor of Nursing
University of Wisconsin, Oshkosh
Oshkosh, Wisconsin

Ellen Frances McCarty, PhD, RN, CS
Professor of Nursing
Salve Regina University
Newport, Rhode Island

Connie M. Metzler, MSN, RN
Instructor of Nursing
Lancaster Institute for Health Education
Lancaster, Pennsylvania

Patricia A. Miller, MSN, RN
Former Director, School of Nursing
Baystate Medical Center School of Nursing
Springfield, Massachusetts

Jo Ann Barnes Mullaney, PhD, RN, CS
Professor of Nursing
Salve Regina University
Newport, Rhode Island

Kathleen Ann Ohman, RN, MS, EdD
Associate Professor of Nursing
College of St. Benedict/St. John's University
St. Joseph, Minnesota

Lynda C. Opdyke, RN, MSN
Facilitator/Academic Affairs
Mercy School of Nursing
Charlotte, North Carolina

MaeDella Perry, RN, MSN
Nurse Educator
Medical College of Georgia
Augusta, Georgia

Lisa A. Ruth-Sahd, MSN, RN, CEN, CCRN
Nursing Instructor
Lancaster Institute for Health Education
Lancaster, Pennsylvania
Adjunct Faculty
York College of Pennsylvania
York, Pennsylvania

Jeanine T. Seguin, MS, RN, CS
Assistant Professor of Nursing
Keuka College
Keuka Park, New York

Alberta Elaine Severs, MSN, MA, RN
Associate Professor of Nursing
Community College of Rhode Island
Lincoln, Rhode Island

Kimberly Sharpe, MS, RN
Instructor of Nursing
Crouse Hospital School of Nursing
Syracuse, New York

Susan Sienkiewicz, MA, RN, CS
Associate Professor of Nursing
Community College of Rhode Island
Lincoln, Rhode Island

Yvonne Marie Smith, MSN, RN, CCRN
Instructor
Aultman Hospital School of Nursing
Canton, Ohio

Judith Stamp MS, RN
Assistant Professor of Nursing
Hudson Valley Community College
Troy, New York

Yvonne Nazareth Stringfield, EdD, RN
Associate Professor of Nursing
BSN Program Director
Tennessee State University
Nashville, Tennessee

Mattie Tolley, RN, MS
Instructor of Nursing
Southwestern Oklahoma State University
Weatherford, Oklahoma

Johanna M. Tracy, MSN, RN, CS
Instructor of Nursing
Mercer Medical Center
Trenton, New Jersey

Joyce I. Turnbull, RN, MN
Nursing Lecturer/Clinical Instructor
San Jose State University
San Jose, California

Paula A. Viau, PhD, RN
Associate Dean of Nursing
University of Rhode Island
Kingston, Rhode Island

Carol Warner, RN, CPN, MSN
Instructor of Nursing
St. Luke's School of Nursing
Bethlehem, Pennsylvania

Deborah Williams, EdD, RN
Associate Professor of Nursing
Western Kentucky University
Bowling Green, Kentucky

REVIEWERS

Ronnette Chereese Langhorne, RN, MS
Instructor of Nursing, Norfolk State University
Norfolk, Virginia

Luanne Linnard-Palmer, EdD, CPON, RN
Professor of Nursing, Dominican University of California
San Rafael, California

Rosemary Macy, RN, PhDc
Assistant Professor of Nursing, Boise State University
Boise, Idaho

Cecilia Jane Maier, MS, RN, CCRN
Assistant Professor, Mount Caramel College of Nursing
Columbus, Ohio

Darrell Spurlock, Jr. MSN, RN, CCRN, CEN
Instructor, Mount Caramel College of Nursing
Columbus, Ohio

STUDENT REVIEWERS

Danielle Darisse
Salve Regina University
Newport, Rhode Island

Kristen Foti
Salve Regina University
Newport, Rhode Island

Stefanie Hall
Salve Regina University
Newport, Rhode Island

Rebecca Hormanski
Salve Regina University
Newport, Rhode Island

Kristin Long
Salve Regina University
Newport, Rhode Island

Nicole Macklin
Salve Regina University
Newport, Rhode Island

Preface

"Success is climbing a mountain, facing the challenge of obstacles, and reaching the top of the mountain."

—Linda Anne Silvestri, MSN, RN

Welcome to Saunders Pyramid to Success! The *Saunders Q&A Review for the NCLEX-RN® Examination* is one of a series of products designed to assist you in achieving your goal of becoming a registered nurse. The *Saunders Q&A Review for the NCLEX-RN Examination* provides you with 5000 practice NCLEX-RN test questions based on the 2004 NCLEX-RN test plan.

The 2004 test plan for NCLEX-RN identifies a framework based on *Client Needs*. These Client Needs categories include Physiological Integrity; Safe, Effective Care Environment; Health Promotion and Maintenance; and Psychosocial Integrity. *Integrated Processes* are also identified as a component of the test plan. These include Caring; Communication and Documentation; Nursing Process; and Teaching/ Learning. This book has been uniquely designed and includes chapters that describe each specific component of the 2004 NCLEX-RN test plan framework and chapters that contain practice questions specific to each component.

CAT NCLEX-RN TEST PREPARATION

This book begins with information regarding NCLEX-RN preparation. Chapter 1 addresses all of the information related to the 2004 NCLEX-RN test plan and the testing procedures related to the examination. This chapter answers all of the questions you may have regarding the testing procedures.

Chapter 2 provides information to the foreign-educated nurse about the process of obtaining a license to practice as a registered nurse in the United States.

Chapter 3 discusses the NCLEX-RN from a nonacademic viewpoint and emphasizes a holistic approach for your individual test preparation. This chapter identifies the components of a structured study plan and pattern, anxiety-reducing techniques, and personal focus issues. Nursing students want to hear what other students have to say about their experiences with NCLEX-RN. Students seek that view with regard to what it is really like to take this examination. Chapter 4 is written by a nursing graduate who recently took the NCLEX-RN, addresses the issue of what NCLEX-RN is all about, and includes the "story of success."

Chapter 5, "Test-Taking Strategies," includes all of the important strategies that will assist in teaching you how to read a question, how not to read into a question, and how to use the process of elimination and various other strategies to select the correct response from the options presented.

CLIENT NEEDS

Chapters 6 to 10 address the 2004 NCLEX-RN test plan component, *Client Needs*. Chapter 6 describes each category of Client Needs as identified by the test plan and lists any subcategories, the percentage of test questions for each category, and some of the content included on NCLEX-RN. Chapters 7 to 10 contain practice test questions related specifically to each category of Client Needs. Chapter 7 contains questions related to Physiological Integrity, Chapter 8 contains Safe, Effective Care Environment questions, Chapter 9 contains Health Promotion and Maintenance questions, and Chapter 10 contains Psychosocial Integrity questions.

INTEGRATED PROCESSES

Chapters 11 and 12 address the *Integrated Processes* as identified in the test plan for NCLEX-RN. Chapter 11 describes each Integrated Process. Chapter 12 contains practice test questions related specifically to each Integrated Process, including Caring; Communication and Documentation; Nursing Process; and Teaching/ Learning.

COMPREHENSIVE TEST

A comprehensive test is included at the end of this book. It consists of 300 practice questions representative of the components of the 2004 test plan framework for NCLEX-RN.

SPECIAL FEATURES OF THE BOOK

Book Design

The book is designed with a unique two-column format. The left column presents the practice questions and options, and the right column provides the corresponding answers, rationales, test-taking strategies, and references. The two-column format makes the review easier so that you do not have to flip through pages in search of answers and rationales.

Practice Questions

While preparing for NCLEX-RN, students have a strong need to review practice test questions. Each chapter contains practice test questions in the NCLEX-RN format. This book contains 1800 practice questions that are in the multiple-choice format or in one of the alternate test question formats used in the NCLEX-RN examination. The accompanying software includes all of the questions from the book, including the alternate test question formats, plus an additional 3200 questions for a total of 5000 test questions.

Multiple-Choice Questions

While you are preparing for NCLEX-RN, it is crucial for you to practice questions. This book contains 1800 practice questions in NCLEX format, most of which are multiple-choice questions to reflect the NCLEX-RN test plan. The accompanying software includes all of the multiple-choice questions from the book, plus an additional 3200 questions for a total of 5000 questions.

Critical Thinking: Alternate Format Questions

Chapters 7, 8, 9, 10, and 12 and the Comprehensive Test contain *Critical Thinking: Alternate Format Questions*. These questions may be presented as a fill-in-the-blank question, a multiple-response question, a prioritizing (ordered response) question, or with an image that relates to the question. These types of questions provide you practice in prioritizing, decision making, and critical thinking skills. The accompanying software includes all of the Critical Thinking: Alternate Format Questions from the book, plus an abundance of additional questions in the alternate format.

Answer Sections for Practice Questions

Each practice question is followed by the correct answer, rationale, test-taking strategy, question categories, and a reference source. The structure of the answer section is unique and provides the following information for every question:

Rationale: The rationale provides you with significant information regarding both correct and incorrect options.

Test-Taking Strategy: The test-taking strategy provides you with the logic for selecting the correct option and assists you in selecting an answer to a question on which you must guess. Specific suggestions for review are identified in the test-taking strategy.

Question Categories: Each question is identified based on the categories used by the NCLEX-RN test plan. Additional content area categories are provided with each question to assist you in identifying areas in need of review. The categories identified with each question include Level of Cognitive Ability, Client Needs, Integrated Process, and the specific nursing Content Area. All categories are identified by their full names so that you do not need to memorize codes or abbreviations.

Reference Source: The reference source and page number are provided for you so that you can easily find the information you need to review in your undergraduate nursing textbooks.

NCLEX-RN REVIEW SOFTWARE

Packaged in this book you will find an NCLEX-RN review CD-ROM. This software contains 5000 questions: 1800 from the book and 3200 additional questions. It contains multiple-choice questions and the Critical Thinking: Alternate Format Questions, including fill-in-the-blank questions, multiple-response questions, prioritizing (ordered response) questions, and image questions. This Windows- and Macintosh-compatible program offers three testing modes for review of the multiple-choice questions.

Quiz: Ten randomly chosen questions on the Client Needs, Integrated Process, or specific Content Area. Results are given and a review of the answer, rationale, and test-taking strategy is provided after you answer all 10 questions.

Study: All questions in a selected Client Needs, Integrated Process, or Content Area. The answer, rationale, test-taking strategy, question categories, and reference source appear after answering each question.

Examination: One hundred randomly chosen questions from the entire pool of 5000 questions. The answer, rationale, test-taking strategy, question categories, reference source, and results appear after you answer all 100 questions.

The CD-ROM allows you to customize your review and determine your areas of strength and weakness. It also provides you with a wealth of practice test questions while simulating the NCLEX-RN experience on computer.

HOW TO USE THIS BOOK

The *Saunders Q&A Review for the NCLEX-RN Examination* is especially designed to help you with your successful journey to the peak of the Pyramid to Success: becoming a registered nurse. As you begin your journey through this book, you will be introduced to all of the important points regarding the CAT NCLEX-RN examination, the process of testing, and the unique and special tips regarding how to prepare yourself both academically and nonacademically for this important examination. Read the chapter from the nursing graduate who recently passed NCLEX-RN, and consider what the graduate had to say about the examination. The test-taking strategy chapter will provide you with important strategies that will guide you in selecting the correct option or assist you in guessing the answer. Read this chapter and practice these strategies as you proceed through your journey with this book.

Once you have completed reading the introductory components of this book, it is time to begin the practice questions. As you read through each question and select an answer, be sure to read the rationale and the test-taking strategy. The rationale provides you with significant information regarding both the correct and incorrect options, and the test-taking strategy provides you with the logic for selecting the correct option. The strategy also identifies the content area that you need to review if you had difficulty with the question. Use the reference source provided so that you can easily find the information you need to review.

As you work your way through the *Saunders Q&A Review for the NCLEX-RN Examination* to identify your areas of strength and weakness, you can return to the companion book, *Saunders Comprehensive Review for the NCLEX-RN Examination,* to focus your study on these areas. The companion book and its accompanying CD-ROM provide you with a comprehensive review of all areas of the nursing content reflected in the 2004 CAT NCLEX-RN test plan.

Another companion book to the *Saunders Q&A Review for the NCLEX-RN Examination* is the *Saunders Strategies for Success for the NCLEX-RN Examination.* This product provides you with all of the test-taking strategies that will help you pass both your nursing examinations and the NCLEX-RN examination. It contains 500 practice test questions in NCLEX format.

To determine your readiness for the NCLEX-RN examination, you will use the next step in the *Saunders Pyramid to Success*: the *Saunders Computerized Review for the NCLEX-RN Examination.* This unique software program contains 2000 NCLEX-RN–style questions. The software provides a detailed analysis similar to that used in standardized nursing examinations.

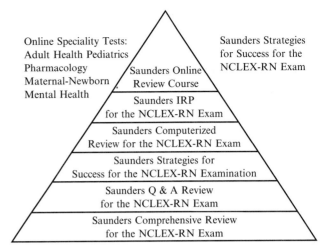

To strengthen your abilities in a specific content area, use the online specialty tests, which are available in the following content areas: Adult Health, Mental Health, Maternal-Newborn, Pediatrics, and Pharmacology. Each specialty test provides you with 100 practice test questions in NCLEX format.

The *Saunders Online Review Course for the NCLEX-RN Examination* is another valuable resource to use in preparing for the examination. This course contains a total of 10 modules and 47 lessons. Every lesson contains content for review, illustrations, practice questions, and a case study followed by questions related to the case study. Each module is followed by a 100-question exam that contains questions representative of the content in the module lessons. There is also a Pretest Exam that generates an individualized plan of study, a Comprehensive (Cumulative) Exam, and a CAT (computerized adaptive testing) Exam. The course provides you with a systematic and individualized method for preparing to take the NCLEX examination.

A final component of the *Saunders Pyramid to Success* is the *Saunders Instructor's Resource Package for the NCLEX-RN Examination.* This manual and CD-ROM accompany the Saunders program of NCLEX-RN review products. Be sure to ask your nursing program director and nursing faculty about this CD-ROM and its use for a review course or a self-paced review in your school's computer laboratory. Good luck with your journey through the Saunders Pyramid to Success. I wish you continued success throughout your new career as a Registered Nurse!

Linda Anne Silvestri MSN, RN

ACKNOWLEDGMENTS

There are many individuals who in their own way have contributed to my success in making my professional dreams become a reality.

First, I want to acknowledge my parents, who opened my door of opportunity in education. I thank my mother, Frances Mary, for all of her love, support, and assistance as I continuously worked to achieve my professional goals. I thank my father, Arnold Lawrence, who always provided insightful words of encouragement. My memories of his love and support will always remain in my heart. I also thank my sister, Dianne Elodia; my brother, Lawrence Peter; and my niece, Gina Marie, who were continuously supportive, giving, and helpful during my research and preparation of this publication.

I sincerely thank Mary Ann Hogan, MSN, RN, who has always encouraged and supported me through my professional endeavors. And a special thank you and acknowledgment goes to two important individuals: Dianne E. Ventrice and Lawrence Fiorentino. They provided continuous support and dedication to my work in both the NCLEX review courses and in reference support for the third edition of this book.

I want to thank all of my nursing students at the Community College of Rhode Island in Warwick, who approached me in 1991 and persuaded me to assist them in preparing to take the NCLEX-RN examination. Their enthusiasm and inspiration led to the commencement of my professional endeavors in conducting NCLEX-RN review courses for nursing students. I also thank the numerous nursing students who have attended my review courses for their willingness to share their needs and ideas. Their input has certainly added a special uniqueness to this publication.

I thank the contributors to this publication and to previous publications who provided practice questions, and the many faculty and student reviewers of this publication. A special thank you to Rebecca S. Blaszczak, RN, for providing a chapter in this publication regarding her experiences with NCLEX-RN, and to Laurent W. Valliere for providing a chapter on the nonacademic preparation strategies for taking the NCLEX-RN examination, for teaching in my NCLEX-RN review courses, and for his commitment and dedication in assisting my nursing students to prepare for NCLEX-RN from a nonacademic point of view. I wish to acknowledge all of the nursing faculty who taught in my NCLEX-RN review courses; their commitment, dedication, and expertise has certainly assisted nursing students in achieving success with the NCLEX-RN.

I sincerely acknowledge and thank two very important individuals from Elsevier Health Sciences. I thank Nancy O'Brien, Managing Editor, for all of her assistance throughout the preparation of this edition and for her continuous enthusiasm, support, and expert professional guidance. And a very special thank you to Charlene Ketchum, Associate Developmental Editor, for her continuous assistance, enthusiasm, and support, and for keeping me on track. Her expert organizational skills maintained order in all of the work that I submitted for manuscript production. I also want to thank Loren Wilson, Director of Review and Testing, and Shelly Hayden, Managing Editor, for all of their guidance and support in preparing the previous edition of this book.

I want to acknowledge all of the staff at Elsevier Health Sciences for their tremendous assistance throughout the preparation and production of this publication. A special thank you to all of them. I thank all of the special people in the production department: Jeff Patterson, Publication Services Manager, Jeanne Genz, Project Manager, Jyotika Shroff, Designer, and Joe Selby, Producer who assisted in finalizing this publication.

I sincerely thank Bob Boehringer, Director of Nursing Marketing, and Andrew Eilers, Marketing Manager, whose support, hard work, and special creativity assisted with this publication.

I would also like to acknowledge Patricia Mieg, Educational Sales Representative, who encouraged me to submit my ideas and initial work to the W.B. Saunders Company and initiated my meeting with Maura Connor, former Senior Acquisitions Editor, to create the first edition of this book. I want to thank Maura for her professional direction that led me to success as I initially created *Saunders Pyramid to Success for NCLEX-RN*.

I also need to thank Salve Regina University for the opportunity to educate nursing students in the baccalaureate nursing program and for its support during my research and writing of this publication. I would like to especially acknowledge my colleagues, Dr. Sandra Solem, Dr. Ellen McCarty, Dr. JoAnn Mullaney, Dr. Jane McCool, Dr. Peggy Matteson, and Dr. Bethany Sykes, for all of their support and encouragement.

I wish to acknowledge the Community College of Rhode Island, which provided me with the opportunity to educate nursing students in the Associate Degree of Nursing Program, and a special thank you to Patricia Miller, MSN, RN, and Michelina McClellan, MS, RN, from Baystate Medical Center, School of Nursing, in Springfield, Massachusetts who were my first mentors in nursing education.

Lastly, a very special thank you to all of my nursing students: you light up my life, and your hearts and minds will shape the future of the profession of nursing!

Linda Anne Silvestri, MSN, RN

Contents

To All Future Registered Nurses,

Congratulations to you!

Whether you are a nursing student in a nursing program completing your studies or a graduate nurse or foreign-educated nurse preparing to take the NCLEX-RN® examination, you should be very proud and pleased with yourself for your many accomplishments. I know that you are working very hard to become successful and that you have proved to yourself that you can achieve your goals.

I have been teaching nursing students for many years and have been conducting NCLEX-RN Review Courses since 1991. Preparing to take an examination can be an anxiety-producing experience. A component of achieving success in examinations is possessing the knowledge and experience needed to answer a question correctly. An additional component of becoming successful in these examinations is to become comfortable and confident with the ability to face the challenge of a question and to answer the question correctly. In my experience working with students, it is evident that students strongly need to review practice questions. The more questions, answers, and rationales with which a student can practice, the more proficient the student becomes with test-taking strategies and the ability to answer a question correctly. Your knowledge, your experience, and the incorporation of test-taking strategies will lead you to success. On NCLEX-RN, the questions require thought and critical analysis. Consistent practice with test questions will assist you in becoming comfortable, confident, and proficient with answering the questions correctly.

I am excited and pleased to be able to provide you with the *Saunders Pyramid to Success* products. These products will prepare you for your most important professional goal of becoming a registered nurse. *Saunders Pyramid to Success* products provide you with everything you need to prepare for NCLEX-RN. These products include material required for examination preparation for all nursing students regardless of educational background, specific strengths, areas in need of improvement, or clinical experience during the nursing program.

Saunders Q&A Review for the NCLEX-RN Examination is designed to provide you with questions specifically representative of the components of the current NCLEX-RN test plan. The framework for the test plan focuses on *Client Needs* and the *Integrated Processes*. Therefore, chapters with practice test questions representative of this framework are included in this book and CD-ROM. There are a total of 5000 practice test questions that are in the multiple-choice format and alternate question format.

So let's get started and begin our journey through the Pyramid to Success, and welcome to the profession of nursing!

Sincerely,

Linda Anne Silvestri MSN, RN

Linda Anne Silvestri MSN, RN

NCLEX-RN® Preparation

NCLEX-RN®

THE PYRAMID TO SUCCESS

Welcome to *Saunders Q&A Review for the NCLEX-RN® Examination*, the second component of the Pyramid to Success! At this time, you have completed your first path toward the peak of the pyramid with *Saunders Comprehensive Review for the NCLEX-RN Examination*. Now it is time to continue that journey to become a registered nurse with *Saunders Q&A Review for the NCLEX-RN Examination!*

As you begin your journey through this book, you will be introduced to all of the important points regarding the NCLEX-RN Examination, the process of testing, and the unique and special tips regarding how to prepare yourself for this very important examination. You will read what a nursing graduate who passed NCLEX-RN has to say about the examination. All of those important test-taking strategies are detailed. These details will guide you in selecting the correct option or in selecting an answer to a question you must guess at.

Saunders Q&A Review for the NCLEX-RN Examination contains 5,000 NCLEX-RN-style practice questions. The chapters have been developed to provide a description of the components of the NCLEX-RN test plan, including the Client Needs and the Integrated Processes. In addition, chapters have been prepared to contain practice questions specific to each category of Client Needs and the Integrated Processes.

In each chapter that contains practice questions, a rationale, test-taking strategy, and reference source containing a page number are provided with each question. Each question is coded on the basis of the Level of Cognitive Ability, Client Needs category, Integrated Process, and the content area being tested. The rationale provides you with significant information regarding both the correct and incorrect options. The test-taking strategy provides you with the logical path to selecting the correct option and identifies the content area to review, if necessary. The reference source and page number provide easy access to the information that you need to review.

After you complete the *Saunders Q&A Review for the NCLEX-RN Examination*, you are ready for the *Saunders Computerized Review for the NCLEX-RN Examination*, a computer disk program that contains more than 2,000 NCLEX-RN-style questions to help you determine your readiness for the NCLEX-RN examination. Additional resources to assist you in preparing for this examination include the online specialty tests titled Adult Health, Mental Health, Maternal-Newborn, Pediatrics, and Pharmacology, and the online NCLEX-RN review course.

The online NCLEX-RN review course addresses all areas of the test plan identified by the National Council of State Boards of Nursing (NCSBN). It contains a pretest that provides feedback regarding your strengths and weaknesses and generates an individualized study schedule in a calendar format. Content review includes practice questions and case studies, figures and illustrations, a glossary, and animations and videos. A cumulative examination and a computerized adaptive exam (CAT) are also key components of the online review course. The types of practice questions in this course include multiple choice, fill in the blank, multiple response, those that require you to prioritize (ordered response), and questions containing figures that may require you to use the computer mouse to answer. These additional products in Saunders Pyramid to Success, including the online specialty tests and the online review course, can be obtained at the Elsevier Web site at www.elsevierhealth.com or by calling Elsevier Health at 1-800-545-2522.

Let's continue our journey through the Pyramid to Success!

THE EXAMINATION PROCESS

An important step in the Pyramid to Success is to become as familiar as possible with the examination process. A significant amount of anxiety can occur in candidates facing the challenge of this examination.

Knowing what the examination is all about and knowing what you will encounter during the process of testing will assist in alleviating fear and anxiety. The information contained in this chapter addresses the procedures related to the development of the NCLEX-RN test plan, the components of the test plan, and the answers to the questions most commonly asked by nursing students and graduates preparing to take the NCLEX-RN examination. The information contained in this chapter related to the test plan was obtained from the National Council of State Boards of Nursing (NCSBN) Web site (www.ncsbn.org) and from the *Test Plan for the National Council Licensure Examination for Registered Nurses* (Effective Date: April 2004), National Council of State Boards of Nursing, Chicago, 2003. Additional information regarding the test and its development can be obtained by accessing the NCSBN web site or by writing to the National Council of State Boards of Nursing at 111 E. Wacker Drive, Suite 2900, Chicago, Illinois 60601.

COMPUTERIZED ADAPTIVE TESTING (CAT)

The abbreviation CAT stands for Computerized Adaptive Testing. This means that the examination is created as the test taker answers each question. All of the test questions are categorized on the basis of the test plan structure and the level of difficulty of the question. As you answer a question, the computer will determine your competency based on the answer you selected. If you selected a correct answer to a question, the computer scans the question bank and selects a more difficult question. If you selected an incorrect answer, the computer scans the question bank and selects an easier question. This process continues until the test plan requirements are met and a reliable pass or fail decision is made.

When a test question is presented on the computer screen, it must be answered or the test will not move on. This means that you will not be able to skip questions, go back and review questions, or go back and change answers. Remember, in a CAT, once an answer is recorded, all subsequent questions administered depend, to an extent, on the answer selected for that question. Skipping and returning to earlier questions are not compatible with the logical methodology of a CAT. The inability to skip questions or go back to change previous answers will not be a disadvantage to you. Actually, you will not fall into that trap of changing a correct answer to an incorrect one with CAT. If you are faced with a question that contains unfamiliar content, you may need to guess at the answer. There is no penalty for guessing on this examination. Remember, with most questions, the answer will be right there in front of you. If you need to guess, use your nursing knowledge to its fullest extent, as well as all of the test-taking strategies you have practiced in this review program.

You do not need any computer experience to take this examination. A keyboard tutorial is provided and administered to all test takers at the start of the examination. The tutorial will instruct you on the use of the on-screen optional calculator, the use of the mouse, and how to record an answer. In addition to the traditional four options of a multiple-choice question, the tutorial also provides instructions on how to respond to different question formats. A proctor is present to assist in explaining the use of the computer to ensure your full understanding of how to proceed.

DEVELOPMENT OF THE TEST PLAN

The test plan for the NCLEX-RN examination is developed by the National Council of State Boards of Nursing (NCSBN). As an initial step in the test development process, the NCSBN considers the legal scope of nursing practice as governed by state laws and regulations, including the nurse practice act, and uses these laws to define the areas on the examination that will assess the competence of a candidate (test taker) for nurse licensure.

The NCSBN also conducts a practice/job analysis study to determine the framework for the test plan for the examination. The participants in this study include newly licensed registered nurses from all types of basic education programs. The participants are provided a list of nursing activities and are asked about the frequency of performing these specific activities, their impact on maintaining client safety, and the setting where the activities were performed. The results of the study are analyzed by a panel of experts at the NCSBN, and decisions are made regarding the test plan framework. Because nursing practice continues to change, this study is conducted every three years. The results of this study, most recently conducted in 2002, provided the structure for the test plan implemented in April 2004.

THE TEST PLAN

The content of NCLEX-RN reflects the activities that a newly licensed entry-level registered nurse must be able to perform in order to provide clients with safe and effective nursing care. The questions are written to address the Levels of Cognitive Ability, Client Needs, and Integrated Processes as identified in the test plan developed by the NCSBN (Box 1-1).

BOX 1-1

Examination Questions

Each examination question addresses:
A Level of Cognitive Ability
A Client Needs category
An Integrated Process

Levels of Cognitive Ability

The examination for licensure as a registered nurse may include questions at the cognitive levels of knowledge, comprehension, application, and analysis. However, most questions are written at the application or higher levels of cognitive ability, such as the analysis level, because the practice of nursing requires critical thinking in decision making. This means that the test taker will be required to analyze and/or apply the information provided in the test question. Box 1-2 presents an example of a question that requires you to analyze data in order to accurately interpret a client's status.

Client Needs

In the test plan implemented in April 2004, the NCSBN has identified a test plan framework based on Client Needs. The NCSBN identifies four major categories of Client Needs. Some of these categories are further divided into subcategories. Table 1-1 identifies these Client Needs and the associated percentage of test questions. Refer to Chapter 6 for a detailed description of the categories of Client Needs and the NCLEX-RN examination.

Integrated Processes

The NCSBN identifies four processes that are fundamental to the practice of nursing. These processes are a component of the test plan and are incorporated throughout the major categories of Client Needs. Box 1-3 identifies these processes. Refer to Chapter 11 for a detailed description of the Integrated Processes and the NCLEX-RN examination.

TYPES OF QUESTIONS ON THE EXAMINATION

The types of questions that may be administered on the examination include multiple choice, fill in the blank, multiple response, prioritizing (ordered response), and questions that contain a figure or illustration. You may also encounter a question that may require you to use the mouse component of the computer system. For example, you may be presented with a visual that displays the arterial vessels of an adult client. In this visual, you may be asked to "point and click" (using the mouse) on the area where the dorsalis pedis pulse could be felt. The NCSBN provides specific directions for you to follow with these questions to guide you in your process of testing. Be sure to read these directions as they appear on the computer screen.

Multiple Choice

Most of the questions you will be asked to answer will be in the multiple-choice format. These questions will

---

BOX 1-2

Level of Cognitive Ability

Question
A client with trigeminal neuralgia who is receiving carbamazepine (Tegretol) 400 mg orally daily has a white blood cell (WBC) count of 2800/uL, blood urea nitrogen (BUN) of 17 mg/dL, sodium level of 141 mEq/L, and uric acid level of 5.0 ng/dL. On the basis of these laboratory values, the nurse determines that the:
1. Sodium level is low, indicating an electrolyte imbalance
2. Uric acid level is elevated, indicating a risk for renal calculi
3. BUN is elevated, indicating nephrotoxicity
4. WBC is low, indicating a blood dyscrasia

Answer: 4

This question requires you to analyze each of the laboratory values identified in the question. You need to know the adverse effects of carbamazepine and the normal laboratory values in order to make an accurate interpretation regarding the client's status. Recall that blood dyscrasias, such as agranulocytosis, is an adverse effect of this medication, and note that the only abnormal laboratory value in the question is the WBC.
Level of Cognitive Ability: Analysis

References:
Hodgson, B., & Kizior, R. (2004). *Saunders nursing drug handbook 2004.* Philadelphia: Saunders, p. 148.
Pagana, K., & Pagana, T. (2003). *Mosby's diagnostic and laboratory test reference* (6th ed.). St. Louis: Mosby, pp. 814; 902; 905; 944.

TABLE 1-1

Client Needs Categories and Percentage of Questions

Physiological Integrity	
Basic Care and Comfort	6%-12%
Pharmacological and Parenteral Therapies	13%-19%
Reduction of Risk Potential	13%-19%
Physiological Adaptation	11%-17%
Safe, Effective Care Environment	
Management of Care	13%-19%
Safety and Infection Control	8%-14%
Health Promotion and Maintenance	6%-12%
Psychosocial Integrity	6%-12%

From National Council of State Boards of Nursing, (eds). (2004). NCLEX-RN Examination Detailed Test Plan for the National Licensure Examination for Registered nurses. Chicago: Author.

BOX 1-3

Integrated Processes

Caring
Communication and documentation
Nursing process (assessment, analysis, planning, implementation, and evaluation)
Teaching/learning

BOX 1-4

Fill in the Blank

Question

A physician's order reads: acetaminophen (Tylenol) liquid, 450 mg orally every 4 hours prn for pain. The medication label reads: 160 mg/5 mL. The nurse prepares how many milliliters to administer one dose? (Round to the nearest whole number)
Answer:_____

Answer: 14

In this question you need to use the formula for calculating a medication dose. Once the dose is determined, you will need to type in your answer. In this particular question, you are asked to round to the nearest whole number. Always follow the specific directions noted on the computer screen when answering the question. Also, remember that there will be an on-screen calculator on the computer for your use if needed.

Reference:
Kee, J., & Marshall, S. (2004). *Clinical calculations: With applications to general and specialty areas* (5th ed.). Philadelphia: Saunders, p. 158.

---

provide you with data about a particular client situation and four answers or options.

Fill in the Blank

These types of questions may ask you to perform a medication calculation, an intravenous calculation, or to calculate an intake or output record on a client. You will need to type in your answer. (See Box 1-4 for an example.)

Multiple Response

For a multiple-response question, you will be asked to select or check all of the options, such as nursing interventions, that relate to the information in the question. No partial credit is given for correct selections. You need to do exactly as the question asks, which will be to select *all* options that apply. (See Box 1-5 for an example.)

Prioritizing (Ordered Response)

These questions may ask you to identify nursing actions in order of priority. Information will be presented in a question, and based on the data, you need to determine what you will do first, second, third, and so forth. On the NCLEX-RN examination, when presented with this type of question, you will use the computer mouse and will be asked to "drag and drop" the nursing actions, placing them in order of priority. (See Box 1-6 for an example of this type of question.)

BOX 1-5

Multiple Response

Question

A nurse is preparing to remove a nasogastric tube from a client. Select all of the actions that the nurse would take to perform this procedure.
X Assess for the presence of bowel sounds
X Untape the nasogastric tube from the client's nose
___Keep the tube attached to the prescribed amount of suction during removal
X Instill 20 mL of air into the nasogastric tube to displace secretions back into the client's stomach
X Ask the client to hold the breath during removal of the tube
___Place the client in a supine position
In a multiple-response question, you will be asked to select or check all of the options, such as nursing actions, that relate to the information in the question. To answer this question, visualize the procedure and think about airway patency, preventing aspiration, and preventing mucosal irritation to identify the correct interventions. After explaining the procedure for tube removal to the client, the nurse would assess for the presence of bowel sounds. The tube would not be removed if bowel sounds are absent. The nurse would don clean gloves, place the client in an upright position, and place a towel across the client's chest. The suction is turned off and the nasogastric tube is disconnected from the suction tube. The nurse instills 20 mL of air into the nasogastric tube to displace secretions back into the client's stomach and decrease the client's risk of aspiration. The nasogastric tube is untaped from the client's nose. The client is instructed to hold the breath during removal of the tube, and the tube is pulled out in one quick, steady motion.

Reference:
Harkreader, H., & Hogan, M.A. (2004). *Fundamentals of nursing: Caring and clinical judgment* (2nd ed.). Philadelphia: Saunders, p. 580.

Figure or Illustration

This type of question will provide you with a figure or illustration and will ask you to answer the question based on it. The question could contain a chart, table, or a figure or illustration. In this type of question, you may also be asked to use the computer mouse and "point and click" on a specific area in the visual. A chart, table, or a figure or illustration may appear in any type of question, including a multiple-choice question. (See Box 1-7 for an example.)

ITEM WRITERS

Question (item) writers are selected by the NCSBN after an extensive application process. The writers are registered nurses who hold a master's degree or a higher degree. Many of the writers are nursing educators; however, a nurse currently employed in clinical nursing practice and working directly with nurses who have entered practice within the last 12 months may be

BOX 1-6

Prioritizing (Ordered Response)

Question

A nurse hears the alarm sound on the telemetry monitor, quickly looks at the monitor, and notes that a client is in ventricular tachycardia. The nurse rushes to the client's room and upon reaching the client's bedside, the nurse performs the following actions in which priority order?

1. Checks for a pulse at the carotid artery
2. Opens the airway
3. Determines unresponsiveness
4. Looks, listens, and feels for breathing

Answer: 3241

This question asks you to prioritize nursing actions. Remember to read the directions on the computer screen to guide you in answering this type of question. Use the steps of basic life support to answer the question. Determining unresponsiveness is the first assessment action to take. When a client is in ventricular tachycardia, there is a significant decrease in cardiac output. However, assessing for unresponsiveness ensures whether the client is affected by the decreased cardiac output. If the client is unresponsive, the nurse proceeds through the ABCs (i.e., airway, breathing, and circulation) of cardiopulmonary resuscitation (CPR).

Reference:

Black, J., & Hawks, J. (2005). *Medical-surgical nursing: Clinical management for positive outcomes* (7th ed.). Philadelphia: Saunders, pp. 1688-1689.

BOX 1-7

Visual or Illustration

Question

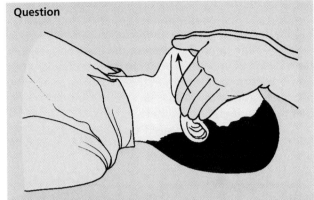

An emergency room nurse initiates cardiopulmonary resuscitation (CPR) on a victim who was in a motor vehicle accident. The nurse uses this method to open the airway in which of the following situations?

1. In all situations requiring CPR
2. If neck trauma is suspected
3. If the client is unconscious
4. If the client has a history of headaches

Answer: 2

In this question, you are provided with a figure and are asked a question about it. The jaw thrust without head-tilt maneuver is used when head and/or neck trauma is suspected. This maneuver opens the airway while maintaining proper head and neck alignment, thus reducing the risk of further damage to the neck. In situations requiring CPR, the client will be unconscious. It is unlikely that the nurse will be able to obtain data regarding the client's history.

Reference:

Harkreader, H., & Hogan, M.A. (2004). *Fundamentals of nursing: Caring and clinical judgment* (2nd ed.). Philadelphia: Saunders, p. 909.

---

selected to participate in this process. Question writers voluntarily submit an application to become a writer and must meet specific established criteria designated by the NCSBN in order to be accepted as a participant in the process.

REGISTERING TO TAKE THE EXAMINATION

The initial step in the registration process is to submit an application to the state board of nursing in the state in which you intend to obtain licensure. You need to obtain information from the board of nursing regarding the specific registration process, because the process may vary from state to state. In most states, you may register for the examination through the Web, by mail, or by telephone. It is very important that you follow the registration instructions and complete the registration forms precisely and accurately. Registration forms that are not properly completed, or not accompanied by the proper fees in the required method of payment, will be returned to you and will delay testing. There is a fee for taking the examination, and you may also have to pay additional fees to the board of nursing in the state in which you are applying. You will be sent a confirmation indicating that your registration was received. If you do not receive a confirmation within four weeks of submitting your registration, you should contact the candidate

services. Information regarding this contact can be obtained at the NCLEX candidate Web site at www.vue.com/nclex.

AUTHORIZATION TO TEST (ATT)

Once your eligibility to test has been determined by the board of nursing in the state in which licensure is requested, your registration form is processed and an Authorization to Test form will be sent to you. You cannot make an appointment until the board of nursing declares eligibility and you receive an Authorization to Test form. The examination will take place at Pearson Professional Centers, and an appointment can be made through the Web or by telephone. First-time test takers will be offered an appointment within 30 days of the call to schedule an appointment, and repeat test takers will be offered an appointment within 45 days. You can schedule an appointment at any Pearson Professional Center. You do not have to take the examination in the same state in which you are seeking licensure. A confirmation of your appointment will be sent to you.

The Authorization to Test form contains important information including your test authorization number, candidate identification number, and an expiration date. Note the expiration date on the form because you must test by this date. You also need to take your Authorization to Test form to the test center on the day of your examination. You will not be admitted to the examination if you do not have it.

If for any reason you need to cancel or reschedule your appointment to test, you can make the change on the candidate Web site or by calling candidate services. The change needs to be made one full business day (24 hours) before your scheduled appointment.

If you fail to arrive for the examination or fail to unschedule your appointment to test without providing appropriate notice, you will forfeit your examination fee and your Authorization to Test will be invalidated. This information will be reported to the board of nursing in the state in which you have applied for licensure, and you will be required to register and pay the testing fees again.

You must arrive at the testing center at least 30 minutes before the test is scheduled. If you arrive late for the scheduled testing appointment, you may be required to forfeit your examination appointment. If it is necessary for the appointment to be forfeited, you will need to re-register for the examination and pay an additional fee. The board of nursing will be notified that you did not test. A few days before your scheduled date of testing, take the time to drive to the testing center to determine its exact location, the length of time required to arrive at that destination, and any potential obstacles that might delay you, such as road construction, traffic, or parking sites.

SPECIAL TESTING CIRCUMSTANCES

A test taker who requires special testing accommodations should contact the board of nursing before submitting a registration form. The board of nursing will provide the procedures for the request. The board of nursing must authorize special testing accommodations. Following board of nursing approval, the NCSBN reviews the requested accommodations and must also approve the request. If the request is approved, the testing appointment must be made by the NCLEX Program Coordinator, who can be contacted by calling NCLEX candidate services. Canceling or rescheduling an appointment must be done through the NCLEX Program Coordinator.

THE TESTING CENTER

The testing center is designed to ensure complete security of the testing process. Strict candidate identification requirements have been established. To be admitted to the testing center, it is imperative that you bring the Authorization to Test form, along with two forms of identification. Both forms of identification must be signed, current or nonexpired, and one must contain a recent photograph of you. The name on the photograph identification must be the same as the name on the Authorization to Test form. A digital fingerprint, signature, and photograph will be taken at the test center and accompany the NCLEX results to confirm your identity. Additionally, if you leave the testing room for any reason, you may be required to have your fingerprint taken again to be readmitted to the room.

Personal belongings are not allowed in the testing room. Secure storage will be provided for the candidate; however, storage space is limited, so you must plan accordingly. In addition, the testing center will not assume responsibility for your personal belongings. The testing waiting areas are generally small; therefore, friends or family members who accompany you are not permitted to wait in the testing center while you are taking the examination.

Once you have completed the admission process and a brief orientation, the proctor will escort you to the assigned computer. You will be seated at an individual table area with an appropriate work space that includes computer equipment, appropriate lighting, an erasable note board, and a marker. No items including unauthorized scratch paper are allowed into the testing room. Electronic devices such as watches, beepers, or cell phones are not allowed in the testing room. Eating, drinking, and the use of tobacco are not allowed in the testing room. You will be observed at all times by the test proctor while taking the examination. Additionally, video and audio recording of all test sessions occurs. Pearson Professional Centers has no control over the sounds made by typing on the computer. If these sounds are distracting, raise your hand to summon the proctor. Earplugs are available upon request.

You must follow the directions given by the test center staff and must remain seated during the test, except when authorized to leave. If you feel that you have a problem with the computer, need an additional note board, need to take a break, or need the test proctor for any reason, you must raise your hand.

TESTING TIME

The maximum testing time is 6 hours, which includes the tutorial, two preprogrammed optional breaks, and any unscheduled breaks that you may take. The first preprogrammed optional break takes place after 2 testing hours, and the second preprogrammed optional break after $3\frac{1}{2}$ hours of testing. The computer screen will notify you of the time for these breaks. You must leave the testing room during breaks, and when you return, you will be required to provide a fingerprint to be readmitted to the testing room.

LENGTH OF THE EXAMINATION

The minimum number of questions that you will need to answer is 75. Of these 75 questions, 60 will be operational (scored) questions and 15 will be pretest (unscored) questions. The maximum number of questions in the test is 265. Fifteen of the total number of questions that you need to answer will be pretest (unscored) questions.

The pretest questions may be presented as scored questions on future examinations. These pretest questions are not identified as such. In other words, you do not know which questions are the pretest (unscored) questions.

PASS OR FAIL DECISIONS

All of the examination questions are categorized by test plan area and level of difficulty. This is an important point to keep in mind when considering how a pass or fail decision is made by the computer, because a pass or fail decision is not based on a percentage of correctly answered questions. After the minimum number of questions have been answered (75 questions), the computer compares the test taker's ability level to the standard required for passing. The standard required for passing is set based on the expert judgment of several individuals appointed by the NCSBN. If the test taker is clearly above the passing standard, then the test taker passes the examination. If the test taker is clearly below the passing standard, then the test taker fails the examination. If the computer is not able to clearly determine if the test taker has passed or failed because the test taker's ability is close to the passing standard, then the computer continues asking questions. After each question, the test taker's ability is determined, and when it becomes clear on which side of the passing standard the test taker falls (above the standard or below the standard), the examination ends. If the test taker is administered the maximum number of questions (265 questions), the computer will make a pass or fail decision by recomputing the test taker's final ability level, based on every question answered, and comparing it with the passing standard. If the ability level is above the passing standard, the test taker passes. If it is not above the passing standard, the test taker fails.

If the examination ends because you have run out of time, the computer may not have enough information to make a clear pass or fail decision. If this is the situation, the computer will review the test taker's performance during testing and specifically at the performance with the last 60 questions answered. If the test taker's ability was consistently above the passing standard, the test taker passes. If the test taker's ability falls at or below the passing standard, even once, the test taker fails.

COMPLETING THE EXAM

Once the test is completed, you will complete a brief computer-delivered questionnaire about your testing experience. After this questionnaire is completed, you need to raise your hand to summon the test proctor. The test proctor will collect and inventory all note boards and then permit you to leave.

PROCESSING RESULTS

Every computerized examination is scored twice: once by the computer at the testing center and then again after the examination is transmitted to Pearson Professional Centers. No results are released at the testing center. The board of nursing will mail your results to you approximately one month after taking the examination. You should not telephone Pearson Professional Centers, the NCSBN, candidate services, or the state board of nursing for results.

CANDIDATE PERFORMANCE REPORT

A candidate performance report is provided to a test taker who failed the examination. This report provides the test taker with information about strengths and weaknesses in relation to the test plan and provides a guide for studying and retaking the examination. The test taker must wait a period of 45 or 91 days before retaking the examination. This time period is established by each board of nursing and the NCSBN.

INTERSTATE ENDORSEMENT

Because the NCLEX-RN examination is a national examination, you can apply to take the examination in any state. Once licensure is received, you can apply for Interstate Endorsement. The procedures and requirements for Interstate Endorsement may vary from state to state, and these procedures can be obtained from the state board of nursing in the state in which endorsement is sought.

STATE BOARDS OF NURSING

Contact information was obtained from the NCSBN Web site (www.ncsbn.org). Because contact information may change, access this Web site for updated information if necessary.

Alabama Board of Nursing
770 Washington Avenue
RSA Plaza, Suite 250
Montgomery, AL 36130-3900
Phone: (334) 242-4060
Fax: (334) 242-4360
Web site: www.abn.state.al.us

Alaska Board of Nursing
550 West Seventh Avenue, Suite 1500
Anchorage, AK 99501-3567
Phone: (907) 269-8161
Fax: (907) 269-8196
Web site: www.dced.state.ak.us/occ/pnur.htm

American Samoa Health Services Regulatory Board
LBJ Tropical Medical Center
Pago Pago, AS 96799
Phone: (684) 633-1222
Fax: (684) 633-1869

Arizona State Board of Nursing
1651 E. Morten Avenue, Suite 210
Phoenix, AZ 85020
Phone: (602) 889-5150
Fax: (602) 889-5155
Web site: www.azboardofnursing.org

Arkansas State Board of Nursing
University Tower Building
1123 S. University, Suite 800
Little Rock, AR 72204-1619
Phone: (501) 686-2700
Fax: (501) 686-2714
Web site: www.state.ar.us/nurse

California Board of Registered Nursing
400 R St., Suite 4030
Sacramento, CA 95814-6239
Phone: (916) 322-3350
Fax: (916) 327-4402
Web site: www.rn.ca.gov

Colorado Board of Nursing
1560 Broadway, Suite 880
Denver, CO 80202
Phone: (303) 894-2430
Fax: (303) 894-2821
Web site: www.dora.state.co.us/nursing

Connecticut Board of Examiners for Nursing
Dept. of Public Health
410 Capitol Avenue, MS# 13PHO
P.O. Box 340308
Hartford, CT 06134-0328
Phone: (860) 509-7624
Fax: (860) 509-7553
Web site: www.state.ct.us/dph

Delaware Board of Nursing
861 Silver Lake Blvd.
Cannon Building, Suite 203
Dover, DE 19904
Phone: (302) 739-4522
Fax: (302) 739-2711
Web site: www.professionallicensing.state. de.us/boards/
nursing/index.shtml

District of Columbia Board of Nursing
Department of Health
825 N. Capitol Street N.E.
2nd Floor, Room 2224
Washington, DC 20002
Fax: (202) 442-9431
Phone: (202) 442-4778
Web site: www.dchealth.dc.gov

Florida Board of Nursing
Mailing Address:
4052 Bald Cypress Way, BIN C02
Tallahassee, FL 32399-3252
Physical Address:
4042 Bald Cypress Way
Room 120
Tallahassee, FL 32399
Phone: (850) 245-4125
Fax: (850) 245-4172
Web site: www.doh.state.fl.us/mqa

Georgia Board of Nursing
237 Coliseum Drive
Macon, GA 31217-3858
Phone: (478) 207-1640
Fax: (478) 207-1660
Web site: www.sos.state.ga.us/plb/rn

Guam Board of Nurse Examiners
Regular mailing address:
P.O. Box 2816
Hagatna, Guam 96932
Street address (for Fed Ex and UPS deliveries):
651 Legacy Square Commercial Complex,
South Route 10, Suite 9
Mangilao, Guam 96913
Phone: (671) 735-7406 or (671) 725-7411
Fax: (671) 735-7413

Hawaii Board of Nursing
King Kalakaua Building
335 Merchant Street, 3rd Floor
Honolulu, HI 96813
Phone: (808) 586-3000
Fax: (808) 586-2689
Web site: www.state.hi.us/dcca/pvl/areas_nurse.html

Idaho Board of Nursing
280 N. 8th Street, Suite 210
P.O. Box 83720
Boise, ID 83720
Phone: (208) 334-3110
Fax: (208) 334-3262
Web site: www.state.id.us/ibn/ibnhome.htm

Illinois Department of Professional Regulation
James R. Thompson Center
100 West Randolph, Suite 9-300
Chicago, IL 60601
Phone: (312) 814-2715
Fax: (312) 814-3145
Web site: www.dpr.state.il.us

Illinois Department of Professional Regulation
320 W. Washington St., 3rd Floor
Springfield, IL 62786
Phone: (217) 782-8556
Fax: (217) 782-7645

Indiana State Board of Nursing
Health Professions Bureau
402 W. Washington Street, Room W066
Indianapolis, IN 46204
Phone: (317) 234-2043
Fax: (317) 233-4236
Web site: www.state.in/us/hpb/boards/isbn

Iowa Board of Nursing
RiverPoint Business Park
400 S.W. 8th Street, Suite B
Des Moines, IA 50309-4685
Phone: (515) 281-3255
Fax: (515) 281-4825
Web site: www.state.ia.us/government/nursing

Kansas State Board of Nursing
Landon State Office Building
900 S.W. Jackson, Suite 1051
Topeka, KS 66612
Phone: (785) 296-4929
Fax: (785) 296-3929
Web site: www.ksbn.org

Kentucky Board of Nursing
312 Whittington Parkway, Suite 300
Louisville, KY 40222
Phone: (502) 329-7000
Fax: (502) 329-7011
Web site: www.kbn.ky.gov

Louisiana State Board of Nursing
3510 N. Causeway Boulevard, Suite 501
Metairie, LA 70002
Phone: (504) 838-5332
Fax: (504) 838-5349
Web site: www.lsbn.state.la.us

Maine State Board of Nursing
158 State House Station
Augusta, ME 04333
Phone: (207) 287-1133
Fax: (207) 287-1149
Web site: www.maine.gov/boardofnursing

Maryland Board of Nursing
4140 Patterson Avenue
Baltimore, MD 21215
Phone: (410) 585-1900
Fax: (410) 358-3530
Web site: www.mbon.org

Massachusetts Board of Registration in Nursing
Commonwealth of Massachusetts
239 Causeway Street
Boston, MA 02114
Phone: (617) 727-9961
Fax: (617) 727-1630
Web site: www.state.ma.us/reg/boards/rn

Michigan DCH/Bureau of Health Professions
Ottawa Towers North
611 W. Ottawa, 1st Floor
Lansing, MI 48933
Phone: (517) 335-0918
Fax: (517) 373-2179
Web site: www.michigan.gov/healthlicense

Minnesota Board of Nursing
2829 University Avenue SE, Suite 500
Minneapolis, MN 55414
Phone: (612) 617-2270
Fax: (612) 617-2190
Web site: www.nursingboard.state.mn.us

Mississippi Board of Nursing
1935 Lakeland Drive, Suite B
Jackson, MS 39216-5014
Phone: (601) 987-4188
Fax: (601) 364-2352
Web site: www.msbn.state.ms.us

Missouri State Board of Nursing
3605 Missouri Blvd.
P.O. Box 656
Jefferson City, MO 65102-0656
Phone: (573) 751-0681
Fax: (573) 751-0075
Web site: http://pr.mo.gov/nursing.asp

Montana State Board of Nursing
301 South Park
P.O. Box 200513
Helena, MT 59620-0513
Phone: (406) 841-2340
Fax: (406) 841-2343
Web site: www.discoveringmontana. com/dli/bsd/
license/bsd_boards/nur_board/board_page.htm

Nebraska Department of Health and Human Services
Regulation and Licensure
Nursing and Nursing Support
301 Centennial Mall South
Lincoln, NE 68509-4986
Phone: (402) 471-4376
Fax: (402) 471-1066
Web site: www.hhs.state.ne.us/crl/nursing/
nursingindex.htm

Nevada State Board of Nursing
Licensure and Certification
2500 West Sahara Avenue, Suite 207
Las Vegas, Nevada 89102-4293
Phone: (702) 486-5800
Fax: (702) 486-5803
Web site: www.nursingboard.state.nv.us

New Hampshire Board of Nursing
21 South Fruit Street, Suite 16
Concord, NH 03301-2341
Phone: (603) 271-2323
Fax: (603) 271-6605
Web site: www.state.nh.us/nursing

New Jersey Board of Nursing
P.O. Box 45010
124 Halsey Street, 6th Floor
Newark, NJ 07101
Phone: (973) 504-6586
Fax: (973) 648-3481
Web site: www.state.nj.us/lps/ca/medical.htm

New Mexico Board of Nursing
6301 Indian School Road NE, Suite 710
Albuquerque, NM 87110
Phone: (505) 841-8340
Fax: (505) 841-8347
Web site: www.state.nm.us/clients/nursing

New York State Board of Nursing
89 Washington Avenue, Education Bldg.
2nd Floor, West Wing
Albany, NY 12234
Phone: (518) 474-3817 Ext. 280
Fax: (518) 474-3706
Web site: www.nysed.gov/prof/nurse.htm

North Carolina Board of Nursing
3724 National Drive, Suite 201
Raleigh, NC 27612
Phone: (919) 782-3211
Fax: (919) 781-9461
Web site: www.ncbon.com

North Dakota Board of Nursing
919 South 7th Street, Suite 504
Bismarck, ND 58504
Phone: (701) 328-9777
Fax: (701) 328-9785
Web site: www.ndbon.org

Northern Mariana Islands
Commonwealth Board of Nurse Examiners
P.O. Box 501458
Saipan, MP 96950
Phone: (670) 664-4812
Fax: (670) 664-4813

Ohio Board of Nursing
17 South High Street, Suite 400
Columbus, OH 43215-3413
Phone: (614) 466-3947
Fax: (614) 466-0388
Web site: www.nursing.ohio.gov

Oklahoma Board of Nursing
2915 N. Classen Boulevard, Suite 524
Oklahoma City, OK 73106
Phone: (405) 962-1800
Fax: (405) 962-1821
Web site: www.youroklahoma.com/nursing

Oregon State Board of Nursing
800 N.E. Oregon Street, Box 25, Suite 465
Portland, OR 97232
Phone: (503) 731-4745
Fax: (503) 731-4755
Web site: www.osbn.state.or.us

Pennsylvania State Board of Nursing
P.O. Box 2649
Harrisburg, PA 17105-2649
Phone: (717) 783-7142
Fax: (717) 783-0822
Web site: www.dos.state.pa.us/bpoa/cwp/view.asp?
a=1104&q=432869

Puerto Rico Board of Nurse Examiners
Commonwealth of Puerto Rico
800 Roberto H. Todd Avenue
Room 202, Stop 18
Santurce, PR 00908
Phone: (787) 725-7506
Fax: (787) 725-7903

Rhode Island Board of Nurse Registration and Nursing
Education
105 Cannon Building
Three Capitol Hill
Providence, RI 02908
Phone: (401) 222-5700
Fax: (401) 222-3352
Web site: www.healthri.org/hsr/professional/nurses.htm

South Carolina State Board of Nursing
110 Centerview Drive, Suite 202
Columbia, SC 29210
Phone: (803) 896-4550
Fax: (803) 896-4525
Web site: www.llr.state.sc.us/pol/nursing

South Dakota Board of Nursing
4305 South Louise Ave., Suite 201
Sioux Falls, SD 57106-3115
Phone: (605) 362-2760
Fax: (605) 362-2768
Web site: www.state.sd.us/dcr/nursing

Tennessee State Board of Nursing
425 Fifth Avenue North
1st Floor, Cordell Hull Building
Nashville, TN 37247
Phone: (615) 532-5166
Fax: (615) 741-7899
Web site: www.tennessee.gov/health

Texas Board of Nurse Examiners
333 Guadalupe, Suite 3-460
Austin, TX 78701
Phone: (512) 305-7400
Fax: (512) 305-7401
Web site: www.bne.state.tx.us

Utah State Board of Nursing
Heber M. Wells Bldg., 4th Floor
160 East 300 South
Salt Lake City, UT 84111
Phone: (801) 530-6628
Fax: (801) 530-6511
Web site: www.commerce.state.ut.us

Vermont State Board of Nursing
81 River Street
Heritage Building
Montpelier, VT 05609-1106
Phone: (802) 828-2396
Fax: (802) 828-2484
Web site: www.vtprofessionals.org/opr1/nurses

Virgin Islands Board of Nurse Licensure
Veterans Drive Station
St. Thomas, VI 00803
Phone: (340) 776-7397
Fax: (340) 777-4003

Virginia Board of Nursing
6603 West Broad Street, 5th Floor
Richmond, VA 23230-1712
Phone: (804) 662-9909
Fax: (804) 662-9512
Web site: www.dhp.state.va.us

Washington State Nursing Care Quality Assurance Commission
Department of Health
HPQA #6
310 Israel Rd. SE
Tumwater, WA 98501-7864
Phone: (360) 236-4700
Fax: (360) 236-4738
Web site: https://wws2.wa.gov/doh/hpqa-licensing/HPS6/Nursing/default.htm

West Virginia Board of Examiners for Registered Professional Nurses
101 Dee Drive
Charleston, WV 25311
Phone: (304) 558-3596
Fax: (304) 558-3666
Web site: www.wvrnboard.com

Wisconsin Department of Regulation and Licensing
1400 E. Washington Avenue, Rm. 173
Madison, WI 53708
Phone: (608) 266-0145
Fax: (608) 261-7083
Web site: www.drl.state.wi.us

Wyoming State Board of Nursing
2020 Carey Avenue, Suite 110
Cheyenne, WY 82001
Phone: (307) 777-7601
Fax: (307) 777-3519
Web site: http://nursing.state.wy.us/

REFERENCES

Black, J., & Hawks, J. (2005). *Medical-surgical nursing: Clinical management for positive outcomes* (7th ed.). Philadelphia: Saunders.

Harkreader, H., & Hogan, M.A. (2004). *Fundamentals of nursing: Caring and clinical judgment.* (2nd ed.). Philadelphia: Saunders.

Hodgson, B., & Kizior, R. (2004). *Saunders nursing drug handbook 2004.* Philadelphia: Saunders.

Ignatavicius, D., & Workman, M. (2005). *Medical surgical nursing: Critical thinking for collaborative care* (5th ed.). Philadelphia: Saunders.

Kee, J., & Marshall, S. (2004). *Clinical calculations: With applications to general and specialty areas* (5th ed.). Philadelphia: Saunders.

National Council of State Boards of Nursing. (2004). *NCLEX® Examination candidate bulletin.* Chicago: Author.

National Council of State Boards of Nursing (eds.). (2003). *Test Plan for the National Council Licensure Examination for Registered Nurses.* (Effective Date: April 2004). Chicago: Author.

Pagana, K., & Pagana, T. (2003). *Mosby's diagnostic and laboratory test reference* (6th ed.). St. Louis: Mosby.

Phipps, W., Monahan, F., Sands, J., Marek, J., & Neighbors, M. (2003). *Medical-surgical nursing: Health and illness perspectives* (7th ed.). St. Louis: Mosby.

Web site: www.ncsbn.org (National Council of State Boards of Nursing, Inc.)

Preparation for the NCLEX®
Examination: Transitional Issues
for the Foreign-Educated Nurse

INTRODUCTION

This chapter is written to provide you with information regarding the certification processes that you will have to pursue to become a registered nurse in the United States. An important factor to consider as you pursue this process is that some of the requirements may vary from state to state. Therefore, as a first step in the process, it is important to contact the board of nursing in the state in which you are planning to obtain licensure. To assist you in making a contact with the state board of nursing, refer to Chapter 1 in this book. At the end of the chapter you will find the address, phone and fax numbers, and Web site address (if available) for each state. You can also access this information through the National Council of State Boards of Nursing (NCSBN) Web site at www. ncsbn.org. Once you have accessed the NCSBN Web site, select the link "Boards of Nursing." Additionally, you can write to the NCSBN regarding the NCLEX examination at 111 E. Wacker Drive, Suite 2900, Chicago, Illinois 60601. The telephone number for the NCSBN is (312) 525-3600; fax number is (312) 279-1032.

VISASCREEN™

U.S. immigration law requires certain health care professionals to successfully complete a screening program before receiving an occupational visa (Section 343 of the Illegal Immigration Reform and Immigration Responsibility Act [IIRIRA] of 1996). Therefore, you are required to obtain a VisaScreen™ certificate. Information on eligibility for the VisaScreening process and the rules of the IIRIRA can be obtained from U.S. Citizen and Immigration Services (USCIS) at http://uscis.gov/graphics/howdoi/HealthCert.htm.

The Commission on Graduates of Foreign Nursing Schools (CGFNS) is the organization that offers this federal screening program. The International Commission on Health Care Professions (ICHP), a division of the CGFNS, administers the VisaScreen™. The VisaScreen™ components include an educational analysis, licensure

verification, assessment of proficiency in the English language, and an exam that tests nursing knowledge. Each of these components is described in the following sections. Once all of the components have been successfully achieved, the applicant is presented with a VisaScreen™ Certificate. Information related to the VisaScreen™ can be obtained through the CGFNS Web site at http://cgfns.org/cgfns/index.html.

Educational Analysis

1. Applicant must present proof of completion of senior secondary school education, separate from any professional certification.
2. Applicant must present proof of completion from a government-approved professional health care program of at least two years in length.
3. Applicant must provide documentation that he or she has completed a minimum number of clock and/or credit hours in specific theoretical and clinical areas while in nursing school.

Licensure Verification

Applicant must present all current and past licensure for review.

Proficiency in the English Language

Applicant must submit proof of a passing score on an English language proficiency exam approved by the U.S. Department of Education and Health and Human Services. (See Box 2-1 for the English proficiency exams and testing organizations.)

Exam to Test Nursing Knowledge

1. The one-day qualifying exam that is administered as part of the process for obtaining a CGFNS Certificate tests nursing knowledge; therefore, a

BOX 2-1

English Language Proficiency Examinations and Testing Organizations

English Language Proficiency Examinations
Test of English as a Foreign Language (TOEFL)
The Test of English for International Communication (TOEIC)

Testing Organizations
Educational Testing Service (ETS)
P.O. Box 6151
Princeton, NJ 08541-6151
Telephone: (609) 771-7100
E-mail: toefl@ets.org

International English Language Testing System (IELTS)
IELTS Administrator
Cambridge Examinations and IELTS International
100 East Corson Street, Suite 200
Pasadena, CA 91103
Telephone: (626) 564-2954
E-mail: ielts@ceii.org
Web site: www.ielts.org

CGFNS Certificate provides proof of adequate nursing knowledge. This qualifying exam is described in the following section, "Components of the CGFNS Certification Program."

2. A foreign-educated nurse who is licensed and practicing nursing in the United States is also required to obtain a VisaScreen™; if the nurse does not have a CGFNS Certificate, the nurse may be granted eligibility to take the NCLEX® examination to provide proof of nursing knowledge.

TAKING THE NCLEX® FOR VISASCREEN™

A foreign-educated nurse who is licensed and practicing nursing in the United States may apply to take the NCLEX examination for VisaScreen™ purposes through NCSBN's test service, Pearson VUE. Information regarding this process and the *NCSBN NCLEX for VisaScreen™ Candidate Bulletin* can be obtained from the NCSBN Web site at www.ncsbn.org/testing/generalinformation_NCLEXforVisaScreen.asp. Information about the NCLEX examination and the NCLEX-RN Test Plan can be located in the Testing Services area of the NCSBN Web site at www.ncsbn.org/testing/index.asp.

STATE REQUIREMENTS

Most states in the United States require that you receive certification from the CGFNS before you can be eligible to take the NCLEX exam. If the state in which you intend to obtain licensure does not require CGFNS certification, it may require submission of some of the same documents that CGFNS requires. Therefore, in addition to what CGFNS requires, a state may require the following:

1. Proof of citizenship or lawful alien status
2. Official transcripts of educational credentials sent directly to the board of nursing from the school of nursing
3. Validation of theoretical instruction and clinical practice in a variety of nursing areas including medical nursing, surgical nursing, pediatric nursing, maternity and newborn nursing, and mental health nursing
4. Copy of nursing license and/or diploma
5. Proof of proficiency in the English language
6. Photographs of the applicant
7. Application fees

THE COMMISSION ON GRADUATES OF FOREIGN NURSING SCHOOLS (CGFNS)

The CGFNS provides a certification program for nurses educated and licensed outside of the United States. The Certification Program offered by the CGFNS is a requirement of most state boards of nursing, and the certificate may be required before you can take the NCLEX examination. The Certification Program ensures that you are eligible and qualified to meet licensure and other practice requirements in the United States, and it also predicts your success on the NCLEX examination. This program also assists you in obtaining your VisaScreen™ Certificate. Additional information relating to CGFNS and its Certification Program can be obtained through its Web site at www.cgfns.org.

ELIGIBILITY FOR THE CGFNS CERTIFICATION PROGRAM

The CGFNS Certification Program is designed for nurses educated outside of the United States who hold both an initial and current registration/licensure as a first-level general registered nurse. According to the CGFNS, a first-level nurse is called a registered nurse or professional nurse in most countries. As a general nurse, the foreign-educated nurse must have obtained theoretical instruction and clinical practice in a variety of nursing areas including medical nursing, surgical nursing, pediatric nursing, maternity and newborn nursing, and mental health nursing. If the nurse educated outside of the United States does not meet these requirements, he or she is not eligible for the Certification Program.

COMPONENTS OF THE CGFNS CERTIFICATION PROGRAM

The CGFNS Certification Program contains three parts and all parts must be successfully completed in order to be awarded a CGFNS Certificate. The three parts include a credentials review, a one-day qualifying exam that tests nursing knowledge, and an English language proficiency exam. The qualifying exam and the English language proficiency exam can be taken at various locations throughout the world. This provides the applicant the opportunity to obtain the CGFNS Certificate before coming to the United States to take the NCLEX exam. These three parts of the Certification Program are described in the following sections.

Credentials Review

The CGFNS requires validation of education and a licensing history of the applicant to ensure that the applicant has the appropriate credentials to seek certification. The CGFNS must receive transcripts and validation documents from the nursing program and licensing agency. Transcripts and validation documents will not be accepted from the applicant. The specific credentialing requirements are similar to those needed for the VisaScreen™ Certificate and include the following:

1. Completed a senior secondary school education
2. Graduated from a government-approved nursing program of at least two years in length
3. Obtained theoretical instruction and clinical practice in the areas of medical nursing, surgical nursing, pediatric nursing, maternity/newborn nursing, and mental health nursing
4. Holds a full and unrestricted license or registration to practice as a first-level general nurse in the country where he or she completed general nursing education
5. Holds a current license or registration as a first-level general nurse

Qualifying Exam

The qualifying exam tests the applicant's knowledge in nursing in the areas of adult health, pediatrics, maternity and newborn, mental health, and community health. The exam is designed to ensure that the applicant has the knowledge to provide nursing care to various client groups at the same level as recent U.S. nursing graduates.

English Language Proficiency Exam

The applicant must take and pass an English language proficiency exam either before or after the qualifying exam. This exam needs to be taken from a testing organization that is approved by the CGFNS, and the applicant must apply directly with the testing organization to take the exam. The exam scores must be sent directly to the CGFNS from the testing organization. The CGFNS will not accept test scores from the applicant. (See Box 2-1 for the types of English proficiency exams, approved testing organizations, and their contact information.)

The CGFNS identifies certain applicants as exempt from the English language proficiency requirement. In order for an applicant to be exempt, he or she must meet all of the following criteria: (1) native language is English; (2) country of nursing education was Australia, Canada (except Quebec), New Zealand, the United Kingdom, Trinidad, or Tobango (3) language of instruction and language of textbooks was English.

Once each of the three required components of the CGFNS Certification Program have been met, the CGFNS will issue a certificate of completion. Unless the state in which you intend to obtain licensure indicates additional requirements, and if you have received your VisaScreen™ Certificate, you will be eligible to take the NCLEX® examination.

REGISTERING TO TAKE THE NCLEX® EXAMINATION

If you are planning to take the examination in the United States, the initial step in the registration process is to submit an application to the state board of nursing in the state in which you intend to obtain licensure. You need to obtain information from the board of nursing regarding the specific registration process, because the process may vary from state to state. In most states, you may register for the examination through the Web, by mail, or by telephone. It is very important that you follow the registration instructions and complete the registration forms precisely and accurately. Registration forms that are not properly completed, or not accompanied by the proper fees in the required method of payment, will be returned to you and will delay testing. There is a fee for taking the examination, and you may also have to pay additional fees to the board of nursing in the state in which you are applying. You will be sent a confirmation indicating that your registration was received. If you do not receive a confirmation within four weeks of submitting your registration, you should contact the candidate services. Information regarding this contact can be obtained at the NCLEX candidate Web site at www.vue.com/nclex.

Once your eligibility to take the NCLEX examination has been verified by the board of nursing in the state in which licensure is requested, your registration form is processed and an Authorization to Test form will be sent to you. You cannot make an appointment until the board of nursing declares eligibility and you receive an Authorization to Test form. The examination will take place at Pearson Professional Centers, and an appointment can be made through the Web or by telephone. You can schedule an appointment at any Pearson Professional Center. You do not have to take the examination in the same state in which you are seeking licensure. A confirmation of your appointment will be sent to you. For additional information regarding the

NCLEX examination and testing procedures, refer to Chapter 1.

According to the NCSBN, NCLEX testing abroad became available in January 2005. The countries that will provide this testing are Seoul, South Korea; London, England; and Hong Kong. This testing service provides the nurse who is interested in becoming a licensed nurse in the United States an opportunity to pass NCLEX before traveling to the United States.

PREPARING TO TAKE THE NCLEX EXAMINATION

The challenge that is presented to you is one that requires patience and endurance. The positive result of your endeavor will certainly reward you professionally and give you the personal satisfaction of knowing you have become part of a family of highly skilled professionals, the Registered Nurse. You have successfully completed the requirements to become eligible to take the NCLEX examination, and now you have one more important goal to achieve: to pass the NCLEX examination.

I highly recommend adequate preparation for the NCLEX examination because it is difficult. An important step that you have taken in preparing is that you are using this book, *Saunders Q&A Review for the NCLEX-RN Examination*. The companion book, *Saunders Comprehensive Review for the NCLEX-RN Examination* provides you with both content review and more than 4,000 practice questions based on the NCLEX-RN test plan. Next, the *Saunders Computerized Review for the NCLEX-RN Examination* is a computer disk program that contains more than 2,000 NCLEX-RN-style questions to help you determine your readiness for NCLEX-RN.

If you prefer to prepare by using online resources, access the *Saunders Online NCLEX-RN Review Course* at www.elsevierhealth.com. Additional online specialty tests titled *Adult Health, Mental Health, Maternal-Newborn, Pediatrics,* and *Pharmacology* are also available.

Lastly, never lose sight of your goal. Patience and dedication will contribute significantly to your achieving the status of Registered Nurse. Remember: success is climbing a mountain, facing the challenge of obstacles, and reaching the top of the mountain. I wish you the best success in your career as a registered nurse in the United States of America!

REFERENCES

Commission on Graduates of Foreign Nursing Schools Web site: www.cgfns.org

International English Language Testing System E-mail: ielts@ceii.org

International English Language Testing System Web site: www.ielts.org

National Council of State Boards of Nursing Web site: www.ncsbn.org

National Council of State Boards of Nursing. (September 2004). *NCLEX for VisaScreen through NCSBN: Frequently asked questions.* Chicago: Author. Retrieved November 14, 2004 from National Council of State Boards of Nursing Web site: www.ncsbn.org.

Test of English as a Foreign Language E-mail: toefl@ets.org

Profiles to Success

LAURENT W. VALLIERE, B.S.

Preparing to take the National Council Licensure Examination for Registered Nurses (NCLEX-RN®) can produce a great deal of anxiety in the nursing graduate. You may be thinking that the NCLEX-RN is the most important examination you will ever have to take and that it reflects the culmination of everything you have worked so hard for. NCLEX-RN is an important examination because achieving that nursing license defines the beginning of your career as a Registered Nurse. A vital ingredient to your success on NCLEX-RN involves avoiding negative thoughts that allow this examination to seem overwhelming and intimidating. Such thoughts will take full control over your destiny (Box 3-1).

Nursing graduates preparing for NCLEX-RN must develop a comprehensive plan. The most important component in developing a plan is to identify the study patterns that guided you to your nursing degree. It is important to begin your planning by reflecting on all of the personal and academic challenges you experienced during your nursing education. Take time to focus on the thoughts, feelings, and emotions you experienced before taking an examination while in your nursing program. Examine the methods you used in preparing for that examination both academically and from the standpoint of how you dealt with the anxiety that parallels the experience of facing an examination. These factors are very important considerations in preparing for NCLEX-RN because they identify the patterns that worked for you. Think about this for a moment. Your own methods of study must have worked, or you would not be at the point of preparing for NCLEX-RN.

Each individual requires his or her own methods of preparing for an examination. Graduate nurses who have taken NCLEX-RN will probably share their experiences and methods of preparing for this challenge with you. It is very helpful to listen to what they may tell you. These graduates will provide you with important strategies they have used. Listen closely to what they have to say, but remember that this examination is all about you. Your identity and what you require in terms of preparation are most important.

Reflect on the methods and strategies that worked for you throughout your nursing program. Do not think that you need to develop new methods and strategies in preparing for NCLEX-RN. Use what has worked for you. Take some time to reflect on these strategies, write them down on a large blank card, sign your name, and write "R.N." after your name. Post this card in a place where you will see it every morning of every day. Commit to your own special strategies. These strategies reflect your profile and identity and will lead you to success!

A frequent concern of graduates preparing for NCLEX-RN relates to deciding whether they should study alone or become part of a study group. Examining your profile will easily direct you with making this decision. Again, reflect on what has worked for you throughout your nursing program as you prepared for examinations. Remember: your needs are most impor-

---

BOX 3-1

Profiles to Success

- Avoid negative thoughts that allow the examination to seem overwhelming and intimidating.
- Develop a comprehensive plan to prepare for the examination.
- Examine the study methods and strategies you used in preparing for examinations during nursing school.
- Develop realistic time goals.
- Select a study time period and study place that will be most conducive to your success.
- Commit to your own special study methods and strategies.
- Incorporate a balance of exercise with adequate rest and relaxation time in your preparation schedule.
- Maintain healthy eating habits.
- Learn to control anxiety.
- Remember that discipline and perseverance will automatically bring control.
- Remember that this examination is all about you.
- Remember that your self-confidence and the belief in yourself will lead you to success!

tant. Address your own needs and do not become pressured by peers who are encouraging you to join a study group, if this is not your normal pattern for study. Remember that additional pressure is not what you need at this important time of your life.

Nursing graduates preparing for NCLEX-RN frequently inquire about the best method of preparing for NCLEX-RN. First, remember that you are prepared. In fact, you began preparing for this examination on the first day that you entered your nursing program.

The task that you are faced with is to review, in a comprehensive manner, all of the nursing content that you learned in your nursing program. It can become totally overwhelming to look at your bookshelf, which is overflowing with the nursing books that you used during nursing school, and your challenge becomes monumental when you look at the boxes of nursing lecture notes you have accumulated. It is unrealistic to even think that you could read all of those nursing books and lecture notes in preparation for NCLEX-RN. These books and lecture notes should be used as a reference source, if needed, during your preparation for NCLEX-RN.

Saunders Comprehensive Review for the NCLEX-RN Examination has identified for you all of the important nursing content areas relevant to the examination. During your review through the comprehensive review, you should have noted the areas that may be unfamiliar or unclear. Be sure that you have taken the necessary time to become familiar with these needed areas. Now, progress through the Pyramid to Success and test your knowledge in this book, *Saunders Q&A Review for the NCLEX-RN Examination.* You may identify nursing content areas that still require further review. Take the time to review, as you are guided to do in this book.

Your profile to success requires that you develop realistic time goals to prepare for NCLEX-RN. It is necessary to take the time to examine your life and all of the commitments you may have. These commitments may include family, work, and friends. As you develop your goals, remember to plan time for fun and exercise. To achieve success, you require a balance of both work time and enjoyment time. If you do not plan for some leisure time, you will become frustrated and perhaps even angry. These sorts of feelings will block your ability to focus and concentrate. Remember that you need time for yourself.

Goal development may be a relatively easy process because you have probably been juggling your life commitments ever since you entered nursing school. Remember that your goal is to identify a daily time frame and time period for you to use in reviewing and preparing for NCLEX-RN. Open your calendar and identify days on which life commitments will not allow you to spend this time preparing. Block those days off and do not consider them as part of your review time. Identify the time that is best for you in terms of your ability to concentrate and focus, so that you can accomplish the most in your identified time frame. Be sure that you consider a time that is quiet and free of distractions. Many individuals find that the morning hours provide the most productive hours, whereas others may find the afternoon and evening hours most productive. Remember that this examination is all about you, and select that time period that will be most conducive to your success.

The place of study is also very important. Select a place that is quiet and comfortable for study and a place where you normally do your studying and preparing. Some individuals prefer to study at home in their own environment; if this is your normal pattern, be sure that you are able to free yourself of distractions during your scheduled preparation time. If you are not able to free yourself of distractions, you may consider spending your preparation time in a library. Reflect on what worked best for you during your nursing program in selecting your place of study.

Selecting the amount of daily preparation time has frequently been a dilemma for many graduates preparing for NCLEX-RN. It is very important to set a realistic time period that can be adhered to on a daily basis. Set a time frame that will provide you with quality time and a time frame that can be achieved. If you set a time frame that is not realistic and cannot be achieved every day, you will become frustrated. This frustration will block your journey toward the peak of the Pyramid to Success.

The best suggestion to you is to spend at least two hours daily for NCLEX-RN preparation. Two hours is a realistic time period both in terms of quality time and a time frame that is achievable. You may find that after two hours your ability to focus and concentrate will diminish. You may, however, find that on some days you are able to spend more than the scheduled two hours; if you can and feel as though your ability to concentrate and focus is still present, then do so.

Discipline and perseverance will automatically bring control. Control will provide you with the momentum that will sweep you to the peak in the Pyramid to Success. Discipline yourself to spend time preparing for NCLEX-RN every day. Daily preparation is very important because it maintains a consistent pattern and keeps you in synchrony with the mind flow needed the day you are scheduled to take the NCLEX-RN examination. Some days you may think about skipping your scheduled preparation time because you are not in the mood for study. On these days, practice discipline and persevere. Stand yourself up, shake off those thoughts of skipping a day of preparation, take a deep breath, and get the oxygen flowing throughout your body. Look in the mirror, smile, and say to yourself "This time is for me and I can do this!" Look at your card that displays your name with "R.N." after it, and get yourself to that special study place. Remember that discipline and perseverance will bring control!

In the profile to success, academic preparation directs the path to the peak of the Pyramid to Success; however, additional factors will influence successful achievement to the peak including your ability to control anxiety, physical stamina, the amount of rest and relaxation you have, your self-confidence, and the belief in yourself that you will achieve success on NCLEX-RN. You need to take time to think about these important factors and incorporate them into your daily preparation schedule.

Anxiety is a common concern among students preparing to take NCLEX-RN. Some anxiety is a normal feeling and will keep your senses sharp and alert. A great deal of anxiety, however, can block your process of thinking and hamper your ability to focus and concentrate. You have already practiced the task of controlling anxiety when you took examinations in nursing school. Now you need to continue with this practice and incorporate this control on a daily basis. Each day, before beginning your scheduled preparation time, sit in your quiet special study place, close your eyes, and take a slow deep breath. Fill your body with oxygen, hold your breath to a count of four, and then exhale slowly through your mouth. Continue with this exercise and repeat it four to six times. This exercise will help relieve your mind of any unnecessary chatter and will deliver oxygen to all of your body tissues and to your brain. On your scheduled day of NCLEX-RN, after the necessary pretesting procedures, you will be escorted to your test computer. Practice this breathing exercise before beginning the examination. Use this exercise during the examination if you feel yourself becoming anxious and distracted and if you are having difficulty focusing or concentrating. Remember that breathing will move that oxygen to your brain!

Physical stamina is a necessary component of readiness for NCLEX-RN. Plan to incorporate a balance of exercise with adequate rest and relaxation time in your preparation schedule. It is also important that you maintain healthy eating habits. Begin to practice these healthy habits now, if you have not already done so. There are a few points to keep in mind each day as you plan your daily meals. Three balanced meals are important, with snacks, such as fruits, included between meals. Remember that food items that contain fat will slow you down and those that contain caffeine will cause nervousness and sometimes shakiness. These items need to be avoided. Healthy foods that are high in complex carbohydrates work best to supply you with your energy needs. Remember that your brain can work like a muscle: it requires those carbohydrates. In addition, be sure that you include those needed fruits and vegetables in your diet (Box 3-2).

If you are the type of individual who does not regularly eat breakfast, work on changing that habit. Practice the habit of eating breakfast now, as you are preparing for NCLEX-RN. Attempt to provide your brain with energy in the morning with some form of carbohydrate

---

BOX 3-2

Healthy Eating Habits

- Eat three balanced meals each day.
- Include snacks, such as fruits and vegetables, between meals.
- Avoid food items that contain fat.
- Avoid food items that contain caffeine.
- Consume healthy foods that are high in complex carbohydrates.

---

food. It will make a difference. On your scheduled day for NCLEX-RN, feed your brain and eat a healthy breakfast. In addition, on this very important day, bring some form of snack such as a fruit or bagel for break time, and feed your brain again so that you will have the energy to concentrate, focus, and complete your examination.

Adequate rest, relaxation, and exercise is important in your preparation process. Many graduates preparing for NCLEX-RN have difficulty sleeping, particularly the night before the examination. Begin now to develop methods that will assist in relaxing your body and mind and allow you to obtain a restful sleep. You may already have a particular method developed to help you sleep. If not, it may be helpful to try the breathing exercise while you lie in bed to assist in eliminating any mind chatter that is present. It is also helpful to visualize your favorite and most peaceful place while you do these breathing exercises. Graduates have also stated that listening to quiet music and relaxation tapes have assisted in helping them relax and sleep. Begin to practice some of these helpful methods now, while you are preparing for NCLEX-RN. Identify those that work best for you. The night before your scheduled examination is an important one. Spend time having some fun, get to bed early, and incorporate the relaxation method that you have been using to help you sleep.

Confidence and belief that you have the ability to achieve success will bring your goals to fruition. Reflect on your profile maintained during your nursing education. Your confidence and belief in yourself, along with your academic achievements, have brought you to the status of graduate nurse. Now you are facing one more important challenge. Can you meet this challenge successfully? Yes, you can! There is no reason to think otherwise, if you have taken all of the necessary steps to ensure that profile to success.

Each morning, place your feet on the floor, stand tall, take a deep breath, and smile. Take both hands and imagine yourself brushing off any negative feelings. Look at your card that bears your name with the letters "R.N." after it, and tell yourself: "Yes, I can do this successfully!" Believe in yourself, and you will reach the peak of the Pyramid to Success! Congratulations, and I wish you continued success in your career as a Registered Nurse!

The NCLEX-RN Examination®: From a Student's Perspective

REBECCA S. BLASZCZAK, RN

"RN!" It's amazing how much time and effort is put into the title "RN." The title represents so much: registered nurse, college graduate, student loans, clinicals, countless hours of studying, and much, much more. When I look back on it all, I find it amazing to think that I survived and can now call myself a registered nurse. As daunting as the task ahead looks, know that with hard work and determination, you too can conquer the NCLEX-RN examination and become a registered nurse.

When I first picked up my *Saunders Comprehensive Review for the NCLEX-RN Examination* book, I took one look at it and thought there was no way I would ever read the entire thing. Now, I simply chuckle and think about how not only did I read the entire text cover to cover, but it became my ultimate study guide and resource for all of my nursing classes! For three years I carried the *Saunders Comprehensive Review for the NCLEX-RN Examination* from class to my dorm room to the library. It became my best friend and the greatest study tool I had when preparing for my boards!

I feel that throughout my nursing education, I was preparing for the NCLEX-RN examination. All of my professors used the *Saunders Comprehensive Review for the NCLEX-RN Examination* as a tool to guide students' study. They would assign certain chapters corresponding with the lesson they were teaching. By the time my senior year came, I already had a strong and wonderful knowledge base to build on and focus my studying.

When it came down to my last year in school, I realized I really needed to buckle down and focus on the NCLEX examination. I had already read and reread the *Saunders Comprehensive Review for the NCLEX-RN Examination*, so I decided it was time to pick up a few more study tools. Now my study selection grew to *Saunders Q&A Review for the NCLEX-RN Examination* and the *Saunders Computerized Review for the NCLEX-RN Examination*. I found it helpful to vary my studying techniques, so I would alternate between reading a chapter and doing practice questions on the computer.

I tried to get through one or two sections in the review books each day, answering all of the questions and reviewing content areas that I found difficult.

Along with studying by myself, I got together with a group of friends to form a small study group. Together we worked our way through the *Saunders Comprehensive Review for the NCLEX-RN Examination* and tackled chapter after chapter. During the study session, we took on the roles of both student and teacher. We each had different areas of weaknesses and strengths, so by working together we were able to help each other understand the material. I also found that by talking aloud with a group of people, I was able to see the information differently and understand it better. Of course, we found ways to make studying fun, and soon our study sessions became something I looked forward to. Our weekly meetings were a way to summarize chapters I had read on my own and obtain answers to any questions I had.

The closer I got to my examination date, the harder I studied. After graduation, I attended a NCLEX-RN review course. It was a weeklong review session designed to help prepare for the boards. I found this to be an extremely helpful part of my preparation. After spending four years learning countless facts, it was difficult at times to know which information was most important to know and which information slightly less important. The review course helped summarize information and offer guidance for studying. In the review course, the first thing we were asked to do was write on a piece of paper our names with "RN" after it. What seemed like a small task turned out to be a wonderful inspiration for me. Every time I was tired of studying or felt overwhelmed, I would take out my piece of paper with my name and the letters "RN" after it, and it helped me maintain stamina and realize that yes, I could do this.

The most helpful part of the review course and the *Saunders Comprehensive Review for the NCLEX-RN Examination* was the review of the chapter on test-taking strategies. As much as I wanted to know everything there is to know about nursing, I knew it was impossible to memorize the countless pieces of information I had picked up over the years. By learning how to take the test, I knew that even if I didn't know a specific fact or situation, I would at least be able to make an educated guess. Learning how to take the test was just as important as learning facts for the test.

If someone were to flip through my *Saunders Comprehensive Review for the NCLEX-RN Examination*, they would notice that it was a well-loved book. In other words, I am probably the only person who can understand and follow along with my book. Over the years, I have highlighted, edited, added, doodled, spilled on, and simply abused my book. When specific topics were discussed in class, I would reference my comprehensive review book, adding notes in the margins or highlighting key areas. I would circle areas where I had questions, so that I would be reminded to look up information or ask someone else for help.

The last week before I took the NCLEX-RN examination, I decided to break my studying down into sections. I redesigned a schedule for myself that broke studying down into two-hour blocks, with breaks in between. After each two-hour session, I would get up and stretch, watch TV, or simply take a nap to allow the information to sink in and my mind to rest. I looked at studying as if it were a full-time job. I knew it was for only one week and that I could get through it because the reward would be priceless. I spent approximately eight hours a day studying during the last week before my boards. I wanted to be sure that I knew how to take the test and wouldn't make any "silly" mistakes. During this last week, I practiced question after question in both the *Saunders Q&A Review for the NCLEX-RN Examination* and the *Saunders Computerized Review for the NCLEX-RN Examination*. After each set of questions, I would read the answers and review any content areas of which I was unsure. This repetition helped me learn both specific pieces of information and the structure of the exam questions.

The final night before my test, I decided to kick back and relax. My nerves were increasing with each hour that passed, and I knew that I needed to get my mind off the exam if I were to get any sleep that night. An evening of friends and TV was just what I needed. I spent a few hours relaxing and doing mindless activities before turning in for a good night's sleep. Surprisingly enough, I was able to sleep soundly and woke the next morning with a fresh set of nerves. I had a light breakfast and then headed to the testing center. I arrived approximately 30 minutes early, knowing that I would need some time to clear my head before I headed into the testing center.

When I walked into the waiting room, I saw three other women looking just as nervous as I was. Oddly enough, that seemed to comfort me. I knew that we were all going through the same thing and that I wasn't alone in this nervous state. When I went through the final checkpoint and was assigned a computer to sit at, I thought: "This is it, the moment I had worked so hard for." The moment I logged onto the computer and began my examination, I seemed to go into a trance. Facts were flying through my head as I broke down each question. After what seemed like days, I finally got to question number 75. I knew this was the infamous number and that depending on how I had done, the test might be over. Once I had picked an answer, I took a deep breath and clicked the button. Much to my surprise, my test shut off. As relieved as I was, I also felt a rise of panic. I knew there was nothing left for me to do except wait and keep my fingers crossed.

Even though it was only two days, it seemed like an eternity waiting for my test results. There was no way I would have been able to wait a couple of weeks or a month that it would take to get the actual letter in the mail. So, I logged onto the state board of nursing Web site. Seeing an RN license number after my name on the state board of nursing Web site was one of the best moments of my life. I was ecstatic and slightly in shock. I started calling and telling people that I had passed, but I don't think it really set in that I was a registered nurse until the letter came with my actual license and license number on it a few weeks later. That was when I truly believed I had done it. My hard work and countless hours of studying over the past four years had paid off.

In conclusion, I want to wish you the best of luck with what lies ahead. Although the task may seem overwhelming at times, know that you can do it. Don't be afraid to ask for help; every question is important. Study hard, but remember to allow for time to relax and enjoy yourself. You too can achieve your dream and become a registered nurse!

Test-Taking Strategies

I. **Pyramid to Success** (Box 5-1)
II. **How to Avoid Reading into the Question** (Box 5-2)
   A. Pyramid Points
   1. Read every word in the question and specifically determine what the question is asking
   2. Focus only on the information in the question and avoid asking yourself "Well, what if . . . ?"
   3. Look for the key words in the question, such as "early signs" *or* "late signs"
   4. In multiple choice questions, multiple response questions, or questions that require you to prioritize nursing actions, read every choice or option presented
   5. Use the process of elimination when choices or options are presented; reread the question and what the question is specifically asking to assist you in determining your final choice or choices
   6. With questions that require you to fill in the blank, focus on the information in the question and determine what the question is asking; if the question requires you to calculate a medication dose, and intravenous flow rate, or intake and output amounts, recheck your work in calculating to verify the answer
   7. Remember, focus on the information in the question and specifically what the question is asking!

   B. The Parts of a Question (Box 5-3)
   1. The question will consist of a Case Situation, Question Stem, and the Options (a Fill-In-The Blank question will not contain options)
   2. The case situation provides you with the information about the client and the information that you need to consider in answering the question
   3. The question stem asks something specific about the case situation
   4. The options are all of the answers
   5. In a multiple choice question, there will be four options and you must select one; read every option carefully and always use the process of elimination
   6. In a multiple response question, there will be several options and you must select all options that apply to the situation in the question; read each option carefully;

BOX 5-1

Pyramid to Success

Read the question and every option thoroughly and carefully!
Ask yourself, "What is the question specifically asking?"
Be alert to key words and true and false response questions!
Eliminate the incorrect options!
Use all of your nursing knowledge, your clinical experiences, and your test-taking skills and strategies to answer the question!

BOX 5-2

Practice Question: Avoid Reading into the Question

A client with metastatic cancer is receiving a continuous intravenous infusion of morphine sulfate to alleviate pain. The nurse monitors the client for which *adverse or toxic effect* of the medication?
1. Dizziness
2. Sedation
3. Skeletal muscle flaccidity
4. Nausea

Answer: 3

Test-Taking Strategy: Read every word in the question and specifically determine what the question is asking. The question is asking about the adverse or toxic effect of morphine sulfate. Dizziness, sedation, and nausea are side effects of morphine sulfate that the client may experience, but are not toxic effects. Remember, focus on the information in the question and what the question is asking!

BOX 5-3

Multiple Choice Question: Case Situation, Question Stem, and Options

Case Situation: A client arrives to the surgical unit following nasal surgery and has nasal packing in place.
Stem: The nurse reviews the physician's orders and anticipates that which client position would be prescribed to reduce swelling?
Options:
1. Sim's
2. Prone
3. Supine
4. Semi-Fowler's position

Answer: 4

BOX 5-4

Common Key Words

Early or late
Best
First
Initial
Immediately
Most likely or least likely
Most appropriate or least appropriate

visualize the situation, and use your nursing knowledge to answer the question

7. In a prioritizing (ordered response) question, you will be required to place in order of priority certain nursing interventions; visualize the situation, and use your nursing knowledge to answer the question

III. **Look for Key Words** (Box 5-4 and Box 5-5)
  1. Key words focus your attention on a specific or critical point to consider when answering the question
  2. Some key words may indicate that all of the options are correct, and that it will be necessary to prioritize in order to select the correct option
  3. As you read the question, look for the key words; key words will make a difference with regard to how you will answer the question.

IV. **The Issue of the Question** (Box 5-6)
  A. The issue of the question is the specific subject content that the question is asking about
  B. Identifying the issue of the question will assist in eliminating the incorrect options and direct you to selecting the correct option
  C. The issue of the question can include
    1. A medication or intravenous (IV) therapy
    2. An intended effect or side effect of a medication
    3. An adverse or toxic effect of a medication
    4. A treatment or procedure
    5. A complication of a health care problem, treatment, or procedure
    6. A specific nursing action

BOX 5-5

Practice Question: Look for the Key Words

A nurse is caring for a client who just returned from the recovery room after undergoing abdominal surgery. The nurse monitors the client for which *early sign* of hypovolemic shock?
1. Increased pulse rate
2. Increased depth of respiration
3. Lethargy
4. Decreased deep tendon reflexes

Answer: 1

Test-Taking Strategy: Note the key words, "early sign". Focusing on these key words and recalling that the earliest clinical signs of hypovolemic shock are cardiovascular changes will direct you to the correct option. Although increased depth of respirations, lethargy, and decreased or absent deep tendon reflexes occur in hypovolemic shock, these are not early signs. Rather, they occur as the shock progresses. Remember to look for key words!

BOX 5-6

The Issue of the Question

A pediatric nurse in the ambulatory care unit is caring for a child following a tonsillectomy. The mother of the child tells the nurse that the child is complaining of a dry throat and would like something to relieve the dryness. Which of the following would the nurse give to the mother for the child?
1. Warm ginger ale
2. A glass of milk
3. Cola with ice
4. Yellow noncitrus Jello

Answer: 4

Test-Taking Strategy: The issue of the question relates to the foods and fluids that should be avoided following tonsillectomy. Carbonated beverages will irritate the throat. Milk can coat the throat and cause coughing. Focusing on the issue and thinking about the food items that irritate the throat will direct you to the correct option. Remember, focus on the issue!

V. **True and False Response Questions** (Box 5-7 and Box 5-8)
  A. True response questions use key words that ask you to select an option that is accurate regarding the information in the question
  B. False response questions use key words that ask you to select an option that is not accurate regarding the information in the question
  C. Read every word in the question and be especially alert in noting key words that ask you to select an option that is not accurate regarding the information in the question

BOX 5-7

Practice Question: True Response

A community health nurse is providing an educational session to community members regarding dietary measures that will assist in reducing the risk of osteoporosis. The nurse instructs the community members to increase dietary intake of which food that would be *most helpful* to minimize this risk?
1. Yogurt
2. Turkey
3. Spaghetti
4. Shell fish

Answer: 1

Test-Taking Strategy: This question identifies an example of a true response question. Note the key words "most helpful". Recall that in the client with osteoporosis, calcium intake should be increased. This will assist in directing you to option 1. Remember true response questions ask you to select an option that is accurate!

BOX 5-8

Practice Question: False Response

The nurse has provided instructions to a client with glaucoma regarding measures that will prevent an increase in intraocular pressure in the eye. Which statement if made by the client indicates *a need for further education*?
1. "I should restrict my fluid intake to prevent an increase in pressure."
2. "I should eat foods that are high in fiber."
3. "I should avoid lifting objects that weigh greater that 20 pounds."
4. "I should move objects by using my feet and pushing them rather than lifting them."

Answer: 1

Test-Taking Strategy: This question identifies an example of a false response question. Note the key words "a need for further education". These key words indicate that you need to select an option that identifies an incorrect client statement. Recall that an increase in intraocular pressure is a concern. Using principles related to activities that will increase intraocular pressure will direct you to option 1. Remember false response questions ask you to select an option that is not accurate regarding the information in the question!

VI. Questions that Require Prioritizing
  A. Questions in the examination may require you to use the skill of prioritizing nursing actions
  B. Look for the key words in the question that indicate the need to prioritize (Box 5-9)
  C. Remember, when a question requires prioritization, all options may be correct and you need to determine the correct order of action
  D. Guidelines to use include the ABCs—airway, breathing, and circulation; Maslow's Hierarchy of Needs theory; and the steps of the nursing process

BOX 5-9

Common Key Words that Indicate the Need to Prioritize

Best
Essential
First
Highest priority
Immediate
Initial
Most important
Next
Primary
Vital

BOX 5-10

Practice Question: Use of the ABCs

A nurse is preparing to suction a client with a tracheostomy tube. The nurse gathers the supplies needed for the procedure and prepares to suction the client. Which of the following is the *initial* nursing action?
1. Lubricate the catheter
2. Hyperoxygenate the client
3. Place the catheter into the tracheostomy tube
4. Place suction on the catheter

Answer: 2

Test-Taking Strategy: Use the ABCs—airway, breathing, and circulation—as a guide to direct you to the correct option. Note the key word "initial" in the stem of the question. Recall that suctioning will remove oxygen from the client. Option 2, the correct option, addresses airway. Remember use the ABCs—airway, breathing, and circulation—to prioritize!

  E. The ABCs (Box 5-10)
    1. Use the ABCs—airway, breathing, and circulation—when selecting an answer or determining the order of priority
    2. Remember the order of priority: airway, breathing, and circulation
    3. Airway is always the first priority!
  F. Maslow's Hierarchy of Needs theory (Box 5-11)
    1. Use Maslow's Hierarchy of Needs theory as a guide to prioritize
    2. Physiological needs are the priority; therefore, select an option or determine the order of priority by addressing physiological needs first
    3. When a physiological need is not addressed in the question or noted in one of the options, continue to use Maslow's Hierarchy of Needs theory as a guide and look for the option that addresses safety
  G. Steps of the nursing process
    1. Use the steps of the nursing process to prioritize
    2. The steps include assessment, analysis, planning, implementation, and evaluation and are followed in this order

BOX 5-11

Practice Question: Maslow's Hierarchy of Needs Theory

A nurse is reviewing the plan of care for a pregnant client with a diagnosis of sickle cell anemia. Which nursing diagnosis, if stated on the plan of care, would the nurse select as receiving the *highest priority*?
1. Anxiety
2. Ineffective coping
3. Disturbed body image
4. Deficient fluid volume

Answer: 4

Test-Taking Strategy: Note the key words, "highest priority". Use Maslow's Hierarchy of Needs theory to prioritize, remembering that physiological needs come first. Using this guideline will direct you to option 4. Deficient fluid volume is a physiological need and is the priority nursing diagnosis. Remember, physiological needs are the priority!

3. Assessment
   a. Remember that assessment is the first step in the nursing process
   b. When you are asked to select your first and initial nursing action, follow the steps of the nursing process to prioritize when selecting the correct option
   c. Assessment questions address the process of gathering subjective and objective data relative to the client, confirming that data, and communicating and documenting the data
   d. Look for key words in the options that reflect assessment (Box 5-12)
   e. If an option contains the concept of assessment or the collection of client data, it is best to select that option (Box 5-13)
   f. If an assessment action is not one of the options, follow the steps of the nursing process as your guide to select your initial or first action.
   g. *Possible exception to the guideline:* If the question presents an emergency situation, read carefully; in an emergency situation, an intervention may be the priority!

BOX 5-12

Assessment: Key Words

Ascertain
Assess
Check
Determine
Find out
Identify
Monitor
Observe
Obtain information

BOX 5-13

Practice Question: The Nursing Process/Assessment

A client with multiple sclerosis tells a home health care nurse that she is having increasing difficulty in transferring from the bed to a chair. The home health care nurse would *initially*:
1. Observe the client demonstrating the transfer technique
2. Document the number of falls that the client has had in recent weeks
3. Discuss potential nursing home placement
4. Start a restorative nursing program before an injury occurs

Answer: 1

Test-Taking Strategy: Use the steps of the nursing process. Assessment is the first step. Options 2, 3, and 4 identify the implementation step of the nursing process. The initial action is to observe the client demonstrating the transfer technique. Remember assessment is the first step of the nursing process!

4. Analysis (Box 5-14)
   a. Analysis questions are the most difficult questions because they require understanding of the principles of physiological responses and require interpretation of the data on the basis of assessment
   b. Analysis questions require critical thinking and determining the rationale for therapeutic interventions that may be addressed in the question
   c. Analysis questions may address the formulation of a nursing diagnosis and the communication and documentation of the results of the process of analysis

BOX 5-14

Practice Question: The Nursing Process/Analysis

A nurse is reviewing the laboratory results of an infant suspected of having hypertrophic pyloric stenosis. Which of the following laboratory findings would the nurse *most likely* expect to note in this infant?
1. A blood pH of 7.50
2. A blood pH of 7.30
3. A blood bicarbonate of 22 mEq/L
4. A blood bicarbonate of 19 mEq/L

Answer: 1

Test-Taking Strategy: It is necessary to understand the physiology associated with hypertrophic pyloric stenosis and that metabolic alkalosis is likely to occur as a result of vomiting. Next, it is necessary to know which laboratory findings would be noted in this acid-base condition. Analysis of this data will direct you to the correct option. Remember analysis is the second step of the nursing process!

BOX 5-15

Practice Question: The Nursing Process/Planning

A nurse develops a plan of care for a client with a cataract. Which nursing diagnosis is the *priority*?
1. Fear Related to loss of eyesight
2. Social Isolation related to decreased ability to mobilize in the community
3. Disturbed Sensory Perception (Visual) related to ocular lens opacity
4. Risk for Injury related to decreased vision

Answer: 3

Test-Taking Strategy: This question relates to planning nursing care and asks you to identify the priority nursing diagnosis. Use Maslow's Hierarchy of Needs theory to answer the question. Remembering that physiological needs are the priority will direct you to option 3. Risk for Injury is a potential rather than an actual problem, and according to Maslow's Hierarchy of Needs theory, safety is the second priority. Fear and Social Isolation are psychosocial needs. Remember planning is the third step of the nursing process!

5. Planning (Box 5-15)
   a. Planning questions require prioritizing nursing diagnoses, determining goals and outcome criteria for goals of care, developing the plan of care, and communicating and documenting the plan of care
   b. With regard to nursing diagnoses, remember that actual client problems rather than potential or at risk client problems will most likely be the priority
   c. Remember that this is a nursing examination and the answer to the question most likely involves something that is included in the nursing care plan, rather than the medical plan
6. Implementation (Box 5-16)
   a. Implementation questions address the process of organizing and managing care, counseling and teaching, providing care to achieve established goals, supervising and coordinating care, and communicating and documenting nursing interventions
   b. This exam is about nursing, so focus on the nursing action rather than on the medical action, unless the question is asking you what prescription (medical order) is anticipated.
   c. The only client whom you need to be concerned about is the client in the question that you are answering; remember that this client is your only assigned client
   d. Answer the question as if the situation was textbook and ideal and the nurse had all the time and resources needed and readily available at the client's bedside
7. Evaluation (Box 5-17)
   a. Evaluation questions focus on comparing the actual outcomes of care with the expected outcomes and focus on how the nurse should monitor or make a judgment concerning a client's response to therapy or to a nursing action
   b. These questions address evaluating the client's ability to implement self-care, health care team members' ability to implement care, and the process of communicating and documenting evaluation findings
   c. In an evaluation question, be alert to false response questions because they are frequently used in evaluation type questions, and the question may ask for a client statement that indicates either accurate or

BOX 5-16

Practice Question: The Nursing Process/Implementation

A client is being admitted to the hospital after receiving a radium implant for bladder cancer. The nurse would take which *priority* action in the care of this client?
1. Encourage the client to take frequent rest periods
2. Admit the client to a private room .
3. Encourage the family to visit
4. Place the client on reverse isolation

Answer: 2

Test-Taking Strategy: Implementation questions address the process of organizing and managing care and providing care to achieve established goals. The client who has a radiation implant is placed in a private room and has limited visitors. This reduces the exposure of others to the radiation. Frequent rest periods are a helpful general intervention, but are not a priority for the client in this situation. Reverse isolation is unnecessary. Remember implementation is the fourth step of the nursing process!

BOX 5-17

Practice Question: The Nursing Process/Evaluation

A home health nurse is reviewing medications with the client receiving colchicine for the treatment of gout. The nurse evaluates that the *medication is* "effective" if the client reports a decrease in:
1. Blood glucose
2. Blood pressure
3. Joint inflammation
4. Headaches

Answer: 3

Test-Taking Strategy: This is an evaluation question and contains a true response stem as identified by the words "medication is effective". In this question, focusing on the client's diagnosis and recalling the pathophysiology associated with gout will direct you to option 3. Remember evaluation is the fifth step of the nursing process!

inaccurate information related to the issue of the question

VII. **Client Needs**

A. Physiological Integrity

1. These questions address the nurse's role in promoting physical health and well-being in the client by providing care and comfort, reducing client risk potential, and managing the client's health alterations

2. Content addressed in these questions relates to basic care and comfort, pharmacological and parenteral therapies, reducing the risk of the development of complications, and managing and providing care to clients with acute, chronic, or life-threatening conditions

3. Remember that physiological needs are a priority and are addressed first

4. Use the ABCs, airway, breathing, and circulation, Maslow's Hierarchy of Needs theory, and the steps of the Nursing Process when selecting an option addressing physiological integrity

B. Safe, Effective Care Environment

1. These questions address the nurse's role in providing and directing care that will ensure an environment that promotes protecting the client, family or significant other(s), and other health care personnel

2. Content addressed in these questions relates to the nursing role of coordinating and integrating cost-effective care, supervising and/or collaborating with members of the multi-disciplinary health care team, and environmental safety

3. Be alert to safety needs addressed in a question and remember the importance of handwashing, call bells, bed positioning, the appropriate use of siderails, and standard precautions

C. Health Promotion and Maintenance

1. These questions address the nurse's role in providing and directing nursing care that prevents health problems, provides early detection of health problems, and provides and directs care that incorporates knowledge of expected growth and development principles

2. Content addressed in these questions relates to assisting the client and significant other(s) through the normal stages of growth and development, and assisting the client and significant other(s) to develop health practices that promote wellness, and to recognize alterations in health care status

3. Use the Teaching/Learning Theory if the question addresses client education, remembering that client motivation and client readiness to learn is the first priority

4. Be alert to false response questions that address health promotion and maintenance and client education

D. Psychosocial Integrity

1. These questions address the nurse's role in providing nursing care that supports and promotes the emotional, mental, and social well-being of the client and significant other(s)

2. Content addressed in these questions relates to promoting the client or significant other(s) ability to cope, adapt, or problem-solve in situations such as illness or stressful events, and providing care to clients with maladaptive behavior or acute or chronic mental illness

3. In this Client Needs category you may be asked communication-type questions that relate to how you would respond to a client, a client's family member or significant other, or to other health care team members

4. Use therapeutic communication techniques to answer communication questions because of their effectiveness in the communication process

5. Remember to select the answer that focuses on the client, client's family member, or significant others' feelings, concerns, anxieties, or fears (Box 5-18)

VIII. **Eliminating Similar Options** (Box 5-19)

A. When answering the question, use the process of elimination and look for similar options

---

BOX 5-18

Practice Question: Communication

A client is admitted to the emergency department with an acute anterior wall myocardial infarction. The nurse discusses streptokinase (Streptase) therapy with the client and the spouse and the spouse verbalizes concerns about the dangers of this treatment. Which statement by the nurse to the spouse is *appropriate*?

1. "Your loved one is very ill. The physician has made the best decision for you."
2. "There is no reason to worry. We use this medication all of the time."
3. "I'm certain you made the correct decision to use this medication."
4. "You have concerns about whether this treatment is the best option."

Answer: 4

Test-Taking Strategy: Paraphrasing is restating the client's or family member's own words. Option 4 is the only option that is therapeutic and addresses feelings. Option 1 denies the person's right to an opinion. Option 2 is offering a false reassurance. In option 3, the nurse is expressing approval, which can be harmful to the client-nurse or family-nurse relationship. Remember focus on feelings, concerns, anxieties, or fears!

BOX 5-19

Practice Question: Eliminate Similar Options

A nurse is assigned to care for a group of clients. On review of the clients' medical records, the nurse determines that which client is *at risk for excess fluid volume*?
1. The client with an ileostomy
2. The client on diuretics
3. The client on gastrointestinal suctioning
4. The client with renal failure

Answer: 4

Test-Taking Strategy: Focus on what the question is asking, *the client at risk for excess fluid volume*. Think about the pathophysiology associated with each condition identified in the options. The only client that retains fluid is the client with renal failure. The client with an ileostomy, the client on diuretics, and the client on gastrointestinal suctioning all lose fluid. Remember: eliminate similar options!

> B. If any of the options include the same idea, then they are incorrect and can be eliminated
> C. Remember that there is only one correct option and the answer to the question is the option that is different

IX. **Eliminate Options that Contain Absolute Words** (Box 5-20)
  A. As you read each option, look for absolute words
  B. Absolute words tend to make an option incorrect and if you note an absolute word in an option, eliminate that option
  C. Some of these absolute words include all, always, every, must, none, never, and only

X. **Look for the Umbrella Option** (Box 5-21)
  A. When answering a question, if you note that more than one option appears to be correct,

BOX 5-20

Practice Question: Eliminate Options that Contain Absolute Words

A nurse is providing safety instructions to the mother of a child with hemophilia and tells the mother to do which of the following to *provide a safe environment* for the child?
1. Remove toys with sharp edges from the child's toy box
2. Allow the child to play with toys only if a parent is present
3. Place a helmet and elbow pads on the child every day
4. Allow the child to play indoors only

Answer: 1

Test-Taking Strategy: Focus on the issue, *provide a safe environment*. Eliminate options that contain absolute words. Options 2 and 4 contain the absolute word *only*. Option 3 contains the absolute word *every*. Remember absolute words tend to make an option incorrect.

BOX 5-21

Practice Question: Look for the Umbrella Option

A nurse in the emergency room receives a telephone call from emergency medical services and is told that several victims who survived a plane crash and are suffering from cold exposure will be transported to the hospital. The *initial* nursing action of the emergency room nurse is which of the following?
1. Supply the trauma rooms with bottles of sterile water and normal saline
2. Call the laundry department and ask the department to send as many warm blankets as possible to the emergency room
3. Call the nursing supervisor to activate the agency disaster plan
4. Call the intensive care unit to request that nurses be sent to the emergency room

Answer: 3

Test-Taking Strategy: Option 3 is the umbrella option. Activating the agency disaster plan will ensure that the interventions in options 1, 2, and 4 will occur. Remember the umbrella option is a general statement and may contain the ideas of the other options within it!

> look for the umbrella option (also known as global option or comprehensive option)
> B. The umbrella option is one that is a general statement and may contain the ideas of the other options within it
> C. The umbrella option will be the correct answer

XI. **Use the Guidelines for Delegating and Assignment-Making** (Box 5-22)
  A. You may be asked a question that will require you to decide how you will delegate a task or assign clients to other health care providers
  B. Focus on the information in the question and what task or assignment is to be delegated
  C. Once you have determined what task or assignment is to be delegated, consider the client's needs and match the client's needs with the scope of practice of the health care providers identified in the question
  D. The Nurse Practice Act and any practice limitations define which aspects of care can be delegated and which must be performed by the registered nurse
  E. Generally noninvasive interventions such as skin care, range-of-motion exercises, ambulation, grooming, and hygiene measures can be assigned to a nursing assistant
  F. A licensed practical nurse (LPN) can perform the tasks that a nursing assistant can perform and can additionally perform certain invasive tasks such as dressings, suctioning, urinary catheterization, and administering medications orally or by subcutaneous or intramuscular injections

BOX 5-22

Practice Question: Use the Guidelines for Delegating and Assignment-Making

A nurse is planning the client assignments for the day and has a licensed practical nurse (LPN) and a nursing assistant on the nursing team. Which client would the nurse most appropriately assign to the LPN?
1. A client with stable congestive heart failure who has early stage Alzheimer's disease
2. A client who was treated for dehydration and is weak and needs assistance with bathing
3. A client with emphysema who is receiving oxygen at 2 liters by nasal cannula and becomes dyspneic on exertion
4. A client who is scheduled for an electrocardiogram and a chest x-ray

Answer: 3

Test-Taking Strategy: The nurse would most appropriately assign the client with emphysema to the LPN. This client has an airway problem and has the highest priority needs from the clients presented in the options. The clients described in option 1, 2, and 4 can appropriately be cared for by the nursing assistant. Remember: match the client's needs with the scope of practice of the health care provider!

BOX 5-23

Practice Question: Answering Pharmacology Questions

Oral levothyroxine (Synthroid) daily is prescribed for a client with hypothyroidism. The nurse provides medication instructions to the client and tells the client to *take the medication*:
1. Just after breakfast
2. With a snack at 3:00 pm
3. In the morning on an empty stomach
4. With food

Answer: 3

Test-Taking Strategy: Note that a medical diagnosis is presented in the question. This will assist you in determining that the medication is used to treat this condition. Additionally, most thyroid replacement medications contain *thy* in their names. Also use the strategy of eliminating similar options. Note that options 1, 2, and 4 are similar and indicate that the medication should be taken with food. Remember with pharmacology questions, focus on the information in the question and the classification of the medication!

G. The registered nurse can perform the tasks that a LPN can perform and is responsible for assessment and planning care, supervising care, initiating teaching, and administering intravenous medications

XII. **Answering Pharmacology Questions** (Box 5-23)
   A. If you are familiar with the medication, use nursing knowledge to answer the question
   B. Remember that the question will identify both the generic name and the trade name of the medication
   C. If the question identifies a medical diagnosis, then try to make a relationship between the medication and the diagnosis; for example, you can determine that cyclophosphamide (Cytoxan) is an antineoplastic medication if the question refers to a client with breast cancer who is taking this medication
   D. Try to determine the classification of the medication being addressed to assist in answering the question; identifying the classification will assist in determining a medication action and/or side effects (Cardizem is a cardiac medication)
   E. Recognize the common side effects associated with each medication classification and then relate the appropriate nursing interventions to each side effect; for example, if a side effect is hypertension then the associated nursing intervention would be to monitor the blood pressure

   F. Learn medications that belong to a classification by commonalities in their medication names; for example, medications that are xanthine bronchodilators end with "line" (theophylline)
   G. Look at the medication name and use medical terminology to assist in determining the medication action; for example, *lopressor* lowers (*lo*) the blood pressure (*pressor*)
   H. If the question requires a medication calculation, remember that a calculator is available on the computer; talk yourself through each step to be sure the answer makes sense and recheck the calculation before answering the question particularly if the answer seems like an unusual dosage
   I. Pyramid Points to Remember
      1. Generally, the client should not take an antacid with medication because the antacid will affect the absorption of the medication
      2. Enteric-coated and sustained-release tablets should not be crushed; additionally, capsules should not be opened
      3. The client should never adjust or change a medication dose or abruptly stop taking a medication
      4. The nurse never adjusts or changes the client's medication dosage or never discontinues a medication
      5. The client needs to avoid taking any over-the-counter medications or any other medications such as herbal preparations unless

they are approved for use by the health care provider

6. The client needs to avoid alcohol and smoking.

7. Medications are never administered if the order is difficult to read, is unclear, or identifies a medication dose that is not a normal one

REFERENCES

Harkreader, H. & Hogan, M.A. (2004) *Fundamentals of nursing: caring and clinical judgment.* (2nd ed.). Philadelphia: Saunders.

Hodgson, B., & Kizior, R. (2004). *Saunders nursing drug handbook 2004.* Philadelphia: Saunders.

Ignatavicius, D. & Workman, M. (2005). *Medical surgical nursing: Critical thinking for collaborative care* (5th ed.). Philadelphia: Saunders.

Keltner, N., Schwecke, L., & Bostrom, C. (2003) *Psychiatric nursing* (4th ed.). St:Louis: Mosby.

Lewis, S., Heitkemper, M., & Dirksen, S. (2004). *Medical-surgical nursing: Assessment and management of clinical problems* (6th ed.). St. Louis: Mosby.

National Council of State Boards of Nursing (eds.) (2003). *Test Plan for the National Council Licensure Examination for Registered Nurses.* (Effective Date: April 2004). Chicago: Author.

Phipps, W., Monahan, F., Sands, J., Marek, J. & Neighbors, M. (2003). *Medical-surgical nursing: health and illness perspectives* (7th ed.). St. Louis: Mosby.

Riley, J. (2004). *Communication in nursing* (5th ed.). St. Louis: Mosby.

Varcarolis, Elizabeth M. (2002). *Foundations of psychiatric mental health nursing.* (4th ed.). Philadelphia: Saunders.

Wong, D., & Hockenberry, M. (2003). *Wong's Nursing care of infants and children* (7th ed.). St. Louis: Mosby.

Client Needs

Client Needs and the NCLEX-RN® Test Plan

In the new test plan implemented in April 2004, the National Council of State Boards of Nursing has identified a test plan framework based on *Client Needs*. This framework was selected on the basis of the findings in a practice analysis study of newly licensed registered nurses in the United States. This study identified the nursing activities performed by entry-level nurses. Also, the Client Needs categories identified by the National Council of State Boards of Nursing provide a structure for defining nursing actions and competencies across all settings for all clients. The National Council of State Boards of Nursing identifies four major categories of Client Needs. Some of these categories are further divided into subcategories, and the percentage of test questions in each subcategory is identified (Table 6-1).

The information contained in this chapter related to the test plan was obtained from the National Council

of State Boards of Nursing (NCSBN) Web site (*www.ncsbn.org*), from the *Test Plan for the National Council Licensure Examination for Registered Nurses* (Effective Date: April 2004), National Council of State Boards of Nursing, Chicago, 2003, and from the *NCLEX-RN Examination Detailed Test Plan for the National Council Licensure Examination for Registered Nurses*, National Council of State Boards of Nursing, Chicago, 2004. Additional information regarding the test and its development can be obtained by accessing the NCSBN Web site at *www.ncsbn.org* or by writing to the National Council of State Boards of Nursing at 111 E. Wacker Drive, Suite 2900, Chicago, Illinois 60601.

PHYSIOLOGICAL INTEGRITY

The Physiological Integrity category includes four subcategories: Basic Care and Comfort, Pharmacological and Parenteral Therapies, Reduction of Risk Potential, and Physiological Adaptation. Basic Care and Comfort (6% to 12%) addresses content that tests the knowledge, skills, and ability required to provide comfort and assistance to the client in the performance of activities of daily living. Pharmacological and Parenteral Therapies (13% to 19%) addresses content that tests the knowledge, skills, and ability required to administer medications and parenteral therapies. Reduction of Risk Potential (13% to 19%) addresses content that tests the knowledge, skills, and ability required to prevent complications or health problems related to the client's condition, or any prescribed treatments or procedures. Physiological Adaptation (11% to 17%) addresses content that tests the knowledge, skills, and ability required to provide care to clients with acute, chronic, or life-threatening conditions.

The National Council of State Boards of Nursing identifies nursing content related to the subcategories of this Client Needs category (Box 6-1). See Box 6-2 for

Table 6-1

Client Needs Categories and Percentage of Questions

Client Needs Category	Percentage of Questions on NCLEX-RN Exam
Safe, Effective Care Environment	
Management of Care	13%-19%
Safety and Infection Control	8%-14%
Health Promotion and Maintenance	6%-12%
Psychosocial Integrity	6%-12%
Physiological Integrity	
Basic Care and Comfort	6%-12%
Pharmacological and Parenteral Therapies	13%-19%
Reduction of Risk Potential	13%-19%
Physiological Adaptation	11%-17%

From National Council of State Boards Nursing (eds). (2004), *NCLEX-RN Examination Detailed Test Plan for the National Licensure Examination for Registered Nurses*. Chicago: Author.

BOX 6-1

NCLEX-RN Content: Physiological Integrity

BASIC CARE AND COMFORT
Alternative therapies
Assistive devices such as canes, walkers, crutches, etc.
Comfort and palliative care including nonpharmacological comfort interventions
Complementary therapies
Elimination
Hydration
Hygiene
Immobility
Mobility
Nutrition
Rest and sleep

PHARMACOLOGICAL AND PARENTERAL THERAPIES
Administration and monitoring of blood and blood products
Administration of intravenous therapy
Adverse effects of medications and parenteral therapies
Care to central venous access devices
Contraindications to medications and parenteral therapies
Expected effects of medications and parenteral therapies
Medication and intravenous administration and dosage calculation

Pain management
Pharmacological agents, actions, interactions, side effects, adverse and toxic effects
Total parenteral nutrition
Types of parenteral fluids

REDUCTION OF RISK POTENTIAL
Diagnostic tests: preprocedure and postprocedure
Monitoring laboratory values
Potential for alterations in body systems
Potential for complications of diagnostic tests, procedures, treatments, and surgery
Therapeutic treatments and procedures

PHYSIOLOGICAL ADAPTATION
Fluid and electrolyte imbalances
Managing illnesses
Infectious diseases
Managing medical emergencies
Pathophysiology related to diseases and conditions
Care to the client receiving radiation therapy
Providing respiratory care
Unexpected responses to therapies, treatments, and procedures

From National Council of State Boards of Nursing (eds.). (2004). *NCLEX-RN Examination Detailed Test Plan for the National Council Licensure Examination for Registered Nurses*. Chicago: Author.

BOX 6-2

Physiological Integrity Questions

BASIC CARE AND COMFORT
A client has been taught to use a walker to aid in mobility following internal fixation of a hip fracture. A nurse determines that the client is using the walker incorrectly if the client:
1. Holds the walker by using the hand grips
2. Leans forward slightly when advancing the walker
3. Advances the walker with reciprocal motion
4. Supports body weight on the hands while advancing the weaker leg

Answer: 3

Rationale: This question addresses the subcategory Basic Care and Comfort, in the Client Needs category of Physiological Integrity, and addresses content related to the use of an assistive device. The client should use the walker by placing the hands on the hand grips for stability. The client lifts the walker to advance it, and leans forward slightly while moving it. The client walks into the walker, supporting the body weight on the hands while moving the weaker leg. A disadvantage of the walker is that it does not allow for reciprocal walking motion. If the client were to try to use reciprocal motion with a walker, the walker would advance forward one side at a time as the client walks; thus the client would not be supporting the weaker leg with the walker during ambulation.

PHARMACOLOGICAL AND PARENTERAL THERAPIES
A nurse is caring for a client who is receiving tacrolimus (Prograf) daily following a liver transplant. Which of the following indicates to the nurse that the client is experiencing an adverse reaction to the medication?
1. A decrease in urine output
2. Hypotension
3. Profuse sweating
4. Photophobia

Answer: 1

Rationale: This question addresses the subcategory Pharmacological and Parenteral Therapies, in the Client Needs category of Physiological Integrity, and addresses content related to the adverse effect of a medication. Tacrolimus (Prograf) is an immunosuppressant medication used in the prophylaxis of organ rejection in clients receiving allogenic liver transplants. Frequent side effects include headache, tremor, insomnia, paresthesia, diarrhea, nausea, constipation, vomiting, abdominal pain, and hypertension. Adverse reactions and toxic effects include nephrotoxicity and pleural effusion. Nephrotoxicity is characterized by an increasing serum creatinine and blood urea nitrogen level and a decrease in urine output.

Continued

BOX 6-2

Physiological Integrity Questions—cont'd

REDUCTION OF RISK POTENTIAL

A nurse is caring for a client who is going to have an arthrogram using a contrast medium. Which of the following assessments by the nurse would be of highest priority?
1. Allergy to iodine or shellfish
2. Ability of the client to remain still during the procedure
3. Whether the client has any remaining questions about the procedure
4. Whether the client wishes to void before the procedure

Answer: 1

Rationale: This question addresses the subcategory Reduction of Risk Potential, in the Client Needs category of Physiological Integrity, and addresses a potential complication of a diagnostic test. Because of the risk of allergy to contrast dye, the nurse places highest priority on assessing whether the client has an allergy to iodine or shellfish. The nurse also reinforces information about the test, tells the client about the need to remain still during the procedure, and encourages the client to void before the procedure for comfort.

PHYSIOLOGICAL ADAPTATION

A pregnant client tells a nurse that she felt wetness on her peri-pad and that she found some clear fluid. The nurse immediately inspects the perineum and notes the presence of the umbilical cord. The nurse's initial action is to:
1. Notify the physician
2. Monitor the fetal heart rate
3. Transfer the client to the delivery room
4. Place the client in Trendelenburg position

Answer: 4

Rationale: This question addresses the subcategory Physiological Adaptation, in the Client Needs category of Physiological Integrity, and addresses an acute and life-threatening physical health condition. On inspection of the perineum, if the umbilical cord is noted, the nurse immediately places the client into Trendelenburg position while pushing the presenting part upward to relieve the cord compression. This position is maintained, the physician is notified, and the nurse monitors the fetal heart rate. The client is transferred to the delivery room when prescribed by the physician.

---

examples of questions in this Client Needs category, and refer to Chapter 7 for practice questions reflective of this Client Needs category.

SAFE, EFFECTIVE CARE ENVIRONMENT

The Safe, Effective Care Environment category includes two subcategories: Management of Care and Safety and Infection Control. Management of Care (13% to 19%) addresses content that tests the knowledge, skills, and ability required to enhance the care delivery setting to protect clients, families, significant others, visitors, and health care personnel. Safety and Infection Control (8% to 14%) addresses content that tests the knowledge, skills, and ability required to protect clients, families, significant others, visitors, and health care personnel from health and environmental hazards.

The National Council of State Boards of Nursing identifies nursing content related to the subcategories of this Client Needs category (Box 6-3). See Box 6-4 for examples of questions in this Client Needs category, and refer to Chapter 8 for practice questions reflective of this Client Needs category.

HEALTH PROMOTION AND MAINTENANCE

The Health Promotion and Maintenance category (6% to 12%) addresses the principles related to growth and development. This Client Needs category also addresses

---

BOX 6-3

NCLEX-RN Content: Safe, Effective Care Environment

MANAGEMENT OF CARE
Advance directives
Case management
Client advocacy and client rights including confidentiality and informed consent
Concepts of management
Consultation with members of the health care team
Continuity of care
Delegation and supervision
Education
Establishing priorities
Ethical practice and legal responsibilities
Performance improvement
Referrals
Resource management

SAFETY AND INFECTION CONTROL
Accident and error prevention
Disaster planning and emergency response planning
Handling hazardous and infectious materials
Injury prevention including home safety
Medical and surgical asepsis
Reporting unusual occurrences
Safe use of equipment, restraints, and safety devices
Standard and other precautions

From National Council of State Boards of Nursing (eds.). (2004). *NCLEX-RN Examination Detailed Test Plan for the National Council Licensure Examination for Registered Nurses.* Chicago: Author.

BOX 6-4

Safe, Effective Care Environment Questions

MANAGEMENT OF CARE
A registered nurse is delegating activities to a nursing staff. Which activity is least appropriate for a nursing assistant?
1. Assisting a child who has difficulty swallowing to eat lunch
2. Obtaining frequent oral temperatures on a client
3. Accompanying a client who is being discharged to home following a bowel resection 8 days ago to his transportation
4. Collecting a urine specimen from a woman admitted 3 days ago

Answer: 1

Rationale: This question addresses the subcategory Management of Care in the Client Needs category of Safe, Effective Care Environment, and specifically addresses content related to delegation. Work that is delegated to others must be done consistent with the individual's level of expertise and licensure or lack of licensure. In this case, the least appropriate activity for a nursing assistant would be assisting with feeding a child who has difficulty swallowing. The child has a high potential for complications, such as choking and aspiration. The remaining three options do not include situations to indicate that these activities carry any risk.

SAFETY AND INFECTION CONTROL
A nurse has given a subcutaneous injection to a client with acquired immunodeficiency syndrome (AIDS). The nurse disposes of the used needle and syringe by:
1. Recapping the needle and discarding the syringe in the disposal unit
2. Placing the uncapped needle and syringe in a labeled, rigid plastic container
3. Breaking the needle before discarding it
4. Placing the uncapped needle and syringe in a labeled cardboard box

Answer: 2

Rationale: This question addresses the subcategory Safety and Infection Control, in the Client Needs category of Safe, Effective Care Environment, and specifically addresses content related to standard precautions. Standard precautions include specific guidelines for handling of needles. Needles should not be recapped, bent, broken, or cut after use. They should be disposed of in a labeled, impermeable container specific for this purpose. Needles should not be discarded in cardboard boxes, because they are not impervious. Needles should never be left lying around after use.

BOX 6-5

NCLEX-RN Content: Health Promotion and Maintenance

Antepartum, intrapartum, and postpartum periods
Care to the newborn
Developmental stages and transitions
Expected body image changes
Family planning and family systems
Growth and development and the aging process
Health and wellness and preventing disease
Health screening and promotion programs
High-risk behaviors
Human sexuality
Immunizations
Lifestyle choices
Physical assessment techniques
Self-care principles
Teaching and learning

From National Council of State Boards of Nursing (eds.). (2004). *NCLEX-RN Examination Detailed Test Plan for the National Council Licensure Examination for Registered Nurses.* Chicago: Author.

BOX 6-6

Health Promotion and Maintenance Questions

A clinic nurse is providing instructions to a client in the third trimester of pregnancy regarding measures to relieve heartburn. The nurse tells the client to:
1. Eat fatty foods only once a day in the morning
2. Avoid milk and hot tea
3. Eat small, frequent meals
4. Use antacids that contain sodium

Answer: 3

Rationale: This question addresses the Client Needs category of Health Promotion and Maintenance, and addresses the antepartum period. Measures to provide relief of heartburn include eating small, frequent meals and avoidance of fatty fried foods, coffee, and cigarettes. Mild antacids may be acceptable if they do not contain aspirin or sodium. Frequent sips of milk, hot tea, or water are helpful. Gum is also helpful in the relief of heartburn.

A client with atherosclerosis asks a nurse about dietary modifications to lower the risk of heart disease. The nurse encourages the client to eat which of the following foods that will lower this risk?
1. Baked chicken with skin
2. Fresh cantaloupe
3. Broiled cheeseburger
4. Mashed potato with gravy

Answer: 2

Rationale: This question addresses the Client Needs category of Health Promotion and Maintenance, and addresses health and wellness. To lower the risk of heart disease, the diet should be low in saturated fat, with the appropriate number of total calories. The diet should include fewer red meats and more white meat, with the skin removed. Dairy products used should be low in fat, and foods with high amounts of empty calories should be avoided. Fresh fruits and vegetables are naturally low in fat.

BOX 6-7

NCLEX-RN Content: Psychosocial Integrity

Abuse and neglect
Behavioral interventions
Chemical dependency
Coping mechanisms
Crisis interventions
Cultural diversity
Domestic violence
Grief and loss and end-of-life issues
Mental health concepts
Religious and spiritual issues
Sensory/perceptual alterations
Sexual abuse
Situational role changes
Stress management
Support systems
Therapeutic interactions
Unexpected body image changes

From National Council of State Boards of Nursing (eds.). (2004). *NCLEX-RN Examination Detailed Test Plan for the National Council Licensure Examination for Registered Nurses.* Chicago: Author.

BOX 6-8

Psychosocial Integrity Questions

A stillborn was delivered in the birthing suite a few hours ago. After the birth, the family has remained together, holding and touching the baby. Which statement by the nurse would further assist them in their initial period of grief?
1. "Don't worry, there is nothing you could do to prevent this from happening."
2. "We need to take the baby from you now so that you can get some sleep."
3. "What have you named your baby?"
4. "We will see to it that you have an early discharge so that you don't have to be reminded of this experience."

Answer: 3

Rationale: This question addresses the Client Needs category of Psychosocial Integrity, and addresses content related to grief and loss. Nurses should be able to explore measures that assist the family to create a memory of the baby so that the existence of the child is confirmed and the parents can complete the grieving process. Option 3 addresses this issue and also demonstrates a caring and empathetic response. Options 1, 2, and 4 are blocks to communication and devalue the parents' feelings.

A nurse in the mental health clinic is performing an initial assessment of a family with a diagnosis of domestic violence. Which of the following factors would the nurse initially want to include in the assessment?
1. The family's anger toward the intrusiveness of the nurse
2. The family's denial of the violent nature of their behavior
3. The family's current ability to use community resources
4. The coping style of each family member

Answer: 4

Rationale: This question addresses the Client Needs category of Psychosocial Integrity, and addresses domestic violence. Note the key word "initially". The initial family assessment includes a careful history of each family member. Options 1, 2, and 3 address the family. Option 4 addresses each family member.

---

content that tests the knowledge, skills, and ability required to assist the client, family members, and/or significant others to prevent health problems, to recognize alterations in health, and to develop health practices that promote and support wellness.

The National Council of State Boards of Nursing identifies nursing content related to this Client Needs category (Box 6-5). See Box 6-6 for examples of questions in this Client Needs category, and refer to Chapter 9 for practice questions reflective of this Client Needs category.

PSYCHOSOCIAL INTEGRITY

The Psychosocial Integrity category (6% to 12%) addresses content that tests the knowledge, skills, and ability required to promote and support the client, family, and/or significant others' ability to cope, adapt, and/or solve problems during stressful events. This Client Needs category also addresses the emotional, mental, and social well-being of the client, family, or significant other, and the knowledge, skills, and ability required to care for the client with an acute or chronic mental illness.

The National Council of State Boards of Nursing identifies nursing content related to this Client Needs category (Box 6-7). See Box 6-8 for examples of questions in this Client Needs category, and refer to Chapter 10 for practice questions reflective of this Client Needs category.

REFERENCES

Black, J., & Hawks, J. (2005). *Medical-surgical nursing: Clinical management for positive outcomes* (7th ed.). Philadelphia: Saunders.

Hodgson, B., & Kizior, R. (2004). *Saunders nursing drug handbook 2004.* Philadelphia: Saunders.

Harkreader, H., & Hogan, M.A. (2004). *Fundamentals of nursing: caring and clinical judgment.* (2nd ed.). Philadelphia: Saunders.

Lewis, S., Heitkemper, M., & Dirksen, S. (2004). *Medical-surgical nursing: Assessment and management of clinical problems* (6th ed.). St. Louis: Mosby.

Lowdermilk, D., & Perry, S. (2003). *Maternity nursing.* (6th ed.). St. Louis: Mosby.

National Council of State Boards of Nursing (NCSBN) Web site: *www.ncsbn.org*

National Council of State Boards of Nursing (eds.). (2003). *Test Plan for the National Council Licensure Examination for Registered Nurses.* (Effective Date: April 2004). Chicago: Author.

National Council of State Boards of Nursing (eds.). (2004). *NCLEX-RN® Examination Detailed Test Plan for the National Council Licensure Examination for Registered Nurses.* Chicago: Author.

Potter, P., & Perry, A. (2005). *Fundamentals of nursing* (6th ed.). St. Louis: Mosby.

Varcarolis, Elizabeth M. (2002). *Foundations of psychiatric mental health nursing.* (4th ed.). Philadelphia: Saunders.

Physiological Integrity

1. During an assessment of a prenatal client with a history of left-sided heart failure, a nurse notes that the client is experiencing unusual episodes of a nonproductive cough on minimal exertion. The nurse interprets that this finding may be an early manifestation of which cardiac problem?
   1 Orthopnea
   2 Decreased blood volume
   3 Right-sided heart failure
   4 Pulmonary edema

Answer: 4
Rationale: Pulmonary edema from heart failure may first be manifested as a cough. The cough occurs in response to fluid filling the alveolar spaces. Pulmonary edema develops as a result of left ventricular failure or acute fluid overload. Orthopnea is an assessment finding. Increased rather than decreased blood volume occurs in heart failure. A nonproductive cough is a late manifestation of right-sided heart failure.

Test-Taking Strategy: Note the key words "early manifestation." Focus on the data: left-sided heart failure. Remember "left" and "lung" to direct you to option 4. Review the complications of left-sided heart failure and the early manifestation of pulmonary edema if you had difficulty with this question.

Level of Cognitive Ability: Analysis
Client Needs: Physiological Integrity
Integrated Process: Nursing Process/Assessment
Content Area: Maternity/Antepartum

Reference:
Lowdermilk, D., & Perry, A. (2004). *Maternity & women's health care* (8th ed.). St. Louis: Mosby, p. 912.

---

2. A nurse is performing an assessment on a client with a diagnosis of chronic angina pectoris who is receiving sotalol (Betapace) 80 mg orally daily. Which assessment finding indicates that the client is experiencing a side effect of the medication?
   1 Difficulty swallowing
   2 Diaphoresis
   3 Dry mouth
   4 Palpitations

Answer: 4
Rationale: Sotalol is a beta-adrenergic blocking agent. Side effects include bradycardia, palpitations, an irregular heartbeat, difficulty breathing, signs of congestive heart failure, and cold hands and feet. Gastrointestinal disturbances, anxiety and nervousness, and unusual tiredness and weakness can also occur. Options 1, 2, and 3 are not side effects of this medication.

Test-Taking Strategy: Note that the question presents a client with chronic angina pectoris, a cardiac disorder. Remember that medication names ending with "lol" (sotalol) are beta-blockers, which are commonly used for cardiac disorders. Note that option 4 is the only option that is directly cardiac related. Review the side effects of sotalol if you had difficulty with this question.

Level of Cognitive Ability: Analysis
Client Needs: Physiological Integrity
Integrated Process: Nursing Process/Assessment
Content Area: Pharmacology

Reference:
Hodgson, B., & Kizior, R. (2004). *Saunders nursing drug handbook 2004*. Philadelphia: Saunders, p. 930.

---

3. Before performing a venipuncture to initiate continuous intravenous (IV) therapy, a nurse should:
   1 Apply a tourniquet below the chosen vein site
   2 Inspect the IV solution for particles or contamination
   3 Secure an armboard to the joint located above the IV site
   4 Place a cool compress over the vein

Answer: 2
Rationale: All IV solutions should be free of particles or precipitates. A tourniquet is applied above the chosen vein site. Cool compresses will cause vasoconstriction, making the vein less visible. Armboards are applied after the IV is started and are used only if necessary.

Test-Taking Strategy: Note the key word "before" and use the steps of the nursing process. Option 2 is the only option that reflects assessment, the first step of the nursing process. Review nursing interventions related to initiating an IV if you had difficulty with this question.

Level of Cognitive Ability: Application
Client Needs: Physiological Integrity
Integrated Process: Nursing Process/Implementation
Content Area: Fundamental Skills

Reference:
Potter, P., & Perry, A. (2005). *Fundamentals of nursing* (6th ed.). St. Louis: Mosby, p. 1164.

---

4. A nurse is caring for a client who had an allogenic liver transplant and is receiving tacrolimus (Prograf) daily. Which finding indicates to the nurse that the client is experiencing an adverse reaction to the medication?
   1 Decrease in urine output
   2 Hypotension
   3 Profuse sweating
   4 Photophobia

Answer: 1
Rationale: Tacrolimus (Prograf) is an immunosuppressant medication used in the prophylaxis of organ rejection in clients receiving allogenic liver transplants. Frequent side effects include headache, tremor, insomnia, paresthesia, diarrhea, nausea, constipation, vomiting, abdominal pain, and hypertension. Adverse reactions and toxic effects include nephrotoxicity and pleural effusion. Nephrotoxicity is characterized by an increasing serum creatinine level and a decrease in urine output.

Test-Taking Strategy: First, determine the medication classification. Note the client's diagnosis and look at the medication name Prograf, "Pro" meaning "for" and "graf" meaning "graft," to identify the action of the medication: to prevent transplant rejection. This will assist in identifying the medication classification as immunosuppressant. Next, recalling that nephrotoxicity is an adverse effect of the medication will direct you to option 1. Review the adverse effects of this medication if you had difficulty with this question.

Level of Cognitive Ability: Analysis
Client Needs: Physiological Integrity

Integrated Process: Nursing Process/Assessment
Content Area: Pharmacology

Reference:
Hodgson, B., & Kizior, R. (2004). *Saunders nursing drug handbook 2004.* Philadelphia: Saunders, p. 950.

---

5. A client was admitted to the hospital 24 hours ago following pulmonary trauma. The nurse monitors for which earliest clinical manifestation of acute respiratory distress syndrome (ARDS)?
1 Increase in respiratory rate
2 Blood-tinged frothy sputum
3 Bronchial breath sounds
4 Diffuse pulmonary infiltrates on the chest X-ray

Answer: 1
Rationale: Acute respiratory distress syndrome usually develops within 24 to 48 hours after an initiating event, such as pulmonary trauma. In most cases, tachypnea and dyspnea are the earliest clinical manifestations. Blood-tinged frothy sputum would present later, after the development of pulmonary edema. Breath sounds in the early stages of ARDS are usually clear but then may progress to bronchial breath sounds when pulmonary edema occurs. Chest X-ray findings may be normal during the early stages but will show infiltrates in the later stages.

Test-Taking Strategy: Note the key words "earliest clinical manifestation." It is important to remember with respiratory conditions that the initial presenting symptoms of a complication are tachypnea and dyspnea along with restlessness, as the hypoxia develops. Review the early clinical manifestations of ARDS if you had difficulty with this question.

Level of Cognitive Ability: Analysis
Client Needs: Physiological Integrity
Integrated Process: Nursing Process/Assessment
Content Area: Adult Health/Respiratory

Reference:
Ignatavicius, D., & Workman, M. (2002). *Medical surgical nursing: Critical for collaborative care* (4th ed.). Philadelphia: Saunders, pp. 599-601.

---

6. A nurse is caring for a client with Buck's traction and is monitoring the client for complications of the traction. Which assessment finding indicates a complication?
1 Weak pedal pulses
2 Drainage at the pin sites
3 Warm toes with brisk capillary refill
4 Complaints of discomfort

Answer: 1
Rationale: Weak pedal pulses are a sign of vascular compromise, which can be caused by pressure on the tissues of the leg by the elastic bandage or boot used to secure this type of traction. This type of traction does not use pins, rather it is secured by elastic bandages or a prefabricated boot. Warm toes with brisk capillary refill is a normal assessment finding. Discomfort is an expected finding.

Test-Taking Strategy: Use the ABCs—airway, breathing, and circulation. Option 1 indicates a sign of vascular compromise. Review care of the client with Buck's traction if you had difficulty with this question.

Level of Cognitive Ability: Analysis
Client Needs: Physiological Integrity
Integrated Process: Nursing Process/Analysis
Content Area: Adult Health/Musculoskeletal

Reference:
Lewis, S., Heitkemper, M., & Dirksen, S. (2004). *Medical-surgical nursing: Assessment and management of clinical problems* (6th ed.). St. Louis: Mosby, p. 1660.

7. A prenatal client has been diagnosed with a vaginal infection from the organism *Candida albicans*. Which finding(s) would the nurse expect to note on assessment of the client?
   1 Absence of any signs and symptoms
   2 Pain, itching, and vaginal discharge
   3 Proteinuria, hematuria, edema, and hypertension
   4 Costovertebral angle pain

Answer: 2
Rationale: Clinical manifestations of a *Candida* infection include pain, itching, and a thick, white vaginal discharge. Proteinuria, edema, and hypertension are signs of pregnancy-induced hypertension. Hematuria, proteinuria, and costovertebral angle pain are clinical manifestations associated with urinary tract infections.

Test-Taking Strategy: Use the process of elimination, focusing on the issue: vaginal infection. Note the relationship between the issue and option 2. Review the signs of a vaginal *Candida* infection if you had difficulty with this question.

Level of Cognitive Ability: Analysis
Client Needs: Physiological Integrity
Integrated Process: Nursing Process/Assessment
Content Area: Maternity/Antepartum

Reference:
Lowdermilk, D., & Perry, A. (2004). *Maternity & women's health care* (8th ed.). St. Louis: Mosby, p. 208.

---

8. A prenatal client is suspected of having iron-deficiency anemia. Which finding would the nurse expect to note regarding the client's status?
   1 A low hemoglobin and hematocrit level
   2 A high hemoglobin and hematocrit level
   3 Excess fluid volume
   4 Deficient fluid volume

Answer: 1
Rationale: When the hemoglobin level is below 11 mg/dL, iron deficiency is suspected. An indirect index of the oxygen-carrying capacity is the packed red blood cell volume or hematocrit level. Pathological anemia of pregnancy is primarily caused by iron deficiency. Options 3 and 4 are nursing diagnoses and are not noted in iron-deficiency anemia.

Test-Taking Strategy: Use the process of elimination. Note the word "deficiency" in the question and the word "low" in option 1. Review the manifestations of iron-deficiency anemia if you had difficulty with this question.

Level of Cognitive Ability: Analysis
Client Needs: Physiological Integrity
Integrated Process: Nursing Process/Assessment
Content Area: Maternity/Antepartum

Reference:
Lowdermilk, D., & Perry, A. (2004). *Maternity & women's health care* (8th ed.). St. Louis: Mosby, pp. 918; 920.

---

9. A nurse is caring for the postpartum client. Which finding would make the nurse suspect endometritis in this client?
   1 Lochia rubra on the second day postpartum
   2 Fever over 38°C, beginning three days postpartum
   3 Elevated white blood cell count
   4 Breast engorgement

Answer: 2
Rationale: Fever on the third or fourth day postpartum should raise concerns about possible endometritis until proven otherwise. A woman with endometritis normally presents with a temperature over 38°C. Lochia rubra on the second day postpartum is a normal finding. The white blood cell count of a postpartum woman is normally elevated. Thus, this method of detecting infection is not of great value in the puerperium. Breast engorgement is also a normal response in the postpartum period and is not associated with endometritis.

Test-Taking Strategy: Use the process of elimination, focusing on the issue: endometritis. Recalling the normal findings in the post-partum period will assist in eliminating options 1, 3, and 4. Review the signs of endometritis if you had difficulty with this question.

Level of Cognitive Ability: Analysis
Client Needs: Physiological Integrity
Integrated Process: Nursing Process/Assessment
Content Area: Maternity/Postpartum

Reference:
Lowdermilk, D., & Perry, A. (2004). *Maternity & women's health care* (8th ed.). St. Louis: Mosby, p. 1047.

---

10. A nurse is performing an assessment on a post-term infant. Which physical characteristic would the nurse expect to observe?
   1 Vernix that covers the body in a thick layer
   2 Peeling of the skin
   3 Smooth soles without creases
   4 Lanugo covering the entire body

Answer: 2
Rationale: The post-term infant (born after the 42nd week of gestation) exhibits dry, peeling, cracked, almost leather-like skin over the body, which is called *desquamation*. The preterm infant (born between 24 to 37 weeks of gestation) exhibits thick vernix covering the body, smooth soles without creases, and lanugo covering the entire body.

Test-Taking Strategy: Use the process of elimination, focusing on the issue: post-term infant. Recalling that the post-term infant is born after the 42nd week of gestation will direct you to option 2. Review the characteristics of preterm and post-term infants if you had difficulty with this question.

Level of Cognitive Ability: Analysis
Client Needs: Physiological Integrity
Integrated Process: Nursing Process/Assessment
Content Area: Maternity/Postpartum

References:
Lowdermilk, D., & Perry, A. (2004). *Maternity & women's health care* (8th ed.). St. Louis: Mosby, pp. 716; 1140.
Murray, S., McKinney, E., & Gorrie, T. (2002). *Foundations of maternal-newborn nursing* (3rd ed.). Philadelphia: Saunders, pp. 538; 834.

---

11. A nurse is performing an admission assessment on a post-term infant and notes that the infant is experiencing tachypnea, grunting, retractions, and nasal flaring. The nurse interprets that these symptoms are indicative of:
   1 Hypoglycemia
   2 Meconium aspiration syndrome
   3 Respiratory distress syndrome
   4 Transient tachypnea of the newborn

Answer: 2
Rationale: Tachypnea, grunting, retractions, and nasal flaring are symptoms of respiratory distress related to meconium aspiration syndrome, which can occur in post-term infants who have decreased amniotic fluid and are prone to cord compression. It develops when meconium in the amniotic fluid enters the lungs during fetal life or during labor. Transient tachypnea of the newborn is primarily found in infants delivered via cesarean section. Respiratory distress syndrome is a complication of preterm infants. The symptoms noted in the question are unrelated to hypoglycemia.

Test-Taking Strategy: Use the process of elimination, focusing on the symptoms identified in the question. Option 1 is eliminated first because hypoglycemia is not a respiratory condition. From the remaining options, recalling the complications that can occur in a post-term infant will direct you to option 2. Review these complications if you had difficulty with this question.

Level of Cognitive Ability: Analysis
Client Needs: Physiological Integrity
Integrated Process: Nursing Process/Analysis
Content Area: Maternity/Postpartum

References:
Lowdermilk, D., & Perry, A. (2004). *Maternity & women's health care* (8th ed.). St. Louis: Mosby, p. 1139.
Murray, S., McKinney, E., & Gorrie, T. (2002). *Foundations of maternal-newborn nursing* (3rd ed.). Philadelphia: Saunders, p. 845.

---

12. A nurse is caring for a client who had an orthopedic injury of the leg requiring surgery. Postoperatively, which nursing assessment is of highest priority?
1 Checking for bladder distention
2 Assessing for Homans' sign
3 Monitoring for extremity shortening
4 Monitoring for heel breakdown

Answer: 2
Rationale: Deep vein thrombosis is a potentially serious complication of orthopedic injuries and surgery. Checking for a positive Homans' sign assesses for this complication. Although bladder distention, extremity lengthening or shortening, or heel breakdown can occur, these complications are not potentially serious complications.

Test-Taking Strategy: Use the ABCs—airway, breathing, and circulation—to answer the question. Assessment for deep vein thrombosis involves circulation. Review postoperative assessment following orthopedic surgery if you had difficulty with this question.

Level of Cognitive Ability: Analysis
Client Needs: Physiological Integrity
Integrated Process: Nursing Process/Assessment
Content Area: Delegating/Prioritizing

Reference:
Black, J., & Hawks, J. (2005). *Medical-surgical nursing: Clinical management for positive outcomes* (7th ed.). Philadelphia: Saunders, p. 630.

---

13. A nurse is caring for a client with hypertension receiving torsemide (Demedex) 5 mg orally daily. Which of the following would indicate to the nurse that the client might be experiencing an adverse reaction related to the medication?
1 A blood urea nitrogen (BUN) of 15 mg/dL
2 A chloride level of 98 mEq/L
3 A sodium level of 135 mEq/L
4 A potassium level of 3.1 mEq/L

Answer: 4
Rationale: Torsemide (Demedex) is a loop diuretic. The medication can produce acute, profound water loss, volume and electrolyte depletion, dehydration, decreased blood volume, and circulatory collapse. Option 4 is the only option that indicates an electrolyte depletion because the normal potassium level is 3.5 to 5.1 mEq/L. The normal sodium level is 135 to 145 mEq/L. The normal chloride level is 98 to 107 mEq/L. The normal blood BUN is 5 to 20 mg/dL.

Test-Taking Strategy: Use the process of elimination and knowledge of normal laboratory values to assist in selecting option 4, because this is the only abnormal laboratory value presented. Review this content if you are unfamiliar with this medication or these normal laboratory values.

Level of Cognitive Ability: Analysis
Client Needs: Physiological Integrity
Integrated Process: Nursing Process/Analysis
Content Area: Pharmacology

References:
Hodgson, B., & Kizior, R. (2004). *Saunders nursing drug handbook 2004.* Philadelphia: Saunders, p. 1005.
McKenry, L., & Salerno, E. (2003). *Mosby's pharmacology in nursing* (21st ed.). St. Louis: Mosby, p. 677.

---

14. A nurse is performing an admission assessment on a client admitted with newly diagnosed Hodgkin's disease. Which of the following would the nurse expect the client to report?
1 Night sweats
2 Severe lymph node pain
3 Weight gain
4 Headache with minor visual changes

Answer: 1
Rationale: Assessment of a client with Hodgkin's disease most often reveals enlarged, painless lymph nodes, fever, malaise, and night sweats. Weight loss may be present if metastatic disease occurs. Headache and visual changes may occur if brain metastasis is present.

Test-Taking Strategy: Use the process of elimination. Eliminate options 2 and 4 first because they are similar in that they relate to discomfort. Weight gain is rarely the symptom of any new cancer diagnosis, so eliminate option 3. Review content related to Hodgkin's disease if you had difficulty with this question.

Level of Cognitive Ability: Analysis
Client Needs: Physiological Integrity
Integrated Process: Nursing Process/Assessment
Content Area: Adult Health/Oncology

Reference:
Black, J., & Hawks, J. (2005). *Medical-surgical nursing: Clinical management for positive outcomes* (7th ed.). Philadelphia: Saunders, p. 2412.

---

15. A nurse is assessing a three-day-old preterm neonate with a diagnosis of respiratory distress syndrome (RDS). Which assessment finding indicates that the neonate's respiratory status is improving?
1 Presence of a systolic murmur
2 Respiratory rate between 60 to 70 breaths per minute
3 Edema of the hands and feet
4 Urine output of 1 to 3 mL/kg/hour

Answer: 4
Rationale: Increased urination is an early sign that the neonate's respiratory condition is improving. Lung fluid, which occurs in RDS, moves from the lungs into the blood stream as the condition improves and the alveoli open. This extra fluid circulates to the kidneys, which results in increased voiding. Systolic murmurs usually indicate the presence of a patent ductus arteriosus, which is a common complication of RDS. Respiratory rates above 60 are indicative of tachypnea, which is a sign of respiratory distress. Edema of the hands and feet occurs within the first 24 hours as a result of low protein concentrations, a decrease in colloidal osmotic pressure, and transudation of fluid from the vascular system to the tissues.

Test-Taking Strategy: Use the process of elimination. Note the issue: respiratory status is improving. Option 4 is the only normal finding and indicates a normal urine output, which would indicate resolution of excess lung fluid. Review RDS if you had difficulty answering the question.

Level of Cognitive Ability: Analysis
Client Needs: Physiological Integrity
Integrated Process: Nursing Process/Evaluation
Content Area: Maternity/Postpartum

Reference:
Lowdermilk, D., & Perry, A. (2004). *Maternity & women's health care* (8th ed.). St. Louis: Mosby, pp. 688; 1133.

---

16. A nurse is caring for a term newborn. Which assessment finding would predispose the newborn to the occurrence of jaundice?
1　A negative direct Coombs' test result
2　Birth weight of 8 pounds 6 ounces
3　Presence of a cephalhematoma
4　Infant blood type of O negative

Answer: 3
Rationale: Enclosed hemorrhage, such as with cephalhematoma, predisposes the newborn to jaundice by producing an increased bilirubin load as the cephalhematoma resolves and is absorbed into the circulatory system. A negative direct Coombs' test result indicates that there are no maternal antibodies on fetal erythrocytes. The birth weight in option 2 is within the acceptable ranges for a term newborn, and therefore does not contribute to an increased bilirubin level. The classic Rh incompatibility situation involves an Rh-negative mother with an Rh-positive fetus/newborn.

Test-Taking Strategy: Use the process of elimination. Recalling the risk factors associated with jaundice and the association between hemorrhage and jaundice will direct you to option 3. Review the risk factors associated with jaundice if you had difficulty with this question.

Level of Cognitive Ability: Analysis
Client Needs: Physiological Integrity
Integrated Process: Nursing Process/Assessment
Content Area: Maternity/Postpartum

References:
Lowdermilk, D., & Perry, A. (2004). *Maternity & women's health care* (8th ed.). St. Louis: Mosby, pp. 691; 771; 1089.
Murray, S., McKinney, E., & Gorrie, T. (2002). *Foundations of maternal-newborn nursing* (3rd ed.). Philadelphia: Saunders, p. 490.

---

17. Which assessment is most important for the nurse to make before advancing a client from liquid to solid food?
1　Food preferences
2　Appetite
3　Presence of bowel sounds
4　Chewing ability

Answer: 4
Rationale: It may be necessary to modify a client's diet to a soft or mechanical chopped diet if the client has difficulty chewing. Food preferences should be ascertained on admission assessment. Appetite will affect the amount of food eaten, but not the type of diet ordered. Bowel sounds should be present before introducing any diet, including liquids.

Test-Taking Strategy: Use the process of elimination. Focusing on the issue, advancing a diet from liquid to solid, will direct you to option 4. Review nursing considerations related to dietary measures if you had difficulty with this question.

Level of Cognitive Ability: Analysis
Client Needs: Physiological Integrity
Integrated Process: Nursing Process/Assessment
Content Area: Fundamental Skills

Reference:
Potter, P., & Perry, A. (2005). *Fundamentals of nursing* (6th ed.). St. Louis: Mosby, pp. 1282; 1285; 1289.

---

18. A nurse is assessing a client who is diagnosed with cystitis. Which assessment finding is inconsistent with the typical clinical manifestations noted in this disorder?
1. Urinary retention
2. Burning on urination
3. Low back pain
4. Hematuria

Answer: 1

Rationale: Clinical manifestations of cystitis usually include urinary frequency, urgency, dysuria, inability to void, or voiding only small amounts. The urine may be cloudy, with hematuria and bacteriuria. The client may complain of pain that is suprapubic or in the lower back. Nonspecific signs include fever, chills, malaise, and nausea and vomiting. Some clients may be asymptomatic, particularly the older client.

Test-Taking Strategy: Use the process of elimination. Noting the key word "inconsistent" guides you to look for an incorrect option. First, eliminate options 2 and 4, because they are commonly associated with cystitis. From the remaining options, recalling that urgency and frequency, not urinary retention, are signs of cystitis directs you to option 1. Review the clinical manifestations of cystitis if you had difficulty with this question.

Level of Cognitive Ability: Analysis
Client Needs: Physiological Integrity
Integrated Process: Nursing Process/Assessment
Content Area: Adult Health/Renal

Reference:
Lewis, S., Heitkemper, M., & Dirksen, S. (2004). *Medical-surgical nursing: Assessment and management of clinical problems* (6th ed.). St. Louis: Mosby, p. 1175.

---

19. What method would the nurse use to most accurately assess the effectiveness of a weight loss diet for an obese client?
1. Checking daily weights
2. Checking serum protein levels
3. Doing daily calorie counts
4. Monitoring daily intake and output

Answer: 1

Rationale: The most accurate measurement of weight loss is daily weighing of the client at the same time of the day, in the same clothes, and using the same scale. Options 2, 3, and 4 measure nutrition and hydration status.

Test-Taking Strategy: Use the process of elimination. Focus on the issue, weight loss, and note the key words "most accurately assess." Assessing weight will most accurately identify weight changes. Review care of the client on a weight loss program if you had difficulty with this question.

Level of Cognitive Ability: Application
Client Needs: Physiological Integrity
Integrated Process: Nursing Process/Implementation
Content Area: Fundamental Skills

Reference:
Lewis, S., Heitkemper, M., & Dirksen, S. (2004). *Medical-surgical nursing: Assessment and management of clinical problems* (6th ed.). St. Louis: Mosby, p. 341.

20. A client has fallen and sustained a leg injury. Which question would the nurse ask the client to help determine if the injury caused a fracture?
   1   "Does the discomfort feel like a cramp?"
   2   "Does the pain feel like the muscle was stretched?"
   3   "Is the pain a dull ache?"
   4   "Is the pain sharp and continuous?"

Answer: 4
Rationale: Fracture pain is generally described as sharp, continuous, and increasing in frequency. Bone pain is often described as a dull, deep ache. Strains result from trauma to a muscle body or to the attachment of a tendon from overstretching or overextension. Muscle injury is often described as an aching or cramping pain, or soreness.

Test-Taking Strategy: Use the process of elimination, focusing on the issue: a fracture. Recalling that a new injury such as a fracture is more likely to be described as sharp will direct you to option 4. Review the clinical manifestations of a fracture if you had difficulty with this question.

Level of Cognitive Ability: Application
Client Needs: Physiological Integrity
Integrated Process: Nursing Process/Assessment
Content Area: Adult Health/Musculoskeletal

Reference:
Black, J., & Hawks, J. (2005). *Medical-surgical nursing: Clinical management for positive outcomes* (7th ed.). Philadelphia: Saunders, pp. 622; 652.

---

21. A nurse obtains a fingerstick glucose reading of 425 mg/dL on a client who was recently started on total parenteral nutrition (TPN). What nursing action is most appropriate at this time?
   1   Stop the TPN
   2   Decrease the flow rate of the TPN
   3   Administer insulin
   4   Notify the physician

Answer: 4
Rationale: Hyperglycemia is a complication of TPN, and the nurse reports abnormalities to the physician. Options 1, 2, and 3 are not done without a physician's order.

Test-Taking Strategy: Use the process of elimination. Note that options 1, 2, and 3 are not within the scope of nursing practice and require a physician's order. A blood glucose greater than 400 mg/dL requires notification of the physician. Review the complications associated with TPN if you had difficulty with this question.

Level of Cognitive Ability: Application
Client Needs: Physiological Integrity
Integrated Process: Nursing Process/Implementation
Content Area: Fundamental Skills

Reference:
Ignatavicius, D., & Workman, M. (2002). *Medical surgical nursing: Critical thinking for collaborative care* (4th ed.). Philadelphia: Saunders, p. 1483.

---

22. A client with urolithiasis is scheduled for extracorporeal shock wave lithotripsy. The nurse assesses to ensure that which of the following items are in place or maintained before sending the client for the procedure?
   1   Signed informed consent and clear liquid restriction preprocedure
   2   Signed informed consent, NPO status, and an intravenous (IV) line
   3   IV line and a Foley catheter
   4   NPO status and a Foley catheter

Answer: 2
Rationale: Extracorporeal shock wave lithotripsy is done with conscious sedation or general anesthesia. The client must sign an informed consent form for the procedure and must be NPO for the procedure. The client needs an IV line for the procedure as well. A Foley catheter is not needed.

Test-Taking Strategy: Use the process of elimination. Begin to answer by eliminating options 3 and 4, because a Foley catheter is not needed for this procedure. From the remaining options, recalling that the procedure is invasive and that the client is premedicated before the procedure will direct you to option 2. Review the preprocedure preparation for extracorporeal shock wave lithotripsy if you had difficulty with this question.

Level of Cognitive Ability: Application
Client Needs: Physiological Integrity
Integrated Process: Nursing Process/Assessment
Content Area: Adult Health/Renal

References:
Black, J., & Hawks, J. (2005). *Medical-surgical nursing: Clinical management for positive outcomes* (7th ed.). Philadelphia: Saunders, p. 888.
Ignatavicius, D., & Workman, M. (2002). *Medical surgical nursing: Critical thinking for collaborative care* (4th ed.). Philadelphia: Saunders, pp. 1336; 1635.

---

23. A client has developed atrial fibrillation and has a ventricular rate of 150 beats per minute. The nurse assesses the client for:
1 Hypotension and dizziness
2 Nausea and vomiting
3 Hypertension and headache
4 Flat neck veins

Answer: 1
Rationale: The client with uncontrolled atrial fibrillation with a ventricular rate over 100 beats per minute is at risk for low cardiac output caused by loss of atrial kick. The nurse assesses the client for palpitations, chest pain or discomfort, hypotension, pulse deficit, fatigue, weakness, dizziness, syncope, shortness of breath, and distended neck veins.

Test-Taking Strategy: Use the process of elimination. Recalling that flat neck veins are normal or indicate hypovolemia will assist in eliminating option 4. Remembering that nausea and vomiting are associated with vagus nerve activity, not a tachycardic state, will assist you in eliminating option 2. From the remaining options, thinking of the effects of a falling cardiac output will direct you to option 1. Review the symptoms related to atrial fibrillation if you had difficulty with this question.

Level of Cognitive Ability: Application
Client Needs: Physiological Integrity
Integrated Process: Nursing Process/Assessment
Content Area: Adult Health/Cardiovascular

Reference:
Ignatavicius, D., & Workman, M. (2002). *Medical surgical nursing: Critical thinking for collaborative care* (4th ed.). Philadelphia: Saunders, p. 674.

---

24. A preschooler with a history of cleft palate repair comes to the clinic for a routine well-child checkup. To determine if this child is experiencing a long-term effect of cleft palate, the nurse asks the parent which question?
1 "Was the child recently treated for pneumonia?"
2 "Does the child play with an imaginary friend?"
3 "Is the child unresponsive when given directions?"
4 "Has the child had any difficulty swallowing food?"

Answer: 3
Rationale: Unresponsiveness may be an indication that the child is experiencing hearing loss. A child who has a history of cleft palate should be routinely checked for hearing loss. Options 1 and 4 are unrelated to cleft palate after repair. Option 2 is normal behavior for a preschool child. Many preschoolers with vivid imaginations have imaginary friends.

Test-Taking Strategy: Use the process of elimination, focusing on the issue: a long-term effect. Recalling that hearing loss can occur in a child with cleft palate will direct you to option 3. Review the long-term effects of cleft palate if you had difficulty with this question.

Level of Cognitive Ability: Application
Client Needs: Physiological Integrity
Integrated Process: Nursing Process/Assessment
Content Area: Child Health

Reference:
James, S., Ashwill, J., & Droske, S. (2002). *Nursing care of children: Principles & practice* (2nd ed.). Philadelphia: Saunders, p. 536.

---

25. A nurse is performing a respiratory assessment on a client being treated for an asthma attack. The nurse determines that the client's respiratory status is worsening if which of the following occurs?

1 Loud wheezing
2 Wheezing during inspiration and expiration
3 Wheezing on expiration
4 Noticeably diminished breath sounds

Answer: 4
Rationale: Wheezing is not a reliable manifestation to determine the severity of an asthma attack. Clients with minor attacks may experience loud wheezes, whereas others with severe attacks may not wheeze. The client with severe asthma attacks may have no audible wheezing because of the decrease of airflow. For wheezing to occur, the client must be able to move sufficient air to produce breath sounds. Wheezing usually occurs first on expiration. As the asthma attack progresses, the client may wheeze during both inspiration and expiration. Noticeably diminished breath sounds are an indication of severe obstruction and impending respiratory failure.

Test-Taking Strategy: Use the ABCs—airway, breathing, and circulation. Note the key words "client's respiratory status is worsening." Remember that diminished breath sounds indicate obstruction and impending respiratory failure. Review care of the client experiencing an asthma attack if you had difficulty with this question.

Level of Cognitive Ability: Analysis
Client Needs: Physiological Integrity
Integrated Process: Nursing Process/Analysis
Content Area: Adult Health/Respiratory

Reference:
Lewis, S., Heitkemper, M., & Dirksen, S. (2004). *Medical-surgical nursing: Assessment and management of clinical problems* (6th ed.). St. Louis: Mosby, p. 640.

---

26. A nurse is assessing the casted extremity of a client for signs of infection. Which of the following findings is indicative of infection?

1 Coolness and pallor of the skin
2 Presence of a "hot spot" on the cast
3 Diminished distal pulse
4 Dependent edema

Answer: 2
Rationale: Signs and symptoms of infection under a casted area include odor or purulent drainage from the cast, or the presence of "hot spots," which are areas on the cast that are warmer than others. The physician should be notified if any of these occur. Signs of impaired circulation in the distal extremity include coolness and pallor of the skin, diminished arterial pulse, and edema.

Test-Taking Strategy: Use the process of elimination and focus on the issue: infection. Thinking about the signs of infection (i.e., redness, swelling, heat, and drainage) will direct you to option 2. The "hot spot" on the cast could signify infection underneath that area. Review the signs and symptoms of infection if you had difficulty with this question.

Level of Cognitive Ability: Application
Client Needs: Physiological Integrity
Integrated Process: Nursing Process/Assessment
Content Area: Adult Health/Musculoskeletal

Reference:
Black, J., & Hawks, J. (2005). *Medical-surgical nursing: Clinical management for positive outcomes* (7th ed.). Philadelphia: Saunders, p. 633.

---

27. A home care nurse assesses a client with chronic obstructive pulmonary disease (COPD) who is complaining of increased dyspnea. The client is on home oxygen via a concentrator at 2 liters per minute, and the client's respiratory rate is 22 breaths per minute. The appropriate nursing action is to:
  1 Determine the need to increase the oxygen
  2 Conduct further assessment of the client's respiratory status
  3 Call emergency services to take the client to the emergency room
  4 Reassure the client that there is no need to worry

Answer: 2
Rationale: Obtaining further assessment data is the appropriate nursing action. Reassuring the client that there is "no need to worry" is inappropriate. Calling emergency services is a premature action. Oxygen is not increased without the approval of the physician, especially because the client with COPD can retain carbon dioxide.

Test-Taking Strategy: Use the process of elimination. Eliminate option 4 because it is an inappropriate communication technique. From the remaining options, remember that assessment is the first step of the nursing process. This will direct you to option 2. Review care of the client with COPD if you had difficulty with this question.

Level of Cognitive Ability: Application
Client Needs: Physiological Integrity
Integrated Process: Nursing Process/Implementation
Content Area: Adult Health/Respiratory

Reference:
Black, J., & Hawks, J. (2005). *Medical-surgical nursing: Clinical management for positive outcomes* (7th ed.). Philadelphia: Saunders, p. 1822.

---

28. A client with schizophrenia tells the nurse, "I stopped taking my chlorpromazine (Thorazine) because of the way it made me feel." Which side effect is the nurse likely to note during further assessment of the client's complaint?
  1 Increased urination
  2 Drowsiness
  3 Hand tremors
  4 Nervousness

Answer: 2
Rationale: Side effects of chlorpromazine can include hypotension, dizziness and fainting especially with parenteral use, drowsiness, blurred vision, dry mouth, lethargy, constipation or diarrhea, nasal congestion, peripheral edema, and urinary retention. Options 1, 3, and 4 are not side effects of chlorpromazine.

Test-Taking Strategy: Use the process of elimination. Eliminate options 3 and 4 first because they are similar. Next, focus on the name of the medication. Recall that most phenothiazine medication names end with "zine" and that a side effect of these medications is drowsiness. Review this information if you are unfamiliar with the side effects of this medication.

Level of Cognitive Ability: Analysis
Client Needs: Physiological Integrity
Integrated Process: Nursing Process/Assessment
Content Area: Pharmacology

Reference:
Hodgson, B., & Kizior, R. (2004). *Saunders nursing drug handbook 2004.* Philadelphia: Saunders, p. 203.

---

29. A home care nurse is making follow-up visits to a client following renal transplant. The nurse assesses the client for which signs of acute graft rejection?
  1 Hypotension, graft tenderness, and anemia
  2 Hypertension, oliguria, thirst, and hypothermia
  3 Fever, vomiting, hypotension, and copious amounts of dilute urine
  4 Fever, hypertension, graft tenderness, and malaise

Answer: 4
Rationale: Acute rejection usually occurs within the first 3 months after transplant, although it can occur for up to 2 years post-transplant. The client exhibits fever, hypertension, malaise, and graft tenderness. Treatment is immediately begun with corticosteroids and possibly also with monoclonal antibodies and antilymphocyte agents.

Test-Taking Strategy: Use the process of elimination. Begin to answer this question by eliminating options 1 and 3, because hypotension is not part of the clinical picture with graft rejection. From the remaining options, recalling that fever rather than hypothermia accompanies this complication will direct you to option 4. Review the signs of acute graft rejection if you had difficulty with this question.

Level of Cognitive Ability: Application
Client Needs: Physiological Integrity
Integrated Process: Nursing Process/Assessment
Content Area: Adult Health/Renal

References:
Black, J., & Hawks, J. (2005). *Medical-surgical nursing: Clinical management for positive outcomes* (7th ed.). Philadelphia: Saunders, p. 969.
Ignatavicius, D., & Workman, M. (2002). *Medical surgical nursing: Critical thinking for collaborative care* (4th ed.). Philadelphia: Saunders, pp. 1699-1700.

---

30. A nurse is caring for a client diagnosed with a skin infection who is receiving tobramycin sulfate (Nebcin) intravenously every 8 hours. Which of the following would indicate to the nurse that the client is experiencing an adverse reaction related to the medication?
  1 A blood urea nitrogen (BUN) of 30 mg/dL
  2 A white blood cell count (WBC) of 6000/ul
  3 A sedimentation rate of 15 mm/hour
  4 A total bilirubin of 0.5 mg/dL

Answer: 1
Rationale: Adverse reactions or toxic effects of tobramycin sulfate include nephrotoxicity as evidenced by an increased BUN and serum creatinine; irreversible ototoxicity as evidenced by tinnitus, dizziness, ringing or roaring in the ears, and reduced hearing; and neurotoxicity as evidenced by headaches, dizziness, lethargy, tremors, and visual disturbances. A normal WBC is 4500 to 11,000/ul. The normal sedimentation rate is 0 to 30 mm/hour. The normal total bilirubin level is less than 1.5 mg/dL. The normal BUN is 5 to 20 mg/dL.

Test-Taking Strategy: Use the process of elimination and knowledge of normal laboratory values to assist in directing you to option 1, because this is the only abnormal laboratory value presented in the options. Review this content if you are unfamiliar with this medication or these laboratory values.

Level of Cognitive Ability: Analysis
Client Needs: Physiological Integrity
Integrated Process: Nursing Process/Analysis
Content Area: Pharmacology

Reference:
Hodgson, B., & Kizior, R. (2004). *Saunders nursing drug handbook 2004.* Philadelphia: Saunders, p. 992.

---

31. A nurse hears the alarm sound on the telemetry monitor. The nurse quickly looks at the monitor and notes that a client is in ventricular tachycardia. The nurse rushes to the client's room. Upon reaching the client's bedside, the nurse would take which action first?
1 Prepare for cardioversion
2 Prepare to defibrillate the client
3 Call a code
4 Check the client's level of consciousness

Answer: 4
Rationale: Determining unresponsiveness is the first assessment action to take. When a client is in ventricular tachycardia, there is a significant decrease in cardiac output. However, assessing for unresponsiveness ensures whether the client is affected by the decreased cardiac output. If the client is unconscious, then the ABCDs—airway, breathing, circulation, defibrillation—of cardiopulmonary resuscitation or basic life support are initiated.

Test-Taking Strategy: Note the key word "first." Use the steps of cardiopulmonary resuscitation or basic life support to answer the question. Remember: determining unresponsiveness is the first action. Review the nursing actions to take if a client experiences ventricular tachycardia if you had difficulty with this question.

Level of Cognitive Ability: Application
Client Needs: Physiological Integrity
Integrated Process: Nursing Process/Implementation
Content Area: Delegating/Prioritizing

Reference:
Black, J., & Hawks, J. (2005). *Medical-surgical nursing: Clinical management for positive outcomes* (7th ed.). Philadelphia: Saunders, pp. 1682-1685.

---

32. A nurse is assessing a preoperative client and asks the client which question to assist in determining the client's risk for developing malignant hyperthermia postoperatively?
1 "What is your normal body temperature?"
2 "Do you experience frequent infections?"
3 "Do you have a family history of problems with general anesthesia?"
4 "Have you ever suffered from heat exhaustion or heat stroke?"

Answer: 3
Rationale: Malignant hyperthermia is a genetic disorder in which a combination of anesthetic agents (succinylcholine and inhalation agents such as halothanes) trigger uncontrolled skeletal muscle contractions. This quickly leads to a potentially fatal hyperthermia. Questioning the client about the family history of general anesthesia problems may reveal this as a possibility for the client. Options 1, 2, and 4 are unrelated to this surgical complication.

Test-Taking Strategy: Use the process of elimination. Recalling that this disorder is genetic will direct you to option 3. Review the characteristics of malignant hypertension if you had difficulty with this question.

Level of Cognitive Ability: Analysis
Client Needs: Physiological Integrity
Integrated Process: Nursing Process/Assessment
Content Area: Fundamental Skills

Reference:
Black, J., & Hawks, J. (2005). *Medical-surgical nursing: Clinical management for positive outcomes* (7th ed.). Philadelphia: Saunders, p. 298.

33. A nursing instructor has taught a student about the protective structures of the brain and asks the student to identify the membranes that envelope the brain and spinal cord. The student responds correctly by stating that these are the:
1 Basal ganglia
2 Corticospinal tract
3 Meninges
4 Gray matter areas

Answer: 3
Rationale: The meninges, three membranes that envelope the brain and spinal cord, are predominantly for protection. Each layer (pia mater, arachnoid, and dura mater) is a separate membrane. The basal ganglia consist of subcortical gray matter buried deep in the cerebral hemispheres. The basal ganglia, along with the corticospinal tract, are important in controlling complex motor activity.

Test-Taking Strategy: Focus on the issue: the membranes that envelope the brain and spinal cord. Eliminate options 1, 2, and 4 because they have a similar function and are important in controlling complex motor activity. Review the anatomy and physiology of the brain if you had difficulty with this question.

Level of Cognitive Ability: Comprehension
Client Needs: Physiological Integrity
Integrated Process: Teaching/Learning
Content Area: Adult Health/Neurological

Reference:
Black, J., & Hawks, J. (2005). *Medical-surgical nursing: Clinical management for positive outcomes* (7th ed.). Philadelphia: Saunders, p. 2001.

34. A client has been taking methyldopa (Aldomet) for approximately 2 months. A home care nurse monitoring the effects of therapy determines that drug tolerance has developed if which of the following were noted in the client?
1 Decrease in weight
2 Decrease in blood pressure
3 Output greater than intake
4 Gradual rise in blood pressure

Answer: 4
Rationale: Methyldopa (Aldomet) is an antihypertensive medication. During the second or third month of therapy with methyldopa, drug tolerance can develop, which is evident by rising blood pressure levels. The physician should be notified, who may then increase the medication dosage or add a diuretic to the medication regimen. The client is also at risk of developing fluid retention, which would be manifested as dependent edema, intake greater than output, and an increase in weight. This would also warrant adding a diuretic to the course of therapy.

Test-Taking Strategy: Use the process of elimination. First, recall that methyldopa is an antihypertensive. Next, recall the definition of drug tolerance; that is, as one adjusts to a medication, the therapeutic effect diminishes. These concepts will direct you to option 4. Review the effects of methyldopa and the definition of tolerance if you had difficulty with this question.

Level of Cognitive Ability: Analysis
Client Needs: Physiological Integrity
Integrated Process: Nursing Process/Assessment
Content Area: Pharmacology

References:
Hodgson, B., & Kizior, R. (2004). *Saunders nursing drug handbook 2004.* Philadelphia: Saunders, p. 654.
McKenry, L., & Salerno, E. (2003). *Mosby's pharmacology in nursing* (21st ed.). St. Louis: Mosby, p. 579.

35. A client with a known history of panic disorder comes to the emergency room and states to the nurse, "Please help me. I think I'm having a heart attack." What is the priority nursing action?
1 Determine what the client's activity involved when the pain started
2 Identify the manifestations related to the panic disorder
3 Check the client's vital signs
4 Encourage the client to use relaxation techniques

Answer: 3

Rationale: Clients with panic disorders can experience acute physical symptoms, such as chest pain and palpitations. The priority is to assess the client's physical condition to rule out a physiological disorder. Although options 1, 2, and 4 may be appropriate at some point in the care of the client, they are not the priority.

Test-Taking Strategy: Use Maslow's hierarchy of needs theory, recalling that physiological needs are the priority. Also, use of the ABCs—airway, breathing, and circulation—will direct you to option 3. Review care of the client with a panic disorder who develops physiological manifestations if you had difficulty with this question.

Level of Cognitive Ability: Application
Client Needs: Physiological Integrity
Integrated Process: Nursing Process/Implementation
Content Area: Mental Health

Reference:
Varcarolis, E.M. (2002). *Foundations of psychiatric mental health nursing* (4th ed.). Philadelphia: Saunders, p. 310.

36. A client with trigeminal neuralgia (Tic Douloureux) asks the nurse for a snack and something to drink. The nurse determines that the appropriate fluid and food items for this client to meet nutritional needs are:
1 Hot herbal tea with graham crackers
2 Iced coffee and peanut butter and crackers
3 Vanilla wafers and lukewarm milk
4 Hot cocoa with honey and toast

Answer: 3

Rationale: Because mild tactile stimulation of the face of clients with trigeminal neuralgia can trigger pain, the client needs to eat or drink lukewarm, nutritious foods that are soft and easy to chew. Extremes of temperature will cause trigeminal pain.

Test-Taking Strategy: Use the process of elimination. Note the similarity between options 1, 2, and 4. These options contain hot or iced items and foods that are mechanically difficult to chew and swallow. Review care of the client with trigeminal neuralgia if you had difficulty with this question.

Level of Cognitive Ability: Application
Client Needs: Physiological Integrity
Integrated Process: Nursing Process/Implementation
Content Area: Adult Health/Neurological

References:
Black, J., & Hawks, J. (2005). *Medical-surgical nursing: Clinical management for positive outcomes* (7th ed.). Philadelphia: Saunders, pp. 2153-2154.
Ignatavicius, D., & Workman, M. (2002). *Medical surgical nursing: Critical thinking for collaborative care* (4th ed.). Philadelphia: Saunders, p. 970.

37. A nurse is performing an assessment on a client with peptic ulcer disease. The nurse understands that which data are unrelated to the client's disorder?
  1 Use of acetaminophen (Tylenol)
  2 A history of tarry black stools
  3 Complaints of gastric pain 2 to 4 hours after meals
  4 A history of alcohol abuse

Answer: 1

Rationale: Unlike aspirin, acetaminophen has little effect on platelet function, doesn't affect bleeding time, and generally produces no gastric bleeding. Therefore, acetaminophen is not a risk factor for bleeding from peptic ulcers. Options 2 and 3 are manifestations of peptic ulcers and bleeding peptic ulcers. Because alcohol may aggravate the stomach mucosa, a history of alcohol abuse is often seen in clients with peptic ulcer disease.

Test-Taking Strategy: Note the key word "unrelated." Use the process of elimination and focus on the client's diagnosis: peptic ulcer disease. Recall that bleeding is a concern and select the option that is not related to this concern. Review assessment of the client with peptic ulcer disease if you had difficulty with this question.

Level of Cognitive Ability: Analysis
Client Needs: Physiological Integrity
Integrated Process: Nursing Process/Assessment
Content Area: Adult Health/Gastrointestinal

Reference:
Lewis, S., Heitkemper, M., & Dirksen, S. (2004). *Medical-surgical nursing: Assessment and management of clinical problems* (6th ed.). St. Louis: Mosby, p. 1036.

---

38. A child is admitted to the orthopedic nursing unit after spinal rod insertion for the treatment of scoliosis. Which assessment is most important in the immediate postoperative period?
  1 Capillary refill, sensation, and motion in all extremities
  2 Pain level
  3 Ability to turn using the logroll technique
  4 Ability to flex and extend the feet

Answer: 1

Rationale: When the spinal column is manipulated during surgery, altered neurovascular status is a possible complication; therefore, neurovascular checks including circulation, sensation, and motion should be checked at least every 2 hours. Level of pain is an important postoperative assessment, but circulatory status is most important. Assessment of flexion and extension of the lower extremities is a component of option 1, which includes checking motion. Logrolling is performed by nurses.

Test-Taking Strategy: Use the ABCs—airway, breathing, and circulation—and the process of elimination. Option 1 addresses circulatory status. Review priority nursing assessments following spinal rod insertion if you had difficulty with this question.

Level of Cognitive Ability: Application
Client Needs: Physiological Integrity
Integrated Process: Nursing Process/Assessment
Content Area: Child Health

Reference:
Wong, D., & Hockenberry, M. (2003). *Wong's nursing care of infants and children* (7th ed.). St. Louis: Mosby, pp. 1814-1816.

39. A nurse has just finished assisting the physician in placing a central intravenous (IV) line. Which of the following is a priority nursing intervention?

1 Obtain a temperature to monitor for infection
2 Monitor the blood pressure (BP) to assess for fluid volume overload
3 Label the dressing with the date and time of catheter insertion
4 Prepare the client for a chest X-ray

Answer: 4

Rationale: A major risk associated with central line placement is the possibility of a pneumothorax developing from an accidental puncture of the lung. Assessing the results of a chest X-ray is one of the best methods to determine if this complication has occurred and to verify catheter tip placement before initiating intravenous (IV) therapy. A temperature elevation would not likely occur immediately after placement. Although BP assessment is always important in assessing a client's status after an invasive procedure, fluid volume overload is not a concern until IV fluids are started. Labeling the dressing site is important but is not the priority.

Test-Taking Strategy: Use the process of elimination and note the key words "has just finished" and "priority nursing intervention." Recall that assessment of accurate placement is essential before initiating IV therapy. Review care of the client following central line placement if you had difficulty with this question.

Level of Cognitive Ability: Application
Client Needs: Physiological Integrity
Integrated Process: Nursing Process/Implementation
Content Area: Delegating/Prioritizing

Reference:
Lewis, S., Heitkemper, M., & Dirksen, S. (2004). *Medical-surgical nursing: Assessment and management of clinical problems* (6th ed.). St. Louis: Mosby, p. 988.

40. A nurse is admitting a client suspected of having tuberculosis (TB) to the hospital. The nurse understands that the most accurate method for confirming the diagnosis is:

1 Obtaining data about the client's long history of hemoptysis
2 A positive purified protein derivative test (PPD)
3 A sputum culture positive for *Mycobacterium tuberculosis*
4 A chest X-ray positive for lung lesions

Answer: 3

Rationale: The most accurate means of confirming the diagnosis of tuberculosis is by sputum culture. Establishing the presence of *Mycobacterium tuberculosis* is essential for a definitive diagnosis. Hemoptysis is not a common finding and is usually associated with more advanced cases of tuberculosis. A positive PPD indicates exposure to tuberculosis. A chest X-ray does not confirm the diagnosis of tuberculosis. Lung lesions may be indicative of diseases other than tuberculosis.

Test-Taking Strategy: Note the key words "confirming the diagnosis." Consider which test or data would be most definitive. The actual presence of *Mycobacterium tuberculosis* in the sputum culture is the most accurate method. Review the diagnostic tests related to tuberculosis if you had difficulty with this question.

Level of Cognitive Ability: Analysis
Client Needs: Physiological Integrity
Integrated Process: Nursing Process/Assessment
Content Area: Adult Health/Respiratory

Reference:
Ignatavicius, D., & Workman, M. (2002). *Medical surgical nursing: Critical thinking for collaborative care* (4th ed.). Philadelphia: Saunders, p. 585.

41. A child has just returned from surgery and has a hip spica cast. A priority nursing action at this time is to:
1 Elevate the head of bed
2 Abduct the hips using pillows
3 Assess circulatory status
4 Turn the child on the right side

Answer: 3

Rationale: During the first few hours after a cast is applied, the chief concern is swelling that may cause the cast to act as a tourniquet and obstruct circulation. Therefore, circulatory assessment is the priority. Elevating the head of the bed of a child in a hip spica cast would cause discomfort. Using pillows to abduct the hips is not necessary because a hip spica cast immobilizes the hip and knee. Turning the child side to side at least every 2 hours is important because it allows the body cast to dry evenly and prevents complications related to immobility; however, it is not a higher priority than checking circulation.

Test-Taking Strategy: Use the process of elimination and the ABCs—airway, breathing, and circulation—to answer this question. Also, use the nursing process to answer this question. Because assessment is the first step in the nursing process, it is likely that the priority is to assess. Review nursing care following application of a spica cast if you had difficulty with this question.

Level of Cognitive Ability: Application
Client Needs: Physiological Integrity
Integrated Process: Nursing Process/Implementation
Content Area: Child Health

Reference:
Wong, D., & Hockenberry, M. (2003). *Wong's nursing care of infants and children* (7th ed.). St. Louis: Mosby, p. 1786.

42. A nurse is assessing a client with a brain stem injury. In addition to performing the Glasgow Coma Scale, the nurse plans to:
1 Check cranial nerve functioning and respiratory rate and rhythm
2 Perform arterial blood gases
3 Assist with a lumbar puncture
4 Perform a pulmonary wedge pressure

Answer: 1

Rationale: Assessment should be specific to the area of the brain involved. Assessing the respiratory status and cranial nerve function is a critical component of the assessment process in a client with a brain stem injury. Options 2, 3, and 4 are not necessary based on the data in the question.

Test-Taking Strategy: Use the process of elimination. Recall the anatomical location of the respiratory center to direct you to option 1. Remember: the respiratory center is located in the brain stem. Review content and nursing care related to brain stem injuries if you had difficulty with this question.

Level of Cognitive Ability: Application
Client Needs: Physiological Integrity
Integrated Process: Nursing Process/Planning
Content Area: Adult Health/Neurological

References:
Ignatavicius, D., & Workman, M. (2002). *Medical surgical nursing: Critical thinking for collaborative care* (4th ed.). Philadelphia: Saunders, pp. 889-890.
Phipps, W., Monahan, F., Sands, J., Marek, J., & Neighbors, M. (2003). *Medical-surgical nursing: Health and illness perspectives* (7th ed.). St. Louis: Mosby, p. 1332.

43. A client has had a Miller-Abbott tube in place for 24 hours. Which assessment finding indicates that the tube is located in the intestine?
1 Aspirate from the tube has a pH of 7
2 The abdominal X-ray report indicates that the end of the tube is above the pylorus
3 Bowel sounds are absent
4 The client is nauseous

Answer: 1
Rationale: The Miller-Abbott tube is a nasoenteric tube that is used to decompress the intestine and to correct a bowel obstruction. The end of the tube should be located in the intestine. The pH of the gastric fluid is acidic and the pH of the intestinal fluid is alkaline (7 or higher). Location of the tube can also be determined by X-ray.

Test-Taking Strategy: Use the process of elimination. Focus on the issue: a Miller-Abbott tube and intestinal location. Recalling that intestinal fluid is alkaline will direct you to option 1. Review the purpose and nursing care of a client with a Miller-Abbott tube if you had difficulty with this question.

Level of Cognitive Ability: Analysis
Client Needs: Physiological Integrity
Integrated Process: Nursing Process/Analysis
Content Area: Adult Health/Gastrointestinal

References:
Black, J., & Hawks, J. (2005). *Medical-surgical nursing: Clinical management for positive outcomes* (7th ed.). Philadelphia: Saunders, p. 745.
Lewis, S., Heitkemper, M., & Dirksen, S. (2004). *Medical-surgical nursing: Assessment and management of clinical problems* (6th ed.). St. Louis: Mosby, pp. 950; 1080.

44. While a client with myxedema is being admitted to the hospital, the client reports having experienced a lack of energy, cold intolerance, and puffiness around the eyes and face. The nurse knows that these symptoms are caused by a lack of production of which hormone(s)?
1 Luteinizing hormone (LH)
2 Adrenocorticotropic hormone (ACTH)
3 Triiodothyronine (T3) and thyroxine (T4)
4 Prolactin (PRL) and growth hormone (GH)

Answer: 3
Rationale: Although all of these hormones originate from the anterior pituitary, only T3 and T4 are associated with the client's symptoms. Myxedema results from inadequate thyroid hormone levels (T3 and T4). Low levels of thyroid hormone result in an overall decrease in the basal metabolic rate, affecting virtually every body system and leading to weakness, fatigue, and a decrease in heat production. A decrease in LH results in the loss of secondary sex characteristics. A decrease in ACTH is seen in Addison's disease. PRL stimulates breast milk production by the mammary glands, and GH affects bone and soft tissue by promoting growth through protein anabolism and lipolysis.

Test-Taking Strategy: Use the process of elimination. Recalling that myxedema is associated with the thyroid gland will assist in making a relationship between what the question is asking about and option 3. Review content and laboratory values related to myxedema if you had difficulty with this question.

Level of Cognitive Ability: Comprehension
Client Needs: Physiological Integrity
Integrated Process: Nursing Process/Analysis
Content Area: Adult Health/Endocrine

Reference:
Lewis, S., Heitkemper, M., & Dirksen, S. (2004). *Medical-surgical nursing: Assessment and management of clinical problems* (6th ed.). St. Louis: Mosby, p. 1320.

45. A 33-year-old female is admitted to the hospital with a suspected diagnosis of Graves' disease. Which symptom related to the client's menstrual cycle would the client most likely report?
1 Dysmenorrhea
2 Metrorrhagia
3 Amenorrhea
4 Menorrhagia

Answer: 3
Rationale: Amenorrhea or a decreased menstrual flow is common in the client with Graves' disease. Dysmenorrhea, metrorrhagia, and menorrhagia are also disorders related to the female reproductive system; however, they do not manifest in the presence of Graves' disease.

Test-Taking Strategy: Focus on the client's suspected diagnosis. Thinking about the pathophysiology associated with Graves' disease will direct you to option 3. Review the clinical manifestations of Graves' disease if you had difficulty with this question.

Level of Cognitive Ability: Analysis
Client Needs: Physiological Integrity
Integrated Process: Nursing Process/Assessment
Content Area: Adult Health/Endocrine

Reference:
Lewis, S., Heitkemper, M., & Dirksen, S. (2004). *Medical-surgical nursing: Assessment and management of clinical problems* (6th ed.). St. Louis: Mosby, p. 1315.
Phipps, W., Monahan, F., Sands, J., Marek, J., & Neighbors, M. (2003). *Medical-surgical nursing: Health and illness perspectives* (7th ed.). St. Louis: Mosby, p. 889.

46. A nurse is performing an assessment on a client with pregnancy-induced hypertension (PIH) who is in labor. The nurse most likely expects to note:
1 Decelerations and increased variability of the fetal heart rate
2 Increased blood pressure
3 Decreased brachial reflexes
4 Increased urine output

Answer: 2
Rationale: The major symptom of PIH is increased blood pressure. As the disease progresses, it is possible that increased brachial reflexes, decreased fetal heart rate and variability, and decreased urine output will occur, particularly during labor.

Test-Taking Strategy: Use the process of elimination. Noting the name of the disorder will easily direct you to option 2. Review the manifestations associated with PIH if you had difficulty with this question.

Level of Cognitive Ability: Analysis
Client Needs: Physiological Integrity
Integrated Process: Nursing Process/Assessment
Content Area: Maternity/Intrapartum

Reference:
Lowdermilk, D., & Perry, A. (2004). *Maternity & women's health care* (8th ed.). St. Louis: Mosby, pp. 416; 838.

47. A nurse has just administered a purified protein derivative (PPD) skin test to a client who is at low risk for developing tuberculosis. The nurse determines that the test is positive if which of the following occurs?
1 An induration of 15 mm
2 A large area of erythema
3 The presence of a wheal
4 Client complains of constant itching

Answer: 1
Rationale: An induration of 15 mm or more is considered positive for clients in low-risk groups. Erythema is not a positive reaction. The presence of a wheal would indicate that the skin test was administered appropriately. Itching is not an indication of a positive PPD.

Test-Taking Strategy: Focus on the issue: a positive test, and note that the client is at low risk for developing tuberculosis. This will direct you to option 1. Review the interpretation of PPD results if you had difficulty with this question.

Level of Cognitive Ability: Analysis
Client Needs: Physiological Integrity
Integrated Process: Nursing Process/Assessment
Content Area: Adult Health/Respiratory

Reference:
Black, J., & Hawks, J. (2005). *Medical-surgical nursing: Clinical management for positive outcomes* (7th ed.). Philadelphia: Saunders, p. 1846.

---

48. A nurse is performing an otoscopic examination on a client with a suspected diagnosis of mastoiditis. The nurse would expect to note which of the following if this disorder was present?
1 A thick and immobile tympanic membrane
2 A pearly colored tympanic membrane
3 A mobile tympanic membrane
4 A transparent tympanic membrane

Answer: 1
Rationale: Otoscopic examination in a client with mastoiditis reveals a red, dull, thick, and immobile tympanic membrane with or without perforation. Options 2, 3, and 4 indicate normal findings in an otoscopic examination.

Test-Taking Strategy: Use the process of elimination and knowledge of normal assessment findings on an ear examination to direct you to option 1, the only abnormal finding. Review the assessment findings associated with this disorder if you had difficulty with this question.

Level of Cognitive Ability: Analysis
Client Needs: Physiological Integrity
Integrated Process: Nursing Process/Assessment
Content Area: Adult Health/Ear

Reference:
Ignatavicius, D., & Workman, M. (2002). *Medical surgical nursing: Critical thinking for collaborative care* (4th ed.). Philadelphia: Saunders, pp. 1053;1066.

---

49. A nurse is reviewing the record of a client with a disorder involving the inner ear. Which of the following would the nurse most likely expect to note documented as an assessment finding in this client?
1 Complaints of itching in the affected ear
2 Complaints of severe pain in the affected ear
3 Complaints of burning in the ear
4 Complaints of tinnitus

Answer: 4
Rationale: Tinnitus is the most common complaint of clients with ear disorders, especially disorders involving the inner ear. Symptoms of tinnitus can range from mild ringing in the ear that can go unnoticed during the day to a loud roaring in the ear that can interfere with the client's thinking process and attention span. The assessment findings noted in options 1, 2, and 3 are not specifically noted in the client with an inner ear disorder.

Test-Taking Strategy: Focus on the issue of the question: inner ear disorder. Recalling the function of the inner ear will direct you to option 4. Review this content if you had difficulty with this question or are unfamiliar with the signs and symptoms associated with an inner ear disorder.

Level of Cognitive Ability: Analysis
Client Needs: Physiological Integrity
Integrated Process: Nursing Process/Assessment
Content Area: Adult Health/Ear

Reference:
Ignatavicius, D., & Workman, M. (2002). *Medical surgical nursing: Critical thinking for collaborative care* (4th ed.). Philadelphia: Saunders, p. 1067.

50. A nurse has an order to administer hydroxyzine (Vistaril) to a client by the intramuscular (IM) route. Before administering the medication, the nurse tells the client that:

1 There will be some pain at the injection site
2 There will be relief from nausea within 5 minutes
3 Excessive salivation is a side effect
4 The client will have increased alertness for about 2 hours

Answer: 1

Rationale: Hydroxyzine is an antiemetic and sedative/hypnotic that may be used in conjunction with narcotic analgesics for added effect. The injection can be extremely painful. Medications administered by the IM route generally take 20 to 30 minutes to become effective. Hydroxyzine causes dry mouth and drowsiness as side effects.

Test-Taking Strategy: Use the process of elimination and read each option carefully. Begin to answer this question by eliminating options 2 and 4, which are the least likely effects. From the remaining options, noting that the medication is administered by the IM route will direct you to option 1. Review the side effects of this medication if you had difficulty with this question.

Level of Cognitive Ability: Application
Client Needs: Physiological Integrity
Integrated Process: Nursing Process/Implementation
Content Area: Pharmacology

Reference:
Hodgson, B., & Kizior, R. (2004). *Saunders nursing drug handbook 2004.* Philadelphia: Saunders, p. 512.

---

51. A client with diabetes mellitus has a blood glucose level of 644 mg/dL. The nurse interprets that this client is most at risk of developing which type of acid-base imbalance?

1 Respiratory acidosis
2 Respiratory alkalosis
3 Metabolic acidosis
4 Metabolic alkalosis

Answer: 3

Rationale: Diabetes mellitus can lead to metabolic acidosis. When the body does not have sufficient circulating insulin, the blood glucose level rises. At the same time, the cells of the body utilize all available glucose. The body then breaks down glycogen and fat for fuel. The by-products of fat metabolism are acidotic and can lead to the condition known as diabetic ketoacidosis. Options 1, 2, and 4 are incorrect.

Test-Taking Strategy: Use the process of elimination. Noting the client's diagnosis will assist in eliminating options 1 and 2. From the remaining options, remember that the client with diabetes mellitus is at risk for developing metabolic acidosis. Review the causes of metabolic acidosis if you had difficulty with this question.

Level of Cognitive Ability: Analysis
Client Needs: Physiological Integrity
Integrated Process: Nursing Process/Analysis
Content Area: Adult Health/Endocrine

Reference:
Black, J., & Hawks, J. (2005). *Medical-surgical nursing: Clinical management for positive outcomes* (7th ed.). Philadelphia: Saunders, p. 1267.

52. A nurse is reviewing the client's most recent blood gas results, and the results indicate a pH of 7.43, P_{CO_2} of 31 mmHg, and HCO_3 of 21 mEq/L. The nurse interprets these results as indicative of which acid-base imbalance?
1 Uncompensated metabolic alkalosis
2 Compensated metabolic acidosis
3 Uncompensated respiratory acidosis
4 Compensated respiratory alkalosis

Answer: 4
Rationale: The normal pH is 7.35 to 7.45, the normal P_{CO_2} is 35 to 45 mmHg, and the normal HCO_3 is 22 to 27 mEq/L. The pH is elevated in alkalosis and low in acidosis. In a respiratory condition, an opposite effect will be seen between the pH and the P_{CO_2}. In a metabolic condition, the pH and the bicarbonate move in the same direction. Because the pH is within the normal range of 7.35 to 7.45, compensation has occurred.

Test-Taking Strategy: Remember that in a respiratory imbalance you will find an opposite response between the pH and the P_{CO_2}, as indicated in the question. Therefore, options 1 and 2 are eliminated first. Next, remember that the pH is elevated with alkalosis, and compensation has occurred as evidenced by a normal pH. Option 4 reflects a respiratory alkalotic condition and compensation, and describes the blood gas values as indicated in the question. Review the steps related to reading blood gas values if you had difficulty with this question.

Level of Cognitive Ability: Analysis
Client Needs: Physiological Integrity
Integrated Process: Nursing Process/Analysis
Content Area: Fundamental Skills

Reference:
Black, J., & Hawks, J. (2005). *Medical-surgical nursing: Clinical management for positive outcomes* (7th ed.). Philadelphia: Saunders, p. 252.

53. A nurse is caring for a client with a nasogastric tube that is attached to low suction. The nurse assesses the client for symptoms of which acid-base disorder?
1 Metabolic acidosis
2 Metabolic alkalosis
3 Respiratory acidosis
4 Respiratory alkalosis

Answer: 2
Rationale: Loss of gastric fluid via nasogastric suction or vomiting causes metabolic alkalosis because of the loss of hydrochloric acid, which is a potent acid in the body. Thus, this situation results in an alkalotic condition. The respiratory system is not involved.

Test-Taking Strategy: Eliminate options 1 and 3 first, because the loss of hydrochloric acid would cause an alkalotic condition. Because the question addresses a situation other than a respiratory one, the acid-base disorder would be metabolic alkalosis. Review the causes of metabolic alkalosis if you had difficulty with this question.

Level of Cognitive Ability: Application
Client Needs: Physiological Integrity
Integrated Process: Nursing Process/Assessment
Content Area: Fundamental Skills

Reference:
Black, J., & Hawks, J. (2005). *Medical-surgical nursing: Clinical management for positive outcomes* (7th ed.). Philadelphia: Saunders, p. 255.

54. A nurse caring for a client with late-stage salicylate poisoning who is experiencing metabolic acidosis reviews the results of the client's blood chemistry profile. The nurse anticipates that which laboratory value is related to the client's acid-base disturbance?
1 Sodium: 145 mEq/L
2 Magnesium: 2.0 mEq/L
3 Potassium: 5.2 mEq/L
4 Phosphorus: 2.3 mEq/L

Answer: 3

Rationale: The client with late-stage salicylate poisoning is at risk for metabolic acidosis because of the effects of acetylsalicylic acid in the body. Clinical manifestations of metabolic acidosis include hyperpnea with Kussmaul's respirations, headache, nausea, vomiting, diarrhea, fruity smelling breath caused by improper fat metabolism, central nervous system depression, twitching, convulsions, and hyperkalemia. The other laboratory values listed are within the normal reference ranges.

Test-Taking Strategy: Knowledge about the clinical manifestations of metabolic acidosis along with normal laboratory values will direct you to option 3. Note that the only abnormal laboratory value is the potassium level. Review normal laboratory values and the clinical manifestations of metabolic acidosis if you had difficulty with this question.

Level of Cognitive Ability: Analysis
Client Needs: Physiological Integrity
Integrated Process: Nursing Process/Analysis
Content Area: Fundamental Skills

References:

Black, J., & Hawks, J. (2005). *Medical-surgical nursing: Clinical management for positive outcomes* (7th ed.). Philadelphia: Saunders, p. 256.
Lewis, S., Heitkemper, M., & Dirksen, S. (2004). *Medical-surgical nursing: Assessment and management of clinical problems* (6th ed.). St. Louis: Mosby, pp. 342-343.

55. An emergency room nurse prepares to treat a child with acetaminophen (Tylenol) overdose. The nurse reviews the physician's orders, expecting that which of the following will be prescribed?
1 Vitamin K (AquaMephyton)
2 Protamine sulfate
3 Succimer (Chemet)
4 N-acetylcysteine (NAC)

Answer: 4

Rationale: N-acetylcysteine (NAC) is the antidote for acetaminophen overdose. It is administered orally with juice or soda or via a nasogastric tube. Vitamin K is the antidote for warfarin (Coumadin). Protamine sulfate is the antidote for heparin. Succimer (Chemet) is used in the treatment of lead poisoning.

Test-Taking Strategy: Knowledge regarding the antidote for acetaminophen overdose is required to answer this question. Learn the major antidotes for medication overdose if you are unfamiliar with them.

Level of Cognitive Ability: Analysis
Client Needs: Physiological Integrity
Integrated Process: Nursing Process/Analysis
Content Area: Child Health

Reference:

Hodgson, B., & Kizior, R. (2004). *Saunders nursing drug handbook 2004.* Philadelphia: Saunders, p. 8.

56. A 1000-mL intravenous (IV) solution of normal saline 0.9% is prescribed for the client. The nurse understands that this type of IV solution:
1 Is isotonic with the plasma and other body fluids
2 Is hypertonic with the plasma and other body fluids
3 Affects the plasma osmolarity
4 Is the same solution as sodium chloride 0.45%

Answer: 1
Rationale: Sodium chloride 0.9% (not sodium chloride 0.45%) is the same solution as normal saline 0.9%. This solution is isotonic (not hypertonic), and isotonic solutions are frequently used for IV infusion because they do not affect the plasma osmolarity.

Test-Taking Strategy: Focus on the percentage of the solution: 0.9%. This will assist in eliminating option 4. From the remaining options, note the relationship between the name of the solution, normal saline, and the word "isotonic." Remember that "normal saline" is isotonic and would not affect plasma osmolarity. Review the tonocity of IV fluids if you had difficulty with this question.

Level of Cognitive Ability: Analysis
Client Needs: Physiological Integrity
Integrated Process: Nursing Process/Analysis
Content Area: Fundamental Skills

Reference:
Black, J., & Hawks, J. (2005). *Medical-surgical nursing: Clinical management for positive outcomes* (7th ed.). Philadelphia: Saunders, p. 210.

---

57. A client who has fallen from a ladder and fractured three ribs has arterial blood gas (ABG) results of pH 7.38, PCO_2 38 mmHg, PO_2 86 mmHg, HCO_3 23 mEq/L. The nurse interprets that the client's ABGs indicate which of the following?
1 Normal results
2 Metabolic alkalosis
3 Metabolic acidosis
4 Respiratory acidosis

Answer: 1
Rationale: Normal ABG results include a pH of 7.35 to 7.45, a PCO_2 of 35 to 45 mmHg, a PO_2 of 80 to 100, and a HCO_3 of 22 to 27 mmHg. The client's results fall in the normal range.

Test-Taking Strategy: Specific knowledge of the normal ABG levels is needed to answer this question. Review these normal levels if you had difficulty with this question.

Level of Cognitive Ability: Analysis
Client Needs: Physiological Integrity
Integrated Process: Nursing Process/Analysis
Content Area: Adult Health/Respiratory

Reference:
Black, J., & Hawks, J. (2005). *Medical-surgical nursing: Clinical management for positive outcomes* (7th ed.). Philadelphia: Saunders, p. 252.

---

58. An adult client has undergone a lumbar puncture to obtain cerebrospinal fluid (CSF) for analysis. The nurse assesses for which of the following values that should be negative if the CSF is normal?
1 Protein
2 Glucose
3 White blood cells
4 Red blood cells

Answer: 4
Rationale: The adult with normal cerebrospinal fluid has no red blood cells in the CSF. The client may have small levels of white blood cells (0 to 5 cells). Protein (15 to 45 mg/dL) and glucose (45 to 80 mg/dL) are normally present in CSF.

Test-Taking Strategy: Use the process of elimination and note the key word "normal" in the question. Recalling that the presence of red blood cells would indicate blood vessel rupture or meningeal irritation will direct you to option 4. Review normal CSF values if you had difficulty with this question.

Level of Cognitive Ability: Analysis
Client Needs: Physiological Integrity
Integrated Process: Nursing Process/Assessment
Content Area: Adult Health/Neurological

Reference:
Lewis, S., Heitkemper, M., & Dirksen, S. (2004). *Medical-surgical nursing: Assessment and management of clinical problems* (6th ed.). St. Louis: Mosby, p. 1487.

---

59. A client with a burn injury is transferred to the nursing unit and a regular diet has been prescribed. Which dietary items should the nurse encourage the client to eat in order to promote wound healing?
1 Veal, potatoes, Jell-O, orange juice
2 Peanut butter and jelly, cantaloupe, tea
3 Chicken breast, broccoli, strawberries, milk
4 Spaghetti with tomato sauce, garlic bread, ginger ale

Answer: 3
Rationale: Protein and vitamin C are necessary for wound healing. Poultry and milk are good sources of protein. Broccoli and strawberries are good sources of vitamin C. Peanut butter is a source of niacin. Jell-O and jelly have no nutrient value. Spaghetti is a complex carbohydrate.

Test-Taking Strategy: Remember that all components of an option must be correct in order for the option to be correct. Knowledge that protein and vitamin C are necessary for wound healing would assist in selecting the option that contains those nutrients. Eliminate options 1 and 2 first because jelly and Jell-O have no nutrient value related to healing. From the remaining options, select option 3 over option 4 because of the greater nutrient value in these food items. Review foods high in protein and vitamin C if you had difficulty with this question.

Level of Cognitive Ability: Application
Client Needs: Physiological Integrity
Integrated Process: Nursing Process/Implementation
Content Area: Fundamental Skills

Reference:
Williams, S. (2001). *Basic nutrition & diet therapy* (11th ed.). St. Louis: Mosby, p. 564.

---

60. A nurse caring for a client with a neurological disorder is planning care to maintain nutritional status. The nurse is concerned about the client's swallowing ability. Which of the following food items would the nurse plan to avoid in this client's diet?
1 Cheese casserole
2 Scrambled eggs
3 Mashed potatoes
4 Spinach

Answer: 4
Rationale: In general, flavorful, warm, or well-chilled foods with texture stimulate the swallow reflex. Moist pastas, casseroles, egg dishes, and potatoes are usually effective. Raw vegetables, chunky vegetables such as diced beets, and stringy vegetables such as spinach, corn, and peas are foods commonly excluded from the diet of a client with a poor swallow reflex.

Test-Taking Strategy: Note the key words "swallowing ability" and "avoid." Use the process of elimination to select option 4 as the food that is stringy and with the least amount of substance or consistency. Review feeding measures for a client with altered swallowing ability if you had difficulty with this question.

Level of Cognitive Ability: Application
Client Needs: Physiological Integrity
Integrated Process: Nursing Process/Planning
Content Area: Adult Health/Neurological

Reference:
Williams, S. (2001). *Basic nutrition & diet therapy* (11th ed.). St. Louis: Mosby, 636.

61. A nurse reviews the assessment data of a client admitted to the hospital with a diagnosis of anxiety. The nurse assigns priority to which assessment finding?
1 Tearful, withdrawn, oriented times four, isolated
2 Blood pressure 160/100 mmHg; pulse 120 beats per minute; respirations 18 breaths per minute
3 Temperature 99.4°F, affect bland
4 Fist clenched, pounding table, fearful

Answer: 4
Rationale: Anxiety symptoms may take a physical harm form, and if these symptoms occur, they are of priority. Tearfulness, withdrawn, isolated, and elevated vital signs are abnormal findings. However, these findings are not life-threatening, although they should be monitored.

Test-Taking Strategy: Note the key word "priority" and focus on the client's diagnosis. Remembering that client safety and safety of others is the priority will direct you to option 4. Review the priority interventions for anxiety if you had difficulty with this question.

Level of Cognitive Ability: Analysis
Client Needs: Physiological Integrity
Integrated Process: Nursing Process/Analysis
Content Area: Delegating/Prioritizing

Reference:
Varcarolis, E.M. (2002). *Foundations of psychiatric mental health nursing* (4th ed.). Philadelphia: Saunders, p.285.

62. A client is resuming a diet after a Billroth II procedure. To minimize complications from eating, the nurse tells the client to avoid doing which of the following?
1 Eating six small meals per day
2 Eating a diet high in protein
3 Lying down after eating
4 Drinking liquids with meals

Answer: 4
Rationale: The client who has had a Billroth II procedure is at risk for dumping syndrome. The client should avoid drinking liquids with meals to prevent this syndrome. The client should be placed on a dry diet that is high in protein, moderate in fat, and low in carbohydrates. Frequent small meals are encouraged, and the client should avoid concentrated sweets.

Test-Taking Strategy: Note the key word "avoid" in the stem of the question. Focusing on the diagnosis (surgical procedure) and recalling that dumping syndrome is a complication of this surgical procedure will direct you to option 4. Review the complications of gastric surgery and the prevention and management of the complications if you had difficulty with this question.

Level of Cognitive Ability: Application
Client Needs: Physiological Integrity
Integrated Process: Teaching/Learning
Content Area: Adult Health/Gastrointestinal

Reference:
Black, J., & Hawks, J. (2005). *Medical-surgical nursing: Clinical management for positive outcomes* (7th ed.). Philadelphia: Saunders, p. 759.

63. A nurse is preparing to administer diazepam (Valium) by the intravenous (IV) route to a client who is having a seizure. The nurse plans to:
1 Dilute the prescribed dose in 50 mL of 5% dextrose in water
2 Administer the prescribed dose at a rate of 5 mg per minute
3 Mix the prescribed dose into the existing IV of 5% dextrose in normal saline
4 Administer the prescribed dose by IV push directly into the vein

Answer: 4
Rationale: Intravenous diazepam is given by IV push directly into a large vein (reduces the risk of thrombophlebitis), at a rate no greater that 1 mg per minute. It should not be mixed with other medications or solutions and can be diluted only with normal saline.

Test-Taking Strategy: Use the process of elimination. Eliminate options 1 and 3 first because they are similar. From the remaining options, it is necessary to know that this medication is administered at a rate no greater than 1 mg per minute. Review the procedure for the administration of IV diazepam if you had difficulty with this question.

Level of Cognitive Ability: Application
Client Needs: Physiological Integrity
Integrated Process: Nursing Process/Planning
Content Area: Pharmacology

Reference:
Hodgson, B., & Kizior, R. (2004). *Saunders nursing drug handbook 2004.* Philadelphia: Saunders, p. 299.

---

64. A nurse is closely monitoring a child with increased intracranial pressure who has been exhibiting decorticate posturing. The nurse notes that the child suddenly exhibits decerebrate posturing and interprets that this change in the child's condition indicates which of the following?
1 An improvement in condition
2 Decreasing intracranial pressure
3 Deteriorating neurological function
4 An insignificant finding

Answer: 3
Rationale: The progression from decorticate to decerebrate posturing usually indicates deteriorating neurological function and warrants physician notification. Options 1, 2, and 4 are inaccurate interpretations.

Test-Taking Strategy: Use the process of elimination. Eliminate options 1 and 2 first because they are similar. From the remaining options, recalling the significance of decerebrate posturing will assist in eliminating option 4. Review the significance of decorticate and decerebrate posturing if you had difficulty with this question.

Level of Cognitive Ability: Analysis
Client Needs: Physiological Integrity
Integrated Process: Nursing Process/Analysis
Content Area: Child Health

Reference:
Wong, D., & Hockenberry, M. (2003). *Wong's nursing care of infants and children* (7th ed.). St. Louis: Mosby, p. 1651.

---

65. A nurse caring for a hospitalized infant is monitoring for increased intracranial pressure (ICP) and notes that the anterior fontanel bulges when the infant cries. Based on this assessment finding, which action would the nurse take?
1 Lower the head of the bed
2 Document the findings
3 Place the infant on NPO status
4 Notify the physician immediately

Answer: 2
Rationale: The anterior fontanel is diamond-shaped and located on the top of the head. It should be soft and flat in a normal infant, and it normally closes by 12 to 18 months of age. The posterior fontanel closes by 2 to 3 months of age. A bulging or tense fontanel may result from crying or increased ICP. Noting a bulging fontanel when the infant cries is a normal finding that should be documented and monitored. It is not necessary to notify the physician. Options 1 and 3 are inappropriate actions.

Test-Taking Strategy: Use the process of elimination and focus on the information in the question. Note the key words "bulges when the infant cries." This should provide you with the clue that this is a normal finding. Remember that a bulging or tense fontanel may result from crying. Review normal assessment findings in an infant if you had difficulty with this question.

Level of Cognitive Ability: Application
Client Needs: Physiological Integrity
Integrated Process: Nursing Process/Implementation
Content Area: Child Health

Reference:
James, S., Ashwill, J., & Droske, S. (2002). *Nursing care of children: Principles & practice* (2nd ed.). Philadelphia: Saunders, pp. 240; 943.

---

66. A nurse is assessing the vital signs of a 3-year-old child hospitalized with a diagnosis of croup and notes that the respiratory rate is 28 breaths per minute. Based on this finding, which nursing action is appropriate?
  1 Reassess the respiratory rate in 15 minutes
  2 Notify the physician
  3 Document the findings
  4 Administer oxygen

Answer: 3
Rationale: The normal respiratory rate for a 3-year-old is approximately 20 to 30 breaths per minute. Because the respiratory rate is normal, options 1, 2, and 4 are unnecessary actions. The nurse would document the findings.

Test-Taking Strategy: Recalling that the normal respiratory rate for a 3-year-old child is approximately 20 to 30 breaths per minute will direct you to option 3. Review the normal vital signs in a 3-year-old if you had difficulty with this question.

Level of Cognitive Ability: Application
Client Needs: Physiological Integrity
Integrated Process: Nursing Process/Implementation
Content Area: Child Health

Reference:
James, S., Ashwill, J., & Droske, S. (2002). *Nursing care of children: Principles & practice* (2nd ed.). Philadelphia: Saunders, p. 235.

---

67. A nurse is performing an assessment on a female client who is suspected of having mittelschmerz. Which of the following would the nurse expect to note on assessment of the client?
  1 Client complains of pain at the beginning of menstruation
  2 Profuse vaginal bleeding
  3 Sharp pelvic pain that occurs at the time of ovulation
  4 Pain that occurs during intercourse

Answer: 3
Rationale: Mittelschmerz (middle pain) refers to pelvic pain that occurs midway between menstrual periods or at the time of ovulation. The pain is caused by growth of the dominant follicle within the ovary, or rupture of the follicle and subsequent spillage of follicular fluid and blood into the peritoneal space. The pain is fairly sharp and is felt on the right or left side of the pelvis. It generally lasts 1 to 3 days, and slight vaginal bleeding may accompany the discomfort.

Test-Taking Strategy: Use the process of elimination. Recalling that mittelschmerz is "middle pain" will direct you to option 3. Review this disorder if you are unfamiliar with it.

Level of Cognitive Ability: Comprehension
Client Needs: Physiological Integrity
Integrated Process: Nursing Process/Assessment
Content Area: Fundamental Skills

Reference:
Lowdermilk, D., & Perry, A. (2004). *Maternity & women's health care* (8th ed.). St. Louis: Mosby, p. 100.

---

68. A client seen in the health care clinic has been diagnosed with endometriosis and asks the nurse to describe this condition. The nurse tells the client that endometriosis:
1. Is the presence of tissue outside the uterus that resembles the endometrium
2. Is pain that occurs during ovulation
3. Is also known as primary dysmenorrhea
4. Causes the cessation of menstruation

Answer: 1
Rationale: Endometriosis is defined as the presence of tissue outside the uterus that resembles the endometruim in both structure and function. The response of this tissue to the stimulation of estrogen and progesterone during the menstrual cycle is identical to that of the endometrium. Primary dysmenorrhea refers to menstrual pain without identified pathology. Mittelschmerz refers to pelvic pain that occurs midway between menstrual periods, and amenorrhea is the cessation of menstruation for a period of at least three cycles or 6 months in a woman who has established a pattern of menstruation and can result from a variety of causes.

Test-Taking Strategy: Use the process of elimination. Note the relationship between "endometriosis" in the question and "endometrium " in the correct option. Review this disorder if you had difficulty with this question.

Level of Cognitive Ability: Application
Client Needs: Physiological Integrity
Integrated Process: Nursing Process/Implementation
Content Area: Fundamental Skills

Reference:
Lowdermilk, D., & Perry, A. (2004). *Maternity & women's health care* (8th ed.). St. Louis: Mosby, p. 162.

---

69. A client calls the physician's office to schedule an appointment because a home pregnancy test was performed and the results were positive. The nurse determines that the home pregnancy test identified the presence of which of the following in the urine?
1. Estrogen
2. Progesterone
3. Human chorionic gonadotropin (hCG)
4. Follicle-stimulating hormone (FSH)

Answer: 3
Rationale: In early pregnancy, hCG is produced by trophoblastic cells that surround the developing embryo. This hormone is responsible for positive pregnancy tests. Options 1, 2, and 4 are incorrect.

Test-Taking Strategy: Knowledge regarding the changes caused by placental hormones in early pregnancy is required to answer this question. Review this pregnancy test if you are unfamiliar with it.

Level of Cognitive Ability: Comprehension
Client Needs: Physiological Integrity
Integrated Process: Nursing Process/Assessment
Content Area: Maternity/Antepartum

Reference:
Chernecky, C., & Berger, B. (2004). *Laboratory tests and diagnostic procedures* (4th ed.). Philadelphia: Saunders, pp. 891-892.

70. A hepatitis B screen is performed on a pregnant client, and the results indicate the presence of antigens in the maternal blood. Which of the following would the nurse anticipate to be prescribed?
1 Repeat hepatitis screen
2 Retesting the mother in 1 week
3 The administration of hepatitis vaccine and hepatitis B immune globulin to the neonate within 12 hours after birth
4 The administration of antibiotics during pregnancy

Answer: 3
Rationale: A hepatitis B screen is performed to detect the presence of antigens in maternal blood. If antigens are present, the neonate needs to receive the hepatitis vaccine and hepatitis B immune globulin within 12 hours after birth. Options 1, 2, and 4 are incorrect actions or treatment measures.

Test-Taking Strategy: Use the process of elimination. Eliminate options 1 and 2 because they are similar. From the remaining options, recalling that the concern is the effect on the fetus and neonate will assist in directing you to the correct option. Review the purpose and the significance of the hepatitis B screen if you had difficulty with this question.

Level of Cognitive Ability: Analysis
Client Needs: Physiological Integrity
Integrated Process: Nursing Process/Analysis
Content Area: Maternity/Antepartum

Reference:
Lowdermilk, D., & Perry, A. (2004). *Maternity & women's health care* (8th ed.). St. Louis: Mosby, p. 1065.

71. During a prenatal visit, the client informs the nurse that she is experiencing pain in the calf when she walks. Which of the following would be the appropriate nursing action?
1 Tell the client that this is normal during pregnancy
2 Instruct the client to restrict walking
3 Assess for the presence of Homans' sign
4 Instruct the client to elevate the legs consistently throughout the day

Answer: 3
Rationale: If a woman complains of calf pain during walking, it could be an indication of venous thrombosis of the lower extremities. The appropriate nursing action would be to assess for Homans' sign, which would assist in determining the presence of venous thrombosis. It is not appropriate to tell the mother that this is normal during pregnancy. Ambulation is an important exercise, and the woman should be encouraged to ambulate during pregnancy. Although it is important to elevate the legs during pregnancy, elevating the legs consistently is not an appropriate nursing action.

Test-Taking Strategy: Note the key word "appropriate" in the stem of the question. Use the steps of the nursing process to assist in answering the question. Option 3 is the only option that addresses assessment. Review normal and abnormal expectations in the prenatal period if you had difficulty with this question.

Level of Cognitive Ability: Application
Client Needs: Physiological Integrity
Integrated Process: Nursing Process/Implementation
Content Area: Maternity/Antepartum

Reference:
Lowdermilk, D., & Perry, A. (2004). *Maternity & women's health care* (8th ed.). St. Louis: Mosby, p. 633.

72. A clinic nurse is performing an assessment on a client seen in the health care clinic for a first prenatal visit. The nurse asks the client when the first day of the last menstrual period (LMP) was, and the client reports February 9, 2007. Using Nagele's rule, the nurse determines that the estimated date of confinement is:

1 October 16, 2007
2 November 16, 2007
3 October 7, 2007
4 November 7, 2007

Answer: 2

Rationale: Accurate use of Nagele's rule requires that the woman have a regular 28-day menstrual cycle. To calculate the estimated date of confinement, the nurse would add 7 days to the first day of the LMP, subtract 3 months, and then add 1 year. First day of last menstrual period: February 9, 2007; add 7 days: February 16, 2007; subtract three months: November 16, 2006; and add 1 year, November 16, 2007.

Test-Taking Strategy: Use Nagele's rule to answer this question. Be careful when following the steps to determine the estimated data of confinement using this rule. Read all of the options carefully, noting the dates and years before selecting an option. Review Nagele's rule if you had difficulty with this question.

Level of Cognitive Ability: Comprehension
Client Needs: Physiological Integrity
Integrated Process: Nursing Process/Assessment
Content Area: Maternity/Antepartum

Reference:
Lowdermilk, D., & Perry, A. (2004). *Maternity & women's health care* (8th ed.). St. Louis: Mosby, p. 398.

73. A nurse is preparing to access an implanted vascular port to administer chemotherapy. The nurse:

1 Anchors the port with the dominant hand
2 Palpates the port to locate the center of the septum
3 Places a warm pack over the area for several minutes to alleviate possible discomfort
4 Cleans the area with alcohol, working from the outside inward

Answer: 2

Rationale: Before accessing an implanted vascular port, the nurse must palpate the port to locate the center of the septum. The port should then be anchored with the nondominant hand. Cool compresses over the site can help alleviate pain upon entry. The site should be cleansed with alcohol, working from the inside out to prevent introducing germs into the access site.

Test-Taking Strategy: Use the process of elimination. Recalling the principles related to the effects of applying cool applications and the principles of aseptic technique will assist in eliminating options 3 and 4. From the remaining options, select option 2 over option 1 because it does not make sense to anchor the port with the dominant hand. The nurse would need the dominant hand to perform the access. Review the concepts related to implanted vascular ports if you had difficulty answering this question.

Level of Cognitive Ability: Application
Client Needs: Physiological Integrity
Integrated Process: Nursing Process/Implementation
Content Area: Fundamental Skills

Reference:
Lewis, S., Heitkemper, M., & Dirksen, S. (2004). *Medical-surgical nursing: Assessment and management of clinical problems* (6th ed.). St. Louis: Mosby, p. 314.

74. A nurse is preparing to measure the fundal height of a client who is 36 weeks' gestation. To perform the procedure, the nurse would:
1 Turn the client onto her left side
2 Instruct the client to lie in a prone position
3 Place the client in a prone position with the head of the bed elevated
4 Assist the client to a standing position

Answer: 1
Rationale: When measuring fundal height, the client lies in a supine position and the nurse should instruct the client to turn onto her left side, or the nurse can elevate the left buttock by placing a pillow under the area. Options 2, 3, and 4 are incorrect client positions for measuring fundal height.

Test-Taking Strategy: Focus on the issue of the question and think about the physiological effects of an enlarged uterus at 36 weeks' gestation. Eliminate options 2 and 3 first because they are similar. Next, recalling the risk for vena cava syndrome or knowing that the standing position is inappropriate for measuring fundal height will assist in directing you to option 1. Review the procedure for measuring fundal height if you had difficulty with this question.

Level of Cognitive Ability: Application
Client Needs: Physiological Integrity
Integrated Process: Nursing Process/Implementation
Content Area: Maternity/Antepartum

References:
Lowdermilk, D., & Perry, A. (2004). *Maternity & women's health care* (8th ed.). St. Louis: Mosby, p. 416.
Murray, S., McKinney, E., & Gorrie, T. (2002). *Foundations of maternal-newborn nursing* (3rd ed.). Philadelphia: Saunders, p. 143.

75. A nurse is measuring the fundal height on a client who is 36 weeks' gestation when the client complains of feeling lightheaded. The nurse determines that the client's complaint is most likely caused by:
1 Fear
2 Compression of the vena cava
3 A full bladder
4 Anemia

Answer: 2
Rationale: Compression of the inferior vena cava and aorta by the uterus may cause supine hypotension syndrome (vena cava syndrome) late in pregnancy. Having the client turn onto her left side or elevating the left buttock during fundal height measurement will correct or prevent the problem. Options 1, 3, and 4 are unrelated to this syndrome.

Test-Taking Strategy: Focus on the information in the question. Recalling that compression of the inferior vena cava and aorta by the uterus may cause supine hypotension syndrome will direct you to option 2. Review vena cava syndrome and its causes if you had difficulty with this question.

Level of Cognitive Ability: Analysis
Client Needs: Physiological Integrity
Integrated Process: Nursing Process/Analysis
Content Area: Maternity/Antepartum

Reference:
Murray, S., McKinney, E., & Gorrie, T. (2002). *Foundations of maternal-newborn nursing* (3rd ed.). Philadelphia: Saunders, p. 124.

76. A nurse in the prenatal clinic is monitoring a client who is pregnant with twins. The nurse monitors the client most closely for which complication that is most likely associated with a twin pregnancy?
1   Maternal anemia
2   Post-term labor
3   Hemorrhoids
4   Gestational diabetes

Answer: 1
Rationale: Maternal anemia often occurs in twin pregnancies because of a greater demand for iron by the fetuses. Option 2 is incorrect because twin pregnancies often end in prematurity. Hemorrhoids occur in pregnancy but are not the most likely occurrence associated with a twin pregnancy. Option 4 is not a complication of a twin pregnancy.

Test-Taking Strategy: Focus on the issue of the question, a twin pregnancy, and note the key words "most likely." Thinking about the physiological occurrences of a twin pregnancy will direct you to option 1. Review the risks associated with a twin pregnancy if you had difficulty with this question.

Level of Cognitive Ability: Application
Client Needs: Physiological Integrity
Integrated Process: Nursing Process/Assessment
Content Area: Maternity/Antepartum

Reference:
Lowdermilk, D., & Perry, A. (2004). *Maternity & women's health care* (8th ed.). St. Louis: Mosby, p. 443.

---

77. A clinic nurse is assessing a prenatal client with heart disease. The nurse carefully assesses the client's vital signs, weight, and fluid and nutritional status to detect for complications caused by:
1   Hypertrophy and increased contractility of the heart
2   The increase in circulating blood volume
3   Fetal cardiomegaly
4   Rh incompatibility

Answer: 2
Rationale: Pregnancy taxes the circulating system of every woman because both the blood volume and cardiac output increase. Options 1, 3, and 4 are not directly associated with pregnancy in a client with a cardiac condition.

Test-Taking Strategy: Use the process of elimination and focus on the client of the question. Eliminate options 3 and 4 first because they address the fetus, not the prenatal client. From the remaining options, recalling the changes that take place in the woman during pregnancy will direct you to option 2. Also, remember that hypertrophy of the heart may occur in cardiac disease, but the outcome would be a decrease in contractility, not an increase. Review the pathophysiology in relation to cardiac disease in the pregnant client if you had difficulty with this question.

Level of Cognitive Ability: Application
Client Needs: Physiological Integrity
Integrated Process: Nursing Process/Assessment
Content Area: Maternity/Antepartum

Reference:
Lowdermilk, D., & Perry, A. (2004). *Maternity & women's health care* (8th ed.). St. Louis: Mosby, p. 911.

78. A nurse has assisted the physician with a liver biopsy that was done at the bedside. Upon completion of the procedure, the nurse assists the client into which of the following positions?
1 Left side-lying with a small pillow or towel under the puncture site
2 Right side-lying with a small pillow or towel under the puncture site
3 Left side-lying with the right arm elevated above the head
4 Right side-lying with the left arm elevated above the head

Answer: 2
Rationale: Following a liver biopsy, the client is assisted to assume a right side-lying position with a small pillow or folded towel under the puncture site for 2 hours. This position compresses the liver against the chest wall at the biopsy site.

Test-Taking Strategy: Use knowledge regarding the anatomy of the body to answer this question. Remember that the liver is on the right side of the body, and that the application of pressure on the right side will minimize the escape of blood or bile through the puncture site. Review care of the client following a liver biopsy if you had difficulty with this question.

Level of Cognitive Ability: Application
Client Needs: Physiological Integrity
Integrated Process: Nursing Process/Implementation
Content Area: Fundamental Skills

Reference:
Chernecky, C., & Berger, B. (2004). *Laboratory tests and diagnostic procedures* (4th ed.). Philadelphia: Saunders, p. 733.

79. A client has an order for "enemas until clear" before major bowel surgery. After preparing the equipment and solution, the nurse assists the client into which of the following positions to administer the enema?
1 Left-lateral Sims' position
2 Right-lateral Sims' position
3 Left side-lying with head of bed elevated 45 degrees
4 Right side-lying with head of bed elevated 45 degrees

Answer: 1
Rationale: When administering an enema, the client is placed in a left Sims' position so that the enema solution can flow by gravity in the natural direction of the colon. The head of the bed is not elevated in the Sims' position.

Test-Taking Strategy: Use knowledge regarding the anatomy of the bowel to answer the question. This will assist in eliminating options 2 and 4. From the remaining options, visualize the procedure for administering an enema and eliminate option 3 because the head of the bed should be flat during enema administration. Review the procedure for administering an enema if you had difficulty with this question.

Level of Cognitive Ability: Application
Client Needs: Physiological Integrity
Integrated Process: Nursing Process/Implementation
Content Area: Fundamental Skills

Reference:
Potter, P., & Perry, A. (2005). *Fundamentals of nursing* (6th ed.). St. Louis: Mosby, p. 1399.

80. A physician has just inserted a Cantor (nasointestinal) tube in a client with a bowel obstruction. When the procedure is complete, the nurse assists the client into which of the following positions initially to maximize the effect of the tube?
1 Right side
2 Left side
3 Prone
4 Supine

Answer: 1
Rationale: The Cantor tube is a single-lumen, mercury-weighted tube. The weight of the mercury tube carries the tube by gravity. Following insertion, to facilitate movement of the tube, the client is positioned on the right side.

Test-Taking Strategy: Note the key word "initially." Recalling the anatomy of the gastrointestinal tract and the purpose of a nasointestinal tube will direct you to option 1. Review nursing care related to the client with a Cantor tube if you had difficulty with this question.

Level of Cognitive Ability: Application
Client Needs: Physiological Integrity
Integrated Process: Nursing Process/Implementation
Content Area: Fundamental Skills

Reference:
Elkin, M., Perry, A., & Potter, P. (2004). *Nursing interventions & clinical skills* (3rd ed.). St. Louis: Mosby, p. 803.

---

81. A nurse is caring for a client following craniotomy who has a supratentorial incision. The nurse places a sign above the client's bed stating that the client should be maintained in which of the following positions?
1 Semi-Fowler's
2 Dorsal recumbent
3 Prone
4 Supine

Answer: 1
Rationale: Following supratentorial surgery (surgery above the brain's tentorium), the client's head is usually elevated 30 degrees to promote venous outflow through the jugular veins. Options 2, 3, and 4 are incorrect positions following this surgery.

Test-Taking Strategy: Use the process of elimination. A helpful strategy is to remember: supra, above the brain's tentorium, head up. Also note that options 2, 3, and 4 are similar in that they are flat positions. Review positioning following craniotomy surgery if you had difficulty with this question.

Level of Cognitive Ability: Application
Client Needs: Physiological Integrity
Integrated Process: Nursing Process/Implementation
Content Area: Fundamental Skills

Reference:
Ignatavicius, D., & Workman, M. (2002). *Medical surgical nursing: Critical thinking for collaborative care* (4th ed.). Philadelphia: Saunders, p. 1004.

---

82. A postpartum nurse is reviewing the records of the new mothers admitted to the postpartum unit. The nurse determines that which new mother would be at least risk for developing a puerperal infection?
1 A mother with a history of previous infections
2 A mother who experienced prolonged rupture of the membranes
3 A mother who had an excessive number of vaginal exams
4 A mother who underwent a vaginal delivery of the newborn

Answer: 4
Rationale: Risk factors associated with puerperal infection include a history of previous infections, cesarean births, trauma, prolonged rupture of the membranes, prolonged labor, excessive number of vaginal exams, and retained placental fragments.

Test-Taking Strategy: Note the key words "at least risk" and focus on the issue, developing a puerperal infection. Eliminate option 1 first because of its relationship to infection. Next, eliminate option 2 because of the word "prolonged" and option 3 because of the word "excessive." Review the risk factors associated with puerperal infection if you had difficulty with this question.

Level of Cognitive Ability: Analysis
Client Needs: Physiological Integrity
Integrated Process: Nursing Process/Assessment
Content Area: Maternity/Antepartum

Reference:
Lowdermilk, D., & Perry, A. (2004). *Maternity & women's health care* (8th ed.). St. Louis: Mosby, pp. 1046-1047.

83. A nurse in the delivery room assists with the delivery of a newborn infant. Following delivery, the nurse prevents heat loss in the newborn infant resulting from conduction by:
1 Wrapping the newborn in a blanket
2 Closing the doors to the delivery room
3 Drying the newborn with a warm blanket
4 Placing a warm pad on the crib before placing the newborn in the crib

Answer: 4
Rationale: Hypothermia caused by conduction occurs when the newborn infant is on a cold surface, such as a cold pad or mattress. Warming the crib pad will assist in preventing hypothermia by conduction. Evaporation of moisture from a wet body dissipates heat along with the moisture. Keeping the newborn infant dry by drying the wet newborn infant at birth will prevent hypothermia via evaporation. Convection occurs as air moves across the newborn infant's skin from an open door and heat is transferred to the air. Radiation occurs when heat from the newborn infant radiates to a colder surface.

Test-Taking Strategy: Note the key word "conduction" in the question to assist in selecting the correct option. Recalling that conduction occurs when a baby is on a cold surface will assist in directing you to option 4. Review these heat loss concepts if you had difficulty with this question.

Level of Cognitive Ability: Application
Client Needs: Physiological Integrity
Integrated Process: Nursing Process/Planning
Content Area: Maternity/Postpartum

Reference:
Lowdermilk, D., & Perry, A. (2004). *Maternity & women's health care* (8th ed.). St. Louis: Mosby, pp. 727-728.

84. A nurse provides a class to new mothers on newborn care. When teaching cord care, the nurse tells the new mothers:
1 If triple dye has been applied to the cord, it is not necessary to do anything else to it
2 To apply alcohol to the cord, ensuring that all areas around the cord are cleaned two to three times a day
3 To apply alcohol thoroughly to the cord, being careful not to move the cord because it will cause the newborn infant pain
4 All that is necessary is to wash the cord with antibacterial soap, allowing it to air dry one time a day

Answer: 2
Rationale: The cord needs to be cleansed with alcohol thoroughly, and the cord and base should be cleaned two to three times per day with alcohol (or per agency protocol). The steps are (1) lift the cord, (2) wipe around the cord starting at the top, (3) clean the base of the cord, and (4) fold the diaper below the umbilical cord to allow the cord to air dry and to prevent contamination from urine. Continuation of cord care is necessary until the cord falls off within 7 to 14 days. The infant does not feel pain in this area. Water and soap are not necessary; in fact, the cord should be kept from getting wet.

Test-Taking Strategy: Use the process of elimination. Simply recalling that the cord should be cleansed two to three times a day will direct you to the correct option. Review the principles related to cord care if you had difficulty with this question.

Level of Cognitive Ability: Application
Client Needs: Physiological Integrity
Integrated Process: Teaching/Learning
Content Area: Maternity/Postpartum

References:
Lowdermilk, D., & Perry, A. (2004). *Maternity & women's health care* (8th ed.). St. Louis: Mosby, p. 728.
Murray, S., McKinney, E., & Gorrie, T. (2002). *Foundations of maternal-newborn nursing* (3rd ed.). Philadelphia: Saunders, pp. 559; 568.

85. A nurse is monitoring a preterm newborn infant for signs of respiratory distress syndrome (RDS). The nurse monitors the infant for:

  1 Cyanosis, tachypnea, retractions, grunting respirations, and nasal flaring
  2 Acrocyanosis, apnea, pneumothorax, and grunting
  3 Barrel shaped chest, hypotension, and bradycardia
  4 Acrocyanosis, emphysema, and interstitial edema

Answer: 1

Rationale: The newborn infant with RDS may present with clinical signs of cyanosis, tachypnea or apnea, nasal flaring, chest wall retractions, or audible grunts. Acrocyanosis is the bluish discoloration of the hands and feet, is associated with immature peripheral circulation, and is not uncommon in the first few hours of life. Options 2, 3, and 4 do not indicate clinical signs of RDS.

Test-Taking Strategy: Use the process of elimination. Recalling that acrocyanosis may be a normal sign in a newborn infant will assist in eliminating options 2 and 4. From the remaining options, it is necessary to be familiar with the signs of RDS. Also, note the relationship between the diagnosis and the signs noted in option 1. Review the signs of RDS if you had difficulty with this question.

Level of Cognitive Ability: Application
Client Needs: Physiological Integrity
Integrated Process: Nursing Process/Assessment
Content Area: Maternity/Postpartum

References:
Lowdermilk, D., & Perry, A. (2004). *Maternity & women's health care* (8th ed.). St. Louis: Mosby, p. 683.
Murray, S., McKinney, E., & Gorrie, T. (2002). *Foundations of maternal-newborn nursing* (3rd ed.). Philadelphia: Saunders, pp. 831-832.

86. A nurse is preparing to assess the apical heart rate of a newborn infant in the newborn nursery. The nurse performs the procedure and notes that the heart rate is normal if which of the following is noted?

  1 A heart rate of 90 beats per minute
  2 A heart rate of 140 beats per minute
  3 A heart rate of 180 beats per minute
  4 A heart rate of 190 beats per minute

Answer: 2

Rationale: The normal heart rate in a newborn infant is 100 to 170 beats per minute. Options 1, 3, and 4 are incorrect. Option 1 indicates bradycardia, and options 3 and 4 indicate tachycardia.

Test-Taking Strategy: Focus on the issue: a newborn infant. Recalling the normal heart rate for a newborn infant will direct you to the correct option. Review this content if you are unfamiliar with this normal finding.

Level of Cognitive Ability: Analysis
Client Needs: Physiological Integrity
Integrated Process: Nursing Process/Assessment
Content Area: Maternity/Postpartum

Reference:
Lowdermilk, D., & Perry, A. (2004). *Maternity & women's health care* (8th ed.). St. Louis: Mosby, pp. 684; 712.

87. A nurse reviews the electrolyte values of a client with congestive heart failure, notes that the potassium level is low, and notifies the physician. The physician prescribes a dose of intravenous (IV) potassium chloride. When administering the IV potassium chloride, the nurse plans to:
1 Inject it as a bolus
2 Dilute it per medication instructions
3 Use a filter in the IV line
4 Apply cool compresses to the IV site during administration

Answer: 2
Rationale: Potassium chloride is very irritating to the vein and needs to be diluted to prevent phlebitis. Potassium chloride is never administered as a bolus injection. A filter is not necessary for potassium solutions. Cool compresses would constrict the blood vessel, which could possibly be more irritating to the vein.

Test-Taking Strategy: Use the process of elimination. Recalling that potassium chloride is always diluted before administration will eliminate option 1. From the remaining options, noting the words "per medication instructions" in option 2 will direct you to this option. Review the procedure for administering IV potassium chloride if you had difficulty with this question.

Level of Cognitive Ability: Application
Client Needs: Physiological Integrity
Integrated Process: Nursing Process/Planning
Content Area: Pharmacology

Reference:
Hodgson, B., & Kizior, R. (2004). *Saunders nursing drug handbook 2004.* Philadelphia: Saunders, p. 823.

88. A childbirth educator tells a class of expectant parents that it is standard routine to instill a medication into the eyes of a newborn infant as a preventive measure against ophthalmia neonatorum. The educator tells the class that the medication currently used for the prophylaxis of ophthalmia neonatorium is:
1 Erythromycin ophthalmic eye ointment
2 Neomycin ophthalmic eye ointment
3 Penicillin ophthalmic eye ointment
4 Vitamin K injection

Answer: 1
Rationale: Ophthalmic erythromycin 0.5% ointment is a broad-spectrum antibiotic and is used prophylactically to prevent ophthalmia neonatorum, an eye infection acquired from the newborn infant's passage through the birth canal. Infection from these organisms can cause blindness or serious eye damage. Erythromycin is effective against *Neisseria gonorrhoeae* and *Chlamydia trachomatis.* Vitamin K is administered to the newborn infant to prevent abnormal bleeding, and it promotes liver formation of the clotting factors II, VII, IX, and X. Options 2 and 3 are incorrect.

Test-Taking Strategy: Focusing on the issue, eye medication, will assist in eliminating option 4. From the remaining options, recalling that erythromycin is a broad-spectrum antibiotic will direct you to option 1. Review initial care of the newborn infant if you had difficulty with this question.

Level of Cognitive Ability: Application
Client Needs: Physiological Integrity
Integrated Process: Teaching/Learning
Content Area: Maternity/Postpartum

Reference:
Lowdermilk, D., & Perry, A. (2004). *Maternity & women's health care* (8th ed.). St. Louis: Mosby, p. 728.

89. A nurse is developing a teaching plan for the mother of a newborn infant who is human immunodeficiency virus (HIV) positive. The nurse includes which specific instruction in the teaching plan?

1 Instruct the mother to provide meticulous skin care to the newborn infant and to change the infant's diaper after each voiding or stool
2 Instruct the mother to feed the newborn infant in an upright position with the head and chest tilted slightly back to avoid aspiration
3 Instruct the mother to feed the newborn infant with a special nipple and burp the infant frequently to decrease the tendency to swallow air
4 Instruct the mother to check the anterior fontanel for bulging and sutures for widening each day

Answer: 1

Rationale: Meticulous skin care helps protect the HIV-infected newborn infant from secondary infections. Feeding the newborn in an upright position, using a special nipple, and bulging fontanels are unrelated to the pathology associated with HIV.

Test-Taking Strategy: Read the question carefully and use the process of elimination. The question specifically asks for instructions to be given to the mother regarding HIV. Although options 2, 3, and 4 may be correct or partially correct, the content does not specifically relate to care of the newborn infant infected with HIV. Review care of an infant infected with HIV if you had difficulty with this question.

Level of Cognitive Ability: Application
Client Needs: Physiological Integrity
Integrated Process: Teaching/Learning
Content Area: Maternity/Postpartum

Reference:
Lowdermilk, D., & Perry, A. (2004). *Maternity & women's health care* (8th ed.). St. Louis: Mosby, pp. 1066-1067.

---

90. Following assessment and diagnostic evaluation, it has been determined that the client has Lyme disease, stage II. The nurse assesses the client for which of the following that is most indicative of this stage?

1 Erythematous rash
2 Neurological deficits
3 Headache
4 Lethargy

Answer: 2

Rationale: Stage II of Lyme disease develops within 1 to 6 months in most untreated individuals. The most serious problems in this stage include cardiac conduction defects and neurological disorders such as Bell's palsy and paralysis. These problems are not usually permanent. Flulike symptoms (headache and lethargy) and a rash appear in stage I.

Test-Taking Strategy: Use the process of elimination. Recalling that a rash and flulike symptoms occur in stage I will direct you to the correct option. Review the clinical manifestations associated with each stage of Lyme disease if you had difficulty with this question.

Level of Cognitive Ability: Analysis
Client Needs: Physiological Integrity
Integrated Process: Nursing Process/Assessment
Content Area: Adult Health/Integumentary

Reference:
Phipps, W., Monahan, F., Sands, J., Marek, J., & Neighbors, M. (2003). *Medical-surgical nursing: Health and illness perspectives* (7th ed.). St. Louis: Mosby, p. 1544.

91. A nurse is caring for a client with a diagnosis of pemphigus. On assessment of the client, the nurse looks for which hallmark sign characteristic of this condition?
1 Homans' sign
2 Chvostek's sign
3 Tousseau's sign
4 Nikolsky's sign

Answer: 4

Rationale: A hallmark sign of pemphigus is Nikolsky's sign, which is when the epidermis can be rubbed off by slight friction or injury. Other characteristics include flaccid bullae that rupture easily and emit a foul-smelling drainage leaving crusted, denuded skin. The lesions are common on the face, back, chest, and umbilicus. Even slight pressure on an intact blister may cause spread to adjacent skin. Trousseau's sign is a sign for tetany, in which carpal spasm can be elicited by compressing the upper arm and causing ischemia to the nerves distally. Chvostek's sign, seen in tetany, is a spasm of the facial muscles elicited by tapping the facial nerve in the region of the parotid gland. Homans' sign, a sign of thrombosis in the leg, is discomfort in the calf on forced dorsiflexion of the foot.

Test-Taking Strategy: Use the process of elimination. Eliminate options 2 and 3 first because they are similar and both relate to tetany. From the remaining options, recalling that Homans' sign is related to thrombophlebitis will direct you to option 4. Review these various signs if you had difficulty with this question.

Level of Cognitive Ability: Analysis
Client Needs: Physiological Integrity
Integrated Process: Nursing Process/Assessment
Content Area: Adult Health/Integumentary

Reference:
Black, J., & Hawks, J. (2005). *Medical-surgical nursing: Clinical management for positive outcomes* (7th ed.). Philadelphia: Saunders, p. 1418.

92. Following tonsillectomy, which of the following fluid or food items is appropriate to offer to the child?
1 Cool Cherry Kool-Aid
2 Vanilla pudding
3 Cold ginger ale
4 Jell-O

Answer: 4

Rationale: Following tonsillectomy, clear, cool liquids should be administered. Citrus, carbonated, and extremely hot or cold liquids need to be avoided because they may irritate the throat. Red liquids need to be avoided because they give the appearance of blood if the child vomits. Milk and milk products (pudding) are avoided because they coat the throat and cause the child to clear the throat, thus increasing the risk of bleeding.

Test-Taking Strategy: Note the key word "appropriate." Avoiding foods and fluids that may irritate or cause bleeding is the concern. This will assist in eliminating options 2 and 3. The word "cherry" in option 1 should be the clue that this is not an appropriate food item. Review dietary measures following tonsillectomy if you had difficulty with this question.

Level of Cognitive Ability: Application
Client Needs: Physiological Integrity
Integrated Process: Nursing Process/Implementation
Content Area: Child Health

Reference:
James, S., Ashwill, J., & Droske, S. (2002). *Nursing care of children: Principles & practice* (2nd ed.). Philadelphia: Saunders, p. 636.

93. A nurse is checking postoperative orders and planning care for a 110-pound child after spinal fusion. Morphine sulfate, 8 mg subcutaneously every 4 hours prn for pain, is prescribed. The pediatric drug reference states that the safe dose is 0.1 to 0.2 mg/kg/dose every 2 to 4 hours. From this information, the nurse determines that:

1 The dose is too low
2 The dose is too high
3 The dose is within the safe dosage range
4 There is not enough information to determine the safe dose

Answer: 3
Rationale: Use the formula to determine the dosage parameters. Convert pounds to kilograms by dividing by 2.2.
110 lbs. divided by 2.2 = 50 kg
Dosage parameters: 0.1 mg/kg/dose × 50 kg = 5 mg
  0.2 mg/kg/dose × 50 kg = 10 mg
Dosage is within the safe dosage range.

Test-Taking Strategy: Identify the key components of the question and what the question is asking. In this case, the question asks for the safe dosage range for medication. Change pounds to kilograms. Calculate the dosage parameters using the safe dose range identified in the question and the child's weight in kg. Review medication calculations if you had difficulty with this question.

Level of Cognitive Ability: Analysis
Client Needs: Physiological Integrity
Integrated Process: Nursing Process/Analysis
Content Area: Child Health

Reference:
Kee, J., & Marshall, S. (2004). *Clinical calculations: With applications to general and specialty areas* (4th ed.). Philadelphia: Saunders, pp. 235-236.

94. A nurse is performing a physical assessment on a client and is testing the client's reflexes. What action would the nurse take to assess the pharyngeal reflex?

1 Shine a light toward the bridge of the nose
2 Stimulate the back of the throat with a tongue depressor
3 Ask the client to swallow
4 Pull down on the lower eyelid

Answer: 2
Rationale: The pharyngeal (gag) reflex is tested by touching the back of the throat with an object, such as a tongue depressor. A positive response to this reflex is considered normal. The corneal light reflex is tested by shining a penlight toward the bridge of the nose at a distance of 12 to 15 inches (light reflection should be symmetrical in both corneas). Asking the client to swallow assesses the swallow reflex. To assess the palpebral conjunctiva, the nurse would pull down and evert the lower eyelid.

Test-Taking Strategy: Focus on the type of reflex addressed in the question. Recalling that "pharyngeal" refers to the pharynx, or back of the throat, will assist in determining how this reflex is tested and direct you to option 2. Review assessment of reflexes if you had difficulty with this question.

Level of Cognitive Ability: Application
Client Needs: Physiological Integrity
Integrated Process: Nursing Process/Assessment
Content Area: Adult Health/Neurological

Reference:
Wilson, S., & Giddens, J. (2005). *Health assessment for nursing practice* (3rd ed.). St. Louis: Mosby, pp. 306; 309; 624.

95. A pediatric nurse specialist provides an educational session to the nursing students about childhood communicable diseases. A nursing student asks the pediatric nurse specialist to describe the signs and symptoms associated with the most common complication of mumps. The pediatric nurse specialist responds knowing that which of the following signs or symptoms is indicative of the most common complication of this communicable disease?

1 A red swollen testicle
2 Nuchal rigidity
3 Pain
4 Deafness

Answer: 2

Rationale: The most common complication of mumps is aseptic meningitis, with the virus being identified in the cerebrospinal fluid. Common signs include nuchal rigidity, lethargy, and vomiting. A red swollen testicle may be indicative of orchitis. Although this complication appears to cause most concern among parents, it is not the most common complication. Although mumps is one of the leading causes of unilateral nerve deafness, it does not occur frequently. Muscular pain, parotid pain, or testicular pain may occur, but pain does not indicate a sign of a common complication.

Test-Taking Strategy: Use the process of elimination. Recalling that aseptic meningitis is the most common complication of mumps will direct you to option 2. Review the complications associated with mumps if you had difficulty with this question.

Level of Cognitive Ability: Analysis
Client Needs: Physiological Integrity
Integrated Process: Teaching/Learning
Content Area: Child Health

Reference:
James, S., Ashwill, J., & Droske, S. (2002). *Nursing care of children: Principles & practice* (2nd ed.). Philadelphia: Saunders, pp. 454-455.

96. A 5-year-old child is hospitalized with Rocky Mountain Spotted Fever (RMSF). The nursing assessment reveals that the child was bitten by a tick 2 weeks ago. The child presents with complaints of headache, fever, and anorexia, and the nurse notes a rash on the palms of the hands and soles of the feet. The nurse reviews the physician's orders and anticipates that which of the following medications will be prescribed?

1 Tetracycline (Achromycin)
2 Amphotericin B (Ketoconazole)
3 Ganciclovir (Foscarnet)
4 Amantadine (Rimantadine)

Answer: 1

Rationale: The nursing care of a child with RMSF will include the administration of tetracycline. An alternative medication is chloramphenicol, a fluoroquinolone. Amphotericin B is used for fungal infections. Ganciclovir is used to treat cytomegalovirus. Amantadine is used to treat influenza A virus.

Test-Taking Strategy: Knowledge regarding the treatment plan associated with RMSF is required to answer this question. Review this content if you are unfamiliar with this treatment plan or with the medications identified in the options.

Level of Cognitive Ability: Analysis
Client Needs: Physiological Integrity
Integrated Process: Nursing Process/Analysis
Content Area: Child Health

Reference:
Wong, D., & Hockenberry, M. (2003). *Wong's nursing care of infants and children* (7th ed.). St. Louis: Mosby, p. 765.

97. A nursing instructor assigns a student nurse to present a clinical conference to the student group about brain tumors in children. The nursing student prepares for the conference and includes which of the following information in the presentation?
  1 Surgery is not normally performed because of the risk of functional deficits occurring as a result of the surgery.
  2 Head shaving is not required before removal of the brain tumor.
  3 Chemotherapy is the treatment of choice.
  4 The most significant symptoms are headaches and vomiting.

Answer: 4
Rationale: The hallmark symptoms of children with brain tumors are headaches and vomiting. The treatment of choice is total surgical removal of the tumor without residual neurological damage. Before surgery, the child's head will be shaved, although every effort is made to shave only as much hair as is necessary. Although chemotherapy may be needed, it is not the treatment of choice.

Test-Taking Strategy: Use the process of elimination. Eliminate options 1 and 2 first because of the absolute word "not." From the remaining options, recalling that the treatment of choice is total surgical removal of the tumor will direct you to option 4. Review this content if you are unfamiliar with the clinical manifestations and interventions associated with a brain tumor.

Level of Cognitive Ability: Application
Client Needs: Physiological Integrity
Integrated Process: Teaching/Learning
Content Area: Child Health

Reference:
Wong, D., & Hockenberry, M. (2003). *Wong's nursing care of infants and children* (7th ed.). St. Louis: Mosby, p. 1619.

---

98. A magnetic resonance imaging (MRI) scan is prescribed for a client with a suspected brain tumor. The nurse anticipates that the physician will prescribe which of the following before the procedure?
  1 An antihistamine
  2 A corticosteroid
  3 A sedative
  4 An antibiotic

Answer: 3
Rationale: An MRI is a noninvasive diagnostic test that visualizes the body's tissues, structure, and blood flow. The client is positioned on a padded table and moved into a cylinder-shaped scanner. Relaxation techniques or a sedative are used before the procedure to reduce claustrophobic effects. There is no useful purpose for administering an antihistamine, corticosteroid, or antibiotic.

Test-Taking Strategy: Focus on the diagnostic test. Recalling that claustrophobia is a concern will direct you to option 3. Review this diagnostic test if you are unfamiliar with it.

Level of Cognitive Ability: Analysis
Client Needs: Physiological Integrity
Integrated Process: Nursing Process/Analysis
Content Area: Fundamental Skills

Reference:
Chernecky, C., & Berger, B. (2004). *Laboratory tests and diagnostic procedures* (4th ed.). Philadelphia: Saunders, p. 758.

99. Tretinoin (Retin-A) is prescribed for a client with acne. The client calls the clinic nurse and tells the nurse that her skin has become very red and is beginning to peel. The nurse makes which statement to the client?
1 "Come to the clinic immediately."
2 "Discontinue the medication."
3 "Notify the physician."
4 "This is a normal occurrence with the use of this medication."

Answer: 4
Rationale: Tretinoin decreases cohesiveness of the epithelial cells, increasing cell mitosis and turnover. It is potentially irritating, particularly when used correctly. Within 48 hours of use, the skin generally becomes red and begins to peel. Options 1, 2, and 3 are incorrect statements to the client.

Test-Taking Strategy: Use the process of elimination. Options 1 and 3 can be eliminated first because they are similar. Eliminate option 2 next because it is not within the scope of nursing practice to advise a client to discontinue a medication. Review the effects of this medication if you had difficulty with this question.

Level of Cognitive Ability: Application
Client Needs: Physiological Integrity
Integrated Process: Nursing Process/Implementation
Content Area: Pharmacology

Reference:
Hodgson, B., & Kizior, R. (2004). *Saunders nursing drug handbook 2004.* Philadelphia: Saunders, p. 1016.

100. A child is hospitalized with a diagnosis of lead poisoning, and chelation therapy is prescribed. The nurse caring for the child would prepare to administer which of the following medications?
1 Activated charcoal
2 Sodium bicarbonate
3 Ipecac syrup
4 Dimercaprol (BAL)

Answer: 4
Rationale: Dimercaprol (BAL) is a chelating agent that is used to treat lead poisoning. Sodium bicarbonate may be used in salicylate poisoning. Ipecac syrup may be prescribed by the physician to induce vomiting in certain poisoning situations. Activated charcoal is used to decrease absorption in certain poisoning situations.

Test-Taking Strategy: Focus on the issue: treatment related to lead poisoning. Think about the classifications of the medications in the options. Recalling that dimercaprol (BAL) is a chelating agent will direct you to option 4. Review this treatment if you are unfamiliar with it.

Level of Cognitive Ability: Application
Client Needs: Physiological Integrity
Integrated Process: Nursing Process/Planning
Content Area: Child Health

Reference:
Hodgson, B., & Kizior, R. (2004). *Saunders nursing drug handbook 2004.* Philadelphia: Saunders, p. 1082.

101. A nurse is performing pin site care on a client in skeletal traction. Which finding would the nurse expect to note when assessing the pin sites?
1 Redness and swelling around the pin sites
2 Loose pin sites
3 Purulent drainage from the pin sites
4 Serous draining from the pin sites

Answer: 4
Rationale: A small amount of serous drainage may be expected after cleaning and removing crusting around the pin sites. Redness and swelling around the pin sites and purulent drainage may be indicative of an infection. Pins should not be loose, and if this is noted, the physician should be notified.

Test-Taking Strategy: Use the process of elimination. Option 2 is not an expected finding and can be eliminated first because loose pins would not provide a secure hold with the traction. Eliminate options 1 and 3 next because they are similar and indicate signs of infection. Review assessment of pin sites in the client with skeletal traction if you had difficulty with this question.

Level of Cognitive Ability: Analysis
Client Needs: Physiological Integrity
Integrated Process: Nursing Process/Assessment
Content Area: Adult Health/Musculoskeletal

References:
Black, J., & Hawks, J. (2005). *Medical-surgical nursing: Clinical management for positive outcomes* (7th ed.). Philadelphia: Saunders, p. 636.
Ignatavicius, D., & Workman, M. (2002). *Medical surgical nursing: Critical thinking for collaborative care* (4th ed.). Philadelphia: Saunders, p. 1137.

---

102. A nurse is caring for a client who has been placed in Buck's extension traction while awaiting surgical repair of a fractured femur. The nurse prepares to perform a complete neurovascular assessment of the affected extremity and plans to assess:
   1 Color, sensation, movement, capillary refill, and pulse of the affected extremity
   2 Warmth of the skin and the temperature in the affected extremity
   3 Vital signs and bilateral lung sounds
   4 Pain level and for the presence of edema in the affected extremity

Answer: 1
Rationale: A complete neurological assessment of an extremity includes color, sensation, movement, capillary refill, and pulse of the affected extremity. Option 2 identifies only some of the components of a neurological assessment. Options 3 and 4 do not identify the components of a neurovascular assessment.

Test-Taking Strategy: Focus on the key words "complete neurovascular assessment of the affected extremity." Use the ABCs—airway, breathing, and circulation—to direct you to option 1. Review the components of a neurovascular assessment if you had difficulty with this question.

Level of Cognitive Ability: Application
Client Needs: Physiological Integrity
Integrated Process: Nursing Process/Assessment
Content Area: Adult Health/Musculoskeletal

Reference:
Phipps, W., Monahan, F., Sands, J., Marek, J., & Neighbors, M. (2003). *Medical-surgical nursing: Health and illness perspectives* (7th ed.). St. Louis: Mosby, pp. 1479; 1481.

---

103. A client in the emergency room has a plaster of Paris cast applied. The client arrives at the nursing unit, and the nurse prepares to transfer the client into the bed by:
   1 Supporting the cast with the fingertips only
   2 Asking the client to support the cast during transfer
   3 Placing ice on top of the cast
   4 Using the palms of the hands and soft pillows to support the cast

Answer: 4
Rationale: The palms or the flat surface of the extended fingers should be used when moving a wet cast to prevent indentations. Pillows are used to support the curves of the cast to prevent cracking or flattening of the cast from the weight of the body. Half-full bags of ice may be placed next to the cast to prevent swelling, but this action would be performed after the client is placed in bed. Asking the client to support the cast during transfer is inappropriate.

Test-Taking Strategy: Focusing on the key words "transfer the client into the bed" will assist in eliminating option 3. Eliminate option 2 next because it is inappropriate to ask the client to support the cast. From the remaining options, eliminate option 1 because of the absolute word "only" in this option. Review care of the client in a newly applied plaster cast if you had difficulty with this question.

Level of Cognitive Ability: Application
Client Needs: Physiological Integrity
Integrated Process: Nursing Process/Planning
Content Area: Adult Health/Musculoskeletal

Reference:
Phipps, W., Monahan, F., Sands, J., Marek, J., & Neighbors, M. (2003). *Medical-surgical nursing: Health and illness perspectives* (7th ed.). St. Louis: Mosby, p. 1481.

---

104. A physician orders the deflation of the esophageal balloon of a Sengstaken-Blakemore tube in a client. The nurse prepares for the procedure knowing that the deflation of the esophageal balloon places the client at risk for:
1. Increased ascites
2. Esophageal necrosis
3. Recurrent hemorrhage from the esophageal varices
4. Gastritis

Answer: 3
Rationale: A Sengstaken-Blakemore tube is inserted in clients with cirrhosis who have ruptured esophageal varices. It has esophageal and gastric balloons. The esophageal balloon exerts pressure on the ruptured esophageal varices and stops the bleeding. The pressure of the esophageal balloon is released at intervals to decrease the risk of trauma to the esophageal tissues, including esophageal rupture or necrosis. When the balloon is deflated, the client may begin to bleed again from the esophageal varices.

Test-Taking Strategy: Focus on the issue and recall the purpose of the esophageal balloon of the Sengstaken-Blakemore tube. Remembering that the esophageal balloon exerts pressure on ruptured esophageal varices and stops the bleeding will assist in directing you to the correct option. Review the complications associated with this type of tube if you are unfamiliar with it.

Level of Cognitive Ability: Analysis
Client Needs: Physiological Integrity
Integrated Process: Nursing Process/Planning
Content Area: Adult Health/Gastrointestinal

Reference:
Black, J., & Hawks, J. (2005). *Medical-surgical nursing: Clinical management for positive outcomes* (7th ed.). Philadelphia: Saunders, pp. 1345-1346.

---

105. A physician tells a nurse that a client can be given droperidol (Inapsine) for the relief of postoperative nausea. The nurse anticipates that the physician will order the medication by which of the following routes?
1. Oral
2. Intravenous
3. Subcutaneous
4. Intranasal

Answer: 2
Rationale: Droperidol may be administered by the intramuscular (IM) or intravenous (IV) routes. The IV route is the route used when relief of nausea is needed. The IM route may be used when the medication is used as an adjunct to anesthesia. Options 1, 3, and 4 are not routes of administration of this medication.

Test-Taking Strategy: Focus on the data in the question. Noting that the client is a postoperative client will assist in directing you to option 2. Review this medication if you had difficulty with this question.

Level of Cognitive Ability: Analysis
Client Needs: Physiological Integrity
Integrated Process: Nursing Process/Analysis
Content Area: Pharmacology

Reference:
Hodgson, B., & Kizior, R. (2004). *Saunders nursing drug handbook 2004.* Philadelphia: Saunders, pp. 345-346.

106. A nurse is teaching the parents of a child with celiac disease about dietary measures. The nurse tells the parents to:

1   Read all label ingredients carefully to avoid hidden sources of gluten
2   Restrict corn and rice in the diet
3   Restrict fresh starchy vegetables in the diet
4   Substitute grain cereals with pasta products

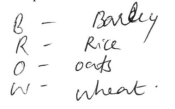

B — Barley
R — Rice
O — oats
W — wheat.

Answer: 1

Rationale: Gluten is found primarily in the grains of wheat and rye. Corn and rice become substitute foods. Gluten is added to many foods as hydrolyzed vegetable protein that is derived from cereal grains, therefore labels need to be read. Corn and rice as well as vegetables are acceptable in a gluten-free diet. Many pasta products contain gluten. Grains are frequently added to processed foods for thickness or fillers.

Test-Taking Strategy: Use the process of elimination, recalling that a gluten-free diet is required in celiac disease. Select option 1 because it is the umbrella (global) option. Review the dietary measures in celiac disease if you had difficulty with this question.

Level of Cognitive Ability: Application
Client Needs: Physiological Integrity
Integrated Process: Teaching/Learning
Content Area: Child Health

Reference:
Wong, D., & Hockenberry, M. (2003). *Wong's nursing care of infants and children* (7th ed.). St. Louis: Mosby, p. 1450.

---

107. A 45-year-old client is admitted to the hospital for evaluation of recurrent runs of ventricular tachycardia noted on Holter monitoring. The client is scheduled for electrophysiology studies (EPS) the following morning. Which statement would the nurse include in a teaching plan for this client?

1   "During the procedure, a special wire is used to increase the heart rate and produce the irregular beats that caused your signs and symptoms."
2   "You will be sedated during the procedure and will not remember what has happened."
3   "This test is a noninvasive method of determining the effectiveness of your medication regime."
4   "You will continue to take your medications until the morning of the test."

Answer: 1

Rationale: The purpose of EPS is to study the heart's electrical system. During this invasive procedure, a special wire is introduced into the heart to produce dysrhythmias. To prepare for this procedure, the client should be NPO for 6 to 8 hours before the test, and all antidysrhythmics are held for at least 24 hours before the test in order to study the dysrhythmias without the influence of medications. Because the client's verbal responses to the rhythm changes are extremely important, sedation is avoided if possible.

Test-Taking Strategy: Note the relationship between the words "recurrent runs of ventricular tachycardia" in the question and "produce the irregular beats" in option 1. Review this procedure if you had difficulty with this question.

Level of Cognitive Ability: Application
Client Needs: Physiological Integrity
Integrated Process: Teaching/Learning
Content Area: Adult Health/Cardiovascular

Reference:
Chernecky, C., & Berger, B. (2004). *Laboratory tests and diagnostic procedures* (4th ed.). Philadelphia: Saunders, pp. 497-499.

108. A nurse is providing diet teaching to a client with congestive heart failure (CHF). The nurse tells the client to avoid:
1 Leafy green vegetables
2 Steak sauce
3 Apple juice
4 Sherbet

Answer: 2
Rationale: Steak sauce is high in sodium. Leafy green vegetables, any juice (except tomato or V8 brand vegetable), and sherbet are all low in sodium. Clients with CHF should monitor sodium intake.

Test-Taking Strategy: Note the key word "avoid." Use the process of elimination, noting that options 1, 3, and 4 are similar in that they are low-sodium foods. Recalling that the client with CHF should limit sodium intake will direct you to option 2. Review dietary measures for the client with CHF if you had difficulty with this question.

Level of Cognitive Ability: Application
Client Needs: Physiological Integrity
Integrated Process: Teaching/Learning
Content Area: Adult Health/Cardiovascular

Reference:
Black, J., & Hawks, J. (2005). *Medical-surgical nursing: Clinical management for positive outcomes* (7th ed.). Philadelphia: Saunders, p. 1662.

109. A home care nurse is developing a plan of care for an older client with diabetes mellitus who has gastroenteritis. In order to maintain food and fluid intake to prevent dehydration, the nurse plans to:
1 Offer water only until the client is able to tolerate solid foods
2 Withhold all fluids until vomiting has ceased for at least 4 hours
3 Encourage the client to take 8 to 12 ounces of fluid every hour while awake
4 Maintain a clear liquid diet for at least 5 days before advancing to solids to allow inflammation of the bowel to dissipate

Answer: 3
Rationale: The client should be offered liquids containing both glucose and electrolytes. Small amounts of fluid may be tolerated even when vomiting is present. The diet should be advanced as tolerated, and include a minimum of 100 to 150 grams of carbohydrates daily. Offering water only and maintaining liquids for 5 days will not prevent dehydration but may promote it in this client.

Test-Taking Strategy: Eliminate options 1 and 2 because of the words "only" and "all" in these options respectively. From the remaining options, note the words "for at least 5 days" in option 4. Thinking about the issue, a client with diabetes mellitus and preventing dehydration, will assist in eliminating this option. Review sick day rules for a client with diabetes mellitus if you had difficulty with this question.

Level of Cognitive Ability: Application
Client Needs: Physiological Integrity
Integrated Process: Nursing Process/Planning
Content Area: Adult Health/Endocrine

Reference:
Ignatavicius, D., & Workman, M. (2002). *Medical surgical nursing: Critical thinking for collaborative care* (4th ed.). Philadelphia: Saunders, p. 1273.

110. A client is unable to expectorate sputum for a sputum sample, and the nurse is preparing to obtain the sample via saline inhalation. The nurse instructs the client to inhale the warm saline vapor via nebulizer by:
1 Holding the nebulizer under the nose
2 Keeping the lips closed lightly over the mouthpiece
3 Keeping the lips closely tightly over the mouthpiece
4 Alternating one vapor breath with one breath from room air

Answer: 2

Rationale: The inhalation of heated vapor helps the client to cough productively because the vapor condenses on the tracheo-bronchial mucosa and stimulates the production of secretions and a cough reflex. The client is told to lightly cover the mouthpiece with the lips and not to form a tight seal. The client inhales vaporized saline until coughing results. Options 1, 3, and 4 are incorrect.

Test-Taking Strategy: Note that options 2 and 3 are opposite actions in that one option reads to keep the lips closely *tightly* over the mouthpiece while the other reads to keep the lips closely *lightly* over the mouthpiece. Visualizing this procedure will direct you to option 2. Review this variation of procedure for obtaining a sputum sample if you had difficulty with the question.

Level of Cognitive Ability: Application
Client Needs: Physiological Integrity
Integrated Process: Nursing Process/Implementation
Content Area: Fundamental Skills

References:
Lewis, S., Heitkemper, M., & Dirksen, S. (2004). *Medical-surgical nursing: Assessment and management of clinical problems* (6th ed.). St. Louis: Mosby, pp. 560-562.
McKenry, L., & Salerno, E. (2003). *Mosby's pharmacology in nursing* (21st ed.). St. Louis: Mosby, p. 705.

111. A nurse has completed tracheostomy care for a client whose tracheostomy tube has a nondisposable inner cannula. The nurse reinserts the inner cannula into the tracheostomy immediately after:
1 Suctioning the client's airway
2 Rinsing it with sterile water
3 Shaking it to dry
4 Drying it thoroughly with a soft tissue

Answer: 3

Rationale: After washing and rinsing the inner cannula, the nurse shakes it to dry. The nurse then inserts the cannula into the tracheostomy and turns it clockwise to lock it into place. Suctioning is not performed without an inner cannula in place. A wet cannula (option 2) should not be inserted into a tracheostomy. A fine-mesh sterile gauze may be used to dry the inner cannula. Using soft tissue to dry the cannula can cause particles of the tissue to gather on the cannula, leading to respiratory problems following insertion. Additionally, the items used for this procedure need to be sterile.

Test-Taking Strategy: Use the process of elimination and focus on the issue, reinserting the inner cannula. Eliminate option 1 first because you would not suction a client without an inner cannula in place. Eliminate option 2 next because a wet cannula should not be inserted. From the remaining options, eliminate option 4 because of the words "soft tissue." Review the procedure for tracheotomy care if you had difficulty with this question.

Level of Cognitive Ability: Application
Client Needs: Physiological Integrity
Integrated Process: Nursing Process/Implementation
Content Area: Fundamental Skills

References:
Lewis, S., Heitkemper, M., & Dirksen, S. (2004). *Medical-surgical nursing: Assessment and management of clinical problems* (6th ed.). St. Louis: Mosby, p. 579.
Phipps, W., Monahan, F., Sands, J., Marek, J., & Neighbors, M. (2003). *Medical-surgical nursing: Health and illness perspectives* (7th ed.). St. Louis: Mosby, p. 520.

112. A nurse suspects that an air embolism has occurred when the client's central venous catheter disconnects from the IV tubing. The nurse immediately turns the client to the:
1 Left side with the head higher than the feet
2 Right side with the head higher than the feet
3 Left side with the feet higher than the head
4 Right side with the feet higher than the head

Answer: 3
Rationale: If the client experiences air embolism, the immediate action is to place the client on the left side with the feet higher than the head. This position traps air in the right atrium. If necessary, the air can then be directly removed by intracardiac aspiration. Options 1, 2, and 4 are incorrect positions.

Test-Taking Strategy: Visualize each position in the options. Recalling that the goal of action is to trap air in the right atrium will direct you to option 3. Review immediate care of a client with an air embolism if you had difficulty with this question.

Level of Cognitive Ability: Application
Client Needs: Physiological Integrity
Integrated Process: Nursing Process/Implementation
Content Area: Fundamental Skills

Reference:
Black, J., & Hawks, J. (2005). *Medical-surgical nursing: Clinical management for positive outcomes* (7th ed.). Philadelphia: Saunders, p. 1833.

---

113. An anxious client enters the emergency room seeking treatment for a laceration of the finger that occurred when using a power tool. The client's vital signs are pulse 96 beats per minute, blood pressure (BP) 148/88 mmHg, and respirations 24 breaths per minute. After cleansing the injury and reassuring the client, the nurse rechecks the vital signs and notes a pulse of 82 beats per minute, BP 130/80 mmHg, and respirations 20 breaths per minute. The nurse determines that the change in vital signs is caused by:
1 Reduced stimulation of the sympathetic nervous system
2 The cooling effects of the cleansing solution
3 The body's physical adaptation to the air conditioning
4 Possible impending cardiovascular collapse

Answer: 1
Rationale: Physical or emotional stress triggers a sympathetic nervous system response. Responses that are reflected in the vital signs include an increased pulse, increased blood pressure, and increased respiratory rate. Stress reduction, then, returns these parameters to baseline. Options 2, 3, and 4 are unrelated to the changes in vital signs.

Test-Taking Strategy: Eliminate options 2 and 3 first because they are similar. Next note the information in the question, that the client is anxious and has an injury. These two pieces of information guide you to think about the body's response to stress. Recalling the relationship of stress to the sympathetic nervous system will direct you to option 1. Review the effects of physical stress on the vital signs if you had difficulty with this question.

Level of Cognitive Ability: Analysis
Client Needs: Physiological Integrity
Integrated Process: Nursing Process/Analysis
Content Area: Fundamental Skills

References:
Black, J., Hawks, J. & Keene, A. (2001). *Medical-surgical nursing: Clinical management for positive outcomes* (6th ed.). Philadelphia: Saunders, pp. 2252-2253.
Phipps, W., Monahan, F., Sands, J., Marek, J., & Neighbors, M. (2003). *Medical-surgical nursing: Health and illness perspectives* (7th ed.). St. Louis: Mosby, p. 465.

114. A nurse is scheduling multiple diagnostic procedures for the client with heart failure who experiences activity intolerance. The procedures ordered include an echocardiogram, chest X-ray, and a computed axial tomography (CAT) scan. The nurse schedules the procedure in which sequence to best meet the needs of this client?

1 Chest X-ray in the morning, echocardiogram in the afternoon, and the CAT scan in the morning of the following day

2 Chest X-ray and echocardiogram together in the morning, and the CAT scan in the afternoon of the same day

3 Echocardiogram in the morning, and the chest X-ray and CAT scan together in the afternoon of the same day

4 CAT scan in the morning, and the chest X-ray and echocardiogram on the following morning

Answer: 1

Rationale: Echocardiograms can be done at the bedside. Chest X-rays and CAT scans are done in the radiology department (unless a portable chest X-ray is ordered). The best sequence for this client would be to have the client go to a procedure in another department in the morning (when most rested); have a rest period; have another procedure on the unit in the afternoon (when more fatigued); and go off the nursing unit again the next morning (when rested again). A client who has activity intolerance will do best when activities are spaced.

Test-Taking Strategy: Focus on the issue: activity intolerance. Recalling that the client will do best if activities are spaced will direct you to option 1. Review interventions for the client with activity tolerance if you had difficulty with this question.

Level of Cognitive Ability: Application
Client Needs: Physiological Integrity
Integrated Process: Nursing Process/Planning
Content Area: Fundamental Skills

Reference:
Black, J., & Hawks, J. (2005). *Medical-surgical nursing: Clinical management for positive outcomes* (7th ed.). Philadelphia: Saunders, p. 1667.

115. A nurse is preparing to initiate an intravenous nitroglycerin drip on a client with acute myocardial infarction. In the absence of an invasive (arterial) monitoring line, the nurse prepares to have which piece of equipment for use at the bedside?

1 Defibrillator

2 Pulse oximeter

3 Central venous pressure (CVP) tray

4 Noninvasive blood pressure monitor

Answer: 4

Rationale: Nitroglycerin dilates both arteries and veins, causing peripheral blood pooling, thus reducing preload, afterload, and myocardial work. This action accounts for the primary side effect of nitroglycerin, which is hypotension. In the absence of an arterial monitoring line, the nurse should have a noninvasive blood pressure monitor for use at the bedside.

Test-Taking Strategy: Use the process of elimination, noting the key words "absence of an invasive (arterial) monitoring line." Recalling the purpose of this type of monitoring device and the action of nitroglycerin will direct you to option 4. Review nursing responsibilities when administering a nitroglycerin drip if you had difficulty with this question.

Level of Cognitive Ability: Application
Client Needs: Physiological Integrity
Integrated Process: Nursing Process/Planning
Content Area: Adult Health/Cardiovascular

Reference:
Phipps, W., Monahan, F., Sands, J., Marek, J., & Neighbors, M. (2003). *Medical-surgical nursing: Health and illness perspectives* (7th ed.). St. Louis: Mosby, p. 671.

116. A client in labor has a concurrent diagnosis of sickle cell anemia. Because the client is at high risk for sickling crisis, which action is the priority to assist in preventing a crisis from occurring during labor?
1 Reassure the client
2 Administer oxygen throughout labor
3 Maintain strict asepsis
4 Prevent bearing down

Answer: 2
Rationale: During the labor process, the client with sickle cell anemia is at high risk for being unable to meet the oxygen demands of labor. Administering oxygen will prevent sickle cell crisis during labor. Options 1 and 3 are appropriate actions but are unrelated to sickle cell crisis. Option 4 is inappropriate.

Test-Taking Strategy: Note the key word "priority." Focus on the client's diagnosis and use the ABCs—airway, breathing, and circulation—to direct you to option 2. Review care of the client with sickle cell anemia in labor if you had difficulty with this question.

Level of Cognitive Ability: Application
Client Needs: Physiological Integrity
Integrated Process: Nursing Process/Implementation
Content Area: Maternity/Intrapartum

Reference:
Lowdermilk, D., & Perry, A. (2004). *Maternity & women's health care* (8th ed.). St. Louis: Mosby, p. 921.

117. A client is scheduled for several diagnostic tests to rule out renal disease. As an essential preprocedure component of the nursing assessment, the nurse plans to ask the client about a history of:
1 Frequent antibiotic use
2 Long-term diuretic therapy
3 Allergy to shellfish or iodine
4 Familial renal disease

Answer: 3
Rationale: The client undergoing any type of diagnostic testing should be questioned about allergy to shellfish, seafood, or iodine. This is essential to identify the risk for potential allergic reaction to contrast dye, which may be used in some diagnostic tests. The other items are also useful as part of the assessment, but are not as critical as the allergy determination in the preprocedure period.

Test-Taking Strategy: Note the key words "essential" and "preprocedure component." Because the question indicates that diagnostic testing is planned, the items in the options are evaluated against their potential connection to this aspect of care. Recalling that contrast dye is used in many diagnostic tests will direct you to option 3. Review client assessment related to diagnostic testing if you had difficulty with this question.

Level of Cognitive Ability: Application
Client Needs: Physiological Integrity
Integrated Process: Nursing Process/Assessment
Content Area: Adult Health/Renal

Reference:
Phipps, W., Monahan, F., Sands, J., Marek, J., & Neighbors, M. (2003). *Medical-surgical nursing: Health and illness perspectives* (7th ed.). St. Louis: Mosby, p. 1198.

118. A nurse has an order to obtain a 24-hour urine collection on a client with a renal disorder. The nurse avoids which of the following to ensure proper collection of the 24-hour specimen?

1   Have the client void at the start time, and place this specimen in the container

2   Discard the first voiding, and save all subsequent voidings during the 24-hour time period

3   Place the container on ice, or in a refrigerator

4   Have the client void at the end time, and place this specimen in the container

Answer: 1

Rationale: The nurse asks the client to void at the beginning of the collection period and discards this urine sample. All subsequent voided urine is saved in a container, which is placed on ice or refrigerated. The client is asked to void at the finish time, and this sample is added to the collection. The container is labeled, placed on fresh ice, and sent to the laboratory immediately.

Test-Taking Strategy: Use the process of elimination and note the key word "avoids." This word indicates a false-response question and that you need to select the option that is an incorrect nursing action. Focusing on the issue, a 24-hour urine collection, will assist in eliminating options 2 and 3. From the remaining options, think about the procedure. Having the client void at the finish time makes sense, because this captures the urine that the bladder has stored between the last time of voiding and the finish time for the specimen. On the other hand, if you save the first specimen, you do not know how long that urine has been stored in the bladder. Therefore, you would not be getting a true "24-hour" collection. Review this procedure if you had difficulty with this question.

Level of Cognitive Ability: Application
Client Needs: Physiological Integrity
Integrated Process: Nursing Process/Implementation
Content Area: Fundamental Skills

Reference:
Phipps, W., Monahan, F., Sands, J., Marek, J., & Neighbors, M. (2003). *Medical-surgical nursing: Health and illness perspectives* (7th ed.). St. Louis: Mosby, p. 1196.

---

119. A nurse is caring for a client in active labor. The nurse performs which of the following to best prevent fetal heart rate decelerations?

1   Increases the rate of the oxytocin (Pitocin) infusion

2   Encourages upright or side-lying maternal positions

3   Monitors the fetal heart rate every 30 minutes

4   Prepares the client for a cesarean delivery

Answer: 2

Rationale: Side-lying and upright positions such as walking, standing, and squatting can improve venous return and encourage effective uterine activity. The nurse should discontinue an oxytocin infusion in the presence of fetal heart rate decelerations, thereby reducing uterine activity and increasing uteroplacental perfusion. Monitoring the fetal heart rate every 30 minutes will not prevent fetal heart rate decelerations. There are many nursing actions to prevent fetal heart rate decelerations, without necessitating surgical intervention.

Test-Taking Strategy: Use the process of elimination and focus on the issue: "best prevent fetal heart rate decelerations." Options 1, 3, and 4 will not "prevent" fetal heart rate decelerations. Side-lying and upright positions will improve venous return and encourage effective uterine activity. Review nursing interventions for the client in labor if you had difficulty with this question.

Level of Cognitive Ability: Application
Client Needs: Physiological Integrity
Integrated Process: Nursing Process/Implementation
Content Area: Maternity/Intrapartum

Reference:
Lowdermilk, D., & Perry, A. (2004). *Maternity & women's health care* (8th ed.). St. Louis: Mosby, p. 530.

120. A client with diabetes mellitus is at 36 weeks' gestation. The client has had weekly nonstress tests for the last 3 weeks, and the results have been reactive. This week, the nonstress test was nonreactive after 40 minutes. Based on these results, the nurse would anticipate the client will be prepared for:

1 Immediate induction of labor
2 Hospitalization with continuous fetal monitoring
3 A return appointment in 2 to 7 days to repeat the nonstress test
4 A contraction stress test

Answer: 4

Rationale: A nonreactive nonstress test needs further assessment. There is not enough data in the question to indicate that the procedures in options 1 and 2 are necessary at this time. To send the client home for 2 to 7 days may place the fetus in jeopardy. A contraction stress test is the next test needed to further assess the fetal status.

Test-Taking Strategy: Use the process of elimination, focusing on the issue: a change in test results from reactive to nonreactive. Options 1 and 2 can be eliminated first because they are unnecessary at this time. Option 3 can be eliminated next because repeating the test at a later time is not a safe intervention, especially considering the fact that previous test results were reactive. Review the meanings of the test results related to a nonstress test if you had difficulty with this question.

Level of Cognitive Ability: Analysis
Client Needs: Physiological Integrity
Integrated Process: Nursing Process/Planning
Content Area: Maternity/Antepartum

Reference:
Lowdermilk, D., & Perry, A. (2004). *Maternity & women's health care* (8th ed.). St. Louis: Mosby, pp. 830-831.

---

121. A nurse is administering magnesium sulfate to a client for severe preeclampsia. During the administration of the medication, the nurse:

1 Assesses for signs and symptoms of labor because the client's level of consciousness will be altered
2 Assesses the client's temperature every 2 hours because the client is at high risk for infection
3 Schedules a nonstress test every 4 hours to assess fetal well-being
4 Schedules a daily ultrasound to assess fetal movement

Answer: 1

Rationale: Because of the sedative effect of the magnesium sulfate, the client may not perceive labor. This client is not at high risk for infection. A nonstress test may be done, but not every 4 hours. Daily ultrasounds are not necessary for this client.

Test-Taking Strategy: Use the nursing process to answer the question. Assessment is the first step, therefore eliminate options 3 and 4. From the remaining options, knowledge that the client is not at high risk for infection will assist in directing you to option 1. Review nursing responsibilities when administering magnesium sulfate if you had difficulty with this question.

Level of Cognitive Ability: Application
Client Needs: Physiological Integrity
Integrated Process: Nursing Process/Implementation
Content Area: Maternity/Antepartum

Reference:
Lowdermilk, D., & Perry, A. (2004). *Maternity & women's health care* (8th ed.). St. Louis: Mosby, p. 853.

122. A client's nasogastric (NG) tube stops draining. The nurse should take which appropriate action?
1   Irrigate the tube
2   Clamp the tube
3   Pull the tube out approximately 2 inches
4   Replace the tube

Answer: 1
Rationale: If a client's nasogastric tube stops draining, the nurse would first check the functioning of the equipment. The nurse would ensure that there was an order for irrigating the tube and would then irrigate the tube with 30 to 60 mL of normal saline (or with another acceptable solution per agency procedure). There is no useful reason to clamp the tube because it is probably clogged. Pulling out the tube could displace the tube, placing the client at risk for aspiration. Replacement of the tube is the last step if other actions are unsuccessful.

Test-Taking Strategy: Focus on the issue: that the tube stops draining. The only action that will resolve this problem is option 1. Review care of the client with an NG tube if you had difficulty with this question.

Level of Cognitive Ability: Application
Client Needs: Physiological Integrity
Integrated Process: Nursing Process/Implementation
Content Area: Fundamental Skills

Reference:
Harkreader, H., & Hogan, M.A. (2004). *Fundamentals of nursing: caring and clinical judgment* (2nd ed.). Philadelphia: Saunders. p. 579.

123. A nurse is planning to give a tepid tub bath to a child who has hyperthermia. The nurse plans to:
1   Obtain isopropyl alcohol to add to the bath water
2   Warm the water to the same body temperature of the child
3   Have cool water available to add to the bath water
4   Allow 5 minutes for the child to soak in the bath water

Answer: 3
Rationale: Adding cool water to an already warm bath allows the water temperature to slowly drop. The child is able to gradually adjust to the changing water temperature and will not experience chilling. Alcohol is toxic and contraindicated for tepid sponge or tub baths. To achieve the best cooling results, the water temperature should be at least 2 degrees lower than the child's body temperature. The child should be in a tepid tub bath for 20 to 30 minutes to achieve maximum results.

Test-Taking Strategy: Use the process of elimination. Eliminate option 1, recalling that alcohol is toxic. Eliminate option 2 because water that is the same as body temperature will not reduce hyperthermia. Eliminate option 4 because of the 5-minute time frame. Review measures for hyperthermia and the procedure for giving a tepid bath to a child if you had difficulty with this question.

Level of Cognitive Ability: Application
Client Needs: Physiological Integrity
Integrated Process: Nursing Process/Planning
Content Area: Child Health

Reference:
Wong, D., & Hockenberry, M. (2003). *Wong's nursing care of infants and children* (7th ed.). St. Louis: Mosby, pp. 771;1130.

124. A nurse is assigned to care for a child who is one day postoperative following a surgical repair of a cleft lip. Which nursing intervention is appropriate when caring for this child's surgical incision?
1 Clean the incision only when serous exudate forms
2 Rub the incision gently with a sterile cotton-tipped swab
3 Rinse the incision with sterile water after feeding
4 Replace the Logan bar carefully after cleaning the incision

Answer: 3
Rationale: The incision should be rinsed with sterile water after every feeding. Rubbing alters the integrity of the suture line. Rather, the incision should be patted or dabbed. The purpose of the Logan bar is to maintain the integrity of the suture line. Removing the Logan bar on the first postoperative day would increase tension on the surgical incision.

Test-Taking Strategy: Use the process of elimination. Eliminate options 1 and 2 first because of the word "only" in option 1 and "rub" in option 2. Focus on the words "one day postoperative." This should assist in eliminating option 4. Review care of a child following surgical repair of a cleft lip if you had difficulty with this question.

Level of Cognitive Ability: Application
Client Needs: Physiological Integrity
Integrated Process: Nursing Process/Implementation
Content Area: Child Health

References:
Wong, D., & Hockenberry, M. (2003). *Wong's nursing care of infants and children* (7th ed.). St. Louis: Mosby, p. 461.
James, S., Ashwill, J., & Droske, S. (2002). *Nursing care of children: Principles & practice* (2nd ed.). Philadelphia: Saunders, p. 538.

125. A client is in ventricular tachycardia and the physician orders intravenous (IV) lidocaine (Xylocaine). The nurse plans to dilute the concentrated solution of lidocaine with:
1 5% dextrose in water
2 Lactated Ringer's
3 Normal saline 0.9%
4 Normal saline 0.45%

Answer: 1
Rationale: Lidocaine for IV administration is dispensed in concentrated and dilute formulations. The concentrated formulation must be diluted with 5% dextrose in water.

Test-Taking Strategy: Use the process of elimination. Eliminate options 3 and 4 first because they are similar solutions. From the remaining options, it is necessary to know that the concentrated formulation must be diluted with 5% dextrose in water. Review the procedure for administering this medication if you had difficulty with this question.

Level of Cognitive Ability: Application
Client Needs: Physiological Integrity
Integrated Process: Nursing Process/Implementation
Content Area: Adult Health/Cardiovascular

Reference:
Lehne, R. (2004). *Pharmacology for nursing care* (5th ed.). Philadelphia: Saunders, pp. 496-497.

126. A client receiving total parenteral nutrition (TPN) via a central venous intravenous (IV) line is scheduled to receive an antibiotic by the IV route. Which action by the nurse is appropriate before hanging the antibiotic solution?

1 Ensure a separate IV access for the antibiotic
2 Turn off the TPN for 30 minutes before administering the antibiotic
3 Check with the pharmacy regarding compatibility of the antibiotic and the TPN solution
4 Flush the central line with 60 mL of normal saline before hanging the antibiotic

Answer: 1

Rationale: The TPN line is used only for the administration of the TPN solution. Any other IV medication must be administered though a separate IV access site. Therefore, options 2, 3, and 4 are incorrect actions.

Test-Taking Strategy: Use the process of elimination. Eliminate options 2, 3, and 4 because they are similar in that they involve using the TPN line for the administration of the antibiotic. Review care of the client receiving TPN if you had difficulty with this question.

Level of Cognitive Ability: Application
Client Needs: Physiological Integrity
Integrated Process: Nursing Process/Implementation
Content Area: Fundamental Skills

Reference:
Phipps, W., Monahan, F., Sands, J., Marek, J., & Neighbors, M. (2003). *Medical-surgical nursing: Health and illness perspectives* (7th ed.). St. Louis: Mosby, p. 1059.

127. A nurse is inserting an indwelling urinary catheter into a male client. As the nurse inflates the balloon with a syringe, the client complains of discomfort. The nurse:

1 Removes the syringe from the balloon because discomfort is normal and temporary
2 Aspirates the fluid from the balloon, advances the catheter farther, then reinflates the balloon
3 Aspirates the fluid from the balloon, waits until the discomfort subsides, then reinflates the balloon
4 Aspirates the fluid from the balloon, removes the catheter, and reinserts a new catheter

Answer: 2

Rationale: If the balloon is positioned in the urethra, inflating the balloon could produce trauma, and pain will occur. If pain occurs, the fluid should be aspirated and the catheter inserted a little farther in order to provide sufficient space to inflate the balloon. The catheter's balloon is behind the opening at the catheter insertion tip. Inserting the catheter the extra distance will ensure that the balloon is inflated inside the bladder and not in the urethra. There is no need to remove the catheter and reinsert a new one. Pain when the balloon is inflated is not normal.

Test-Taking Strategy: Note the issue: client's complaint of discomfort on balloon inflation. Use the process of elimination and attempt to visualize the procedure to direct you to option 2. Review the complications associated with insertion of a urinary catheter if you had difficulty with this question.

Level of Cognitive Ability: Application
Client Needs: Physiological Integrity
Integrated Process: Nursing Process/Implementation
Content Area: Fundamental Skills

Reference:
Potter, P., & Perry, A. (2005). *Fundamentals of nursing* (6th ed.). St. Louis: Mosby, p. 1355.

128. A client with acquired immunodeficiency syndrome (AIDS) who has cytomegalovirus retinitis (CMV) is receiving ganciclovir sodium (Cytovene). The nurse implements which of the following in the care of this client?

1 Monitors blood glucose levels for elevation
2 Administers the medication on an empty stomach only
3 Tells the client to use a soft toothbrush and an electric razor
4 Applies pressure to venipuncture sites for 2 minutes

Answer: 3

Rationale: Ganciclovir causes neutropenia and thrombocytopenia as the most frequent side effects. For this reason, the nurse monitors the client for signs and symptoms of bleeding, and implements the same precautions that are used for a client receiving anticoagulant therapy. Thus, venipuncture sites should be held for approximately 10 minutes. The medication does not have to be taken on an empty stomach. The medication may cause hypoglycemia, but not hyperglycemia.

Test-Taking Strategy: Use the process of elimination. Recalling that this medication causes thrombocytopenia will direct you to option 3. Review the nursing considerations related to this medication if you had difficulty with this question.

Level of Cognitive Ability: Application
Client Needs: Physiological Integrity
Integrated Process: Nursing Process/Implementation
Content Area: Adult Health/Immune

Reference:
Hodgson, B., & Kizior, R. (2004). *Saunders nursing drug handbook 2004.* Philadelphia: Saunders, p. 457.

129. A client without history of respiratory disease has experienced sudden onset of chest pain and dyspnea, and is diagnosed with pulmonary embolus. The nurse immediately implements which expected orders prescribed for this client?

1 Semi-Fowler's position, oxygen, and the administration of morphine sulfate intravenously (IV)
2 Supine position, oxygen, and meperidine hydrochloride (Demerol) intramuscularly (IM)
3 High-Fowler's position, oxygen, and two tablets acetaminophen with codeine (Tylenol #3)
4 High-Fowler's position, oxygen, and morphine sulfate IV

Answer: 1

Rationale: Standard therapeutic intervention for the client with pulmonary embolus includes proper positioning, oxygen, and intravenous analgesics. The head of the bed is placed in semi-Fowler's position. High-Fowler's is avoided because extreme hip flexure slows venous return from the legs and increases the risk of new thrombi. The supine position will increase the dyspnea that occurs with pulmonary embolism. The usual analgesic of choice is morphine sulfate administered IV. This medication reduces pain, alleviates anxiety, and can diminish congestion of blood in the pulmonary vessels because it causes peripheral venous dilatation.

Test-Taking Strategy: Use the process of elimination. Eliminate option 2 first because a supine position will exacerbate the dyspnea. From the remaining options, recall that a high-Fowler's is avoided because extreme hip flexure slows venous return from the legs and increases the risk of new thrombi. This will assist in eliminating options 3 and 4. Review immediate care of the client with pulmonary embolus if you had difficulty with this question.

Level of Cognitive Ability: Application
Client Needs: Physiological Integrity
Integrated Process: Nursing Process/Implementation
Content Area: Adult Health/Respiratory

Reference:
Black, J., & Hawks, J. (2005). *Medical-surgical nursing: Clinical management for positive outcomes* (7th ed.). Philadelphia: Saunders, p. 1183.

130. A client who recently experienced myocardial infarction is scheduled to have a percutaneous transluminal coronary angioplasty (PTCA). The nurse plans to teach the client that during this procedure, a balloon-tipped catheter will:

1 Cut away the plaque from the coronary vessel wall using a cutting blade
2 Be used to compress the plaque against the coronary blood vessel wall
3 Inflate a mesh-like device that will spring open
4 Be positioned in a coronary artery to take pressure measurements in the vessel

Answer: 2

Rationale: In PTCA a balloon-tipped catheter is used to compress the plaque against the coronary blood vessel wall. Option 1 describes coronary atherectomy, option 3 describes placement of a coronary stent, and option 4 describes part of the process used in cardiac catheterization.

Test-Taking Strategy: Look at the name of the procedure. "Angioplasty" refers to repair of a blood vessel; this will assist in eliminating options 3 and 4. From the remaining options, recalling that a procedure that cuts something away would have the suffix "-ectomy" will assist in eliminating option 1. Review this procedure if you had difficulty with this question.

Level of Cognitive Ability: Application
Client Needs: Physiological Integrity
Integrated Process: Teaching/Learning
Content Area: Adult Health/Cardiovascular

Reference:
Lewis, S., Heitkemper, M., & Dirksen, S. (2004). *Medical-surgical nursing: Assessment and management of clinical problems* (6th ed.). St. Louis: Mosby, pp. 922-923.

---

131. A nurse is caring for a client who has been placed in Buck's extension traction. The nurse provides for countertraction to reduce shear and friction by:

1 Slightly elevating the head of the bed
2 Slightly elevating the foot of the bed
3 Providing an overhead trapeze
4 Using a footboard

Answer: 2

Rationale: The part of the bed under an area in traction is usually elevated to aid in countertraction. For the client in Buck's extension traction (which is applied to a leg), the foot of the bed is elevated. An overhead trapeze or footboard is not used to provide countertraction. Option 2 provides a force that opposes the traction force effectively without harming the client.

Test-Taking Strategy: Use the process of elimination. Eliminate option 1, recalling that Buck's extension traction is applied to the leg. From the remaining options, focus on the issue, providing countertraction, to eliminate options 3 and 4. Review Buck's extension traction if you had difficulty with this question.

Level of Cognitive Ability: Application
Client Needs: Physiological Integrity
Integrated Process: Nursing Process/Implementation
Content Area: Adult Health/Musculoskeletal

Reference:
Ignatavicius, D., & Workman, M. (2002). *Medical surgical nursing: Critical thinking for collaborative care* (4th ed.). Philadelphia: Saunders, p. 1136.

132. A nurse has inserted a nasogastric (NG) tube to the level of the oropharynx and has repositioned the client's head in a flexed-forward position. The client has been asked to begin swallowing, and as the nurse starts to slowly advance the NG tube with each swallow, the client begins to gag. Which nursing action would least likely result in proper tube insertion and promote client relaxation?

1 Continuing to advance the tube to the desired distance
2 Pulling the tube back slightly
3 Checking the back of the pharynx using a tongue blade and flashlight
4 Instructing the client to breathe slowly

Answer: 1

Rationale: As the NG tube is passed through the oropharynx, the gag reflex is stimulated, which may cause gagging. Instead of passing through to the esophagus, the NG tube may coil around itself in the oropharynx, or it may enter the larynx and obstruct the airway. Because the tube may enter the larynx, advancing the tube may position it in the trachea. Slow breathing helps the client relax to reduce the gag response. The tube may be advanced after the client relaxes.

Test-Taking Strategy: Note the key words "least likely." Focusing on these key words and noting that the client is gagging will direct you to option 1. Review this procedure if you had difficulty with this question.

Level of Cognitive Ability: Application
Client Needs: Physiological Integrity
Integrated Process: Nursing Process/Implementation
Content Area: Adult Health/Gastrointestinal

Reference:
Harkreader, H., & Hogan, M.A. (2004). *Fundamentals of nursing: caring and clinical judgment* (2nd ed.). Philadelphia: Saunders. p. 578.

133. A nurse is planning care for the client with heart failure. The nurse asks the dietary department to remove which item from all meal trays before delivering them to the client?

1 Salt packets
2 1% milk
3 Margarine
4 Decaffeinated tea

Answer: 1

Rationale: Sodium restriction reduces water retention and improves cardiac efficiency. A standard dietary modification for the client with heart failure is sodium restriction.

Test-Taking Strategy: Focusing on the client's diagnosis will assist in recalling the need for sodium restriction and direct you to option 1. Review care of the client with heart failure if you had difficulty with this question.

Level of Cognitive Ability: Application
Client Needs: Physiological Integrity
Integrated Process: Nursing Process/Implementation
Content Area: Adult Health/Cardiovascular

Reference:
Black, J., & Hawks, J. (2005). *Medical-surgical nursing: Clinical management for positive outcomes* (7th ed.). Philadelphia: Saunders, p. 1662.

134. A nurse is caring for an infant with spina bifida (meningomyelocele type) who had the gibbus (sac on the back containing cerebrospinal fluid, the meninges, and the spinal cord) surgically removed. The nurse plans which of the following in the postoperative period to maintain the infant's safety?

1 Elevating the head with the infant in the prone position
2 Covering the back dressing with a binder
3 Placing the infant in a head-down position
4 Strapping the infant in a baby seat sitting up

Answer: 1

Rationale: Elevating the head will decrease the chance of cerebrospinal fluid collecting in the cranial cavity. The infant needs to be prone for several days to decrease the pressure on the surgical site on the back. Binders and a baby seat should not be used because of the pressure they would exert on the surgical site.

Test-Taking Strategy: Use the process of elimination. Recall that preventing pressure on the surgical site and preventing intracranial cerebrospinal fluid collection are goals for the postoperative period. Options 2 and 4 would increase pressure on the surgical site, and option 3 would not promote drainage of cerebrospinal fluid from the cranial cavity. Review postoperative nursing care following this procedure if you had difficulty with this question.

Level of Cognitive Ability: Application
Client Needs: Physiological Integrity
Integrated Process: Nursing Process/Planning
Content Area: Child Health

Reference:
James, S., Ashwill, J., & Droske, S. (2002). *Nursing care of children: Principles & practice* (2nd ed.). Philadelphia: Saunders, p. 957.

135. A client is experiencing signs and symptoms of acute iron intoxication. The nurse checks the medication supply closet to ensure that which medication that is an antidote to the iron is available for use?

1 Deferoxamine (Desferal)
2 Dirithromycin (Dynabac)
3 Ferrous fumarate (Feostat)
4 Ferrous sulfate (Slow Fe)

Answer: 1

Rationale: The antidote to iron dextran is deferoxamine, which is a heavy metal antagonist. This medication chelates unbound iron in the circulation and forms a water-soluble complex that can be eliminated by the kidneys. Dirithromycin is a macrolide antiinfective. Ferrous sulfate and ferrous fumarate are forms of iron supplements.

Test-Taking Strategy: Eliminate options 3 and 4 first because they are similar and are both iron supplements. From the remaining options, it is necessary to know that the antidote to iron dextran is deferoxamine. Review this antidote if you had difficulty with this question.

Level of Cognitive Ability: Application
Client Needs: Physiological Integrity
Integrated Process: Nursing Process/Planning
Content Area: Pharmacology

References:
Hodgson, B., & Kizior, R. (2004). *Saunders nursing drug handbook 2004.* Philadelphia: Saunders, p. 1085.
McKenry, L., & Salerno, E. (2003). *Mosby's pharmacology in nursing* (21st ed.). St. Louis: Mosby, p. 1164.

136. A client with pulmonary edema is receiving oxygen via nasal cannula at 6 liters per minute. Arterial blood gas (ABG) results indicate: pH 7.29, Pco_2 49 mm Hg, pO_2 58 mm Hg, HcO_3^- 18 mEq/L. The nurse anticipates that the physician will order which of the following for respiratory support?

1 Lowering the oxygen to 4 liters per minute via nasal cannula
2 Keeping the oxygen at 6 liters per minute via nasal cannula
3 Adding a partial rebreather mask to the current order
4 Intubation and mechanical ventilation

Answer: 4

Rationale: If respiratory failure occurs, endotracheal intubation and mechanical ventilation are necessary. The client is exhibiting respiratory acidosis, metabolic acidosis, and hypoxemia. Lowering or keeping the oxygen at the same liter flow will not improve the client's condition. A partial rebreather mask will raise CO_2 levels even further.

Test-Taking Strategy: Use the process of elimination, noting the ABG values. Noting that the oxygen level is low will eliminate options 1 and 2. Knowing that the Pco_2 is high will eliminate option 3, because a partial rebreather mask will raise CO_2 levels even further. Review ABG values and the treatment for respiratory failure if you had difficulty with this question.

Level of Cognitive Ability: Analysis
Client Needs: Physiological Integrity
Integrated Process: Nursing Process/Analysis
Content Area: Adult Health/Respiratory

Reference:
Black, J., & Hawks, J. (2005). *Medical-surgical nursing: Clinical management for positive outcomes* (7th ed.). Philadelphia: Saunders, p. 1879.

137. A client with an arteriovenous (AV) shunt in place for hemodialysis is at risk for bleeding. The nurse does which of the following as a priority action to prevent this complication?

1 Monitors the results of partial thromboplastin time (PTT) tests as they are ordered
2 Checks the shunt once per shift
3 Assesses the shunt for the presence of a bruit and thrill
4 Ensures that small clamps are attached to the AV shunt dressing

Answer: 4

Rationale: An AV shunt is a less common form of access site, but carries a risk for bleeding when it is used. This is because two ends of a cannula are tunneled subcutaneously into an artery and a vein, and the ends of the cannula are joined. If accidental disconnection occurs, the client could lose blood rapidly. For this reason, small clamps are attached to the dressing that covers the insertion site for use if needed. The shunt should be checked at least every 4 hours. Checking the results of the PTT does not prevent bleeding. Checking for the presence of a bruit and thrill assesses the patency.

Test-Taking Strategy: Use the process of elimination, focusing on the issue: preventing bleeding. The only option that relates to this issue is option 4. Review care of the client with an AV shunt if you had difficulty with this question.

Level of Cognitive Ability: Application
Client Needs: Physiological Integrity
Integrated Process: Nursing Process/Implementation
Content Area: Adult Health/Renal

Reference:
Ignatavicius, D., & Workman, M. (2002). *Medical surgical nursing: Critical thinking for collaborative care* (4th ed.). Philadelphia: Saunders, p. 1692.

138. A client is due in hydrotherapy for a burn dressing change. To ensure that the procedure is most tolerable for the client, the nurse takes which of the following actions?
1 Sends dressing supplies with the client to hydrotherapy
2 Ensures that the client has a robe and slippers
3 Administers an analgesic 20 minutes before therapy
4 Administers the intravenous antibiotic 30 minutes before therapy

Answer: 3
Rationale: The client should receive pain medication approximately 20 minutes before a burn dressing change. This will help the client tolerate an otherwise painful procedure. Antibiotics are timed evenly around the clock and not necessarily in relation to timing of burn dressing changes. Dressing supplies are generally available in the hydrotherapy area and do not need to be sent with the client. A robe and slippers are beneficial for the client's comfort if traveling by wheelchair, but pain medication is more essential.

Test-Taking Strategy: Use Maslow's hierarchy of needs theory and focus on the key words "most tolerable." This will direct you to option 3. Review care of the burn client if you had difficulty with this question.

Level of Cognitive Ability: Application
Client Needs: Physiological Integrity
Integrated Process: Nursing Process/Implementation
Content Area: Adult Health/Integumentary

Reference:
Black, J., & Hawks, J. (2005). *Medical-surgical nursing: Clinical management for positive outcomes* (7th ed.). Philadelphia: Saunders, p. 1451.

---

139. A nurse caring for a client with heart failure receives a telephone call from the laboratory and is told that the client has a magnesium level of 1.4 mg/dL. The nurse plans to:
1 Encourage increased intake of phosphate antacids
2 Monitor the client for dysrhythmias
3 Instruct the client to avoid foods that contain magnesium
4 Encourage intake of foods such as ground beef, eggs, or chicken breast

Answer: 2
Rationale: The normal magnesium ranges from 1.8 to 3.0 mg/dL. Phosphate use should be limited in the presence of hypomagnesemia because it worsens the condition. The client should be monitored for dysrhythmias, because the client is at risk for ventricular dysrhythmias. Ground beef, eggs, and chicken breast are examples of foods that are low in magnesium. The client would be advised to consume foods high in magnesium.

Test-Taking Strategy: Recalling the normal magnesium level and noting that the client is experiencing hypomagnesemia will direct you to option 2. Also, use of the ABCs—airway, breathing, and circulation—will direct you to the correct option. Review this electrolyte disorder and its treatment if you had difficulty with this question.

Level of Cognitive Ability: Application
Client Needs: Physiological Integrity
Integrated Process: Nursing Process/Planning
Content Area: Fundamental Skills

References:
Black, J., & Hawks, J. (2005). *Medical-surgical nursing: Clinical management for positive outcomes* (7th ed.). Philadelphia: Saunders, p. 1582.
Chernecky, C., & Berger, B. (2004). *Laboratory tests and diagnostic procedures* (4th ed.). Philadelphia: Saunders, p. 752.

140. A nurse is preparing to care for a client following parathyroidectomy. The nurse plans care anticipating which postoperative order?
  1 Place in a flat position with the head and neck immobilized
  2 Take a rectal temperature only until discharge
  3 Maintain endotracheal tube for 36 hours
  4 Ensure that intravenous calcium preparations are available

Answer: 4
Rationale: Hypocalcemia is a potentially life-threatening complication following parathyroidectomy, and the nurse should ensure that intravenous calcium preparations are readily available. Semi-Fowler's position is the position of choice to assist in lung expansion and prevent edema. Rectal temperatures are not required. Tympanic temperatures can be taken. The client will not necessarily have an endotracheal tube.

Test-Taking Strategy: Eliminate option 2 first because of the absolute word "only." Next, focusing on the anatomical location of the surgical procedure will assist in eliminating option 1. From the remaining options, recalling that the client will not necessarily have an endotracheal tube and noting the words "36 hours" in option 3 will assist in eliminating this option. Review care of the client following parathyroidectomy if you had difficulty with this question.

Level of Cognitive Ability: Application
Client Needs: Physiological Integrity
Integrated Process: Nursing Process/Planning
Content Area: Adult Health/Endocrine

References:
Black, J., & Hawks, J. (2005). *Medical-surgical nursing: Clinical management for positive outcomes* (7th ed.). Philadelphia: Saunders, p. 1212.
Phipps, W., Monahan, F., Sands, J., Marek, J., & Neighbors, M. (2003). *Medical-surgical nursing: Health and illness perspectives* (7th ed.). St. Louis: Mosby, p. 911.

141. A client with a wound infection and osteomyelitis is to receive hyperbaric oxygen therapy. During the therapy, the nurse implements which priority intervention?
  1 Ensures that oxygen is being delivered
  2 Maintains an intravenous access
  3 Administers sedation to prevent claustrophobia
  4 Provides emotional support to the client's family

Answer: 1
Rationale: Hyperbaric oxygen therapy is a process by which oxygen is administered at greater than atmospheric pressure. When oxygen is inhaled under pressure, the level of tissue oxygen is greatly increased. The high levels of oxygen promote the action of phagocytes and promote healing of the wound. Because the client is placed in a closed chamber, the administration of oxygen is of primary importance. Although options 2, 3, and 4 may be appropriate interventions, option 1 is the priority.

Test-Taking Strategy: Note the key word "priority." Use the ABCs—airway, breathing, and circulation—to direct you to option 1. Review nursing care related to this therapy if you had difficulty with this question.

Level of Cognitive Ability: Application
Client Needs: Physiological Integrity
Integrated Process: Nursing Process/Implementation
Content Area: Delegating/Prioritizing

References:
Black, J., & Hawks, J. (2005). *Medical-surgical nursing: Clinical management for positive outcomes* (7th ed.). Philadelphia: Saunders, p. 414.
Lewis, S., Heitkemper, M., & Dirksen, S. (2004). *Medical-surgical nursing: Assessment and management of clinical problems* (6th ed.). St. Louis: Mosby, p. 222.

142. A nurse is caring for a client with a herniated lumbar intervertebral disc. The nurse plans to place the client in which position to minimize the pain?
1 High-Fowler's position with the foot of the bed flat
2 Semi-Fowler's position with the knees slightly raised
3 Semi-Fowler's position with the foot of the bed flat
4 Flat with the knees raised

Answer: 2
Rationale: Clients with low back pain are often more comfortable when placed in semi-Fowler's position with the knees raised sufficiently to flex the knees. This relaxes the muscles of the lower back and relieves pressure on the spinal nerve root. Keeping the foot of the bed flat will enhance extension of the spine. Keeping the bed flat with the knees raised would excessively stretch the lower back and would also put the client at risk for thrombophlebitis.

Test-Taking Strategy: Use the process of elimination. Focus on the client's diagnosis and the issue: the position that will minimize pain. Visualize each of the positions, noting that option 2 places the least amount of pressure on the spine. Review care of the client with a herniated lumbar intervertebral disc if you had difficulty with this question.

Level of Cognitive Ability: Application
Client Needs: Physiological Integrity
Integrated Process: Nursing Process/Planning
Content Area: Adult Health/Neurological

Reference:
Lewis, S., Heitkemper, M., & Dirksen, S. (2004). *Medical-surgical nursing: Assessment and management of clinical problems* (6th ed.). St. Louis: Mosby, p. 1700.

143. A mother arrives at the emergency room with her child, stating that she just found the child sitting on the floor next to an empty bottle of aspirin. On assessment, the nurse notes that the child is drowsy but conscious. The nurse anticipates that the physician will prescribe which of the following?
1 Ipecac syrup
2 Activated charcoal
3 Magnesium citrate
4 Magnesium sulfate

Answer: 1
Rationale: Ipecac is administered to induce vomiting in certain poisoning situations. In this situation, the child is conscious and the ingested substance (aspirin) will not damage the esophagus or lungs from vomiting. Activated charcoal may be prescribed as an antidote in some poisoning situations, but its action is to absorb ingested toxic substances. Options 3 and 4 are unrelated to treatment for this occurrence.

Test-Taking Strategy: Use the process of elimination. Eliminate options 3 and 4 first because they are unrelated to the issue of poisoning. From the remaining options, note that the child is conscious. Also, think about the effect that the specific poison may have on the esophagus if vomited. Noting that the question states that the child was "just" found, and considering that aspirin will not harm the esophagus will direct you to option 1. Review measures to treat aspirin poisoning if you had difficulty with this question.

Level of Cognitive Ability: Application
Client Needs: Physiological Integrity
Integrated Process: Nursing Process/Planning
Content Area: Child Health

Reference:
Wong, D., & Hockenberry, M. (2003). *Wong's nursing care of infants and children* (7th ed.). St. Louis: Mosby, pp. 622; 671; 673.

144. A client with myasthenia gravis is admitted to the hospital, and the nursing history reveals that the client is taking pyridostigmine (Mestinon). The nurse assesses the client for side effects of the medication and asks the client about the presence of:
1 Muscle cramps
2 Mouth ulcers
3 Feelings of depression
4 Unexplained weight gain

Answer: 1
Rationale: Mestinon is an acetylcholinesterase inhibitor. Muscle cramps and small muscle contractions are side effects and occur as a result of overstimulation of neuromuscular receptors. Options 2, 3, and 4 are not associated with this medication.

Test-Taking Strategy: Recall that myasthenia gravis is a neuromuscular disorder. Select the option that is most closely associated with this disorder. This will direct you to option 1. Review the side effects associated with this medication if you had difficulty with this question.

Level of Cognitive Ability: Application
Client Needs: Physiological Integrity
Integrated Process: Nursing Process/Assessment
Content Area: Pharmacology

Reference:
Hodgson, B., & Kizior, R. (2004). *Saunders nursing drug handbook 2004.* Philadelphia: Saunders, p. 858.

145. A client with a fractured right ankle has a short leg plaster cast applied in the emergency department. During discharge teaching, the nurse provides which information to the client to prevent complications?
1 Keep the right ankle elevated above the heart level with pillows for 24 hours
2 Weight-bearing on the right leg is allowed once the cast feels dry
3 Expect burning and tingling sensations under the cast for 3 to 4 days
4 Trim the rough edges of the cast after it is dry

Answer: 1
Rationale: Leg elevation is important to increase venous return and decrease edema, which can cause compartment syndrome, a major complication of fractures and casting. Weight-bearing on a fractured extremity is prescribed by the physician during follow-up examination, after an X-ray is taken. Additionally, a walking heel or cast shoe may be added to the cast if the client is allowed to bear weight and walk on the affected leg. Although the client may feel heat after the cast is applied, burning and/or tingling sensations indicate nerve damage or ischemia and are not expected. These complaints should be reported immediately. Option 4 is incorrect. The client and/or family may be taught how to "petal" the cast to prevent skin irritation and breakdown, but rough edges, if trimmed, can fall into the cast and cause a break in skin integrity.

Test-Taking Strategy: Focus on the issue: to prevent complications. Use the process of elimination and the ABCs—airway, breathing and circulation. Option 1 is associated with maintenance of circulation. Review client teaching points related to cast care if you had difficulty with this question.

Level of Cognitive Ability: Application
Client Needs: Physiological Integrity
Integrated Process: Teaching/Learning
Content Area: Adult Health/Musculoskeletal

Reference:
Lewis, S., Heitkemper, M., & Dirksen, S. (2004). *Medical-surgical nursing: Assessment and management of clinical problems* (6th ed.). St. Louis: Mosby, p. 1663.

146. An older adult female client with a fractured left tibia has a long leg cast and is using crutches to ambulate. In caring for the client, the nurse assesses for which sign or symptom that indicates a complication associated with crutch walking?
1 Forearm muscle weakness
2 Left leg discomfort
3 Tricep muscle spasms
4 Weak biceps brachii

Answer: 1
Rationale: Forearm muscle weakness is a sign of radial nerve injury caused by crutch pressure on the axillae. When a client lacks upper body strength, especially in the flexor and extensor muscles of the arms, he or she frequently allows weight to rest on the axillae and on the crutch pads instead of using the arms for support while ambulating with crutches. Leg discomfort is expected as a result of the injury. Tricep muscle spasms may occur as a result of increased muscle use, but is not a complication of crutch walking. Weak biceps brachii is a common physical assessment finding in older adults and is not a complication of crutch walking.

Test-Taking Strategy: Focus on the issue: a complication of crutch walking. When asked about a complication of the use of crutches, think about nerve injury caused by crutch pressure on the axillae. This will direct you to option 1. Review this complication if you had difficulty with this question.

Level of Cognitive Ability: Analysis
Client Needs: Physiological Integrity
Integrated Process: Nursing Process/Assessment
Content Area: Adult Health/Musculoskeletal

Reference:
Potter, P., & Perry, A. (2005). *Fundamentals of nursing* (6th ed.). St. Louis: Mosby, p. 949.

147. A client with myasthenia gravis is experiencing prolonged periods of weakness, and the physician orders an edrophonium (Tensilon) test. A test dose is administered and the client becomes weaker. The nurse interprets this test result as:
1 Normal
2 Positive
3 Myasthenia crisis
4 Cholinergic crisis

Answer: 4
Rationale: A Tensilon test may be performed to determine whether increasing weakness in a previously diagnosed myasthenic client is a result of cholinergic crisis (overmedication with anticholinesterase drugs) or myasthenic crisis (under medication with cholinesterase inhibitors). Worsening of the symptoms after the test dose of medication is administered indicates a cholinergic crisis.

Test-Taking Strategy: Focus on the issue: the client becomes weaker after edrophonium is administered. Recalling that edrophonium is a short-acting anticholinesterase and that the treatment for myasthenia gravis includes administration of an anticholinesterase will assist in answering the question. If the client's symptoms worsen after administration of edrophonium, then the client is likely experiencing overmedication. Review this test and the interpretation of results if you had difficulty with this question.

Level of Cognitive Ability: Analysis
Client Needs: Physiological Integrity
Integrated Process: Nursing Process/Analysis
Content Area: Adult Health/Neurological

Reference:
Lewis, S., Heitkemper, M., & Dirksen, S. (2004). *Medical-surgical nursing: Assessment and management of clinical problems* (6th ed.). St. Louis: Mosby, p. 1575.

148. A nurse notes an isolated premature ventricular contraction (PVC) on the cardiac monitor. The appropriate nursing action is to:
1 Continue to monitor the rhythm
2 Notify the physician immediately
3 Prepare for defibrillation
4 Prepare to administer lidocaine hydrochloride (LidoPen)

Answer: 1

Rationale: As an isolated occurrence, the PVC is not life-threatening. In this situation, the nurse should continue to monitor the client. Frequent PVCs, however, may be precursors of more life-threatening rhythms, such as ventricular tachycardia and ventricular fibrillation. If this occurred, the physician needs to be notified.

Test-Taking Strategy: Focus on the information in the question and note the key word "isolated." This should direct you to the option that addresses continued monitoring. Also, use of the ABCs—airway, breathing, and circulation—will direct you to option 1. Review the implications of PVCs and the associated interventions if you had difficulty with this question.

Level of Cognitive Ability: Application
Client Needs: Physiological Integrity
Integrated Process: Nursing Process/Implementation
Content Area: Adult Health/Cardiovascular

Reference:
Black, J., & Hawks, J. (2005). *Medical-surgical nursing: Clinical management for positive outcomes* (7th ed.). Philadelphia: Saunders, pp. 1682-1683.

149. A nurse is caring for a client admitted to the hospital with the diagnosis of active tuberculosis. This nurse determines that the diagnosis was confirmed by a:
1 Mantoux test
2 Sputum culture
3 Tine test
4 Chest x-ray

Answer: 2

Rationale: A sputum culture showing *Mycobacterium tuberculosis* confirms the diagnosis of tuberculosis. Usually three sputum samples are obtained for the acid-fast smear. After the initiation of medication therapy, sputum samples are obtained again to determine the effectiveness of therapy. A positive Tine or Mantoux test indicates exposure to tuberculosis but does not confirm the presence of *Mycobacterium tuberculosis*. A positive chest X-ray may indicate the presence of tuberculosis lesions, but again does not confirm active disease.

Test-Taking Strategy: Note the key words "active" and "confirmed" in the stem of the question. Active tuberculosis can only be confirmed by the presence of the bacilli. The sputum culture is the only method of determining the presence of this organism. Review tests associated with diagnosing tuberculosis if you had difficulty with this question.

Level of Cognitive Ability: Analysis
Client Needs: Physiological Integrity
Integrated Process: Nursing Process/Assessment
Content Area: Adult Health/Respiratory

Reference:
Lewis, S., Heitkemper, M., & Dirksen, S. (2004). *Medical-surgical nursing: Assessment and management of clinical problems* (6th ed.). St. Louis: Mosby, p. 603.

150. A clinic nurse prepares to assess the fundal height in a client in the second trimester of pregnancy. When measuring the fundal height, the nurse will most likely expect the measurement to:

1 Correlate with gestational age
2 Be greater than gestational age
3 Be lesser than gestational age
4 Have no correlation to gestational age

Answer: 1

Rationale: Up until the third trimester, the measurement of fundal height will, on average, correlate with the gestational age. Options 2, 3, and 4 are incorrect.

Test-Taking Strategy: Note the key words "most likely." Focus on the issue: second trimester and fundal height. Recall the correlation of fundal height and gestational age to direct you to option 1. Review this prenatal assessment if you had difficulty with this question.

Level of Cognitive Ability: Analysis
Client Needs: Physiological Integrity
Integrated Process: Nursing Process/Assessment
Content Area: Maternity/Antepartum

References:
Lowdermilk, D., & Perry, A. (2004). *Maternity & women's health care* (8th ed.). St. Louis: Mosby, pp. 416-417.
Murray, S., McKinney, E., & Gorrie, T. (2002). *Foundations of maternal-newborn nursing* (3rd ed.). Philadelphia: Saunders, p. 533.

151. A pregnant client tells a nurse that she felt wetness on her peri-pad and that she found some clear fluid. The nurse immediately inspects the perineum and notes the presence of the umbilical cord. The nurse's initial action is to:

1 Notify the physician
2 Monitor the fetal heart rate
3 Transfer the client to the delivery room
4 Place the client in Trendelenburg's position

Answer: 4

Rationale: On inspection of the perineum, if the umbilical cord is noted, the nurse immediately places the client into Trendelenburg's position while pushing the presenting part upward to relieve the cord compression. This position is maintained and the physician is notified. The nurse monitors the fetal heart rate. The client is transferred to the delivery room when prescribed by the physician.

Test-Taking Strategy: Note the key words "presence of umbilical cord," which indicates the need for an immediate action on the nurse's part to prevent or relieve cord compression. The only action that will achieve this is option 4. The physician is notified after positioning the client. Review nursing actions for this complication if you had difficulty with this question.

Level of Cognitive Ability: Application
Client Needs: Physiological Integrity
Integrated Process: Nursing Process/Implementation
Content Area: Maternity/Intrapartum

Reference:
Lowdermilk, D., & Perry, A. (2004). *Maternity & women's health care* (8th ed.). St. Louis: Mosby, p. 1028.

152. A nurse admits a newborn infant to the nursery. On assessment of the infant, the nurse palpates the anterior fontanel and notes that it feels soft. The nurse determines that this finding indicates:

1   Increased intracranial pressure
2   Dehydration
3   Decreased intracranial pressure
4   A normal finding

Answer: 4

Rationale: The anterior fontanel is normally 2 to 3 cm in width, 3 to 4 cm in length, and diamond-like in shape. It can be described as soft, which is normal, or full and bulging, which could indicate increased intracranial pressure. Conversely, a depressed fontanel could mean that the infant is dehydrated.

Test-Taking Strategy: Use the process of elimination. Focusing on the key word "soft" will direct you to option 4. Review the normal findings related to the fontanels if you had difficulty with this question.

Level of Cognitive Ability: Analysis
Client Needs: Physiological Integrity
Integrated Process: Nursing Process/Assessment
Content Area: Maternity/Postpartum

Reference:
Lowdermilk, D., & Perry, A. (2004). *Maternity & women's health care* (8th ed.). St. Louis: Mosby, pp. 468; 718.

153. A client with acquired immunodeficiency syndrome (AIDS) is admitted to the hospital for chills, fever, nonproductive cough, and pleuritic chest pain. A diagnosis of pneumocystis carinii pneumonia is made and the client is started on intravenous (IV) pentamidine (Pentam-300). The nurse plans to infuse the medication over:

1   1 hour with the client in a supine position
2   30 minutes with the client in a reclining position
3   1 hour and the client may be ambulatory
4   15 minutes with the client in a supine position

Answer: 1

Rationale: Intravenous pentamidine is infused over 1 hour with the client supine to minimize severe hypotension and dysrhythmias. Options 2, 3, and 4 are inaccurate in either the length of time that pentamidine is administered or the client's position.

Test-Taking Strategy: Use the process of elimination. Eliminate option 4 first because this time frame is very short for an IV medication. From the remaining options, recalling that the medication causes hypotension will direct you to option 1, which addresses both the supine position and the longest time of administration. Review this medication if you had difficulty with this question.

Level of Cognitive Ability: Application
Client Needs: Physiological Integrity
Integrated Process: Nursing Process/Planning
Content Area: Adult Health/Immune

Reference:
Hodgson, B., & Kizior, R. (2004). *Saunders nursing drug handbook 2004.* Philadelphia: Saunders, p. 793.

154. A nurse is caring for a client who has been transferred to the surgical unit after having a pelvic exenteration. During the postoperative period, if the client complains of pain in the calf area, the nurse would:
1 Administer prn meperidine hydrochloride (Demerol) as prescribed for postoperative pain
2 Check the calf area for temperature, color, and size
3 Lightly massage the calf area to relieve the pain
4 Ask the client to walk and observe the gait

Answer: 2
Rationale: The nurse monitors for postoperative complications such as deep vein thrombosis, pulmonary emboli, and wound infection. Pain in the calf area could indicate a deep vein thrombosis. Change in color, temperature, or size of the client's calf could also indicate this complication. Options 3 and 4 could result in an embolus if in fact the client had a deep vein thrombosis. Administering pain medication for this client complaint is not the appropriate nursing action. Further assessment needs to be obtained.

Test-Taking Strategy: Focus on the information in the question and use the steps of the nursing process. Assessment is the first step. Option 2 is the only option that addresses assessment. Review postoperative complications and appropriate interventions if you had difficulty with this question.

Level of Cognitive Ability: Application
Client Needs: Physiological Integrity
Integrated Process: Nursing Process/Implementation
Content Area: Adult Health/Cardiovascular

Reference:
Ignatavicius, D., & Workman, M. (2002). *Medical surgical nursing: Critical thinking for collaborative care* (4th ed.). Philadelphia: Saunders, p. 1775.

155. A nurse is preparing to assess the respirations of a newborn infant just admitted to the newborn nursery. The nurse performs the procedure and determines that the respiratory rate is normal if which of the following are noted?
1 A respiratory rate of 20 breaths per minute
2 A respiratory rate of 40 breaths per minute
3 A respiratory rate of 90 breaths per minute
4 A respiratory rate of 100 breaths per minute

Answer: 2
Rationale: Normal respiratory rate varies from 30 to 80 breaths per minute when the infant is not crying. Respirations should be counted for 1 full minute to ensure an accurate measurement because the newborn infant may be a periodic breather. Observing and palpating respirations while the infant is quiet promotes accurate assessment. Palpation aids observation in determining the respiratory rate. Option 1 indicates bradypnea and options 3 and 4 indicate tachypnea.

Test-Taking Strategy: Use the process of elimination and knowledge regarding the normal respiratory rate for a newborn infant to answer this question. If you are unfamiliar with this normal finding, review this content.

Level of Cognitive Ability: Analysis
Client Needs: Physiological Integrity
Integrated Process: Nursing Process/Assessment
Content Area: Maternity/Postpartum

Reference:
Lowdermilk, D., & Perry, A. (2004). *Maternity & women's health care* (8th ed.). St. Louis: Mosby, p. 713.

156. A client is in her second trimester of pregnancy. During her routine prenatal visit, she states that she frequently has calf pain when she walks. The nurse checks for which sign to assist in identifying the origin of the discomfort?
1 Chadwick's sign
2 Brudzinski's sign
3 Homans' sign
4 Kernig's sign

Answer: 3

Rationale: Homans' sign tests for venous thrombosis of the lower extremity. Pain in the calf during walking could indicate venous thrombosis. Chadwick's sign is a cervical change and is a probable sign of pregnancy. Brudzinski's sign and Kernig's sign test for meningeal irritability.

Test-Taking Strategy: Use the process of elimination. Eliminate options 2 and 4 first because they both test for meningeal irritation. From the remaining options, focus on the key words "frequently has calf pain when she walks" to assist in directing you to option 3. Review the signs identified in the options if you had difficulty with this question.

Level of Cognitive Ability: Analysis
Client Needs: Physiological Integrity
Integrated Process: Nursing Process/Assessment
Content Area: Maternity/Antepartum

Reference:
Lowdermilk, D., & Perry, A. (2004). *Maternity & women's health care* (8th ed.). St. Louis: Mosby, p. 633.

---

157. A nurse is evaluating the patency of a peripheral intravenous (IV) site and suspects an infiltration. The nurse does which of the following to determine if the IV has infiltrated?
1 Gently palpates the surrounding tissue for edema and coolness
2 Strips the tubing quickly while assessing for a rapid blood return
3 Increases the IV flow rate and observes the site for immediate tightening of tissue
4 Checks the area around the IV site for discomfort, redness, and warmth

Answer: 1

Rationale: When assessing an IV for signs and symptoms of infiltration, it is important to assess the site for edema and coolness, signifying leakage of the IV fluid into the surrounding tissues. Stripping the tubing will not cause a blood return but will force IV fluid into the vein or surrounding tissues, which could cause more tissue damage. Increasing the IV flow rate can further damage the tissues if the IV has infiltrated. The IV site will feel cool if the IV fluid has infiltrated into the surrounding tissues. Redness and warmth may indicate phlebitis.

Test-Taking Strategy: Use the process of elimination, focusing on the issue: infiltration. Recalling that the site will feel cool will direct you to option 1. Review the signs of infiltration if you had difficulty with this question.

Level of Cognitive Ability: Application
Client Needs: Physiological Integrity
Integrated Process: Nursing Process/Implementation
Content Area: Fundamental Skills

Reference:
Potter, P., & Perry, A. (2005). *Fundamentals of nursing* (6th ed.). St. Louis: Mosby, p. 1189.

158. An unresponsive and pulseless client is brought into the emergency room after being in a car accident, and a neck injury is suspected. The nurse opens the client's airway by which method?
1 Head tilt/chin lift
2 Lift the head up and place the head on two pillows and attempt to ventilate
3 Jaw-thrust maneuver
4 Keeping the client flat and grasping the tongue

Answer: 3
Rationale: In suspected neck injuries, the appropriate way to open the airway is the jaw-thrust maneuver. If a neck injury is present, this maneuver will prevent further injury. Options 1, 2, and 4 are incorrect.

Test-Taking Strategy: Note the key words "neck injury is suspected." Recalling the principles related to airway management will assist in eliminating options 2 and 4. From the remaining options, visualize each and eliminate option 1 because this method would cause further damage to a neck injury. Review basic life support measures if you had difficulty with this question.

Level of Cognitive Ability: Application
Client Needs: Physiological Integrity
Integrated Process: Nursing Process/Implementation
Content Area: Fundamental Skills

Reference:
Harkreader, H., & Hogan, M.A. (2004). *Fundamentals of nursing: caring and clinical judgment* (2nd ed.). Philadelphia: Saunders. p. 909.

---

159. A nurse is caring for a child with Reye's syndrome. The nurse monitors for signs of which major problem associated with this syndrome?
1 Increased intracranial pressure
2 Protein in the urine
3 A history of a staphylococcus infection
4 Symptoms of hyperglycemia

Answer: 1
Rationale: Intracranial pressure and encephalopathy are major problems associated with Reye's syndrome. Protein is not present in the urine. Reye's syndrome is related to a history of viral infections, and hypoglycemia is a symptom of this disease.

Test-Taking Strategy: Use the process of elimination and note the key words, "major problem." This will assist in directing you to option 1. Review the manifestations and problems associated with Reye's syndrome if you had difficulty with this question.

Level of Cognitive Ability: Application
Client Needs: Physiological Integrity
Integrated Process: Nursing Process/Assessment
Content Area: Child Health

Reference:
Wong, D., & Hockenberry, M. (2003). *Wong's nursing care of infants and children* (7th ed.). St. Louis: Mosby, p. 1683.

---

160. A child is admitted to the hospital with a suspected diagnosis of pneumococcus pneumonia. The nurse prepares to implement which of the following?
1 Have a chest X-ray done to determine how much consolidation there is in the lungs
2 Allow the child to go to the playroom to play with other children
3 Monitor the child's respiratory rate and breath sounds
4 Start antibiotic therapy immediately

Answer: 3
Rationale: A complication of pneumococcus pneumonia is pleural effusion, so the respiratory status of the child needs to be monitored. Antibiotic therapy is not started until cultures are obtained. The child should not be allowed in the playroom at this time. A chest X-ray needs to be prescribed by the physician.

Test-Taking Strategy: Use the steps of the nursing process. Option 3 addresses assessment. This option also addresses the ABCs—airway, breathing, and circulation. It is also the option that is directly related to the child's diagnosis. Review care of the child with pneumonia if you had difficulty with this question.

Level of Cognitive Ability: Application
Client Needs: Physiological Integrity
Integrated Process: Nursing Process/Implementation
Content Area: Child Health

Reference:
Wong, D., & Hockenberry, M. (2003). *Wong's nursing care of infants and children* (7th ed.). St. Louis: Mosby, p. 1370.

---

161. A nurse admits a client to the hospital with a suspected diagnosis of bulimia nervosa. When performing the admission assessment, the nurse elicits data knowing that the client with bulimia:
1 Overeats for the enjoyment of food
2 Binge eats then purges
3 Overeats in response to losing control over a weight loss diet
4 Is accepting of body size

Answer: 2
Rationale: Individuals with bulimia nervosa develop cycles of binge eating, followed by purging. They seldom attempt to diet and have no sense of loss of control. Options 1, 3, and 4 are true of the obese person who may binge eat (not purge).

Test-Taking Strategy: Use the process of elimination. Eliminate options 1 and 3 because they are similar. From the remaining options, recalling the definition of bulimia will direct you to option 2. Review the characteristics associated with this disorder if you had difficulty with this question.

Level of Cognitive Ability: Analysis
Client Needs: Physiological Integrity
Integrated Process: Nursing Process/Assessment
Content Area: Mental Health

Reference:
Stuart, G., & Laraia, M. (2005). *Principles and practice of psychiatric nursing* (8th ed.). St. Louis: Mosby, pp. 527-529.

---

162. A nurse is caring for the client who develops compartment syndrome from a severely fractured arm. The client asks the nurse how this can happen. The nurse's response is based on the understanding that:
1 An injured artery causes impaired arterial perfusion through the compartment
2 The fascia expands with injury, causing pressure on underlying nerves and muscles
3 A bone fragment has injured the nerve supply in the area
4 Bleeding and swelling cause increased pressure in an area that cannot expand

Answer: 4
Rationale: Compartment syndrome is caused by bleeding and swelling within a compartment, which is lined by fascia that does not expand. The bleeding and swelling places pressure on the nerves, muscles, and blood vessels in the compartment, triggering the symptoms.

Test-Taking Strategy: Use the process of elimination. Option 1 is eliminated first because this syndrome is not caused by an arterial injury. Knowing that the fascia cannot expand eliminates option 2. From the remaining options, it is necessary to know that bleeding and swelling (not a nerve injury) cause the symptoms. Review the physiology associated with compartment syndrome if you had difficulty with this question.

Level of Cognitive Ability: Analysis
Client Needs: Physiological Integrity
Integrated Process: Nursing Process/Implementation
Content Area: Adult Health/Musculoskeletal

Reference:
Black, J., & Hawks, J. (2005). *Medical-surgical nursing: Clinical management for positive outcomes* (7th ed.). Philadelphia: Saunders, p. 628.

163. A client has undergone fasciotomy to treat compartment syndrome of the leg. The nurse prepares to provide which type of wound care to the fasciotomy site?
1 Dry sterile dressings
2 Wet sterile saline dressings
3 Hydrocolloid dressings
4 One-half strength betadine dressings

Answer: 2
Rationale: The fasciotomy site is not sutured, but is left open to relieve pressure and edema. The site is covered with wet sterile saline dressings. After 3 to 5 days, when perfusion is adequate and edema subsides, the wound is debrided and closed. A hydrocolloid dressing is not indicated for use with clean, open incisions. The incision is clean, not dirty, so there should be no reason to require betadine. Additionally, betadine can be irritating to normal tissues.

Test-Taking Strategy: Use the process of elimination and knowledge of what a fasciotomy involves and the basics of wound care. Recall that the skin is not sutured closed, but left open for pressure relief. Remembering that moist tissue needs to remain moist will direct you to option 2. Review care of a fasciotomy site if you had difficulty with this question.

Level of Cognitive Ability: Application
Client Needs: Physiological Integrity
Integrated Process: Nursing Process/Planning
Content Area: Adult Health/Musculoskeletal

Reference:
Phipps, W., Monahan, F., Sands, J., Marek, J., & Neighbors, M. (2003). *Medical-surgical nursing: Health and illness perspectives* (7th ed.). St. Louis: Mosby, p. 1489.

164. A nurse is caring for a female client who was recently admitted to the hospital with a diagnosis of anorexia nervosa. When the nurse enters the room, the client is engaged in rigorous push-ups. Which nursing action would be best?
1 Allow the client to complete the exercise program
2 Tell the client that she is not allowed to exercise rigorously
3 Interrupt the client and offer to take the client for a walk
4 Interrupt the client and weigh the client immediately

Answer: 3
Rationale: Clients with anorexia nervosa are frequently preoccupied with rigorous exercise and push themselves beyond normal limits to work off caloric intake. The nurse must provide for appropriate exercise as well as place limits on rigorous activities.

Test-Taking Strategy: Use the process of elimination, noting the key word "best." Focus on the need for the nurse to set firm limits with clients who have this disorder. Also, recalling that the nurse needs to provide and guide the client to perform appropriate exercise will direct you to option 3. Review interventions for clients with this disorder if you had difficulty with this question.

Level of Cognitive Ability: Application
Client Needs: Physiological Integrity
Integrated Process: Nursing Process/Implementation
Content Area: Mental Health

Reference:
Stuart, G., & Laraia, M. (2005). *Principles and practice of psychiatric nursing* (8th ed.). St. Louis: Mosby, p. 530.

165. A nurse assesses the peripheral intravenous (IV) site dressing and notes that it is damp and that the tape is loose. The appropriate nursing action is to:
  1 Stop the infusion immediately and notify the physician
  2 Check that the tubing is securely attached to the catheter and redress the site
  3 Increase the IV flow rate to determine if the leaking increases
  4 Remove the tape around the IV site, slow the IV rate, and then discontinue the IV

Answer: 2
Rationale: If there is leakage at the IV site, the nurse should first locate the source. The nurse should assess the site further to be certain that all connections are secure. The nurse should not increase the flow rate. Although it may leak more, it may also cause tissue damage if the IV was infiltrating. The infusion most likely will need to be stopped, but the physician would not need to be notified. Slowing and discontinuing the IV is also premature. The IV must first be assessed for the cause of the leaking.

Test-Taking Strategy: Note the key word " appropriate" and recall that the nurse needs to determine the cause of the leaking. Use the steps of the nursing process and remember that assessment is the first step. This will direct you to option 2. Review care of the client with an IV if you had difficulty with this question.

Level of Cognitive Ability: Application
Client Needs: Physiological Integrity
Integrated Process: Nursing Process/Implementation
Content Area: Fundamental Skills

Reference:
Potter, P., & Perry, A. (2005). *Fundamentals of nursing* (6th ed.). St. Louis: Mosby, pp. 1180-1181.

166. A nurse assists the physician with the removal of a chest tube. During removal of the chest tube, the nurse instructs the client to:
  1 Breathe out forcefully
  2 Breathe in deeply
  3 Exhale and bear down
  4 Breathe normally

Answer: 3
Rationale: The client is instructed to perform the Valsalva maneuver (take a deep breath, exhale, and bear down) for chest tube removal. This maneuver will increase intrathoracic pressure, thereby lessening the potential for air to enter the pleural space. Options 1, 2, and 4 are incorrect.

Test-Taking Strategy: Use the process of elimination. Eliminate options 2 and 4 because they are similar in that breathing will cause air to enter the pleural space. From the remaining options, eliminate option 1 because of the word "forcefully." Review the procedure for the removal of chest tubes if you had difficulty with this question.

Level of Cognitive Ability: Application
Client Needs: Physiological Integrity
Integrated Process: Nursing Process/Implementation
Content Area: Adult Health/Respiratory

Reference:
Lewis, S., Heitkemper, M., & Dirksen, S. (2004). *Medical-surgical nursing: Assessment and management of clinical problems* (6th ed.). St. Louis: Mosby, p. 625.

167. A nurse assesses the water seal chamber of a closed chest drainage system and notes fluctuations in the chamber. The nurse determines that this finding indicates that:
1 An air leak is present
2 The tubing is kinked
3 The lung has reexpanded
4 The system is functioning as expected

Answer: 4
Rationale: Fluctuations (tidaling) in the water seal chamber are normal during inhalation and exhalation until the lung reexpands and the client no longer requires chest drainage. If fluctuations are absent, it could indicate an air leak, kinking, or that the lung has reexpanded.

Test-Taking Strategy: Note the key words "water seal chamber" and "fluctuations." Recalling the normal expectations related to the functioning of chest tube drainage systems will direct you to option 4. Review care of the client with a chest tube if you had difficulty with this question.

Level of Cognitive Ability: Analysis
Client Needs: Physiological Integrity
Integrated Process: Nursing Process/Analysis
Content Area: Adult Health/Respiratory

Reference:
Black, J., & Hawks, J. (2005). *Medical-surgical nursing: Clinical management for positive outcomes* (7th ed.). Philadelphia: Saunders, p. 1863.

168. A nurse is caring for a client with depression who has not responded to antidepressant medication. The nurse anticipates that what treatment modality may be prescribed?
1 Electroconvulsive therapy
2 Psychosurgery
3 Short-term seclusion
4 Neuroleptic medication

Answer: 1
Rationale: Electroconvulsive therapy is an effective treatment for depression that has not responded to medication. Psychosurgery is invasive, rarely performed, and would not treat depression. Seclusion is not used to treat depression. Neuroleptics are not effective in the treatment of depression.

Test-Taking Strategy: Use the process of elimination. Eliminate option 2 first because it is the most invasive of the options given. Next eliminate option 3 because seclusion would isolate the client and further exacerbate the client's feelings of depression. From the remaining options, recalling that neuroleptics are not used to treat depression will direct you to option 1. Review treatment measures for depression if you had difficulty with this question.

Level of Cognitive Ability: Analysis
Client Needs: Physiological Integrity
Integrated Process: Nursing Process/Analysis
Content Area: Mental Health

Reference:
Varcarolis, E.M. (2002). *Foundations of psychiatric mental health nursing* (4th ed.). Philadelphia: Saunders, p. 478.

169. A client arrives in the emergency department after being in an automobile accident. The client was physically unharmed yet was hyperventilating and complaining of dizziness and nausea. In addition, the client appeared confused and had difficulty focusing on what was going on. The nurse assesses the client's level of anxiety as:

1 Mild
2 Moderate
3 Severe
4 Panic

Answer: 3

Rationale: The person whose anxiety is assessed as severe is unable to solve problems and has difficulty focusing on what is happening in the environment. Somatic symptoms are usually present. The individual with mild anxiety is only mildly uncomfortable and may even find performance enhanced. The individual with moderate anxiety grasps less information about a situation and has some difficulty problem solving. The individual in panic will demonstrate markedly disturbed behavior and may lose touch with reality.

Test-Taking Strategy: Use the process of elimination. Focus on the signs and symptoms presented in the question to eliminate options 1 and 4. Noting the fact that the client has difficulty focusing on what was going on should direct you to option 3 from the remaining options. Review the characteristics related to the levels of anxiety if you had difficulty with this question.

Level of Cognitive Ability: Analysis
Client Needs: Physiological Integrity
Integrated Process: Nursing Process/Assessment
Content Area: Mental Health

Reference:
Stuart, G., & Laraia, M. (2005). *Principles and practice of psychiatric nursing* (8th ed.). St. Louis: Mosby, p. 261.

170. A child is admitted to the hospital with a diagnosis of acute rheumatic fever. The nurse reviews the blood laboratory findings knowing that which of the following will confirm the likelihood of this disorder?

1 Increased leukocyte count
2 Decreased hemoglobin count
3 Increased antistreptolysin-0 (ASO)
4 Decreased erythrocyte sedimentation rate

Answer: 3

Rationale: Children suspected of having rheumatic fever are tested for streptococcal antibodies. The most reliable and best standardized test to confirm the diagnosis is the ASO titer. An elevated level indicates the presence of rheumatic fever.

Test-Taking Strategy: Use the process of elimination and note the key word "confirm." Focusing on the diagnosis will assist in eliminating options 2 and 4. From the remaining options, recall that an increased leukocyte count indicates the presence of infection, but is not specific in confirming a particular diagnosis. Review the diagnostic tests for rheumatic fever if you had difficulty with this question.

Level of Cognitive Ability: Analysis
Client Needs: Physiological Integrity
Integrated Process: Nursing Process/Assessment
Content Area: Child Health

Reference:
Wong, D., & Hockenberry, M. (2003). *Wong's nursing care of infants and children* (7th ed.). St. Louis: Mosby, p.1512.

171. A 5-year-old child is admitted to the hospital for heart surgery to repair the tetralogy of Fallot. The nurse reviews the child's record and notes that the child has clubbed fingers. The nurse understands that the clubbing is most likely caused by:
1 Peripheral hypoxia
2 Delayed physical growth
3 Chronic hypertension
4 Destruction of bone marrow

Answer: 1
Rationale: Clubbing, a thickening and flattening of the tips of the fingers and toes, is thought to occur because of a chronic tissue hypoxia and polycythemia. Options 2, 3, and 4 do not cause clubbing.

Test-Taking Strategy: Use the ABCs—airway, breathing, and circulation. Hypoxia relates to oxygenation, which is a concern with this disorder. Review the manifestations associated with tetralogy of Fallot if you had difficulty with this question.

Level of Cognitive Ability: Analysis
Client Needs: Physiological Integrity
Integrated Process: Nursing Process/Analysis
Content Area: Child Health

References:
Wong, D., & Hockenberry, M. (2003). *Wong's nursing care of infants and children* (7th ed.). St. Louis: Mosby, pp. 452; 1474; 1486; 1497.
James, S., Ashwill, J., & Droske, S. (2002). *Nursing care of children: Principles & practice* (2nd ed.). Philadelphia: Saunders, p. 238.

172. An older client admitted to the hospital with a hip fracture is placed in Buck's extension traction. The nurse plans to frequently monitor which specific item?
1 Temperature
2 Mental state
3 Range of motion ability
4 Neurovascular status

Answer: 4
Rationale: The neurovascular status of the extremity of the client in Buck's extension traction must be assessed frequently. Older clients are especially at risk for neurovascular compromise because many older clients already have disorders that affect the peripheral vascular system. Although the client's temperature is monitored, it is not specific to the use of Buck's extension traction. Although clients in some types of traction do become depressed after a few days or weeks, Buck's extension traction is usually used preoperatively, which typically involves a few hours or 1 to 2 days at the most. Range of motion of the involved leg is contraindicated in hip fractures.

Test-Taking Strategy: Use the process of elimination, focusing on the issue: Buck's extension traction. Recalling the purpose of this traction and visualizing its use will direct you to option 4. Also, use of the ABCs—airway, breathing, and circulation—will direct you to option 4. Review nursing care of the client in Buck's extension traction if you had difficulty with this question.

Level of Cognitive Ability: Application
Client Needs: Physiological Integrity
Integrated Process: Nursing Process/Assessment
Content Area: Adult Health/Musculoskeletal

Reference:
Lewis, S., Heitkemper, M., & Dirksen, S. (2004). *Medical-surgical nursing: Assessment and management of clinical problems* (6th ed.). St. Louis: Mosby, p. 1660.

173. A client who has a renal mass asks the nurse why an ultrasound has been scheduled, as opposed to other diagnostic tests that may be ordered. The nurse formulates a response based on the understanding that:

1 An ultrasound can differentiate a solid mass from a fluid-filled cyst
2 An ultrasound is much more cost effective than other diagnostic tests
3 (All) other tests are more invasive than an ultrasound
4 (All) other tests require more elaborate post-procedure care

Answer: 1

Rationale: A significant advantage of an ultrasound is that it can differentiate a solid mass from a fluid-filled cyst. It is noninvasive, and does not require any special after care. Other diagnostic tests, such as magnetic resonance imaging and computed tomography scanning, are also noninvasive (unless contrast is used) and require no special after care either. However, the ultrasound can discriminate between solid and fluid masses most optimally.

Test-Taking Strategy: Eliminate options 3 and 4 first because of the absolute word "all." From the remaining options, focus on the client's diagnosis to direct you to option 1. Review the purpose of an ultrasound if you had difficulty with this question.

Level of Cognitive Ability: Application
Client Needs: Physiological Integrity
Integrated Process: Nursing Process/Implementation
Content Area: Adult Health/Renal

Reference:
Lewis, S., Heitkemper, M., & Dirksen, S. (2004). *Medical-surgical nursing: Assessment and management of clinical problems* (6th ed.). St. Louis: Mosby, p. 1165.

174. A client has been admitted to the hospital with a diagnosis of primary acute glomerulonephritis. On assessment, the nurse first asks the client about a recent history of:

1 Bleeding ulcer
2 Hypertension
3 Fungal infection
4 Streptococcal infection

Answer: 4

Rationale: The predominant cause of acute glomerulonephritis is infection with beta-hemolytic streptococcus 3 weeks before the onset of symptoms. In addition to bacteria, other infectious agents that could trigger the disorder include viruses or parasites. Hypertension and bleeding ulcer are not precipitating causes.

Test-Taking Strategy: Use the process of elimination. Recalling that infection is a common trigger for glomerulonephritis assists in eliminating options 1 and 2 first. From the remaining options, it is necessary to know that streptococcal infections, rather than fungal infections, are a common cause of this problem. Review the causes of acute glomerulonephritis if you had difficulty with this question.

Level of Cognitive Ability: Application
Client Needs: Physiological Integrity
Integrated Process: Nursing Process/Assessment
Content Area: Adult Health/Renal

Reference:
Black, J., & Hawks, J. (2005). *Medical-surgical nursing: Clinical management for positive outcomes* (7th ed.). Philadelphia: Saunders, p. 927.

175. A client has just been admitted to the emergency room with chest pain. Serum enzyme levels are drawn, and the results indicate an elevated serum creatine kinase (CK)-MB isoenzyme, troponin T, and troponin I. The nurse concludes that these results are compatible with:
1 New-onset myocardial infarction (MI)
2 Stable angina
3 Unstable angina
4 Prinzmetal's angina

Answer: 1

Rationale: Creatine kinase (CK)-MB isoenzyme is a sensitive indicator of myocardial damage. Levels begin to rise 3 to 6 hours after the onset of chest pain, peak at approximately 24 hours, and return to normal in about 3 days. Troponin is a regulatory protein found in striated muscle (skeletal and myocardial). Increased amounts of troponins are released into the bloodstream when an infarction causes damage to the myocardium. Therefore, the client's results are compatible with new-onset MI. Options 2, 3, and 4 all refer to angina. These levels would not be elevated in angina.

Test-Taking Strategy: Use the process of elimination. Eliminate options 2, 3, and 4 because they are similar and all refer to angina. Review the diagnostic laboratory values related to MI if you had difficulty with this question.

Level of Cognitive Ability: Analysis
Client Needs: Physiological Integrity
Integrated Process: Nursing Process/Analysis
Content Area: Adult Health/Cardiovascular

Reference:

Black, J., & Hawks, J. (2005). *Medical-surgical nursing: Clinical management for positive outcomes* (7th ed.). Philadelphia: Saunders, p. 1709.

176. As part of cardiac assessment, the nurse palpates the apical pulse. To perform this assessment, the nurse places the fingertips:
1 To the right of the midclavicular line at the third intercostal space
2 To the right of the midclavicular line at the fifth intercostal space
3 At the left midclavicular line at the third intercostal space
4 At the left midclavicular line at the fifth intercostal space

Answer: 4

Rationale: The point of maximal impulse (PMI), where the apical pulse is palpated, is normally located in the fourth or fifth intercostal space, at the left midclavicular line. The client is placed in a sitting position.

Test-Taking Strategy: Use the process of elimination. Recalling that the PMI corresponds to the left ventricular apex and visualizing each position in the options will direct you to option 4. Review thoracic landmarks if you had difficulty with this question.

Level of Cognitive Ability: Application
Client Needs: Physiological Integrity
Integrated Process: Nursing Process/Assessment
Content Area: Adult Health/Cardiovascular

Reference:

Wilson, S., & Giddens, J. (2005). *Health assessment for nursing practice* (3rd ed.). St. Louis: Mosby, p. 384.

177. A nurse is caring for a client receiving bolus feedings via a Levin-type nasogastric tube. The nurse places the client in which position to administer the feeding?
1 Head of the bed flat
2 Semi-Fowler's to Fowler's
3 Supine
4 Lateral recumbent

Answer: 2
Rationale: Aspiration is a possible complication associated with nasogastric tube feeding. The head of the bed is elevated 35 to 40 degrees to prevent this complication. The positions in options 1, 3, and 4 are flat positions and would place the client at risk for aspiration of the feeding.

Test-Taking Strategy: Use the process of elimination. Eliminate options 1, 3, and 4 because they are similar and are flat positions. Review care of the client receiving tube feedings if you had difficulty with this question.

Level of Cognitive Ability: Application
Client Needs: Physiological Integrity
Integrated Process: Nursing Process/Implementation
Content Area: Fundamental Skills

Reference:
Harkreader, H., & Hogan, M.A. (2004). *Fundamentals of nursing: caring and clinical judgment* (2nd ed.). Philadelphia: Saunders, p. 551.

178. A nurse is caring for a client with acute pancreatitis who has a history of alcoholism. The nurse closely monitors the client for paralytic ileus, knowing that which assessment data indicates this complication of pancreatitis?
1 Firm, nontender mass palpable at the lower right costal margin
2 Severe, constant pain with rapid onset
3 Inability to pass flatus
4 Loss of anal sphincter control

Answer: 3
Rationale: An inflammatory reaction such as acute pancreatitis can cause paralytic ileus, the most common form of nonmechanical obstruction. Inability to pass flatus is a clinical manifestation of paralytic ileus. Option 1 is the description of the physical finding of liver enlargement. The liver is usually enlarged in the client with cirrhosis or hepatitis. Although this client may have an enlarged liver, an enlarged liver is not a sign of paralytic ileus. Pain is associated with paralytic ileus, but the pain usually presents as a more constant generalized discomfort. Pain that is severe, constant, and rapid in onset is more likely caused by strangulation of the bowel. Loss of sphincter control is not a sign of paralytic ileus.

Test-Taking Strategy: Focus on the issue: a sign of paralytic ileus. Recalling the definition of this complication will direct you to option 3. Review the signs of paralytic ileus if you had difficulty with this question.

Level of Cognitive Ability: Application
Client Needs: Physiological Integrity
Integrated Process: Nursing Process/Assessment
Content Area: Adult Health/Gastrointestinal

Reference:
Black, J., & Hawks, J. (2005). *Medical-surgical nursing: Clinical management for positive outcomes* (7th ed.). Philadelphia: Saunders, pp. 845; 1293.

179. After performing an initial abdominal assessment on a client with a diagnosis of cholelithiasis, the nurse documents that the bowel sounds are normal. Which of the following descriptions best describes this assessment finding?
  1 Waves of loud gurgles auscultated in all four quadrants
  2 Very high-pitched loud rushes auscultated especially in one or two quadrants
  3 Soft gurgling or clicking sounds auscultated in all four quadrants
  4 Low-pitched swishing sounds auscultated in one or two quadrants

Answer: 3
Rationale: Although frequency and intensity of bowel sounds will vary depending on the phase of digestion, normal bowel sounds are relatively soft gurgling or clicking sounds that occur irregularly 5 to 35 times per minute. Loud gurgles (Borborygmi) indicate hyperperistalsis. Bowel sounds will be higher pitched and loud (hyperresonance) when the intestines are under tension, such as in intestinal obstruction. A swishing or buzzing sound represents turbulent blood flow associated with a bruit. No aortic bruits should be heard.

Test-Taking Strategy: Use the process of elimination. Normally, bowel sounds should be audible in all four quadrants, therefore options 2 and option 4 can be eliminated. From the remaining options, select option 3 because of the word "soft" in this option. Review normal abdominal assessment findings if you had difficulty with this question.

Level of Cognitive Ability: Analysis
Client Needs: Physiological Integrity
Integrated Process: Nursing Process/Assessment
Content Area: Adult Health/Gastrointestinal

Reference:
Potter, P., & Perry, A. (2005). *Fundamentals of nursing* (6th ed.). St. Louis: Mosby, p. 743.

180. A nurse is assigned to care for a client with nephrotic syndrome. The nurse assesses which most important parameter on a daily basis?
  1 Albumin levels
  2 Weight
  3 Blood urea nitrogen (BUN) level
  4 Activity tolerance

Answer: 2
Rationale: The client with nephrotic syndrome typically presents with edema, hypoalbuminemia, and proteinuria. The nurse carefully assesses the fluid balance of the client, which includes daily monitoring of weight, intake and output, edema, and girth measurements. Albumin levels are monitored as they are prescribed, as are the BUN and creatinine levels. The client's activity level is adjusted according to the amount of edema and water retention. As edema increases, the client's activity level should be restricted.

Test-Taking Strategy: Use the process of elimination, noting the key words "daily basis." Recalling the typical signs of nephrotic syndrome will direct you to option 2. Review these signs if you had difficulty with this question.

Level of Cognitive Ability: Application
Client Needs: Physiological Integrity
Integrated Process: Nursing Process/Assessment
Content Area: Adult Health/Renal

Reference:
Black, J., & Hawks, J. (2005). *Medical-surgical nursing: Clinical management for positive outcomes* (7th ed.). Philadelphia: Saunders, p. 926.

181. A client is being admitted to the hospital with a diagnosis of urolithiasis and ureteral colic. The nurse assesses the client for pain that is:

1 Dull and aching in the costovertebral area
2 Sharp and radiating posteriorly to the spinal column
3 Excruciating, wavelike, and radiating toward the genitalia
4 Aching and cramplike throughout the abdomen

Answer: 3

Rationale: The pain of ureteral colic is caused by movement of a stone through the ureter, and is sharp, excruciating, and wavelike, radiating to the genitalia and thigh. The stone causes reduced flow of urine, and the urine also contains blood because of its abrasive action on urinary tract mucosa. Stones in the renal pelvis cause pain that is a deep ache in the costovertebral area. Renal colic is characterized by pain that is acute, with tenderness over the costovertebral area.

Test-Taking Strategy: Use the process of elimination, focusing on the diagnosis: urolithiasis and ureteral colic. Recall the anatomical location of the kidneys and the ureters. Because the kidneys are located in the posterior abdomen near the ribcage, pain in the costovertebral area is more likely to be associated with stones in the renal pelvis. On the other hand, sharp wavelike pain that radiates toward the genitalia is more consistent with the location of the ureters in the abdomen. Review the assessment findings for this disorder if you had difficulty with this question.

Level of Cognitive Ability: Analysis
Client Needs: Physiological Integrity
Integrated Process: Nursing Process/Assessment
Content Area: Adult Health/Renal

Reference:
Black, J., & Hawks, J. (2005). *Medical-surgical nursing: Clinical management for positive outcomes* (7th ed.). Philadelphia: Saunders, p. 884.

182. A nurse is assessing the client with left-sided heart failure. The client states that he needs to use three pillows under the head and chest at night to be able to breathe comfortably while sleeping. The nurse documents that the client is experiencing:

1 Dyspnea on exertion
2 Dyspnea at rest
3 Orthopnea
4 Paroxysmal nocturnal dyspnea

Answer: 3

Rationale: Dyspnea is a subjective complaint that can range from an awareness of breathing to physical distress and does not necessarily correlate with the degree of heart failure. Dyspnea can be exertional or at rest. Orthopnea is a more severe form of dyspnea, requiring the client to assume a "three-point" position while upright and use pillows to support the head and thorax at night. Paroxysmal nocturnal dyspnea is a severe form of dyspnea occurring suddenly at night because of rapid fluid reentry into the vasculature from the interstitium during sleep.

Test-Taking Strategy: Use the process of elimination and knowledge of the different degrees of dyspnea. Eliminate options 1 and 4 because the question mentions nothing about exertion or a sudden (paroxysmal) event. From the remaining options, select option 3 because the client is breathing "comfortably" with the use of pillows. Review the various descriptions of dyspnea if you had difficulty with this question.

Level of Cognitive Ability: Analysis
Client Needs: Physiological Integrity
Integrated Process: Communication and Documentation
Content Area: Adult Health/Cardiovascular

Reference:
Black, J., & Hawks, J. (2005). *Medical-surgical nursing: Clinical management for positive outcomes* (7th ed.). Philadelphia: Saunders, p. 1563.

183. A nurse is notified that a client will be admitted to the nursing unit in sickle cell crisis. In preparing for the admission, the nurse anticipates that which of the following will be prescribed as a priority in the management of the current crisis?
1 Administration of oxygen
2 Fluid administration
3 Red blood cell transfusion
4 Genetic counseling

Answer: 2

Rationale: The priority items in the management of sickle cell crisis are hydration therapy and pain relief. To achieve this goal, the client is given IV fluids to promote hydration and reverse the agglutination of sickled cells in small blood vessels. Narcotic analgesics may be given to relieve the pain that accompanies the crisis. Oxygen would be given based on individual need. Red blood cell transfusion may also be done in selected circumstances, such as aplastic crisis or when the episode is refractive to other therapy. Genetic counseling is recommended, but not during the acute phase of illness.

Test-Taking Strategy: Focus on the client's diagnosis. Recalling that clumping of sickled cells occurs in this disorder will assist in directing you to the option that would reverse this process. Review the treatment for sickle cell crisis if you had difficulty with this question.

Level of Cognitive Ability: Analysis
Client Needs: Physiological Integrity
Integrated Process: Nursing Process/Planning
Content Area: Fundamental Skills

Reference:
Black, J., & Hawks, J. (2005). *Medical-surgical nursing: Clinical management for positive outcomes.* (7th ed.). Philadelphia: Saunders, pp. 2297; 2299.

184. A nurse suspects that a client who had a myocardial infarction is developing cardiogenic shock. The nurse assesses for which peripheral vascular manifestation of this complication?
1 Flushed, dry skin with bounding pedal pulses
2 Warm, moist skin with irregular pedal pulses
3 Cool, dry skin with alternating weak and strong pedal pulses
4 Cool, clammy skin with weak or thready pedal pulses

Answer: 4

Rationale: Classic signs of cardiogenic shock include increased pulse (weak and thready), decreased blood pressure, decreasing urinary output, signs of cerebral ischemia (confusion, agitation), and cool, clammy skin.

Test-Taking Strategy: Use the process of elimination and recall the signs and symptoms of shock. The word "clammy" in option 4 should direct you to this option. Review the signs of cardiogenic shock if you had difficulty with this question.

Level of Cognitive Ability: Analysis
Client Needs: Physiological Integrity
Integrated Process: Nursing Process/Assessment
Content Area: Adult Health/Cardiovascular

Reference:
Ignatavicius, D., & Workman, M. (2002). *Medical surgical nursing: Critical thinking for collaborative care* (4th ed.). Philadelphia: Saunders, p. 804.

185. A nurse is caring for a client who returns from cardiac surgery with chest tubes in place. The nurse assesses the drainage on an hourly basis and determines that the client is stable as long as drainage does not exceed how many milliliters over the first 24 hours?

1 100
2 200
3 500
4 1000

Answer: 3

Rationale: Chest tube drainage should not exceed 100 mL per hour during the first 2 hours postoperatively, and approximately 500 mL of drainage is expected in the first 24 hours after cardiac surgery. The nurse measures and records the drainage on an hourly basis. The drainage is initially dark red and becomes more serous over time.

Test-Taking Strategy: Focus on the issue: a postoperative client. Eliminate options 1 and 2 because the values are so small. From the remaining options, try converting the drainage to liters recalling that 1000 mL equals 1 liter and 500 mL equals 1/2 liter. Knowing that there are only about 6 liters of blood circulating in the body will direct you to option 3. Review the expected postoperative findings following cardiac surgery if you had difficulty with this question.

Level of Cognitive Ability: Analysis
Client Needs: Physiological Integrity
Integrated Process: Nursing Process/Analysis
Content Area: Adult Health/Cardiovascular

Reference:
Phipps, W., Monahan, F., Sands, J., Marek, J., & Neighbors, M. (2003). *Medical-surgical nursing: Health and illness perspectives* (7th ed.). St. Louis: Mosby, p. 755.

186. A client with renal cancer is being treated preoperatively with radiation therapy. The nurse evaluates that the client has an understanding of proper care of the skin over the treatment field if the client states to:

1 Avoid skin exposure to direct sunlight
2 Apply lotion to the affected skin
3 Wash the ink marks off the skin
4 Wear tight clothing over the skin site to provide support

Answer: 1

Rationale: The client undergoing radiation therapy should wash the site using mild soap and warm or cool water, and pat the area dry. No lotions, creams, alcohol, or deodorants should be placed on the skin over the treatment site. Lines or ink marks that are placed on the skin to guide the radiation therapy should be left in place. The affected skin should be protected from temperature extremes, direct sunlight, and chlorinated water (as from swimming pools). The client should wear cotton clothing over the skin site and guard against irritation from tight or rough clothing such as belts or bras.

Test-Taking Strategy: Use the process of elimination, noting the key words "understanding of proper care." Recalling that the goal of care is to prevent skin irritation will direct you to option 1. Review client teaching related to radiation therapy if you had difficulty with this question.

Level of Cognitive Ability: Analysis
Client Needs: Physiological Integrity
Integrated Process: Teaching/Learning
Content Area: Adult Health/Oncology

Reference:
Phipps, W., Monahan, F., Sands, J., Marek, J., & Neighbors, M. (2003). *Medical-surgical nursing: Health and illness perspectives* (7th ed.). St. Louis: Mosby, p. 336.

187. A client with renal failure is receiving epoetin alfa (Epogen) to support erythropoiesis. The nurse questions the client about compliance with taking which of the following medications that supports red blood cell (RBC) production?
1 Calcium supplement
2 Iron supplement
3 Magnesium supplement
4 Zinc supplement

Answer: 2

Rationale: Iron is needed for RBC production. Otherwise, the body cannot produce sufficient erythrocytes. In either case, the client is not receiving the full benefit of epoetin alfa therapy if iron is not taken.

Test-Taking Strategy: Use the process of elimination. Note the relationship of RBC production in the question and iron in the correct option. Review the concepts related to epoetin alfa and RBC production if you had difficulty with this question.

Level of Cognitive Ability: Application
Client Needs: Physiological Integrity
Integrated Process: Nursing Process/Assessment
Content Area: Adult Health/Renal

Reference:
McKenry, L., & Salerno, E. (2003). *Mosby's pharmacology in nursing* (21st ed.). St. Louis: Mosby, p. 695.

188. A home health nurse is performing an initial assessment on a client who has arrived home with a permanent pacemaker following cardiac surgery. The nurse determines the client's ability regarding self-care related to the pacemaker when the nurse:
1 Asks the client to take the pulse in the wrist or neck and checks the accuracy of the client's reading
2 Determines if the client knows not to operate a microwave oven
3 Determines if the client knows to expect feelings of dizziness and fatigue
4 Asks the client to move the arms and shoulders vigorously to check pacemaker functioning

Answer: 1

Rationale: Clients with permanent pacemakers must be able to take their pulse in the wrist and/or neck accurately in order to note any variation in the pulse rate or rhythm that may need to be reported to the physician. Clients can safely operate most appliances and tools, such as microwave ovens, video recorders, AM-FM radios, electric blankets, lawn mowers, and leaf blowers, as long as the devices are grounded and in good repair. If the client experiences any feelings of dizziness, fatigue, or an irregular heartbeat, the physician is notified. The arms and shoulders should not be moved vigorously for 6 weeks after insertion.

Test-Taking Strategy: Use the process of elimination. Recalling that a pacemaker assists in controlling cardiac rate and rhythm will direct you to option 1. Review client teaching points related to a pacemaker if you had difficulty with this question.

Level of Cognitive Ability: Analysis
Client Needs: Physiological Integrity
Integrated Process: Teaching/Learning
Content Area: Adult Health/Cardiovascular

Reference:
Black, J., & Hawks, J. (2005). *Medical-surgical nursing: Clinical management for positive outcomes* (7th ed.). Philadelphia: Saunders, p. 1697.

189. A client with a severe major depressive episode is unable to address activities of daily living. The appropriate nursing intervention would be to:
1 Feed, bathe, and dress the client as needed until the client can perform these activities independently
2 Structure the client's day so that adequate time can be devoted to the client's assuming responsibility for activities of daily living
3 Offer the client choices and describe the consequences for the failure to comply with the expectation of maintaining activities of daily living
4 Have the client's peers confront the client about how the noncompliance in addressing activities of daily living affects the milieu

Answer: 1
Rationale: The symptoms of major depression include depressed mood, loss of interest or pleasure, changes in appetite and sleep patterns, psychomotor agitation or retardation, fatigue, feelings of worthlessness or guilt, diminished ability to think or concentrate, and recurrent thoughts of death. Often, the client does not have the energy or interest to complete activities of daily living. Option 2 is incorrect because the client still lacks the energy and motivation to do these independently. Option 3 may lead to increased feelings of worthlessness as the client fails to meet expectations. Option 4 will increase the client's feelings of poor self-esteem and unworthiness.

Test-Taking Strategy: Focus on the client's diagnosis and the issue of the question. Use Maslow's hierarchy of needs theory. Remember: physiological needs are the priority. Review care of the client with depression if you had difficulty with this question.

Level of Cognitive Ability: Application
Client Needs: Physiological Integrity
Integrated Process: Nursing Process/Implementation
Content Area: Mental Health

Reference:
Stuart, G., & Laraia, M. (2005). *Principles and practice of psychiatric nursing* (8th ed.). St. Louis: Mosby, p. 358.

190. A pregnant woman of 32 weeks' gestation is admitted to the obstetric unit for observation after an automobile accident. The client is experiencing slight vaginal bleeding and mild cramps. The nurse does which of the following to determine the viability of the fetus?
1 Inserts an intravenous line and begins an infusion at 125 mL per hour
2 Administers oxygen to the woman via a face mask at 7 to 10 liters per minute
3 Positions and connects the ultrasound transducer and the tocotransducer to the external fetal monitor
4 Positions and connects a spiral electrode to the fetal monitor for internal fetal monitoring

Answer: 3
Rationale: External fetal monitoring will allow the nurse to determine any change in the fetal heart rate and rhythm that would indicate that the fetus is in jeopardy. Internal monitoring is contraindicated when there is vaginal bleeding of an unstated cause, especially in preterm labor. Because fetal distress has not been determined at this time, oxygen administration is premature. The amount of bleeding described is insufficient to require intravenous fluid replacement.

Test-Taking Strategy: Focus on the client of the question: the fetus. Next, use the steps of the nursing process, and note that option 3 is an assessment and a noninvasive measure. Review fetal assessment techniques if you had difficulty with this question.

Level of Cognitive Ability: Application
Client Needs: Physiological Integrity
Integrated Process: Nursing Process/Implementation
Content Area: Maternity/Antepartum

Reference:
Lowdermilk, D., & Perry, A. (2004). *Maternity & women's health care* (8th ed.). St. Louis: Mosby, pp. 520-521.

191. A nurse is reviewing the results of a sweat test performed on a child with cystic fibrosis (CF). The nurse would expect to note which finding?

  1 A sweat sodium concentration less than 40 mEq/L

  2 A sweat potassium concentration less than 40 mEq/L

  3 A sweat potassium concentration greater than 40 mEq/L

  4 A sweat chloride concentration greater than 60 mEq/L

Answer: 4

Rationale: A consistent finding of abnormally high sodium and chloride concentrations in the sweat is a unique characteristic of CF. Normally, the sweat chloride concentration is less than 40 mEq/L. A sweat chloride concentration greater than 60 mEq/L is diagnostic of CF. Potassium concentration is unrelated to the sweat test.

Test-Taking Strategy: Use the process of elimination. Eliminate options 2 and 3 first because the potassium level is unrelated to the sweat test. From the remaining options, note that option 4 indicates a "greater" value. Review this test if you had difficulty with this question.

Level of Cognitive Ability: Analysis
Client Needs: Physiological Integrity
Integrated Process: Nursing Process/Analysis
Content Area: Child Health

Reference:
Wong, D., & Hockenberry, M. (2003). *Wong's nursing care of infants and children* (7th ed.). St. Louis: Mosby, p. 1896.

---

192. A nurse is assessing a client with a Cantor tube. Which finding indicates correct placement of the tube?

  1 A pH of aspirate of 7.0 or greater

  2 A pH of aspirate less than 7.0

  3 The presence of gastric contents when checking residuals

  4 The auscultation of air when inserted into the abdomen

Answer: 1

Rationale: The Cantor tube is an intestinal tube and is used for aspirating intestinal contents. For intestinal intubation the tube is threaded through the nose into the stomach and then through the pylorus, where peristaltic activity of the bowel carries it to the desired intestinal area. The nurse ensures intestinal placement by checking the pH of aspirate. A pH reading greater than 7 indicates intestinal contents; a reading less than 7 indicates gastric contents.

Test-Taking Strategy: Use the process of elimination. Recalling that the Cantor tube is an intestinal tube will assist in eliminating options 3 and 4. From the remaining options, recalling that intestinal fluid is alkaline will assist in directing you to option 1. Review the principles associated with the care of a client with a Cantor tube if you had difficulty with this question.

Level of Cognitive Ability: Analysis
Client Needs: Physiological Integrity
Integrated Process: Nursing Process/Analysis
Content Area: Adult Health/Gastrointestinal

References:
Black, J., & Hawks, J. (2005). *Medical-surgical nursing: Clinical management for positive outcomes* (7th ed.). Philadelphia: Saunders, p. 745.
Lewis, S., Heitkemper, M., & Dirksen, S. (2004). *Medical-surgical nursing: Assessment and management of clinical problems* (6th ed.). St. Louis: Mosby, pp. 950; 1080.

193. A nurse performs a neurovascular assessment on a client with a newly applied cast. Close observation and further evaluation would be required if the nurse notes:

1 Capillary refill less than 6 seconds
2 Palpable pulses distal to the cast
3 Sensation when the area distal to the cast is pinched
4 Blanching of the nail bed when depressed

Answer: 1

Rationale: To assess for adequate circulation, the nail bed of each finger or toe is depressed until it blanches, and then the pressure is released. Optimally, the color will change from white to pink rapidly (less than 3 seconds). If this does not occur, the toes or fingers will require close observation and further evaluation. Palpable pulses and sensations distal to the cast are expected. However, if pulses could not be palpated or if the client complained of numbness or tingling, the physician should be notified.

Test-Taking Strategy: Use the process of elimination. Note the key words "close observation and further evaluation." Eliminate options 2, 3, and 4 because these options identify normal expected findings. Option 1 identifies an abnormal or unexpected finding. Review assessment of capillary refill if you had difficulty with this question.

Level of Cognitive Ability: Analysis
Client Needs: Physiological Integrity
Integrated Process: Nursing Process/Assessment
Content Area: Adult Health/Neurological

References:
Black, J., & Hawks, J. (2005). *Medical-surgical nursing: Clinical management for positive outcomes* (7th ed.). Philadelphia: Saunders, p. 633.
Wilson, S., & Giddens, J. (2005). *Health assessment for nursing practice* (3rd ed.). St. Louis: Mosby, p. 381.

194. A nurse is caring for a client with a head injury and is monitoring the client for decerebrate posturing. Which of the following is characteristic of this type of posturing?

1 Extension of the extremities after a stimulus
2 Flexion of the extremities after a stimulus
3 Upper extremity flexion with lower extremity extension
4 Upper extremity extension with lower extremity flexion

Answer: 1

Rationale: Decerebrate posturing, which can occur with upper brain stem injury, is the extension of the extremities after a stimulus. Options 2, 3, and 4 are incorrect descriptions of this type of posturing.

Test-Taking Strategy: Use the process of elimination. Remember that decerebrate may also be known as extension. Recalling this concept will direct you to option 1. Review posturing and its relationship to neurological disorders if you had difficulty with this question.

Level of Cognitive Ability: Analysis
Client Needs: Physiological Integrity
Integrated Process: Nursing Process/Assessment
Content Area: Adult Health/Neurological

References:
Ignatavicius, D., & Workman, M. (2002). *Medical surgical nursing: Critical thinking for collaborative care* (4th ed.). Philadelphia: Saunders, pp. 889-890.
Phipps, W., Monahan, F., Sands, J., Marek, J., & Neighbors, M. (2003). *Medical-surgical nursing: Health and illness perspectives* (7th ed.). St. Louis: Mosby, pp. 1320-1321

195. A nurse is caring for a client admitted to the surgical nursing unit following right modified radical mastectomy. The nurse includes which of the following in the nursing plan of care for this client?
1 Position the client supine with right arm elevated on a pillow
2 Take blood pressures in the right arm only
3 Draw serum laboratory samples from the right arm only
4 Check the right posterior axilla area when assessing the surgical dressing

Answer: 4

Rationale: If there is drainage or bleeding from the surgical site after mastectomy, gravity will cause the drainage to seep down and soak the posterior axillary portion of the dressing first. The nurse checks this area to detect early bleeding. The client should be positioned with the head in semi-Fowler's position and the arm elevated on pillows to decrease edema. Edema is likely to occur because lymph drainage channels have been resected during the surgical procedure. Blood pressure measurement, venipuncture, and IV sites should not involve use of the operative arm.

Test-Taking Strategy: Use the process of elimination. Eliminate options 2 and 3 first because of the words "right arm only." From the remaining options, use knowledge of the effects of gravity to direct you to option 4. Review care of the client following mastectomy if you had difficulty with this question.

Level of Cognitive Ability: Application
Client Needs: Physiological Integrity
Integrated Process: Nursing Process/Planning
Content Area: Adult Health/Oncology

Reference:
Ignatavicius, D., & Workman, M. (2002). *Medical surgical nursing: Critical thinking for collaborative care* (4th ed.). Philadelphia: Saunders, pp. 1743-1744.

196. A nurse is assisting the client with hepatic encephalopathy to fill out the dietary menu. The nurse advises the client to avoid which of the following entree items that could aggravate the client's condition?
1 Fresh fruit plate
2 Tomato soup
3 Vegetable lasagna
4 Ground beef patty

Answer: 4

Rationale: Clients with hepatic encephalopathy have impaired ability to convert ammonia to urea and must limit intake of protein and ammonia-containing foods in the diet. The client should avoid foods such as chicken, beef, ham, cheese, buttermilk, onions, peanut butter, and gelatin.

Test-Taking Strategy: Use the process of elimination, focusing on the client's diagnosis and note the key word "avoid." Note that options 1, 2, and 3 are similar in that they address food items of a fruit and vegetable nature. Review dietary measures for the client with hepatic encephalopathy if you had difficulty with this question.

Level of Cognitive Ability: Application
Client Needs: Physiological Integrity
Integrated Process: Teaching/Learning
Content Area: Adult Health/Gastrointestinal

Reference:
Ignatavicius, D., & Workman, M. (2002). *Medical surgical nursing: Critical thinking for collaborative care* (4th ed.). Philadelphia: Saunders, p. 1312.

197. A client with a colostomy is complaining of gas building up in the colostomy bag. The nurse instructs the client that which of the following food items can be consumed to prevent this problem?

1 Beans
2 Cauliflower
3 Potatoes
4 Corn

Answer: 3

Rationale: Gas-forming foods include corn, cauliflower, onions, beans, and cabbage. These should be avoided by the client with a colostomy until tolerance to them is determined.

Test-Taking Strategy: Focus on the issue: gas-forming foods. Note the similarity between options 1, 2, and 4 in terms of their food substance. Review those food items that are gas-forming if you had difficulty with this question.

Level of Cognitive Ability: Application
Client Needs: Physiological Integrity
Integrated Process: Teaching/Learning
Content Area: Adult Health/Gastrointestinal

Reference:
Ignatavicius, D., & Workman, M. (2002). *Medical surgical nursing: Critical thinking for collaborative care* (4th ed.). Philadelphia: Saunders, p. 1253.

---

198. A client receiving total parenteral nutrition (TPN) complains of nausea, excessive thirst, and increased frequency of voiding. The nurse initially assesses which of the following client data?

1 Serum blood urea nitrogen and creatinine
2 Capillary blood glucose
3 Last serum potassium
4 Rectal temperature

Answer: 2

Rationale: The symptoms exhibited by the client are consistent with hyperglycemia. The nurse would need to assess the client's blood glucose level to verify this data. Clients receiving TPN are at risk for hyperglycemia related to the increased glucose load of the solution. The other options would not provide any information that would correlate with the client symptoms.

Test-Taking Strategy: Focus on the client's symptoms and think about the complications of TPN. Recalling that hyperglycemia is a complication will direct you to option 2. Review the complications associated with TPN and the signs of hyperglycemia if you had difficulty with this question.

Level of Cognitive Ability: Analysis
Client Needs: Physiological Integrity
Integrated Process: Nursing Process/Assessment
Content Area: Adult Health/Gastrointestinal

Reference:
Ignatavicius, D., & Workman, M. (2002). *Medical surgical nursing: Critical thinking for collaborative care* (4th ed.). Philadelphia: Saunders, p. 1372.

---

199. A client admitted to the hospital with a diagnosis of cirrhosis has massive ascites and difficulty breathing. The nurse performs which intervention as a priority measure to assist the client with breathing?

1 Auscultates the lung fields every 4 hours
2 Repositions side to side every 2 hours
3 Encourages deep breathing exercises every 2 hours
4 Elevates the head of the bed 60 degrees

Answer: 4

Rationale: The client is having difficulty breathing because of upward pressure on the diaphragm from the ascitic fluid. Elevating the head of the bed enlists the aid of gravity in relieving pressure on the diaphragm. The other options are general measures to promote lung expansion in the client with ascites, but the priority measure is the one that relieves diaphragmatic pressure.

Test-Taking Strategy: Note the key words "priority measure" and the issue: assist with breathing. Recalling that elevating the head will provide immediate relief of symptoms will direct you to option 4. Review care of the client with ascites who is having difficulty breathing if you had difficulty with this question.

Level of Cognitive Ability: Application
Client Needs: Physiological Integrity
Integrated Process: Nursing Process/Implementation
Content Area: Delegating/Prioritizing

Reference:
Ignatavicius, D., & Workman, M. (2002). *Medical surgical nursing: Critical thinking for collaborative care* (4th ed.). Philadelphia: Saunders, p. 1313.

---

200. A nurse provides dietary measures to a client with mild diverticulitis. The nurse encourages the client to eat foods that are:
1 Low in fiber
2 High in fiber
3 High in fat
4 Low roughage

Answer: 2
Rationale: Mild diverticular disease is treated with a high-fiber diet and prevention of constipation with bran and bulk laxatives. A diet high in fat should be avoided because high-fat foods tend to be low in fiber. A low-roughage diet is similar to a low-fiber diet.

Test-Taking Strategy: Use the process of elimination. Eliminate options 1 and 4 first because they are similar. From the remaining options, recalling that the goal in mild diverticular disease is to prevent constipation will direct you to option 2. Review the diet prescribed for this disorder if you had difficulty with this question.

Level of Cognitive Ability: Application
Client Needs: Physiological Integrity
Integrated Process: Nursing Process/Implementation
Content Area: Adult Health/Gastrointestinal

Reference:
Black, J., & Hawks, J. (2005). *Medical-surgical nursing: Clinical management for positive outcomes* (7th ed.). Philadelphia: Saunders, p. 842.

---

201. A client with Cushing's disease is being admitted to the hospital after a stab wound to the abdomen. The nurse places highest priority on which of the following nursing diagnoses developed for this client?
1 Risk for Deficient Fluid Volume
2 Risk for Infection
3 Disturbed Body Image
4 Ineffective Health Maintenance

Answer: 2
Rationale: The client with a stab wound has a break in the body's first line of defense against infection. The client with Cushing's disease is at great risk for infection caused by excess cortisol secretion, subsequent impaired antibody function, and decreased proliferation of lymphocytes. The client may also have an Ineffective Health Maintenance and Disturbed Body Image, but these are not the highest priority at this time. The client would be at risk for Excess Fluid Volume, not Deficient Fluid Volume, with Cushing's disease.

Test-Taking Strategy: Note the key words "highest priority." Use Maslow's hierarchy of needs theory to eliminate options 3 and 4. From the remaining options, focus on the client's diagnosis. Eliminate option 1 because it is the opposite of what is expected with this disorder. Review the needs of a client with Cushing's disease if you had difficulty with this question.

Level of Cognitive Ability: Analysis
Client Needs: Physiological Integrity
Integrated Process: Nursing Process/Analysis
Content Area: Adult Health/Endocrine

Reference:
Black, J., & Hawks, J. (2005). *Medical-surgical nursing: Clinical management for positive outcomes* (7th ed.). Philadelphia: Saunders, p. 1222.

202. A female adolescent client is admitted to the mental health unit after medical stabilization for an overdose of acetaminophen (Tylenol). The client's boyfriend broke up with her 2 weeks ago and the client stopped eating at that time and has lost 15 pounds. The nurse avoids which intervention when caring for a client?
1 Offer frequent, nutritious snacks
2 Provide meals on an isolation tray that contains no glass or metal utensils
3 Stand the client in front of a mirror to show her how thin she is
4 Offer bland, easily digestible foods

Answer: 3
Rationale: The client has been denying herself food as a means of self-harm. Reinforcing her success at this is not therapeutic. Meeting her nutritional needs is the nursing care priority. Options 1 and 4 meet the client's nutritional needs. Option 2 is a necessary safety measure.

Test-Taking Strategy: Note the key word "avoids." This word indicates a false-response question and that you need to select the option that is an incorrect nursing action. Use Maslow's hierarchy of needs theory. Options 1 and 4 address a physiological need. Option 2 addresses both a physiological and safety need. Option 3 addresses a psychosocial need. Review care of the client at risk for self-harm if you had difficulty with this question.

Level of Cognitive Ability: Application
Client Needs: Physiological Integrity
Integrated Process: Nursing Process/Implementation
Content Area: Mental Health

Reference:
Varcarolis, E.M. (2002). *Foundations of psychiatric mental health nursing* (4th ed.). Philadelphia: Saunders, p. 643.

203. A nurse evaluates a client following treatment for carbon monoxide poisoning. The nurse would document that the treatment was effective when the:
1 Client is awake and talking
2 Carboxyhemoglobin levels are less than 5%
3 Heart monitor shows sinus tachycardia
4 Client is sleeping soundly

Answer: 2
Rationale: Normal carboxyhemoglobin levels are less than 5% for an adult (0.05 to 2.5% for a nonsmoker and 5 to 10% for a heavy smoker). Clients can be awake and talking with abnormally high levels. The symptoms of carbon monoxide poisoning are tachycardia, tachypnea, and central nervous system depression.

Test-Taking Strategy: Note the relationship between the words "carbon monoxide poisoning" in the question and option 2. Option 2 is the only option that specifically addresses this issue. Review the normal carboxyhemoglobin levels if you had difficulty with this question.

Level of Cognitive Ability: Analysis
Client Needs: Physiological Integrity
Integrated Process: Nursing Process/Evaluation
Content Area: Adult Health/Respiratory

References:
Black, J., & Hawks, J. (2005). *Medical-surgical nursing: Clinical management for positive outcomes* (7th ed.). Philadelphia: Saunders, p. 1906.
Chernecky, C., & Berger, B. (2004). *Laboratory tests and diagnostic procedures* (4th ed.). Philadelphia: Saunders, p. 324.

204. A nurse instructs a preoperative client in the proper use of an incentive spirometer. Postoperative assessment of the effectiveness of its use is determined if the client exhibits:
1 Coughing
2 Shallow breaths
3 Wheezing in one lung field
4 Unilateral chest expansion

Answer: 1
Rationale: Incentive devices have many desired and positive effects. Incentive devices provide the stimulus for a spontaneous deep breath. Spontaneous deep breathing, using the sustained maximal inspiration concept, reduces atelectasis, opens airways, stimulates coughing, and actively encourages individual participation in recovery. Shallow breaths, wheezing, and unilateral chest expansion would indicate that the incentive spirometry was not effective. Wheezing indicates narrowing or obstruction of the airway and unilateral chest expansion could indicate atelectasis.

Test-Taking Strategy: Focus on the issue: the effectiveness of an incentive spirometer. Eliminate options 2, 3, and 4, which indicate abnormal findings. Review the purpose of an incentive spirometer if you had difficulty with this question.

Level of Cognitive Ability: Analysis
Client Needs: Physiological Integrity
Integrated Process: Nursing Process/Evaluation
Content Area: Fundamental Skills

Reference:
Potter, P., & Perry, A. (2005). *Fundamentals of nursing* (6th ed.). St. Louis: Mosby, pp. 1109; 1117; 1614.

205. A client is to be started on prazosin hydrochloride (Minipress). The client asks the nurse why the first dose must be taken at bedtime. The nurse's response is based on the understanding that during early use, prazosin:
1 Can cause dizziness, lightheadedness, or possible syncope
2 Results in extreme drowsiness
3 Should be taken when the stomach is empty
4 Can cause significant dependent edema

Answer: 1
Rationale: Prazosin is an alpha-adrenergic blocking agent. "First-dose hypotensive reaction" may occur during early therapy, which is characterized by dizziness, lightheadedness, and possible loss of consciousness. This can also occur when the dosage is increased. This effect usually disappears with continued use or when the dosage is decreased. Options 2, 3 and 4 are not characteristics of the medication.

Test-Taking Strategy: Note the name of the medication, *Minipress*. This will assist in determining that the medication is an antihypertensive agent. Recalling that orthostatic hypotension occurs with the use of antihypertensives will direct you to option 1. Review the effects of this medication if you had difficulty with this question.

Level of Cognitive Ability: Application
Client Needs: Physiological Integrity
Integrated Process: Teaching/Learning
Content Area: Pharmacology

Reference:
Hodgson, B., & Kizior, R. (2004). *Saunders nursing drug handbook 2004.* Philadelphia: Saunders, p. 828.

206. A nurse has applied the prescribed dressing to the leg of a client with an ischemic arterial leg ulcer. The nurse would use which of the following methods to cover the dressing?
1 Apply a large, soft pad, and tape it to the skin
2 Apply a Kerlix roll and tape it to the skin
3 Apply small Montgomery straps and tie the edges together
4 Apply a Kling roll and tape the edge of the roll onto the bandage

Answer: 4
Rationale: With an arterial ulcer, the nurse applies tape only to the bandage. Tape is never used directly on the skin because it could cause further tissue damage. For the same reason, Montgomery straps could not be applied to the skin (although these are generally intended for use on abdominal wounds, anyway). Standard dressing technique includes the use of Kling rolls on circumferential dressings.

Test-Taking Strategy: Use the process of elimination, noting that options 1, 2, and 3 are similar. Eliminate options 1 and 2 recalling that tape is not applied to the skin. For the same reason, eliminate option 3, because the Montgomery straps would need to be adhered to the skin as well. Review care of the client with an arterial leg ulcer if you had difficulty with this question.

Level of Cognitive Ability: Application
Client Needs: Physiological Integrity
Integrated Process: Nursing Process/Implementation
Content Area: Adult Health/Cardiovascular

References:
Black, J., & Hawks, J. (2005). *Medical-surgical nursing: Clinical management for positive outcomes* (7th ed.). Philadelphia: Saunders, p. 1528.
Potter, P., & Perry, A. (2005). *Fundamentals of nursing* (6th ed.). St. Louis: Mosby, pp. 1537; 1542.

207. A child is admitted to the pediatric unit with a diagnosis of celiac disease. Based on this diagnosis, the nurse expects that the child's stools will be:
1 Dark in color
2 Abnormally small in amount
3 Unusually hard
4 Malorodous

Answer: 4
Rationale: The stools of a child with celiac disease are characteristically malodorous, pale, large (bulky), and soft (loose). Excessive flatus is common, and bouts of diarrhea may occur.

Test-Taking Strategy: Use the process of elimination. Thinking about the pathophysiology that occurs in celiac disease will direct you to option 4. Review these manifestations if you had difficulty with this question.

Level of Cognitive Ability: Analysis
Client Needs: Physiological Integrity
Integrated Process: Nursing Process/Assessment
Content Area: Child Health

Reference:
James, S., Ashwill, J., & Droske, S. (2002). *Nursing care of children: Principles & practice* (2nd ed.). Philadelphia: Saunders, pp. 577-578,

208. A clinic nurse is caring for a client with a suspected diagnosis of pregnancy-induced hypertension (PIH). The nurse assesses the client, expecting to note which of the following if PIH is present?
1 Glycosuria, hypertension, and obesity
2 Edema, ketonuria, and obesity
3 Edema, tachycardia, and ketonuria
4 Hypertension, edema, and proteinuria

Answer: 4
Rationale: Pregnancy-induced hypertension is the most common hypertensive disorder in pregnancy. It is characterized by the development of hypertension, proteinuria, and edema. Glycosuria and ketonuria occur in diabetes mellitus. Tachycardia and obesity are not specifically related to diagnosing PIH.

Test-Taking Strategy: Use the process of elimination. Eliminate options 2 and 3 because they do not address hypertension. From the remaining options, recalling that glycosuria is an indication of diabetes mellitus will assist in directing you to option 4. Review the clinical manifestations associated with PIH if you had difficulty with this question.

Level of Cognitive Ability: Application
Client Needs: Physiological Integrity
Integrated Process: Nursing Process/Assessment
Content Area: Maternity/Antepartum

Reference:
Lowdermilk, D., & Perry, A. (2004). *Maternity & women's health care* (8th ed.). St. Louis: Mosby, p. 838.

---

209. A client who undergoes a gastric resection is at risk for developing dumping syndrome. The nurse monitors the client for:
1 Extreme thirst
2 Bradycardia
3 Dizziness
4 Constipation

Answer: 3
Rationale: Early manifestations of dumping syndrome occur 5 to 30 minutes after eating. Symptoms include vasomotor disturbances such as dizziness, tachycardia, syncope, sweating, pallor, palpitations, and the desire to lie down.

Test-Taking Strategy: Use the process of elimination. Recalling that the symptoms of this disorder are vasomotor in nature will direct you to option 3. Review this disorder and the appropriate treatment measures if you had difficulty with this question.

Level of Cognitive Ability: Application
Client Needs: Physiological Integrity
Integrated Process: Nursing Process/Assessment
Content Area: Adult Health/Gastrointestinal

Reference:
Ignatavicius, D., & Workman, M. (2002). *Medical surgical nursing: Critical thinking for collaborative care* (4th ed.). Philadelphia: Saunders, p. 1230.

---

210. A nurse is caring for a client who had a craniotomy (supratentorial surgery). When assessing the client for the major postoperative complication following craniotomy, the nurse monitors for:
1 Restlessness
2 Bleeding
3 Hypotension
4 Bradycardia

Answer: 1
Rationale: The major postoperative complication following craniotomy (supratentorial surgery) is increased intracranial pressure (ICP) from cerebral edema, hemorrhage, or obstruction of the normal flow of cerebrospinal fluid (CSF). Symptoms of increased ICP include severe headache, deteriorating level of consciousness, restlessness, irritability, and dilated or pinpoint pupils that are slow to react or nonreactive to light. Without prompt recognition and treatment, herniation syndromes develop and death can occur. Options 2, 3, and 4 are not associated with increased ICP.

Test-Taking Strategy: Note the client's diagnosis. Always monitor the neurological client for increased ICP. Remember that changes in the level of consciousness is the first key indicator of increased ICP. Option 1 is the only option that addresses level of consciousness. Review the signs of increased ICP and postoperative complications following craniotomy if you had difficulty with this question.

Level of Cognitive Ability: Analysis
Client Needs: Physiological Integrity
Integrated Process: Nursing Process/Assessment
Content Area: Adult Health/Neurological

Reference:
Ignatavicius, D., & Workman, M. (2002). *Medical surgical nursing: Critical thinking for collaborative care* (4th ed.). Philadelphia: Saunders, p. 1003.

---

211. Buck's extension traction is applied to an older client following a hip fracture. The nurse explains to the client that this type of traction is:
1 Skin traction involving the use of traction attached to the skin and soft tissues
2 Skeletal traction involving the use of surgically inserted pins
3 Circumferential traction involving the use of a belt around the body
4 Plaster traction involving the use of a cast

Answer: 1
Rationale: Buck's extension traction is a form of skin traction and involves the use of a belt or boot that is attached to the skin and soft tissues. The purpose of this type of traction is to decrease painful muscle spasms that accompany fractures. The weight that is used as a pulling force is limited (usually 5 to 10 pounds) to prevent injury to the skin. Options 2, 3, and 4 are incorrect descriptions.

Test-Taking Strategy: Recalling that Buck's extension traction is a skin traction will assist in eliminating options 2, 3 and 4. Review the purpose and principles related to this type of traction if you had difficulty with this question.

Level of Cognitive Ability: Application
Client Needs: Physiological Integrity
Integrated Process: Nursing Process/Implementation
Content Area: Adult Health/Musculoskeletal

Reference:
Black, J., & Hawks, J. (2005). *Medical-surgical nursing: Clinical management for positive outcomes* (7th ed.). Philadelphia: Saunders, p. 628.

---

212. A client is taking cascara sagrada. The nurse tells the client that which of the following may be experienced as a side effect of this medication?
1 Gastrointestinal (GI) bleeding
2 Peptic ulcer disease
3 Abdominal cramps
4 Partial bowel obstruction

Answer: 3
Rationale: Cascara sagrada is a laxative that causes nausea and abdominal cramps as the most frequent side effects. The problems identified in options 1, 2, and 4 are not side effects of this medication.

Test-Taking Strategy: Use the process of elimination. Remember that options that are similar are not likely to be correct. Therefore, eliminate options 1,2, and 4 because they are GI disorders. Also recalling that cascara sagrada is a laxative and that laxatives can cause cramping will direct you to option 3. Review the action and side effects of this medication if you had difficulty with this question.

Level of Cognitive Ability: Application
Client Needs: Physiological Integrity
Integrated Process: Teaching/Learning
Content Area: Pharmacology

Reference:
Hodgson, B., & Kizior, R. (2004). *Saunders nursing drug handbook 2004.* Philadelphia: W. B. Saunders, p. 157.

---

213. Skin closure with heterograft will be performed on a client with a burn injury, and the client asks the nurse about the meaning of a heterograft. The nurse tells the client that a heterograft is skin from:

1   Another species
2   A cadaver
3   The burned client
4   A skin bank

Answer: 1

Rationale: Biologic dressings are usually heterograft or homograft material. Heterograft is skin from another species. The most commonly used type of heterograft is pigskin because of its availability and its relative compatibility with human skin. Homograft is skin from another human, which is usually obtained from a cadaver and is provided through a skin bank. Autograft is skin from the client.

Test-Taking Strategy: Focus on the key word "heterograft." Options 2, 3, and 4 are similar and all relate to grafts from human skin. Review the various types of skin closure grafts if you had difficulty with this question.

Level of Cognitive Ability: Application
Client Needs: Physiological Integrity
Integrated Process: Nursing Process/Implementation
Content Area: Adult Health/Integumentary

Reference:
Ignatavicius, D., & Workman, M. (2002). *Medical surgical nursing: Critical thinking for collaborative care* (4th ed.). Philadelphia: Saunders, p. 1578.

---

214. A nurse is caring for a client admitted to the hospital after sustaining a head injury. The nurse appropriately positions the client:

1   With the head elevated on a pillow
2   In left Sims' position
3   In reverse Trendelenburg
4   With the head of the bed elevated 30 to 45 degrees

Answer: 4

Rationale: The client with a head injury is positioned to avoid extreme flexion or extension of the neck and to maintain the head in the midline, neutral position. The client is logrolled when turned to avoid extreme hip flexion. The head of the bed is elevated 30 to 45 degrees. All of these measures are used to enhance venous drainage, which helps prevent increased intracranial pressure (ICP).

Test-Taking Strategy: Use the process of elimination, recalling that the client with a head injury is at risk for increased ICP. Bearing this in mind and considering the principles of gravity will direct you to option 4. Review care of the client following a head injury if you had difficulty with this question.

Level of Cognitive Ability: Application
Client Needs: Physiological Integrity
Integrated Process: Nursing Process/Implementation
Content Area: Adult Health/Neurological

Reference:
Ignatavicius, D., & Workman, M. (2002). *Medical surgical nursing: Critical thinking for collaborative care* (4th ed.). Philadelphia: Saunders, p. 996.

215. A newborn infant is diagnosed with esophageal atresia. The nurse assesses the infant, knowing that a typical finding in this disorder is:
1. Continuous drooling
2. Diaphragmatic breathing
3. Slowed reflexes
4. Passage of large amounts of frothy stool

Answer: 1

Rationale: Esophageal atresia prevents the passage of swallowed mucus and saliva into the stomach. After fluid has accumulated in the pouch, it flows from the mouth and the infant then drools continuously. The inability to swallow amniotic fluid in utero prevents the accumulation of normal meconium, and lack of stools results. Responsiveness of the infant to stimulus would depend on the overall condition of the infant and is not considered a classic sign of esophageal atresia. Diaphragmatic breathing is not associated with this disorder.

Test-Taking Strategy: Focus on the anatomical location of the disorder to eliminate options 3 and 4 first. From the remaining options, recalling the pathophysiology associated with esophageal atresia and recalling that the word "atresia" indicates narrowing will direct you to option 1. Review the manifestations associated with this disorder if you had difficulty with this question.

Level of Cognitive Ability: Analysis
Client Needs: Physiological Integrity
Integrated Process: Nursing Process/Assessment
Content Area: Child Health

Reference:
Wong, D., & Hockenberry, M. (2003). *Wong's nursing care of infants and children* (7th ed.). St. Louis: Mosby, p. 463.

216. A nurse is determining the need for suctioning in a client with an endotracheal (ET) tube attached to a mechanical ventilator. Which observation by the nurse indicates this need?
1. Low peak inspiratory pressure on the ventilator
2. Visible mucus bubbling in the ET tube
3. Apical pulse rate of 72 beats per minute
4. Clear breath sounds

Answer: 2

Rationale: Indications for suctioning include moist, wet respirations, restlessness, rhonchi on auscultation of the lungs, visible mucus bubbling in the ET tube, increased pulse and respiratory rates, and increased peak inspiratory pressures on the ventilator. A low peak inspiratory pressure would indicate a leak in the mechanical ventilation system.

Test-Taking Strategy: Focus on the issue: the need for suctioning. Eliminate options 3 and 4 first because they are normal findings. From the remaining options, focus on the issue and note the word "mucus" in option 2. Review assessment of the client being mechanically ventilated and the indications for the need for suctioning if you had difficulty with this question.

Level of Cognitive Ability: Analysis
Client Needs: Physiological Integrity
Integrated Process: Nursing Process/Assessment
Content Area: Adult Health/Respiratory

Reference:
Ignatavicius, D., & Workman, M. (2002). *Medical surgical nursing: Critical thinking for collaborative care* (4th ed.). Philadelphia: Saunders, p. 605.

217. A client is intubated and receiving mechanical ventilation. The physician has added 7 cm of positive end expiratory pressure (PEEP) to the ventilator settings of the client. The nurse assesses for which of the following expected but adverse effects of PEEP?

1 Systolic blood pressure decrease from 122 to 98 mmHg
2 Decreased heart rate from 78 beats per minute to 64
3 Decreased peak pressure on the ventilator
4 Increased temperature from 98°F to 100°F rectally

Answer: 1

Rationale: PEEP leads to increased intrathoracic pressure, which in turn leads to decreased cardiac output. This is manifested in the client by decreased blood pressure and increased pulse (compensatory). Peak pressures on the ventilator should not be affected, although the pressure at the end of expiration remains positive at the level set for the PEEP. Fever would indicate respiratory infection or infection from another source.

Test-Taking Strategy: Note the key words "expected but adverse." Knowing that PEEP increases intrathoracic pressure leads you to look for the option that reflects a consequence of this event. Fever is irrelevant, and option 4 is eliminated first. From the remaining options, think about the effects of PEEP to direct you to option 1. Review the effects of PEEP if you had difficulty with this question.

Level of Cognitive Ability: Analysis
Client Needs: Physiological Integrity
Integrated Process: Nursing Process/Assessment
Content Area: Adult Health/Respiratory

Reference:
Ignatavicius, D., & Workman, M. (2002). *Medical surgical nursing: Critical thinking for collaborative care* (4th ed.). Philadelphia: Saunders, p. 605.

218. A nurse is assessing the respiratory status of the client following thoracentesis. The nurse would become most concerned with which of the following assessment findings?

1 Respiratory rate of 22 breaths per minute
2 Equal bilateral chest expansion
3 Few scattered wheezes, unchanged from baseline
4 Diminished breath sounds on the affected side

Answer: 4

Rationale: Following thoracentesis, the nurse assesses vital signs and breath sounds. The nurse especially notes increased respiratory rates, dyspnea, retractions, diminished breath sounds, or cyanosis, which could indicate pneumothorax. Any of these signs should be reported to the physician. Options 1 and 2 are normal findings. Option 3 indicates a finding that is unchanged from the baseline.

Test-Taking Strategy: Use the process of elimination, noting the key words "most concerned." Eliminate options 1 and 2 first because they are normal findings. Option 3 is an abnormality, but note that the wheezes are unchanged from the client's baseline. Option 4 is the abnormal finding. Review the signs of complications following a thoracentesis if you had difficulty with this question.

Level of Cognitive Ability: Analysis
Client Needs: Physiological Integrity
Integrated Process: Nursing Process/Analysis
Content Area: Adult Health/Respiratory

Reference:
Ignatavicius, D., & Workman, M. (2002). *Medical surgical nursing: Critical thinking for collaborative care* (4th ed.). Philadelphia: Saunders, p. 485.

219. A nurse is preparing to administer a Mantoux skin test to a client. The nurse determines that which area is most appropriate for injection of the medication?
1 Inner aspect of the forearm that is not heavily pigmented
2 Inner aspect of the forearm that is close to a burn scar
3 Dorsal aspect of the upper arm near a mole
4 Dorsal aspect of the upper arm that has a small amount of hair

Answer: 1
Rationale: Intradermal injections are most commonly given in the inner surface of the forearm. Other sites include the dorsal area of the upper arm or the upper back beneath the scapulae. The nurse finds an area that is not heavily pigmented and is clear of hairy areas or lesions that could interfere with reading the results.

Test-Taking Strategy: Use the process of elimination. Note that options 2, 3, and 4 are similar in that they indicate areas that are not clear of lesions or hair. Review the basics of intradermal injection techniques if you had difficulty with this question.

Level of Cognitive Ability: Application
Client Needs: Physiological Integrity
Integrated Process: Nursing Process/Assessment
Content Area: Adult Health/Respiratory

Reference:
Potter, P., & Perry, A. (2005). *Fundamentals of nursing* (6th ed.). St. Louis: Mosby, p. 882.

---

220. A home care nurse is planning therapeutic measures for the client who experienced a rib fracture 2 days earlier. The nurse tells the client to avoid which of the following?
1 Ambulation
2 Coughing and deep breathing
3 Strapping the ribs
4 Analgesics

Answer: 3
Rationale: Fractured ribs are treated with good pulmonary therapy techniques such as coughing and deep breathing, rapid mobilization, and adequate pain control. Strapping of the ribs is not a treatment measure because it restricts deep breathing and can increase the incidence of atelectasis and pneumonia.

Test-Taking Strategy: Use the process of elimination, focusing on the client's injury and noting the key word "avoid." Recalling that rib strapping restricts deep breathing will direct you to option 3. Review client teaching points related to measures in treating a rib fracture if you had difficulty with this question.

Level of Cognitive Ability: Application
Client Needs: Physiological Integrity
Integrated Process: Nursing Process/Implementation
Content Area: Adult Health/Respiratory

Reference:
Black, J., & Hawks, J. (2005). *Medical-surgical nursing: Clinical management for positive outcomes* (7th ed.). Philadelphia: Saunders, p. 1901.

---

221. A hospitalized client is dyspneic and has been diagnosed with left pneumothorax by chest X-ray. Which of the following observed by the nurse indicates that the pneumothorax is rapidly worsening?
1 Pain with respiration
2 Hypertension
3 Tracheal deviation to the right
4 Tracheal deviation to the left

Answer: 3
Rationale: A pneumothorax is characterized by distended neck veins, displaced point of maximal impulse (PMI), subcutaneous emphysema, tracheal deviation to the unaffected side, decreased fremitus, and worsening cyanosis. The client could have pain with respiration. The increased intrathoracic pressure would cause the blood pressure to fall, not rise.

Test-Taking Strategy: Focus on the client's diagnosis and the key words "rapidly worsening." Pain and hypertension are the least specific indicators and are eliminated first. From the remaining options, remember that a large pneumothorax causes the trachea to be pushed in the opposite direction, to the unaffected side. Review the complications of pneumothorax if you had difficulty with this question.

Level of Cognitive Ability: Analysis
Client Needs: Physiological Integrity
Integrated Process: Nursing Process/Assessment
Content Area: Adult Health/Respiratory

Reference:
Ignatavicius, D., & Workman, M. (2002). *Medical surgical nursing: Critical thinking for collaborative care* (4th ed.). Philadelphia: Saunders, p. 613.

---

222. A client is admitted to the hospital with a diagnosis of right lower lobe pneumonia. The nurse auscultates the right lower lobe, expecting to note which of the following types of breath sounds?
1 Bronchial
2 Bronchovesicular
3 Vesicular
4 Absent

Answer: 1
Rationale: Bronchial sounds are normally heard over the main bronchi. The client with pneumonia will have bronchial breath sounds over area(s) of consolidation, because the consolidated tissue carries bronchial sounds to the peripheral lung fields. The client may also have crackles in the affected area resulting from fluid in the interstitium and alveoli. Absent breath sounds are not likely to occur unless a serious complication of the pneumonia occurs. Bronchovesicular sounds are normally heard over the main bronchi. Vesicular sounds are normally heard over the lesser bronchi, bronchioles, and lobes.

Test-Taking Strategy: Use the process of elimination. Recalling that bronchovesicular sounds are normally heard over the main bronchi and vesicular breath sounds are normal in the lung periphery helps eliminate options 2 and 3. From the remaining options, recall that the pneumonia transmits bronchial breath sounds, so they are heard over the area of consolidation. Review assessment findings in pneumonia if you had difficulty with this question.

Level of Cognitive Ability: Analysis
Client Needs: Physiological Integrity
Integrated Process: Nursing Process/Assessment
Content Area: Adult Health/Respiratory

Reference:
Lewis, S., Heitkemper, M., & Dirksen, S. (2004). *Medical-surgical nursing: Assessment and management of clinical problems* (6th ed.). St. Louis: Mosby, p. 597.

223. A nurse assesses the client with acquired immunodeficiency syndrome (AIDS) for early signs of Kaposi's sarcoma. The nurse observes the client for lesion(s) that are:

1 Unilateral, raised, and bluish-purple in color
2 Bilateral, flat, and pink, turning to dark violet or black in color
3 Unilateral, red, raised, and resembling a blister
4 Bilateral, flat, and brownish and scaly in appearance

Answer: 2

Rationale: Kaposi's sarcoma generally starts with an area that is flat and pink that changes to a dark violet or black color. The lesions are usually present bilaterally. They may appear in many areas of the body and are treated with radiation, chemotherapy, and cryotherapy.

Test-Taking Strategy: Use the process of elimination. Recalling that Kaposi's sarcoma occurs in a bilateral pattern eliminates options 1 and 3. From the remaining options, recalling the character of the lesions will direct you to option 2. Review the characteristics of this disorder if you had difficulty with this question.

Level of Cognitive Ability: Analysis
Client Needs: Physiological Integrity
Integrated Process: Nursing Process/Assessment
Content Area: Adult Health/Immune

Reference:
Black, J., & Hawks, J. (2005). *Medical-surgical nursing: Clinical management for positive outcomes* (7th ed.). Philadelphia: Saunders, p. 2393.

---

224. A client is suspected of having a pleural effusion. The nurse assesses the client for which typical manifestations of this respiratory problem?

1 Dyspnea at rest and moist, productive cough
2 Dyspnea on exertion and moist, productive cough
3 Dyspnea at rest and dry, nonproductive cough
4 Dyspnea on exertion and dry, nonproductive cough

Answer: 4

Rationale: Typical assessment findings in the client with a pleural effusion include dyspnea, which usually occurs with exertion, and a dry, nonproductive cough. The cough is caused by bronchial irritation and possible mediastinal shift.

Test-Taking Strategy: Use the process of elimination. Recalling that a pleural effusion is in the pleural space and not the airway helps to eliminate options 1 and 2. Remembering that dyspnea occurs on exertion before it occurs at rest will direct you to option 4 from the remaining options. Review the manifestations of pleural effusion if you had difficulty with this question.

Level of Cognitive Ability: Application
Client Needs: Physiological Integrity
Integrated Process: Nursing Process/Assessment
Content Area: Adult Health/Respiratory

Reference:
Black, J., & Hawks, J. (2005). *Medical-surgical nursing: Clinical management for positive outcomes* (7th ed.). Philadelphia: Saunders, p. 1873.

---

225. A client with pleural effusion had a thoracentesis, and a sample of fluid was sent to the laboratory. Analysis of the fluid reveals a high red blood cell count. The nurse interprets that this result is most consistent with:

1 Trauma
2 Infection
3 Heart failure
4 Liver failure

Answer: 1

Rationale: Pleural effusion that has a high red blood cell count may result from trauma and may be treated with placement of a chest tube for drainage. Other causes of pleural effusion include infection, heart failure, liver or renal failure, malignancy, or inflammatory processes. Infection would be accompanied by white blood cells. The fluid portion of the serum would accumulate with liver failure and heart failure.

Test-Taking Strategy: Use the process of elimination. Noting the key words "red blood cell count" will direct you to option 1. Review the causes of pleural effusion if you had difficulty with this question.

Level of Cognitive Ability: Analysis
Client Needs: Physiological Integrity
Integrated Process: Nursing Process/Analysis
Content Area: Adult Health/Respiratory

Reference:
Black, J., & Hawks, J. (2005). *Medical-surgical nursing: Clinical management for positive outcomes* (7th ed.). Philadelphia: Saunders, p. 1873.

---

226. A nurse is scheduling a client for diagnostic studies of the gastrointestinal (GI) system. Which of the following studies, if ordered, should the nurse schedule last?
1 Abdominal computerized tomography scan
2 Ultrasound
3 Colonoscopy
4 Barium enema

Answer: 4
Rationale: Barium is instilled into the lower GI tract during a barium enema and may take up to 72 hours to clear the GI tract. The presence of barium could cause interference with obtaining clear visualization and accurate results of the other tests listed, if performed before the client has fully excreted the barium. For this reason, diagnostic studies that involve barium contrast are scheduled at the conclusion of other diagnostic studies.

Test-Taking Strategy: Use the process of elimination. Note the key word "last." Recall that barium shows up on X-ray as opaque and that this substance would impair visualization during other tests. Review the procedure for the diagnostic tests listed in the options if you had difficulty with this question.

Level of Cognitive Ability: Application
Client Needs: Physiological Integrity
Integrated Process: Nursing Process/Planning
Content Area: Delegating/Prioritizing

Reference:
Black, J., & Hawks, J. (2005). *Medical-surgical nursing: Clinical management for positive outcomes* (7th ed.). Philadelphia: Saunders, p. 783.

---

227. A nurse is caring for a client who is scheduled to have a liver biopsy. Before the procedure, it is most important for the nurse to assess the client's:
1 History of nausea and vomiting
2 Tolerance for pain
3 Allergy to iodine or shellfish
4 Ability to lie still and hold the breath

Answer: 4
Rationale: It is most important for the nurse to assess the client's ability to lie still and hold the breath for the procedure. This helps the physician avoid complications, such as puncturing the lung or other organs. Assessment of allergy to iodine or shellfish is unnecessary for this procedure, because no contrast dye is used. Knowledge of the history related to nausea and vomiting is generally a part of assessment of the gastrointestinal system, but has no relationship to the procedure. The client's tolerance for pain is a useful item to know. However, the area will receive a local anesthetic.

Test-Taking Strategy: Use the process of elimination. Visualizing this procedure and thinking about its complications will direct you to option 4. Review this procedure if you had difficulty with this question.

Level of Cognitive Ability: Application
Client Needs: Physiological Integrity
Integrated Process: Nursing Process/Assessment
Content Area: Adult Health/Gastrointestinal

Reference:
Chernecky, C., & Berger, B. (2004). *Laboratory tests and diagnostic procedures* (4th ed.). Philadelphia: Saunders, p. 733.

---

228. A nurse is caring for a client diagnosed with pneumonia. The nurse plans which of the following as the best time to take the client for a short walk?
1   After the client uses the metered-dose inhaler
2   After recording oxygen saturation on the bedside flow sheet
3   After the client eats lunch
4   After the client has a brief nap

Answer: 1
Rationale: The nurse should schedule activities for the client with pneumonia after the client has received respiratory treatments or medications. After the administration of bronchodilators (often administered by metered-dose inhaler), the client has the best oxygen exchange possible and would tolerate the activity best. Still, the nurse implements activity cautiously, so as not to increase the client's dyspnea. The client would become fatigued after eating; therefore, this is not a good time to ambulate the client. Although the client may be rested somewhat after a nap, from the options provided this is not the best time to ambulate. Option 2 is unrelated to the client's ability to tolerate ambulation.

Test-Taking Strategy: Note the key word "best." Use the ABCs—airway, breathing, and circulation. The use of bronchodilator medication would widen the air passages, allowing for more air to enter the client's lungs. Review care of the client with pneumonia if you had difficulty with this question.

Level of Cognitive Ability: Application
Client Needs: Physiological Integrity
Integrated Process: Nursing Process/Planning
Content Area: Adult Health/Respiratory

Reference:
Black, J., & Hawks, J. (2005). *Medical-surgical nursing: Clinical management for positive outcomes* (7th ed.). Philadelphia: Saunders, pp. 1842-1843.

---

229. A nurse has just inserted an indwelling Foley catheter into the bladder of a postoperative client who has not voided for 6 hours and has a distended bladder. After the tubing is secured and the collection bag is hung on the bed frame, the nurse notices that 800 mL of urine has drained into the collection bag. The appropriate nursing action for the safety of the client is to:
1   Clamp the tubing for 30 minutes and then release
2   Provide suprapubic pressure to maintain a steady flow of urine
3   Check the specific gravity of the urine
4   Raise the collection bag high enough to slow the rate of drainage

Answer: 1
Rationale: Rapid emptying of a large volume of urine may cause engorgement of pelvic blood vessels and hypovolemic shock. Clamping the tubing for 30 minutes allows for equilibration to prevent complications. Option 2 would increase the flow of urine, which would lead to hypovolemic shock. Option 3 is an assessment and would not affect the flow of urine or prevent possible hypovolemic shock. Option 4 could cause backflow of urine. Infection is likely to develop if urine is allowed to flow back into the bladder.

Test-Taking Strategy: Note the key words "800 mL." Recall the physiology of the hemodynamic changes following the rapid collapse of an overdistended bladder. Eliminate options 2 and 4 because slowing the rate of urine drainage is the issue. Note that option 3 is an assessment action rather than an action that affects the amount of urine drainage. Review the complications associated with inserting a Foley catheter in a client with a distended bladder if you had difficulty with this question.

Level of Cognitive Ability: Application
Client Needs: Physiological Integrity
Integrated Process: Nursing Process/ Implementation
Content Area: Fundamental Skills

References:
Elkin, M., Perry, A., & Potter, P. (2004). *Nursing interventions & clinical skills* (3rd ed.). St. Louis: Mosby, p. 847.
Potter, P., & Perry, A. (2005). *Fundamentals of nursing* (6th ed.). St. Louis: Mosby, p. 1357.

---

230. A nurse has an order to administer Amphotericin B (Fungizone) intravenously to the client with histoplasmosis. The nurse plans to do which of the following during administration of the medication?
1 Monitor for hypothermia
2 Administer a concurrent fluid challenge
3 Assess the intravenous infusion site
4 Monitor for an excessive urine output

Answer: 3
Rationale: Amphotericin B is a toxic medication, which can produce symptoms during administration such as chills, fever (hyperthermia), headache, vomiting, and impaired renal function (decreased urine output). The medication is also very irritating to the IV site, commonly causing thrombophlebitis. The nurse administering this medication monitors for these complications. Administering a concurrent fluid challenge is not necessary.

Test-Taking Strategy: Use the process of elimination, recalling the toxic effects of this medication. Knowing that fever and chills can occur eliminates option 1. Recalling that the medication can be toxic to the kidneys eliminates option 4. From the remaining options, knowing that there is no rationale for giving concurrent fluids will direct you to option 3. Review nursing care related to the administration of this medication if you had difficulty with this question.

Level of Cognitive Ability: Application
Client Needs: Physiological Integrity
Integrated Process: Nursing Process/Planning
Content Area: Adult Health/Immune

Reference:
McKenry, L., & Salerno, E. (2003). *Mosby's pharmacology in nursing* (21st ed.). St. Louis: Mosby, p. 1015.

---

231. A client who experiences repeated pleural effusions from inoperable lung cancer is to undergo pleurodesis. The nurse plans to assist with which of the following after the physician injects the sclerosing agent through the chest tube?
1 Clamp the chest tube
2 Ambulate the client
3 Ask the client to cough and deep breathe
4 Ask the client to remain in one position only

Answer: 1
Rationale: After injection of the sclerosing agent, the chest tube is clamped to prevent the agent from draining back out of the pleural space. A repositioning schedule is used by some physicians, but its usefulness in dispersing the substance is controversial. Ambulation, coughing, and deep breathing have no specific purpose in the immediate period after injection.

Test-Taking Strategy: Note that the client is having a pleurodesis. This will assist in eliminating option 2. Eliminate option 4 because of the word "only." From the remaining options, recall the purpose of the procedure. It is most reasonable to clamp the chest tube so that the sclerosing agent cannot flow back out of the tube. Coughing and deep breathing have no specific purpose in this situation. Review this procedure if you had difficulty with this question.

Level of Cognitive Ability: Application
Client Needs: Physiological Integrity
Integrated Process: Nursing Process/Planning
Content Area: Adult Health/Respiratory

Reference:
Ignatavicius, D., & Workman, M. (2002). *Medical surgical nursing: Critical thinking for collaborative care* (4th ed.). Philadelphia: Saunders, p. 569.

---

232. A client with a bladder injury has had surgical repair of the injured area and placement of a suprapubic catheter. The nurse plans to do which of the following to prevent complications with the use of this catheter?
   1 Monitor urine output every shift
   2 Encourage a high intake of oral fluids
   3 Prevent kinking of the catheter tubing
   4 Measure specific gravity once a shift

Answer: 3
Rationale: A complication after surgical repair of the bladder is disruption of sutures caused by tension on them from urine buildup. The nurse prevents this from happening by ensuring that the catheter is able to drain freely. This involves basic catheter care, including keeping the tubing free from kinks, keeping the tubing below the level of the bladder, and monitoring the flow of urine frequently. Measurement of urine specific gravity and a high oral fluid intake do not prevent complications of bladder surgery. Monitoring urine output every shift is insufficient to detect decreased flow from catheter kinking.

Test-Taking Strategy: Use the process of elimination. Eliminate option 4 first because specific gravity measurement is not a preventive action. Eliminate option 1 next, because once-a-shift measurement is not a preventive action and is also insufficient in frequency. From the remaining options, knowing that a high oral fluid intake will not prevent complications with the catheter directs you to option 3. Review care of the client with a suprapubic catheter if you had difficulty with this question.

Level of Cognitive Ability: Application
Client Needs: Physiological Integrity
Integrated Process: Nursing Process/Planning
Content Area: Adult Health/Renal

Reference:
Ignatavicius, D., & Workman, M. (2002). *Medical surgical nursing: Critical thinking for collaborative care* (4th ed.). Philadelphia: Saunders, p. 1788.

---

233. A client with benign prostatic hyperplasia undergoes transurethral resection of the prostate (TURP). The nurse orders which of the following solutions from the pharmacy so it is available postoperatively for continuous bladder irrigation (CBI)?
   1 Sterile water
   2 Sterile normal saline
   3 Sterile Dakin's solution
   4 Sterile water with 5% dextrose

Answer: 2
Rationale: Continuous bladder irrigation is done following TURP using sterile normal saline, which is isotonic. Sterile water is not used because the solution could be absorbed systemically, precipitating hemolysis and possibly renal failure. Dakin's solution contains hypochlorite and is used only for wound irrigation in selected circumstances. Solutions containing dextrose are not introduced into the bladder.

Test-Taking Strategy: Use the process of elimination, noting the issue: a continuous bladder irrigation. Recalling that normal saline is isotonic will direct you to option 2. Review the procedure for CBI if you had difficulty with this question.

Level of Cognitive Ability: Application
Client Needs: Physiological Integrity
Integrated Process: Nursing Process/Implementation
Content Area: Adult Health/Renal

Reference:
Ignatavicius, D., & Workman, M. (2002). *Medical surgical nursing: Critical thinking for collaborative care* (4th ed.). Philadelphia: Saunders, p. 1787.

---

234. A client with acquired immunodeficiency syndrome (AIDS) is being admitted to the hospital for treatment of pneumocystis carinii infection. Which of the following activities does the nurse plan to include in the care of this client that assists in maintaining comfort?
1 Assess respiratory rate, rhythm, depth, and breath sounds
2 Evaluate arterial blood gas results
3 Keep the head of the bed elevated
4 Monitor vital signs

Answer: 3
Rationale: Clients with respiratory difficulties are often more comfortable with the head of the bed elevated. Options 1, 2, and 4 are appropriate measures to evaluate respiratory function and to avoid complications. Option 3 is the only option that addresses planning for client comfort.

Test-Taking Strategy: Use the process of elimination. Focusing on the issue, maintaining comfort, will direct you to option 3. Also, note that options 1, 2, and 4 are similar and are all measures to evaluate respiratory function. Review measures to promote comfort in a client with a respiratory infection if you had difficulty with this question.

Level of Cognitive Ability: Application
Client Needs: Physiological Integrity
Integrated Process: Nursing Process/Planning
Content Area: Adult Health/Immune

Reference:
Ignatavicius, D., & Workman, M. (2002). *Medical surgical nursing: Critical thinking for collaborative care* (4th ed.). Philadelphia: Saunders, p. 382.

---

235. A client with significant flail chest has arterial blood gases (ABGs) that reveal a Pao_2 of 68 and a $Paco_2$ of 51. Two hours ago the Pao_2 was 82 and the $Paco_2$ was 44. Based on these changes, the nurse obtains which of the following items?
1 Injectable Lidocaine (Xylocaine)
2 Portable chest X-ray machine
3 Intubation tray
4 Chest tube insertion set

Answer: 3
Rationale: The client with flail chest has painful, rapid, shallow respirations while experiencing severe dyspnea. The effort of breathing and the paradoxical chest movement have the net effect of producing hypoxia and hypercapnea. The client develops respiratory failure and requires intubation and mechanical ventilation, usually with positive end expiratory pressure (PEEP). Therefore, an intubation tray is necessary.

Test-Taking Strategy: Use the process of elimination, noting the changes in the ABG values. Recall that a falling arterial oxygen level and a rising carbon dioxide level indicate respiratory failure. The usual treatment for respiratory failure is intubation, which makes option 3 correct. Review the complications of flail chest and the signs of respiratory failure if you had difficulty with this question.

Level of Cognitive Ability: Application
Client Needs: Physiological Integrity
Integrated Process: Nursing Process/Implementation
Content Area: Adult Health/Respiratory

Reference:
Black, J., & Hawks, J. (2005). *Medical-surgical nursing: Clinical management for positive outcomes* (7th ed.). Philadelphia: Saunders, p. 2493.

---

236. A client with empyema is to have a thoracentesis performed at the bedside. The nurse plans to have which of the following available in the event that the procedure is not effective?

1 Code cart
2 Chest tube and drainage system
3 Extra-large drainage bottle
4 A small-bore needle

Answer: 2

Rationale: If the exudate is too thick for drainage via thoracentesis, the client may require placement of a chest tube to adequately drain the purulent effusion. A small-bore needle would not effectively allow exudate to drain. Options 1 and 3 are also unnecessary.

Test-Taking Strategy: Note the client's diagnosis. In this condition, the exudate is often very thick. Recalling that the purpose of thoracentesis is to provide drainage of the pleura will direct you to option 2. Review care of the client undergoing a thoracentesis if you difficulty with this question.

Level of Cognitive Ability: Application
Client Needs: Physiological Integrity
Integrated Process: Nursing Process/Planning
Content Area: Adult Health/Respiratory

References:
Black, J., & Hawks, J. (2005). *Medical-surgical nursing: Clinical management for positive outcomes* (7th ed.). Philadelphia: Saunders, p. 1772.
Ignatavicius, D., & Workman, M. (2002). *Medical surgical nursing: Critical thinking for collaborative care* (4th ed.). Philadelphia: Saunders, p. 569.

---

237. A nurse is preparing to administer an opioid to a client via an epidural catheter. Before administering the medication, the nurse aspirates and obtains 5 mL of clear fluid. The nurse takes which action?

1 Injects the opioid slowly
2 Notifies the anesthesiologist
3 Injects the aspirate (6 mL of clear fluid) back into the catheter and administers the opioid
4 Flushes the catheter with 6 mL of sterile water before injecting the opioid

Answer: 2

Rationale: Aspiration of clear fluid of less than 1 mL is indicative of epidural catheter placement. More than 1 mL of clear fluid or bloody return means that the catheter may be in the subarachnoid space or in a vessel. Therefore, the nurse would not inject the medication and would notify the anesthesiologist. Options 1, 3, and 4 are incorrect actions.

Test-Taking Strategy: Use the process of elimination, focusing on the key word "epidural." Eliminate options 1, 3, and 4 first because they are similar and indicate administering the opioid. Review the procedure for administrating medication through an epidural catheter if you had difficulty with this question.

Level of Cognitive Ability: Application
Client Needs: Physiological Integrity
Integrated Process: Nursing Process/Implementation
Content Area: Pharmacology

Reference:
Elkin, M., Perry, A., & Potter, P. (2004). *Nursing interventions & clinical skills* (3rd ed.). St. Louis: Mosby, p. 256.

238. A nurse is planning care for a client with a chest tube attached to a Pleurevac drainage system. The nurse avoids which of the following activities to prevent a tension pneumothorax?
1. Adding water to the suction chamber as it evaporates
2. Taping the connection between the chest tube and the drainage system
3. Maintaining the collection chamber below the client's waist
4. Clamping the chest tube

Answer: 4

Rationale: To prevent a tension pneumothorax, the nurse avoids clamping the chest tube, unless specifically ordered. In many facilities, clamping of the chest tube is contraindicated by agency policy. Adding water to the suction control chamber is an appropriate nursing action and is done as needed to maintain the full suction level ordered. Taping the connection between the chest tube and system is also indicated to prevent accidental disconnection. Maintaining the system below waist level is indicated to prevent fluid from reentering the pleural space.

Test-Taking Strategy: Use the process of elimination, noting the key word "avoids." This word indicates a false-response question and that you need to select the option that is an incorrect nursing action. Recall that tension pneumothorax occurs when air is trapped in the pleural space and has no exit. Therefore, it is necessary to evaluate each of the options in terms of relative risk for air trapping in the pleural space. Clamping the chest tube could trap air in the pleural space. Review the causes of tension pneumothorax and care of the client with a chest tube if you had difficulty with this question.

Level of Cognitive Ability: Application
Client Needs: Physiological Integrity
Integrated Process: Nursing Process/Implementation
Content Area: Adult Health/Respiratory

References:

Lewis, S., Heitkemper, M., & Dirksen, S. (2004). *Medical-surgical nursing: Assessment and management of clinical problems* (6th ed.). St. Louis: Mosby, p. 624.
Phipps, W., Monahan, F., Sands, J., Marek, J., & Neighbors, M. (2003). *Medical-surgical nursing: Health and illness perspectives* (7th ed.). St. Louis: Mosby, pp. 556-557.

239. A nurse is assisting a client with a chest tube to get out of bed, and the chest tubing accidentally gets caught in the bed rail and disconnects. While trying to reestablish the connection, the Pleur-Evac drainage system falls over and cracks. The nurse takes which immediate action?
1. Calls the physician
2. Immerses the chest tube in a bottle of sterile normal saline
3. Applies a petrolatum gauze over the end of the chest tube
4. Clamps the chest tube

Answer: 2

Rationale: If a chest tube accidentally disconnects from the tubing of the drainage apparatus, the nurse should first reestablish an underwater seal to prevent tension pneumothorax and mediastinal shift. This can be accomplished by reconnecting the chest tube, or in this case, immersing the end of the chest tube in a bottle of sterile normal saline or water. The physician should be notified after taking corrective action. If the physician is called first, tension pneumothorax has time to develop. Clamping the chest tube could also cause tension pneumothorax. A petrolatum gauze would be applied to the skin over the chest tube insertion site if the entire chest tube was accidentally removed from the chest.

Test-Taking Strategy: Use the process of elimination, noting the key word "immediate." Eliminate option 1 as too time consuming to be the "immediate" action. Option 4 would create a tension pneumothorax, because this action does not reestablish an underwater seal. From the remaining options, noting that an underwater seal must be established will direct you to option 2. Review care of the client with a chest tube if you had difficulty with this question.

Level of Cognitive Ability: Application
Client Needs: Physiological Integrity
Integrated Process: Nursing Process/Implementation
Content Area: Adult Health/Respiratory

Reference:
Black, J., & Hawks, J. (2005). *Medical-surgical nursing: Clinical management for positive outcomes* (7th ed.). Philadelphia: Saunders, p. 1865.

---

240. A nurse is caring for a client with a diagnosis of Cushing's syndrome. The nurse plans which of these measures to prevent complications from this medical condition?

1 Monitoring glucose levels
2 Monitoring epinephrine levels
3 Encouraging daily jogging
4 Encouraging visits from friends

Answer: 1
Rationale: In the client with Cushing's syndrome, increased levels of glucocorticoids can result in hyperglycemia and signs and symptoms of diabetes mellitus. Epinephrine levels are not affected. Clients experience activity intolerance related to muscle weakness and fatigue, therefore option 3 is incorrect. Visitors should be limited because of the client's impaired immune response.

Test-Taking Strategy: Focus on complications of Cushing's syndrome. Recalling that increased levels of glucocorticoids can result in hyperglycemia will direct you to option 1. Review the clinical manifestations associated with Cushing's syndrome if you had difficulty with this question.

Level of Cognitive Ability: Analysis
Client Needs: Physiological Integrity
Integrated Process: Nursing Process/Planning
Content Area: Adult Health/Endocrine

Reference:
Ignatavicius, D., & Workman, M. (2002). *Medical surgical nursing: Critical thinking for collaborative care* (4th ed.). Philadelphia: Saunders, p. 1418.

---

241. A client with a central venous catheter who is receiving total parenteral nutrition (TPN) suddenly becomes short of breath, complains of chest pain, and is tachycardic, pale, and anxious. The nurse, suspecting an air embolism, places the client in lateral Trendelenburg position on the left side and then:

1 Slows the rate of the TPN after checking the lines for air
2 Clamps the catheter and notifies the physician
3 Monitors vital signs every 30 minutes
4 Boluses the client with 500 mL normal saline to break up the air embolus

Answer: 2
Rationale: If the client experiences air embolus, the nurse should clamp the catheter immediately and notify the physician. The client is placed in the lateral Trendelenburg position on the left side to trap the air in the right atrium. The other options are incorrect. Although vital signs are monitored, they are monitored continuously.

Test-Taking Strategy: Note the key words "suspecting an air embolism." Recall that air embolism is a life-threatening condition and that the physician needs to be notified if a life-threatening condition exists. This will direct you to option 2. Review the interventions for an air embolism if you had difficulty with this question.

Level of Cognitive Ability: Application
Client Needs: Physiological Integrity
Integrated Process: Nursing Process/Implementation
Content Area: Adult Health/Renal

Reference:
Ignatavicius, D., & Workman, M. (2002). *Medical surgical nursing: Critical thinking for collaborative care* (4th ed.). Philadelphia: Saunders, pp. 207.

242. A nurse notes on the cardiac monitor that a client with aldosteronism is experiencing a dysrhythmia. The nurse immediately assesses the client's:

1 Plasma potassium level
2 Intake and output
3 Peripheral pulses
4 Superficial reflexes

Answer: 1

Rationale: Aldosteronism can lead to hypokalemia, which in turn can cause life-threatening dysrhythmias. Options 2, 3, and 4 are not immediate priorities for this client.

Test-Taking Strategy: Note the key word "immediately." Recalling the complications associated with this disorder and that altered potassium levels can cause dysrhythmias will direct you to option 1. Review the complications of aldosteronism if you had difficulty with this question.

Level of Cognitive Ability: Application
Client Needs: Physiological Integrity
Integrated Process: Nursing Process/Implementation
Content Area: Adult Health/Endocrine

Reference:
Ignatavicius, D., & Workman, M. (2002). *Medical surgical nursing: Critical thinking for collaborative care* (4th ed.). Philadelphia: Saunders, pp. 735-736.

---

243. A nurse is monitoring the results of serial arterial blood gases for the client who has been diagnosed with carbon monoxide poisoning and is asking for the oxygen mask to be removed. The nurse determines that the oxygen may be safely removed once the carboxyhemoglobin level decreases to less than:

1 5%
2 10%
3 15%
4 25%

Answer: 1

Rationale: Oxygen may be removed safely from the client with carbon monoxide poisoning once carboxyhemoglobin levels are less than 5%. Options 2, 3, and 4 are elevated levels.

Test-Taking Strategy: Focus on the issue: safely removing the oxygen. If you are unsure, it would be best to select the lowest level as identified in option 1. Review the normal carboxyhemoglobin levels if you had difficulty with this question.

Level of Cognitive Ability: Analysis
Client Needs: Physiological Integrity
Integrated Process: Teaching/Learning
Content Area: Adult Health/Respiratory

References:
Chernecky, C., & Berger, B. (2004). *Laboratory tests and diagnostic procedures* (4th ed.). Philadelphia: Saunders, p. 324.
Ignatavicius, D., & Workman, M. (2002). *Medical surgical nursing: Critical thinking for collaborative care* (4th ed.). Philadelphia: Saunders, p. 1566.

---

244. A nurse is teaching a pregnant client about nutrition. The nurse includes which information in the client's teaching plan?

1 The nutritional status of the mother significantly influences fetal growth and development
2 All mothers are at high risk for nutritional deficiencies
3 Calcium is not important until the third trimester
4 Iron supplements are not necessary unless the mother has iron-deficiency anemia

Answer: 1

Rationale: Poor nutrition during pregnancy can negatively influence fetal growth and development. Although pregnancy poses some nutritional risk for the mother, not all clients are at high risk. Calcium is critical during the third trimester but must be increased from the onset of pregnancy. Intake of dietary iron is insufficient for the majority of pregnant women, and iron supplements are routinely prescribed.

Test-Taking Strategy: Use the process of elimination. Option 2 uses the absolute word "all," therefore eliminate this option. Options 3 and 4 offer specific time frames or conditions for interventions; therefore, eliminate these options. Option 1 is a general or umbrella (global) option that is true for any stage of pregnancy. Review the importance of nutrition during pregnancy if you had difficulty with this question.

Level of Cognitive Ability: Application
Client Needs: Physiological Integrity
Integrated Process: Nursing Process/Implementation
Content Area: Maternity/Antepartum

Reference:
Lowdermilk, D., & Perry, A. (2004). *Maternity & women's health care* (8th ed.). St. Louis: Mosby, pp. 420-421.

---

245. A nurse is formulating a plan of care for a client receiving enteral feedings. The nurse identifies which nursing diagnosis as the highest priority for this client?
1 Imbalanced Nutrition, Less Than Body Requirements
2 Risk for Aspiration
3 Risk for Deficient Fluid Volume
4 Diarrhea

Answer: 2
Rationale: Any condition in which gastrointestinal motility is slowed or esophageal reflux is possible places a client at risk for aspiration. Although options 1, 3, and 4 may be a concern, these are not the priority.

Test-Taking Strategy: Note the key words "highest priority." Use the ABCs—airway, breathing, circulation. Option 2 addresses airway management. Options 1, 3, and 4 are possible problems, but not as high a priority as airway maintenance. Review care of the client receiving enteral feedings if you had difficulty with this question.

Level of Cognitive Ability: Analysis
Client Needs: Physiological Integrity
Integrated Process: Nursing Process/Analysis
Content Area: Delegating/Prioritizing

Reference:
Ignatavicius, D., & Workman, M. (2002). *Medical surgical nursing: Critical thinking for collaborative care* (4th ed.). Philadelphia: Saunders, p. 1370.

---

246. A client is admitted to the hospital with a diagnosis of Cushing's syndrome. The nurse monitors the client for which of the following that is most likely to occur in this client?
1 Deficient fluid volume
2 Hypoglycemia
3 Hypovolemia
4 Mental status changes

Answer: 4
Rationale: When Cushing's syndrome develops, the normal function of the glucocorticoids becomes exaggerated and the classic picture of the syndrome emerges. This exaggerated physiological action can cause mental status changes, including memory loss, poor concentration and cognition, euphoria, and depression. It can also cause persistent hyperglycemia along with sodium and water retention, producing edema and hypertension.

Test-Taking Strategy: Use the process of elimination. Eliminate options 1 and 3 first because they are similar. Recalling that hyperglycemia rather than hypoglycemia occurs in this condition will direct you to option 4. Review the manifestations of Cushing's syndrome if you had difficulty with this question.

Level of Cognitive Ability: Application
Client Needs: Physiological Integrity
Integrated Process: Nursing Process/Assessment
Content Area: Adult Health/Endocrine

Reference:
Ignatavicius, D., & Workman, M. (2002). *Medical surgical nursing: Critical thinking for collaborative care* (4th ed.). Philadelphia: Saunders, p. 1417.

247. A physician is performing indirect visualization of the larynx on a client to assess the function of the vocal cords. The nurse tells the client to do which of the following during the procedure?
1   Try to swallow
2   Hold the breath
3   Breathe normally
4   Roll the tongue to the back of the mouth

Answer: 3

Rationale: Indirect laryngoscopy is done to assess the function of the vocal cords or to obtain tissue for biopsy. Observations are made during rest and phonation by using a laryngeal mirror, head mirror, and light source. The client is placed in an upright position to facilitate passage of the laryngeal mirror into the mouth and is instructed to breathe normally. The tongue cannot be moved back because it would occlude the airway. Swallowing cannot be done with the mirror in place. The procedure takes longer than the time the client would be able to hold the breath, and this action is ineffective anyway.

Test-Taking Strategy: Use the process of elimination. Option 4 is eliminated first because it is not possible to move the tongue back with the mirror in place. It would also cause the airway to become occluded. Given the length of time needed to do the procedure, the client could not realistically hold the breath, so option 2 is eliminated next. Trying to swallow would actually cause the larynx to move against the mirror and could cause gagging. Review care of the client during indirect laryngoscopy if you had difficulty with this question.

Level of Cognitive Ability: Application
Client Needs: Physiological Integrity
Integrated Process: Nursing Process/Implementation
Content Area: Adult Health/Respiratory

Reference:
Ignatavicius, D., & Workman, M. (2002). *Medical surgical nursing: Critical thinking for collaborative care* (4th ed.). Philadelphia: Saunders, p. 486.

---

248. A nurse is caring for a client scheduled for a bilateral adrenalectomy for treatment of an adrenal tumor that is producing excessive aldosterone (primary hyperaldosteronism). The nurse most appropriately tells the client which of the following?
1   "You will most likely need to undergo chemotherapy after surgery."
2   "You will need to take hormone replacements for the rest of your life."
3   "You will need to wear an abdominal binder after surgery."
4   "You will not require any special long-term treatment after surgery."

Answer: 2

Rationale: The major cause of primary hyperaldosteronism is an aldosterone-secreting tumor called an aldosteronoma. Surgery is the treatment of choice. Clients undergoing a bilateral adrenalectomy will need permanent replacement of adrenal hormones. Option 1, 3, and 4 are inaccurate.

Test-Taking Strategy: Note the key word "bilateral." Recalling the function of the adrenal glands and that glucocorticoids and mineralocorticoids are essential to sustain life will direct you to option 2. Review care following bilateral adrenalectomy if you had difficulty with this question.

Level of Cognitive Ability: Application
Client Needs: Physiological Integrity
Integrated Process: Teaching/Learning
Content Area: Adult Health/Endocrine

Reference:
Ignatavicius, D., & Workman, M. (2002). *Medical surgical nursing: Critical thinking for collaborative care* (4th ed.). Philadelphia: Saunders, p. 1419.

249. A nurse is caring for a client who is scheduled for an adrenalectomy. The nurse plans to administer which medication in the preoperative period to prevent Addison's crisis?
1 Spironolactone (Aldactone) intramuscularly
2 Methylprednisolone sodium succinate (Solu-Medrol) intravenously
3 Prednisone (Deltasone) orally
4 Fludrocortisone (Florinef) subcutaneously

Answer: 2
Rationale: A glucocorticoid preparation will be administered intravenously or intramuscularly in the immediate preoperative period to a client scheduled for an adrenalectomy. Methylprednisolone sodium succinate protects the client from developing acute adrenal insufficiency (Addison's crisis) that occurs as a result of the adrenalectomy. Aldactone is a potassium-sparing diuretic. Prednisone is an oral corticosteroid. Fludrocortisone is a mineralocorticoid.

Test-Taking Strategy: Focus on the issue: preventing Addison's crisis in a client scheduled for adrenalectomy. Recalling the function of the adrenals will assist in eliminating options 1 and 4. From the remaining options, select option 2 because the client is preoperative and should receive medications via routes other than orally. Review preoperative care for the client scheduled for adrenalectomy if you had difficulty with this question.

Level of Cognitive Ability: Application
Client Needs: Physiological Integrity
Integrated Process: Nursing Process/Planning
Content Area: Adult Health/Endocrine

Reference:
Ignatavicius, D., & Workman, M. (2002). *Medical surgical nursing: Critical thinking for collaborative care* (4th ed.). Philadelphia: Saunders, p. 1418.

---

250. A nurse is preparing a client with Graves' disease to receive radioactive iodine therapy. The nurse tells the client which of the following about the therapy?
1 The radioactive iodine is designed to destroy the entire thyroid gland with just one dose
2 It takes 6 to 8 weeks after treatment to experience relief from the symptoms of the disease
3 The high levels of radioactivity prohibit contact with family for 4 weeks after initial treatment
4 Following the initial dose, subsequent treatments must continue lifelong

Answer: 2
Rationale: Following treatment with radioactive iodine therapy, a decrease in thyroid hormone level should be noted, which would help alleviate symptoms. Relief of symptoms does not occur until 6 to 8 weeks after initial treatment. This form of therapy is not designed to destroy the entire gland; rather, some of the cells that synthesize thyroid hormone will be destroyed by the local radiation. The nurse needs to reassure the client and family that unless the dosage is extremely high, clients are not required to observe radiation precautions. The rationale for this is that the radioactivity quickly dissipates. Occasionally, a client may require a second or third dose, but treatments are not lifelong.

Test-Taking Strategy: Use the process of elimination and knowledge regarding this treatment. Note the absolute words "entire," "prohibit," and "must" in the incorrect options. Review this treatment if you had difficulty with this question.

Level of Cognitive Ability: Application
Client Needs: Physiological Integrity
Integrated Process: Nursing Process/Implementation
Content Area: Adult Health/Endocrine

Reference:
Ignatavicius, D., & Workman, M. (2002). *Medical surgical nursing: Critical thinking for collaborative care* (4th ed.). Philadelphia: Saunders, pp. 1427-1428.

251. A client arrives at the emergency department with upper gastrointestinal (GI) bleeding and is in moderate distress. The priority nursing action is to:

1 Ask the client about the precipitating events
2 Insert a nasogastric (NG) tube and hematest the emesis
3 Complete an abdominal physical examination
4 Obtain vital signs

Answer: 4

Rationale: The priority action is to obtain vital signs to determine whether the client is in shock from blood loss and to obtain a baseline by which to monitor the progress of treatment. The client may not be able to provide subjective data until the immediate physical needs are met. Insertion of an NG tube may be prescribed but is not the priority action. A complete abdominal physical examination needs to be performed but is not the priority.

Test-Taking Strategy: Use the process of elimination, noting the key word "priority." Recall that the client with a GI bleed is at risk for shock. Also, option 4 addresses the ABCs—airway, breathing, and circulation. Review care of the client with a GI bleed if you had difficulty with this question

Level of Cognitive Ability: Application
Client Needs: Physiological Integrity
Integrated Process: Nursing Process/Implementation
Content Area: Delegating/Prioritizing

Reference:
Ignatavicius, D., & Workman, M. (2002). *Medical surgical nursing: Critical thinking for collaborative care* (4th ed.). Philadelphia: Saunders, p. 1341.

---

252. A client with acute renal failure is ordered to be on a fluid restriction of 1500 mL per day. The nurse best plans to assist the client with maintaining the restriction by:

1 Prohibiting beverages with sugar to minimize thirst
2 Using mouthwash with alcohol for mouth care
3 Asking the client to calculate the IV fluids into the total daily allotment
4 Removing the water pitcher from the bedside

Answer: 4

Rationale: The nurse can help the client maintain fluid restriction through a variety of means. One way is to provide frequent mouth care; however, alcohol-based products should be avoided because they are drying to mucous membranes. The use of ice chips and lip ointments are other interventions that may be helpful to the client on fluid restriction. Beverages that the client enjoys are provided and are not restricted based on sugar content. The client is not asked to keep track of IV fluid intake; this is the nurse's responsibility. The water pitcher should be removed from the bedside to aid in compliance.

Test-Taking Strategy: Use the process of elimination. Eliminate option 3 because this is a nursing responsibility. Eliminate option 2 next, because alcohol-based products are drying to oral mucous membranes and could exacerbate thirst. From the remaining options, focus on the key word "best" to direct you to option 4. Review measures to promote compliance with fluid restrictions if you had difficulty with this question.

Level of Cognitive Ability: Application
Client Needs: Physiological Integrity
Integrated Process: Nursing Process/Implementation
Content Area: Adult Health/Renal

Reference:
Ignatavicius, D., & Workman, M. (2002). *Medical surgical nursing: Critical thinking for collaborative care* (4th ed.). Philadelphia: Saunders, pp. 1684-1685.

253. A nurse has administered approximately half of a high cleansing enema when the client complains of pain and cramping. Which nursing action is appropriate?
  1 Raising the enema bag so that the solution can be completed quickly
  2 Clamping the tubing for 30 seconds and restarting the flow at a slower rate
  3 Reassuring the client and continuing the flow
  4 Discontinuing the enema and notifying the physician

Answer: 2
Rationale: The enema fluid should be administered slowly. If the client complains of pain or cramping, the flow is stopped for 30 seconds and restarted at a slower rate. Slow enema administration and stopping the flow temporarily, if necessary, will decrease the likelihood of intestinal spasm and premature ejection of the solution. The higher the solution container is held above the rectum, the faster the flow and the greater the force in the rectum. There is no need to discontinue the enema and notify the physician at this time.

Test-Taking Strategy: Use the process of elimination, focusing on the issue: alleviating pain and cramping. Eliminate options 1 and 3 first because they are similar. From the remaining options, noting that there is no need to notify the physician will direct you to option 2. Review the procedure for enema administration if you had difficulty with this question.

Level of Cognitive Ability: Application
Client Needs: Physiological Integrity
Integrated Process: Nursing Process/Implementation
Content Area: Fundamental Skills

Reference:
Potter, P., & Perry, A. (2005). *Fundamentals of nursing* (6th ed.). St. Louis: Mosby, p. 1401.

254. The client with chronic renal failure who is scheduled for hemodialysis this morning is due to receive a daily dose of enalapril (Vasotec). The nurse plans to administer this medication:
  1 Just before dialysis
  2 During dialysis
  3 Upon return from dialysis
  4 The day after dialysis

Answer: 3
Rationale: Antihypertensive medications, such as enalapril, are administered to the client following hemodialysis. This prevents the client from becoming hypotensive during dialysis and also from having the medication removed from the bloodstream by dialysis. There is no rationale for waiting a full day to resume the medication. This would lead to ineffective control of the blood pressure.

Test-Taking Strategy: Use the process of elimination. Think about the effects of an antihypertensive medication on the blood pressure when fluid is being removed from the body. Because hypotension is much more likely to occur in this circumstance, eliminate options 1 and 2. Most clients are hemodialyzed three times a week, so if the medication were held for dialysis until the following day, the client would miss three of the seven doses that would usually be given in a week. This would lead to ineffective blood pressure control. Therefore, eliminate option 4. Review the procedure for preparing a client for dialysis if you had difficulty with this question.

Level of Cognitive Ability: Application
Client Needs: Physiological Integrity
Integrated Process: Nursing Process/Planning
Content Area: Pharmacology

References:
Black, J., & Hawks, J. (2005). *Medical-surgical nursing: Clinical management for positive outcomes* (7th ed.). Philadelphia: Saunders, p. 961.
McKenry, L., & Salerno, E. (2003). *Mosby's pharmacology in nursing* (21st ed.). St. Louis: Mosby, pp. 586-587.

---

255. A nurse is preparing to administer a cleansing enema. The nurse positions the client in the:
  1 Left lateral position with the right leg acutely flexed
  2 Supine position with the legs elevated
  3 Dorsal recumbent position
  4 Right lateral position with the left leg acutely flexed

Answer: 1

Rationale: The sigmoid and descending colon are located on the left side. Therefore, the left lateral position uses gravity to facilitate the flow of solution into the sigmoid and descending colon. Acute flexion of the right leg allows for adequate exposure of the anus. Options 2, 3, and 4 are incorrect positions.

Test-Taking Strategy: Use the process of elimination. Visualize this procedure and think about the anatomy of the colon to direct you to option 1. Review this procedure if you had difficulty with this question.

Level of Cognitive Ability: Application
Client Needs: Physiological Integrity
Integrated Process: Nursing Process/Implementation
Content Area: Fundamental Skills

Reference:
Potter, P., & Perry, A. (2005). *Fundamentals of nursing* (6th ed.). St. Louis: Mosby, p. 1399.

---

256. A nurse is preparing to care for a client returning from the operating room following a subtotal thyroidectomy. The nurse anticipates the need for which of the following items to be placed at the bedside?
  1 Emergency tracheostomy kit
  2 Ampule of Saturated Solution of Potassium Iodide (SSKI)
  3 Hypothermia blanket
  4 Magnesium sulfate in a ready-to-inject vial

Answer: 1

Rationale: Respiratory distress can occur following thyroidectomy as a result of swelling in the tracheal area. The nurse would ensure that an emergency tracheostomy kit is available. SSKI is typically administered preoperatively to block thyroid hormone synthesis and release, as well as place the client in a euthyroid state. Surgery on the thyroid does not alter the heat control mechanism of the body. Magnesium sulfate would not be indicated because the incidence of hypomagnesemia is not a common problem post-thyroidectomy.

Test-Taking Strategy: Recall the anatomical location of the thyroid gland to direct you to option 1. Also, use the ABCs—airway, breathing, and circulation. Maintaining a patent airway is critical. Review care of the client following thyroidectomy if you had difficulty with this question.

Level of Cognitive Ability: Application
Client Needs: Physiological Integrity
Integrated Process: Nursing Process/Planning
Content Area: Adult Health/Endocrine

Reference:
Ignatavicius, D., & Workman, M. (2002). *Medical surgical nursing: Critical thinking for collaborative care* (4th ed.). Philadelphia: Saunders, p. 1429.

257. Sodium nitroprusside (Nipride) is prescribed for a client with a diagnosis of cardiogenic shock. The nurse plans to do which of the following when preparing to administer this medication?
1 Protect the solution from light
2 Add potassium to the infusion bag
3 Administer only through a central venous line
4 Obtain a baseline thiocyanate level

Answer: 1
Rationale: Sodium nitroprusside becomes unstable when exposed to light and must be protected. No other medications are added to the infusion bag. It can be given through a peripheral line. The level of thiocyanate (a nitroprusside metabolite similar to cyanide) is usually drawn if the client is maintained on this therapy for several days.

Test-Taking Strategy: Use the process of elimination and knowledge of the principles related to administering IV medications. Options 2 and 3 can be eliminated even without knowledge of this medication using these basic principles. Usually, levels of any medication or their by-products are drawn after administration has been ongoing, so eliminate option 4. Review this medication if you had difficulty with this question.

Level of Cognitive Ability: Application
Client Needs: Physiological Integrity
Integrated Process: Nursing Process/Planning
Content Area: Pharmacology

Reference:
Hodgson, B., & Kizior, R. (2004). *Saunders nursing drug handbook 2004.* Philadelphia: Saunders, p. 736.

---

258. A nurse is encouraging the client to cough and deep breathe after cardiac surgery. The nurse ensures that which of the following items is available to maximize the effectiveness of this procedure?
1 Ambu bag
2 Incisional splinting pillow
3 Suction equipment
4 Nebulizer

Answer: 2
Rationale: The use of an incisional splint such as a "cough pillow" can ease discomfort during coughing and deep breathing. The client who is comfortable will do more effective deep breathing and coughing exercises. Use of an incentive spirometer is also indicated. Options 1, 3, and 4 will not encourage the client to cough and deep breathe.

Test-Taking Strategy: Use the process of elimination. Focus on the issue: an item that will maximize effectiveness. This issue eliminates options 1 and 3, which are items used by the nurse. A nebulizer (option 4) is used to deliver medication. Review measures that will assist the postoperative client to cough and deep breathe if you had difficulty with this question.

Level of Cognitive Ability: Application
Client Needs: Physiological Integrity
Integrated Process: Nursing Process/Implementation
Content Area: Adult Health/Respiratory

Reference:
Potter, P., & Perry, A. (2005). *Fundamentals of nursing* (6th ed.). St. Louis: Mosby, p. 1616.

259. A nurse is preparing to administer an intermittent tube feeding through a nasogastric tube. The nurse assesses gastric residual before administering the tube feeding to:
1 Confirm proper nasogastric tube placement
2 Determine patency of the tube
3 Assess fluid and electrolyte status
4 Evaluate absorption of the last feeding

Answer: 4

Rationale: All stomach contents are aspirated and measured before administering a tube feeding. This procedure measures the gastric residual, which is determined in order to evaluate whether undigested formula from a previous feeding remains. It is important to assess gastric residual because administration of a tube feeding to a full stomach could result in overdistention, thus predisposing the client to regurgitation and possible aspiration. Assessing residual does not confirm placement, determine patency, or assess fluid and electrolyte status.

Test-Taking Strategy: Focus on the issue: the purpose for assessing the residual. Note the relationship between the issue and option 4. Review the purpose of assessing residual if you had difficulty with this question.

Level of Cognitive Ability: Application
Client Needs: Physiological Integrity
Integrated Process: Nursing Process/Assessment
Content Area: Fundamental Skills

Reference:
Ignatavicius, D., & Workman, M. (2002). *Medical surgical nursing: Critical thinking for collaborative care* (4th ed.). Philadelphia: Saunders, p. 1370.

260. A nurse is caring for a client scheduled to undergo a renal biopsy. To minimize the risk of post-procedure complications, the nurse reports which of the following laboratory results to the physician before the procedure?
1 Blood urea nitrogen (BUN): 18 mg/dL
2 Serum creatinine: 1.2 mg/dL
3 Bleeding time: 13 minutes
4 Potassium: 3.8 mEq/L

Answer: 3

Rationale: Post-procedure hemorrhage is a complication after renal biopsy. Because of this, bleeding times are assessed before the procedure. The normal bleeding time is 1 to 6 minutes depending on the type of test performed by the laboratory. The nurse ensures that these results are available and reports abnormalities promptly. Options 1, 2, and 4 identify normal values. The normal BUN is 5 to 20 mg/dL, the normal serum creatinine is 0.6 to 1.3 mg/dL, and the normal potassium is 3.5 to 5.1 mEq/L.

Test-Taking Strategy: When a client is to have a biopsy, remember that bleeding is a concern. This will direct you to option 3. Also note that options 1, 2, and 4 identify normal values. Review the complications of renal biopsy and normal laboratory values if you had difficulty with this question.

Level of Cognitive Ability: Analysis
Client Needs: Physiological Integrity
Integrated Process: Nursing Process/Implementation
Content Area: Adult Health/Renal

Reference:
Ignatavicius, D., & Workman, M. (2002). *Medical surgical nursing: Critical thinking for collaborative care* (4th ed.). Philadelphia: Saunders, p. 1610.

261. A client involved in a house fire is experiencing respiratory distress, and an inhalation injury is suspected. The nurse monitors which of the following for the presence of carbon monoxide poisoning?
1 Pulse oximetry
2 Urine myoglobin
3 Sputum carbon levels
4 Serum carboxyhemoglobin levels

Answer: 4
Rationale: Serum carboxyhemoglobin levels are the most direct measure of carbon monoxide poisoning, provide the level of poisoning, and thus determine the appropriate treatment measures. The carbon monoxide molecule has a 200 times greater affinity for binding with hemoglobin than an oxygen molecule, causing decreased availability of oxygen to the cells. Clients are treated with 100% oxygen. Options 1, 2, and 3 would not identify carbon monoxide poisoning.

Test-Taking Strategy: Use the process of elimination. Note the relationship between "carbon monoxide" and option 4. Review carbon monoxide poisoning if you had difficulty with this question.

Level of Cognitive Ability: Application
Client Needs: Physiological Integrity
Integrated Process: Nursing Process/Assessment
Content Area: Adult Health/Respiratory

References:
Black, J., & Hawks, J. (2005). *Medical-surgical nursing: Clinical management for positive outcomes* (7th ed.). Philadelphia: Saunders, p. 1906.
Chernecky, C., & Berger, B. (2004). *Laboratory tests and diagnostic procedures* (4th ed.). Philadelphia: Saunders, p. 324.

262. A nurse is assigned to care for a client with hypertonic labor contractions. The nurse plans to conserve the client's energy and promote rest by:
1 Avoiding uncomfortable procedures such as intravenous infusions or epidural anesthesia
2 Assisting the client with breathing and relaxation techniques
3 Keeping the room brightly lit so the client can watch her monitor
4 Keeping the television (TV) or radio on to provide distraction

Answer: 2
Rationale: Breathing and relaxation techniques aid the client in coping with the discomfort of labor and in conserving energy. Intravenous or epidural pain relief can be useful. Intravenous hydration can increase perfusion and oxygenation of maternal and fetal tissues and provide glucose for energy needs. Noise from a TV or radio and light stimulation does not promote rest. A quiet, dim environment would be more advantageous.

Test-Taking Strategy: Focus on the issue: conserving energy and promoting rest for the client. Noting the key word "assisting" in option 2 will direct you to this option. Review care of the client with hypertonic labor contractions if you had difficulty with this question.

Level of Cognitive Ability: Application
Client Needs: Physiological Integrity
Integrated Process: Nursing Process/Planning
Content Area: Maternity/Antepartum

Reference:
Lowdermilk, D., & Perry, A. (2004). *Maternity & women's health care* (8th ed.). St. Louis: Mosby, p. 577.

263. A client with acute pyelonephritis has nausea and is vomiting and is scheduled for an intravenous pyelogram. The nurse places highest priority on which action?
1 Place the client on hourly intake and output measurements
2 Request an order for an intravenous infusion from the physician
3 Ask the client to sign the informed consent
4 Explain the procedure thoroughly to the client

Answer: 2
Rationale: The highest priority of the nurse would be to request an order for an intravenous infusion. This is needed to replace fluid lost with vomiting, will be necessary for dye injection for the procedure, and will assist with the elimination of the dye following the procedure. The intake and output should be measured, but this will not assist in preventing dehydration. Explanation of the procedure and obtaining the signed informed consent are done once the client's physiological needs are met.

Test-Taking Strategy: Using Maslow's hierarchy of needs theory will assist in eliminating options 3 and 4. From the remaining options, noting that the client is vomiting will direct you to option 2. Review care of the client who is vomiting if you had difficulty with this question.

Level of Cognitive Ability: Application
Client Needs: Physiological Integrity
Integrated Process: Nursing Process/Implementation
Content Area: Adult Health/Renal

Reference:
Ignatavicius, D., & Workman, M. (2002). *Medical surgical nursing: Critical thinking for collaborative care* (4th ed.). Philadelphia: Saunders, pp. 163; 165.

264. A nurse is planning care for a client with a T-3 spinal cord injury. The nurse includes which intervention in the plan to prevent autonomic dysreflexia (hyperreflexia)?
1 Assess vital signs and observe for hypotension, tachycardia, and tachypnea
2 Teach the client that this condition is relatively minor with few symptoms
3 Assist the client to develop a daily bowel routine to prevent constipation
4 Administer dexamethasone (Decadron) as per physician's order

Answer: 3
Rationale: Autonomic dysreflexia (hyperreflexia) is a potentially life-threatening condition and may be triggered by bladder distention, bowel distention, visceral distention, or stimulation of pain receptors in the skin. A daily bowel program eliminates this trigger. A client with autonomic dysreflexia would be hypertensive and bradycardic. Removal of the stimuli results in prompt resolution of the signs and symptoms. Option 4 is unrelated to this specific condition.

Test-Taking Strategy: Focus on the key word "prevent" to eliminate options 1 and 2. From the remaining options, remembering that this condition may be triggered by bowel distention will direct you to option 3. Review the causes if you are unfamiliar with this syndrome.

Level of Cognitive Ability: Application
Client Needs: Physiological Integrity
Integrated Process: Nursing Process/Planning
Content Area: Adult Health/Neurological

References:
Black, J., & Hawks, J. (2005). *Medical-surgical nursing: Clinical management for positive outcomes* (7th ed.). Philadelphia: Saunders, p. 904.
Ignatavicius, D., & Workman, M. (2002). *Medical surgical nursing: Critical thinking for collaborative care* (4th ed.). Philadelphia: Saunders, pp. 931; 935.

265. A client in cardiogenic shock has an order for an intravenous (IV) nitroglycerin (Nitrostat) drip for control of chest pain and to increase myocardial tissue perfusion. The nurse understands that the nitroglycerin must be prepared by mixing the medication:

1 In a solution that is in a plastic bag
2 In a solution that is in a glass bottle
3 Every hour because of its unstable chemical structure
4 Under a laminar flow hood

Answer: 2

Rationale: IV nitroglycerin is prepared only in glass bottles, using the administration sets provided. Standard plastic (polyvinyl chloride) tubing will adsorb the nitroglycerin, thus reducing the potency and reliability of the medication. It should also be protected from extremes of light and temperature. It should be remixed every 4 hours. It does not require mixture under a laminar flow hood.

Test-Taking Strategy: Use the process of elimination. Eliminate option 3 because "every hour" is much too frequent. From the remaining options, note that options 1 and 2 provide opposite methods of administration. This should provide a clue that one of these methods may be accurate. Remember: standard plastic will absorb the nitroglycerin. Review the procedure for preparing IV nitroglycerin if you had difficulty with this question.

Level of Cognitive Ability: Analysis
Client Needs: Physiological Integrity
Integrated Process: Nursing Process/Implementation
Content Area: Pharmacology

Reference:
McKenry, L., & Salerno, E. (2003). *Mosby's pharmacology in nursing* (21st ed.). St. Louis: Mosby, p. 609.

---

266. A client has a left pleural effusion that has not yet been treated. The nurse plans to have which of the following items available for immediate use?

1 Thoracentesis tray
2 Paracentesis tray
3 Intubation tray
4 Central venous line insertion tray

Answer: 1

Rationale: The client with a significant pleural effusion is usually treated by thoracentesis. This procedure allows drainage of the fluid, which may then be analyzed to determine the precise cause of the effusion. The nurse ensures that a thoracentesis tray is readily available in case the client's symptoms should rapidly become more severe. A paracentesis tray is needed for the removal of abdominal effusion. Options 3 and 4 are not specifically indicated for this procedure.

Test-Taking Strategy: Use the process of elimination and knowledge regarding the usual treatment for pleural effusion. Note the relationship between the word "pleural" in the question and "thoracentesis" in the correct option. Review the treatment for pleural effusion if you had difficulty with this question.

Level of Cognitive Ability: Application
Client Needs: Physiological Integrity
Integrated Process: Nursing Process/Planning
Content Area: Adult Health/Respiratory

Reference:
Black, J., & Hawks, J. (2005). *Medical-surgical nursing: Clinical management for positive outcomes* (7th ed.). Philadelphia: Saunders, p. 1873.

267. A client has been taking procainamide (Pronestyl) 750 mg orally twice a day. The nurse prepares to administer the medication and implements which of the following before giving the medication?
1 Nothing, because this is a nontoxic medication
2 Checks the blood pressure and pulse
3 Schedules the client for a drug level to be drawn 1 hour after the dose
4 Obtains a complete blood cell count and liver function studies

Answer: 2
Rationale: Procainamide is an antidysrhythmic medication. Before the medication is administered, the client's blood pressure and pulse are checked. This medication can cause toxic effects, and serum blood levels would be checked before administering the medication (therapeutic serum level is 3 to 10 mcg/mL). Obtaining a complete blood cell count and liver function studies is unnecessary.

Test-Taking Strategy: Use the steps of the nursing process. This will direct you to option 2 because it is the only assessment action. Also recalling that this medication is an antidysrhythmic will direct you to the correct option. Review this medication if you had difficulty with this question.

Level of Cognitive Ability: Application
Client Needs: Physiological Integrity
Integrated Process: Nursing Process/Implementation
Content Area: Pharmacology

Reference:
Hodgson, B., & Kizior, R. (2004). *Saunders nursing drug handbook 2004.* Philadelphia: Saunders, p. 836.

---

268. A client with urolithiasis is being evaluated to determine the type of stone that is being formed. The nurse plans to keep which of the following items available in the client's room to assist in this process?
1 A calorie count sheet
2 A strainer
3 An intake and output record
4 A vital signs graphic sheet

Answer: 2
Rationale: The urine is strained until the stone is passed and obtained and analyzed. Straining the urine will catch small stones that may be sent to the laboratory for analysis. Once the type of stone is determined, an individualized plan of care for prevention and treatment is developed. Options 1, 3, and 4 are unrelated to the question.

Test-Taking Strategy: Focus on the issue: an item that will help determine the type of stone. Eliminate options 1, 3, and 4 because these items give information about food intake, vital signs, and fluid balance, but will not provide data that will help determine the type of stone. Review care of the client with urolithiasis if you had difficulty with this question.

Level of Cognitive Ability: Application
Client Needs: Physiological Integrity
Integrated Process: Nursing Process/Planning
Content Area: Adult Health/Renal

Reference:
Black, J., & Hawks, J. (2005). *Medical-surgical nursing: Clinical management for positive outcomes* (7th ed.). Philadelphia: Saunders, p. 887.

269. A client develops bilateral wheezes, orthopnea, and tachypnea, and the nurse notes the presence of 2+ pitting edema. The nurse suspects pulmonary edema and notifies the physician. While awaiting the physician's arrival, the nurse avoids which action?
  1 Preparing to administer IV morphine sulfate
  2 Placing the client in the high-Fowler's position
  3 Elevating the client's legs
  4 Preparing to administer IV furosemide (Lasix)

Answer: 3
Rationale: Elevating the client's legs would rapidly increase venous return to the right side of the heart and worsen the client's condition. The feet should be in the horizontal position, or the client could dangle at the bedside if the client's condition permits. Anxiety causes an increase in the oxygen demands on the heart. Morphine sulfate reduces anxiety and causes peripheral vasodilation and is likely to be prescribed. A high-Fowler's position increases the thoracic capacity, allowing for improved ventilation. Furosemide will be prescribed because of its diuretic action.

Test-Taking Strategy: Use the process of elimination and note the key word "avoids." This word indicates a false-response question and that you need to select the option that is an incorrect nursing action. Recalling that the pulmonary system is congested will direct you to option 3 because this action would cause further congestion of the pulmonary system. Review care of the client with pulmonary edema if you had difficulty with this question.

Level of Cognitive Ability: Application
Client Needs: Physiological Integrity
Integrated Process: Nursing Process/Implementation
Content Area: Adult Health/Cardiovascular

Reference:
Black, J., & Hawks, J. (2005). *Medical-surgical nursing: Clinical management for positive outcomes* (7th ed.). Philadelphia: Saunders, p. 1880.

270. A nurse is preparing to care for a client following ureterolithotomy who has a ureteral catheter in place. The nurse plans to implement which action in the management of this catheter when the client arrives from the recovery room?
  1 Irrigates the catheter using 10 mL sterile normal saline
  2 Places tension on the catheter
  3 Clamps the catheter
  4 Checks the drainage from the catheter

Answer: 4
Rationale: Drainage from the ureteral catheter should be checked when the client returns from the recovery room and at least every 1 to 2 hours thereafter. The catheter drains urine from the renal pelvis, which has a capacity of 3 to 5 mL. If the volume of urine or fluid in the renal pelvis increases, tissue damage to the pelvis will result from pressure. Therefore, the ureteral tube is never clamped. Additionally, irrigation is not performed unless there is a specific physician's order to do so.

Test-Taking Strategy: Focus on the issue, a ureteral catheter, and think about the anatomy of the kidney. Recalling that the ureteral catheter is placed in the renal pelvis and recalling the anatomy of this anatomical location will assist in eliminating options 1, 2, and 3. Review care of the client with a ureteral catheter if you had difficulty with this question.

Level of Cognitive Ability: Application
Client Needs: Physiological Integrity
Integrated Process: Nursing Process/Implementation
Content Area: Adult Health/Renal

Reference:
Lewis, S., Heitkemper, M., & Dirksen, S. (2004). *Medical-surgical nursing: Assessment and management of clinical problems* (6th ed.). St. Louis: Mosby, p. 1201.

271. Before administering a tube feeding, a nurse aspirates 40 mL of undigested formula from the client's nasogastric tube. The nurse understands that before administering the tube feeding, the 40 mL of gastric aspirate should be:

1 Discarded properly and recorded as output on the client's I & O record
2 Poured into the nasogastric tube through a syringe with the plunger removed
3 Mixed with the formula and poured into the nasogastric tube through a syringe without a plunger
4 Diluted with water and injected into the nasogastric tube using a syringe and putting pressure on the plunger

Answer: 2

Rationale: After checking residual feeding contents, the nurse reinstills the gastric contents into the stomach by removing the syringe bulb or plunger and pouring the gastric contents via the syringe into the nasogastric tube. Gastric contents should be reinstilled (unless they exceed an amount of 100 mL or as defined by agency policy) in order to maintain the client's electrolyte balance. It does not need to be mixed with water, nor should it be discarded or mixed with formula.

Test-Taking Strategy: Use the process of elimination. Remembering that the removal of the gastric contents could disturb the client's electrolyte balance will assist in eliminating option 1. Eliminate option 4 next because of the word "pressure." From the remaining options, recalling that gastric contents aspirated are not mixed with formula will assist in directing you to the correct option. Review this procedure if you had difficulty with this question.

Level of Cognitive Ability: Application
Client Needs: Physiological Integrity
Integrated Process: Nursing Process/Implementation
Content Area: Fundamental Skills

Reference:
Elkin, M., Perry, A., & Potter, P. (2004). *Nursing interventions & clinical skills* (3rd ed.). St. Louis: Mosby, p. 810.

272. A client is beginning to take oral bisacodyl (Dulcolax). To achieve a rapid effect from the medication, the nurse tells the client to take the medication:

1 At bedtime
2 With two glasses of milk
3 With a large meal
4 On an empty stomach

Answer: 4

Rationale: The most rapid effect from dulcolax occurs when it is taken on an empty stomach. It will not have a rapid effect if taken with a large meal. If it is taken at bedtime, the client will have a bowel movement in the morning. Taking the medication with two glasses of milk will not speed up its effect.

Test-Taking Strategy: Focus on the issue: achieving a rapid effect. Recalling that medications generally are more effective if taken on an empty stomach will direct you to option 4. Review the concepts related to administering this medication if you had difficulty with this question.

Level of Cognitive Ability: Application
Client Needs: Physiological Integrity
Integrated Process: Teaching/Learning
Content Area: Pharmacology

Reference:
Hodgson, B., & Kizior, R. (2004). *Saunders nursing drug handbook 2004.* Philadelphia: W. B. Saunders, p. 111.

273. A client with acute respiratory distress syndrome has an order to be placed on a continuous positive airway pressure (CPAP) face mask. The nurse implements which of the following for this procedure to be most effective?
1 Applies the mask to the face with a snug fit
2 Obtains baseline arterial blood gases
3 Obtains baseline pulse oximetry levels
4 Encourages the client to remove the mask frequently for coughing and deep breathing exercises

Answer: 1
Rationale: The face mask must be applied over the nose and mouth with a snug fit, which is necessary to maintain positive pressure in the client's airways. The nurse obtains baseline respiratory assessments and arterial blood gases to evaluate the effectiveness of therapy, but these are not done to increase the effectiveness of the procedure. A disadvantage of the CPAP face mask is that the client must remove it for coughing, eating, or drinking. This removes the benefit of positive pressure in the airway each time it is removed.

Test-Taking Strategy: Focus on the issue: a nursing action that will make the procedure most effective. Options 2 and 3 do not make the therapy more effective and are eliminated. From the remaining options, knowing that positive pressure must be maintained to be effective will direct you to option 1. Review care of the client with a CPAP face mask if you had difficulty with this question.

Level of Cognitive Ability: Application
Client Needs: Physiological Integrity
Integrated Process: Nursing Process/Implementation
Content Area: Adult Health/Respiratory

References:
Elkin, M., Perry, A., & Potter, P. (2004). *Nursing interventions & clinical skills* (3rd ed.). St. Louis: Mosby, p. 758.
Lewis, S., Heitkemper, M., & Dirksen, S. (2004). *Medical-surgical nursing: Assessment and management of clinical problems* (6th ed.). St. Louis: Mosby, p. 1785.

274. A nurse is caring for a client scheduled to undergo a cardiac catheterization for the first time. The nurse tells the client that the:
1 Procedure is performed in the operating room
2 Client may feel fatigue and have various aches, because it is necessary to lie quietly on a hard X-ray table for about 4 hours
3 Client may feel certain sensations at various points during the procedure, such as a fluttery feeling, flushed warm feeling, desire to cough, or palpitations
4 Initial catheter insertion is quite painful; after that, there is little or no pain

Answer: 3
Rationale: Preprocedure teaching points include that the procedure is done in a darkened cardiac catheterization room and that ECG leads are attached to the client. A local anesthetic is used so there is little to no pain with catheter insertion. The X-ray table is hard and may be tilted periodically. The procedure may take up to 2 hours, and the client may feel various sensations with catheter passage and dye injection.
Test-Taking Strategy: Use the process of elimination. The location (operating room) eliminates option 1. The duration of the procedure, 4 hours, eliminates option 2. From the remaining options, noting the words "quite painful" in option 4 will assist in eliminating this option. Review client preparation for this procedure if you had difficulty with this question.

Level of Cognitive Ability: Application
Client Needs: Physiological Integrity
Integrated Process: Teaching/Learning
Content Area: Adult Health/Cardiovascular

Reference:
Ignatavicius, D., & Workman, M. (2002). *Medical surgical nursing: Critical thinking for collaborative care* (4th ed.). Philadelphia: Saunders, p. 642.

275. A client with acquired immunodeficiency syndrome (AIDS) will be receiving aerosolized pentamidine isethionate (NebuPent) prophylactically once every 4 weeks. The home health nurse visits and instructs the client about the medication. Which statement by the client indicates a need for further teaching?

1 "If I develop a cough or shortness of breath after receiving the inhalation therapy, I need to let a doctor or nurse know."
2 "If I have any visual disturbances, I need to let the doctor know."
3 "There are no known side effects of this therapy."
4 "I may experience some nausea with the inhalation therapy."

Answer: 3

Rationale: Side effects associated with this therapy include nausea, visual disturbances, or shortness of breath. The client needs to inform the health care provider if these side effects occur.

Test-Taking Strategy: Note the key words "indicates a need for further teaching." These words indicate a false-response question and that you need to select the option that indicates an incorrect client statement. Noting the words "no known side effects" in option 3 will direct you to this option. Review this medication if you had difficulty with this question.

Level of Cognitive Ability: Analysis
Client Needs: Physiological Integrity
Integrated Process: Teaching/Learning
Content Area: Adult Health/Immune

References:
Hodgson, B., & Kizior, R. (2004). *Saunders nursing drug handbook 2004.* Philadelphia: Saunders, p. 793.

---

276. A nurse admits a client with myocardial infarction (MI) to the coronary care unit (CCU). The nurse plans to do which of the following in delivering care to this client?

1 Administer oxygen at a rate of 6 liters per minute by nasal cannula
2 Infuse intravenous (IV) fluid at a rate of 150 mL per hour
3 Begin thrombolytic therapy
4 Place the client on continuous cardiac monitoring

Answer: 4

Rationale: Standard interventions upon admittance to the CCU as they relate to this question include continuous cardiac monitoring, administering oxygen at a rate of 2 to 4 liters per minute unless otherwise ordered, and ensuring an adequate IV line insertion of an intermittent lock. If an IV infusion is administered, it is maintained at a keep vein open rate to prevent fluid overload and heart failure. Thrombolytic therapy may or may not be prescribed by the physician. Thrombolytic agents are most effective if administered within the first 6 hours of the coronary event.

Test-Taking Strategy: Use the process of elimination. Eliminate options 1 and 2 because the values related to the rates of oxygen and IV fluid are high. From the remaining options, note the relationship between the client's diagnosis and option 4. Review care of the client following MI if you had difficulty with this question.

Level of Cognitive Ability: Application
Client Needs: Physiological Integrity
Integrated Process: Nursing Process/Planning
Content Area: Adult Health/Cardiovascular

Reference:
Ignatavicius, D., & Workman, M. (2002). *Medical surgical nursing: Critical thinking for collaborative care* (4th ed.). Philadelphia: Saunders, pp. 795-796; 798.

277. A nurse is trying to analyze an ECG rhythm strip on an assigned client and asks another nurse how much time each small box on the ECG paper represents. The second nurse responds that each small box measures:

1 0.02 second
2 0.04 second
3 0.20 second
4 0.40 second

Answer: 2

Rationale: Standard ECG graph paper measurements are 0.04 seconds for each small box on the horizontal axis (measuring time) and 1 mm (measuring voltage) for each small box on the vertical axis.

Test-Taking Strategy: Knowledge regarding ECG basics is necessary to answer this question. Review these basics because they will be helpful in answering questions related to dysrhythmias.

Level of Cognitive Ability: Comprehension
Client Needs: Physiological Integrity
Integrated Process: Teaching/Learning
Content Area: Adult Health/Cardiovascular

Reference:
Black, J., & Hawks, J. (2005). *Medical-surgical nursing: Clinical management for positive outcomes* (7th ed.). Philadelphia: Saunders, pp. 1583-1584.

---

278. A nurse is applying ECG electrodes to a diaphoretic client. The nurse does which of the following to keep the electrodes from coming loose?

1 Secures the electrodes with adhesive tape
2 Places clear, transparent dressings over the electrodes
3 Applies lanolin to the skin before applying the electrodes
4 Cleanses the skin with alcohol before applying the electrodes

Answer: 4

Rationale: Alcohol defats the skin and will help the electrodes adhere to the skin. Placing adhesive tape or a clear dressing over the electrodes will not help the adhesive gel of the actual electrode to make better contact with the diaphoretic skin. Lanolin or any other lotion makes the skin slippery and prevents good initial adherence.

Test-Taking Strategy: Use the process of elimination. Note that options 1 and 2 are similar in that they both provide an external form of providing security of the electrodes. From the remaining options, note that option 4 addresses cleansing the skin. Review the procedure for attaching ECG electrodes if you had difficulty with this question.

Level of Cognitive Ability: Application
Client Needs: Physiological Integrity
Integrated Process: Nursing Process/Implementation
Content Area: Adult Health/Cardiovascular

Reference:
Elkin, M., Perry, A., & Potter, P. (2004). *Nursing interventions & clinical skills* (3rd ed.). St. Louis: Mosby, p. 405.

279. A nurse has developed a plan of care for a client with a diagnosis of anterior cord syndrome. Which intervention would the nurse include in the plan of care?

1 Assess the client's sensation of vibration
2 Remind the client to change positions slowly
3 Assess the client's sensation of touch
4 Teach the client about loss of motor function and decreased pain sensation

Answer: 4

Rationale: Clinical findings related to anterior cord syndrome include loss of motor function and decreased pain sensation below the level of injury. The syndrome does not affect sensations of touch, motion, position, and vibration.

Test-Taking Strategy: Specific knowledge of anterior cord syndrome is necessary to answer this question. Remember that this type of injury involves complete motor function loss and decreased pain sensation. If you are unfamiliar with this syndrome, review the nursing interventions related to the disorder.

Level of Cognitive Ability: Application
Client Needs: Physiological Integrity
Integrated Process: Nursing Process/Planning
Content Area: Adult Health/Neurological

Reference:
Black, J., & Hawks, J. (2005). *Medical-surgical nursing: Clinical management for positive outcomes* (7th ed.). Philadelphia: Saunders, p. 2215.

---

280. A nurse is caring for a client with a thoracic spinal cord injury. As part of the nursing care plan, the nurse monitors for spinal shock. In the event that spinal shock occurs, the nurse anticipates that the most likely intravenous (IV) fluid to be prescribed would be:

1 5% dextrose in water
2 Dextran
3 5% dextrose in 0.9% normal saline
4 0.9% normal saline

Answer: 4

Rationale: Normal saline 0.9% is an isotonic solution that primarily remains in the intravascular space, increasing intravascular volume. This IV fluid would increase the client's blood pressure. Dextran is rarely used in spinal shock because isotonic fluid administration is usually sufficient. Additionally, Dextran has potentially serious side effects. Dextrose 5% in water is a hypotonic solution that pulls fluid out of the intravascular space and is not indicated for shock. Dextrose 5% in normal saline 0.9% is hypertonic and indicated for shock resulting from hemorrhage or burns.

Test-Taking Strategy: Focus on the issue: spinal shock. Knowledge of the treatment for spinal shock and the purpose of the various IV fluids will direct you to option 4. Review the IV therapy associated with this disorder if you had difficulty with this question.

Level of Cognitive Ability: Analysis
Client Needs: Physiological Integrity
Integrated Process: Nursing Process/Planning
Content Area: Adult Health/Neurological

Reference:
Black, J., & Hawks, J. (2005). *Medical-surgical nursing: Clinical management for positive outcomes* (7th ed.). Philadelphia: Saunders, pp. 210; 2218.

281. A nurse is preparing to teach a client how to ambulate with a cane. Before teaching cane-assisted ambulation, the priority nursing assessment is to determine:
1 That the client has full range of motion ability
2 The client's balance, strength, and confidence
3 If the client is self-conscious about using a cane
4 That the client has a high level of stamina

Answer: 2

Rationale: Assessing the client's balance, strength, and confidence helps determine if the appropriate assistive device has been chosen. Full range of motion and a high level of stamina are not needed for walking with a cane. Although body image (self-consciousness) is a component of the assessment, it is not the priority.

Test-Taking Strategy: Note the key word "priority" in the stem of the question. Eliminate options 1 and 4 first because they are not required for the use of a cane. Use Maslow's hierarchy of needs theory to assist in directing you to option 2. Review teaching points related to the use of a cane if you had difficulty with this question.

Level of Cognitive Ability: Analysis
Client Needs: Physiological Integrity
Integrated Process: Nursing Process/Assessment
Content Area: Fundamental Skills

Reference:
Potter, P., & Perry, A. (2005). *Fundamentals of nursing* (6th ed.). St. Louis: Mosby, pp. 948-949.

282. A client has Buck's extension traction applied to the right leg. The nurse plans which of the following interventions to prevent complications of the device?
1 Massage the skin of the right leg with lotion every 8 hours
2 Provide pin care once a shift
3 Inspect the skin on the right leg at least once every 8 hours
4 Release the weights on the right leg for range of motion exercises daily

Answer: 3

Rationale: Buck's extension traction is a type of skin traction. The nurse inspects the skin of the limb in traction at least once every 8 hours for irritation or inflammation. Massaging the skin with lotion is not indicated. The nurse never releases the weights of traction unless specifically ordered by the physician. There are no pins to care for with skin traction.

Test-Taking Strategy: Focus on the issue: Buck's extension traction. Recalling that there are no pins in Buck's traction and that the nurse never removes weights without a specific order to do so eliminates options 2 and 4. From the remaining options, noting that the device would have to be removed to apply lotion will direct you to option 3. Also, use of the nursing process will direct you to option 3 because it is the only assessment action. Review care of the client in Buck's extension traction if you had difficulty with this question.

Level of Cognitive Ability: Application
Client Needs: Physiological Integrity
Integrated Process: Nursing Process/Planning
Content Area: Adult Health/Musculoskeletal

Reference:
Ignatavicius, D., & Workman, M. (2002). *Medical surgical nursing: Critical thinking for collaborative care* (4th ed.). Philadelphia: Saunders, p. 1137.

283. A nurse is assessing a client with cardiac disease at the 30-week gestation antenatal visit. The nurse assesses lung sounds in the lower lobes following a routine blood pressure screening. The nurse performs this assessment to:

1 Identify cardiac dysrhythmias
2 Rule out the possibility of pneumonia
3 Assess for early signs of congestive heart failure (CHF)
4 Identify mitral valve prolapse

Answer: 3

Rationale: Fluid volume during pregnancy peaks between 18 to 32 weeks' gestation. During this period, it is essential to observe and record maternal data that would indicate further signs of cardiac decompensation or CHF in the pregnant client. By assessing lung sounds in the lower lobes, the nurse may identify early symptoms of diminished oxygen exchange and potential CHF. Options 1, 2, and 4 are not related to the issue of the question.

Test-Taking Strategy: Focus on the data provided in the question. Note the relationship between cardiac disease and lung sounds in the question and the words "congestive heart failure" in the correct option. Review the complications associated with pregnancy in the client with cardiac disease if you had difficulty with this question.

Level of Cognitive Ability: Analysis
Client Needs: Physiological Integrity
Integrated Process: Nursing Process/Assessment
Content Area: Maternity/Antepartum

References:
McKinney, E., James, S., Murray, S., & Ashwill, J. (2005). *Maternal-child nursing* (2nd ed.). St. Louis: Elsevier, p. 655.
Lowdermilk, D., & Perry, A. (2004). *Maternity &woman's health care* (8th ed.). St. Louis: Mosby, p. 911.

284. A nurse is caring for a client with a newly applied plaster leg cast. The nurse prevents the development of compartment syndrome by:

1 Elevating the limb and applying ice to the affected leg
2 Elevating the limb and covering the limb with bath blankets
3 Placing the leg in a slightly dependent position and applying ice
4 Keeping the leg horizontal and applying ice to the affected leg

Answer: 1

Rationale: Compartment syndrome is prevented by controlling edema. This is achieved most optimally with the use of elevation and the application of ice. The use of bath blankets or a dependent or horizontal leg position will not prevent this syndrome.

Test-Taking Strategy: Use the process of elimination. Recalling that edema is controlled or prevented with limb elevation helps eliminate options 3 and 4. From the remaining options, think about the effects of ice versus bath blankets. Ice will further control edema, whereas bath blankets will produce heat and prevent air circulation needed for the cast to dry. Review interventions to prevent complications following cast application if you had difficulty with this question.

Level of Cognitive Ability: Application
Client Needs: Physiological Integrity
Integrated Process: Nursing Process/Implementation
Content Area: Adult Health/Musculoskeletal

Reference:
Ignatavicius, D., & Workman, M. (2002). *Medical surgical nursing: Critical thinking for collaborative care* (4th ed.). Philadelphia: Saunders, p. 1135.

285. A client undergoing hemodialysis becomes hypotensive. The nurse avoids taking which of the following contraindicated actions?
1 Checking the client's weight and reassessing blood pressure
2 Preparing to administer a 250 mL normal saline bolus
3 Increasing the blood flow from the client into the dialyzer
4 Raising the client's legs and feet

Answer: 3

Rationale: To treat hypotension during hemodialysis, the nurse raises the client's feet and legs to enhance cardiac return. A normal saline bolus of up to 500 mL may be given to increase circulating volume. The nurse would check the client's weight and reassess the blood pressure. Finally, the transmembrane hydrostatic pressure or the blood flow rate into the dialyzer may be decreased. All of these measures should improve the circulating volume and blood pressure.

Test-Taking Strategy: Note the key word "avoids." This word indicates a false-response question and that you need to select the option that is an incorrect nursing action. Focus on the issue, hypotension, and note that the client is being dialyzed. Thinking about each action in the options and how it may affect the blood pressure will direct you to option 3. Review the treatment for this complication of dialysis if you had difficulty with this question.

Level of Cognitive Ability: Application
Client Needs: Physiological Integrity
Integrated Process: Nursing Process/Implementation
Content Area: Adult Health/Renal

Reference:
Lewis, S., Heitkemper, M., & Dirksen, S. (2004). *Medical-surgical nursing: Assessment and management of clinical problems* (6th ed.). St. Louis: Mosby, p. 1236.

286. A nurse is preparing a client for cardioversion using anterolateral paddle placement. The nurse places the conductive gel pads at which areas on the client's chest in preparation for this procedure?
1 Right second intercostal space and left fifth intercostal space at anterior axillary line
2 Left second intercostal space and left fifth intercostal space at midaxillary line
3 Right fourth intercostal space and left fifth intercostal space at anterior axillary line
4 Left fourth intercostal space and left fifth intercostal space at midaxillary line

Answer: 1

Rationale: Anterolateral paddle placement for external countershock involves placing one paddle at the right second intercostal space and the other at the fifth intercostal space at the anterior axillary line.

Test-Taking Strategy: Use the process of elimination. Remember that the paddles are positioned so the electric shock travels through as much myocardium as possible. Visualize each of the placements as described and use knowledge of cardiothoracic landmarks, remembering the position of the heart in the chest. This will direct you to option 1. Review the procedure for cardioversion if you had difficulty with this question.

Level of Cognitive Ability: Application
Client Needs: Physiological Integrity
Integrated Process: Nursing Process/Implementation
Content Area: Adult Health/Cardiovascular

Reference:
Black, J., & Hawks, J. (2005). *Medical-surgical nursing: Clinical management for positive outcomes* (7th ed.). Philadelphia: Saunders, p. 1689.

287. A nurse is preparing a client for venography. The nurse understands that which of the following is unnecessary before this procedure?
1 Asking the client about allergies to iodine or shellfish
2 Obtaining a signed informed consent
3 Determining the location and strength of peripheral pulses
4 Placing the client on an NPO after midnight status on the night before the test

Answer: 4

Rationale: Venography is similar to arteriography, except it evaluates the venous system. A radiopaque dye is injected into selected veins to evaluate patency and blood flow characteristics. The client signs an informed consent because it is an invasive procedure. Allergies to shellfish or iodine must be noted. Peripheral pulses are assessed so comparisons can be made after the procedure. The client is usually given clear liquids for 3 to 4 hours before the procedure to help with dye excretion afterward.

Test-Taking Strategy: Use the process of elimination, noting the key word "unnecessary." Because venography is an invasive procedure using a contrast agent, options 1 and 2 are eliminated first, because they must be done. From the remaining options, recall that an NPO status will promote dehydration rather than dye clearance and that assessing peripheral pulses is necessary to identify potential complications. Review preprocedure care for venography if you had difficulty with this question.

Level of Cognitive Ability: Application
Client Needs: Physiological Integrity
Integrated Process: Nursing Process/Planning
Content Area: Adult Health/Cardiovascular

References:
Chernecky, C., & Berger, B. (2004). *Laboratory tests and diagnostic procedures* (4th ed.). Philadelphia: Saunders, p. 1136.
Lewis, S., Heitkemper, M., & Dirksen, S. (2004). *Medical-surgical nursing: Assessment and management of clinical problems* (6th ed.). St. Louis: Mosby, p. 771

288. A physician writes an order to obtain a 12-lead ECG on a client, and the nurse informs the client of the procedure. Which client statement indicates that the client understands the procedure?
1 "I should not breathe while the ECG is running."
2 "When the ECG begins, I must take a deep breath."
3 "I need to lie still while the ECG is being done."
4 "If I move when the ECG begins, I will be shocked."

Answer: 3

Rationale: Good contact between the skin and electrodes are necessary to obtain a clear 12-lead ECG tracing. Therefore, the electrodes are placed on the flat surfaces of the skin just above the ankles and wrists. Movement may cause a disruption in that contact. The client does not need to hold the breath or take a deep breath during the procedure. The client needs to be reassured that a shock will not be received. Options 1, 2, and 4 are incorrect client statements.

Test-Taking Strategy: Use the process of elimination, focusing on the issue: performing an ECG. Recalling that good contact is required to obtain a clear ECG will direct you to option 3. Review this procedure if you had difficulty with this question.

Level of Cognitive Ability: Analysis
Client Needs: Physiological Integrity
Integrated Process: Nursing Process/Evaluation
Content Area: Adult Health/Cardiovascular

Reference:
Ignatavicius, D., & Workman, M. (2002). *Medical surgical nursing: Critical thinking for collaborative care* (4th ed.). Philadelphia: Saunders, p. 645.

289. A nurse is giving a bed bath to a client who is on strict bed rest. In order to increase venous return from the extremities, the nurse bathes the client's extremities by using:
1 Long, firm strokes from distal to proximal areas
2 Firm circular strokes from proximal to distal areas
3 Short, patting strokes from distal to proximal areas
4 Smooth, light strokes back and forth from proximal to distal areas

Answer: 1
Rationale: Long, firm strokes in the direction of venous flow promote venous return when bathing the extremities. Circular strokes are used on the face. Short, patting strokes and light strokes are not as comfortable for the client and they do not promote venous return.

Test-Taking Strategy: Use the process of elimination, focusing on the issue: increase venous return. Eliminate options 2 and 4 first because a stroke from proximal to distal will not promote venous return. From the remaining options, focusing on the issue will direct you to option 1. Review the principles related to a bed bath if you had difficulty with this question.

Level of Cognitive Ability: Application
Client Needs: Physiological Integrity
Integrated Process: Nursing Process/Implementation
Content Area: Fundamental Skills

Reference:
Potter, P., & Perry, A. (2005). *Fundamentals of nursing* (6th ed.). St. Louis: Mosby, pp. 1025; 1027.

290. A nurse is preparing to give an intramuscular injection that is irritating to the subcutaneous tissues. The drug reference recommends that it be given using the Z-track technique. The nurse avoids which of the following with this administration technique?
1 Selects a large deep muscle for the injection site
2 Injects the medication quickly after the needle is inserted
3 Attaches a new sterile needle to the syringe after drawing up the medication
4 Retracts the skin to the side before piercing the skin with the needle

Answer: 2
Rationale: The Z-track variation of the standard intramuscular technique is used to administer intramuscular medications that are highly irritating to subcutaneous and skin tissues. The nurse selects an intramuscular site for injection, preferably in a large deep muscle such as the ventrogluteal muscle. A new sterile needle is attached because the new needle will not have any medication adhering to the outside that could be irritating to the tissues. Retracting the skin provides a seal over the injected medication to prevent tracking through the subcutaneous tissues. The medication is injected slowly after aspiration, if there is no blood return on aspiration. The needle remains inserted for 10 seconds to allow the medication to disperse evenly. The nurse then releases the skin after withdrawing the needle.

Test-Taking Strategy: Focus on the issue, Z-track injection, and note the key word "avoids." This word indicates a false-response question and that you need to select the option that is an incorrect nursing action. Recalling the purpose of using the Z-track technique and noting the word "quickly" in option 2 will direct you to this option. Review this procedure for administering medications using the Z-track method if you had difficulty with this question.
Level of Cognitive Ability: Application
Client Needs: Physiological Integrity
Integrated Process: Nursing Process/Implementation
Content Area: Fundamental Skills

Reference:
Potter, P., & Perry, A. (2005). *Fundamentals of nursing* (6th ed.). St. Louis: Mosby, p. 890.

291. A nurse is preparing to suction a client's tracheostomy. In order to promote deep breathing and coughing, the client should be positioned in the:
1 Supine position
2 Lateral position
3 Sims' position
4 Semi-Fowler's position

Answer: 4
Rationale: If not contraindicated, before suctioning a tracheostomy, the client is placed in semi-Fowler's position to promote deep breathing, maximum lung expansion, and productive coughing. In this position, gravity pulls downward on the diaphragm, which allows greater chest expansion and lung volume. The lateral position, the supine position, or the Sims' position would not allow for easy visualization of the tracheostomy or easy access of the suction catheter.

Test-Taking Strategy: Use the process of elimination and focus on the issue: the position that will promote deep breathing and coughing during suctioning. Visualize each position and note that options 1, 2, and 3 are similar positions in that the client lies flat. The semi-Fowler's position promotes deep breathing, maximum lung expansion, and productive coughing. Review this procedure if you had difficulty with this question.

Level of Cognitive Ability: Application
Client Needs: Physiological Integrity
Integrated Process: Nursing Process/Implementation
Content Area: Fundamental Skills

Reference:
Potter, P., & Perry, A. (2005). *Fundamentals of nursing* (6th ed.). St. Louis: Mosby, p. 1102.

292. A client in labor is at 40 weeks' gestation, and the nurse checks the fetal heart rate (FHR) for a baseline rate. The nurse is satisfied with the results and tells the client that the baby's heart rate is within normal limits. The nurse then documents which FHR finding?
1 90 beats per minute
2 140 beats per minute
3 180 beats per minute
4 200 beats per minute

Answer: 2
Rationale: The normal FHR ranges from 110 to 160 beats per minute; therefore, option 2 is the only correct option.

Test-Taking Strategy: Knowledge of the normal fetal heart rate is required to answer this question. Review this normal rate if you are unfamiliar with it.

Level of Cognitive Ability: Application
Client Needs: Physiological Integrity
Integrated Process: Communication and Documentation
Content Area: Maternity/Intrapartum

Reference:
Lowdermilk, D., & Perry, A. (2004). *Maternity & women's health care* (8th ed.). St. Louis: Mosby, pp. 416; 712

293. A client receiving chemotherapy has an infiltrated intravenous line and extravasation at the site. The nurse avoids doing which of the following in the management of this situation?
1 Stopping the administration of the medication
2 Leaving the needle in place and aspirating any residual medication
3 Administering an available antidote as prescribed
4 Applying direct manual pressure to the site

Answer: 4
Rationale: General recommendations for managing extravasation of a chemotherapeutic agent include stopping the infusion, leaving the needle in place and attempting to aspirate any residual medication from the site, administering an antidote if available, and assessing the site for complications. Direct pressure is not applied to the site because it could further injure tissues exposed to the chemotherapeutic agent.

Test-Taking Strategy: Use the process of elimination, noting the key word "avoids." This word indicates a false-response question and that you need to select the option that is an incorrect nursing action. Noting that the client was receiving chemotherapy and recalling the damaging effects of extravasation will direct you to option 4. Review treatment measures for extravasation if you had difficulty with this question.

Level of Cognitive Ability: Application
Client Needs: Physiological Integrity
Integrated Process: Nursing Process/Implementation
Content Area: Adult Health/Oncology

Reference:
Black, J., & Hawks, J. (2005). *Medical-surgical nursing: Clinical management for positive outcomes* (7th ed.). Philadelphia: Saunders, p. 374.

---

294. A nurse is suctioning the airway of a client with a tracheostomy. To properly perform the procedure, the nurse:
1 Turns on the wall suction to 180 mmHg
2 Inserts the catheter until coughing or resistance is felt
3 Withdraws the catheter while continuously suctioning
4 Reenters the tracheostomy after suctioning the mouth

Answer: 2
Rationale: The wall suction unit is usually set to 80 to 120 mmHg pressure. This allows adequate removal of secretions while protecting the airway from trauma. The nurse inserts the catheter until resistance is felt, and then withdraws it 1 cm to move away from mucosa. The nurse suctions intermittently during withdrawal of the catheter, and does not reenter the tracheostomy after suctioning the client's mouth.

Test-Taking Strategy: Use the process of elimination. Eliminate option 3 because of the word "continuously" and option 4 because the trachea is not reentered. From the remaining options, it is necessary to know that 180 mmHg pressure would cause trauma to the mucosa. Review this procedure if you had difficulty with this question.

Level of Cognitive Ability: Application
Client Needs: Physiological Integrity
Integrated Process: Nursing Process/Implementation
Content Area: Adult Health/Respiratory

Reference:
Potter, P., & Perry, A. (2005). *Fundamentals of nursing* (6th ed.). St. Louis: Mosby, pp. 1102-1108.

295. A nurse has prepared a client for an intravenous pyelogram. The nurse determines that the client understands the procedure if the client states to report which sensation immediately, if it occurs during the procedure?

1 Nausea
2 Difficulty breathing
3 Warm, flushed feeling in the body
4 Salty taste in the mouth

Answer: 2

Rationale: Intravenous pyelography is a contrast study of the kidneys to determine a variety of disorders of the kidneys, ureters, and bladder. Normal sensations during injection of the iodine-based radiopaque dye include a warm, flushed feeling, salty taste in the mouth, and transient nausea. Difficulty breathing, wheezing, hives, or itching indicate an allergic response and should be reported immediately. This complication is prevented by inquiring about allergies to iodine or shellfish before the procedure.

Test-Taking Strategy: Use the process of elimination and recall that this diagnostic test may involve injection of iodine-based contrast medium. Use of the ABCs—airway, breathing, and circulation—will direct you to option 2. Review this diagnostic procedure if you had difficulty with this question.

Level of Cognitive Ability: Analysis
Client Needs: Physiological Integrity
Integrated Process: Nursing Process/Evaluation
Content Area: Adult Health/Renal

Reference:
Chernecky, C., & Berger, B. (2004). *Laboratory tests and diagnostic procedures* (4th ed.). Philadelphia: Saunders, pp. 696-697.

296. A 15-year-old pregnant client is being treated by a dermatologist for acne. The clinic nurse asks the client about the treatment prescribed for the acne, knowing that which treatment is contraindicated during pregnancy?

1 Topical erythromycin cream
2 Exfoliation
3 Cleansing with antibacterial soap
4 Oral tetracycline (Achromycin)

Answer: 4

Rationale: Tetracycline use during pregnancy may lead to discoloration of the child's teeth when they erupt. This treatment for acne is contraindicated during pregnancy. Options 1, 2, and 3 are appropriate treatments.

Test-Taking Strategy: Use the process of elimination. Focus on the safety factor for the unseen client (fetus) and note the key word "contraindicated." Eliminate options 1, 2, and 3 because they are similar and are all topical treatments. Review the concepts related to medications and safety during pregnancy if you had difficulty with this question.

Level of Cognitive Ability: Analysis
Client Needs: Physiological Integrity
Integrated Process: Nursing Process/Assessment
Content Area: Maternity/Antepartum

Reference:
Hodgson, B., & Kizior, R. (2004). *Saunders nursing drug handbook 2004.* Philadelphia: Saunders, pp. 969-970.

297. The client with a bone infection is to have indium imaging done. The client asks the nurse to explain how the procedure is done. The nurse's response is based on the understanding that:
1 Indium is injected into the bloodstream and collects in normal bone, but not in infected areas.
2 Indium is injected into the bloodstream and highlights the vascular supply to the bone.
3 A sample of the client's leukocytes is tagged with indium, and will subsequently accumulate in infected bone.
4 A sample of the client's red blood cells is tagged with indium, and will subsequently accumulate in normal bone.

Answer: 3
Rationale: A sample of the client's blood is collected, and the leukocytes are tagged with indium. The leukocytes are then reinjected into the client. They accumulate in infected areas of bone and can be detected with scanning. No special preparation or after care is necessary. Options 1, 2, and 4 are incorrect descriptions.

Test-Taking Strategy: Use the process of elimination, focusing on the information in the question. Note that the client has a bone infection. Recall that with any type of infection, leukocytes migrate to the area. This will direct you to option 3. Review this test if you had difficulty with this question.

Level of Cognitive Ability: Application
Client Needs: Physiological Integrity
Integrated Process: Teaching/Learning
Content Area: Fundamental Skills

Reference:
Pagana, K., & Pagana, T. (2003). *Mosby's diagnostic and laboratory test reference* (6th ed.). St. Louis: Mosby, p. 947.

298. A client with repeated episodes of pulmonary emboli from thromboembolism is scheduled for insertion of an inferior vena cava filter (Greenfield filter). The nurse determines that the client has an adequate understanding of the procedure if the client makes which of the following statements?
1 "The filter will keep new blood clots from forming in my legs."
2 "I don't mind having a filter in my artery if it means I won't have any more trouble."
3 "The filter will be like a catcher's mitt and keep the clots from going to my lungs."
4 "It's too bad I have to continue anticoagulant therapy after the surgery."

Answer: 3
Rationale: Insertion of an inferior vena cava filter is indicated for clients with recurrent deep vein thrombosis and/or pulmonary emboli who do not respond to medical therapy, and when anticoagulant therapy is ineffective or contraindicated. The filter device or "umbrella" is inserted percutaneously in the inferior vena cava, where it springs open and attaches to the vena caval wall. The device has holes to allow blood flow, but traps larger clots, thus preventing pulmonary emboli. The filter does not prevent blood clots from forming and is not placed in an artery. Vena cava filters are less effective than anticoagulation and may lead to deep vein thrombosis, so they are generally used only when anticoagulant therapy is ineffective or contraindicated.

Test-Taking Strategy: Specific knowledge regarding this filter is required to answer this question. Thinking about the purpose and the action of a filter will direct you to option 3. Review this content if you had difficulty with this question.

Level of Cognitive Ability: Analysis
Client Needs: Physiological Integrity
Integrated Process: Nursing Process/Evaluation
Content Area: Adult Health/Cardiovascular

Reference:
Black, J., & Hawks, J. (2005). *Medical-surgical nursing: Clinical management for positive outcomes* (7th ed.). Philadelphia: Saunders, p. 1833.

299. A client is admitted to the hospital with a diagnosis of infective endocarditis from *Streptococcus viridans*. The client asks the nurse about the antibiotic therapy that will be given. Knowing that the client has no medication allergies, the nurse prepares the client to receive:
1 Penicillin G benzathine (Bicillin) intravenously (IV) for 10 days, followed by oral doses for 2 weeks
2 Penicillin G benzathine (Bicillin) IV for 4 to 6 weeks, continuing at home after hospital discharge
3 Amphotericin B (Fungizone) IV for 10 days, followed by oral doses for 3 weeks
4 Amphotericin B (Fungizone) IV for 4 to 6 weeks, continuing at home after hospital discharge

Answer: 2
Rationale: Penicillin is frequently the medication of choice for treating endocarditis of bacterial origin. The standard duration of therapy is 4 to 6 weeks, with home care support after hospital discharge, which is usually in 7 to 10 days. Amphotericin B is an antifungal agent and would not be effective with this type of infection.

Test-Taking Strategy: Use the process of elimination. Recalling that amphotericin B is an antifungal agent eliminates options 3 and 4. From the remaining options, note that the severity and nature of the infection makes continued IV therapy necessary; therefore, option 2 is the best option. Review the treatment for this disorder if you had difficulty with this question.

Level of Cognitive Ability: Analysis
Client Needs: Physiological Integrity
Integrated Process: Nursing Process/Planning
Content Area: Adult Health/Cardiovascular

Reference:
Black, J., & Hawks, J. (2005). *Medical-surgical nursing: Clinical management for positive outcomes* (7th ed.). Philadelphia: Saunders, p. 1618.

---

300. A nurse is doing a dressing change on a venous stasis ulcer that is clean and has a growing bed of granulation tissue. The nurse avoids using which of the following dressing materials on this wound?
1 Wet-to-dry saline dressing
2 Wet-to-wet saline dressing
3 Hydrocolloid dressing
4 Vaseline gauze dressing

Answer: 1
Rationale: The use of wet-to-dry saline dressings provides a nonselective mechanical debridement, whereby both devitalized and viable tissue are removed. This method should not be used on a clean, granulating wound. Granulation tissue in a venous stasis ulcer is protected through the use of wet-to-wet saline dressings, Vaseline gauze, or moist occlusive dressings, such as hydrocolloid dressings.

Test-Taking Strategy: Use the process of elimination and note the key word "avoids." This word indicates a false-response question and that you need to select the option that is an incorrect nursing action. Note that the question specifically tells you that the wound is clean with granulation tissue (which needs protection). Next, look at the options and note that options 2, 3, and 4 are similar and have one thing in common: continuous moisture. The wet-to-dry saline dressing could disrupt the healing tissue. Review care of a venous stasis ulcer if you had difficulty with this question.

Level of Cognitive Ability: Application
Client Needs: Physiological Integrity
Integrated Process: Nursing Process/Implementation
Content Area: Fundamental Skills

References:
Ignatavicius, D., & Workman, M. (2002). *Medical surgical nursing: Critical thinking for collaborative care* (4th ed.). Philadelphia: Saunders, p. 767.
Lewis, S., Heitkemper, M., & Dirksen, S. (2004). *Medical-surgical nursing: Assessment and management of clinical problems* (6th ed.). St. Louis: Mosby, p. 937.

301. A nurse is preparing to admit an older client to the hospital who has severe digitalis toxicity from accidental ingestion of a week's supply of the medication. The nurse calls the hospital pharmacy and requests that which medication be brought to the nursing unit?

1 Digoxin immune fab (Digibind)
2 Potassium chloride (K-Dur)
3 Protamine sulfate (Protamine)
4 Furosemide (Lasix)

Answer: 1

Rationale: Digoxin immune fab is an antidote for severe digitalis toxicity. It contains an antibody produced in sheep, which antigenically binds any unbound digitalis in the serum and removes it. As more digoxin reenters the bloodstream from the tissues, it binds that also for excretion by the kidneys. Potassium chloride is a potassium supplement. Protamine sulfate is the antidote for heparin. Furosemide is a diuretic.

Test-Taking Strategy: Note the client's diagnosis and the names of the medications in the options. Noting the relationship between the diagnosis and option 1 will direct you to this option. Review the treatment for digitalis toxicity if you had difficulty with this question.

Level of Cognitive Ability: Application
Client Needs: Physiological Integrity
Integrated Process: Nursing Process/Implementation
Content Area: Pharmacology

References:
Hodgson, B., & Kizior, R. (2004). *Saunders nursing drug handbook 2004.* Philadelphia: Saunders, p. 311.
McKenry, L., & Salerno, E. (2003). *Mosby's pharmacology in nursing* (21st ed.). St. Louis: Mosby, p. 536.

302. The parents of a 6-month-old male report that the infant has been screaming and drawing the knees up to the chest and has passed stools mixed with blood and mucus that are jelly-like. A nurse recognizes these signs and symptoms as indicative of:

1 Hirschsprung's disease
2 Peritonitis
3 Intussusception
4 Appendicitis

Answer: 3

Rationale: The classic signs and symptoms of intussusception are acute, colicky abdominal pain with currant jelly-like stools. Clinical manifestations of Hirschsprung's disease include constipation, abdominal distention, and ribbon-like, foul-smelling stools. Peritonitis is a serious complication that may follow intestinal obstruction and perforation. The most common symptom of appendicitis is colicky, periumbilical or lower abdominal pain in the right quadrant.

Test-Taking Strategy: Use the process of elimination. Eliminate options 2 and 4 because they are similar. Recalling that in Hirschsprung's disease the stools are ribbon-like will assist in eliminating option 1. Review the clinical manifestations of intussusception if you had difficulty with this question.

Level of Cognitive Ability: Analysis
Client Needs: Physiological Integrity
Integrated Process: Nursing Process/Assessment
Content Area: Child Health

Reference:
Wong, D., & Hockenberry, M. (2003). *Wong's nursing care of infants and children* (7th ed.). St. Louis: Mosby, p. 1448.

303. A nurse is caring for a client who has been placed in seclusion. The nurse is documenting care provided to the client and addresses which items in the client's record?

1 Vital signs, toileting, and checking the client based on protocol time frame, such as every 15 minutes

2 Ambulating, toileting, and checking the client based on protocol time frame, such as every 15 minutes

3 Vital signs, toileting, feeding and fluid intake, and checking the client based on protocol time frame, such as every 15 minutes

4 Vital signs, reason for the procedure, date and time

Answer: 3

Rationale: The client in seclusion is assessed continuously or at least every 15 minutes, or according to agency protocol. Vital signs, food and fluid intake, and toileting needs are assessed. Options 1 and 2 are not complete in terms of identification of physiological needs. Option 4 contains client documentation that would precede seclusion.

Test-Taking Strategy: Use Maslow's hierarchy of needs theory and the process of elimination. Note that option 3 is the most complete in terms of the client's basic needs. Review care of the client in seclusion if you had difficulty with this question.

Level of Cognitive Ability: Application
Client Needs: Physiological Integrity
Integrated Process: Communication and Documentation
Content Area: Mental Health

Reference:
Stuart, G., & Laraia, M. (2005). *Principles and practice of psychiatric nursing* (8th ed.). St. Louis: Mosby, p. 645.

---

304. During the admission assessment, the nurse asks the client to run the heel of one foot down the lower anterior surface of the other leg. The nurse notices rhythmic tremors of the leg being tested and concludes that the client has an alteration in the area of:

1 Muscle strength and flexibility
2 Balance and coordination
3 Sensation and reflexes
4 Bowel and bladder function

Answer: 2

Rationale: In this situation, the nurse is performing one test of cerebellar function and is testing for ataxia. Alterations in the cerebellar function are noted by alterations in balance and coordination. Options 1, 3, and 4 are not associated with this assessment technique.

Test-Taking Strategy: Use the process of elimination. Note the relationship between the word "tremors" in the question and "coordination" in option 2. Review assessment for cerebellar function and coordination if you had difficulty with this question.

Level of Cognitive Ability: Analysis
Client Needs: Physiological Integrity
Integrated Process: Nursing Process/Assessment
Content Area: Adult Health/Musculoskeletal

References:
Lewis, S., Heitkemper, M., & Dirksen, S. (2004). *Medical-surgical nursing: Assessment and management of clinical problems* (6th ed.). St. Louis: Mosby, p. 1484.
Phipps, W., Monahan, F., Sands, J., Marek, J., & Neighbors, M. (2003). *Medical-surgical nursing: Health and illness perspectives* (7th ed.). St. Louis: Mosby, p. 1930.

305. A nurse is monitoring the intracranial pressure (ICP) of a client with a head injury and notes that the cerebrospinal fluid pressure (CSF) is averaging 25 mmHg. The nurse analyzes these results as:

1 Normal
2 Compensated, indicating adequate brain adaptation
3 Borderline in elevation, indicating the initial stage of decompensation
4 Increased, indicating a serious compromise in cerebral perfusion

Answer: 4

Rationale: The normal CSF pressure is 5 to 15 mmHg. A pressure of 25 mmHg is increased.

Test-Taking Strategy: Use the process of elimination. Eliminate options 1 and 2 because they are similar. From the remaining options, focusing on the level identified in the question will direct you to option 4. Review intracranial pressure and the normal CSF pressure if you had difficulty with this question.

Level of Cognitive Ability: Analysis
Client Needs: Physiological Integrity
Integrated Process: Nursing Process/Analysis
Content Area: Adult Health/Neurological

Reference:
Ignatavicius, D., & Workman, M. (2002). *Medical surgical nursing: Critical thinking for collaborative care* (4th ed.). Philadelphia: Saunders, p. 894.

---

306. A woman at 32 weeks' gestation is brought into the emergency room after an automobile accident. The client is bleeding vaginally and fetal assessment indicates moderate fetal distress. Which of the following will the nurse do first in an attempt to reduce the stress on the fetus?

1 Start intravenous (IV) fluids at a keep open rate
2 Administer oxygen via a face mask at 7 to 10 liters per minute
3 Elevate the head of the bed to a semi-Fowler's position
4 Set up for an immediate cesarean section delivery

Answer: 2

Rationale: Administering oxygen will increase the amount of oxygen for transport to the fetus, partially compensating for the loss of circulating blood volume. This action is essential regardless of the cause or amount of bleeding. IV fluids will also be initiated. The client will be positioned per physician's order. Although a cesarean delivery may be needed, there is no data that it is necessary at this time.

Test-Taking Strategy: Note the key word "first" in the stem of the question. Using the ABCs—airway, breathing, circulation—will direct you to option 2. Review care of the pregnant client when fetal distress occurs if you had difficulty with this question.

Level of Cognitive Ability: Application
Client Needs: Physiological Integrity
Integrated Process: Nursing Process/Implementation
Content Area: Maternity/Antepartum

Reference:
Murray, S., McKinney, E., & Gorrie, T. (2002). *Foundations of maternal-newborn nursing* (3rd ed.). Philadelphia: Saunders, p. 352.

---

307. A client with a Sengstaken-Blakemore tube in place is admitted to the nursing unit from the emergency room. The nurse plans care knowing that the purpose of this tube is to:

1 Control bleeding from gastritis
2 Apply pressure to esophageal varices
3 Control ascites
4 Remove ammonia-forming bacteria from the gastrointestinal tract

Answer: 2

Rationale: A Sengstaken-Blakemore tube is inserted in clients with cirrhosis who have ruptured esophageal varices. It has esophageal and gastric balloons. The esophageal balloon exerts pressure on the ruptured esophageal varices and stops the bleeding. The gastric balloon holds the tube in correct position and prevents migration of the esophageal balloon. Options 1, 3, and 4 are not the purpose of this tube.

Test-Taking Strategy: Focus on the issue: the purpose of a Sengstaken-Blakemore tube. Recalling the relationship between this tube and ruptured esophageal varices will direct you to option 2. Review the concepts related to this type of tube if you are unfamiliar with them.

Level of Cognitive Ability: Application
Client Needs: Physiological Integrity
Integrated Process: Nursing Process/Planning
Content Area: Adult Health/Gastrointestinal

Reference:
Lewis, S., Heitkemper, M., & Dirksen, S. (2004). *Medical-surgical nursing: Assessment and management of clinical problems* (6th ed.). St. Louis: Mosby, pp. 1122-1123.

---

308. A home health care nurse is instructing a client with chronic obstructive pulmonary disorder (COPD) how to perform breathing techniques that will assist in exhaling carbon dioxide and open the airways. The nurse teaches the client which technique?
1 Pursed-lip breathing
2 Intercostal chest expansion
3 Abdominal breathing
4 Chest physical therapy

Answer: 1
Rationale: Pursed-lip breathing allows the client to slowly exhale carbon dioxide while keeping the airways open. Abdominal breathing is recommended for clients with dyspnea. Intercostal chest expansion and chest physical therapy are not breathing techniques.

Test-Taking Strategy: Use the process of elimination and focus on the issue: a breathing technique for the client with COPD. Eliminate options 2 and 4 first because these are not breathing techniques. From the remaining options, remembering that pursed-lip breathing is associated with the COPD client will assist in directing you to the correct option. Review pursed-lip breathing and abdominal breathing if you are unfamiliar with the purposes and techniques.

Level of Cognitive Ability: Application
Client Needs: Physiological Integrity
Integrated Process: Teaching/Learning
Content Area: Adult Health/Respiratory

Reference:
Potter, P., & Perry, A. (2005). *Fundamentals of nursing* (6th ed.). St. Louis: Mosby, p. 1130.

---

309. A physician has ordered a partial rebreather face mask for a client who has terminal lung cancer. The nurse prepares to implement the order knowing that the mask:
1 Delivers accurate fraction of inspired oxygen (FIO_2) to the client
2 Conserves oxygen by having the client rebreathe his or her own exhaled air
3 Requires that the reservoir bag deflate during inspiration to work effectively
4 Requires a low liter flow to prevent rebreathing of carbon dioxide

Answer: 2
Rationale: Rebreathing masks have a reservoir bag that conserves oxygen and requires a high liter flow to achieve concentrations of 40% to 60%. It does not deliver accurate FIO_2 to the client. The bag should not deflate during inspiration. Rebreathing bags conserve oxygen by having the client rebreathe his or her own exhaled air.

Test-Taking Strategy: Use the process of elimination. Note the relationship between "partial rebreather" in the question and "rebreathe his or her own exhaled air" in the correct option. Review the oxygen delivery system if you had difficulty with this question.

Level of Cognitive Ability: Application
Client Needs: Physiological Integrity
Integrated Process: Nursing Process/Planning
Content Area: Adult Health/Respiratory

References:
Ignatavicius, D., & Workman, M. (2002). *Medical surgical nursing: Critical thinking for collaborative care* (4th ed.). Philadelphia: Saunders, p. 492-493.
Lewis, S., Heitkemper, M., & Dirksen, S. (2004). *Medical-surgical nursing: Assessment and management of clinical problems* (6th ed.). St. Louis: Mosby, p. 667.

---

310. A client has a slow, regular pulse. On the monitor, the nurse notes regular QRS complexes with no associated P waves, and a ventricular rate of 50 beats per minute. The nurse suspects that there is a problem at which part of the cardiac conduction system?
1 The sinoatrial (SA) node
2 The atrioventricular (AV) node
3 The bundle of His
4 The left ventricle

Answer: 1
Rationale: A normal P wave indicates that the impulse that depolarized the atrium was initiated in the SA node. A change in the form or the absence of a P wave can indicate a problem at this part of the conduction system, with the resulting impulse originating from an alternate site lower in the conduction pathway. Options 2, 3, and 4 are incorrect.

Test-Taking Strategy: Use the process of elimination. Option 4 can be eliminated first because it does not identify a mechanism of the conduction system. The question also identifies a regular QRS complex and a ventricular rate of 50 beats per minute indicating an intact AV node, thus the problem lies higher in the conduction system. Correlate a P wave with the SA node. Review the conduction system of the heart if you had difficulty with this question.

Level of Cognitive Ability: Analysis
Client Needs: Physiological Integrity
Integrated Process: Nursing Process/Analysis
Content Area: Adult Health/Cardiovascular

Reference:
Ignatavicius, D., & Workman, M. (2002). *Medical surgical nursing: Critical thinking for collaborative care* (4th ed.). Philadelphia: Saunders, p. 865.

---

311. A client is hospitalized with a diagnosis of thrombophlebitis and is being treated with heparin infusion therapy. About 24 hours after the infusion has begun, the nurse notes that the client's partial thromboplastin time (PTT) is 65 seconds with a control of 30 seconds. What is the appropriate initial nursing action?
1 Discontinue the heparin infusion
2 Do nothing because the client is adequately anticoagulated
3 Notify the physician of the laboratory results
4 Prepare to administrate protamine sulfate

Answer: 2
Rationale: The effectiveness of heparin therapy is monitored by the results of the partial thoromboplastin time (PTT). Desired ranges for therapeutic anticoagulation are 1.5 to 2.5 times the control. A PTT of 65 seconds is within the therapeutic range.

Test-Taking Strategy: Use the process of elimination. Remember that the desired ranges for therapeutic anticoagulation is 1.5 to 2.5 times the control. Noting that the control is 30 and that 1.5 to 2.5 times the control is a range of 45 to 75 will direct you to option 2. Review care of the client receiving a heparin infusion if you had difficulty with this question.

Level of Cognitive Ability: Application
Client Needs: Physiological Integrity
Integrated Process: Nursing Process/Implementation
Content Area: Pharmacology

Reference:
McKenry, L., & Salerno, E. (2003). *Mosby's pharmacology in nursing* (21st ed.). St. Louis: Mosby, p. 624.

---

312. A man is brought to the emergency room complaining of chest pain. His vital signs are blood pressure (BP) 150/90 mmHg, pulse (P) 88 beats per minute (BPM), and respirations (R) 20 breaths per minute. The nurse administers nitroglycerin 0.4 mg sublingually. To evaluate the effectiveness of this medication, the nurse assesses for the relief of chest pain and expects to note which of the following changes in the vital signs?

1 BP 160/100 mmHg, P 120 BPM, R 16 breaths per minute
2 BP 150/90 mmHg, P 70 BPM, R 24 breaths per minute
3 BP 100/60 mmHg, P 96 BPM, R 20 breaths per minute
4 BP 100/60 mmHg, P 70 BPM, R 24 breaths per minute

Answer: 3

Rationale: Nitroglycerin dilates both arteries and veins, causing blood to pool in the periphery. This causes a reduced preload and therefore a drop in cardiac output. This vasodilation causes the blood pressure to fall. The drop in cardiac output causes the sympathetic nervous system to respond and attempt to maintain cardiac output by increasing the pulse. Beta-blockers, such as propranolol (Inderal), are often used in conjunction with nitroglycerin to prevent this rise in heart rate.

Test-Taking Strategy: Use the process of elimination. Knowing that nitroglycerin is a vasodilator and that it causes the BP to drop will assist in eliminating options 1 and 2. Next recall that if chest pain is reduced and cardiac workload is reduced, the client will be more comfortable; therefore, a rise in respirations should not be seen. This assists in eliminating option 4. Review the effects of nitroglycerin if you had difficulty with this question.

Level of Cognitive Ability: Analysis
Client Needs: Physiological Integrity
Integrated Process: Nursing Process/Evaluation
Content Area: Pharmacology

Reference:
Hodgson, B., & Kizior, R. (2004). *Saunders nursing drug handbook 2004.* Philadelphia: Saunders, p. 733.

---

313. A client who has had an abdominal aortic aneurysm repair is one day postoperative. The nurse performs an abdominal assessment and notes the absence of bowel sounds. The nurse should:

1 Call the physician immediately
2 Remove the nasogastric (NG) tube
3 Feed the client
4 Document the finding and continue to assess for bowel sounds

Answer: 4

Rationale: Bowel sounds may be absent for 3 to 4 days postoperative due to bowel manipulation during surgery. The nurse should document the finding and continue to monitor the client. The NG tube should stay in place if present, and the client is kept NPO until after the onset of bowel sounds. There is no need to call the physician immediately at this time.

Test-Taking Strategy: Use the process of elimination. Note the key words "one day postoperative." Eliminate option 2 because there is no data in the question regarding the presence of an NG tube. Additionally, an NG tube would not be removed and the client would not be fed (option 3) if bowel sounds are absent. Recalling that bowel sounds may not return for 3 to 4 days postoperative will direct you to option 4 from the remaining options. Review normal postoperative assessment findings if you had difficulty with this question.

Level of Cognitive Ability: Application
Client Needs: Physiological Integrity
Integrated Process: Nursing Process/Implementation
Content Area: Adult Health/Gastrointestinal

References:
Lewis, S., Heitkemper, M., & Dirksen, S. (2004). *Medical-surgical nursing: Assessment and management of clinical problems* (6th ed.). St. Louis: Mosby, p. 402.
Potter, P., & Perry, A. (2005). *Fundamentals of nursing* (6th ed.). St. Louis: Mosby, pp. 1633-1634; 1639-1640.

---

314. A nurse is caring for a client with pregnancy-induced hypertension (PIH) who is in labor. The nurse monitors the client closely for which complication of PIH?
  1 Seizures
  2 Placenta previa
  3 Hallucinations
  4 Altered respiratory status

Answer: 1
Rationale: The major complication of PIH is seizures. Placenta previa, hallucinations, and altered respiratory status are not directly associated with PIH.

Test-Taking Strategy: Use the process of elimination. Remember that seizures are a concern with PIH to direct you to option 1. Review the complications associated with PIH if you had difficulty with this question.

Level of Cognitive Ability: Analysis
Client Needs: Physiological Integrity
Integrated Process: Nursing Process/Assessment
Content Area: Maternity/Intrapartum

Reference:
Lowdermilk, D., & Perry, A. (2004). *Maternity & women's health care* (8th ed.). St. Louis: Mosby, p. 840.

---

315. A nurse is evaluating the outcomes of care for a client who experienced an acute myocardial infarction. Which of the following findings indicate that an expected outcome for the nursing diagnosis of decreased cardiac output has been met?
  1 Cardiac output of 3 liters per minute when measured with a pulmonary artery catheter
  2 Cardiac monitor shows a heart rate of 50 beats per minute after the client has eaten dinner
  3 The client complains of symptoms that require immediate action
  4 The client reports absence of dyspnea and anginal pain with activity

Answer: 4
Rationale: Dyspnea and angina are signs of altered cardiac output. The absence of these with activity indicates that cardiac output is adequate. Normal adult cardiac output is 4 to 8 liters per minute. Option 1 identifies a low reading. A low heart rate affects cardiac output. The client's heart rate should be between 60 to 100 beats per minute. Complaints of symptoms that require immediate action is not an expected outcome.

Test-Taking Strategy: Focus on the issue: an expected outcome. Use the ABCs—airway, breathing, and circulation. Note the key words "absence of dyspnea and anginal pain" in the correct option. Review normal cardiac output and heart rate if you had difficulty with this question.

Level of Cognitive Ability: Analysis
Client Needs: Physiological Integrity
Integrated Process: Nursing Process/Evaluation
Content Area: Adult Health/Cardiovascular

Reference:
Black, J., & Hawks, J. (2005). *Medical-surgical nursing: Clinical management for positive outcomes* (7th ed.). Philadelphia: Saunders, p. 1720.

316. During the initial prenatal visit of a client in the first trimester of pregnancy, the client's hemoglobin level is drawn and the results are recorded in the client's record. The nurse reviews the results and determines the findings to be abnormal and indicative of iron-deficiency anemia. The nurse performs an assessment on the client expecting to note which of the following in this type of anemia?
 1 Pink, mucous membranes
 2 Complaints of headaches and fatigue
 3 Increased vaginal secretions
 4 Complaints of increased frequency of voiding

Answer: 2
Rationale: Iron-deficiency anemia is described as a hemoglobin blood concentration of less than 10.5 to 11.0 g/dL. Complaints of headaches and fatigue are abnormal findings and may reflect complications of this type of anemia caused by the decreased oxygen supply to vital organs. Options 1, 3, and 4 are normal findings in the first trimester of pregnancy.

Test-Taking Strategy: Note the key words "first trimester of pregnancy" in the question. Options 1, 3, and 4 are normal findings during the first trimester of pregnancy. Option 2 is abnormal and may reflect complications caused by the decreased oxygen supply to vital organs. Review the clinical manifestations associated with anemia if you had difficulty with this question.

Level of Cognitive Ability: Analysis
Client Needs: Physiological Integrity
Integrated Process: Nursing Process/Assessment
Content Area: Maternity/Antepartum

Reference:
Lowdermilk, D. & Perry, A. (2004). *Maternity & women's health care* (8th ed.) St. Louis: Mosby, p. 919.
McKinney, E., James, S., Murray, S., & Ashwill, J. (2005). *Maternal-child nursing* (2nd ed.). St. Louis: Elsevier, p. 657.

317. A nurse is caring for a client with multiple myeloma who is receiving intravenous hydration at 100 mL per hour. Which assessment finding would indicate a positive response to the treatment plan?
 1 Weight increase of 1 kilogram
 2 White blood cell count of 6,000 mm^3
 3 Respirations of 18 breaths per minute
 4 Creatinine of 1.0 mg/dL

Answer: 4
Rationale: Renal failure is a concern in the client with multiple myeloma. In multiple myeloma, hydration is essential to prevent renal damage resulting from precipitation of protein in the renal tubules and from excessive calcium and uric acid in the blood. Creatinine is the most accurate measure of renal status. Options 2 and 3 are unrelated to the issue of hydration. Weight gain is not a positive sign when concerned with renal status.

Test-Taking Strategy: Use the process of elimination and focus on the issue: hydration status. Recalling that renal failure is a concern in multiple myeloma will direct you to option 4. Review care of the client with multiple myeloma if you had difficulty with this question.

Level of Cognitive Ability: Analysis
Client Needs: Physiological Integrity
Integrated Process: Nursing Process/Evaluation
Content Area: Adult Health/Oncology

References:
Lewis, S., Heitkemper, M., & Dirksen, S. (2004). *Medical-surgical nursing: Assessment and management of clinical problems* (6th ed.). St. Louis: Mosby, p. 745.
Phipps, W., Monahan, F., Sands, J., Marek, J., & Neighbors, M. (2003). *Medical-surgical nursing: Health and illness perspectives* (7th ed.). St. Louis: Mosby, pp. 1628-1629.

318. A nurse provides discharge instructions to a client with testicular cancer who had testicular surgery. The nurse tells the client:

1 To report any elevation in temperature to the physician
2 To avoid driving a car for at least 8 weeks
3 Not to be fitted for a prosthesis for at least 6 months
4 To avoid sitting for long periods for at least 6 weeks

Answer: 1
Rationale: For the client who has had testicular surgery, the nurse should emphasize the importance of notifying the physician if chills, fever, drainage, redness, or discharge occurs. These symptoms may indicate the presence of an infection. One week after testicular surgery, the client may drive. Often, a prosthesis is inserted during surgery. Sitting needs to be avoided with prostrate surgery because of the risk of hemorrhage, but this risk is not as high with testicular surgery.

Test-Taking Strategy: Use Maslow's hierarchy of needs theory and principles related to prioritizing. Infection is a priority. After any surgical procedure, elevation of temperature could signal an infection and should be reported. Also note the lengthy time periods in options 2, 3, and 4. These will assist in eliminating these options. Review post-testicular surgical teaching points if you had difficulty with this question.

Level of Cognitive Ability: Application
Client Needs: Physiological Integrity
Integrated Process: Teaching/Learning
Content Area: Adult Health/Oncology

Reference:
Ignatavicius, D., & Workman, M. (2002). *Medical surgical nursing: Critical thinking for collaborative care* (4th ed.). Philadelphia: Saunders, p. 1799.

---

319. A multidisciplinary team has been working with the spouse of a home care client who has end-stage liver failure and has been teaching the spouse interventions for pain management. Which statement by the spouse indicates the need for further teaching?

1 "If the pain increases, I must let the nurse know immediately."
2 "I should have my husband try the breathing exercises to control pain."
3 "This narcotic will cause very deep sleep, which is what my husband needs."
4 "If constipation is a problem, increased fluids will help."

Answer: 3
Rationale: Changes in level of consciousness are a potential indicator of narcotic overdose, as well as an indicator of fluid, electrolyte, and oxygenation deficits. It is important to teach the spouse the differences between sleep related to relief of pain and changes in neurological status related to a deficit. Options 1, 2, and 4 all indicate an understanding of appropriate steps to be taken in pain management.

Test-Taking Strategy: Use the process of elimination and note the key words "need for further teaching." These words indicate a false-response question and that you need to select the option that is an incorrect client statement. Note that the client has end-stage liver disease. Focusing on the issue, pain management, will direct you to option 3. Review pain management if you had difficulty with this question.

Level of Cognitive Ability: Analysis
Client Needs: Physiological Integrity
Integrated Process: Teaching/Learning
Content Area: Fundamental Skills

Reference:
Lewis, S., Heitkemper, M., & Dirksen, S. (2004). *Medical-surgical nursing: Assessment and management of clinical problems* (6th ed.). St. Louis: Mosby, pp. 88; 152.

320. A nurse is reviewing the antenatal history of a client in early labor. The nurse recognizes which of the following factors documented in the history as having the greatest potential for causing neonatal sepsis following delivery?

1 Adequate prenatal care
2 Appropriate maternal nutrition and weight gain
3 Spontaneous rupture of membranes 2 hours ago
4 History of substance abuse during pregnancy

Answer: 4

Rationale: Risk factors for neonatal sepsis can arise from maternal, intrapartal, or neonatal conditions. Maternal risk factors before delivery include low socioeconomic status, poor prenatal care and nutrition, and a history of substance abuse during pregnancy. Premature rupture of the membranes or prolonged rupture of membranes greater than 18 hours before birth is also a risk factor for neonatal acquisition of infection.

Test-Taking Strategy: Use the process of elimination. Options 1 and 2 are optimal findings and can be eliminated. From the remaining options, note the key words "2 hours ago" to assist in eliminating option 3. Review potential maternal physiological and psychosocial risk factors that may cause neonatal infections if you had difficulty with this question.

Level of Cognitive Ability: Analysis
Clients Needs: Physiological Integrity
Integrated Process: Nursing Process/Assessment
Content Area: Maternity/Intrapartum

Reference:
Lowdermilk, D., & Perry, A. (2004). *Maternity & women's health care* (8th ed.). St. Louis: Mosby, p. 1072.

321. A nurse performs a prenatal assessment on a client in the first trimester of pregnancy and discovers that the client frequently consumes alcohol beverages. The nurse initiates interventions to assist the client to avoid alcohol consumption in order to:

1 Promote the normal psychosocial adaptation of the mother to pregnancy
2 Reduce the potential for fetal growth restriction in utero
3 Minimize the potential for placental abruptions during the intrapartum period
4 Reduce the risk of teratogenic effects to developing fetal organs, tissues, and structures

Answer: 4

Rationale: The first trimester, "organogenesis," is characterized by the differentiation and development of fetal organs, systems, and structures. The effects of alcohol on the developing fetus during this critical period depend not only on the amount of alcohol consumed, but also on the interaction of quantity, frequency, type of alcohol, and other drugs that may be abused during this period by the pregnant woman. Eliminating consumption of alcohol during this time may promote normal fetal organ development.

Test-Taking Strategy: Use the process of elimination and focus on the key words "first trimester." Recall that during this trimester, development of fetal organs, tissues, and structures take place. Review the effects of alcohol on the fetus in the first trimester of pregnancy if you had difficulty with this question.

Level of Cognitive Ability: Application
Client Needs: Physiological Integrity
Integrated Process: Teaching/Learning
Content Area: Maternity/Antepartum

Reference:
Murray, S., McKinney, E., & Gorrie, T. (2002). *Foundations of maternal-newborn nursing* (3rd ed.). Philadelphia: Saunders, p. 639.

322. A nurse is admitting a client with a diagnosis of myxedema to the hospital. The nurse performs which of the following that will provide data related to this diagnosis?
1 Inspects facial features
2 Palpates the adrenal glands
3 Percusses the thyroid gland
4 Auscultates lung sounds

Answer: 1

Rationale: Inspection of facial features will reveal the characteristic coarse features, presence of edema around the eyes and face, and the blank expression that are characteristic of myxedema. The assessment techniques in options 2, 3, and 4 will not reveal information related to the diagnosis of myxedema.

Test-Taking Strategy: Use the process of elimination. Eliminate options 2 and 4 because they do not relate to the thyroid gland. From the remaining options, recall that palpation, rather than percussion of the thyroid, is the assessment technique used to evaluate the thyroid gland. Review the clinical manifestations associated with myxedema if you had difficulty with this question.

Level of Cognitive Ability: Application
Client Needs: Physiological Integrity
Integrated Process: Nursing Process/Assessment
Content Area: Adult Health/Endocrine

Reference:
Ignatavicius, D., & Workman, M. (2002). *Medical surgical nursing: Critical thinking for collaborative care* (4th ed.). Philadelphia: Saunders, pp. 1431-1432.

323. A nurse is teaching a client with chronic obstructive pulmonary disease (COPD) how to purse-lip breathe. The nurse tells the client:
1 To breathe in and then hold the breath for 30 seconds
2 To loosen the abdominal muscles while breathing out
3 To breathe so that expiration is twice as long as inspiration
4 To inhale with pursed lips and to exhale with the mouth open wide

Answer: 3

Rationale: Prolonging expiration time reduces air trapping caused by airway narrowing that occurs in COPD. Tightening (not loosening) the abdominal muscles aids in expelling air. Exhaling through pursed lips (not with the mouth wide open) increases the intraluminal pressure and prevents the airways from collapsing. The client is not instructed to breathe in and hold the breath for 30 seconds; this action has no useful purpose for the client with COPD.

Test-Taking Strategy: Focus on the issue, pursed-lip breathing, and visualize each of the actions in the options. Recalling that a major purpose of pursed-lip breathing is to prevent air trapping during exhalation will direct you to the correct option. Review the principles of pursed-lip breathing if you are unfamiliar with this technique.

Level of Cognitive Ability: Application
Client Needs: Physiological Integrity
Integrated Process: Teaching/Learning
Content Area: Adult Health/Respiratory

Reference:
Lewis, S., Heitkemper, M., & Dirksen, S. (2004). *Medical-surgical nursing: Assessment and management of clinical problems* (6th ed.). St. Louis: Mosby, pp. 557; 672.

324. A nurse is caring for a pregnant client with a history of human immunodeficiency virus (HIV). Which nursing diagnosis formulated by the nurse has the highest priority for this client?
1 Self-Care Deficit
2 Risk for Infection
3 Imbalanced Nutrition
4 Activity Intolerance

Answer: 2

Rationale: Clients with HIV often show some evidence of immune dysfunction and may have increased vulnerability to common infections. HIV infection impairs cellular and humoral immune function; therefore, individuals with HIV are vulnerable to common bacterial infections. Not every client with HIV will have problems with activity, self-care, or nutrition. Although nutritional deficit is a concern, infection is specifically related to HIV and is a priority because it is more life-threatening.

Test-Taking Strategy: Use the process of elimination, noting the key words "highest priority." Focus on the physiology related to HIV to direct you to option 2. Also, recall that infection is a life-threatening condition in the client with HIV. Review the risks associated with HIV infection if you had difficulty with this question.

Level of Cognitive Ability: Analysis
Client Needs: Physiological Integrity
Integrated Process: Nursing Process/Analysis
Content Area: Maternity/Antepartum

Reference:
Lowdermilk, D., & Perry, A. (2004). *Maternity & women's health care* (8th ed.). St. Louis: Mosby, p. 205.

325. A client is taking lithium carbonate (Lithium) for the treatment of bipolar disorder. Which assessment question would the nurse ask the client to determine signs of early lithium toxicity?
1 "Have you been experiencing leg aches over the past few days?"
2 "Do you have frequent headaches?"
3 "Have you been experiencing any nausea, vomiting, or diarrhea?"
4 "Have you noted excessive urination?"

Answer: 3

Rationale: One of the most common early signs of lithium toxicity is gastrointestinal (GI) disturbances such as nausea, vomiting, or diarrhea. The assessment questions in options 1, 2, and 4 are unrelated to the findings in lithium toxicity.

Test-Taking Strategy: Use the process of elimination and knowledge regarding the "early" signs of toxicity. Recalling that GI disturbances are early manifestations will direct you to option 3. Review these signs if you had difficulty with this question.

Level of Cognitive Ability: Analysis
Client Needs: Physiological Integrity
Integrated Process: Nursing Process/Assessment
Content Area: Pharmacology

References:
Hodgson, B., & Kizior, R. (2004). *Saunders nursing drug handbook 2004.* Philadelphia: Saunders, p. 608.
McKenry, L., & Salerno, E. (2003). *Mosby's pharmacology in nursing* (21st ed.). St. Louis: Mosby, p. 696.

326. A postpartum nurse is caring for a client who delivered a viable newborn infant 2 hours ago. The nurse palpates the fundus and notes the character of the lochia. Which characteristic of the lochia would the nurse expect to note at this time?
1 White-colored lochia
2 Pink-colored lochia
3 Serosanguinous lochia
4 Dark red–colored lochia

Answer: 4
Rationale: When checking the perineum, the lochia is monitored for amount, color, and the presence of clots. The color of the lochia during the fourth stage of labor (the first 1 to 4 hours after birth) is a dark red color. Options 1, 2, and 3 are not the expected characteristics of lochia at this time period.

Test-Taking Strategy: Use the process of elimination. Noting that the question refers to a client who delivered 2 hours ago will direct you to option 4. Review postpartum assessments if you had difficulty with this question.

Level of Cognitive Ability: Analysis
Client Needs: Physiological Integrity
Integrated Process: Nursing Process/Assessment
Content Area: Maternity/Antepartum

References:
Lowdermilk, D. & Perry, A. (2004). *Maternity & women's health care* (8th ed.). St. Louis: Mosby, p. 627;630.
McKinney, E., James, S., Murray, S., & Ashwill, J. (2005). *Maternal-child nursing* (2nd ed.). St. Louis: Elsevier, pp. 386; 480.

---

327. A nurse is performing a prenatal examination on a client in the third trimester. The nurse begins an abdominal examination and performs Leopold maneuvers. The nurse determines which of the following after performing the first maneuver?
1 Fetal lie and presentation
2 Fetal descent
3 Strength of uterine contractions
4 Placenta previa

Answer: 1
Rationale: The first maneuver determines the contents of the fundus (either the fetal head or breech) and thereby the fetal lie. Leopold maneuvers are not performed during a contraction. Placenta previa is diagnosed by ultrasound and not by palpation. Fetal descent is determined with the fourth maneuver.

Test-Taking Strategy: Use the process of elimination. Recalling the purpose and procedure of Leopold maneuvers will assist in eliminating options 3 and 4. From the remaining options, it is necessary to know that the first maneuver determines fetal lie. Review Leopold maneuvers if you had difficulty with this question.

Level of Cognitive Ability: Analysis
Client Needs: Physiological Integrity
Integrated Process: Nursing Process/Assessment
Content Area: Maternity/Antepartum

Reference:
Lowdermilk, D., & Perry, A. (2004). *Maternity & women's health care* (8th ed.). St. Louis: Mosby, pp. 556; 562.

---

328. A nurse is caring for a client with a spinal cord injury who has spinal shock. The nurse performs an assessment on the client, knowing that which assessment will provide the best information about recovery from spinal shock?
1 Blood pressure
2 Pulse rate
3 Reflexes
4 Temperature

Answer: 3
Rationale: Areflexia characterizes spinal shock. Therefore, reflexes would provide the best information about recovery. Vital sign changes (options 1, 2, and 4) are not consistently affected by spinal shock. Because vital signs are affected by many factors, they do not give reliable information about spinal shock recovery. Blood pressure would provide good information about recovery from other types of shock, but not spinal shock.

Test-Taking Strategy: Use the process of elimination. Note that options 1, 2, and 4 are similar and are all vital signs. Option 3 is the different option. Review spinal shock if you are unfamiliar with this content.

Level of Cognitive Ability: Analysis
Client Needs: Physiological Integrity
Integrated Process: Nursing Process/Assessment
Content Area: Adult Health/Neurological

Reference:
Lewis, S., Heitkemper, M., & Dirksen, S. (2004). *Medical-surgical nursing: Assessment and management of clinical problems* (6th ed.). St. Louis: Mosby, pp. 1611-1612; 1620.

---

329. A client is admitted to the hospital for repair of an unruptured cerebral aneurysm. Before surgery, the nurse performs frequent assessments on the client. Which assessment finding would be noted first if the aneurysm ruptures?
1 Widened pulse pressure
2 Unilateral slowing of pupil response
3 Unilateral motor weakness
4 A decline in the level of consciousness

Answer: 4
Rationale: Rupture of a cerebral aneurysm usually results in increased intracranial pressure (ICP). The first sign of pressure in the brain on the brain stem is a change in the level of consciousness. This change in consciousness can be as subtle as drowsiness or restlessness. Because centers that control blood pressure are located lower in the brain stem than those that control consciousness, pulse pressure alteration is a later sign. Slowing of pupil response and motor weakness are also late signs.

Test-Taking Strategy: Note the key word "first." Remember that changes in level of consciousness are the first indication of increased ICP. Review the clinical manifestations associated with a cerebral aneurysm and ICP if you had difficulty with this question.

Level of Cognitive Ability: Analysis
Client Needs: Physiological Integrity
Integrated Process: Nursing Process/Assessment
Content Area: Adult Health/Neurological

Reference:
Ignatavicius, D., & Workman, M. (2002). *Medical surgical nursing: Critical thinking for collaborative care* (4th ed.). Philadelphia: Saunders, pp. 975-976.

---

330. An emergency room staff calls the mental health unit and tells the nurse that a severely depressed client is being transported to the unit. The nurse in the mental health unit expects to note which of the following on assessment of this client?
1 Reports of weight gain, hypersomnia, and a blunted affect
2 Reports of increased crying spells, normal weight, and normal sleep patterns
3 Hesitancy to participate in the activities, but a normal affect
4 Reports of weight loss, insomnia, and decreased crying spells

Answer: 4
Rationale: In the severely depressed client, loss of weight is typical, while the mildly depressed client may experience a gain in weight. Sleep is generally affected in a similar way, with hypersomnia in the mildly depressed client and insomnia in the severely depressed client. The severely depressed client may report that no tears are left for crying.

Test-Taking Strategy: Use the process of elimination and note the key words "severely depressed." Options 2 and 3 identify some degree of normalcy and can be eliminated. From the remaining options, focusing on the key words will direct you to option 4. Review assessment findings associated with the severely depressed client if you had difficulty with this question.

Level of Cognitive Ability: Analysis
Client Needs: Physiological Integrity
Integrated Process: Nursing Process/Assessment
Content Area: Mental Health

Reference:
Stuart, G., & Laraia, M. (2005). *Principles and practice of psychiatric nursing* (8th ed.).
St. Louis: Mosby, p. 334.

---

331. A client with a prior history of suicide attempts is admitted to the mental health unit with the diagnosis of depression. The client's therapist reports to the nurse that the client had called earlier and reported having severe suicidal thoughts. Keeping this information in mind, the priority of the nurse is to assess for:
1   The presence of suicidal thoughts
2   Interaction with peers
3   The amount of food intake for the past 24 hours
4   Information regarding the past treatment regimen

Answer: 1
Rationale: The critical information from the therapist is that the client is having thoughts of self-harm; therefore, the nurse needs further information about present thoughts of suicide so that the treatment plan may be as appropriate as possible. The nurse must make sure the client is safe. The items in options 2, 3, and 4 should be assessed; however, assessment of suicide potential is most important.

Test-Taking Strategy: Use the process of elimination and note the key word "priority." Note the relationship between "severe suicidal thoughts" in the question and in the correct option. Review assessment of the client at risk for self-harm if you had difficulty with this question.

Level of Cognitive Ability: Analysis
Client Needs: Physiological Integrity
Integrated Process: Nursing Process/Assessment
Content Area: Delegating/Prioritizing

Reference:
Stuart, G., & Laraia, M. (2005). *Principles and practice of psychiatric nursing* (8th ed.).
St. Louis: Mosby, p. 348.

---

332. A home care nurse finds a client in the bedroom, unconscious, with a pill bottle in hand. The pill bottle contained the selective serotonin reuptake inhibitor, sertraline (Zoloft). The nurse immediately assesses the client's:
1   Blood pressure
2   Respirations
3   Pulse
4   Urinary output

Answer: 2
Rationale: In an emergency situation, the nurse should determine breathlessness first, then pulselessness. Blood pressure would be assessed after these assessments were determined. Urinary output is also important, but not the priority at this time.

Test-Taking Strategy: Use the ABCs—airway, breathing, and circulation—as the guide for answering this question. Respirations specifically relate to breathing and airway. Review priority assessments in an unconscious client suspected of an overdose from sertraline if you had difficulty with this question.

Level of Cognitive Ability: Analysis
Client Needs: Physiological Integrity
Integrated Process: Nursing Process/Assessment
Content Area: Delegating/Prioritizing

Reference:
Kee, J., & Hayes, E. (2003). *Pharmacology: A nursing process approach* (4th ed.).
Philadelphia: Saunders, p. 312.

333. A nurse is checking a unit of blood received from the blood bank and notes the presence of gas bubbles in the bag. The nurse should take which of the following actions?
  1 Add 10 mL normal saline to the bag
  2 Agitate the bag gently to mix contents
  3 Add 100 units of heparin to the bag
  4 Return the bag to the blood bank

Answer: 4
Rationale: The nurse should return the unit of blood to the blood bank. The presence of gas bubbles in the bag indicates possible bacterial growth, and the unit is considered contaminated. Options 1, 2, and 3 are incorrect actions. Additionally, normal saline, heparin, or any other substance should never be mixed with the blood in a blood bag.

Test-Taking Strategy: Use the process of elimination. Recalling that the presence of gas bubbles indicates bacterial growth will direct you to option 4. Remember, when in doubt, consult with the blood bank. Review concepts related to transfusion of blood if you had difficulty with this question.

Level of Cognitive Ability: Application
Client Needs: Physiological Integrity
Integrated Process: Nursing Process/Implementation
Content Area: Fundamental Skills

Reference:
Phipps, W., Monahan, F., Sands, J., Marek, J., & Neighbors, M. (2003). *Medical-surgical nursing: Health and illness perspectives* (7th ed.). St. Louis: Mosby, p. 1646.

334. A nurse has an order to infuse a unit of blood. The nurse checks the client's intravenous line to make sure that the gauge of the intravenous catheter is at least:
  1 14-gauge
  2 19-gauge
  3 22-gauge
  4 24-gauge

Answer: 2
Rationale: An intravenous line used to infuse blood should be at least 19-gauge or larger. This allows infusion of the blood elements without clogging the line or the IV access site. A 22-gauge or 24-gauge is too small to infuse blood.

Test-Taking Strategy: Focus on the issue: infusion of blood. This focus will assist in eliminating options 3 and 4. From the remaining options, think about the gauge of IV catheters to direct you to option 2. Review IV lines and blood transfusions if you had difficulty with this question.

Level of Cognitive Ability: Application
Client Needs: Physiological Integrity
Integrated Process: Nursing Process/Implementation
Content Area: Fundamental Skills

Reference:
Potter, P., & Perry, A. (2005). *Fundamentals of nursing* (6th ed.). St. Louis: Mosby, p. 1190.

335. A client began receiving a unit of blood 30 minutes ago. The client rings the call bell and complains of difficulty breathing, itching, and a tight sensation in the chest. Which of the following is the first action of the nurse?
1 Recheck the unit of blood for compatibility
2 Check the client's temperature
3 Stop the transfusion
4 Call the physician

Answer: 3
Rationale: The symptoms reported by the client are compatible with transfusion reaction. The first action of the nurse when a transfusion reaction is suspected is to discontinue the transfusion. The IV line is kept open with normal saline and the physician is notified. The nurse then checks the client's vital signs and rechecks the unit of blood for compatibility. Depending on agency protocol, the nurse may also obtain a urinalysis, draw a sample of blood, and return the unit of blood and tubing to the blood bank. The nurse also institutes supportive care for the client, which may include administration of antihistamines, crystalloids, epinephrine, or vasopressors as prescribed.

Test-Taking Strategy: Focus on the data in the question to determine that the client is experiencing a transfusion reaction. Noting that the question asks for the "first action" will direct you to option 3. Review the nursing actions if a transfusion reaction occurs if you had difficulty with this question.

Level of Cognitive Ability: Application
Client Needs: Physiological Integrity
Integrated Process: Nursing Process/Implementation
Content Area: Delegating/Prioritizing

Reference:
Potter, P., & Perry, A. (2005). *Fundamentals of nursing* (6th ed.). St. Louis: Mosby, p. 1193.

336. A client has not eaten or had anything to drink for 4 hours following two episodes of nausea and vomiting. Which of the following items would be best to offer the client who is ready to try resuming oral intake?
1 Ginger ale
2 Gelatin
3 Toast
4 Dry cereal

Answer: 1
Rationale: Clear liquids are best tolerated first after episodes of nausea and vomiting. If the client tolerates sips (20 to 30 mL at a time) of clear liquids, such as water or ginger ale, then the amounts may be increased and gelatin, tea, and broth may be added. Once these are tolerated, solid foods such as toast, cereal, chicken, and other easily digested foods may be tried.

Test-Taking Strategy: Use the process of elimination. Begin to answer this question by eliminating options 3 and 4, which identify solid foods and are less well tolerated than liquids. Choose ginger ale over gelatin because it is a liquid at all temperatures. Review care to the client with nausea and vomiting if you had difficulty with this question.

Level of Cognitive Ability: Application
Client Needs: Physiological Integrity
Integrated Process: Nursing Process/Implementation
Content Area: Adult Health/Gastrointestinal

Reference:
Lewis, S., Heitkemper, M., & Dirksen, S. (2004). *Medical-surgical nursing: Assessment and management of clinical problems* (6th ed.). St. Louis: Mosby, p. 1005.

337. A client has just undergone an upper gastrointestinal (GI) series. The nurse provides which of the following upon the client's return to the unit as an important part of routine post-procedure care?
1   Decreased fluids
2   Bland diet
3   NPO status
4   Mild laxative

Answer: 4
Rationale: Barium sulfate, which is used as a contrast material during an upper GI series, is constipating. If it is not eliminated from the GI tract, it can cause obstruction. Therefore, laxatives or cathartics are administered as part of routine post-procedure care. Increased (not decreased) fluids are also helpful but do not act in the same way as a laxative to eliminate the barium. Options 2 and 3 are not routine post-procedure measures.

Test-Taking Strategy: Focus on the diagnostic test and the key words "routine post-procedure." Recalling that barium is used in this diagnostic test will direct you to option 4. Review post-procedure care following an upper GI series if you had difficulty with this question.

Level of Cognitive Ability: Application
Client Needs: Physiological Integrity
Integrated Process: Nursing Process/Implementation
Content Area: Adult Health/Gastrointestinal

Reference:
Chernecky, C., & Berger, B. (2004). *Laboratory tests and diagnostic procedures* (4th ed.). Philadelphia: Saunders, p. 220.

---

338. A nurse has an order to discontinue the nasogastric tube of an assigned client. After explaining the procedure to the client, the nurse raises the bed to a semi-Fowler's position, places a towel across the chest, clears the tube with normal saline, clamps the tube, and removes the tube:
1   During inspiration
2   After the client takes a deep breath and holds it
3   As the client breathes out
4   After expiration, but before inspiration

Answer: 2
Rationale: Just before removing the tube, the client is asked to take a deep breath and hold it. This action is important because the airway is partially occluded during tube removal. Also, breath-holding minimizes the risk of aspirating gastric contents if spilled from the tube during removal. The nurse pulls the tube out steadily and smoothly while the client holds the breath. Options 1, 3, and 4 are incorrect.

Test-Taking Strategy: Use the process of elimination and visualize this procedure. Recalling that the airway is partially occluded during tube removal will direct you to option 2. Review this procedure if you had difficulty with this question.

Level of Cognitive Ability: Application
Client Needs: Physiological Integrity
Integrated Process: Nursing Process/Implementation
Content Area: Fundamental Skills

Reference:
Elkin, M., Perry, A., & Potter, P. (2004). *Nursing interventions & clinical skills* (3rd ed.). St. Louis: Mosby, pp. 795-796.

339. A nurse is caring for a client who is receiving total parenteral nutrition and has an order to receive an intravenous intralipid infusion. Which of the following actions does the nurse take as part of proper procedure before hanging the intralipid infusion?
1 Adds 100 mL normal saline to the bottle
2 Attaches an in-line filter to the intralipid infusion tubing
3 Removes the bottle of intralipids from the refrigerator
4 Checks the solution for separation or an oily appearance

Answer: 4

Rationale: Intralipid solutions should not be refrigerated. No additives should be placed in the bottle because this could affect the stability of the solution. The solution should be checked for separation or an oily appearance. If found, it should not be used. An in-line filter is not used because it could disturb the flow of solution or become clogged.

Test-Taking Strategy: Use the process of elimination and focus on the name of the solution: intralipids. Think about the consistency of this solution to direct you to option 4. Review this content if you are unfamiliar with the procedure for infusing intralipid solutions.

Level of Cognitive Ability: Application
Client Needs: Physiological Integrity
Integrated Process: Nursing Process/Implementation
Content Area: Fundamental Skills

Reference:
McKenry, L., & Salerno, E. (2003). *Mosby's pharmacology in nursing* (21st ed.). St. Louis: Mosby, p. 1196.

---

340. A nurse is administering a continuous tube feeding to a client. The nurse takes which of the following actions as part of routine care for this client?
1 Checks the residual every 4 hours
2 Changes the feeding bag and tubing every 48 hours
3 Pours additional feeding into the bag when 25 mL are left
4 Holds the feeding if greater than 200 mL are aspirated.

Answer: 1

Rationale: The nasogastric feeding tube is checked at least every 4 hours for residual when administering continuous tube feedings. The residual is also checked before each bolus with intermittent feedings or before administering medications. If the residual exceeds an amount of 100 mL (or as defined by agency policy), the feeding is held. The bag and tubing are completely changed every 24 hours. The bag should be rinsed before adding new formula to the bag that is hanging.

Test-Taking Strategy: Note the key words "continuous tube feedings." Use the steps of the nursing process to answer the question. Option 1 is the only option that addresses assessment. Review the nursing care associated with this procedure if you had difficulty with this question.

Level of Cognitive Ability: Application
Client Needs: Physiological Integrity
Integrated Process: Nursing Process/Implementation
Content Area: Fundamental Skills

References:
Elkin, M., Perry, A., & Potter, P. (2004). *Nursing interventions & clinical skills* (3rd ed.). St. Louis: Mosby, p. 810.
Lewis, S., Heitkemper, M., & Dirksen, S. (2004). *Medical-surgical nursing: Assessment and management of clinical problems* (6th ed.). St. Louis: Mosby, pp. 982-986.

341. A physician is inserting a chest tube. The nurse selects which of the following materials to be used as the first layer of the dressing at the chest tube insertion site?

1 Sterile 4 x 4 gauze pad
2 Absorbent Kerlix dressing
3 Gauze impregnated with povidone-iodine
4 Petrolatum jelly gauze

Answer: 4

Rationale: The first layer of the chest tube dressing is petrolatum gauze, which allows for an occlusive seal at the chest tube insertion site. Additional layers of gauze cover this layer, and the dressing is secured with a strong adhesive tape or elastoplast tape.

Test-Taking Strategy: Use the process of elimination noting the key words "first layer." Recall that an occlusive seal at the site is needed and think about which dressing material will help achieve this seal. Review care of the client requiring chest tube insertion if you had difficulty with this question.

Level of Cognitive Ability: Application
Client Needs: Physiological Integrity
Integrated Process: Nursing Process/Implementation
Content Area: Adult Health/Respiratory

Reference:
Elkin, M., Perry, A., & Potter, P. (2004). *Nursing interventions & clinical skills* (3rd ed.). St. Louis: Mosby, p. 778.

342. A client being seen in the physician's office for follow-up 2 weeks after pneumonectomy complains of numbness and tenderness at the surgical site. The nurse tells the client that this is:

1 A severe problem and the client will probably be rehospitalized
2 Often the first sign of a wound infection and checks the client's temperature
3 Probably caused by permanent nerve damage as a result of surgery
4 Not likely to be permanent, but may last for some months

Answer: 4

Rationale: Clients who undergo pneumonectomy may experience numbness, altered sensation, or tenderness in the area that surrounds the incision. These sensations may last for months. It is not considered to be a severe problem and is not indicative of a wound infection.

Test-Taking Strategy: Use the process of elimination. Eliminate option 1 because of the word "severe." Eliminate option 2 because numbness and tenderness are not signs of infection. Eliminate option 3 because of the word "permanent." Review this surgical procedure and the expected postoperative occurrences if you are not familiar with it.

Level of Cognitive Ability: Application
Client Needs: Physiological Integrity
Integrated Process: Nursing Process/Implementation
Content Area: Adult Health/Respiratory

References:
Lewis, S., Heitkemper, M., & Dirksen, S. (2004). *Medical-surgical nursing: Assessment and management of clinical problems* (6th ed.). St. Louis: Mosby, p. 625.
Phipps, W., Monahan, F., Sands, J., Marek, J., & Neighbors, M. (2003). *Medical-surgical nursing: Health and illness perspectives* (7th ed.). St. Louis: Mosby, p. 558.

343. A client scheduled for pneumonectomy tells the nurse that a friend of his had lung surgery and had chest tubes. The client asks the nurse about how long his chest tubes will be in place after surgery. The nurse responds that:

1 They will be in place for 24 to 48 hours.
2 They will be removed after 3 to 4 days.
3 They usually function for a full week after surgery.
4 Most likely, there will be no chest tubes in place after surgery.

Answer: 4

Rationale: Pneumonectomy involves removal of the entire lung, usually caused by extensive disease such as bronchogenic carcinoma, unilateral tuberculosis, or lung abscess. Chest tubes are not inserted because the cavity is left to fill with serosanguinous fluid, which later solidifies. The phrenic nerve is severed or crushed to elevate the diaphragm, further decreasing the size of the chest cavity on the operative side.

Test-Taking Strategy: Focus on the surgical procedure. Recall that the entire lung is removed with this procedure. This would guide you to reason that chest tubes are unnecessary, because there is no lung remaining to reinflate to fill the pleural space. Review care of the client following pneumonectomy if you had difficulty with this question.

Level of Cognitive Ability: Application
Client Needs: Physiological Integrity
Integrated Process: Nursing Process/Implementation
Content Area: Adult Health/Respiratory

Reference:
Phipps, W., Monahan, F., Sands, J., Marek, J., & Neighbors, M. (2003). *Medical-surgical nursing: Health and illness perspectives* (7th ed.). St. Louis: Mosby, p. 556.

---

344. A nurse is caring for the client with a dissecting abdominal aortic aneurysm. The nurse avoids which of the following while caring for a client?

1 Turns the client to the side to look for ecchymoses on the lower back
2 Auscultates the arteries for bruits
3 Performs deep palpation of the abdomen
4 Tells the client to report back, shoulder, or neck pain

Answer: 3

Rationale: The nurse avoids deep palpation in the client in which a dissecting abdominal aortic aneurysm is known or suspected. Doing so could place the client at risk for rupture. The nurse looks for ecchymoses on the lower back to determine if the aneurysm is leaking and tells the client to report back, neck, shoulder, or extremity pain. The nurse may auscultate the arteries for bruits.

Test-Taking Strategy: Note the key word "avoids" in the stem of the question. This indicates a false-response question and tells you that the correct option will be an incorrect nursing action or one that is contraindicated. With the diagnosis presented, the only option that could cause harm is the option related to deep palpation. Review care of the client with a dissecting abdominal aortic aneurysm if you had difficulty with this question.

Level of Cognitive Ability: Application
Client Needs: Physiological Integrity
Integrated Process: Nursing Process/Implementation
Content Area: Adult Health/Cardiovascular

References:
Ignatavicius, D., & Workman, M. (2002). *Medical surgical nursing: Critical thinking for collaborative care* (4th ed.). Philadelphia: Saunders, p. 757.
Phipps, W., Monahan, F., Sands, J., Marek, J., & Neighbors, M. (2003). *Medical-surgical nursing: Health and illness perspectives* (7th ed.). St. Louis: Mosby, pp. 790-791.

345. A client has undergone angioplasty of the iliac artery. The nurse best detects bleeding from the angioplasty in the region of the iliac artery by:
1. Measuring abdominal girth
2. Auscultating over the area with a Doppler
3. Asking the client about mild pain in the area
4. Palpating the pedal pulses

Answer: 1

Rationale: Bleeding after iliac artery angioplasty causes blood to accumulate in the retroperitoneal area. This can most directly be detected by measuring abdominal girth. Palpation and auscultation of pulses determines patency. Assessment of pain is routinely done, and mild regional discomfort is expected.

Test-Taking Strategy: Use the process of elimination. Focus on the key words "bleeding" and "iliac artery." Select the option that addresses an abdominal assessment because the iliac arteries are located in the peritoneal cavity. This will direct you to option 1. Review this procedure if you had difficulty with this question.

Level of Cognitive Ability: Analysis
Client Needs: Physiological Integrity
Integrated Process: Nursing Process/Assessment
Content Area: Adult Health/Cardiovascular

References:
Ignatavicius, D., & Workman, M. (2002). *Medical surgical nursing: Critical thinking for collaborative care* (4th ed.). Philadelphia: Saunders, p. 747.
Phipps, W., Monahan, F., Sands, J., Marek, J., & Neighbors, M. (2003). *Medical-surgical nursing: Health and illness perspectives* (7th ed.). St. Louis: Mosby, p. 661.

346. A client is scheduled for a right femoral-popliteal bypass graft. The client has a nursing diagnosis of Ineffective Tissue Perfusion. The nurse takes which of the following actions before surgery to address this nursing diagnosis?
1. Completes a preoperative checklist
2. Marks the location of pedal pulses on the right leg
3. Has the client void before surgery
4. Checks the results of any baseline coagulation studies

Answer: 2

Rationale: A nursing diagnosis of Ineffective Tissue Perfusion in the client scheduled for femoral-popliteal bypass grafting indicates that the client is likely to have diminished peripheral pulses. It is important to mark the location of any pulses that are palpated or auscultated. This provides a baseline for comparison in the postoperative period. The other options are part of routine preoperative care.

Test-Taking Strategy: Note the key words "to address this nursing diagnosis." In this case, each of the incorrect options is an action that is part of routine preoperative care and are not specific to this nursing diagnosis. Review care of the client with ineffective tissue perfusion if you had difficulty with this question.

Level of Cognitive Ability: Application
Client Needs: Physiological Integrity
Integrated Process: Nursing Process/Implementation
Content Area: Adult Health/Cardiovascular

References:
Gulanick, M., Myers, J., Klopp, A., Gradishar, D., Galanes, S., & Puzas, M. (2003). *Nursing care plans: Nursing diagnosis and intervention* (5th ed.). St. Louis: Mosby, p. 172.
Lewis, S., Heitkemper, M., & Dirksen, S. (2004). *Medical-surgical nursing: Assessment and management of clinical problems* (6th ed.). St. Louis: Mosby, p. 923.

347. A client who underwent peripheral arterial bypass surgery 16 hours ago complains of increasing pain in the leg at rest, which worsens with movement and is accompanied by paresthesias. The nurse should take which of the following actions?
1 Administer a narcotic analgesic
2 Apply warm moist heat for comfort
3 Apply ice to minimize any developing swelling
4 Call the physician

Answer: 4
Rationale: The classic signs of compartment syndrome are pain at rest that intensifies with movement and the development of paresthesias. Compartment syndrome is characterized by increased pressure within a muscle compartment caused by bleeding or excessive edema. It compresses the nerves in the area and can cause vascular compromise. The physician is notified immediately because the client could require an emergency fasciotomy. Options 1, 2, and 3 are incorrect actions.

Test-Taking Strategy: Use the process of elimination. Note the key words "increasing pain." Also note that the surgery was 16 hours ago. The signs and symptoms described indicate a new problem. These factors should indicate that the physician needs to be notified. Review the complications of this type of surgery if you had difficulty with this question.

Level of Cognitive Ability: Application
Client Needs: Physiological Integrity
Integrated Process: Nursing Process/Implementation
Content Area: Adult Health/Cardiovascular

Reference:
Black, J., & Hawks, J. (2005). *Medical-surgical nursing: Clinical management for positive outcomes* (7th ed.). Philadelphia: Saunders, p. 1518.

348. A nurse in an ambulatory care clinic takes a client's blood pressure (BP) in the left arm and notes that it is 200/118 mmHg. The nurse would:
1 Notify the physician
2 Inquire about the presence of kidney disorders
3 Check the client's blood pressure in the right arm
4 Recheck the pressure in the same arm within 30 seconds

Answer: 3
Rationale: When a high BP reading is noted, the nurse takes the pressure in the opposite arm to see if the blood pressure is elevated in one extremity only. The nurse would also recheck the blood pressure in the same arm, but would wait at least 2 minutes between readings. The nurse would inquire about the presence of kidney disorders that could contribute to the elevated blood pressure. The nurse would notify the physician because immediate treatment may be required, but this would not be done without obtaining verification of the elevation.

Test-Taking Strategy: Use the process of elimination. Eliminate option 4 first because of the time frame, 30 seconds. From the remaining options, select option 3 because it provides verification of the initial reading. Review the procedures for BP measurement if you had difficulty with this question.

Level of Cognitive Ability: Application
Client Needs: Physiological Integrity
Integrated Process: Nursing Process/Implementation
Content Area: Adult Health/Cardiovascular

Reference:
Potter, P., & Perry, A. (2005). *Fundamentals of nursing* (6th ed.). St. Louis: Mosby, p. 660.

349. A hospitalized client has been diagnosed with thrombophlebitis. The nurse would avoid doing which of the following during the care of this client?
1 Applying compression stockings
2 Applying moist heat to the leg
3 Elevating the feet above heart level
4 Adjust the bed to provide a comfortable knee bend

Answer: 4
Rationale: The nurse avoids placing the client in a position that allows a knee bend because it places pressure on the popliteal area, obstructs venous return to the heart, and exacerbates impairment of blood flow. The feet are elevated above heart level to aid in venous return, and warm moist heat may be used to aid in comfort and reduce venospasm. Compression stockings are applied to assist in promoting venous return.

Test-Taking Strategy: Note the key word "avoid." This indicates a false-response question and tells you that the correct option will be an incorrect nursing action. Use principles related to gravity and relief of inflammation to direct you to option 4. Review care of the client with thrombophlebitis if you had difficulty with this question.

Level of Cognitive Ability: Application
Client Needs: Physiological Integrity
Integrated Process: Nursing Process/Implementation
Content Area: Adult Health/Cardiovascular

References:
Black, J., & Hawks, J. (2005). *Medical-surgical nursing: Clinical management for positive outcomes* (7th ed.). Philadelphia: Saunders, p. 1537.
Phipps, W., Monahan, F., Sands, J., Marek, J., & Neighbors, M. (2003). *Medical-surgical nursing: Health and illness perspectives* (7th ed.). St. Louis: Mosby, pp. 793; 797.

350. A new prenatal client is 6 months pregnant. On the first prenatal visit, the nurse notes that the client is gravida 4, para 0, aborta 3. The client is 5′6′′ tall, weighs 130 pounds, and is 25 years old. The client states, "I get really tired after working all day and I can't keep up with my housework." Which factor in the above data would lead the nurse to suspect gestational diabetes?
1 Fatigue
2 Obesity
3 Maternal age
4 Previous fetal demise

Answer: 4
Rationale: Fatigue is a normal occurrence during pregnancy. Five feet, six inches tall and 130 pounds does not meet the criteria of 20% over ideal weight. Therefore, the client is not obese. To be at high risk for gestational diabetes, the maternal age should be greater than 30 years. A previous history of unexplained stillbirths or miscarriages puts the client at high risk for gestational diabetes.

Test-Taking Strategy: Use the process of elimination. Option 1 can be eliminated because fatigue is a normal occurrence during pregnancy. Recalling the risk factors associated with gestational diabetes will indicate that options 2 and 3 do not apply to this client. Review the risk factors associated with gestational diabetes if you had difficulty with this question.

Level of Cognitive Ability: Analysis
Client Needs: Physiological Integrity
Integrated Process: Nursing Process/Analysis
Content Area: Maternity/Antepartum

References:
Lowdermilk, D., & Perry, A. (2004). *Maternity & women's health care* (8th ed.). St. Louis: Mosby, p. 895.
Matteson, P. (2001). *Women's health during the childbearing years: A community-based approach.* St. Louis: Mosby, p. 736.

Hirschsprung's disease – Ribbon-like stools.
Intussusception – Current jelly like.

416. A nurse is preparing to administer ear drops to an infant. The nurse plans to:
1 Pull up and back on the auricle and direct the solution toward the wall of the ear canal
2 Pull down and back on the auricle and direct the solution onto the eardrum
3 Pull down and back on the ear lobe and direct the solution toward the wall of the canal
4 Pull up and back on the ear lobe and direct the solution toward the wall of the canal

Answer: 3
Rationale: The infant should be turned on the side with the affected ear uppermost. With the nondominant hand, the nurse pulls down and back on the ear lobe. The wrist of the dominant hand is rested on the infant's head. The medication is administered by aiming it at the wall of the canal rather than directly onto the eardrum. The infant should be held or positioned with the affected ear uppermost for 10 to 15 minutes to retain the solution. In the adult, the auricle is pulled up and back to straighten the auditory canal.

Test-Taking Strategy: Basic safety principles related to the administration of ear medications should assist in eliminating option 2. Option 1 is eliminated because it is the adult procedure. It would be difficult to pull up and back on an earlobe; therefore, eliminate option 4. Review the procedure for administering ear medications in an infant and adult if you had difficulty with this question.

Level of Cognitive Ability: Application
Client Needs: Physiological Integrity
Integrated Process: Nursing Process/Implementation
Content Area: Pharmacology

Reference:
McKenry, L., & Salerno, E. (2003). *Mosby's pharmacology in nursing* (21st ed.). St. Louis: Mosby, p. 143.

---

417. A client seeks treatment in an ambulatory clinic for a complaint of hoarseness that has persisted for 8 weeks. Based on the symptom, the nurse interprets that the client is at risk of having:
1 Laryngeal cancer
2 Acute laryngitis
3 Bronchogenic cancer
4 Thyroid cancer

Answer: 1
Rationale: Hoarseness is a common early sign of laryngeal cancer, but not of bronchogenic or thyroid cancer. Hoarseness that persists for 8 weeks is not associated with an acute problem, such as laryngitis.

Test-Taking Strategy: Use the process of elimination. Begin to answer this question by eliminating option 2, because an acute problem would not generally last for 8 weeks. From the remaining options, recalling that the vocal cords are in the larynx makes option 1 preferable to any of the other options. Review the signs of laryngeal cancer if you had difficulty with this question.

Level of Cognitive Ability: Analysis
Client Needs: Physiological Integrity
Integrated Process: Nursing Process/Analysis
Content Area: Adult Health/Respiratory

Reference:
Ignatavicius, D., & Workman, M. (2002). *Medical surgical nursing: Critical thinking for collaborative care* (4th ed.). Philadelphia: Saunders, p. 517.

418. A client is admitted to the cardiac intensive care unit following cardiac surgery. The nurse notes that in the first hour after admission, the chest tube drainage was 75 mL. During the second hour, the drainage has dropped to 5 mL. The nurse interprets that:
1 The lung has fully reexpanded
2 This is normal
3 The client needs to cough and deep breathe
4 The tube may be occluded

Answer: 4
Rationale: Chest tube drainage should not exceed 100 mL per hour during the first 2 hours postoperatively, and approximately 500 mL of drainage is expected in the first 24 hours after cardiac surgery. The sudden drop in drainage between the first and second hour indicates that the tube is possibly occluded and requires further assessment by the nurse. Options 1, 2, and 3 are incorrect interpretations.

Test-Taking Strategy: Use the process of elimination. Eliminate option 1 first because it is unlikely that the lung would reexpand in the immediate postoperative period. Needing to cough and deep breathe is a response that is unrelated to the client's problem, so option 3 is eliminated next. From the remaining options, knowing that the drainage would not drop so radically in 1 hour in the immediate postoperative period directs you to option 4. Review the concepts related to chest tube drainage systems in the postoperative client if you had difficulty with this question.

Level of Cognitive Ability: Analysis
Client Needs: Physiological Integrity
Integrated Process: Nursing Process/Analysis
Content Area: Adult Health/Cardiovascular

Reference:
Phipps, W., Monahan, F., Sands, J., Marek, J., & Neighbors, M. (2003). *Medical-surgical nursing: Health and illness perspectives* (7th ed.). St. Louis: Mosby, p. 755.

---

419. A nurse is auscultating the chest of a client who was diagnosed with pleurisy 48 hours ago. The client does not have a pleural friction rub, which was auscultated the previous day. The nurse interprets that this is most likely the result of:
1 Decreased inflammatory reaction at the site
2 The deep breaths that the client is taking
3 Accumulation of pleural fluid in the inflamed area
4 Effectiveness of medication therapy

Answer: 3
Rationale: Pleural friction rub is auscultated early in the course of pleurisy, before pleural fluid accumulates. Once fluid accumulates in the inflamed area, there is less friction between the visceral and parietal lung surfaces, and the pleural friction rub disappears. Options 1, 2, and 4 are incorrect interpretations.

Test-Taking Strategy: Use the process of elimination. Eliminate option 2 first, which would intensify the pain. Options 1 and 4 are similar, and because the question states that the problem was diagnosed 48 hours ago, these should be eliminated next. Remember: fluid accumulation in the area provides a buffer between the lung and chest wall surfaces, which eliminates the friction rub. Review assessment findings in the client with pleurisy if you had difficulty with this question.

Level of Cognitive Ability: Analysis
Client Needs: Physiological Integrity
Integrated Process: Nursing Process/Analysis
Content Area: Adult Health/Respiratory

References:
Ignatavicius, D., & Workman, M. (2002). *Medical surgical nursing: Critical thinking for collaborative care* (4th ed.). Philadelphia: Saunders, p. 578.
Phipps, W., Monahan, F., Sands, J., Marek, J., & Neighbors, M. (2003). *Medical-surgical nursing: Health and illness perspectives* (7th ed.). St. Louis: Mosby, p. 470.

420. A client is admitted to the nursing unit with a diagnosis of pleurisy. The nurse assesses the client for which characteristic symptom of this disorder?

1 Early morning fatigue

2 Dyspnea that is relieved by lying flat

3 Pain that worsens when the breath is held

4 Knife-like pain that worsens on inspiration

Answer: 4

Rationale: A typical symptom of pleurisy is knife-like pain that worsens on inspiration caused by the friction created by rubbing together inflamed pleural surfaces. This pain usually disappears when the breath is held, because these surfaces stop moving. The client does not experience early morning fatigue or dyspnea relieved by lying flat.

Test-Taking Strategy: Use the process of elimination. Option 2 is eliminated first because dyspnea is not relieved by lying flat. Option 1 is eliminated next because fatigue, if it were to occur, would not be present in the morning when the client is most well rested. From the remaining options, keep in mind that pleurisy results from inflammation of the pleura. Because the visceral and parietal lung pleura glide over one another with respiration, it is expected that chest movement precipitates or intensifies the pain. Review the symptoms associated with pleurisy if you had difficulty with this question.

Level of Cognitive Ability: Application
Client Needs: Physiological Integrity
Integrated Process: Nursing Process/Assessment
Content Area: Adult Health/Respiratory

Reference:
Lewis, S., Heitkemper, M., & Dirksen, S. (2004). *Medical-surgical nursing: Assessment and management of clinical problems* (6th ed.). St. Louis: Mosby, p. 629.

---

421. A client has frequent runs of ventricular tachycardia, and the physician prescribes tambocor (Flecanide). Because of the effects of the medications, the nurse does which of the following?

1 Assesses the client for neurological problems

2 Monitors the client's vital signs (BP) and ECG frequently

3 Ensures that the bed rails remain in the up position

4 Monitors the client's urinary output

Answer: 2

Rationale: Tambocor (Flecanide) is an antidysrhythmic medication that slows conduction and decreases excitability, conduction velocity, and automaticity. The nurse needs to monitor for the development of a new or a worsening dysrhythmia. Options 1, 3, and 4 are components of standard care but are not specific to this medication.

Test-Taking Strategy: Use the process of elimination. Note the relation of the information in the question (client has a dysrhythmia) and the nursing action in the correct option. Option 2 is the only option that relates to cardiac status monitoring. Review this medication if you had difficulty with this question.

Level of Cognitive Ability: Analysis
Client Needs: Physiological Integrity
Integrated Process: Nursing Process/Implementation
Content Area: Pharmacology

References:
Lehne, R. (2004). *Pharmacology for nursing care* (5th ed.). Philadelphia: Saunders, p. 504.
McKenry, L., & Salerno, E. (2003). *Mosby's pharmacology in nursing* (21st ed.). St. Louis: Mosby, p. 559.

422. A nurse is performing an assessment on a client with the diagnosis of Brown-Séquard's syndrome. Which finding should the nurse expect to note?
1   Ipsilateral paralysis and loss of touch and vibration
2   Bilateral loss of pain and temperature sensation
3   Contralateral paralysis and loss of touch sensation and vibration
4   Complete paraplegia or quadriplegia, depending on the level of injury

Answer: 1

Rationale: Brown-Séquard's syndrome results from hemisection of the spinal cord, resulting in ipsilateral paralysis and loss of touch, pressure, vibration, and proprioception. Contralaterally, pain and temperature sensation is lost because these fibers decussate after entering the cord. Options 2, 3, and 4 are not assessment findings in this syndrome.

Test-Taking Strategy: Recalling that Brown-Séquard's syndrome results from hemisection of the spinal cord will assist in eliminating options 2 and 4. From the remaining options, it is necessary to know that it results in ipsilateral paralysis and loss of touch, pressure, vibration, and proprioception. Review the assessment findings and the nursing care if you are unfamiliar with this syndrome.

Level of Cognitive Ability: Analysis
Client Needs: Physiological Integrity
Integrated Process: Nursing Process/Assessment
Content Area: Adult Health/Neurological

Reference:
Ignatavicius, D., & Workman, M. (2002). *Medical surgical nursing: Critical thinking for collaborative care* (4th ed.). Philadelphia: Saunders, p. 934.

---

423. A nurse is performing an assessment on a client who has a suspected spinal cord injury. Which of the following is the priority nursing assessment?
1   Pupillary response
2   Respiratory status
3   Mobility level
4   Pain level

Answer: 2

Rationale: All of these assessments would be performed on a client with a suspected spinal cord injury. However, respiratory status is the priority.

Test-Taking Strategy: Use the ABCs—airway, breathing, and circulation—to answer the question. Option 2 addresses airway. Review care of the client with a suspected spinal cord injury if you had difficulty with this question.

Level of Cognitive Ability: Application
Client Needs: Physiological Integrity
Integrated Process: Nursing Process/Assessment
Content Area: Delegating/Prioritizing

Reference:
Ignatavicius, D., & Workman, M. (2002). *Medical surgical nursing: Critical thinking for collaborative care* (4th ed.). Philadelphia: Saunders, p. 933.

---

424. A nurse is caring for a client who is newly diagnosed with a spinal cord injury. The nurse would anticipate that the most likely medication to be prescribed would be:
1   Propranolol (Inderal)
2   Dexamethasone (Decadron)
3   Furosemide (Lasix)
4   Morphine sulfate

Answer: 2

Rationale: The most likely medication to be prescribed for a client with a newly diagnosed spinal cord injury is dexamethasone (Decadron). This medication is a short-acting glucocorticoid and would be administered to reduce traumatic edema. The use of propranolol (a beta-blocker), furosemide (a diuretic), or morphine sulfate (an opioid analgesic) would not be indicated based on the information in this question.

Test-Taking Strategy: Note the key words "newly diagnosed" and the diagnosis "spinal cord injury." Recalling the association between injury and edema and that dexamethasone is used to reduce traumatic edema will assist you in answering the question. Review this content if you are unfamiliar with these medications or the treatment for spinal cord injury.

Level of Cognitive Ability: Analysis
Client Needs: Physiological Integrity
Integrated Process: Nursing Process/Analysis
Content Area: Adult Health/Neurological

References:
McKenry, L., & Salerno, E. (2003). *Mosby's pharmacology in nursing* (21st ed.). St. Louis: Mosby, p. 959.
Phipps, W., Monahan, F., Sands, J., Marek, J., & Neighbors, M. (2003). *Medical-surgical nursing: Health and illness perspectives* (7th ed.). St. Louis: Mosby, p. 1332.

---

425. A nurse is admitting a client with a diagnosis of acquired immunodeficiency syndrome (AIDS) to the medical-surgical unit. The nurse most importantly assesses for which of the following?
1 Jaundiced skin
2 White patches in the oral cavity
3 Bradypnea
4 Urine specific gravity of 1.010

Answer: 2
Rationale: Clients with AIDS frequently develop opportunistic infections. *Candida albicans*, the causative organism of thrush, is a common opportunistic infection. Thrush presents as white patches in the oral cavity. Hairy leukoplakia also presents as white patches in the oral cavity. Jaundice is a symptom of hepatic disease. Clients with AIDS frequently acquire pneumonia and may present with tachypnea, not bradypnea. Clients with AIDS frequently have inadequate nutrition and hydration and may present with dehydration, resulting in a high specific gravity rather than a low specific gravity.

Test-Taking Strategy: Focus on the client's diagnosis. Recalling that the client with AIDS is at risk for developing an infection will direct you to option 2. Review the manifestations associated with AIDS if you had difficulty with this question.

Level of Cognitive Ability: Analysis
Client Needs: Physiological Integrity
Integrated Process: Nursing Process/Assessment
Content Area: Adult Health/Immune

References:
Black, J., & Hawks, J. (2005). *Medical-surgical nursing: Clinical management for positive outcomes* (7th ed.). Philadelphia: Saunders, p. 2389.
Ignatavicius, D., & Workman, M. (2002). *Medical surgical nursing: Critical thinking for collaborative care* (4th ed.). Philadelphia: Saunders, pp. 371; 373.

426. A nurse assesses a client who was involved in a motor vehicle accident. The nurse determines the need to prepare for chest tube insertion if the client exhibits:

1 Shortness of breath and tracheal deviation
2 Chest pain and shortness of breath
3 Decreasing oxygen saturation and bradypnea
4 Peripheral cyanosis and hypotension

Answer: 1

Rationale: Shortness of breath and tracheal deviation results when lung tissue and alveoli have collapsed. The trachea deviates to the unaffected side in the presence of a tension pneumothorax. Air entering the pleural cavity causes the lung to lose its normal negative pressure. The increasing pressure in the affected side displaces contents to the unaffected side. Shortness of breath results from a decreased area available for diffusion of gases. Chest pain and shortness of breath are more commonly associated with myocardial ischemia or infarction. Clients requiring chest tubes exhibit decreasing oxygen saturation but will more likely experience tachypnea related to the hypoxia. Peripheral cyanosis is caused by circulatory disorders. Hypotension may be a result of tracheal shift and impedance of venous return to the heart. However, it may also be the result of other problems such as a failing heart.

Test-Taking Strategy: Focus on the issue: preparation for chest tube insertion. Recalling the signs of a tension pneumothorax and noting the words "tracheal deviation" will direct you to option 1. Review the signs associated with tension pneumothorax and the conditions that require chest tube drainage if you had difficulty with this question.

Level of Cognitive Ability: Analysis
Client Needs: Physiological Integrity
Integrated Process: Nursing Process/Analysis
Content Area: Adult Health/Respiratory

Reference:
Black, J., & Hawks, J. (2005). *Medical-surgical nursing: Clinical management for positive outcomes* (7th ed.). Philadelphia: Saunders, p. 1904.

---

427. A nurse is admitting a client to the mental health unit who has a diagnosis of bipolar disorder, manic phase. In assessing the client regarding sleep patterns and the need for rest, the nurse knows that the most reliable information may be obtained by:

1 Asking the client how many hours of sleep were obtained last night
2 Observing the facial appearance of the client
3 Asking the significant other about the sleep patterns
4 Asking the client to describe the level of fatigue

Answer: 3

Rationale: Option 3 would provide the most reliable information because the client may not be able to report sleep patterns accurately. The client may report that sleep has not been a problem when in fact only 3 hours of sleep have been obtained for the last several days. Rest needs are very important because the manic client may be at the point of exhaustion by the time hospitalization occurs. Facial expressions may be an indicator of fatigue, but they are not quantifiable. The client may not be able to describe the level of fatigue accurately.

Test-Taking Strategy: Use the process of elimination, focusing on the words "most reliable." Eliminate options 1 and 4 because they are similar and require data collection from the client. From the remaining options, focus on the key words. In this situation, the significant other is the only one who can provide accurate information. Review assessment of the client with bipolar disorder if you had difficulty with this question.

Level of Cognitive Ability: Analysis
Client Needs: Physiological Integrity

Integrated Process: Nursing Process/Assessment
Content Area: Mental Health

Reference:
Stuart, G., & Laraia, M. (2005). *Principles and practice of psychiatric nursing* (8th ed.). St. Louis: Mosby, p. 244.

---

428. The parents of a male newborn who is not circumcised request information on how to clean the newborn's penis. The nurse tells the parents to:

1 Retract the foreskin and cleanse the glans when bathing the newborn
2 Avoid retracting the foreskin to cleanse the glans because this may cause adhesions
3 Retract the foreskin no farther than it will go and replace it over the glans after cleaning
4 Retract the foreskin and cleanse the glans with every diaper change

Answer: 2

Rationale: In newborn males, prepuce is continuous with the epidermis of the glans and is nonretractable. Forced retraction may cause adhesions to develop. It is best to allow separation to occur naturally, which will happen between 3 years and puberty. Most foreskins are retractable by 3 years of age and should be pushed back gently for cleaning once a week. Therefore, option 2 is correct.

Test-Taking Strategy: Eliminate options 1, 3, and 4 because they are similar and are incorrect because retracting the foreskin is not recommended in an uncircumcised newborn male. Option 2 is the different option, stating that the foreskin should not be retracted. Review parent teaching points related to the care of an uncircumcised newborn if you had difficulty with this question.

Level of Cognitive Ability: Application
Client Needs: Physiological Integrity
Integrated Process: Teaching/Learning
Content Area: Child Health

Reference:
Lowdermilk, D., & Perry, A. (2004). *Maternity & women's health care* (8th ed.). St. Louis: Mosby, p. 695.

---

429. The client who has been receiving intravenous (IV) aminophylline (Theophylline) has been prescribed an immediate-release oral form of the medication. The IV medication is to be discontinued. The nurse should administer the first dose of the oral medication:

1 Immediately upon discontinuing the IV form
2 In 4 to 6 hours after discontinuing the IV form
3 Just before the next meal
4 Just after the next meal

Answer: 2

Rationale: With an immediate-release preparation, the oral aminophylline should be administered in 4 to 6 hours after discontinuing the IV form of the medication. If the sustained-release form is used, the first oral dose should be administered immediately upon discontinuation of the IV infusion.

Test-Taking Strategy: Use the process of elimination. Eliminate options 3 and 4 because they do not provide information about when the client will eat his or her next meal. Next, note the key words "immediate-release." It then makes sense to wait 4 to 6 hours before administration of the oral form. Review this medication and its methods of administration if you had difficulty with this question.

Level of Cognitive Ability: Application
Client Needs: Physiological Integrity
Integrated Process: Nursing Process/Implementation
Content Area: Pharmacology

Reference:
McKenry, L., & Salerno, E. (2003). *Mosby's pharmacology in nursing* (21st ed.). St. Louis: Mosby, p. 723.

430. A client has a serum sodium level of 129 mEq/L resulting from hypervolemia. The nurse consults with the physician to determine whether which measure should be instituted?

1 Providing a 2-gram sodium diet
2 Providing a 4-gram sodium diet
3 Fluid restriction
4 Administering intravenous hypertonic saline

Answer: 3

Rationale: Hyponatremia is defined as a serum sodium level of less than 135 mEq/L. When it is caused by hypervolemia, it may be treated with fluid restriction. The low serum sodium value is a result of hemodilution. Intravenous hypertonic saline is reserved for hyponatremia when the serum sodium level is lower than 125 mEq/L. A 4-gram sodium diet is a no-added-salt diet. A 2-gram sodium restriction would not raise the serum sodium level.

Test-Taking Strategy: Use the process of elimination. Note that the serum sodium level is low. With this in mind, you would eliminate options 1 and 2. Next, note the key word "hypervolemia." Knowing that hypervolemia causes hemodilution of the serum sodium would guide you to select option 3. Review treatment measures for hyponatremia if you had difficulty with this question.

Level of Cognitive Ability: Application
Client Needs: Physiological Integrity
Integrated Process: Nursing Process/Implementation
Content Area: Fundamental Skills

Reference:
Black, J., & Hawks, J. (2005). *Medical-surgical nursing: Clinical management for positive outcomes* (7th ed.). Philadelphia: Saunders, p. 226.

431. A nurse is planning care for a client whose oxygenation is being monitored by a pulse oximeter. The nurse includes which intervention in the plan to ensure accurate monitoring of the client's oxygenation status?

1 Notify the physician immediately of O_2 saturation less than 90%
2 Instruct the client not to move the sensor
3 Tape the sensor tightly to the client's finger
4 Place the sensor on a finger below the blood pressure cuff

Answer: 2

Rationale: The pulse oximeter passes a beam of light through the tissue, and a sensor attached to the fingertip, toe, or ear lobe measures the amount of light absorbed by the oxygen-saturated hemoglobin. The oximeter then gives a reading of the percentage of hemoglobin that is saturated with oxygen (Sao_2). Motion at the sensor site changes light absorption. The motion mimics the pulsatile motion of blood, and because the detector cannot distinguish between movement of blood and movement of the finger, results can be inaccurate. The sensor should not be placed distal to blood pressure cuffs, pressure dressings, arterial lines, or any invasive catheters. The sensor should not be taped to the client's finger. If values fall below preset norms (usually 90%), the client should be instructed to deep breathe, if this is appropriate. It is not necessary to call the physician immediately unless measures such as deep breathing do not raise the level back to normal.

Test-Taking Strategy: Focus on the issue: "to ensure accurate monitoring." Eliminate option 1 because of the word "immediately." Additionally, it is unrelated to ensuring accurate monitoring with a pulse oximeter. Option 4 is inappropriate; therefore, eliminate this option. From the remaining options, recalling that motion at the sensor site changes light absorption and noting the word "tightly" in option 3 will direct you to the correct option. Review the principles associated with pulse oximetry if you had difficulty with this question.

Level of Cognitive Ability: Application
Client Needs: Physiological Integrity
Integrated Process: Nursing Process/Planning
Content Area: Adult Health/Respiratory

References:
Elkin, M., Perry, A., & Potter, P. (2004). *Nursing interventions & clinical skills* (3rd ed.). St. Louis: Mosby, pp. 290-292.
Potter, P., & Perry, A. (2005). *Fundamentals of nursing* (6th ed.). St. Louis: Mosby, pp. 651-652.

---

432. A nurse teaches a client with thromboangiitis obliterans (Buerger's disease) about measures to control the disease process. The nurse determines that the client needs further instructions about these measures if the client states which of the following?
  1 "I need to stop smoking immediately."
  2 "I will need to take nifedipine (Procardia) as directed."
  3 "I need to keep my legs and arms cool."
  4 "I need to watch for signs and symptoms of skin breakdown."

Answer: 3
Rationale: Interventions are directed at preventing the progression of thromboangiitis obliterans and include conveying the need for immediate smoking cessation, providing medications prescribed for vasodilation, such as nifedipine (Procardia) a calcium channel blocker, or prazosin (Minipress) an alpha-adrenergic blocker. The client should maintain warmth to the extremities, especially by avoiding exposure to cold. The client should inspect the extremities and report signs of infection or ulceration.

Test-Taking Strategy: Note the key words "needs further instructions." These words indicate a false-response question and that you need to select the option that is an incorrect client statement. Because the goals of care for thromboangiitis obliterans are the same as for peripheral arterial disease, the answer to this question is the one that does not promote vasodilation, option 3. Review home care measures for the client with thromboangiitis obliterans if you had difficulty with this question.

Level of Cognitive Ability: Analysis
Client Needs: Physiological Integrity
Integrated Process: Teaching/Learning
Content Area: Adult Health/Cardiovascular

Reference:
Ignatavicius, D., & Workman, M. (2002). *Medical surgical nursing: Critical thinking for collaborative care* (4th ed.). Philadelphia: Saunders, p. 761.

---

433. A client has been admitted to the mental health unit with a diagnosis of social phobia disorder. Which behavior would the nurse expect the client to report during the assessment?
  1 Panic attack when leaving the house
  2 Shortness of breath and palpitations when riding the elevator
  3 Persistent handwashing before eating
  4 Fear of being humiliated in public and embarrassing self in front of others

Answer: 4
Rationale: A social phobia is characterized by a fear of appearing incompetent or inept in the presence of others and of doing something embarrassing. Thus, the client becomes anxious when the attention is on them. Option 1 identifies agoraphobia. Option 2 identifies claustrophobia. Option 3 identifies obsessive-compulsive behavior.

Test-Taking Strategy: Focus on the key words "social phobia." Note the relationship between these words and option 4. Review the characteristics of the various phobias if you had difficulty with this question.

Level of Cognitive Ability: Analysis
Client Needs: Physiological Integrity

Integrated Process: Nursing Process/Assessment
Content Area: Mental Health

Reference:
Stuart, G., & Laraia, M. (2005). *Principles and practice of psychiatric nursing* (8th ed.). St. Louis: Mosby, p. 271.

---

434. A nurse is caring for a client with Parkinson's disease who is taking benztropine mesylate (Cogentin) orally daily. The nurse does which of the following to assess for a side effect of the medication?
1 Checks pupillary response
2 Checks the partial thromboplastin time (PTT)
3 Monitors intake and output
4 Monitors the prothrombin time (PT)

Answer: 3
Rationale: Urinary retention is a side effect of benztropine mesylate. The nurse needs to monitor the client's intake and output and observe for dysuria, distended abdomen, infrequent voiding of small amounts, and overflow incontinence. Options 1, 2, and 4 are unrelated to the side effects of this medication.

Test-Taking Strategy: Use the process of elimination. Eliminate options 2 and 4 first because they are similar. From the remaining options, it is necessary to know that urinary retention is a concern with this medication. Review this medication and its side effects if you had difficulty with this question.

Level of Cognitive Ability: Application
Client Needs: Physiological Integrity
Integrated Process: Nursing Process/Assessment
Content Area: Pharmacology

Reference:
Hodgson, B., & Kizior, R. (2004). *Saunders nursing drug handbook 2004.* Philadelphia: Saunders, p. 101.

---

435. A home care nurse is assessing a client who has begun using peritoneal dialysis. The nurse determines that which manifestation noted in the client would most likely indicate the onset of peritonitis?
1 Temperature of 99.0°F oral
2 History of gastrointestinal (GI) upset 1 week ago
3 Cloudy dialysate output
4 Presence of crystals in dialysate output

Answer: 3
Rationale: Typical symptoms of peritonitis include fever, nausea, malaise, rebound abdominal tenderness, and cloudy dialysate output. The very slight temperature elevation in option 1 is not the clearest indicator of infection. The complaint of GI upset is too vague to indicate peritonitis. Peritonitis would cause cloudy dialysate, but would not cause crystals to appear in the dialysate.

Test-Taking Strategy: Note the key words "most likely" and the issue: indicator of peritonitis. Begin to answer this question by eliminating options 1 and 2 because both of these manifestations are nonspecific. From the remaining options, recall that infection would cause white blood cells to be present in the dialysate, which would yield cloudiness, not crystals, in the dialysate output. Review the signs of peritonitis in the client receiving peritoneal dialysis if you had difficulty with this question.

Level of Cognitive Ability: Analysis
Client Needs: Physiological Integrity
Integrated Process: Nursing Process/Assessment
Content Area: Adult Health/Renal

References:
Ignatavicius, D., & Workman, M. (2002). *Medical surgical nursing: Critical thinking for collaborative care* (4th ed.). Philadelphia: Saunders, p. 1269.
Phipps, W., Monahan, F., Sands, J., Marek, J., & Neighbors, M. (2003). *Medical-surgical nursing: Health and illness perspectives* (7th ed.). St. Louis: Mosby, p. 1286.

---

436. A nurse is working on a medical-surgical nursing unit and is caring for several clients with renal failure. The nurse interprets that which of the following clients is best suited for peritoneal dialysis as a treatment option?
1 A client with severe congestive heart failure
2 A client with a history of ruptured diverticuli
3 A client with a history of herniated lumbar disk
4 A client with a history of three previous abdominal surgeries

Answer: 1
Rationale: Peritoneal dialysis may be the treatment option of choice for clients with severe cardiovascular disease. Severe cardiac disease can be worsened by the rapid shifts in fluid, electrolytes, urea, and glucose that occurs with hemodialysis. For the same reason, peritoneal dialysis may be indicated for the client with diabetes mellitus. Contraindications to peritoneal dialysis include diseases of the abdomen such as ruptured diverticuli or malignancies; extensive abdominal surgeries; history of peritonitis; obesity; and those with a history of back problems, which could be aggravated by the fluid weight of the dialysate. Severe disease of the vascular system may also be a contraindication.

Test-Taking Strategy: Note the issue: the client who would be the best candidate for peritoneal dialysis. Eliminate options 2 and 4 first because they are similar and indicate clients with an abdominal condition. From the remaining options, recall the concepts related to fluid shifts in the body to direct you to option 1. Review the indications for peritoneal dialysis if you had difficulty with this question.

Level of Cognitive Ability: Analysis
Client Needs: Physiological Integrity
Integrated Process: Nursing Process/Analysis
Content Area: Adult Health/Renal

Reference:
Black, J., & Hawks, J. (2005). *Medical-surgical nursing: Clinical management for positive outcomes* (7th ed.). Philadelphia: Saunders, p. 956.

---

437. A client undergoing long-term peritoneal dialysis at home is currently experiencing a problem with reduced outflow from the dialysis catheter. The home care nurse inquires whether the client has had a recent problem with:
1 Vomiting
2 Diarrhea
3 Constipation
4 Flatulence

Answer: 3
Rationale: Reduced outflow may be caused by catheter position and adherence to the omentum, infection, or constipation. Constipation may contribute to reduced outflow in part because peristalsis seems to aid in drainage. For this reason, bisacodyl (Dulcolax) suppositories are sometimes used prophylactically, even without a history of constipation. The other options are unrelated to impaired catheter drainage.

Test-Taking Strategy: Use the process of elimination and focus on the issue: reduced outflow. Evaluate each option in terms of its effect on gut motility, which affects catheter outflow. Each of the incorrect options involves hypermotility of the gastrointestinal tract, which should theoretically facilitate outflow. Constipation is related to decreased gut motility, which could then impair fluid drainage. Review the causes of reduced outflow in peritoneal dialysis if you had difficulty with this question.

Level of Cognitive Ability: Analysis
Client Needs: Physiological Integrity
Integrated Process: Nursing Process/Assessment
Content Area: Adult Health/Renal

Reference:
Black, J., & Hawks, J. (2005). *Medical-surgical nursing: Clinical management for positive outcomes* (7th ed.). Philadelphia: Saunders, p. 958.

---

438. A client with a history of heart failure who is undergoing peritoneal dialysis has developed crackles in the lower lung fields. The nurse interprets that this finding is most likely related to:
1 Compliance with dietary sodium restriction
2 Adherence to digoxin (Lanoxin) therapy schedule
3 Natural progression of the renal failure
4 Intake greater than output on the dialysis record

Answer: 4
Rationale: Crackles in the lung fields of the peritoneal dialysis client result from overhydration or from insufficient fluid removal during dialysis. An intake that is greater than the output of peritoneal dialysis fluid would overhydrate the client, resulting in lung crackles. Adherence to medication and diet therapy should control this sign, not exacerbate it. If dialysis is effective, there is no connection between the progression of renal failure and the development of signs of overhydration.

Test-Taking Strategy: Note the key words "developed crackles." Begin to answer this question by eliminating options 1 and 2. Because adherence to standard therapy should control the signs of heart failure, not exacerbate them, these options are incorrect. From the remaining options, recalling that crackles are caused by excess fluid in the body directs you to option 4. Review complications of peritoneal dialysis if you had difficulty with this question.

Level of Cognitive Ability: Analysis
Client Needs: Physiological Integrity
Integrated Process: Nursing Process/Analysis
Content Area: Adult Health/Renal

Reference:
Black, J., & Hawks, J. (2005). *Medical-surgical nursing: Clinical management for positive outcomes* (7th ed.). Philadelphia: Saunders, p. 958.

---

439. A nurse is teaching the client with asthma how to perform a peak expiratory flow rate measurement. The nurse tells the client to:
1 Inhale an average-size breath
2 Form a loose seal with the mouth around the mouthpiece
3 Blow out as slowly as possible
4 Record the final position of the indicator

Answer: 4
Rationale: A peak expiratory flow rate meter is used to provide an objective measure of the client's peak expiratory flow. The client is instructed to take the deepest possible breath, form a tight seal around the mouthpiece with the lips, and exhale forcefully and rapidly. The final position of the indicator on the meter is recorded.

Test-Taking Strategy: Knowledge regarding this piece of equipment and its use is needed to answer this question. Visualizing this piece of equipment and how it is used will assist in directing you to option 4. Review this commonly used device, which may be used to determine when medication adjustments are needed, if you had difficulty with this question.

Level of Cognitive Ability: Application
Client Needs: Physiological Integrity
Integrated Process: Teaching/Learning
Content Area: Adult Health/Respiratory

Reference:
Elkin, M., Perry, A., & Potter, P. (2004). *Nursing interventions & clinical skills* (3rd ed.). St. Louis: Mosby, p. 759.

---

440. A nurse is teaching the client taking medications by inhalation about the advantages of a newly prescribed spacer device. The nurse determines the need for further teaching if the client states that the spacer device:

1 Reduces the frequency of medication to only once per day
2 Reduces the chance of yeast infection because large drops aren't deposited on the oral tissues
3 Disperses medication more deeply and uniformly
4 Reduces the need to coordinate timing between pressing the inhaler and inspiration

Answer: 1

Rationale: There are key advantages to the use of a spacer device for medications administered by inhalation. One is that it reduces the incidence of yeast infections, because large medication droplets are not deposited on oral tissues. The medication is also dispersed more deeply and uniformly than without a spacer. There is less need to coordinate the effort of inhalation with pressing on the canister of the inhaler. Finally, the use of a spacer may decrease either the number or the volume of the puffs taken. Option 1 is too absolute and limiting by description.

Test-Taking Strategy: Use the process of elimination and note the key words "the need for further teaching." These words indicate a false-response question and that you need to select the client statement that is incorrect. Note the absolute word "only" in option 1. The use of absolute words such as "only" is likely to make the option incorrect. Review the advantages of the use of the spacer device with inhaled medications if you had difficulty with this question.

Level of Cognitive Ability: Analysis
Client Needs: Physiological Integrity
Integrated Process: Teaching/Learning
Content Area: Adult Health/Respiratory

Reference:
Phipps, W., Monahan, F., Sands, J., Marek, J., & Neighbors, M. (2003). *Medical-surgical nursing: Health and illness perspectives* (7th ed.). St. Louis: Mosby, pp. 527-528.

---

441. A nurse is assessing a client with a suspected diagnosis of pulmonary emphysema. The nurse assesses the client for which sign that distinguishes emphysema from chronic bronchitis?

1 Copious sputum production
2 Marked dyspnea
3 Minimal weight loss
4 Cough that began before the onset of dyspnea

Answer: 2

Rationale: Key features of pulmonary emphysema include dyspnea that is often marked, late cough (after the onset of dyspnea), scant mucus production, and marked weight loss. By contrast, chronic bronchitis is characterized by early onset of cough (before dyspnea), copious purulent sputum production, minimal weight loss, and milder severity of dyspnea.

Test-Taking Strategy: Focus on the issue: the differences between these two respiratory disorders and their associated manifestations. Recalling that marked dyspnea is associated with emphysema will direct you to option 2. Review the manifestations of emphysema and chronic bronchitis if you had difficulty with this question.

Level of Cognitive Ability: Analysis
Client Needs: Physiological Integrity
Integrated Process: Nursing Process/Assessment
Content Area: Adult Health/Respiratory

Reference:
Black, J., & Hawks, J. (2005). *Medical-surgical nursing: Clinical management for positive outcomes* (7th ed.). Philadelphia: Saunders, p. 1819.

442. A client with late-stage emphysema becomes confused and is experiencing tremors. The nurse interprets that these symptoms are indicative of which complication of emphysema?
1 Encephalopathy
2 Carbon dioxide narcosis
3 Carbon monoxide poisoning
4 Cerebral embolism

Answer: 2
Rationale: With late-stage emphysema, the retention of carbon dioxide can lead to carbon dioxide narcosis. This is manifested by occipital headache, drowsiness, inability to concentrate, confusion, and tremors. Other signs are a bounding pulse and an arterial carbon dioxide level greater than 75 mmHg.

Test-Taking Strategy: Focus on the issue, a complication of emphysema, and on the client's complaints. Recalling that emphysema is characterized by high carbon dioxide levels will direct you to option 2. Review the manifestations and complications associated with emphysema if you had difficulty with this question.

Level of Cognitive Ability: Analysis
Client Needs: Physiological Integrity
Integrated Process: Nursing Process/Analysis
Content Area: Adult Health/Respiratory

References:
Lewis, S., Heitkemper, M., & Dirksen, S. (2004). *Medical-surgical nursing: Assessment and management of clinical problems* (6th ed.). St. Louis: Mosby, pp. 669; 1833.
Mosby's medical, nursing, & allied health dictionary (6th ed.). St. Louis: Mosby, p. 278.

---

443. A nurse witnesses an accident whereby a pedestrian is hit by an automobile. The nurse stops at the scene and assesses the victim and notes that the client is responsive and has suffered a flail chest involving at least three ribs. The nurse does which of the following to assist the client's respiratory status until help arrives?
1 Assists the victim to sit up
2 Turns the client onto the side with the flail chest
3 Removes the victim's shirt
4 Applies firm but gentle pressure with the hands to the flail segment

Answer: 4
Rationale: If flail chest is present, the nurse applies firm yet gentle pressure to the flail segments of the ribs to stabilize the chest wall, which will ultimately help the client's respiratory status. The nurse does not move an injured person because of the risk of worsening an undetected spinal cord injury. Removing the victim's shirt is of no value in this situation and could in fact chill the victim, which is counterproductive. Injured persons should be kept warm until help arrives at the scene.

Test-Taking Strategy: Use knowledge of the principles of respiration and emergency nursing to answer this question. Eliminate options 1 and 2 because the client should not be moved. From the remaining options, recalling that the client should be kept warm will direct you to option 4. Review emergency care of the client with flail chest if you had difficulty with this question.

Level of Cognitive Ability: Application
Client Needs: Physiological Integrity
Integrated Process: Nursing Process/Implementation
Content Area: Adult Health/Respiratory

Reference:
Lewis, S., Heitkemper, M., & Dirksen, S. (2004). *Medical-surgical nursing: Assessment and management of clinical problems* (6th ed.). St. Louis: Mosby, p. 620.

444. A mental health nurse is assigned to care for a manic client. The nurse reviews the activity schedule for the day and determines that the best activity this client could participate in is:
1 A brown-bag luncheon and a book review
2 Tetherball
3 Paint-by-number activity
4 Deep breathing and a progressive relaxation group

Answer: 2
Rationale: A person who is experiencing mania is overactive, full of energy, lacks concentration, and has poor impulse control. The client needs an activity that will allow him or her to utilize excess energy, yet not endanger others during the process. Options 1, 3, and 4 are relatively sedate activities that require concentration, a quality that is lacking in the manic state. Such activities may lead to increased frustration and anxiety for the client. Tetherball is an exercise that uses the large muscle groups of the body and is a great way to expend the increased energy this client is experiencing.

Test-Taking Strategy: Use the process of elimination and focus on the diagnosis of the client. Eliminate options 1, 3, and 4 because they are similar and are sedate activities. Review care of the client with mania if you had difficulty with this question.

Level of Cognitive Ability: Analysis
Client Needs: Physiological Integrity
Integrated Process: Nursing Process/Planning
Content Area: Mental Health

References:
Stuart, G., & Laraia, M. (2005). *Principles and practice of psychiatric nursing* (8th ed.). St. Louis: Mosby, p. 355.
Varcarolis, E.M. (2002). *Foundations of psychiatric mental health nursing* (4th ed.). Philadelphia: Saunders, p. 480.

445. A client is brought to the emergency room by the police after having seriously lacerated both wrists. The initial action that the nurse will take is to:
1 Assess and treat the wound sites
2 Secure and record a detailed history
3 Encourage and assist the client to ventilate feelings
4 Administer an antianxiety agent

Answer: 1
Rationale: The initial action when a client has attempted suicide is to assess and treat any injuries. Although options 2, 3, and 4 may be appropriate at some point, the initial action would be to treat the wounds.

Test-Taking Strategy: Use Maslow's hierarchy of needs theory to prioritize. Physiological needs come first. Option 1 is the only option that addresses a physiological need. Review initial care of the client who has attempted suicide if you had difficulty with this question.

Level of Cognitive Ability: Application
Client Needs: Physiological Integrity
Integrated Process: Nursing Process/Implementation
Content Area: Mental Health

References:
Fortinash, K., & Holoday-Worret, P. (2004). *Psychiatric mental health nursing* (3rd ed.). St. Louis: Mosby, p. 562.
Stuart, G., & Laraia, M. (2005). *Principles and practice of psychiatric nursing* (8th ed.). St. Louis: Mosby, p. 367.

446. A nurse notes bilateral 2+ edema in the lower extremities of a client with known coronary artery disease who was admitted to the hospital 2 days ago. The nurse plans to do which of the following next after noting this finding?

1 Review the intake and output records for the last 2 days
2 Change the time of diuretic administration from morning to evening
3 Request a sodium restriction of 1 gram per day from the physician
4 Order daily weights starting on the following morning

Answer: 1

Rationale: Edema is the accumulation of excess fluid in the interstitial spaces, which can be measured by intake greater than output and by a sudden increase in weight (2.2 pounds = 1 kilogram). Diuretics should be administered in the morning whenever possible to avoid nocturia. Strict sodium restrictions are reserved for clients with severe symptoms. Obtaining a weight on the following day does not provide the nurse with immediate information.

Test-Taking Strategy: Note the key word "next" and use the steps of the nursing process. Option 1 can give the nurse immediate information about fluid balance. Review the manifestations associated with the complications of coronary artery disease if you had difficulty with this question.

Level of Cognitive Ability: Application
Client Needs: Physiological Integrity
Integrated Process: Nursing Process/Planning
Content Area: Adult Health/Cardiovascular

References:
Black, J., & Hawks, J. (2005). *Medical-surgical nursing: Clinical management for positive outcomes* (7th ed.). Philadelphia: Saunders, pp. 1656; 1664-1665.
Phipps, W., Monahan, F., Sands, J., Marek, J., & Neighbors, M. (2003). *Medical-surgical nursing: Health and illness perspectives* (7th ed.). St. Louis: Mosby, p. 627.

447. A nurse in the emergency room is assessing a client with chest pain. Which finding helps determine that the pain is caused by myocardial infarction (MI)?

1 The pain, unrelieved by nitroglycerin, was relieved with morphine sulfate.
2 The pain was described as burning and gnawing.
3 The client experienced no nausea or vomiting.
4 The client reports that the pain began while pushing a lawnmower.

Answer: 1

Rationale: The pain of angina may radiate to the left arm, is often precipitated by exertion or stress, has few associated symptoms, and is relieved by rest and nitroglycerin. The pain of MI may radiate to the left arm, shoulder, jaw, and neck. It typically begins spontaneously, lasts longer than 30 minutes, is frequently accompanied by associated symptoms (nausea, vomiting, dyspnea, diaphoresis, anxiety), and requires opioid analgesics for relief. A burning and gnawing pain is more likely noted in a upper gastrointestinal disorder.

Test-Taking Strategy: Note the issue: pain caused by an MI. Recall that a classic hallmark of the pain from MI is that it is unrelieved by rest and nitroglycerin. Review the differences between angina and MI if you had difficulty with this question.

Level of Cognitive Ability: Analysis
Client Needs: Physiological Integrity
Integrated Process: Nursing Process/Analysis
Content Area: Adult Health/Cardiovascular

Reference:
Ignatavicius, D., & Workman, M. (2002). *Medical surgical nursing: Critical thinking for collaborative care* (4th ed.). Philadelphia: Saunders, pp. 794; 796.

448. A nurse is assessing a client who has been hospitalized with acute pericarditis. The nurse monitors the client for cardiac tamponade, knowing that which of the following is a manifestation of this complication of pericarditis?
1 Paradoxical pulse
2 Bounding heart sounds
3 Flattened jugular veins
4 Bradycardia

Answer: 1
Rationale: Assessment findings with cardiac tamponade include tachycardia, distant or muffled heart sounds, jugular vein distention, and a falling blood pressure (BP), accompanied by paradoxical pulse (a drop in inspiratory BP by greater than 10 mmHg).

Test-Taking Strategy: Use the process of elimination. Think of the consequences of the pressure dynamics in the chest when the pericardial sac is rapidly filling with blood or fluid. This will assist in directing you to option 1. Review the signs of cardiac tamponade if you had difficulty with this question.

Level of Cognitive Ability: Analysis
Client Needs: Physiological Integrity
Integrated Process: Nursing Process/Assessment
Content Area: Adult Health/Cardiovascular

Reference:
Black, J., & Hawks, J. (2005). *Medical-surgical nursing: Clinical management for positive outcomes* (7th ed.). Philadelphia: Saunders, p. 1623.

449. A nurse is assisting to position the client for pericardiocentesis to treat cardiac tamponade. The nurse positions the client:
1 Lying on left side with a pillow under the chest wall
2 Lying on right side with a pillow under the head
3 Supine with the head of bed elevated at a 30- to 60-degree angle
4 Supine with slight Trendelenburg position

Answer: 3
Rationale: The client undergoing pericardiocentesis is positioned supine with the head of the bed raised to a 30- to 60-degree angle. This places the heart in proximity to the chest wall for easier insertion of the needle into the pericardial sac. Options 1, 2, and 4 are incorrect positions.

Test-Taking Strategy: If you are uncertain how to proceed with this question, visualize each of the positions described. Evaluate how the heart is sitting in the chest with each position and how easily the pericardial sac could be accessed with a needle. This will direct you to option 3. Review this procedure if you had difficulty with this question.

Level of Cognitive Ability: Application
Client Needs: Physiological Integrity
Integrated Process: Nursing Process/Implementation
Content Area: Adult Health/Cardiovascular

Reference:
Chernecky, C., & Berger, B. (2004). *Laboratory tests and diagnostic procedures* (4th ed.). Philadelphia: Saunders, p. 860.

450. A client with multiple sclerosis is treated with diazepam (Valium) for painful muscle spasms. The nurse assesses the client for side effects of the medication and monitors the client for:
1 Urinary frequency
2 Headache
3 Increased salivation
4 Incoordination

Answer: 4
Rationale: Valium is a centrally acting skeletal muscle relaxant. Incoordination and drowsiness are common side effects resulting from the large doses of the medication that must be used to achieve desired effects. Options 1, 2, and 3 are not side effects.

Test-Taking Strategy: Use the process of elimination. Recalling that diazepam is used for muscle spasms will direct you to think that this medication relaxes muscles. The only option that directly relates to this medication action is option 4. Review the action and side effects of this medication if you had difficulty with this question.

Level of Cognitive Ability: Analysis
Client Needs: Physiological Integrity
Integrated Process: Nursing Process/Assessment
Content Area: Pharmacology

Reference:
Hodgson, B., & Kizior, R. (2004). *Saunders nursing drug handbook 2004.* Philadelphia: Saunders, p. 298.

---

451. A client with epilepsy is taking the prescribed dose of phenytoin (Dilantin) to control seizures. A phenytoin (Dilantin) blood level is drawn, and the results reveal a level of 35 mcg/mL. Which effect(s) would be expected as a result of this laboratory result?
   1 No effects because this is a therapeutic phenytoin (Dilantin) level
   2 Slurred speech
   3 Tachycardia
   4 Diarrhea

Answer: 2
Rationale: The therapeutic phenytoin (Dilantin) level is 10 to 20 mcg/mL. Blood levels above 30 mcg/mL produce slurred speech. Options 1, 3, and 4 are incorrect.

Test-Taking Strategy: Knowledge regarding the therapeutic phenytoin (Dilantin) level and the signs that occur in the client when the level rises is required to answer this question. Review the signs associated with an elevated level if you had difficulty with this question.

Level of Cognitive Ability: Analysis
Client Needs: Physiological Integrity
Integrated Process: Nursing Process/Assessment
Content Area: Pharmacology

Reference:
Hodgson, B., & Kizior, R. (2004). *Saunders nursing drug handbook 2004.* Philadelphia: Saunders, pp. 806-807.

---

452. A nurse is caring for a child following cleft palate repair. To reduce the risk of aspiration after feeding the child, the nurse places the child in which best position?
   1 Right side
   2 Sims'
   3 Supine
   4 Prone

Answer: 1
Rationale: The child with cleft palate repair is placed on the right side after feeding to reduce the chance of aspirating regurgitated formula. Options 2, 3, and 4 are positions that would place the child at risk for aspiration.

Test-Taking Strategy: Visualize the anatomical location of the stomach in answering this question and focus on the issue: to reduce the risk of aspiration. Eliminate options 2, 3, and 4 because they are similar and are flat positions. Also remember that positioning on the right side will aid in absorption and reduce the risk of aspiration. Review care of the child following cleft palate repair if you had difficulty with this question.

Level of Cognitive Ability: Application
Client Needs: Physiological Integrity
Integrated Process: Nursing Process/Implementation
Content Area: Child Health

References:
James, S., Ashwill, J., & Droske, S. (2002). *Nursing care of children: Principles & practice* (2nd ed.). Philadelphia: Saunders, p. 538.
Wong, D., & Hockenberry, M. (2003). *Wong's nursing care of infants and children* (7th ed.). St. Louis: Mosby, p. 461.

453. A nurse is monitoring drainage from a nasogastric (NG) tube in a client who had a gastric resection. No drainage is noted during the past 4 hours, and the client complains of severe nausea. The appropriate nursing action would be to:
1 Reposition the tube
2 Irrigate the tube
3 Notify the physician
4 Medicate for nausea

Answer: 3

Rationale: Nausea and vomiting should not occur if the NG tube is patent. The NG tube should not be repositioned or irrigated after gastric surgery because it is placed directly over the suture line. The NG tube is irrigated gently with normal saline only with a physician's order. The client may need medication for the nausea, but in this situation, the physician should be notified.

Test-Taking Strategy: Note that the client had a surgical procedure that involved the gastric area and that an NG tube is placed in this surgical area. This will assist in eliminating options 1 and 2. From the remaining options, noting the key words "severe nausea" should alert you that the physician needs to be notified. Review postoperative nursing care following gastric surgery if you had difficulty with this question.

Level of Cognitive Ability: Application
Client Needs: Physiological Integrity
Integrated Process: Nursing Process/Implementation
Content Area: Adult Health/Gastrointestinal

References:
Black, J., & Hawks, J. (2005). *Medical-surgical nursing: Clinical management for positive outcomes* (7th ed.). Philadelphia: Saunders, p. 760.
Ignatavicius, D., & Workman, M. (2002). *Medical surgical nursing: Critical thinking for collaborative care* (4th ed.). Philadelphia: Saunders, pp. 290-291.

454. A nurse explains to a mother that her newborn infant is being admitted to the neonatal intensive care unit with a probable diagnosis of fetal alcohol syndrome (FAS). The nurse explains the expected effects of FAS to the mother and tells the mother that:
1 Withdrawal symptoms will occur after 6 days.
2 Mental retardation is unlikely to happen.
3 Withdrawal symptoms include tremors, crying, seizures, and abnormal reflexes.
4 The reason the newborn infant is so large is because of the fetal alcohol syndrome.

Answer: 3

Rationale: The long-term prognosis for newborns with FAS is poor. Symptoms of withdrawal include tremors, sleeplessness, seizures, abdominal distention, hyperactivity, abnormal reflexes, and uncontrollable crying. Central nervous system (CNS) disorders are the most common problems associated with FAS. Because of the CNS disorders, children born with FAS are often hyperactive and have a high incidence of speech and language disorders. Symptoms of withdrawal often occur within 6 to 12 hours after life or at the latest, within the first 3 days of life. Most neonates with FAS are mildly to severely mentally retarded. The newborn is usually growth deficient at birth.

Test-Taking Strategy: Use the process of elimination. Focus on the diagnosis to eliminate options 2 and 4. From the remaining options, eliminate option 1 because of the words "after 6 days." Remember that withdrawal symptoms can appear within 6 to 12 hours after life or at the latest, within the first 3 days of life. Review the manifestations associated with FAS if you had difficulty with this question.

Level of Cognitive Ability: Analysis
Client Needs: Physiological Integrity
Integrated Process: Nursing Process/Implementation
Content Area: Maternity/Postpartum

Reference:
Lowdermilk, D., & Perry, A. (2004). *Maternity & women's health care* (8th ed.). St. Louis: Mosby, p. 1072-1073.

455. A client who has type 1 diabetes mellitus is at 10 weeks' gestation and is receiving prenatal care at a high-risk clinic. The nurse tells the client about the early signs of hyperglycemia and determines that the client understands if the client states that an early sign of hyperglycemia is:

1 Increased urination
2 Nervousness
3 Shakiness
4 Hunger

Answer: 1
Rationale: Polyuria (increased urination) is an early sign of hyperglycemia. Other signs can include polydipsia, dry mouth, increased appetite, fatigue, nausea, hot flushed skin, rapid deep breathing, abdominal cramps, acetone breath, headache, drowsiness, depressed reflexes, oliguria or anuria, stupor, and coma.

Test-Taking Strategy: Use the process of elimination. Options 2 and 3 are similar and are eliminated first. From the remaining options, recalling that hunger is a sign of hypoglycemia will assist in eliminating option 4. Review the signs of both hypoglycemia and hyperglycemia if you had difficulty with this question.

Level of Cognitive Ability: Analysis
Client Needs: Physiological Integrity
Integrated Process: Teaching/Learning
Content Area: Maternity/Antepartum

Reference:
Lowdermilk, D., & Perry, A. (2004). *Maternity & women's health care* (8th ed.). St. Louis: Mosby, pp. 1072-1073.

---

456. A client recovering from a craniotomy complains of a "runny nose." The most important nursing action is to:

1 Provide the client with soft tissues
2 Tell the client to use soft tissues to soak up the drainage
3 Monitor the client for signs of a cold
4 Notify the physician

Answer: 4
Rationale: If the client has sustained a craniocerebral injury or is recovering from a craniotomy, careful observation of any drainage from the eyes, ears, nose, or traumatic area is critical. Cerebrospinal fluid is colorless and generally nonpurulent, and its presence indicates a serious breach of cranial integrity. Any suspicious drainage should be reported immediately.

Test-Taking Strategy: Note the key words "most important." This should provide you with the clue that there is a serious nature to the situation presented. Eliminate options 1 and 2 first because they are similar. From the remaining options, recalling the signs of complications associated with crainotomy will direct you to option 4. Review postoperative nursing care following crainiotomy if you had difficulty with this question.

Level of Cognitive Ability: Application
Client Needs: Physiological Integrity
Integrated Process: Nursing Process/Implementation
Content Area: Adult Health/Neurological

Reference:
Ignatavicius, D., & Workman, M. (2002). *Medical surgical nursing: Critical thinking for collaborative care* (4th ed.). Philadelphia: Saunders, p. 1004.

457. A nurse is caring for a client who has returned from the post-anesthesia care unit following prostatectomy. The client has a three-way Foley catheter with infusion of continuous bladder irrigation solution. The nurse assesses that the flow rate is adequate if the color of the urinary drainage is:

1 Dark cherry colored
2 Concentrated yellow with small clots
3 Clear as water
4 Pale yellow or slightly pink

Answer: 4

Rationale: The infusion of bladder irrigant is not at a preset rate, but rather it is increased or decreased to maintain urine that is a clear, pale yellow color, or that has just a slight pink tinge. The infusion rate should be increased if the drainage is cherry colored or if clots are seen. Correspondingly, the rate can be slowed down slightly if the returns are as clear as water.

Test-Taking Strategy: Use the process of elimination. Eliminate option 2 as the least realistic or expected occurrence of all the urine characteristics described in the options. Next, eliminate options 1 and 3 as reflecting inadequate and excessive flow, respectively. With proper flow rate of bladder irrigant, the urine should be pale yellow or slightly pink. Review care of the client following prostatectomy if you had difficulty with this question.

Level of Cognitive Ability: Analysis
Client Needs: Physiological Integrity
Integrated Process: Nursing Process/Assessment
Content Area: Adult Health /Renal

Reference:
Phipps, W., Monahan, F., Sands, J., Marek, J., & Neighbors, M. (2003). *Medical-surgical nursing: Health and illness perspectives* (7th ed.). St. Louis: Mosby, p. 1846.

458. A nurse is assessing a client who is at risk of developing acute renal failure (ARF). The nurse would become most concerned if which of the following assessments was made?

1 Urine output 30 mL/hour (hr) for the last 3 hours, blood urea nitrogen (BUN) 10 mg/dL, creatinine 1.2 mg/dL
2 Urine output 40 mL/hr for the last 3 hours, BUN 15 mg/dL, creatinine 0.8 mg/dL
3 Urine output 20 mL/hr for the last 3 hours, BUN 35 mg/dL, creatinine 2.1 mg/dL
4 Urine output 60 mL/hr for the last 3 hours, BUN 40 mg/dL, creatinine 1.1 mg/dL

Answer: 3

Rationale: With acute renal failure, the client is often oliguric or anuric, although the client may have nonoliguric renal failure. The BUN and serum creatinine levels also rise, indicating defective kidney function. Normal serum BUN levels are usually 5 to 20 mg/dL. Normal creatinine levels range from 0.6 to 1.3 mg/dL. The client who has the greatest abnormality in urine output and laboratory values is the client in option 3. This is the client who is most at risk for developing renal failure.

Test-Taking Strategy: Focus on the issue: developing renal failure. Recalling the normal BUN and creatinine levels and that the minimum required hourly urine output is 30 mL will direct you to option 3. Review these normal values and the signs of renal failure if you had difficulty with this question.

Level of Cognitive Ability: Analysis
Client Needs: Physiological Integrity
Integrated Process: Nursing Process/Assessment
Content Area: Adult Health/Renal

Reference:
Phipps, W., Monahan, F., Sands, J., Marek, J., & Neighbors, M. (2003). *Medical-surgical nursing: Health and illness perspectives* (7th ed.). St. Louis: Mosby, pp. 1262; 1264.

459. A client with acute renal failure has been treated with sodium polystyrene sulfonate (Kayexalate) by mouth. The nurse would evaluate this therapy as effective if which of the following values was noted on follow-up laboratory testing?
  1 Potassium: 4.9 mEq/L
  2 Sodium: 142 mEq/L
  3 Phosphorus: 3.9 mg/dL
  4 Calcium: 9.8 mg/dL

Answer: 1
Rationale: Of all the electrolyte imbalances that accompany renal failure, hyperkalemia is the most dangerous because it can lead to cardiac dysrhythmias and death. If the potassium level rises too high, sodium polystyrene sulfonate (Kayexalate) may be administered to cause excretion of potassium through the gastrointestinal tract. Each of the electrolyte levels noted in the options fall within the normal reference range for that electrolyte. The potassium level, however, is measured following administration of this medication to note the extent of its effectiveness.

Test-Taking Strategy: Use the process of elimination. Note the name of the medication (*Kayex*alate) and its relationship to the laboratory test in option 1. Review this medication if you had difficulty with this question.

Level of Cognitive Ability: Analysis
Client Needs: Physiological Integrity
Integrated Process: Nursing Process/Evaluation
Content Area: Adult Health/Renal

Reference:
Phipps, W., Monahan, F., Sands, J., Marek, J., & Neighbors, M. (2003). *Medical-surgical nursing: Health and illness perspectives* (7th ed.). St. Louis: Mosby, p. 1265.

460. A nurse is admitting a client with chronic renal failure to the nursing unit. The nurse assesses for which most frequent cardiovascular sign that occurs in the client with chronic renal failure?
  1 Hypertension
  2 Hypotension
  3 Tachycardia
  4 Bradycardia

Answer: 1
Rationale: Hypertension is the most common cardiovascular finding in the client with chronic renal failure. It is caused by several mechanisms, including volume overload, renin-angiotensin system stimulation, vasoconstriction from sympathetic stimulation, and the absence of prostaglandins. Hypertension may also be the cause of the renal failure. It is an important item to assess because hypertension can lead to heart failure in the chronic renal failure client, because of increased cardiac workload in conjunction with fluid overload. The client may experience tachycardia or bradycardia or may have a normal pulse rate; these cardiovascular manifestations will depend on a variety of physiological events such as fluid overload, fluid deficit, or normal fluid volume.

Test-Taking Strategy: Use the process of elimination. Recalling that the blood pressure is the key item to assess helps you eliminate options 3 and 4. From the remaining options, recall the functions of the renal system and the kidneys to direct you to option 1. Review the manifestations of chronic renal failure if you had difficulty with this question.

Level of Cognitive Ability: Analysis
Client Needs: Physiological Integrity
Integrated Process: Nursing Process/Assessment
Content Area: Adult Health/Renal

Reference:
Black, J., & Hawks, J. (2005). *Medical-surgical nursing: Clinical management for positive outcomes* (7th ed.). Philadelphia: Saunders, p. 953.

461. A client has sustained a closed fracture and has just had a cast applied to the affected arm. The client is complaining of intense pain. The nurse has elevated the limb, applied an ice bag, and administered an analgesic, which has provided very little pain relief. The nurse interprets that this pain may be caused by:
1 Impaired tissue perfusion
2 The newness of the fracture
3 The anxiety of the client
4 Infection under the cast

Answer: 1
Rationale: Most pain associated with fractures can be minimized with rest, elevation, application of cold, and administration of analgesics. Pain that is not relieved from these measures should be reported to the physician, because it may be caused by impaired tissue perfusion, tissue breakdown, or necrosis. Because this is a new closed fracture and cast, infection would not have had time to set in.

Test-Taking Strategy: Use the process of elimination. Focus on the information in the question to eliminate options 2 and 3. Because the fracture and cast are so new, it is extremely unlikely that infection could have possibly set in. Therefore, eliminate option 4. Review the complications associated with a casted extremity if you had difficulty with this question.

Level of Cognitive Ability: Analysis
Client Needs: Physiological Integrity
Integrated Process: Nursing Process/Analysis
Content Area: Adult Health/Musculoskeletal

Reference:
Ignatavicius, D., & Workman, M. (2002). *Medical surgical nursing: Critical thinking for collaborative care* (4th ed.). Philadelphia: Saunders, p. 1136.

462. The client with a fractured femur experiences sudden dyspnea. A set of arterial blood gases reveal the following: pH is 7.32, $Paco_2$ is 43, Pao_2 is 58, Hco_3 is 20. The nurse interprets that the client probably has experienced fat embolus because of the:
1 $Paco_2$
2 Pao_2
3 Hco_3
4 pH

Answer: 2
Rationale: A key feature of fat embolism is a significant degree of hypoxemia with a Pao_2 often less than 60 mmHg. Other features that distinguish fat embolism from pulmonary embolism are an elevated temperature and the presence of fat in the blood with fat embolus.

Test-Taking Strategy: Use the process of elimination. Recalling that fat embolus causes significant hypoxemia will direct you to option 2. Review the manifestations associated with this disorder if you had difficulty with this question.

Level of Cognitive Ability: Analysis
Client Needs: Physiological Integrity
Integrated Process: Nursing Process/Analysis
Content Area: Adult Health/Musculoskeletal

References:
Lewis, S., Heitkemper, M., & Dirksen, S. (2004). *Medical-surgical nursing: Assessment and management of clinical problems* (6th ed.). St. Louis: Mosby, pp. 1672-1673.
Phipps, W., Monahan, F., Sands, J., Marek, J., & Neighbors, M. (2003). *Medical-surgical nursing: Health and illness perspectives* (7th ed.). St. Louis: Mosby, p. 1486.

463. Mannitol (Osmitrol) is administered intravenously to a client admitted to the hospital with loss of consciousness and a closed head injury. The nurse determines that the medication was most effective if which of the following outcomes was noted?

1 Diuresis of 500 mL in 2 hours and a blood urea nitrogen (BUN) of 15 mg/dL
2 Improved level of consciousness and normal intracranial pressure
3 Weight loss of 1 kilogram and a serum creatinine of 0.8 mg/dL
4 Serum creatinine of 1.2 mg/dL and normal intracranial pressure

Answer: 2

Rationale: Mannitol (Osmitrol) is an osmotic diuretic that can be administered parenterally to treat cerebral edema. Lowering of intracranial pressure occurs within 15 minutes of administration, and diuresis occurs within 1 to 3 hours. Expected effects of the medication include rapid diuresis and fluid loss. For the client with cerebral edema (as in closed head injury), effectiveness is measured by assessing neurological status and intracranial pressure readings.

Test-Taking Strategy: Note the key words "most effective" in the stem of the question. This tells you that more than one option is partially or totally correct. Next note the key words "loss of consciousness and a closed head injury." Note the relationship between these words and the correct option. Review this medication and its expected effect if you had difficulty with this question.

Level of Cognitive Ability: Analysis
Client Needs: Physiological Integrity
Integrated Process: Nursing Process/Evaluation
Content Area: Pharmacology

Reference:
Hodgson, B., & Kizior, R. (2004). *Saunders nursing drug handbook 2004.* Philadelphia: Saunders, p. 625.

---

464. A nurse is caring for a client with a history of renal insufficiency who is having captopril (Capoten) added to the medication regimen. Before administering the first dose, the nurse reviews the medical record for the results of the urinalysis, especially noting for the presence of:

1 Casts
2 Red blood cells (RBCs)
3 Protein
4 White blood cells (WBCs)

Answer: 3

Rationale: Captopril is an angiotensin-converting enzyme (ACE) inhibitor, which may be used for clients who do not respond to the first-line antihypertensive agents. ACE inhibitors are used cautiously in clients with renal impairment. Before beginning treatment, baseline assessment of blood pressure, complete white cell count, and urine protein is performed. Clients with renal insufficiency may develop nephrotic syndrome, so the client may be monitored for proteinuria on a monthly basis for 9 months, and periodically afterward.

Test-Taking Strategy: Note the information in the question. The question tells you that the client has renal insufficiency and directs you to look at urinalysis results. RBCs and WBCs could be indications of trauma and/or infection, so these options can be eliminated first. Eliminate option 1 because casts are mineral deposits that form along the renal tubules and occasionally appear in the urine. Normally the kidneys conserve large protein molecules, which makes the presence of protein in the urine abnormal. Review this medication if you had difficulty with this question.

Level of Cognitive Ability: Analysis
Client Needs: Physiological Integrity
Integrated Process: Nursing Process/Assessment
Content Area: Pharmacology

References:
Hodgson, B., & Kizior, R. (2004). *Saunders nursing drug handbook 2004*. Philadelphia: Saunders, p. 146.
McKenry, L., & Salerno, E. (2003). *Mosby's pharmacology in nursing* (21st ed.). St. Louis: Mosby, p. 587.

---

465. A nurse assesses a client with chronic arterial insufficiency. The client complains of leg pain and cramping after walking three blocks, which is relieved when the client stops and rests. The nurse documents that the client is experiencing:
1 Arterial-venous shunting
2 Deep vein thrombosis
3 Intermittent claudication
4 Venous insufficiency

Answer: 3
Rationale: Intermittent claudication is a classic symptom of peripheral vascular disease, also known by other names, including peripheral arterial disease and chronic arterial insufficiency. Intermittent claudication is described as a cramp-like pain that occurs with exercise and is relieved by rest. Intermittent claudication is caused by ischemia and is reproducible; that is, a predictable amount of exercise causes the pain each time. Options 1, 2, and 4 are incorrect.

Test-Taking Strategy: Use the process of elimination. Note that the question indicates that the client has an arterial disorder. This eliminates option 2 and 4. From the remaining options, noting the relationship between the timing in the question and the word "intermittent" in option 3 will direct you to this option. Review intermittent claudication if you had difficulty with this question.

Level of Cognitive Ability: Application
Client Needs: Physiological Integrity
Integrated Process: Communication and Documentation
Content Area: Adult Health/Cardiovascular

Reference:
Lewis, S., Heitkemper, M., & Dirksen, S. (2004). *Medical-surgical nursing: Assessment and management of clinical problems* (6th ed.). St. Louis: Mosby, pp. 782; 920.

---

466. A nurse is caring for a client with cancer who is receiving daunorubicin (Cerubidine) intravenously. The nurse monitors the client for which side effect of the medication?
1 Hypertension
2 Polycythemia
3 Nausea and vomiting
4 Hypovolemia

Answer: 3
Rationale: Daunorubicin is an antineoplastic medication. The major gastrointestinal (GI) side effects include nausea, vomiting, stomatitis, and esophagitis. Cardiovascular side effects include congestive heart failure and dysrhythmias. Other frequently occurring side effects are alopecia and bone marrow depression. Options 1, 2, and 4 are not side effects of this medication.

Test-Taking Strategy: Focusing on the client's diagnosis will assist in determining that the medication is an antineoplastic. Recalling that antineoplastics commonly cause GI side effects will direct you to option 3. Review the side effects of this medication if you had difficulty with this question.

Level of Cognitive Ability: Application
Client Needs: Physiological Integrity
Integrated Process: Nursing Process/Assessment
Content Area: Pharmacology

Reference:
Hodgson, B., & Kizior, R. (2004). *Saunders nursing drug handbook 2004*. Philadelphia: Saunders, p. 278.

467. A home care nurse is visiting a client who was discharged to home with orders for continued administration of enoxaparin (Lovenox) 30 mg twice daily subcutaneously. On assessment, the nurse questions the client about which highest priority item?
1 Fear of needles
2 Bleeding gums or bruising
3 Constipation
4 Nausea or vomiting

Answer: 2
Rationale: Enoxaparin is an anticoagulant. A common side effect of anticoagulant therapy is bleeding. Because of this, the nurse questions the client about symptoms that could indicate bleeding, such as bleeding gums, bruising, hematuria, or dark tarry stools.

Test-Taking Strategy: Use the process of elimination. Recalling that this medication is an anticoagulant will assist in eliminating options 3 and 4 first. From the remaining options, noting the key words "highest priority" will direct you to option 2. Review this medication if you had difficulty with this question.

Level of Cognitive Ability: Application
Client Needs: Physiological Integrity
Integrated Process: Nursing Process/Assessment
Content Area: Pharmacology

Reference:
Hodgson, B., & Kizior, R. (2004). *Saunders nursing drug handbook 2004.* Philadelphia: Saunders, p. 355.

468. A client has been given a prescription for sulfasalazine (Azulfidine) for the treatment of ulcerative colitis. Before teaching the client about the medication, the nurse asks the client about a history of allergy to:
1 Salicylates or acetaminophen
2 Sulfonamides or salicylates
3 Shellfish or calcium channel blockers
4 Histamine receptor antagonists or beta-blockers

Answer: 2
Rationale: The client who has been prescribed sulfasalazine should be checked for history of allergy to either sulfonamides or salicylates because the chemical composition of sulfasalazine and these medications are similar. The other options are incorrect.

Test-Taking Strategy: Focus on the issue: history of allergy. Note the relationship of "sulfasalazine" in the question and "sulfonamides" in the correct option. Review information about this medication if you had difficulty with this question.

Level of Cognitive Ability: Application
Client Needs: Physiological Integrity
Integrated Process: Nursing Process/Assessment
Content Area: Pharmacology

Reference:
Hodgson, B., & Kizior, R. (2004). *Saunders nursing drug handbook 2004.* Philadelphia: Saunders, pp. 942-943.

469. A nurse is caring for a client with a nursing diagnosis of Impaired Oral Mucous Membranes. The nurse would avoid using which of the following items when giving mouth care to this client?
1 Nonalcoholic mouthwash
2 Soft toothbrush
3 Lip moistener
4 Lemon-glycerin swabs

Answer: 4
Rationale: The nurse avoids using lemon-glycerin swabs for the client with impaired oral mucous membranes because they dry the membranes further and could cause pain. Items that are helpful include a soft toothbrush to prevent trauma, lip moistener to prevent lip cracking, and soothing cleansing rinses, such as nonalcoholic mouthwash or a saline and hydrogen peroxide mixture.

Test-Taking Strategy: Note the key word "avoid." This indicates a false-response question and that you need to select the option that is an incorrect item to use for mouth care. Focus on the nursing diagnosis and evaluate each item in the options in terms of the likelihood of causing trauma to the oral mucous membranes. This will direct you to option 4. Review care of the client with impaired oral mucous membranes if you had difficulty with this question.

Level of Cognitive Ability: Application
Client Needs: Physiological Integrity
Integrated Process: Nursing Process/Implementation
Content Area: Fundamental Skills

Reference:
Ignatavicius, D., & Workman, M. (2002). *Medical surgical nursing: Critical thinking for collaborative care* (4th ed.). Philadelphia: Saunders, p. 167.

---

470. A nurse has an order to administer 20 mEq of potassium to a client with a potassium level of 3.0 mEq/L. The nurse draws up this medication knowing it will be administered:
1 After dilution in an intravenous solution
2 Directly by IV push
3 Intramuscularly
4 Subcutaneously

Answer: 1
Rationale: Potassium chloride may be administered by the intravenous route when the client has moderate to severe hypokalemia. It is always diluted in intravenous solution; administration by IV push could cause death by cardiac arrest. It is not administered intramuscularly or subcutaneously. Intravenous potassium should be administered through an infusion pump. A cardiac monitor should also be in use when administering intravenous potassium.

Test-Taking Strategy: Use basic knowledge of electrolyte replacement and medication administration to answer this question. Recalling the physiology of the cardiac conduction system and the effects of potassium on the heart will direct you to the correct option. Review the procedure for administering potassium if you had difficulty with this question.

Level of Cognitive Ability: Application
Client Needs: Physiological Integrity
Integrated Process: Nursing Process/Implementation
Content Area: Pharmacology

Reference:
Hodgson, B., & Kizior, R. (2004). *Saunders nursing drug handbook 2004.* Philadelphia: Saunders, p. 823.

---

471. A nurse has an order to administer two ophthalmic medications to the client who has undergone eye surgery. The nurse waits how many minutes after administering the first medication before giving the second?
1 It is not necessary to wait, and the second medication can be administered immediately.
2 One to two
3 Three to five
4 Eight to ten

Answer: 3
Rationale: The nurse waits 3 to 5 minutes between administration of the two separate ophthalmic medications. This allows for adequate ocular absorption of the medication and prevents the second medication from flushing out the first.

Test-Taking Strategy: Use the process of elimination. Eliminate option 1 because it does not address the issue of the question. Next, eliminate option 4 because of the lengthy time frame. From the remaining options, recalling that time is needed for ocular absorption of the medication will direct you to option 3. If needed, review the principles of ocular medication administration.

Level of Cognitive Ability: Application
Client Needs: Physiological Integrity
Integrated Process: Nursing Process/Implementation
Content Area: Adult Health/Eye

Reference:
McKenry, L., & Salerno, E. (2003). *Mosby's pharmacology in nursing* (21st ed.). St. Louis: Mosby, p. 801.

---

472. A client has a pH of 7.51 with a bicarbonate level of 29 mEq/L. The nurse prepares to administer which of the following medications that would be prescribed to treat this acid-base disorder?
1 Sodium bicarbonate
2 Furosemide (Lasix)
3 Acetazolamide (Diamox)
4 Spironolactone (Aldactone)

Answer: 3
Rationale: Acetazolamide is a diuretic used in the treatment of metabolic alkalosis. This medication causes excretion of sodium, potassium, bicarbonate, and water by inhibiting the action of carbonic anhydrase. Administration of sodium bicarbonate would aggravate the already existing condition and is contraindicated. Furosemide and spironolactone are loop and potassium-sparing diuretics, respectively. These are of no value when there is a need to excrete bicarbonate.

Test-Taking Strategy: Begin to answer this question by interpreting that the acid-base disorder is metabolic alkalosis. Eliminate option 1 first based on this interpretation. From the remaining options, it is necessary to know which diuretic is used to treat metabolic alkalosis. Review the treatment for this acid-base disorder if you had difficulty with this question.

Level of Cognitive Ability: Application
Client Needs: Physiological Integrity
Integrated Process: Nursing Process/Planning
Content Area: Pharmacology

References:
McKenry, L., & Salerno, E. (2003). *Mosby's pharmacology in nursing* (21st ed.). St. Louis: Mosby, p. 673.
Phipps, W., Monahan, F., Sands, J., Marek, J., & Neighbors, M. (2003). *Medical-surgical nursing: Health and illness perspectives* (7th ed.). St. Louis: Mosby, pp. 277;1895.

---

473. A client is admitted to the hospital in metabolic acidosis caused by diabetic ketoacidosis (DKA). The nurse prepares to administer which of the following medications as a primary initial treatment for this problem?
1 Sodium bicarbonate
2 Calcium gluconate
3 Potassium
4 Regular insulin

Answer: 4
Rationale: The primary treatment for any acid-base imbalance is treatment of the underlying disorder that caused the problem. In this case, the underlying cause of the metabolic acidosis is anaerobic metabolism caused by lack of ability by the body to use circulating glucose. Administration of insulin corrects this problem. Potassium may be added to the treatment regimen if serum potassium levels indicate its need. Options 1 and 2 would not be used to treat this disorder.

Test-Taking Strategy: Focus on the client's diagnosis: diabetic ketoacidosis. Noting the diagnosis and the key words "primary initial treatment" will direct you to option 4. Review the treatment for DKA if you had difficulty with this question.

Level of Cognitive Ability: Application
Client Needs: Physiological Integrity
Integrated Process: Nursing Process/Planning
Content Area: Adult Health/Endocrine

Reference:
Black, J., & Hawks, J. (2005). *Medical-surgical nursing: Clinical management for positive outcomes* (7th ed.). Philadelphia: Saunders, p. 1277.

474. A client is diagnosed with respiratory alkalosis induced by gram-negative sepsis. The nurse prepares to implement which prescribed measure as the most effective means to treat the problem?
1 Administer prescribed antibiotics
2 Administer prn antipyretics
3 Have the client breathe into a paper bag
4 Request an order for a partial rebreather oxygen mask

Answer: 1
Rationale: The most effective way to treat an acid-base disorder is to treat the underlying cause of the disorder. In this case, the problem is sepsis, which is most effectively treated with antibiotic therapy. Antipyretics will control fever secondary to sepsis but do nothing to treat the acid-base balance. The paper bag and partial rebreather mask will assist the client to rebreathe exhaled carbon dioxide, but again, these do not treat the primary cause of the imbalance.

Test-Taking Strategy: Note the key words "sepsis" and "most effective." Recalling that the most effective treatment of acid-base imbalances involves treatment of the primary cause will direct you to option 1. Remember: sepsis is a systemic infection and is treated with antibiotics. Review the treatment for respiratory alkalosis and sepsis if you had difficulty with this question.

Level of Cognitive Ability: Application
Client Needs: Physiological Integrity
Integrated Process: Nursing Process/Planning
Content Area: Adult Health/Immune

References:
Ignatavicius, D., & Workman, M. (2002). *Medical surgical nursing: Critical thinking for collaborative care* (4th ed.). Philadelphia: Saunders, p. 841.
Phipps, W., Monahan, F., Sands, J., Marek, J., & Neighbors, M. (2003). *Medical-surgical nursing: Health and illness perspectives* (7th ed.). St. Louis: Mosby, pp. 276-277.

475. The nurse notes that a client receiving lithium therapy is drowsy, has slurred speech, and is experiencing muscle twitching and impaired coordination. The nurse takes which of the following actions?
1 Doubles the next lithium dose
2 Increases fluids to 2000 mL per day
3 Holds one dose of lithium
4 Calls the physician

Answer: 4
Rationale: Signs and symptoms of lithium toxicity include vomiting and diarrhea, and nervous system changes such as slurred speech, incoordination, drowsiness, muscle weakness, or twitching. Before administering any further doses, the nurse should notify the physician. As long as there are no contraindications, the client should routinely take in between 2000 to 3000 mL of fluid per day while taking this medication.

Test-Taking Strategy: Use the process of elimination. Eliminate options 1 and 3 first because it is not common practice to either hold one dose or double a medication dose without a specific order to do so. From the remaining options, focusing on the client's symptoms will direct you to option 4. Review the signs of toxicity of this medication if you had difficulty with this question.

Level of Cognitive Ability: Application
Client Needs: Physiological Integrity
Integrated Process: Nursing Process/Implementation
Content Area: Pharmacology

References:
Hodgson, B., & Kizior, R. (2004). *Saunders nursing drug handbook 2004.* Philadelphia: Saunders, p. 607.
Kee, J., & Hayes, E. (2003). *Pharmacology: A nursing process approach* (4th ed.). Philadelphia: Saunders, p. 314.

---

476. A client has been started on medication therapy with metoclopramide (Reglan). The nurse monitors which item to determine effectiveness of therapy?
1 Urine output
2 Breath sounds
3 Complaints of headache
4 Episodes of vomiting

Answer: 4
Rationale: Metoclopramide is an antiemetic. The nurse would monitor to see whether the client has experienced a decrease or absence of vomiting to determine the effectiveness of therapy. Options 1, 2, and 3 are unrelated to the action of this medication.

Test-Taking Strategy: Use the process of elimination. Recalling that metoclopramide is an antiemetic will direct you to option 4. Review the action of this medication if you had difficulty with this question.

Level of Cognitive Ability: Analysis
Client Needs: Physiological Integrity
Integrated Process: Nursing Process/Evaluation
Content Area: Pharmacology

Reference:
Hodgson, B., & Kizior, R. (2004). *Saunders nursing drug handbook 2004.* Philadelphia: Saunders, p. 660.

---

477. A nurse is preparing to administer an intramuscular injection to a 2-year-old child. The best site to select for the injection is the:
1 Ventral gluteal muscle
2 Dorsal gluteal muscle
3 Deltoid muscle
4 Vastus lateralis muscle

Answer: 4
Rationale: The vastus lateralis muscle is well developed at birth. It is the best choice for all age groups, but should always be used in children younger than 3 years of age. This muscle is able to tolerate larger volumes and is not located near vital structures such as nerves and blood vessels.

Test-Taking Strategy: Use the process of elimination. Eliminate options 1 and 2 because they are similar. From the remaining options, recall that the deltoid is a smaller muscle close to important nerves and is generally not a preferred site for intramuscular injection. Review the procedure for administering intramuscular injections in a 2-year-old if you had difficulty with this question.

Level of Cognitive Ability: Application
Client Needs: Physiological Integrity
Integrated Process: Nursing Process/Implementation
Content Area: Fundamental Skills

Reference:
Wong, D., & Hockenberry, M. (2003). *Wong's nursing care of infants and children* (7th ed.). St. Louis: Mosby, p. 540.

478. A nurse is developing a plan of care for a school-aged child with a knowledge deficit related to the use of inhalers and peak flow meters. The best expected outcome to be included in the plan of care is that the child will:
1 Express feelings of mastery and competence with the breathing devices
2 Have regular respirations at a rate of 18 to 22 breaths per minute
3 Deny shortness of breath or difficulty breathing
4 Watch the educational video and read printed information provided

Answer: 1
Rationale: School-aged children strive for mastery and competence to achieve the developmental task of industry and accomplishment. Options 2 and 3 do not relate to the knowledge deficit. Option 4 may be a component of the teaching-learning process, but it is a passive process. Option 1 indicates more active participation on the part of the child, and expressing feelings of mastery and competence with the breathing devices indicates that learning took place.

Test-Taking Strategy: Focus on the issue: the best expected outcome. Eliminate options 2 and 3 first because they are similar. From the remaining options, focus on the issue and eliminate option 4 because it does not indicate that learning took place. Also noting that the child is school-aged will direct you to option 1. Review development tasks of the school-aged child if you had difficulty with this question.

Level of Cognitive Ability: Analysis
Client Needs: Physiological Integrity
Integrated Process: Nursing Process/Planning
Content Area: Child Health

Reference:
James, S., Ashwill, J., & Droske, S. (2002). *Nursing care of children: Principles & practice* (2nd ed.). Philadelphia: Saunders, pp. 678-679.

---

479. A nurse is caring for a client with acute mania who is receiving lithium carbonate (Eskalith) and had a serum lithium level drawn. The results of the lithium level are 2.0 mEq /L, and the nurse analyzes these results as:
1 Within normal limits
2 Higher than normal limits indicating toxicity
3 Lower than normal limits
4 Insignificant

Answer: 2
Rationale: The therapeutic level for lithium for the treatment of acute mania is 0.8 to 1.6 mEq/L. A level of 2.0 mEq/L indicates toxicity and requires that the medication be withheld and the blood work repeated. The physician also needs to be notified.

Test-Taking Strategy: Use the process of elimination. Eliminate options 1 and 4 first because they are similar. From the remaining options, recalling the therapeutic lithium level will direct you to option 2. Review this content if you are unfamiliar with this level.

Level of Cognitive Ability: Analysis
Client Needs: Physiological Integrity
Integrated Process: Nursing Process/Analysis
Content Area: Pharmacology

References:
Chernecky, C., & Berger, B. (2004). *Laboratory tests and diagnostic procedures* (4th ed.). Philadelphia: Saunders, p. 728.
Hodgson, B., & Kizior, R. (2004). *Saunders nursing drug handbook 2004.* Philadelphia: Saunders, p. 607.

480. A client calls the ambulatory care clinic and tells the nurse that she found an area that looks like the peel of an orange when performing breast self-examination (BSE), but found no other changes. The nurse should:
1 Tell the client there is nothing to worry about
2 Arrange for the client to be seen at the clinic as soon as possible
3 Tell the client to take her temperature and call back if she has a fever
4 Tell the client to point the area out to the physician at her next regularly scheduled appointment

Answer: 2
Rationale: Peau d'orange or the orange peel appearance of the skin over the breast is associated with late breast cancer. Therefore, the nurse would arrange for the client to come to the clinic at the earliest time possible. Peau d'orange is not indicative of an infection.

Test-Taking Strategy: Use the process of elimination. Eliminate options 1 and 4 because they are similar. From the remaining options, focus on the client's description to direct you to option 2. Review the signs of breast cancer if you had difficulty with this question.

Level of Cognitive Ability: Application
Client Needs: Physiological Integrity
Integrated Process: Nursing Process/Implementation
Content Area: Adult Health/Oncology

Reference:
Ignatavicius, D., & Workman, M. (2002). *Medical surgical nursing: Critical thinking for collaborative care* (4th ed.). Philadelphia: Saunders, p. 1739.

---

481. A nurse instructs a client about the procedure to perform the breast self-examination (BSE). Which client statement indicates a need for further instructions?
1 "I don't need to do that. I'm too old for that."
2 "I do BSE 7 days after I get my period."
3 "I examine my breasts in the shower."
4 "I lie on my back to examine my breasts."

Answer: 1
Rationale: BSE should still be done even after menopause. No one is "too old" to get breast cancer. Options 2, 3, and 4 identify correct components of performing BSE.

Test-Taking Strategy: Use the process of elimination, noting the key words "need for further instructions." These words indicate a false-response question and that you need to select the incorrect client statement. Recalling that BSE should be performed even after menopause will direct you to option 1. Review this content if you had difficulty with this question or are unfamiliar with this procedure.

Level of Cognitive Ability: Analysis
Client Needs: Physiological Integrity
Integrated Process: Teaching/Learning
Content Area: Fundamental Skills

References:
Ignatavicius, D., & Workman, M. (2002). *Medical surgical nursing: Critical thinking for collaborative care* (4th ed.). Philadelphia: Saunders, p. 1732.
Potter, P., & Perry, A. (2005). *Fundamentals of nursing* (6th ed.). St. Louis: Mosby, pp. 735-736.

482. A client with Cushing's syndrome is being instructed by the nurse on follow-up care. Which statement by the client would indicate a need for further instructions?
1 "I should avoid contact sports."
2 "I need to avoid foods high in potassium."
3 "I should check my ankles for swelling."
4 "I need to check my blood glucose regularly."

Answer: 2
Rationale: Hypokalemia is a common characteristic of Cushing's syndrome, and the client is instructed to consume foods high in potassium. Clients also experience activity intolerance, osteoporosis, and frequent bruising. Excess fluid volume results from water and sodium retention. Hyperglycemia is caused by an increased cortisol secretion.

Test-Taking Strategy: Note the key words "need for further instructions." This indicates a false-response question and that you need to select the option that indicates an incorrect client statement. Thinking about the pathophysiology associated with Cushing's syndrome and recalling that hypokalemia is a concern will direct you to option 2. Review this disorder if you had difficulty with this question.

Level of Cognitive Ability: Analysis
Client Needs: Physiological Integrity
Integrated Process: Teaching/Learning
Content Area: Adult Health/Endocrine

References:
Black, J., & Hawks, J. (2005). *Medical-surgical nursing: Clinical management for positive outcomes* (7th ed.). Philadelphia: Saunders, p. 1222.
Ignatavicius, D., & Workman, M. (2002). *Medical surgical nursing: Critical thinking for collaborative care* (4th ed.). Philadelphia: Saunders, pp. 1418-1419.

---

483. A client with aldosteronism is being treated with spironolactone (Aldactone). Which of the following indicates to the nurse that the medication is effective?
1 A decrease in blood pressure
2 A decrease in sodium excretion
3 A decrease in plasma potassium
4 A decrease in body metabolism

Answer: 1
Rationale: Aldactone antagonizes the effect of aldosterone and decreases circulating volume by inhibiting tubular reabsorption of sodium and water. Thus, it produces a decrease in blood pressure. It increases the excretion of sodium and water and increases potassium retention. It has no effect on body metabolism.

Test-Taking Strategy: Note the key words "medication is effective." Think about the action of this medication. Recalling that this medication is also used in hypertensive conditions will direct you to option 1. Review the effects of this medication if you had difficulty with this question.

Level of Cognitive Ability: Analysis
Client Needs: Physiological Integrity
Integrated Process: Nursing Process/Evaluation
Content Area: Adult Health/Endocrine

References:
Hodgson, B., & Kizior, R. (2004). *Saunders nursing drug handbook 2004.* Philadelphia: Saunders, p. 931.
McKenry, L., & Salerno, E. (2003). *Mosby's pharmacology in nursing* (21st ed.). St. Louis: Mosby, p. 679.

484. A nurse is caring for a client with neuroleptic malignant syndrome that resulted from the use of antipsychotic medications. On assessment, the nurse would expect to note:

1 Bradycardia
2 Dysphagia
3 Hypotension
4 Hyperpyrexia

Answer: 4

Rationale: Hyperpyrexia up to 107° F may be present in neuroleptic malignant syndrome. Symptoms develop suddenly and may include respiratory distress and muscle rigidity. As the condition progresses, there is evidence of tachycardia, hypertension, increasing respiratory distress, confusion, and delirium. The presence and severity of symptoms is compounded when two or more antipsychotics are taken concurrently.

Test-Taking Strategy: Consider the physiological responses that occur in neuroleptic malignant syndrome to answer this question. Recalling that hyperpyrexia occurs in this disorder will direct you to the correct option. Review the physiological manifestations that occur in neuroleptic malignant syndrome if you had difficulty with this question.

Level of Cognitive Ability: Analysis
Client Needs: Physiological Integrity
Integrated Process: Nursing Process/Assessment
Content Area: Pharmacology

References:
Kee, J., & Hayes, E. (2003). *Pharmacology: A nursing process approach* (4th ed.). Philadelphia: Saunders, pp. 288-289.
McKenry, L., & Salerno, E. (2003). *Mosby's pharmacology in nursing* (21st ed.). St. Louis: Mosby, p. 400.

485. A client with cancer who is receiving chemotherapy tells the nurse that the food on the meal tray "tastes funny." Which intervention by the nurse is appropriate?

1 Keep the client NPO
2 Administer an antiemetic as ordered
3 Provide oral hygiene care
4 Obtain an order for total parenteral nutrition (TPN)

Answer: 3

Rationale: Cancer treatments may cause distortion of taste. Frequent oral hygiene aids in preserving taste function. Keeping a client NPO increases nutritional risks. Antiemetics are used when nausea and vomiting are a problem. TPN is used when oral intake is not possible.

Test-Taking Strategy: Focus on the issue: taste sensation. Only option 3 addresses this issue. Also note the relationship between the words "tastes" in the question and "oral hygiene care" in the correct option. Review the effects of cancer treatments and the appropriate nursing interventions if you had difficulty with this question.

Level of Cognitive Ability: Application
Client Needs: Physiological Integrity
Integrated Process: Nursing Process/Implementation
Content Area: Adult Health/Oncology

Reference:
Black, J., & Hawks, J. (2005). *Medical-surgical nursing: Clinical management for positive outcomes* (7th ed.). Philadelphia: Saunders, p. 370.

486. A nurse notes redness, warmth, and a purulent drainage at the insertion site of a central venous catheter in a client receiving total parenteral nutrition (TPN). The nurse notifies the physician of this finding because:
1 Infections of a central venous catheter site can lead to septicemia
2 The client is experiencing an allergy to the TPN solution
3 The TPN solution has infiltrated and must be stopped
4 The client is allergic to the dressing material covering the site

Answer: 1

Rationale: Redness, warmth, and purulent drainage are signs of an infection, not an allergic reaction. Infiltration causes the surrounding tissue to become cool and pale.

Test-Taking Strategy: Note the key words "redness, warmth, and a purulent drainage" and focus on the issue: signs of infection. Eliminate options 2 and 4 because they are similar and indicate an allergy. From the remaining options, note that option 1 addresses septicemia, which can be life-threatening to the client. Review nursing interventions related to monitoring for complications of TPN if you had difficulty with this question.

Level of Cognitive Ability: Application
Client Needs: Physiological Integrity
Integrated Process: Nursing Process/Implementation
Content Area: Fundamental Skills

References:
Ignatavicius, D., & Workman, M. (2002). *Medical surgical nursing: Critical thinking for collaborative care* (4th ed.). Philadelphia: Saunders, pp. 212; 1372.
Potter, P., & Perry, A. (2005). *Fundamentals of nursing* (6th ed.). St. Louis: Mosby, p. 1315.

---

487. A nurse is performing a health history on a client with chronic calcifying pancreatitis. The nurse expects to most likely note which of the following when obtaining information regarding the client's health history?
1 Abdominal pain relieved with food or antacids
2 Exposure to occupational chemicals
3 Weight gain
4 Chronic use of alcohol

Answer: 4

Rationale: Chronic use of alcohol is the most frequent cause of chronic calcifying pancreatitis. Abstinence from alcohol is important to prevent the client from developing chronic pancreatitis. Clients usually experience malabsorption with weight loss. Pain will not be relieved with food or antacids. Chemical exposure is associated with cancer of the pancreas.

Test-Taking Strategy: Focus on the issue: the cause of chronic calcifying pancreatitis. Recalling the relationship between alcohol use and pancreatitis will direct you to option 4. Review the causes of pancreatitis if you had difficulty with this question.

Level of Cognitive Ability: Analysis
Client Needs: Physiological Integrity
Integrated Process: Nursing Process/Assessment
Content Area: Adult Health/Gastrointestinal

Reference:
Black, J., & Hawks, J. (2005). *Medical-surgical nursing: Clinical management for positive outcomes* (7th ed.). Philadelphia: Saunders, p. 1297.

488. A client has been taking glucocorticoids to control rheumatoid arthritis. The nurse monitors the client for which adverse effect of this pharmacological therapy?
1 Elevated serum potassium
2 Decreased serum sodium
3 Increased serum glucose
4 Increased white blood cells

Answer: 3
Rationale: Glucocorticoids have three primary uses: replacement therapy for adrenal insufficiency, immunosuppressive therapy, and antiinflammatory therapy. Exogenous glucocorticoids cause the same effects on cellular activity as the naturally produced glucocorticoids; however, exogenous glucocorticoids may produce undesired effects. The glucocorticoids stimulate appetite and increase caloric intake. They also increase the availability of glucose for energy. These combined effects cause the blood glucose levels to rise, making the client prone to hyperglycemia. Options 1, 2, and 4 do not occur as a result of the use of glucocorticoids.

Test-Taking Strategy: Use the process of elimination. First, eliminate options 1 and 2 because they are similar in that they both relate to electrolytes. From the remaining options, recalling that glucocorticoids increase the availability of glucose for energy will direct you to option 3. Review this content if you are unfamiliar with these type of medications, their uses, side effects and adverse effects, and contraindications.

Level of Cognitive Ability: Analysis
Client Needs: Physiological Integrity
Integrated Process: Nursing Process/Analysis
Content Area: Pharmacology

Reference:
Kee, J., & Hayes, E. (2003). *Pharmacology: A nursing process approach* (4th ed.). Philadelphia: Saunders, p. 730.

489. A client with a diagnosis of Cushing's syndrome is undergoing a dexamethasone suppression test. The nurse plans to implement which steps during this test?
1 Administer 1 mg of dexamethasone orally at night and obtain serum cortisol levels the next morning
2 Collect a 24-hour urine specimen to measure serum cortisol levels
3 Draw blood samples before and after exercise to evaluate the effect of exercise on serum cortisol levels
4 Administer an injection of adrenocorticotropic hormone (ACTH) 30 minutes before drawing blood to measure serum cortisol levels

Answer: 1
Rationale: The dexamethasone suppression test is performed to evaluate the function of the adrenal cortex. The procedure for this test is to administer 1 mg of dexamethasone at 11:00 PM to suppress ACTH formation and then to obtain 8:00 AM serum cortisol levels on the following day.

Test-Taking Strategy: Recall that Cushing's syndrome is a disorder caused by excessive amounts of cortisol. Because the test is a dexamethasone suppression test, you would expect that something is given to suppress cortisol production. Keeping this in mind, options 2 and 3 can be eliminated. From the remaining options, focusing on the description of Cushing's syndrome and the purpose of this test will direct you to option 1. Review this test if you had difficulty with this question.

Level of Cognitive Ability: Application
Client Needs: Physiological Integrity
Integrated Process: Nursing Process/Planning
Content Area: Adult Health/Endocrine

Reference:
Chernecky, C., & Berger, B. (2004). *Laboratory tests and diagnostic procedures* (4th ed.). Philadelphia: Saunders, p. 464.

490. A nurse is performing an abdominal assessment on a client. The nurse determines that which of the following findings should be reported to the physician?
1 Concave, midline umbilicus
2 Pulsation between the umbilicus and pubis
3 Bowel sound frequency of 15 sounds per minute
4 Absence of a bruit

Answer: 2
Rationale: The umbilicus should be in the midline, with a concave appearance. The presence of pulsation between the umbilicus and the pubis could indicate abdominal aortic aneurysm and should be reported to the physician. Bowel sounds vary according to the timing of the last meal and usually range in frequency from 5 to 35 per minute. Bruits are not normally present.

Test-Taking Strategy: Use basic nursing knowledge related to physical assessment to answer this question. Note that the wording of the question guides you to look for an abnormal finding. This will direct you to option 2. Review abdominal assessment if you had difficulty with this question.

Level of Cognitive Ability: Analysis
Client Needs: Physiological Integrity
Integrated Process: Nursing Process/Assessment
Content Area: Adult Health/Gastrointestinal

Reference:
Ignatavicius, D., & Workman, M. (2002). *Medical surgical nursing: Critical thinking for collaborative care* (4th ed.). Philadelphia: Saunders, p. 1168.

491. A nurse is performing a cardiovascular assessment on a client. Which of the following items would the nurse assess to gain the best information about the client's left-sided heart function?
1 Breath sounds
2 Peripheral edema
3 Jugular vein distention
4 Hepatojugular reflux

Answer: 1
Rationale: The client with heart failure may present with different symptoms depending on whether the right or the left side of the heart is failing. Peripheral edema, jugular vein distention, and hepatojugular reflux are all indicators of right-sided heart function. Breath sounds are an accurate indicator of left-sided heart function.

Test-Taking Strategy: Focus on the issue: left-sided heart failure. Remember: "left and lungs." Left-sided heart failure leads to respiratory signs and symptoms. Review the signs of right- and left-sided heart failure if you had difficulty with this question.

Level of Cognitive Ability: Application
Client Needs: Physiological Integrity
Integrated Process: Nursing Process/Assessment
Content Area: Adult Health/Respiratory

Reference:
Ignatavicius, D., & Workman, M. (2002). *Medical surgical nursing: Critical thinking for collaborative care* (4th ed.). Philadelphia: Saunders, p. 701.

492. A nurse is caring for the following group of clients on the clinical nursing unit. The nurse interprets that which of these clients is most at risk for the development of pulmonary embolism?

1   A 65-year-old man out of bed one day after prostate resection

2   A 73-year-old woman who has just had a pinning of a hip fracture

3   A 25-year-old woman with diabetic ketoacidosis

4   A 38-year-old man with pulmonary contusion after an auto accident

Answer: 2

Rationale: Clients frequently at risk for pulmonary embolism include those who are immobilized, especially postoperative clients. Other causes include those with conditions that are characterized by hypercoagulability, endothelial disease, and advancing age.

Test-Taking Strategy: The options can best be compared by evaluating the degree of immobility that each client has, and also the age of the client, which is provided in each option. The clients in options 1 and 3 have the least long-term anticipated immobility, and therefore should be eliminated first. From the remaining options, the younger client with the pulmonary contusion would be expected to be less immobile than the older woman with hip fracture. Review the causes of pulmonary embolism if you had difficulty with this question.

Level of Cognitive Ability: Analysis
Client Needs: Physiological Integrity
Integrated Process: Nursing Process/Assessment
Content Area: Adult Health/Respiratory

Reference:
Ignatavicius, D., & Workman, M. (2002). *Medical surgical nursing: Critical thinking for collaborative care* (4th ed.). Philadelphia: Saunders, pp. 591-592.

493. A graduate nurse is assigned to admit a client with a diagnosis of anorexia nervosa to the nursing unit. The nurse preceptor would remind the graduate nurse that assessment findings may indicate:

1   Elevated potassium levels

2   Low blood urea nitrogen

3   Weight loss of at 4% of original weight over a short period

4   That the client is knowledgeable about nutrition

Answer: 4

Rationale: The potassium level is usually low and the blood urea nitrogen is usually high in clients with anorexia nervosa. These clients lose at least 15% of their original body weight in a short period of time. They are very knowledgeable about nutrition and the caloric value of food.

Test-Taking Strategy: Use the process of elimination, focusing on the client's diagnosis. Option 3 is eliminated because the small amount of weight loss (4% of original weight) may not be a cause of concern for too many people. Eliminate options 1 and 2 because these findings do not occur in starvation or in the fluid or electrolyte deficiency typical of anorexia nervosa. Review the typical assessment findings in the client with anorexia nervosa if you had difficulty with this question.

Level of Cognitive Ability: Analysis
Client Needs: Physiological Integrity
Integrated Process: Nursing Process/Assessment
Content Area: Mental Health

Reference:
Stuart, G., & Laraia, M. (2005). *Principles and practice of psychiatric nursing* (8th ed.). St. Louis: Mosby, p. 520.

494. A physician has inserted a nasointestinal tube into a client. Following insertion, the nurse tells the client to lie in which position to help the tube advance into the duodenum, past the pyloric sphincter?
1 Supine with the head of the bed flat
2 Supine with the head elevated 30 degrees
3 On the right side
4 On the left side

Answer: 3

Rationale: Following insertion of a nasoenteric tube, the client is instructed to lie on the right side to aid in the passage of the tube from the stomach into the duodenum, past the pyloric sphincter. Options 1, 2, and 4 are incorrect positions.

Test-Taking Strategy: Use knowledge of basic anatomy and the position of the stomach in the abdomen to help eliminate options 1, 2, and 4. Knowledge of this position can be applied to the management of a client with any type of nasoenteric tube. Review care of the client with a nasoenteric tube if you had difficulty with this question.

Level of Cognitive Ability: Application
Client Needs: Physiological Integrity
Integrated Process: Nursing Process/Implementation
Content Area: Adult Health/Gastrointestinal

Reference:
Elkin, M., Perry, A., & Potter, P. (2004). *Nursing interventions & clinical skills* (3rd ed.). St. Louis: Mosby, p. 803.

---

495. A client with coronary artery disease suddenly complains of palpitations and an irregular heartbeat. The nurse would assess for which of the following to determine if the client is experiencing an inadequate stroke volume?
1 Pulse pressure
2 Pulse deficit
3 Pulsus alternans
4 Water hammer pulse

Answer: 2

Rationale: Palpitations are often a subjective complaint that accompanies dysrhythmias. Irregular rhythms produce varying strengths of stroke volume because of irregular ventricular filling times, and therefore arterial pulsations may become weakened or intermittently absent. The nurse determines this by assessing an apical-radial pulse. An apical rate that is greater than the radial rate is called a "pulse deficit." The pulse pressure is an indirect indicator of overall cardiac output. A water hammer pulse (Corrigan's pulse) is a bounding pulse in which a great surge is felt, followed by a sudden and complete absence of force or fullness in the artery. This type of pulse is associated with aortic regurgitation. Pulsus alternans has a regular rhythm accompanied by pulse volume that alternates strong with weak.

Test-Taking Strategy: Use the process of elimination. Remember that "stroke volume × heart rate = cardiac output." Measures that give a general indication of cardiac output are not specific enough to answer this question, therefore eliminate options 1 and 4. Pulsus alternans (option 3) occurs with a regular rhythm. Review the definition of pulse deficit if you had difficulty with this question.

Level of Cognitive Ability: Analysis
Client Needs: Physiological Integrity
Integrated Process: Nursing Process/Assessment
Content Area: Adult Health/Cardiovascular

References:
Mosby's medical, nursing, & allied health dictionary (6th ed.). St. Louis: Mosby, p. 436; 1438-1439; 1825.
Potter, P., & Perry, A. (2005). *Fundamentals of nursing* (6th ed.). St. Louis: Mosby, p. 725.

496. A nurse is listening to the client's breath sounds and hears a creaking, grating sound on inspiration and expiration over the posterior right lower lobe. The nurse documents that this client has:
1   Crackles
2   Wheezes
3   Rhonchi
4   Pleural friction rub

Answer: 4
Rationale: The nurse is hearing a pleural friction rub, which is characterized by sounds that are described as creaking, groaning, or grating in quality. The sounds are localized over an area of inflammation of the pleura and may be heard in both the inspiratory and expiratory phases of the respiratory cycle. Crackles have the sound that is heard when a few strands of hair are rubbed together near the ear and indicate fluid in the alveoli. Wheezes are musical noises heard on inspiration, expiration, or both. They are the result of narrowed air passages. Rhonchi are usually heard on expiration when there is excessive production of mucus, which accumulates in the air passages.

Test-Taking Strategy: Note the key words "creaking, grating sound." The image called to mind by these sounds is most compatible with the words "friction rub," and that may be sufficient to help you answer the question correctly. In addition, knowing that these sounds are not the classic descriptors for crackles, wheezes, or rhonchi helps you eliminate each of the other options. Review the characteristics of a pleural friction rub if you had difficulty with this question.

Level of Cognitive Ability: Analysis
Client Needs: Physiological Integrity
Integrated Process: Communication and Documentation
Content Area: Adult Health/Respiratory

Reference:
Potter, P., & Perry, A. (2005). *Fundamentals of nursing* (6th ed.). St. Louis: Mosby, p. 721.

497. A nurse is assessing the renal function of a client. After directly noting urine volume and characteristics, the nurse assesses which item as the best indirect indicator of renal function?
1   Bladder distention
2   Level of consciousness
3   Pulse rate
4   Blood pressure

Answer: 4
Rationale: The kidneys normally receive 20% to 25% of the cardiac output, even under conditions of rest. In order for kidney function to be optimal, adequate renal perfusion is necessary. Perfusion can best be estimated by the blood pressure, which is an indirect reflection of the adequacy of cardiac output. The pulse rate affects the cardiac output, but it can be altered by factors unrelated to kidney function. Bladder distention reflects a problem or obstruction that is most often distal to the kidneys. Level of consciousness is an unrelated item.

Test-Taking Strategy: Focus on the issue: renal function. Eliminate option 2 first as the item most unrelated to kidney function. Because bladder distention can be affected by several other factors besides renal function, this is eliminated next. From the remaining options, remember that the cardiac output equals heart rate times stroke volume. The cardiac output overall helps determine the blood pressure and renal perfusion. Thus, blood pressure is the more global or comprehensive option and the one more directly related to kidney perfusion. Review assessment of renal function if you had difficulty with this question.

Level of Cognitive Ability: Application
Client Needs: Physiological Integrity
Integrated Process: Nursing Process/Assessment
Content Area: Adult Health/Renal

References:
Black, J., & Hawks, J. (2005). *Medical-surgical nursing: Clinical management for positive outcomes* (7th ed.). Philadelphia: Saunders, pp. 767; 914.
Ignatavicius, D., & Workman, M. (2002). *Medical surgical nursing: Critical thinking for collaborative care* (4th ed.). Philadelphia: Saunders, p. 1598.

---

498. A nurse notes that the infusion bag of a client receiving total parenteral nutrition (TPN) has become empty. The nurse calls the pharmacy, but the next bag will not be delivered for another 30 minutes. The nurse hangs which of the following solutions until the TPN arrives?
1 5% dextrose in water
2 10% dextrose in water
3 50% dextrose in saline
4 5% dextrose in 0.45% saline

Answer: 2
Rationale: If a TPN solution bag stops running or becomes empty, the nurse should hang an infusion of 10% dextrose in water until another TPN solution arrives or the problem is fixed. This minimizes the chance of the client developing hypoglycemia, because the body produces more insulin in the presence of the high TPN glucose load.

Test-Taking Strategy: Use the process of elimination, recalling that the glucose concentration of TPN is high. Eliminate option 3 because there is no such solution of this type. Remember that options that are similar are not likely to be correct. This guides you to eliminate options 1 and 4, because the percentage of dextrose is the same. Review care of the client receiving TPN if you had difficulty with this question.

Level of Cognitive Ability: Application
Client Needs: Physiological Integrity
Integrated Process: Nursing Process/Implementation
Content Area: Adult Health/Gastrointestinal

Reference:
Ignatavicius, D., & Workman, M. (2002). *Medical surgical nursing: Critical thinking for collaborative care* (4th ed.). Philadelphia: Saunders, p. 1372.

---

499. A client seen in the ambulatory care clinic has ascites and slight jaundice. The nurse assesses the client for a history of chronic use of which of the following medications?
1 Acetaminophen (Tylenol)
2 Acetylsalicylic acid (aspirin)
3 Ibuprofen (Advil)
4 Ranitidine (Zantac)

Answer: 1
Rationale: Acetaminophen is a potentially hepatotoxic medication. Use of this medication and other hepatotoxic agents should be investigated whenever a client presents with symptoms compatible with liver disease (such as ascites and jaundice). Hepatotoxicity is not an adverse effect of the medications identified in options 2, 3, and 4.

Test-Taking Strategy: Focus on the signs noted in the question and recall that these symptoms are compatible with liver disease. With this in mind, evaluate each of the options in relation to their relative ability to be toxic to the liver. Recalling that acetaminophen is hepatotoxic will direct you to option 1. Review these medications if you are unfamiliar with them.

Level of Cognitive Ability: Analysis
Client Needs: Physiological Integrity
Integrated Process: Nursing Process/Assessment
Content Area: Adult Health/Gastrointestinal

Reference:
McKenry, L., & Salerno, E. (2003). *Mosby's pharmacology in nursing* (21st ed.). St. Louis: Mosby, p. 289.

---

500. A nurse is assigned to care for a client who has just undergone eye surgery. The nurse plans to instruct the client that which of the following activities is permitted in the postoperative period?
1 Reading
2 Watching television
3 Bending over
4 Lifting objects

Answer: 2

Rationale: The client is taught to avoid activities that raise intraocular pressure and could cause complications in the postoperative period. The client is also taught to avoid activities that cause rapid eye movements that are irritating in the presence of postoperative inflammation. For these reasons, the client is taught to avoid bending over, lifting heavy objects, straining, sneezing, making sudden movements, or reading. Watching television is permissible because the eye does not need to move rapidly with this activity, and it does not increase the intraocular pressure.

Test-Taking Strategy: Focus on the issue of intraocular pressure when answering this question. Eliminate options 3 and 4 first, because they increase intraocular pressure. From the remaining options, select option 2 because it is less taxing on the eyes. Review postoperative client instructions following eye surgery if you had difficulty with this question.

Level of Cognitive Ability: Application
Client Needs: Physiological Integrity
Integrated Process: Teaching/Learning
Content Area: Adult Health/Eye

Reference:
Lewis, S., Heitkemper, M., & Dirksen, S. (2004). *Medical-surgical nursing: Assessment and management of clinical problems* (6th ed.). St. Louis: Mosby, p. 452.

---

501. A nurse is listening to the lungs of a client who has left lower lobe pneumonia. The nurse interprets that the pneumonia is resolving if which of the following is heard over the affected lung area?
1 Bronchophony
2 Egophony
3 Vesicular breath sounds
4 Whispered pectoriloquy

Answer: 3

Rationale: Vesicular breath sounds are normal sounds that are heard over peripheral lung fields where the air enters the alveoli. A return of breath sounds to normal is consistent with a resolving pneumonia. Bronchophony is an abnormal finding indicative of lung consolidation, and is identified if the nurse can clearly hear the client say "ninety-nine" through the stethoscope when auscultating the lungs. (Normally the client's words are unintelligible if heard through a stethoscope.) Egophony occurs when the sound of the letter "e" is heard as an "a" with auscultation, and also indicates lung consolidation. Finally, whispered pectoriloquy is present if the nurse hears the client when "one-two-three" is whispered. This is an abnormal finding, again heard over an area of consolidation. Consolidation typically occurs with pneumonia.

Test-Taking Strategy: Use knowledge regarding respiratory assessment findings to answer the question. Knowing the anatomical areas where bronchial, vesicular, and bronchovesicular breath sounds are heard will direct you to option 3. Review these types of breath sounds if you had difficulty with this question.

Level of Cognitive Ability: Analysis
Client Needs: Physiological Integrity

Integrated Process: Nursing Process/Evaluation
Content Area: Adult Health/Respiratory

Reference:
Wilson, S., & Giddens, J. (2005). *Health assessment for nursing practice* (3rd ed.). St. Louis: Mosby, pp. 347-348.

---

502. A female client with a history of chronic infection of the urinary system complains of burning and urinary frequency. To determine whether the current problem is of renal origin, the nurse would assess whether the client has pain or discomfort in the:
1 Suprapubic area
2 Right or left costovertebral angle
3 Urinary meatus
4 Pain in the labium

Answer: 2
Rationale: Pain or discomfort from a problem that originates in the kidney is felt at the costovertebral angle on the affected side. Ureteral pain is felt in the ipsilateral labium in the female client or the ipsilateral scrotum in the male client. Bladder infection is often accompanied by suprapubic pain and pain or burning at the urinary meatus when voiding.

Test-Taking Strategy: Focus on the issue: a renal problem. Note the similarity between options 1, 3, and 4 in that they relate to the lower urinary tract. Recalling that the kidneys sit higher than the level of the bladder and retroperitoneally will also direct you to option 2. Review the signs of both renal and bladder infections if you had difficulty with this question.

Level of Cognitive Ability: Analysis
Client Needs: Physiological Integrity
Integrated Process: Nursing Process/Assessment
Content Area: Adult Health/Renal

Reference:
Wilson, S., & Giddens, J. (2005). *Health assessment for nursing practice* (3rd ed.). St. Louis: Mosby, pp. 450-451.

---

503. During a routine visit to the physician's office for monitoring of diabetic control, an older client with diabetes mellitus complains to the nurse of vision changes. The client describes blurring of the vision with difficulty in reading and with driving at night. Given the client's history, the nurse interprets that the client is probably developing:
1 Detached retina
2 Papilledema
3 Glaucoma
4 Cataracts

Answer: 4
Rationale: Although the incidence of cataracts increases with age, the older client with diabetes mellitus is at greater risk for developing cataracts. The most frequent complaint is blurred vision that is not accompanied by pain. The client may also experience difficulty with reading, night driving, and glare. Options 1, 2, and 3 are not directly associated with this client's history or complaints.

Test-Taking Strategy: Note that the client has diabetes mellitus. Use knowledge related to the risks for and signs and symptoms of common eye disorders to answer this question. Review the signs and symptoms of cataracts and the associated risk factors if you had difficulty with this question.

Level of Cognitive Ability: Analysis
Client Needs: Physiological Integrity
Integrated Process: Nursing Process/Analysis
Content Area: Adult Health/Eye

Reference:
Ignatavicius, D., & Workman, M. (2002). *Medical surgical nursing: Critical thinking for collaborative care* (4th ed.). Philadelphia: Saunders, p. 1032.

504. A nurse inquires about a smoking history while conducting a hospital admission assessment for a client with coronary artery disease (CAD). The most important item for the nurse to assess is the:
1   Number of pack-years
2   Brand of cigarettes used
3   Desire to quit smoking
4   Number of past attempts to quit smoking

Answer: 1
Rationale: The number of cigarettes smoked daily and the duration of the habit are used to calculate the number of pack-years, which is the standard method of documenting smoking history. The brand of cigarettes may give a general indication of tar and nicotine levels, but the information has no immediate clinical use. Desire to quit and number of past attempts to quit smoking may be useful when the nurse develops a smoking cessation plan with the client.

Test-Taking Strategy: Note the key words "most important item." The option that would most closely predict the degree of added risk of CAD is the number of pack-years. Review the technique to assess smoking history if you had difficulty with this question.

Level of Cognitive Ability: Analysis
Client Needs: Physiological Integrity
Integrated Process: Nursing Process/Assessment
Content Area: Adult Health/Cardiovascular

Reference:
Ignatavicius, D., & Workman, M. (2002). *Medical surgical nursing: Critical thinking for collaborative care* (4th ed.). Philadelphia: Saunders, pp. 471; 517.

---

505. A client with primary open-angle glaucoma has been prescribed timolol acetate (Timoptic) ophthalmic drops. The client asks the nurse how this medication works. The nurse tells the client that the medication lowers intraocular pressure by:
1   Reducing intracranial pressure
2   Increasing contractions of the ciliary muscle
3   Constricting the pupil
4   Decreasing the production of aqueous humor

Answer: 4
Rationale: Beta-adrenergic blocking agents, such as timolol acetate, reduce intraocular pressure by decreasing the production of aqueous humor. Miotic agents (such as pilocarpine) increase contractions of the ciliary muscle and constrict the pupil, thereby increasing the outflow of aqueous humor. This medication does not affect intracranial pressure.

Test-Taking Strategy: Specific knowledge about the action of this medication is needed to answer this question. Review the action of this medication if you are unfamiliar with it.

Level of Cognitive Ability: Application
Client Needs: Physiological Integrity
Integrated Process: Teaching/Learning
Content Area: Pharmacology

Reference:
Hodgson, B., & Kizior, R. (2004). *Saunders nursing drug handbook 2004.* Philadelphia: Saunders, p. 983.

---

506. A client arrives at the clinic complaining of knee pain. On assessment the nurse notes that the knee area is swollen. The nurse interprets that the client's signs and symptoms most likely indicate:
1   Osteoporosis
2   Degenerative joint disease
3   Rheumatoid arthritis
4   A recent injury

Answer: 4
Rationale: Pain and swelling are associated with musculoskeletal inflammation, infection, or a recent injury. Degenerative joint disease, osteoporosis, and rheumatoid arthritis may be accompanied by pain, but swelling may or may not be present.

Test-Taking Strategy: Focus on the signs and symptoms in the question and note the key words "most likely," which indicates that more than one option may be correct. Swelling and pain are signs of injury or inflammation. This should direct you to option 4. Review the signs associated with a musculoskeletal injury and the signs of degenerative disease if you had difficulty with this question.

Level of Cognitive Ability: Analysis
Client Needs: Physiological Integrity
Integrated Process: Nursing Process/Analysis
Content Area: Adult Health/Musculoskeletal

Reference:
Ignatavicius, D., & Workman, M. (2002). *Medical surgical nursing: Critical thinking for collaborative care* (4th ed.). Philadelphia: Saunders, p. 329.

---

507. A client seeks treatment in the emergency room for a lower leg injury. There is visible deformity to the lower aspect of the leg, and the injured leg appears shorter than the other leg. The area is painful, swollen, and beginning to become ecchymotic. The nurse interprets that this client has experienced a:
1 Contusion
2 Fracture
3 Sprain
4 Strain

Answer: 2
Rationale: Typical signs and symptoms of fracture include pain, loss of function in the area, deformity, shortening of the extremity, crepitus, swelling, and ecchymosis. Not all fractures lead to the development of every sign. A contusion results from a blow to soft tissue and causes pain, swelling, and ecchymosis. A sprain is an injury to a ligament caused by a wrenching or twisting motion. Symptoms include pain, swelling, and inability to use the joint or bear weight normally. A strain results from a pulling force on the muscle. Symptoms include soreness and pain with muscle use.

Test-Taking Strategy: Use the process of elimination and focus on the signs and symptoms in the question. Within the list of signs and symptoms, note the one that states one leg is shorter than another. Only a fractured bone (which shortens with displacement) could cause this sign. This makes it easy to eliminate each of the incorrect options. Review the signs and symptoms of a fracture if you had difficulty with this question.

Level of Cognitive Ability: Analysis
Client Needs: Physiological Integrity
Integrated Process: Nursing Process/Assessment
Content Area: Adult Health/Musculoskeletal

Reference:
Ignatavicius, D., & Workman, M. (2002). *Medical surgical nursing: Critical thinking for collaborative care* (4th ed.). Philadelphia: Saunders, pp. 1130-1131.

---

508. A client arrives at the emergency room with a chemical burn of the left eye. The nurse immediately:
1 Flushes the eye continuously with a sterile solution
2 Applies a cold compress to the injured eye
3 Applies a light bandage to the eye
4 Performs an assessment on the client

Answer: 1
Rationale: When the client has suffered a chemical burn of the eye, the nurse immediately flushes the site with a sterile solution continuously for 15 minutes. If a sterile eye irrigation solution is not available, running water may be used. Performing an assessment may be helpful but is not the priority action. Applying compresses or bandages is incorrect, because they do not rid the eye of the damaging chemical. Cold compresses are used for blows to the eye, whereas light bandages may be placed over cuts of the eye or eyelid.

Test-Taking Strategy: Focus on the injury described in the question: a chemical burn. Next, note the key word "immediately." This focus will direct you to option 1. Review emergency care related to chemical burns to the eye if you had difficulty with this question.

Level of Cognitive Ability: Application
Client Needs: Physiological Integrity
Integrated Process: Nursing Process/Implementation
Content Area: Adult Health/Eye

Reference:
Black, J., & Hawks, J. (2005). *Medical-surgical nursing: Clinical management for positive outcomes* (7th ed.). Philadelphia: Saunders, p. 1446.

---

509. A client tells the nurse about a pattern of getting a strong urge to void, which is followed by incontinence before the client can get to the bathroom. The nurse formulates which of the following nursing diagnoses for this client?
1 Reflex Urinary Incontinence
2 Stress Urinary Incontinence
3 Urge Urinary Incontinence
4 Total Urinary Incontinence

Answer: 3
Rationale: Urge incontinence occurs when the client has urinary incontinence soon after experiencing urgency. Reflex incontinence occurs when incontinence occurs at rather predictable times that correspond to when a certain bladder volume is attained. Stress incontinence occurs when the client voids in increments that are less than 50 mL and has increased abdominal pressure. Total incontinence occurs when there is an unpredictable and continuous loss of urine.

Test-Taking Strategy: Use the process of elimination. Eliminate option 4 first as having the least degree of relationship with the information in the question. Note that the question includes the word "urge." This will direct you to option 3 from the remaining options. Review nursing diagnoses related to incontinence if you had difficulty with this question.

Level of Cognitive Ability: Analysis
Client Needs: Physiological Integrity
Integrated Process: Nursing Process/Analysis
Content Area: Adult Health/Renal

Reference:
Black, J., & Hawks, J. (2005). *Medical-surgical nursing: Clinical management for positive outcomes* (7th ed.). Philadelphia: Saunders, p. 895.

510. A 52-year-old male client is seen in the physician's office for a physical examination after experiencing unusual fatigue over the last several weeks. The client's height is 5 feet, 8 inches, and weight is 220 pounds. Vital signs are temperature 98°F orally, pulse 86 beats per minute, and respirations 18 breaths per minute. The blood pressure (BP) is 184/100 mmHg. Random blood glucose is 122 mg/dL. Which of the following questions should the nurse ask the client first?
1 "Do you exercise regularly?"
2 "Are you considering trying to lose weight?"
3 "Is there a history of diabetes mellitus in your family?"
4 "When was the last time you had your blood pressure checked?"

Answer: 4
Rationale: The client is hypertensive, which is a known major modifiable risk factor for coronary artery disease (CAD). The other major modifiable risk factors not exhibited by this client include smoking and hypercholesterolemia. The client is overweight, which is a contributing risk factor. The client's nonmodifiable risk factors are age and gender. Because the client presents with several risk factors, the nurse places priority of attention on the client's major modifiable risk factors.

Test-Taking Strategy: Use the process of elimination, noting the key word "first." Eliminate options 1 and 2 first because they are similar. From the remaining options, note the client's blood pressure and its relationship to option 4. Review the risk factors for CAD if you had difficulty with this question.

Level of Cognitive Ability: Analysis
Client Needs: Physiological Integrity
Integrated Process: Nursing Process/Assessment
Content Area: Delegating/Prioritizing

Reference:
Ignatavicius, D., & Workman, M. (2002). *Medical surgical nursing: Critical thinking for collaborative care* (4th ed.). Philadelphia: Saunders, p. 792.

511. A nurse is instilling an otic solution into the adult client's left ear. The nurse avoids doing which of the following as part of this procedure?
1 Warming the solution to room temperature
2 Placing the client in a side-lying position with the ear facing up
3 Pulling the auricle backward and upward
4 Placing the tip of the dropper on the edge of the ear canal

Answer: 4
Rationale: The dropper is not allowed to touch any object or any part of the client's skin. The solution is warmed before use. The client is placed on the side with the affected ear upward. The nurse pulls the auricle backward and upward and instills the medication by holding the dropper about 1 cm above the ear canal.

Test-Taking Strategy: Note the key word "avoids." This word indicates a false-response question and that you need to select the option that is an incorrect nursing action. Basic knowledge of proper procedure for administering otic solutions and the principles related to aseptic technique will direct you to option 4. Review this basic nursing procedure if you had difficulty with this question.

Level of Cognitive Ability: Application
Client Needs: Physiological Integrity
Integrated Process: Nursing Process/Implementation
Content Area: Adult Health/Ear

Reference:
Potter, P., & Perry, A. (2005). *Fundamentals of nursing* (6th ed.). St. Louis: Mosby, pp. 862-863.

512. Levothyroxine sodium (Synthroid) is administered to a hospitalized child with congenital hypothyroidism. The child vomits 10 minutes after administration of the dose. The most appropriate nursing action is to:

1 Repeat the prescribed dose
2 Give two doses of the prescribed medicine on the next day
3 Contact the physician immediately
4 Hold the dose for today

Answer: 1

Rationale: Levothyroxine sodium (Synthroid) is the medication of choice for hypothyroidism. The most significant factor adversely affecting the eventual intelligence of children born with congenital hypothyroidism is inadequate treatment. Therefore, compliance with the medication regimen is essential. If the infant or child vomits within 1 hour of taking medication, the dose should be administered again.

Test-Taking Strategy: Use the process of elimination. General principles related to medication administration will assist in eliminating option 2. Eliminate option 3 because it is not necessary. From the remaining options, recalling the importance of the medication to treat this disorder will direct you to option 1. Review the administration of this medication in congenital hypothyroidism if you had difficulty with this question.

Level of Cognitive Ability: Application
Client Needs: Physiological Integrity
Integrated Process: Nursing Process/Implementation
Content Area: Child Health

Reference:
Wong, D., & Hockenberry, M. (2003). *Wong's nursing care of infants and children* (7th ed.). St. Louis: Mosby, p. 321.

---

513. A client diagnosed as having catatonic excitement has been pacing rapidly nonstop for several hours and is not eating or drinking. The nurse recognizes that in this situation:

1 There is an urgent need for physical and medical control
2 There is an urgent need for restraint
3 There is a need to encourage verbalization of feelings
4 The client will soon become catatonic stuporous

Answer: 1

Rationale: Catatonic excitement is manifested by a state of extreme psychomotor agitation. Clients urgently require physical and medical control because they are often destructive and violent to others, and their excitement can cause them to injure themselves or to collapse from complete exhaustion. Options 2, 3, and 4 are incorrect.

Test-Taking Strategy: Use Maslow's hierarchy of needs theory to answer the question. Physiological needs are the priority. Noting the client's behavior described in the question will direct you to option 1. Review care of the client with catatonic excitement if you had difficulty with this question.

Level of Cognitive Ability: Analysis
Client Needs: Physiological Integrity
Integrated Process: Nursing Process/Analysis
Content Area: Mental Health

Reference:
Varcarolis, E.M. (2002). *Foundations of psychiatric mental health nursing* (4th ed.). Philadelphia: Saunders, pp. 534;559.

514. A nurse is caring for a client with type 1 diabetes mellitus. Which of the following laboratory results would indicate a potential complication associated with this disorder?
1 Blood glucose: 112 mg/dL
2 Ketonuria
3 Blood urea nitrogen (BUN): 18 mg/dL
4 Potassium: 4.2 mEq

Answer: 2
Rationale: Ketonuria is an abnormal finding in the client with diabetes mellitus indicating ketosis. Ketosis is a metabolic effect from the lack of insulin on fat metabolism and occurs in type 1 diabetes mellitus. It is associated with the severe complication of diabetic ketoacidosis (hyperglycemia, ketosis, and acidosis). Options 1, 3, and 4 are all normal laboratory findings.

Test-Taking Strategy: Note the key words "indicate a potential complication." Options 1, 3, and 4 are all normal values, so eliminate these options. Review the complications of type 1 diabetes mellitus and normal laboratory values if you had difficulty with this question.

Level of Cognitive Ability: Analysis
Client Needs: Physiological Integrity
Integrated Process: Nursing Process/Analysis
Content Area: Adult Health/Endocrine

Reference:
Ignatavicius, D., & Workman, M. (2002). *Medical surgical nursing: Critical thinking for collaborative care* (4th ed.). Philadelphia: Saunders, p. 1483.

515. A nurse employed in a diabetes mellitus clinic is caring for a client on insulin pump therapy. Which statement by the client indicates that a knowledge deficit exists regarding insulin pump therapy?
1 "If my blood glucose is elevated, I can bolus myself with additional insulin as ordered."
2 "I'll need to check my blood glucose before meals in case I need a premeal insulin bolus."
3 "Now that I have this pump, I don't have to worry about insulin reactions or ketoacidosis ever happening again."
4 "I still need to follow a diet and exercise plan even though I don't inject myself daily anymore."

Answer: 3
Rationale: Hypoglycemic reactions can occur if there is an error in calculating the insulin dose or if the pump malfunctions. Ketoacidosis can occur if too little insulin is used or if there is an increase in metabolic need. The pump does not have a built-in blood glucose monitoring feedback system, so the client is subject to the usual complications associated with insulin administration without the use of a pump. Options 1, 2, and 4 are accurate regarding the use of the insulin pump.

Test-Taking Strategy: Knowledge of the basics of insulin therapy is helpful to answer this question even if you know little about insulin pump therapy. Options 1, 2, and 4 are logical statements regarding the use of endogenous insulin. Option 3, however, presumes a guarantee from a complication of insulin therapy. No biomedical equipment is capable of being 100% safe. Review the principles related to an insulin pump if you had difficulty with this question.

Level of Cognitive Ability: Analysis
Client Needs: Physiological Integrity
Integrated Process: Nursing Process/Evaluation
Content Area: Adult Health/Endocrine

Reference:
Lewis, S., Heitkemper, M., & Dirksen, S. (2004). *Medical-surgical nursing: Assessment and management of clinical problems* (6th ed.). St. Louis: Mosby, pp. 1276-1277.

516. A client with Graves' disease has exophthalmos and is experiencing photophobia. Which of the following interventions would best assist the client with this problem?

1 Administer methimazole (Tapazole) every 8 hours around the clock
2 Lubricate the eyes with tap water every 2 to 4 hours
3 Instruct the client to avoid straining or heavy lifting because this can increase eye pressure
4 Obtain dark glasses for the client

Answer: 4

Rationale: Medical therapy for Graves' disease does not help alleviate the clinical manifestation of exophthalmos. Because photophobia (light intolerance) accompanies this disorder, dark glasses are helpful in alleviating the problem. Tap water, which is hypotonic, could actually cause more swelling to the eye because it could pull fluid into the interstitial space. In addition, the client is at risk for developing an eye infection because the solution is not sterile. There is no need to avoid straining with exophthalmos. Methimazole inhibits the synthesis of thyroid hormone and is used to treat hyperthyroidism but will not alleviate exophthalmos or photophobia.

Test-Taking Strategy: Focus on the issue: photophobia. Recalling the definition of photophobia will direct you to option 4. Review the measures to treat this problem if you had difficulty with this question.

Level of Cognitive Ability: Application
Client Needs: Physiological Integrity
Integrated Process: Nursing Process/Implementation
Content Area: Adult Health/Endocrine

Reference:
Ignatavicius, D., & Workman, M. (2002). *Medical surgical nursing: Critical thinking for collaborative care* (4th ed.). Philadelphia: Saunders, pp. 1424-1425; 1429.

517. A nurse is caring for a client with pneumonia who suddenly becomes restless and has a PaO_2 of 60 mmHg. Which of the following nursing diagnoses would be most appropriate for this client?

1 Fatigue related to a debilitated state
2 Impaired gas exchange related to increased pulmonary secretions
3 Ineffective airway clearance related to dilated bronchioles
4 Impaired gas exchange related to pneumonia

Answer: 2

Rationale: Restlessness and a low PaO_2 are hallmark signs of impaired gas exchange. Although many clients with pneumonia experience fatigue, this nursing diagnosis is not the most appropriate based on the PaO_2 level. Dilated bronchioles would be a goal for treatment and not part of the nursing diagnosis. Pneumonia is a medical diagnosis.

Test-Taking Strategy: Eliminate option 4 because it is a medical diagnosis. Focus on the data in the question to eliminate option 1 next because it is unrelated to this data. From the remaining options, recalling that the bronchioles are not dilated in pneumonia will direct you to option 2. Review care of the client with pneumonia if you had difficulty with this question.

Level of Cognitive Ability: Analysis
Client Needs: Physiological Integrity
Integrated Process: Nursing Process/Analysis
Content Area: Adult Health/Respiratory

Reference:
Ignatavicius, D., & Workman, M. (2002). *Medical surgical nursing: Critical thinking for collaborative care* (4th ed.). Philadelphia: Saunders, p. 581.

518. A client with tuberculosis (TB) is to be started on rifampin (Rifadin). The nurse provides instructions to the client and tells the client:
1 That yellow-colored skin is common
2 To wear glasses instead of soft contact lenses
3 To always take the medication on an empty stomach
4 That as soon as the cultures come back negative, the medication may be stopped

Answer: 2
Rationale: Soft contacts may be permanently damaged by the orange discoloration that rifampin causes in body fluids. Any sign of jaundice (yellow-colored skin) should always be reported. If rifampin is not tolerated on an empty stomach, it may be taken with food. The client may be on the medication for 12 months even if cultures are negative.

Test-Taking Strategy: Use the process of elimination. Eliminate option 3 because of the absolute word "always." Eliminate option 1 because it is an indication of jaundice. From the remaining options, recalling the side effects of rifampin will direct you to option 2. Review this medication if you are unfamiliar with it.

Level of Cognitive Ability: Application
Client Needs: Physiological Integrity
Integrated Process: Teaching/Learning
Content Area: Pharmacology

Reference:
Hodgson, B., & Kizior, R. (2004). *Saunders nursing drug handbook 2004.* Philadelphia: Saunders, p. 886.

519. A nurse reviews the physician's orders for a client with Guillain-Barré syndrome. Which order written by the physician should the nurse question?
1 Assess vital signs frequently
2 Provide a clear liquid diet
3 Perform passive range of motion exercises three times daily
4 Obtain bilateral calf measurements daily

Answer: 2
Rationale: Clients with Guillain-Barré syndrome have dysphagia. Clients with dysphagia are more likely to aspirate clear liquids than thick or semi-solid foods. Because clients with Guillain-Barré syndrome are at risk for hypotension or hypertension, bradycardia, and respiratory depression, frequent monitoring of vital signs is required. Passive range of motion exercises can help prevent contractures, and assessing calf measurements can help detect deep vein thrombosis, for which these clients are at risk.

Test-Taking Strategy: Use the process of elimination, recalling that the client with Guillain-Barré syndrome is at risk for dysphagia. Even if you are unaware that dysphagia is a problem, note that options 1, 3, and 4 are generally part of routine nursing care. Review the manifestations associated with this disorder if you had difficulty with this question.

Level of Cognitive Ability: Analysis
Client Needs: Physiological Integrity
Integrated Process: Nursing Process/Implementation
Content Area: Adult Health/Neurological

References:
Ignatavicius, D., & Workman, M. (2002). *Medical surgical nursing: Critical thinking for collaborative care* (4th ed.). Philadelphia: Saunders, p. 954.
Lewis, S., Heitkemper, M., & Dirksen, S. (2004). *Medical-surgical nursing: Assessment and management of clinical problems* (6th ed.). St. Louis: Mosby, p. 1607.

520. A client with myasthenia gravis arrives at the emergency room and crisis is suspected. The physician plans to administer edrophonium (Tensilon) to differentiate between myasthenic and cholinergic crisis. The nurse prepares to administer which medication if the client is in cholinergic crisis?

1 Atropine sulfate
2 Morphine sulfate
3 Pyridostigmine bromide (Mestinon)
4 Isoproterenol (Isuprel)

[handwritten: Cholinergic crisis – over medication / myasthenic crisis – Under medication]

Answer: 1

Rationale: Clients with cholinergic crisis have experienced overdosage of medication. Tensilon will exacerbate symptoms in cholinergic crisis to the point where the client may need intubation and mechanical ventilation. Intravenous atropine sulfate is used to reverse the effects of these anticholinesterase medications. Morphine sulfate and pyridostigmine bromide would worsen the symptoms of cholinergic crisis. Isuprel is not indicated for cholinergic crisis.

Test-Taking Strategy: Focus on the issue: cholinergic crisis. Recalling the antidote for anticholinesterase medications will direct you to option 1. Memorize this antidote if you had difficulty with this question.

Level of Cognitive Ability: Application
Client Needs: Physiological Integrity
Integrated Process: Nursing Process/Planning
Content Area: Adult Health/Neurological

Reference:
Ignatavicius, D., & Workman, M. (2002). *Medical surgical nursing: Critical thinking for collaborative care* (4th ed.). Philadelphia: Saunders, p. 961.

---

521. A nurse is completing a health history on a client with diabetes mellitus who has been taking insulin for many years. At present the client states that he is experiencing periods of hypoglycemia followed by periods of hyperglycemia. The most likely cause for this occurrence is which of the following?

1 Injecting insulin at a site of lipodystrophy
2 Adjusting insulin according to blood glucose levels
3 Eating snacks between meals
4 Initiating the use of the insulin pump

Answer: 1

Rationale: Tissue hypertrophy (lipodystrophy) involves thickening of the subcutaneous tissue at the injection sites. This can interfere with the absorption of insulin, resulting in erratic blood glucose levels. Because the client has been on insulin for many years, this is the most likely cause of poor control. Options 2, 3, and 4 are appropriate techniques to use in order to regulate blood glucose levels.

Test-Taking Strategy: Note the key words "taking insulin for many years." This indicates that you must consider a long-term complication of insulin administration as the answer to the question. Options 2, 3, and 4 are eliminated because they are actually appropriate techniques to use in order to regulate blood glucose levels. Review lipodystrophy if you had difficulty with this question.

Level of Cognitive Ability: Analysis
Client Needs: Physiological Integrity
Integrated Process: Nursing Process/Analysis
Content Area: Adult Health/Endocrine

Reference:
Ignatavicius, D., & Workman, M. (2002). *Medical surgical nursing: Critical thinking for collaborative care* (4th ed.). Philadelphia: Saunders, pp. 1460-1461.

fetal death

522. A nurse receives a report at the beginning of the shift regarding a client with an intrauterine fetal demise. On assessment of the client, the nurse expects to note which of the following?
1 Elevated blood pressure, proteinuria, and edema
2 Regression of pregnancy symptoms and absence of fetal heart tones
3 Uterine size greater than expected for gestational age
4 Intractable vomiting and dehydration

Answer: 2
Rationale: Symptoms of a fetal demise include a decrease in fetal movement, no change or a decrease in fundal height, and absent fetal heart tones. Additionally, many symptoms of the pregnancy may diminish, such as breast size and tenderness. Option 1 is associated with preeclampsia. Option 4 is associated with hyperemesis gravidarum.

Test-Taking Strategy: Focus on the issue: intrauterine fetal demise. Recalling that fetal demise means fetal death will direct you to option 2. Review the signs associated with fetal demise if you had difficulty with this question.

Level of Cognitive Ability: Analysis
Client Needs: Physiological Integrity
Integrated Process: Nursing Process/Assessment
Content Area: Maternity/Intrapartum

Reference:
Lowdermilk, D., & Perry, A. (2004). *Maternity & women's health care* (8th ed.). St. Louis: Mosby, pp. 876-877.

523. A client admitted to the nursing unit from the emergency department has a C-4 spinal cord injury. Which assessment should the nurse perform first when admitting the client to the nursing unit?
1 Take the client's temperature
2 Assess extremity muscle strength
3 Observe for dyskinesias
4 Listen to breath sounds

Answer: 4
Rationale: Because compromise of respiration is a leading cause of death in cervical cord injury, respiratory assessment is the highest priority. Assessment of temperature and strength can be done after adequate oxygenation is assured. Dyskinesias occur in cerebellar disorders, so they are not as important in cord-injured clients, unless head injury is suspected.

Test-Taking Strategy: Remembering that a cord injury, particularly at the level of C-4, can affect respiratory status will direct you to the correct option. Also, use of the ABCs—airway, breathing, and circulation—can guide assessment priorities in this situation. Breath sounds will be diminished if respiratory muscles are weakened or paralyzed. Review priority care of the client with a C-4 spinal cord injury if you had difficulty with this question.

Level of Cognitive Ability: Application
Client Needs: Physiological Integrity
Integrated Process: Nursing Process/Assessment
Content Area: Delegating/Prioritizing

Reference:
Ignatavicius, D., & Workman, M. (2002). *Medical surgical nursing: Critical thinking for collaborative care* (4th ed.). Philadelphia: Saunders, pp. 933-934.

524. A nurse is assisting in positioning a client for a surgical procedure. The nurse knows that the respiratory system is most vulnerable to which of the following positions?
1 Lithotomy
2 Supine
3 Lateral
4 Sims'

Answer: 1
Rationale: The thoracic cage normally expands in all directions except posteriorly. In the lithotomy position, the expansion of the lungs is restricted at the ribs or sternum, and there is a reduction in the ability of the diaphragm to push down against the abdominal muscles. Respiratory function is impaired because of this interference with normal movements. The volume of air that can be inspired is reduced. The positions identified in options 2, 3, and 4 will not cause this impairment.

Test-Taking Strategy: Use the process of elimination. Options 3 and 4 are similar and are eliminated first. From the remaining options, visualize each of these positions and their effect on the process of respiration. The supine position would not interfere with the expansion of the lungs, as the lithotomy position would. Review these positions if you had difficulty with this question.

Level of Cognitive Ability: Analysis
Client Needs: Physiological Integrity
Integrated Process: Nursing Process/Analysis
Content Area: Fundamental Skills

Reference:
Potter, P., & Perry, A. (2005). *Fundamentals of nursing* (6th ed.). St. Louis: Mosby, pp. 746; 681; 1109; 1457; 1464; 1627.

---

525. A nurse is caring for a client who is receiving an intravenous infusion of theophylline. The nurse checks which of the following to determine medication effectiveness?
1 Pupillary response
2 Pulse rate
3 Temperature
4 Lung sounds

Answer: 4
Rationale: Theophylline is a bronchodilator used to treat bronchial asthma or to reverse bronchospasm caused by chronic bronchitis, emphysema, or chronic obstructive pulmonary disease. To determine medication effectiveness, the nurse would auscultate lung sounds for the absence of rhonchi, crackles, or wheezes. Although the client's temperature would be monitored for signs of respiratory infection in a client with a respiratory disorder, temperature is unrelated to medication effectiveness. Although the pulse rate would be monitored because tachycardia is a sign of toxicity, pulse rate is unrelated to medication effectiveness. Pupillary response is a neurological assessment and is unrelated to this medication.

Test-Taking Strategy: Note the key words "to determine medication effectiveness." Focus on the name of the medication and recall that medication names that end with "line" are bronchodilators. This will direct you to option 4. Also, use of the ABCs—airway, breathing, and circulation—will direct you to the correct option. Review the expected effects of this medication if you had difficulty with this question.

Level of Cognitive Ability: Analysis
Client Needs: Physiological Integrity
Integrated Process: Nursing Process/Evaluation
Content Area: Pharmacology

Reference:
Hodgson, B., & Kizior, R. (2004). *Saunders nursing drug handbook 2004.* Philadelphia: Saunders, pp. 44-46.

526. A nurse is monitoring a client with frequent premature ventricular contractions (PVCs) of more than 6 per minute and is preparing to administer a bolus of lidocaine (Xylocaine). The nurse monitors which of the following after administering the medication?
1 Skin temperature and neurological status
2 Vital signs, ECG, and neurological status
3 Kidney and liver function, and neurological status
4 Visual changes, and kidney and liver function

Answer: 2
Rationale: Lidocaine can cause atrioventricular block with conduction defects. It can also cause paresthesia, numbness, disorientation, and agitation. Monitoring the vital signs, ECG, and neurological status is the priority.

Test-Taking Strategy: Focus on the client's diagnosis: premature ventricular contractions. Note that option 2 is the only option that addresses direct cardiac monitoring. Review this medication if you had difficulty with this question.

Level of Cognitive Ability: Application
Client Needs: Physiological Integrity
Integrated Process: Nursing Process/Implementation
Content Area: Pharmacology

References:
Lehne, R. (2004). *Pharmacology for nursing care* (5th ed.). Philadelphia: Saunders, p. 496; 504.
McKenry, L., & Salerno, E. (2003). *Mosby's pharmacology in nursing* (21st ed.). St. Louis: Mosby, p. 557.

527. A nurse is caring for a client experiencing hypertensive crisis. The physician tells the nurse that medication will be prescribed to help reduce both preload and afterload. The nurse anticipates that the physician will prescribe which medication?
1 Digoxin (Lanoxin)
2 Nitroprusside sodium (Nipride)
3 Morphine sulfate
4 Furosemide (Lasix)

Answer: 2
Rationale: Intravenous nitroprusside (Nipride) is a potent vasodilator that reduces preload and afterload. Digoxin (Lanoxin) is a cardiac glycoside that increases cardiac contractility. Morphine sulfate is a narcotic analgesic. Furosemide (Lasix) is a loop diuretic and can reduce preload by enhancing the renal excretion of sodium and water, which reduces circulating blood volume.

Test-Taking Strategy: Focus on the issue: reducing preload and afterload and the client's diagnosis (hypertensive crisis). Use the process of elimination and recall that nitroprusside sodium is a vasodilator. Review the effects of the medications in the options if you had difficulty with this question.

Level of Cognitive Ability: Analysis
Client Needs: Physiological Integrity
Integrated Process: Nursing Process/Analysis
Content Area: Pharmacology

Reference:
Hodgson, B., & Kizior, R. (2004). *Saunders nursing drug handbook 2004.* Philadelphia: Saunders, p. 736.

528. Streptokinase (Streptase) is being administered to a client following an acute inferior myocardial infarction. The nurse understands that the primary purpose of this medication is to:
1 Inhibit further clot formation
2 Reduce myocardial oxygen demand
3 Prevent platelet aggregation
4 Dissolve the thrombus

Answer: 4
Rationale: Streptokinase is a thrombolytic medication that causes lysis of blood clots. Anticoagulants prevent further clot formation. Beta-blockers, nitrates, and calcium channel blockers are used to reduce myocardial oxygen demand. Streptokinase does not prevent platelet aggregation.

Test-Taking Strategy: Recalling that streptokinase is a thrombolytic medication and that these medications dissolve clots will direct you to option 4. Review this medication if you had difficulty with this question.

Level of Cognitive Ability: Analysis
Client Needs: Physiological Integrity
Integrated Process: Nursing Process/Analysis
Content Area: Pharmacology

Reference:
Hodgson, B., & Kizior, R. (2004). *Saunders nursing drug handbook 2004.* Philadelphia: Saunders, p. 936.

---

529. A nurse is planning to care for a client with pulmonary edema. The nurse establishes a goal to have the client participate in activities that reduce cardiac workload. The nurse identifies which client action as contributing to this goal?
1 Elevating the legs when in bed
2 Sleeping in the supine position
3 Using seasonings to improve the taste of food
4 Using a bedside commode for stools

Answer: 4
Rationale: Using a bedside commode decreases the work of getting to the bathroom or struggling to use the bedpan. Elevating the client's legs increases venous return to the heart, thus increasing cardiac workload. The supine position increases respiratory effort and decreases oxygenation. This increases cardiac workload. Seasonings are high in sodium.

Test-Taking Strategy: Use the process of elimination, focusing on the issue: reducing cardiac overload. Keeping this issue in mind will direct you to option 4. Review measures that will reduce cardiac workload if you had difficulty with this question.

Level of Cognitive Ability: Analysis
Client Needs: Physiological Integrity
Integrated Process: Nursing Process/Analysis
Content Area: Adult Health/Cardiovascular

Reference:
Ignatavicius, D., & Workman, M. (2002). *Medical surgical nursing: Critical thinking for collaborative care* (4th ed.). Philadelphia: Saunders, p. 801.

---

530. A child is sent to the school nurse by the teacher. On assessment, the school nurse notes that the child has a rash. The nurse suspects that the child has erythema infectiosum (fifth disease) because the skin assessment revealed a rash that is:
1 A discrete rose-pink maculopapular rash on the trunk
2 A highly pruritic, profuse macule to papule rash on the trunk
3 A discrete pinkish red maculopapular rash that is spreading to the trunk
4 An erythema on the face that has a "slapped face" appearance

Answer: 4
Rationale: The classic rash of erythema infectiosum, or fifth disease, is the erythema on the face. The discrete rose-pink maculopapular rash is the rash of exanthema subitum (roseola). The highly pruritic, profuse macule to papule rash is the rash of varicella (chickenpox). The discrete pinkish red maculopapular rash is the rash of rubella (German measles).

Test-Taking Strategy: Knowledge regarding the characteristics associated with erythema infectiosum is required to answer the question. If you were unfamiliar with this disorder, note that in options 1, 2, and 3, a similarity exists in that the rash is on the trunk. Option 4 addresses a rash on the face. Review this disorder if you had difficulty with this question.

Level of Cognitive Ability: Analysis
Client Needs: Physiological Integrity
Integrated Process: Nursing Process/Assessment
Content Area: Child Health

Reference:
Wong, D., & Hockenberry, M. (2003). *Wong's nursing care of infants and children* (7th ed.). St. Louis: Mosby, pp. 654-655.

531. A client is taking a monoamine oxidase inhibitor (MAOI). The nurse assesses the client closely because:
1 These medications increase the amount of MAOI in the liver
2 Hypotensive crisis may be precipitated by foods rich in tyramine and tryptophan
3 Headache, hypertension, and nausea and vomiting may indicate toxicity
4 Hypotension may indicate toxicity

Answer: 3
Rationale: Headache, hypertension, tachycardia, nausea, and vomiting are precursors to hypertensive crisis brought about by the ingestion of foods rich in tyramine and tryptophan while the client is taking an MAOI. These medications act by decreasing the amount of MAOI in the liver, which is necessary for the breakdown and utilization of tyramine and tryptophan. Hypertensive crisis may lead to circulatory collapse, intracranial hemorrhage, and death.

Test-Taking Strategy: Use the process of elimination. Eliminate options 2 and 4 first because they are similar. From the remaining options, recalling the relationship between MAOIs and toxicity will direct you to option 3. Review the actions and side effects of MAOIs if you had difficulty with this question.

Level of Cognitive Ability: Application
Client Needs: Physiological Integrity
Integrated Process: Nursing Process/Assessment
Content Area: Pharmacology

References:
Kee, J., & Hayes, E. (2003). *Pharmacology: A nursing process approach* (4th ed.). Philadelphia: Saunders, p. 311.
McKenry, L., & Salerno, E. (2003). *Mosby's pharmacology in nursing* (21st ed.). St. Louis: Mosby, p. 421.

532. A client has returned to the nursing unit following an abdominal hysterectomy and is lying in the supine position. To completely assess the client for postoperative bleeding, the nurse should do which of the following?
1 Check the abdominal dressing
2 Check the perineal pad
3 Ask the client about sensation of moistness
4 Roll the client to one side after checking the perineal pad and the abdominal dressing

Answer: 4
Rationale: The nurse should roll the client to one side after checking the perineal pad and the abdominal dressing. This allows the nurse to check the rectal area, where blood may pool by gravity if the client is lying supine. Asking the client about a sensation of moistness is not a complete assessment.

Test-Taking Strategy: Use the process of elimination. Eliminate option 3 first because it relies on the client. From the remaining options, note that option 4 addresses rolling the client. It is also the most comprehensive option. Review care of the client following hysterectomy if you had difficulty with this question.

Level of Cognitive Ability: Application
Client Needs: Physiological Integrity
Integrated Process: Nursing Process/Implementation
Content Area: Fundamental Skills

Reference:
Ignatavicius, D., & Workman, M. (2002). *Medical surgical nursing: Critical thinking for collaborative care* (4th ed.). Philadelphia: Saunders, p. 1767.

533. A nurse is caring for the client who returned to the nursing unit following suprapubic prostatectomy. The nurse monitors the continuous bladder irrigation to detect which of the following signs of catheter blockage?
1 Drainage that is pale pink
2 Drainage that is bright red
3 Urine leakage around the three-way catheter at the meatus
4 True urine output of 50 mL per hr

Answer: 3
Rationale: Catheter blockage or occlusion by clots following prostatectomy can result in urine backup and leakage around the urethral meatus. This would be accompanied by a stoppage of outflow through the catheter into the drainage bag. Drainage that is bright red indicates that the irrigant is running too slowly; drainage that is pale pink indicates sufficient flow. A true urine output of 50 mL per hr indicates catheter patency.

Test-Taking Strategy: Use the process of elimination, focusing on the issue: catheter blockage. Eliminate options 1 and 2 first because of the word "drainage." This implies catheter patency. From the remaining options, apply basic principles related to Foley catheter management. A leakage around the catheter at the meatus indicates blockage. Review care of the client following prostatectomy if you had difficulty with this question.

Level of Cognitive Ability: Analysis
Client Needs: Physiological Integrity
Integrated Process: Nursing Process/Assessment
Content Area: Adult Health/Renal

Reference:
Ignatavicius, D., & Workman, M. (2002). *Medical surgical nursing: Critical thinking for collaborative care* (4th ed.). Philadelphia: Saunders, p. 1788.

534. A nurse is assigned to a client returning from the post-anesthesia care unit following transurethral prostatectomy. The nurse avoids doing which of the following after this procedure?
1 Reporting signs of confusion
2 Administering a B&O (belladonna & opium) suppository at room temperature
3 Removing the traction tape on the three-way catheter
4 Monitoring hourly urine output

Answer: 3
Rationale: The nurse would avoid removing the traction tape applied by the surgeon in the operating room. The purpose of this tape is to place pressure on the prostate and reduce hemorrhage. B&O suppositories, ordered on a prn basis for bladder spasm, should be warmed to room temperature before administration. The nurse routinely monitors hourly urine output because the client has a three-way bladder irrigation running. The nurse also assesses for confusion, which could result from hyponatremia secondary to the hypotonic irrigant used during the surgical procedure.

Test-Taking Strategy: Use the process of elimination, noting the key word "avoids." This word indicates a false-response question and that you need to select the incorrect nursing action. Eliminate options 1 and 4 first because they are part of routine nursing care and would not be contraindicated in the care of this client. From the remaining options, recalling the need to reduce hemorrhage will direct you to option 3. Review care of the client following prostatectomy if you had difficulty with this question.

Level of Cognitive Ability: Application
Client Needs: Physiological Integrity
Integrated Process: Nursing Process/Implementation
Content Area: Adult Health/Renal

Reference:
Ignatavicius, D., & Workman, M. (2002). *Medical surgical nursing: Critical thinking for collaborative care* (4th ed.). Philadelphia: Saunders, pp. 1787-1788.

535. A client is due for a dose of bumetanide (Bumex). The nurse would temporarily withhold the dose and notify the physician if which of the following laboratory results was noted?
1 Sodium: 137 mEq/L
2 Potassium: 2.9 mEq/L
3 Magnesium: 2.6 mg/dL
4 Chloride: 106 mEq/L

Answer: 2
Rationale: Bumetanide is a loop diuretic that is not potassium-sparing. The value given for potassium is below the therapeutic range of 3.5 to 5.1 mEq/L for this electrolyte. The nurse should notify the physician before giving the dose so that potassium may be ordered. Options 1, 3, and 4 identify normal values.

Test-Taking Strategy: Note the key words "notify the physician." Use the process of elimination and knowledge of the normal laboratory values. Option 2 is the only abnormal value. Review this medication if you had difficulty with this question.

Level of Cognitive Ability: Application
Client Needs: Physiological Integrity
Integrated Process: Nursing Process/Implementation
Content Area: Pharmacology

Reference:
Hodgson, B., & Kizior, R. (2004). *Saunders nursing drug handbook 2004.* Philadelphia: Saunders, p. 127.

---

536. A client with heart failure is receiving furosemide (Lasix) and digoxin (Lanoxin) daily. When the nurse enters the room to administer the morning doses, the client complains of anorexia, nausea, and yellow vision. The nurse should do which of the following first?
1 Administer the medications
2 Give the digoxin only
3 Check the morning serum potassium level
4 Check the morning serum digoxin level

Answer: 4
Rationale: The nurse should check for the result of the digoxin level that was drawn, because the symptoms are compatible with digitalis toxicity. Knowing that a low potassium level may contribute to digitalis toxicity, checking the serum potassium level may give useful additive information, but the digoxin level is checked first. The digoxin should be withheld until the level is known, making options 1 and 2 incorrect.

Test-Taking Strategy: Note the key word "first." Eliminate options 1 and 2 first, because it is not prudent to administer the medication(s) without doing further investigation. From the remaining options, recalling the signs of digoxin toxicity will direct you to option 4. Review the signs of digoxin toxicity if you had difficulty with this question.

Level of Cognitive Ability: Application
Client Needs: Physiological Integrity
Integrated Process: Nursing Process/Implementation
Content Area: Pharmacology

Reference:
Lehne, R. (2004). *Pharmacology for nursing care* (5th ed.). Philadelphia: Saunders, pp. 479-480.

---

537. A nurse is administering an oral dose of erythromycin (E-mycin) to an assigned client. The nurse administers this medication with a:
1 Full glass of milk
2 Full glass of water
3 Sip of orange juice
4 Any citrus beverage

Answer: 2
Rationale: Erythromycin is a macrolide antibiotic that should be taken with a full glass of water. Sufficient volume is needed to obtain the maximal effect of the medication. Depending on the specific type of erythromycin, it may need to be administered on an empty stomach, with meals, or regardless of timing of meals. The nurse should verify the best method of administration for the type of erythromycin ordered. Options 1, 3, and 4 are incorrect.

Test-Taking Strategy: Use the process of elimination. Eliminate options 3 and 4 first because they are similar. From the remaining options, recalling that medication administered with milk affects absorption will direct you to option 2. Review this medication if you had difficulty with this question.

Level of Cognitive Ability: Application
Client Needs: Physiological Integrity
Integrated Process: Nursing Process/Implementation
Content Area: Pharmacology

Reference:
Hodgson, B., & Kizior, R. (2004). *Saunders nursing drug handbook 2004.* Philadelphia: Saunders, p. 373.

---

538. A nurse has given the client a dose of intravenous hydralazine (Apresoline). The nurse evaluates the effectiveness of the medication by monitoring which of the following client parameters?
1 Blood pressure
2 Muscle strength
3 Urine output
4 Blood glucose level

Answer: 1
Rationale: Hydralazine is an antihypertensive medication used in the management of moderate to severe hypertension. It is a vasodilator medication that decreases afterload. The blood pressure needs to be monitored. Options 2, 3, and 4 are not specifically associated with the use of this medication.

Test-Taking Strategy: Use the process of elimination. Note the name of the medication, *Apresoline,* to assist you in determining that the medication is an antihypertensive. This will direct you to option 1. Review this medication if it is unfamiliar to you.

Level of Cognitive Ability: Analysis
Client Needs: Physiological Integrity
Integrated Process: Nursing Process/Evaluation
Content Area: Pharmacology

Reference:
Hodgson, B., & Kizior, R. (2004). *Saunders nursing drug handbook 2004.* Philadelphia: Saunders, p. 498.

---

539. A client arrives in the emergency room and carbon monoxide (CO) poisoning is suspected. The nurse expects the physician to prescribe which of the following to confirm the diagnosis?
1 Carboxyhemoglobin level
2 Complete blood cell count
3 Pulse oximetry
4 Computerized tomography (CT) scan of the head

Answer: 1
Rationale: The diagnosis of carbon monoxide poisoning is confirmed by measurement of carboxyhemoglobin levels in the client's blood. Pulse oximetry readings are unreliable because of the detection of CO-hemoglobin as oxyhemoglobin. The neurological system may be affected by carbon monoxide poisoning, but this will be detected by assessment of clinical manifestations. A CT scan of the head will not confirm the diagnosis or provide any useful information unless a structural defect or injury in the head is a concern. A complete blood cell count may provide useful information but will not confirm the diagnosis.

Test-Taking Strategy: Note the key word "confirm." Note the relationship between the words "carbon monoxide (CO) poisoning" in the question and option 1. Review content related to carbon monoxide poisoning if you had difficulty with this question.

Level of Cognitive Ability: Application
Client Needs: Physiological Integrity
Integrated Process: Nursing Process/Assessment
Content Area: Adult Health/Respiratory

Reference:

Black, J., & Hawks, J. (2005). *Medical-surgical nursing: Clinical management for positive outcomes* (7th ed.). Philadelphia: Saunders, p. 1907.

---

540. A client receiving a dose of intravenous vancomycin (Vancocin) develops chills, tachycardia, syncope, and flushing of the face and trunk. The nurse interprets that:

1 The client is allergic to the medication
2 The medication has interacted with another medication the client is receiving
3 The medication is infusing too rapidly
4 The client is experiencing upper airway obstruction

Answer: 3

Rationale: The client is experiencing signs and symptoms of what is called "red man" or "red neck" syndrome. This is a response caused by histamine release that occurs with rapid or bolus injection. The client may experience chills, fever, flushing of the face and/or trunk, tachycardia, syncope, tingling, and an unpleasant taste in the mouth. The corrective action is to administer the medication more slowly. An antihistamine such as diphenhydramine (Benadryl) may be administered as well. Options 1, 2, and 4 are incorrect interpretations.

Test-Taking Strategy: This question may be difficult and you may want to quickly select option 1. Remember that options that are similar are not likely to be correct. For this reason, begin to answer this question by eliminating options 1 and 4 first. From the remaining options, recalling the adverse effect of "red neck" syndrome associated with the use of this medication will direct you to option 3. Review the adverse effects of this medication if you had difficulty with this question.

Level of Cognitive Ability: Analysis
Client Needs: Physiological Integrity
Integrated Process: Nursing Process/Analysis
Content Area: Pharmacology

References:

Hodgson, B., & Kizior, R. (2004). *Saunders nursing drug handbook 2004.* Philadelphia: Saunders, p. 1042.
McKenry, L., & Salerno, E. (2003). *Mosby's pharmacology in nursing* (21st ed.). St. Louis: Mosby, p. 995.

---

541. A client has an order for beclomethasone (Beclovent) by the intranasal route. The client also has an order for a nasal decongestant. The nurse plans to:

1 Administer the beclomethasone 15 minutes before the decongestant
2 Administer the decongestant 15 minutes before the beclomethasone
3 Administer the beclomethasone immediately before the decongestant
4 Administer the decongestant immediately before the beclomethasone

Answer: 2

Rationale: The nasal decongestant should be administered 15 minutes before the beclomethasone (a glucocorticoid) to clear the nasal passages and enhance absorption of the glucocorticoid. Options 1, 3, and 4 are incorrect methods of administration.

Test-Taking Strategy: Use the same principles in answering this question that you would use when administering bronchodilators and corticosteroids (glucocorticoids) together. Remember: the glucocorticoid is administered last. Review the procedure for administering intranasal medications if you had difficulty with this question.

Level of Cognitive Ability: Application
Client Needs: Physiological Integrity
Integrated Process: Nursing Process/Implementation
Content Area: Pharmacology

References:
Hodgson, B., & Kizior, R. (2004). *Saunders nursing drug handbook 2004*. Philadelphia: Saunders, p. 97.
McKenry, L., & Salerno, E. (2003). *Mosby's pharmacology in nursing* (21st ed.). St. Louis: Mosby, p. 727.

---

542. A client suddenly experiences a seizure, and the nurse notes that the client exhibits uncontrollable jerking movements. The nurse documents that the client experienced which type of seizure?
1 Absence seizure
2 Myoclonic seizure
3 Clonic seizure
4 Tonic seizure

Answer: 2
Rationale: A myoclonic seizure is characterized by sudden uncontrollable jerking movements of a single muscle group or multiple muscle groups. Absence seizures occur in childhood and adolescence and are characterized by a vacant facial expression. A clonic seizure is characterized by rhythmic muscular contraction and relaxation lasting several minutes. A tonic seizure is characterized by an abrupt increase in muscle tone and contraction and the presence of autonomic manifestations.

Test-Taking Strategy: Focus on the data in the question and use knowledge regarding the characteristics of the various types of seizures to answer this question. Review the types of seizures and their characteristics if you had difficulty with this question.

Level of Cognitive Ability: Analysis
Client Needs: Physiological Integrity
Integrated Process: Nursing Process/Assessment
Content Area: Adult Health/Neurological

Reference:
Black, J., & Hawks, J. (2005). *Medical-surgical nursing: Clinical management for positive outcomes* (7th ed.). Philadelphia: Saunders, p. 2076.

---

543. A client is receiving tobramycin (Tobrex). The nurse evaluates that the client is responding well to the medication therapy if which of the following laboratory results is noted?
1 White blood cell (WBC) count of 8,000/cu mm and creatinine level of 0.9 mg/dL
2 WBC count of 15,000/cu mm and a blood urea nitrogen (BUN) of 38 mg/dL
3 Sodium of 140 mEq/L and potassium of 3.9 mEq/L
4 Sodium of 145 mEq/L and chloride of 106 mEq/L

Answer: 1
Rationale: Tobramycin is an antibiotic (aminoglycoside) that causes nephrotoxicity and ototoxicity. The medication is therapeutic if the WBC count drops back into the normal range and the kidney function remains normal. Option 2 indicates an abnormal WBC count, and options 3 and 4 are unrelated to the use of this medication.

Test-Taking Strategy: Use the process of elimination. Begin to answer this question by eliminating options 3 and 4 first, knowing that tobramycin is an antibiotic. Recalling that aminoglycosides cause nephrotoxicity, select option 1 using laboratory values as your guide. Review this medication and normal laboratory values if you had difficulty with this question.

Level of Cognitive Ability: Analysis
Client Needs: Physiological Integrity
Integrated Process: Nursing Process/Evaluation
Content Area: Pharmacology

Reference:
Hodgson, B., & Kizior, R. (2004). *Saunders nursing drug handbook 2004.* Philadelphia: Saunders, p. 992.

---

544. A nurse is caring for a client who is taking a maintenance dosage of lithium carbonate (Eskalith). The nurse plans to:
  1 Monitor daily serum lithium levels
  2 Perform a weekly ECG
  3 Observe for remission of depressive states
  4 Monitor intake and output

Answer: 4
Rationale: Lithium is used to treat manic disorders, not depression. Side effects of lithium are nausea, tremors, polyuria, and polydypsia. Serum lithium concentration is assessed approximately every 2 to 4 days during initial therapy and at longer intervals thereafter. Toxic levels of lithium may induce electrocardiogram changes, but there is no need to perform weekly ECGs if maintenance levels are maintained.

Test-Taking Strategy: Use the process of elimination. Eliminate options 1 and 2 first because of the words "daily" and "weekly" in these options. From the remaining options, recalling that this medication is used to treat manic disorders will direct you to option 4. Review the nursing interventions associated with administering this medication if you had difficulty with this question.

Level of Cognitive Ability: Application
Client Needs: Physiological Integrity
Integrated Process: Nursing Process/Planning
Content Area: Pharmacology

Reference:
McKenry, L., & Salerno, E. (2003). *Mosby's pharmacology in nursing* (21st ed.). St. Louis: Mosby, pp. 426-427.

---

545. A nurse is caring for a client with chronic obstructive pulmonary disease (COPD) who is receiving aminophylline (Theophylline) intravenously. A theophylline blood serum level is drawn on the client. The nurse monitors the results of this blood test and expects the findings to be at which therapeutic level?
  1 5 mcg/mL
  2 8 mcg/mL
  3 18 mcg/mL
  4 25 mcg/mL

Answer: 3
Rationale: Aminophylline (Theophylline) is a bronchodilator. The therapeutic serum level range of theophylline is 10 to 20 mcg/mL. It is critical that the nurse monitor theophylline blood serum levels daily when a client is on this medication to ensure that a therapeutic range is present and to monitor for the potential for toxicity. Options 1 and 2 indicate low levels. Option 4 is a toxic level, indicating the need to stop the medication and notify the physician.

Test-Taking Strategy: Specific knowledge of this medication and the therapeutic serum level range is required to answer this question. Remember that this therapeutic serum level range is the same as the therapeutic serum level range for phenytoin (Dilantin). Review this medication if you had difficulty with this question.

Level of Cognitive Ability: Analysis
Client Needs: Physiological Integrity
Integrated Process: Nursing Process/Assessment
Content Area: Pharmacology

Reference:
Chernecky, C., & Berger, B. (2004). *Laboratory tests and diagnostic procedures* (4th ed.). Philadelphia: Saunders, p. 1040.

546. A nurse is caring for a client with a closed chest drainage system. On assessment of the client, the nurse notes a rise and fall (fluctuation) of fluid in the water seal chamber. Based on this finding, what action will the nurse take?

1 Contacts the physician
2 Adds water to the suction control chamber
3 Documents that the system is functioning accurately
4 Adds water to the water seal chamber

Answer: 3

Rationale: Fluid in the water seal compartment should rise with inspiration and fall with expiration (fluctuations). When fluctuations occur, the drainage tubes are patent and the apparatus is functioning properly. Fluctuations stop when the lung has reexpanded or if the chest drainage tubes are kinked or obstructed. Therefore, the nurse would document that the system is functioning accurately. There is no need to call the physician because this is an expected finding. There is no data in the question indicating the need to add fluid to the chambers.

Test-Taking Strategy: Focus on the nurse's assessment finding: a rise and fall (fluctuation) of fluid in the water seal chamber. Visualize the chest tube drainage system and think about the function of each chamber to assist in determining the nurse's action. Review the functioning of chest tube drainage systems if you had difficulty with this question.

Level of Cognitive Ability: Analysis
Client Needs: Physiological Integrity
Integrated Process: Nursing Process/Implementation
Content Area: Adult Health/Respiratory

Reference:
Black, J., & Hawks, J. (2005). *Medical-surgical nursing: Clinical management for positive outcomes* (7th ed.). Philadelphia: Saunders, p. 1863.

547. A nurse is performing an admission assessment on a client admitted to the hospital with a diagnosis of pheochromocytoma. The nurse prepares to implement what action to assess for the principal manifestation associated with this disorder?

1 Assesses for the presence of peripheral edema
2 Checks the client's pupils
3 Takes the client's blood pressure
4 Checks the peripheral pulses

Answer: 3

Rationale: Pheochromocytoma is a catecholamine-secreting tumor that is usually located in the adrenal medulla. Hypertension is the principal manifestation associated with pheochromocytoma, and it can be persistent, fluctuating, intermittent, or paroxysmal. The blood pressure status would be assessed by taking the client's blood pressure. The assessments in options 1, 2, and 4 are not associated with this disorder.

Test-Taking Strategy: Note the key words "principal manifestation." Recalling that pheochromocytoma is a tumor of the adrenal gland and recalling the function of the adrenal gland will direct you to option 3. Review the principal manifestations of pheochromocytoma if you had difficulty with this question.

Level of Cognitive Ability: Application
Client Needs: Physiological Integrity
Integrated Process: Nursing Process/Assessment
Content Area: Adult Health/Endocrine

Reference:
Black, J., & Hawks, J. (2005). *Medical-surgical nursing: Clinical management for positive outcomes* (7th ed.). Philadelphia: Saunders, p. 1231.

548. A client received a thermal burn caused by the inhalation of steam. The client's mouth is edematous and the nurse notes blisters in the client's mouth. The nurse first assesses which priority item(s)?
1 Temperature via the rectal route
2 Respiratory status and lung sounds
3 Neurological status
4 Level of consciousness

Answer: 2
Rationale: Thermal burns to the lower airways can occur with the inhalation of steam or explosive gases or with the aspiration of scalding liquids. Thermal burns to the upper airways are more common and generally appear erythematous and edematous with mucosal blisters or ulcerations. The mucosal edema can lead to upper airway obstruction, particularly during the first 24 to 48 hours after burn injury. Assessment of respiratory status is the priority. Although the nurse would check the client's temperature and the client's neurological status, respiratory status is the priority.

Test-Taking Strategy: Focus on the type of burn injury described in the question and note the key words "mouth is edematous." Eliminate options 3 and 4 first because they are similar. Use the ABCs—airway, breathing, and circulation—to assist you in answering this question. Review care of the client with a burn injury if you had difficulty with this question.

Level of Cognitive Ability: Analysis
Client Needs: Physiological Integrity
Integrated Process: Nursing Process/Assessment
Content Area: Delegating/Prioritizing

Reference:
Black, J., & Hawks, J. (2005). *Medical-surgical nursing: Clinical management for positive outcomes* (7th ed.). Philadelphia: Saunders, p. 1440.

549. A client with late-stage chronic obstructive pulmonary disease (COPD) is admitted to the hospital with acute exacerbation. Which of the following blood gas results would the nurse most likely expect to note?
1 Po_2 of 68 and Pco_2 of 40
2 Po_2 of 55 and Pco_2 of 40
3 Po_2 of 70 and Pco_2 of 50
4 Po_2 of 60 and Pco_2 of 50

Answer: 4
Rationale: During an acute exacerbation, the arterial blood gases deteriorate with a decreasing Po_2 and an increasing Pco_2. In early stages of COPD, arterial blood gases demonstrate mild to moderate hypoxemia with the Po_2 in the high 60s to high 70s and a normal arterial Pco_2. As the condition advances, hypoxemia increases and hypercapnia may result.

Test-Taking Strategy: Note the key words "acute exacerbation" and "most likely." Recall the physiological manifestations that occur in COPD. Remembering that in COPD a low Po_2 and an elevated Pco_2 is the likely occurrence will direct you to the correct option. Review the clinical manifestations that are likely to occur in an acute exacerbation if you had difficulty with this question.

Level of Cognitive Ability: Analysis
Client Needs: Physiological Integrity
Integrated Process: Nursing Process/Analysis
Content Area: Adult Health/Respiratory

Reference:
Black, J., & Hawks, J. (2005). *Medical-surgical nursing: Clinical management for positive outcomes* (7th ed.). Philadelphia: Saunders, p. 1819.

550. A nurse monitors the respiratory status of the client being treated for acute exacerbation of chronic obstructive pulmonary disease (COPD). Which assessment finding would indicate a deterioration in ventilation?
1 Cyanosis
2 Rapid, shallow respirations
3 Hyperinflated chest
4 Coarse crackles bilaterally

Answer: 2

Rationale: An increase in the rate of respirations and a decrease in the depth of respirations indicates a deterioration in ventilation. Cyanosis is not a good indicator of oxygenation in the client with COPD. Cyanosis may be present with some clients but not all clients. A hyperinflated chest (barrel-chest) and hypertrophy of the accessory muscles of the upper chest and neck may normally be found in clients with severe COPD. During an exacerbation, coarse crackles are expected to be heard bilateral throughout the lungs but do not indicate deterioration in ventilation.

Test-Taking Strategy: Note the key words "deterioration in ventilation." Eliminate options 3 and 4, recalling the normal clinical signs seen in COPD and the signs of exacerbation. Because cyanosis is not a good indicator of oxygenation in the client with COPD, eliminate option 1. Review the clinical manifestations associated with COPD and a deterioration in ventilation if you had difficulty with this question.

Level of Cognitive Ability: Analysis
Client Needs: Physiological Integrity
Integrated Process: Nursing Process/Assessment
Content Area: Adult Health/Respiratory

References:
Ignatavicius, D., & Workman, M. (2002). *Medical surgical nursing: Critical thinking for collaborative care* (4th ed.). Philadelphia: Saunders, p. 542.
Phipps, W., Monahan, F., Sands, J., Marek, J., & Neighbors, M. (2003). *Medical-surgical nursing: health and illness perspectives* (7th ed.). St. Louis: Mosby, p. 569.

CRITICAL THINKING: ALTERNATE FORMAT QUESTIONS

1. A client is admitted to the hospital with a diagnosis of acute bacterial pericarditis, and the nurse prepares to perform an assessment on the client. Select the manifestations and findings that are associated with this inflammatory heart disease:
___ Pericardial friction rub
___ Severe precordial chest pain that intensifies when in the supine position
___ Leukopenia
___ Decreased erythrocyte sedimentation rate
___ Fever
___ Bradycardia

Answer:
Pericardial friction rub
Severe precordial chest pain that intensifies when in the supine position
Fever
Rationale: In acute pericarditis, the membranes surrounding the heart become inflamed and rub against each other, producing the classic pericardial friction rub. The client complains of severe precordial chest pain that intensifies when lying supine and decreases in a sitting position. The pain also intensifies when the client breathes deeply. Fever typically occurs and is accompanied by leukocytosis and an elevated erythrocyte sedimentation rate. Malaise, myalgias, and tachycardia are common.

Test-Taking Strategy: Focusing on the diagnosis will assist in determining that the client would have a fever; the compensatory response to fever is an increased metabolic rate and tachycardia. Also remember that when the client has an inflammatory disease, the erythrocyte sedimentation rate would increase, as would the white blood cell count (leukocytosis not leukopenia). Lastly, focusing on the diagnosis will assist in determining that a pericardial friction rub and severe precordial chest pain will be present. Review the characteristics associated with acute bacterial pericarditis if you had difficulty with this question.

Level of Cognitive Ability: Analysis
Client Needs: Physiological Integrity
Integrated Process: Nursing Process/Assessment
Content Area: Adult Health/Cardiovascular

Reference:
Phipps, W., Monahan, F., Sands, J., Marek, J., & Neighbors, M. (2003). *Medical-surgical nursing: Health and illness perspectives* (7th ed.). St. Louis: Mosby, p. 707.

---

2. A nurse is assessing a client's cigarette smoking habit, and the client states that he smokes three-quarter pack per day over the last 10 years. The nurse calculates that the client has a smoking history of how many pack-years?

Answer: _____

Answer: 7.5
Rationale: The standard method for quantifying smoking history is to multiply the number of packs smoked per day by the number of years of smoking. The number is recorded as the number of pack-years. The calculation for the number of pack-years for the client who has smoked three-quarter pack per day for 10 years is: 0.75 packs × 10 years = 7.5 pack years.

Test-Taking Strategy: Focus on the information in the question and multiply the number of packs of cigarettes smoked per day by the number of years of smoking. Review this calculation if you had difficulty with this question.

Level of Cognitive Ability: Application
Client Needs: Physiological Integrity
Integrated Process: Nursing Process/Assessment
Content Area: Adult Health/Respiratory

Reference:
Ignatavicius, D., & Workman, M. (2002). *Medical surgical nursing: Critical thinking for collaborative care* (4th ed.). Philadelphia: Saunders, p. 471.

---

3. A physician's order reads: acetaminophen (Tylenol) liquid, 450 mg PO every 4 hours prn for pain. The medication label reads: 160 mg/5 mL. The nurse prepares how many milliliters to administer one dose?

Answer: _____

Answer: 14
Rationale: Use the formula for calculating medication dosages.

Formula:

$$\frac{\text{Desired}}{\text{Available}} \times \text{Volume} = \text{mL per dose}$$

$$\frac{450 \text{ mg}}{160 \text{ mg}} \times 5 \text{ mL} = 14 \text{ mL}$$

Test-Taking Strategy: Identify the key components of the question and what the question is asking. In this case, the question asks for mL per one dose. Set up the formula knowing that the desired dose is 450 mg, available is 160 mg per 5 mL. Review medication calculations if you had difficulty with this question.

Level of Cognitive Ability: Application
Client Needs: Physiological Integrity
Integrated Process: Nursing Process/Planning
Content Area: Fundamental Skills

Reference:
Kee, J., & Marshall, S. (2004). *Clinical calculations: With applications to general and specialty areas* (4th ed.). Philadelphia: Saunders, pp. 80-81.

---

4. A nurse witnesses a client going into pulmonary edema. The client's exhibits respiratory distress, but the blood pressure is stable at this time. While waiting for help to arrive, the nurse performs the following actions in which order of priority? (Number 1 is the first action.)
   ___ Rechecks the vital signs
   ___ Places the client in high Fowler's position
   ___ Places the client on a pulse oximeter and cardiac monitor
   ___ Calls the respiratory therapy department for a ventilator

Answer: 3124
Rationale: The client in pulmonary edema is immediately placed in high Fowler's position, if the blood pressure is stable. The nurse would also place the client on a pulse oximeter and a cardiac monitor to monitor cardiopulmonary status. The nurse would also monitor the client's vital signs closely. Because a ventilator may or may not be needed, calling the respiratory therapy department would be the final action from the actions provided. Additional interventions include the administration of oxygen by mask or nasal catheter, the administration of diuretics, insertion of a Foley catheter, and the administration of morphine sulfate.

Test-Taking Strategy: Remember: in a respiratory emergency situation, client positioning may be the first action because it will alleviate dyspnea. Next use the ABCs—airway, breathing, and circulation—to determine that placing the client on a pulse oximeter and cardiac monitor would be the next action. From the remaining options, recall that mechanical ventilation may or may not be needed. This will assist in determining that rechecking the vital signs would be the third action. Review the immediate nursing actions for a client in pulmonary edema if you had difficulty with this question.

Level of Cognitive Ability: Application
Client Needs: Physiological Integrity
Integrated Process: Nursing Process/Implementation
Content Area: Delegating/Prioritizing

Reference:
Lewis, S., Heitkemper, M., & Dirksen, S. (2004). *Medical-surgical nursing: Assessment and management of clinical problems* (6th ed.). St. Louis: Mosby, p. 843.

5. An adult client arrives in the emergency unit with burns to both legs and perineal areas. Using the Rule of Nines, the nurse would determine that approximately what percentage of the client's body surface has been burned?

Answer: _____

Answer: 37

Rationale: The most rapid method used to calculate the size of a burn injury in adult clients whose weights are in normal proportion to their heights is the Rule of Nines. This method divides the body into areas that are in multiples of 9%. Each leg is 18%, each arm is 9%, and the head is 9%. The trunk is 36% and the perineal area is 1%. Both legs and perineal area equal 37%.

Test-Taking Strategy: Knowledge regarding the percentages associated with this method of calculating burn injuries is required to answer this question. Memorize these percentages if you had difficulty with this question.

Level of Cognitive Ability: Analysis
Client Needs: Physiological Integrity
Integrated Process: Nursing Process/Assessment
Content Area: Adult Health/Integumentary

Reference:
Ignatavicius, D., & Workman, M. (2002). *Medical surgical nursing: Critical thinking for collaborative care* (4th ed.). Philadelphia: Saunders, p. 1567.

---

6. A client who works as a security guard at night in an industrial building is brought to the emergency room with suspected carbon monoxide poisoning. List in order of priority the actions that the nurse takes on arrival of the client. (Number 1 is the first action.)
___ Notifies the local health department and requests an inspection at the industrial building
___ Draws blood for carboxyhemoglobin levels
___ Assesses the client
___ Administers 100% oxygen

Answer: 4321

Rationale: On arrival of the client, 100% oxygen is administered at atmospheric pressure or hyperbaric pressure to speed up the elimination of carbon monoxide from the hemoglobin and to reverse hypoxia. The next most important action is assessment of the client. Then blood is drawn (initially and serially) to monitor carboxyhemoglobin levels; once they drop below 5%, oxygen may be discontinued. If the episode was unintentional and precipitated by conditions in a dwelling, the health department is notified.

Test-Taking Strategy: Note that the data in the question indicates an emergency situation and recall that in an emergency an action is usually the first step. Use the ABCs—airway, breathing, and circulation—to direct you to the action that indicates to administer 100% oxygen. Next use the steps of the nursing process; assessment of the client is the second action. From the remaining actions listed, use Maslow's hierarchy of needs theory, recalling that physiological needs are the priority. This will assist you in determining that drawing blood for carboxyhemoglobin levels is the third action. Review care of the client with carbon monoxide poisoning if you had difficulty with this question.

Level of Cognitive Ability: Application
Client Needs: Physiological Integrity
Integrated Process: Nursing Process/Implementation
Content Area: Adult Health/Respiratory

References:
Black, J., & Hawks, J. (2005). *Medical-surgical nursing: Clinical management for positive outcomes* (7th ed.). Philadelphia: Saunders, p. 1906.
Chernecky, C., & Berger, B. (2004). *Laboratory tests and diagnostic procedures* (4th ed.). Philadelphia: Saunders, p. 324.

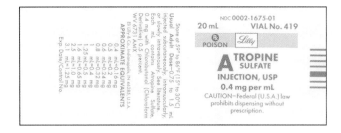

7. A physician has prescribed atropine sulfate gr 1/100, intramuscularly. The nurse reads the label on the medication vial and administers how many mL to the client?

1 0.5
2 1.0
3 1.5
4 2.0

Answer: 3

Rationale: In this medication problem, both the apothecary (grains) and the metric (milligrams) systems are involved. Because the drug preparation is in milligrams (as noted on the medication label), it is necessary to convert grains (gr) to milligrams (mg).

Formula for converting grains to milligrams:

gr:mg :: gr:mg

1:60 :: 1/100:X

X = 60/100

X = 0.6 mg

Formula:

$$\frac{\text{Desired}}{\text{Available}} \times mL = mL \text{ per dose}$$

$$\frac{0.6 \text{ mg}}{0.4 \text{ mg}} \times 1 \text{ mL} = 1.5 \text{ mL}$$

Test-Taking Strategy: Read the physician's order and the medication label, noting that it is first necessary to convert grains to milligrams. Next, follow the formula for the calculation of the correct dose. Use a calculator to verify your answer and make sure that the answer makes sense. Review medication calculation problems if you had difficulty with this question.

Level of Cognitive Ability: Application
Client Needs: Physiological Integrity
Integrated Process: Nursing Process/Implementation
Content Area: Fundamental Skills

Reference:
Kee, J., & Marshall, S. (2004). *Clinical calculations: With applications to general and specialty areas* (5th ed.). Philadelphia: Saunders, pp. 84-85.

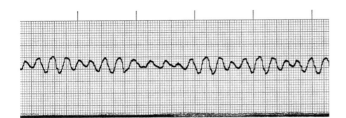

8. A nurse is in the room of a client on a cardiac monitor who suddenly becomes unconscious and exhibits this cardiac rhythm (see figure). The nurse calls for help, knowing that which of the following items will be needed immediately?
1 Pacemaker insertion tray
2 Ventilator
3 Defibrillator
4 Lidocaine hydrochloride (Xylocaine)

Answer: 3

Rationale: This cardiac rhythm indicates coarse ventricular fibrillation. A defibrillator is needed to correct ventricular fibrillation. Options 1 and 2 will do nothing to correct this rhythm. Lidocaine may be used to treat other ventricular dysrhythmias, such as ventricular tachycardia (an organized, although potentially deadly rhythm).

Test-Taking Strategy: Focus on the cardiac rhythm, noting that the client is exhibiting ventricular fibrillation. Note the relationship between this cardiac rhythm and defibrillation in the correct option. Review the characteristics of and treatment for ventricular fibrillation if you had difficulty with this question.

Level of Cognitive Ability: Application
Client Needs: Physiological Integrity
Integrated Process: Nursing Process/Implementation
Content Area: Adult Health/Cardiovascular

References:
Black, J., & Hawks, J. (2005). *Medical-surgical nursing: Clinical management for positive outcomes* (7th ed.). Philadelphia: Saunders, p. 1686.
Ignatavicius, D., & Workman, M. (2002). *Medical surgical nursing: Critical thinking for collaborative care* (4th ed.). Philadelphia: Saunders, p. 678.

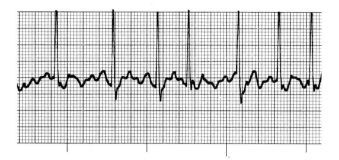

9. A nurse analyzed an ECG strip (see figure) for a client with left-sided heart failure, as follows: atrial rate: no identifiable P waves; baseline irregular ventricular rate: 160 beats per minute (BPM); rhythm: irregular PR interval and indiscernible, QRS at 0.08. The nurse interprets the rhythm strip as:
   1 Sinus dysrhythmia
   2 Atrial fibrillation
   3 Ventricular fibrillation
   4 Third-degree heart block

Answer: 2
Rationale: Atrial fibrillation is characterized by rapid, chaotic atrial depolarization, with ventricular rates ranging from 160 to 180 BPM. The ECG reveals chaotic or no identifiable P waves and a baseline that is irregular. The PR interval is irregular. A sinus dysrhythmia has a normal P wave, PR interval, and QRS complex. In ventricular fibrillation, there are no identifiable P waves, QRS complexes, or T waves. In third-degree heart block, the atria and ventricles beat independently.

Test-Taking Strategy: Recall that in atrial fibrillation the P wave is absent or chaotic. This will direct you to option 2. Review this content if you are unfamiliar with the cardiac dysrhythmias identified in the options.

Level of Cognitive Ability: Analysis
Client Needs: Physiological Integrity
Integrated Process: Nursing Process/Analysis
Content Area: Adult Health/Cardiovascular

Reference:
Black, J., & Hawks, J. (2005). *Medical-surgical nursing: Clinical management for positive outcomes* (7th ed.). Philadelphia: Saunders, p. 1677.

---

10. A physician's order reads "haloperidol decanoate (Haldol) 175 mg intramuscularly." The medication is available in 100 mg per mL. How many mL of the medication would the nurse draw into the syringe for injection?

    Answer: _____

Answer: 1.75
Rationale: Use the formula for calculating medication dosages.

Formula:
Desired dose is 175 mg; Medication available is 1mL = 100 mg

Ratio: 175 mg : X mL :: 100 mg : 1 mL

175 : 100X = 1.75 mL

Test-Taking Strategy: When reading math calculation questions, identify the dosage or concentration on hand and the dosage or concentration needed. Once these are identified, set up the mathematical problem and solve for X. Use a calculator to verify your answer and make sure the answer makes sense. Review the formula for calculating medication dosages if you had difficulty with this question.

Level of Cognitive Ability: Application
Client Needs: Physiological Integrity

Integrated Process: Nursing Process/Implementation
Content Area: Pharmacology

Reference:
Kee, J., & Marshall, S. (2004). *Clinical calculations: With applications to general and specialty areas* (4th ed.). Philadelphia: Saunders, pp. 80-81.

---

11. A nurse is sending an arterial blood gas (ABG) specimen to the laboratory for analysis. Select the pieces of information that the nurse writes on the laboratory requisition:

___ The date and time the specimen was drawn

___ A list of client allergies

___ Any supplemental oxygen the client is receiving

___ The client's temperature

___ Ventilator settings

Answer:
The date and time the specimen was drawn
Any supplemental oxygen the client is receiving
The client's temperature
Ventilator settings

Rationale: An ABG requisition usually contains information about the date and time the specimen was drawn, the client's temperature, whether the specimen was drawn on room air or using supplemental oxygen, and the ventilator settings if the client is on a mechanical ventilator. The client's allergies do not have a direct bearing on the laboratory results.

Test-Taking Strategy: Review the pieces of information from the viewpoint of the relevance of the item to the client's airway status or oxygen utilization. The only piece of information that does not relate to airway status or oxygen utilization is the client's allergies. Review the procedure related to drawing ABGs if you had difficulty with this question.

Level of Cognitive Ability: Application
Client Needs: Physiological Integrity
Integrated Process: Communication and Documentation
Content Area: Adult Health/Respiratory

Reference:
Chernecky, C., & Berger, B. (2004). *Laboratory tests and diagnostic procedures* (4th ed.). Philadelphia: Saunders, p. 249

REFERENCES

Black, J., & Hawks, J. (2005). *Medical-surgical nursing: Clinical management for positive outcomes* (7th ed.). Philadelphia: Saunders.

Chernecky, C., & Berger, B. (2004). *Laboratory tests and diagnostic procedures* (4th ed.). Philadelphia: Saunders.

Elkin, M., Perry, A., & Potter, P. (2004). *Nursing interventions & clinical skills* (3rd ed.). St. Louis: Mosby.

Fortinash, K., & Holoday-Worret, P. (2004). *Psychiatric mental health nursing* (3rd ed.). St. Louis: Mosby.

Gulanick, M., Myers, J., Klopp, A., Gradishar, D., Galanes, S., & Puzas, M. (2003). *Nursing care plans: Nursing diagnosis and intervention* (5th ed.). St. Louis: Mosby.

Harkreader, H., & Hogan, M.A. (2004). *Fundamentals of nursing: Caring and clinical judgment* (2nd ed.). Philadelphia: Saunders.

Hodgson, B., & Kizior, R. (2004). *Saunders nursing drug handbook 2004*. Philadelphia: Saunders.

Ignatavicius, D., & Workman, M. (2005). *Medical surgical nursing: Critical thinking for collaborative care* (5th ed.). Philadelphia: Saunders.

James, S., Ashwill, J., & Droske, S. (2002). *Nursing care of children: Principles & practice* (2nd ed.). Philadelphia: Saunders.

Kee, J., & Hayes, E. (2003). *Pharmacology: A nursing process approach* (4th ed.). Philadelphia: Saunders.

Kee, J., & Marshall, S. (2004). *Clinical calculations: With applications to general and specialty areas* (5th ed.). Philadelphia: Saunders.

Lehne, R. (2004). *Pharmacology for nursing care* (5th ed.). Philadelphia: Saunders.

Lewis, S., Heitkemper, M., & Dirksen, S. (2004). *Medical-surgical nursing: Assessment and management of clinical problems* (6th ed.). St. Louis: Mosby.

Lowdermilk, D., & Perry, A. (2004). *Maternity & women's health care* (8th ed.). St. Louis: Mosby.

Matteson, P. (2001). *Women's health during the childbearing years: A community-based approach*. St. Louis: Mosby.

McKenry, L., & Salerno, E. (2003). *Mosby's pharmacology in nursing* (21st ed.). St. Louis: Mosby.

McKinney, E., James, S., Murray, S., & Ashwill, J. (2005). *Maternal-child nursing* (2nd ed.). St. Louis: Elsevier.

Mosby's medical, nursing, & allied health dictionary (6th ed.). St. Louis: Mosby.

Murray, S., McKinney, E., & Gorrie, T. (2002). *Foundations of maternal-newborn nursing* (3rd ed.). Philadelphia: Saunders.

Pagana, K., & Pagana, T. (2003). *Mosby's diagnostic and laboratory test reference* (6th ed.). St. Louis: Mosby.

Phipps, W., Monahan, F., Sands, J., Marek, J., & Neighbors, M. (2003). *Medical-surgical nursing: Health and illness perspectives* (7th ed.). St. Louis: Mosby.

Potter, P., & Perry, A. (2005). *Fundamentals of nursing* (6th ed.). St. Louis: Mosby.

Stuart, G., & Laraia, M. (2005). *Principles and practice of psychiatric nursing* (8th ed.). St. Louis: Mosby.

Varcarolis, E.M. (2002). *Foundations of psychiatric mental health nursing* (4th ed.). Philadelphia: Saunders.

Williams, S. (2001). *Basic nutrition & diet therapy* (11th ed.). St. Louis: Mosby.

Wilson, S., & Giddens, J. (2005). *Health assessment for nursing practice* (3rd ed.). St. Louis: Mosby.

Wong, D., & Hockenberry, M. (2003). *Wong's nursing care of infants and children* (7th ed.). St. Louis: Mosby.

Safe, Effective Care Environment

1. A nurse is planning the client assignments for the shift. Which client would the nurse assign to the nursing assistant?
   1. A client requiring dressing changes
   2. A client requiring frequent ambulation
   3. A client on a bowel management program requiring rectal suppositories and a daily enema
   4. A client with diabetes mellitus requiring daily insulin and reinforcement of dietary measures

Answer: 2
Rationale: Assignment of tasks to the nursing assistant needs to be made based on job description, level of clinical competence, and state law. Options 1, 3, and 4 involve care that requires the skill of a licensed nurse. The client described in option 2 has needs that can be met by a nursing assistant.

Test-Taking Strategy: Focus on the issue: the assignment to a nursing assistant. Think about the tasks that the nursing assistant can safely perform and match the client's needs with these tasks. Eliminate options 1, 3, and 4 because these clients require care that needs to be provided by a licensed nurse. Review the guidelines regarding assignment making and delegating if you had difficulty with this question.

Level of Cognitive Ability: Application
Client Needs: Safe, Effective Care Environment
Integrated Process: Nursing Process/Planning
Content Area: Delegating/Prioritizing

References:
Elkin, M., Perry, A., & Potter, P. (2004). *Nursing interventions & clinical skills* (3rd ed.). St. Louis: Mosby, pp. 6-8.
Potter, P., & Perry, A. (2005). *Fundamentals of nursing* (6th ed.). St. Louis: Mosby, pp. 42; 378-379; 418.

2. A psychotic client is pacing, agitated, and presenting with aggressive gestures. The client's speech pattern is rapid, and the client's affect is belligerent. Based on this objective data, the immediate priority of care is to:
   1. Provide safety for the client and other clients on the unit
   2. Bring the client to a less stimulated area to calm down and gain control
   3. Provide the clients on the unit with a sense of comfort and safety
   4. Assist the staff in caring for the client in a controlled environment

Answer: 1
Rationale: If a client is exhibiting signs that indicate loss of control, the nurse's immediate priority is to ensure safety for all clients. Option 1 is the only option that addresses the client and other clients' safety needs. Option 2 addresses the client's needs. Option 3 addresses other clients' needs. Option 4 is not client centered.

Test-Taking Strategy: Focus on the data in the question. Note the issue of the question: safety. Option 1 is an umbrella (global) option and addresses the safety of all. Review nursing care for the client who is agitated and out of control if you had difficulty with this question.

Level of Cognitive Ability: Application
Client Needs: Safe, Effective Care Environment
Integrated Process: Nursing Process/Implementation
Content Area: Mental Health

Reference:

Stuart, G., & Laraia, M. (2005). *Principles and practice of psychiatric nursing* (8th ed.). St. Louis: Mosby, pp. 378; 721.

---

3. A magnetic resonance imaging (MRI) test is prescribed for a client with Bell's palsy. Which nursing action is included in the client's plan of care to prepare for this test?

1 Keep the client NPO for 6 hours before the test

2 Remove all metal-containing objects from the client

3 Shave the groin for insertion of a femoral catheter

4 Instruct the client in inhalation techniques for the administration of gas

Answer: 2

Rationale: In an MRI, radio-frequency pulses in a magnetic field are converted into pictures. All metal objects, such as rings, bracelets, hairpins, watches, etc., should be removed. In addition, a history should be taken to ascertain whether the client has any internal metallic devices, such as orthopedic hardware, pacemakers, shrapnel, etc. For an abdominal MRI, the client is usually NPO. An NPO status is not necessary for an MRI of the head. The groin may be shaved for an angiogram, and inhalation of gas may be prescribed with a positron emission tomography (PET).

Test-Taking Strategy: Focus on the name of the test and the client's diagnosis. Note the relation between "magnetic" in the question and "metal" in the correct option. If you are unfamiliar with client preparation for an MRI, review this content.

Level of Cognitive Ability: Application
Client Needs: Safe, Effective Care Environment
Integrated Process: Nursing Process/Planning
Content Area: Adult Health/Neurological

Reference:

Chernecky, C., & Berger, B. (2004). *Laboratory tests and diagnostic procedures* (4th ed.). Philadelphia: Saunders, p. 754.

---

4. A physician asks a nurse to discontinue the feeding tube in a client who is in a chronic debilitated and comatose state. The physician tells the nurse that the request was made by the client's spouse and children. The nurse understands the legal basis for carrying out the order and first checks the client's record for documentation of:

1 A court approval to discontinue the treatment

2 A written order by the physician to remove the tube

3 Authorization by the family to discontinue the treatment

4 Approval by the institutional Ethics Committee

Answer: 3

Rationale: The family or a legal guardian can make treatment decisions for the client who is unable to do so. Once the decision is made, the physician writes the order. Generally, the family makes decisions in collaboration with physicians, other health care workers, and other trusted advisors. Although a written order by the physician is necessary, the nurse first checks for documentation of the family's request. Unless special circumstances exist, a court order is not necessary. Although some health care agencies may require reviewing such requests via the Ethics Committee, this is not the nurse's first action.

Test-Taking Strategy: Note the key word "first" to determine the sequence of decision making in this situation. No data in the question indicates the need for court approval. Therefore, assessment for family authorization is the nurse's first action. Review these ethical and legal principles if you had difficulty with this question.

Level of Cognitive Ability: Application
Client Needs: Safe, Effective Care Environment
Integrated Process: Communication and Documentation
Content Area: Leadership/Management

Reference:
Potter, P., & Perry, A. (2005). *Fundamentals of nursing* (6th ed.). St. Louis: Mosby, p. 416.

---

5. A nurse is assisting the physician with the insertion of a Miller-Abbott tube. The nurse understands that the procedure puts the client at risk for aspiration and implements which action to decrease this risk?
   1   Inserts the tube with the balloon inflated
   2   Instructs the client to cough when the tube reaches the nasal pharynx
   3   Places the client in a high-Fowler's position
   4   Instructs the client to perform a Valsalva maneuver if the impulse to gag and vomit occurs

Answer: 3
Rationale: The Miller-Abbott tube is a nasoenteric tube that is used to decompress the intestine, as in correcting a bowel obstruction. Initial insertion of the tube is a physician responsibility. The tube is inserted with the balloon deflated in a manner similar to the proper procedure for inserting a nasogastric tube. The client is usually given water to drink to facilitate passage of the tube through the nasopharynx and esophagus. A high-Fowler's position decreases the risk of aspiration if vomiting occurs.

Test-Taking Strategy: Focus on the issue: decreasing the risk of aspiration for the client undergoing insertion of a Miller-Abbott tube. Option 1 can be eliminated because a tube could not be inserted if the balloon was inflated. Eliminate option 2 because coughing can cause the tube to be expelled. A Valsalva maneuver is not used if the impulse to gag occurs. Review this procedure if you had difficulty with this question.

Level of Cognitive Ability: Application
Client Needs: Safe, Effective Care Environment
Integrated Process: Nursing Process/Implementation
Content Area: Adult Health/Gastrointestinal

References:
Black, J., & Hawks, J. (2005). *Medical-surgical nursing: Clinical management for positive outcomes* (7th ed.). Philadelphia: Saunders, p. 745.
Lewis, S., Heitkemper, M., & Dirksen, S. (2004). *Medical-surgical nursing: Assessment and management of clinical problems* (6th ed.). St. Louis: Mosby, p. 1080.
Potter, P., & Perry, A. (2005). *Fundamentals of nursing* (6th ed.). St. Louis: Mosby, p. 1300.

---

6. A nurse is caring for a client receiving total parenteral nutrition (TPN). The nurse implements which action to decrease the risk of infection?
   1   Assesses vital signs at four-hour intervals
   2   Instructs the client to perform a Valsalva maneuver during intravenous tubing changes
   3   Administers acetaminophen (Tylenol) before changing the central line dressing
   4   Uses aseptic technique in handling the TPN solution and tubing

Answer: 4
Rationale: Clients receiving TPN are at high risk for developing infection. Concentrated glucose solutions are an excellent medium for bacterial growth. Using aseptic technique in handling all equipment and solutions is paramount to prevention of infection. Option 1 will detect signs of an infection but is not associated with prevention. Options 2 and 3 are unrelated to decreasing the risk of infection.

Test-Taking Strategy: Note the key words "decrease the risk of infection." Option 1 relates to early detection of infection, not decreasing the risk. Options 2 and 3 do not relate to the issue of the question. Remember, aseptic technique is critical to prevent infection. Review care of the client receiving TPN and the measures to prevent infection if you had difficulty with this question.

Level of Cognitive Ability: Application
Client Needs: Safe, Effective Care Environment
Integrated Process: Nursing Process/Implementation
Content Area: Fundamental Skills

References:

Black, J., & Hawks, J. (2005). *Medical-surgical nursing: Clinical management for positive outcomes* (7th ed.). Philadelphia: Saunders, pp. 708-709.
Potter, P., & Perry, A. (2005). *Fundamentals of nursing* (6th ed.). St. Louis: Mosby, p. 1167.

---

7. A home care nurse is assisting a client in managing cancer pain. To ensure that the client has adequate and safe pain control, the nurse plans to:

1 Try multiple medication modalities for pain relief to get the maximum pain relief effect
2 Start with low doses of medication and gradually increase to a dose that relieves pain, not exceeding the maximal daily dose
3 Rely totally on prescription and over-the-counter medications to relieve pain
4 Keep a baseline level of pain so that the client does not become sedated or addicted

Answer: 2

Rationale: Safe pain control includes starting with low doses and working up to a dose of medication that relieves the pain. Multiple medication modalities interventions can be unsafe and ineffective. Option 3 does not take into account other nursing interventions that may relieve pain, such as massage, therapeutic touch, or music. Maintaining a baseline level of pain to avoid sedation or addiction is not appropriate practice, unless the client requests this, and this information has not been provided in the case situation.

Test-Taking Strategy: Use the process of elimination and focus on safety issues. Option 1 uses the word "multiple" and option 3 uses the word "totally." Therefore, eliminate these options. Option 4 can be eliminated next because it is inaccurate information. Review safe pain control management if you had difficulty with this question.

Level of Cognitive Ability: Application
Client Needs: Safe, Effective Care Environment
Integrated Process: Caring
Content Area: Adult Health/Oncology

Reference:

Black, J., & Hawks, J. (2005). *Medical-surgical nursing: Clinical management for positive outcomes* (7th ed.). Philadelphia: Saunders, pp. 450; 454; 460.

---

8. A home care nurse provides medication instructions to a client. To ensure safe administration of medication in the home, the nurse:

1 Demonstrates the proper procedure to take prescribed medications
2 Allows the client to verbalize and demonstrate correct administration procedures
3 Instructs the client that it is all right to double up on medications if a dose has been missed
4 Conducts pill counts on each home visit

Answer: 2

Rationale: To ensure safe administration of medication, the nurse allows the client to verbalize and demonstrate correct procedure and administration of medications. Demonstrating the proper procedure for the client does not ensure that the client can safely perform this procedure. It is not acceptable to double up on medication, and conducting a pill count on each visit is not realistic or appropriate.

Test-Taking Strategy: Focus on the issue: safe administration of medication. Options 3 and 4 can be eliminated first because these are not appropriate practices. From the remaining options, note that option 2 is client centered. Review the principles of teaching and learning and the methods of ensuring safe administration of medication if you had difficulty with this question.

Level of Cognitive Ability: Application
Client Needs: Safe, Effective Care Environment
Integrated Process: Teaching/Learning
Content Area: Fundamental Skills

Reference:
Potter, P., & Perry, A. (2005). *Fundamentals of nursing* (6th ed.). St. Louis: Mosby, pp. 844-845.

---

9. A client remains in atrial fibrillation with rapid ventricular response despite pharmacological intervention. Synchronous cardioversion is scheduled to convert the rapid rhythm. The nurse plans to implement which important action to ensure safety and prevent complications of this procedure?
   1 Sedate the client before cardioversion
   2 Ensure that emergency equipment is available
   3 Ensure that the defibrillator is set on the synchronous mode
   4 Cardiovert the client at 360 joules

Answer: 3
Rationale: Cardioversion is similar to defibrillation with two major exceptions: (1) the countershock is synchronized to occur during ventricular depolarization (QRS complex), and (2) less energy is used for the countershock. The rationale for delivering the shock during the QRS complex is to prevent the shock from being delivered during repolarization (T wave), often termed the "vulnerable period." If the shock is delivered during this period, the resulting complication is ventricular fibrillation. It is crucial that the defibrillator is set on the "synchronous" mode for a successful cardioversion. Options 1 and 2 will not prevent complications. Cardioversion usually begins with 50 to 100 joules.

Test-Taking Strategy: Focus on the issue of the question: ensure safety and prevent complications. Noting the key word "synchronous" in the question will direct you to option 3. Review this procedure if you had difficulty with this question.

Level of Cognitive Ability: Application
Client Needs: Safe, Effective Care Environment
Integrated Process: Nursing Process/Implementation
Content Area: Adult Health/Cardiovascular

Reference:
Lewis, S., Heitkemper, M., & Dirksen, S. (2004). *Medical-surgical nursing: Assessment and management of clinical problems* (6th ed.). St. Louis: Mosby, p. 875.

---

10. A client with a diagnosis of thrombophlebitis is being treated with heparin sodium therapy. In planning a safe environment, the nurse ensures that which medication is available if the client develops a significant bleeding problem?
   1 Fresh frozen plasma
   2 Protamine sulfate
   3 Streptokinase (Streptase)
   4 Phytonadione (Vitamin K)

Answer: 2
Rationale: Protamine sulfate is the antidote for heparin sodium. Phytonadione is the antidote for warfarin (Coumadin). Fresh frozen plasma may also be used for bleeding related to warfarin (Coumadin) therapy. Streptokinase is a thrombolytic agent used to dissolve blood clots.

Test-Taking Strategy: Focus on the issue: planning a safe environment, and note the name of the medication. Recalling that the antidote for heparin sodium is protamine sulfate will direct you to the correct option. Review the antidotes for commonly administered medications if you had difficulty with this question.

Level of Cognitive Ability: Application
Client Needs: Safe, Effective Care Environment
Integrated Process: Nursing Process/Planning
Content Area: Pharmacology

Reference:
Hodgson, B., & Kizior, R. (2004). *Saunders nursing drug handbook 2004.* Philadelphia: Saunders, p. 853.

---

11. A nurse is teaching a client with cardiomyopathy about home care safety measures. The nurse addresses which most important measure to ensure client safety?
1   Assessing pain
2   Avoiding over-the-counter medications
3   Administering vasodilators
4   Moving slowly from a sitting to a standing position

Answer: 4
Rationale: Orthostatic changes can occur in the client with cardiomyopathy as a result of venous return obstruction. Sudden changes in blood pressure may lead to falls. Vasodilators are not normally prescribed for the client with cardiomyopathy. Options 1 and 2, although important, are not directly related to the issue of safety.

Test-Taking Strategy: Focus on the issue: to ensure client safety at home, and note the key words "most important." Recalling that blood pressure changes occur in cardiomyopathy will direct you to option 4. Review client teaching related to cardiomyopathy if you had difficulty with this question.

Level of Cognitive Ability: Application
Client Needs: Safe, Effective Care Environment
Integrated Process: Teaching/Learning
Content Area: Adult Health/Cardiovascular

Reference:
Black, J., & Hawks, J. (2005). *Medical-surgical nursing: Clinical management for positive outcomes* (7th ed.). Philadelphia: Saunders, p. 1607.

---

12. A nurse instructs a client with a diagnosis of valvular disease to use an electric razor for shaving. The nurse tells the client that the importance of its use is that:
1   Any cut may cause infection
2   Electric razors can be disinfected
3   All straight razors contain bacteria
4   Cuts need to be avoided

Answer: 4
Rationale: Clients with valvular disease are placed on anticoagulants to prevent thrombus formation and possible stroke. The importance of use of an electric razor is to prevent cuts and possible bleeding. Options 1, 2, and 3 are all unrelated to the issue of bleeding; rather, they relate to infection.

Test-Taking Strategy: Recalling that the client with valvular disease will be placed on anticoagulants will assist in answering the question. Note that options 1, 2, and 3 are similar and relate to infection. Option 4 relates to bleeding. Review care of the client with valvular disease if you had difficulty with this question.

Level of Cognitive Ability: Application
Client Needs: Safe, Effective Care Environment.
Integrated Process: Teaching/Learning
Content Area: Adult Health/Cardiovascular

Reference:
Phipps, W., Monahan, F., Sands, J., Marek, J., & Neighbors, M. (2003). *Medical-surgical nursing: Health and illness perspectives* (7th ed.). St. Louis: Mosby, p. 736.

13. A nurse is caring for a client during the recovery phase following a myocardial infarction. A cardiac catheterization, using the femoral artery approach, is performed to assess the degree of coronary artery thrombosis. Which nursing action following the procedure is unsafe for the client?
1 Placing the client's bed in the Fowler's position
2 Encouraging the client to increase fluid intake
3 Instructing the client to move the toes when checking circulation, motion, and sensation
4 Resuming prescribed precatheterization medications

Answer: 1

Rationale: Immediately following a cardiac catheterization with the femoral artery approach, the client should not flex or hyperextend the affected leg to avoid blood vessel occlusion or hemorrhage. Placing the client in the Fowler's position (flexion) increases the risk of occlusion or hemorrhage. Fluids are encouraged to assist in removing the contrast medium from the body. Asking the client to move the toes is done to assess motion, which could be impaired if a hematoma or thrombus were developing. The precatheterization medications are needed to treat acute and chronic conditions.

Test-Taking Strategy: Note the key word "unsafe" in the stem of the question. This key word indicates a false-response question and tells you that you need to select the option that indicates an incorrect nursing action. Also note the words "femoral artery approach." Recalling that flexion or hyperextension is avoided following this procedure will direct you to option 1. Review postcardiac catheterization care if you had difficulty with this question.

Level of Cognitive Ability: Application
Client Needs: Safe, Effective Care Environment
Integrated Process: Nursing Process/Implementation
Content Area: Adult Health/Cardiovascular

Reference:
Phipps, W., Monahan, F., Sands, J., Marek, J., & Neighbors, M. (2003). *Medical-surgical nursing: Health and illness perspectives* (7th ed.). St. Louis: Mosby, p. 640.

14. A nurse plans to carry out a multidisciplinary research project on the effects of immobility on clients' stress levels. The nurse understands that which principle is most important when planning this project?
1 Collaboration with other disciplines is essential to the successful practice of nursing.
2 The Corporate Nurse Executive should be consulted, because the project will take nursing time.
3 All clients have the right to refuse to participate in research using human subjects.
4 The cooperation of the physicians on staff must be ensured in order for the project to succeed.

Answer: 3

Rationale: The proposed project is research and includes human subjects. Although options 1, 2, and 4 need to be considered, they are all secondary to the overriding principle of the legal and ethical practice of nursing that any client has the right to refuse to participate in research using human subjects.

Test-Taking Strategy: Focus on the issue: the most important principle. Recalling that the client has the right to refuse to participate in research will direct you to option 3. Review the ethical and legal guidelines related to research if you had difficulty with this question.

Level of Cognitive Ability: Application
Client Needs: Safe, Effective Care Environment
Integrated Process: Nursing Process/Planning
Content Area: Leadership/Management

Reference:
Potter, P., & Perry, A. (2005). *Fundamentals of nursing* (6th ed.). St. Louis: Mosby, pp. 81-82.

15. A nurse has an order to obtain a sputum culture from a client admitted to the hospital with a diagnosis of pneumonia. The nurse avoids which action when obtaining the specimen?
1 Placing the lid of the culture container face down on the bedside table
2 Obtaining the specimen early in the morning
3 Having the client brush his teeth before expectoration
4 Instructing the client to take deep breaths before coughing

Answer: 1

Rationale: Placing the lid face down on the bedside table contaminates the lid and could result in inaccurate findings. The specimen is obtained early in the morning whenever possible, because increased amounts of sputum collect in the airways during sleep. The client should rinse the mouth or brush the teeth before specimen collection to avoid contaminating the specimen. The client should take deep breaths before expectoration for best sputum production.

Test-Taking Strategy: Use the process of elimination, noting the key word "avoids." This key word indicates a false-response question and tells you that you need to select the option that indicates an incorrect nursing action. Begin by eliminating options 2 and 4, which are helpful in obtaining a specimen of sufficient volume. From the remaining options, using the basic principles of aseptic technique will direct you to option 1. Review the procedure for sputum collection if you had difficulty with this question.

Level of Cognitive Ability: Application
Client Needs: Safe, Effective Care Environment
Integrated Process: Nursing Process/Implementation
Content Area: Fundamental Skills

References:
Black, J., & Hawks, J. (2005). *Medical-surgical nursing: Clinical management for positive outcomes* (7th ed.). Philadelphia: Saunders, pp. 92-94.
Chernecky, C., & Berger, B. (2004). *Laboratory tests and diagnostic procedures* (4th ed.). Philadelphia: Saunders, pp. 1018-1019.
Phipps, W., Monahan, F., Sands, J., Marek, J., & Neighbors, M. (2003). *Medical-surgical nursing: Health and illness perspectives* (7th ed.). St. Louis: Mosby, p. 473.

16. A multidisciplinary health care team is planning care for a client with hyperparathyroidism. The nurse identifies which client outcome to the health care team?
1 Describes how to take antacids
2 Restricts fluids to 1000 mL per day
3 Walks down the hall for 15 minutes, three times a day
4 Describes how to take antidiarrheal medications

Answer: 3

Rationale: Mobility of the client with hyperparathyroidism should be encouraged as much as possible because of the calcium imbalance that occurs in this disorder and the predisposition to the formation of renal calculi. Fluids should not be restricted. Options 1 and 4 are not specifically associated with this disorder.

Test-Taking Strategy: Use the process of elimination. Eliminate options 1 and 4 first because they are similar. From the remaining options, recalling that the client is predisposed to the formation of renal calculi will direct you to option 3. Review care of the client with hyperparathyroidism if you had difficulty with this question.

Level of Cognitive Ability: Analysis
Client Needs: Safe, Effective Care Environment
Integrated Process: Nursing Process/Planning
Content Area: Leadership/Management

Reference:
Phipps, W., Monahan, F., Sands, J., Marek, J., & Neighbors, M. (2003). *Medical-surgical nursing: Health and illness perspectives* (7th ed.). St. Louis: Mosby, p. 910.

17. A nurse has inserted a nasogastric tube (NG) into the stomach of a client and prepares to check for accurate tube placement. The nurse avoids which least reliable method for checking tube placement?
1 Aspirating the tube with a 50-mL syringe to obtain gastric contents
2 Measuring the pH of gastric aspirate
3 Placing the end of the tube in water to check for bubbling
4 Instilling 10 to 20 mL of air into the tube while auscultating over the stomach

Answer: 3
Rationale: The least reliable method for determining accurate placement of the NG tube is to place the end of the tube in water to observe for bubbling. Options 1, 2, and 4 are accurate methods to determine placement. The best method, however, is to verify placement by X-ray.

Test-Taking Strategy: Use the process of elimination. Note the key words "avoids" and "least reliable." These key words indicate a false-response question and tell you that you need to select the option that is an unreliable method. Visualize this procedure and focus on the issue, accurate tube placement, to direct you to option 3. Review this procedure if you had difficulty with this question.

Level of Cognitive Ability: Application
Client Needs: Safe, Effective Care Environment
Integrated Process: Nursing Process/Implementation
Content Area: Fundamental Skills

Reference:
Ignatavicius, D., & Workman, M. (2002). *Medical surgical nursing: Critical thinking for collaborative care* (4th ed.). Philadelphia: Saunders, p. 1228.

18. A nurse employed in a preschool agency is planning a staff education program to prevent the spread of an outbreak of an intestinal parasitic disease. The nurse includes which priority prevention measure in the educational session?
1 Staff will practice standard precautions when changing diapers and assisting children with toileting
2 All toileting areas will be cleansed daily with soap and water
3 Only bottled water will be used for drinking
4 All food will be cooked before eating

Answer: 1
Rationale: The fecal-oral route is the mode of transmission of an intestinal parasitic disease. Standard precautions prevent the transmission of infection. Cleaning with soap and water is not as effective as the use of bleach. Water and fresh foods can be vehicles for transmission, but municipal water sources are usually safe. Some fresh foods do not need to be cooked as long as they are washed well and provided that they weren't grown in soil contaminated with human feces.

Test-Taking Strategy: Focus on the issue, preventing the spread of infection. Option 1 addresses the issue of the question and is the most umbrella (global) option, addressing standard precautions. Also, note that options 2, 3, and 4 contain the absolute words "all" and "only." Review measures that will prevent the spread of an intestinal parasitic infection if you had difficulty with this question.

Level of Cognitive Ability: Application
Client Needs: Safe, Effective Care Environment
Integrated Process: Teaching/Learning
Content Area: Child Health

Reference:
McKinney, E., James, S., Murray, S., & Ashwill, J. (2005). *Maternal-child nursing* (2nd ed.). St. Louis: Elsevier, p. 1039.

19. A client has arrived at the labor and delivery unit in active labor. The nursing assessment reveals a history of recurrent genital herpes and the presence of lesions in the genital tract. The nurse plans to:
1 Prepare the client for a cesarean delivery
2 Limit visitors and maintain reverse isolation
3 Prepare the client for a spontaneous vaginal delivery
4 Rupture the membranes artificially, looking for meconium-stained fluid

Answer: 1

Rationale: A cesarean delivery can reduce the risk of neonatal infection with a mother in labor who has herpetic genital tract lesions. Intact membranes provide another barrier to transmitting the disease to the neonate. There is no need to limit visitors or maintain isolation, although standard precautions should be maintained.

Test-Taking Strategy: Use the process of elimination, focusing on the issue: presence of genital herpes lesions. Eliminate options 3 and 4 first because they are similar and would place the neonate in contact with the lesions. From the remaining options, consider the risks to the neonate to direct you to option 1. Review care of the client in labor who has genital herpes lesions if you had difficulty with this question.

Level of Cognitive Ability: Application
Client Needs: Safe, Effective Care Environment
Integrated Process: Nursing Process/Planning
Content Area: Maternity/Intrapartum

Reference:
Lowdermilk, D., & Perry, A. (2004). *Maternity & women's health care* (8th ed.). St. Louis: Mosby, p. 675.

---

20. A nurse is performing a bladder catheterization and is inserting an indwelling Foley catheter. The nurse understands that which of the following represents an unsafe action when performing this procedure?
1 Inflating the balloon to test patency before catheter insertion
2 Advancing the catheter an additional 2.5 to 5 cm (1 to 2 inches) once urine appears in the catheter tubing
3 Inflating the balloon with 4 to 5 mL more than the balloon capacity
4 Placing the drainage bag lower than bladder level, with no kinks in the tubing

Answer: 3

Rationale: The nurse would test the patency of the balloon before insertion. If the balloon is not patent and the catheter was inserted without checking patency, it would need to be removed and replaced (remember this procedure places the client at risk for infection, and repeated insertions need to be avoided). The catheter should be advanced for 1 to 2 more inches beyond the point where the flow of urine is first noted. This ensures that the catheter balloon is fully in the bladder before it is inflated. The drainage bag is placed lower than bladder level (without kinks) in the tubing to ensure drainage and prevent backflow of urine. The balloon is inflated per the manufacturer's instructions and is not overinflated.

Test-Taking Strategy: Note the key word "unsafe." This key word indicates a false-response question and tells you that you need to select the option that indicates an incorrect nursing action. Visualize the procedure to assist in answering the question. Basic principles related to this procedure will assist in eliminating options 1 and 4. From the remaining options, noting the words "more than" in option 3 will direct you to this option. Review this procedure if you had difficulty with this question.

Level of Cognitive Ability: Application
Client Needs: Safe, Effective Care Environment
Integrated Process: Nursing Process/Implementation
Content Area: Fundamental skills

Reference:
Potter, P., & Perry, A. (2005). *Fundamentals of nursing* (6th ed.). St. Louis: Mosby, pp. 1348-1350.

21. A moderately depressed client who was admitted to the mental health unit 2 days ago suddenly begins smiling and reporting that the crisis is over. The client says to the nurse, "Call the doctor. I'm finally cured." The nurse interprets this behavior as a cue to modify the treatment plan by:

1 Allowing off-unit privileges prn
2 Suggesting a reduction of medication
3 Allowing increased "in-room" activities
4 Increasing the level of suicide precautions

Answer: 4

Rationale: A client who is moderately depressed and has only been hospitalized 2 days is unlikely to have such a dramatic cure. When a mood suddenly lifts, it is likely that the client may have made the decision to harm him or herself. Suicide precautions are necessary to keep the client safe.

Test-Taking Strategy: Use the process of elimination, focusing on the data in the question and recalling that depression does not resolve in 2 days. Options 1 and 2 support the client's notion that a cure has occurred. Option 3 allows the client to increase isolation. Recalling that safety is of the utmost importance will direct you to option 4. Review care of the client with depression if you had difficulty with this question.

Level of Cognitive Ability: Analysis
Client Needs: Safe, Effective Care Environment
Integrated Process: Nursing Process/Planning
Content Area: Mental Health

References:
Fortinash, K., & Holoday-Worret, P. (2004). *Psychiatric mental health nursing* (3rd ed.). St. Louis: Mosby. p. 218.
Stuart, G., & Laraia, M. (2005). *Principles and practice of psychiatric nursing* (8th ed.). St. Louis: Mosby, p. 348.

22. A nurse is planning care for a suicidal client. The nurse implements additional precautions at which of the following times?

1 During the day shift
2 On weekdays
3 Between 8 AM to 10 AM
4 During shift change

Answer: 4

Rationale: At shift change, there is often less availability of staff. The psychiatric nurse and staff should increase precautions for suicidal clients at that time. Weekends are also high-risk times, not weekdays. The night shift also presents a high-risk time.

Test-Taking Strategy: Use the process of elimination. Options 1, 2, and 3 are similar and can be eliminated. Remember that the nurse could anticipate that times with less supervision of the client could be times of increased risks. Review care of the suicidal client if you had difficulty with this question.

Level of Cognitive Ability: Application
Client Needs: Safe, Effective Care Environment
Integrated Process: Nursing Process/Planning
Content Area: Mental Health

Reference:
Fortinash, K., & Holoday-Worret, P. (2004). *Psychiatric mental health nursing* (3rd ed.). St. Louis: Mosby. p. 565.

23. A nurse is assisting with transferring a client from the operating room table to a stretcher. To provide safety to the client, the nurse:

1 Moves the client rapidly from the table to the stretcher
2 Uncovers the client completely before transferring to the stretcher
3 Secures the client with safety belts after transferring to the stretcher
4 Instructs the client to move self from the table to the stretcher

Answer: 3

Rationale: During the transfer of the client after the surgical procedure is complete, the nurse should avoid exposure of the client because of the risk for potential heat loss. Hurried movements and rapid changes in position should be avoided because these predispose the client to hypotension. At the time of the transfer from the surgery table to the stretcher, the client is still affected by the effects of the anesthesia; therefore, the client should not move self. Safety belts can prevent the client from falling off the stretcher.

Test-Taking Strategy: Use the process of elimination and focus on the issue: safety. Options 1 and 2 are unsafe techniques for the client. Note the word "rapidly" in option 1 and the words "uncover the client completely" in option 2. Option 4 is not appropriate because of the effects of the anesthesia. Review care of the postoperative client if you had difficulty with this question.

Level of Cognitive Ability: Application
Client Needs: Safe, Effective Care Environment
Integrated Process: Nursing Process/Implementation
Content Area: Fundamental Skills

Reference:
Ignatavicius, D., & Workman, M. (2002). *Medical surgical nursing: Critical thinking for collaborative care* (4th ed.). Philadelphia: Saunders, pp. 281; 286.

24. A nurse is planning care for a hallucinating and delusional client who has been rescued from a suicide attempt. The nurse plans to:

1 Check the whereabouts of the client every 15 minutes
2 Initiate suicide precautions with 30-minute checks
3 Initiate one-to-one suicide precautions
4 Ask that the client report suicidal thoughts immediately

Answer: 3

Rationale: One-to-one suicide precautions are required for the client rescued from a suicide attempt. In this situation, additional key information is that the client is delusional and hallucinating. Both of these factors increase the risk of unpredictable behavior, decreased judgment, and the risk of suicide. Options 1, 2, and 4 do not provide the constant supervision necessary for this client.

Test-Taking Strategy: Use the process of elimination. Focusing on the data in question will direct you to option 3, the intervention that will provide the most supervision. Review suicide precautions if you had difficulty with this question.

Level of Cognitive Ability: Application
Client Needs: Safe, Effective Care Environment
Integrated Process: Nursing Process/Planning
Content Area: Mental Health

Reference:
Stuart, G., & Laraia, M. (2001). *Principles and practice of psychiatric nursing* (7th ed.). St. Louis: Mosby, p. 379.

25. A nurse is developing a plan of care for a client receiving anticoagulant agents. The nurse identifies which priority nursing diagnosis for the client?
  1 Deficient fluid volume
  2 Risk for activity intolerance
  3 Risk for injury
  4 Risk for infection

Answer: 3

Rationale: Anticoagulant therapy predisposes the client to injury because of the agent's inhibitory effects on the body's normal blood-clotting mechanism. Bruising, bleeding, and hemorrhage may occur in the course of activities of daily living and with other activities. Options 1, 2, and 4 are unrelated to this form of therapy.

Test-Taking Strategy: Use the process of elimination. Recalling that anticoagulants present a risk for bleeding will assist in directing you to option 3. Review the effects of anticoagulants if you had difficulty with this question.

Level of Cognitive Ability: Analysis
Client Needs: Safe, Effective Care Environment
Integrated Process: Nursing Process/Analysis
Content Area: Pharmacology

References:
Ignatavicius, D., & Workman, M. (2002). *Medical surgical nursing: Critical thinking for collaborative care* (4th ed.). Philadelphia: Saunders, p. 764.
McKenry, L., & Salerno, E. (2003). *Mosby's pharmacology in nursing* (21st ed.). St. Louis: Mosby, p. 621.

26. A client being seen in the emergency department with complaints of abdominal pain has a diagnosis of acute abdomen and the cause has not been determined. The nurse would question an order for which of the following at this time?
  1 Insertion of a nasogastric tube
  2 Insertion of an intravenous (IV) line
  3 Administration of a narcotic analgesic
  4 Institution of an NPO diet status

Answer: 3

Rationale: Until the cause of the acute abdomen is determined and a decision about the need for surgery is made, the nurse would question an order to give a narcotic analgesic because it could mask the client's symptoms. The nurse can expect the client to be placed on NPO status and to have an IV line inserted. Insertion of a nasogastric tube may be helpful to provide decompression of the stomach.

Test-Taking Strategy: Note the key words "cause has not been determined" and "would question an order." Think about the client's diagnosis. Recalling that surgery may be a necessary intervention should direct you to option 3. Review interventions for the client with acute abdomen if you had difficulty with this question.

Level of Cognitive Ability: Application
Client Needs: Safe, Effective Care Environment
Integrated Process: Communication and Documentation
Content Area: Adult Health/Gastrointestinal

References:
Lewis, S., Heitkemper, M., & Dirksen, S. (2004). *Medical-surgical nursing: Assessment and management of clinical problems* (6th ed.). St. Louis: Mosby, p. 1062.
Phipps, W., Monahan, F., Sands, J., Marek, J., & Neighbors, M. (2003). *Medical-surgical nursing: Health and illness perspectives* (7th ed.). St. Louis: Mosby, p. 231.

27. A home care nurse is working with a family to assist them in caring for a newborn with congenital tracheoesophageal fistula who is receiving enteral feedings. A woman identifying herself as a family friend telephones the nurse to inquire if there is anything she can do to assist the parents. The best nursing action is to:
1 Request that the friend come to the client's home, where she can be taught to administer the feedings
2 Inform the friend to directly contact the family and offer her assistance to them
3 Report the friend's telephone call to the nurse manager for referral to the client's social worker
4 Inform the friend that the family has no need for assistance at this time because the nurse is making daily visits

Answer: 2
Rationale: A nurse must uphold the client's rights and does not give any information regarding a client's care needs to anyone who is not directly involved in the client's care. To request that the friend come for teaching is a direct violation of the client's right to privacy. There is no information in the question to indicate that the family desires assistance from the friend. To refer the call to the nurse manager and social worker again assumes that the friend's assistance and involvement is desired by the family. Informing the friend that the nurse is visiting daily is providing information that is considered confidential. Option 2 directly refers the friend to the family.

Test-Taking Strategy: Use the process of elimination and focus on the issue: confidentiality and the client's right to privacy. Option 2 is the only option that upholds the client's rights. Review these rights if you had difficulty with this question.

Level of Cognitive Ability: Application
Client Needs: Safe, Effective Care Environment
Integrated Process: Caring
Content Area: Leadership/Management

References:
Elkin, M., Perry, A., & Potter, P. (2004). *Nursing interventions & clinical skills* (3rd ed.). St. Louis: Mosby, pp. 4-5.
Potter, P., & Perry, A. (2005). *Fundamentals of nursing* (6th ed.). St. Louis: Mosby, pp. 391-392.

28. A nurse has been assigned to care for a young man recovering at home from a disabling lung infection. While obtaining a nursing history, the nurse learns that the infection is probably the result of human immunodeficiency virus (HIV). The nurse informs the client that she is morally opposed to homosexuality and cannot care for him. The nurse then leaves the client's home. Which of the following is true regarding the nurse's actions?
1 The nurse has a duty to protect self from client care situations that are morally repellent.
2 The nurse has a legal right to inform the client of any barriers to providing care.
3 The nurse has the right to refuse to care for any client without justifying that refusal.
4 The nurse has a duty to provide competent care to assigned clients in a nondiscriminatory manner.

Answer: 4
Rationale: The nurse has a duty to provide care to all clients in a nondiscriminatory manner. Personal autonomy does not apply if it interferes with the rights of the client. There is no legal obligation to inform the client of the nurse's personal objections to the client. Refusal to provide care may be acceptable if that refusal does not put the client's safety at risk and the refusal is primarily associated with religious objections, not personal objection to lifestyle or medical diagnosis. The nurse also has an obligation to observe the principle of nonmaleficence (causing nor allowing harm to befall the client).

Test-Taking Strategy: Use the process of elimination, thinking about the client's rights and the nurse's ethical and legal responsibilities. Note the key words "provide competent care" and "nondiscriminatory" in the correct option. Review client rights if you had difficulty with this question.

Level of Cognitive Ability: Analysis
Client Needs: Safe, Effective Care Environment
Integrated Process: Caring
Content Area: Adult Health/Immune

Reference:
Elkin, M., Perry, A., & Potter, P. (2004). *Nursing interventions & clinical skills* (3rd ed.). St. Louis: Mosby, pp. 4-5.

29. A nurse is preparing to administer heparin sodium (Liquaemin) 5000 units subcutaneously. The nurse takes which action to safely administer the medication?
1 Injects within 1 inch of the umbilicus
2 Massages the injection site following administration
3 Injects via an infusion device
4 Changes the needle on the syringe after withdrawing the medication from the vial

Answer: 4
Rationale: The injection site is located in the abdominal fat layer. It is not injected within 2 inches of the umbilicus or into any scar tissue. The needle is withdrawn rapidly, pressure is applied, and the area is not massaged. Injection sites are rotated. Heparin administered subcutaneously does not require an infusion device. After withdrawal of heparin from the vial, the needle is changed before injection to prevent leakage of medication along the needle tract.

Test-Taking Strategy: Use the process of elimination. Noting the key word "subcutaneously" will assist in eliminating option 3. From the remaining options, recall that heparin is an anticoagulant. This will assist in eliminating options 1 and 2. Review this procedure if you had difficulty with this question.

Level of Cognitive Ability: Application
Client Needs: Safe, Effective Care Environment
Integrated Process: Nursing Process/Planning
Content Area: Pharmacology

Reference:
Hodgson, B., & Kizior, R. (2004). *Saunders nursing drug handbook 2004.* Philadelphia: Saunders, p. 492.

---

30. A nurse is caring for a client with cancer. The client tells the nurse that a lawyer will be arriving today to prepare a living will. The client asks the nurse to act as one of the witnesses for the will. The nurse takes which action?
1 Agrees to act as a witness
2 Refuses to help the client
3 Informs the client that a nurse caring for a client cannot serve as a witness to a living will
4 Calls the physician

Answer: 3
Rationale: A living will addresses the withdrawal or withholding of life sustaining interventions that unnaturally prolong life. It identifies the person who will make care decisions if the client is unable to take action. It is witnessed and signed by two people who are unrelated to the client. Nurses or employees of a facility in which the client is receiving care and beneficiaries of the client should not serve as a witness. There is no reason to call the physician.

Test-Taking Strategy: Use the process of elimination. Eliminate option 2 because of the word "refuses." From the remaining options, it is necessary to recall the nurse's role regarding witnessing a legal document. Review the concepts surrounding a living will if you are unfamiliar with them.

Level of Cognitive Ability: Application
Client Needs: Safe, Effective Care Environment
Integrated Process: Nursing Process/Implementation
Content Area: Fundamental Skills

References:
Harkreader, H., & Hogan, M.A. (2004). *Fundamentals of nursing: Caring and clinical judgment* (2nd ed.). Philadelphia: Saunders. p. 36.
Potter, P., & Perry, A. (2005). *Fundamentals of nursing* (6th ed.). St. Louis: Mosby, pp. 409-410.

31. A home care nurse visits a 3-year-old child with chickenpox. The child's mother tells the nurse that the child keeps scratching the skin at night and asks the nurse what to do. The nurse tells the mother to:

1 Apply generous amounts of a cortisone cream to prevent itching
2 Place soft cotton gloves on the child's hands at night
3 Keep the child in a warm room at night so the covers will not cause the child to scratch
4 Give the child a glass of warm milk at bedtime to help the child to sleep

Answer: 2

Rationale: Gloves will keep the child from scratching the open lesions from chickenpox. Generous amounts of any topical cream can lead to drug toxicity. A warm room will increase the child's skin temperature and make itching worse. Warm milk will have no effect on itching.

Test-Taking Strategy: Use the process of elimination. Eliminate option 3 first because this action will promote scratching and itching. Option 4 should be eliminated next because it is unrelated to scratching. From the remaining options, the words "generous amounts" in option 1 should provide you with the clue that this option is incorrect. Review home care measures for the child with chickenpox if you had difficulty with this question.

Level of Cognitive Ability: Application
Client Needs: Safe, Effective Care Environment
Integrated Process: Teaching/Learning
Content Area: Child Health

Reference:
Wong, D., & Hockenberry, M. (2003). *Wong's nursing care of infants and children* (7th ed.). St. Louis: Mosby, p. 653.

---

32. An older client has been identified as a victim of physical abuse. In planning care, the nurse places highest priority on:

1 Obtaining treatment for the abusing family member
2 Adhering to the mandatory abuse reporting laws
3 Notifying the caseworker to intervene in the family situation
4 Removing the client from any immediate danger

Answer: 4

Rationale: The priority nursing intervention is to remove the abused victim from the abusive environment. Options 1, 2, and 3 may be appropriate interventions but are not the priority.

Test-Taking Strategy: Note the key words "highest priority." Use Maslow's hierarchy of needs theory, remembering that if a physiological need is not present, then safety is the priority. Option 4 is the only option that directly addresses client safety. Review care of the abused older client if you had difficulty with this question.

Level of Cognitive Ability: Application
Client Needs: Safe, Effective Care Environment
Integrated Process: Nursing Process/Planning
Content Area: Mental Health

Reference:
Varcarolis, E.M. (2002). *Foundations of psychiatric mental health nursing* (4th ed.). Philadelphia: Saunders, pp. 713-715.

---

33. A client diagnosed with leukemia asks the nurse questions about preparing a living will. The nurse informs the client that the initial step in preparing this document is to:

1 Consult with the American Cancer Society
2 Talk to the hospital chaplain
3 Contact a lawyer
4 Discuss the request with the physician

Answer: 4

Rationale: The client should discuss the request for a living will with the physician. The client should also discuss this desire with the family. Wills should be prepared with legal counsel and should identify the executor of the estate, address distribution and use of property, and the specific plans for burial. Although options 1 and 2 may be helpful, their contact would not be the initial step. The lawyer would be contacted following discussion with the physician and family.

Test-Taking Strategy: Use the process of elimination and note the key words "initial step." Remembering that the physician is the primary care provider will assist in directing you to the correct option. Contacts addressed in options 1, 2, and 3 may follow the discussion with the physician. Review the concepts related to living wills if you had difficulty with this question.

Level of Cognitive Ability: Application
Client Needs: Safe, Effective Care Environment
Integrated Process: Nursing Process/Implementation
Content Area: Fundamental Skills

References:
Harkreader, H., & Hogan, M.A. (2004). *Fundamentals of nursing: Caring and clinical judgment* (2nd ed.). Philadelphia: Saunders. p. 36.
Potter, P., & Perry, A. (2005). *Fundamentals of nursing* (6th ed.). St. Louis: Mosby, pp. 409-410.

---

34. A hospitalized client occasionally becomes disoriented. The appropriate nursing action to ensure safety for this client would be to:
1 Raise the head of the bed to 45 degrees
2 Keep the side rails on the bed in the up position and the call light within reach
3 Keep the over-the-bed light in the client's room on
4 Request that only two visitors visit at a time

Answer: 2
Rationale: Keeping the side rails up prevents the disoriented client from accidentally falling out of bed. Providing the call light to the client gives access to the health care team when assistance is needed. Raising the head of the bed will not ensure safety. Keeping the over-the-bed light on may be disruptive. Limiting visitors will not ensure safety.

Test-Taking Strategy: Focus on the issue of safety. Eliminate options 1 and 4 because these actions do not provide safety for the client. Eliminate option 3 because this option may be disruptive and lead to further disorientation. Review basic safety measures for the disoriented client if you had difficulty with this question.

Level of Cognitive Ability: Application
Client Needs: Safe, Effective Care Environment
Integrated Process: Nursing Process/Implementation
Content Area: Fundamental Skills

Reference:
Elkin, M., Perry, A., & Potter, P. (2004). *Nursing interventions & clinical skills* (3rd ed.). St. Louis: Mosby, p. 84.

---

35. A client with a subarachnoid hemorrhage has been placed on subarachnoid (aneurysm) precautions. To provide a safe environment, the nurse ensures that the client is provided with which of the following?
1 Daily stool softeners
2 Bright lights
3 Television and radio
4 Enemas as needed

Answer: 1
Rationale: Subarachnoid (aneurysm) precautions include a variety of measures designed to decrease stimuli that could increase the client's intracranial pressure. These include instituting dim lighting and reducing environmental noise and stimuli. Enemas should be avoided, but stool softeners should be provided. Straining at stool is contraindicated because it increases intracranial pressure.

Test-Taking Strategy: Focus on the client's diagnosis and the need to reduce environmental stimuli and prevent increased intracranial pressure. Options 2 and 3 can be eliminated first because these items will stimulate the client. From the remaining options, eliminate option 4 because administration of an enema will increase intracranial pressure. Review the nursing interventions for the client on aneurysm precautions if you had difficulty with this question.

Level of Cognitive Ability: Application
Client Needs: Safe, Effective Care Environment
Integrated Process: Nursing Process/Implementation
Content Area: Adult Health/Neurological

Reference:
Phipps, W., Monahan, F., Sands, J., Marek, J., & Neighbors, M. (2003). *Medical-surgical nursing: Health and illness perspectives* (7th ed.). St. Louis: Mosby, p. 1385.

---

36. A nurse is about to administer an intravenous dose of tobramycin (Tobrex) when the client complains of vertigo and ringing in the ears. The nurse should:
    1 Hang the dose of medication immediately
    2 Give a dose of droperidol (Inapsine) with the tobramycin
    3 Hold the dose and call the physician
    4 Check the client's pupillary responses

Answer: 3
Rationale: Ringing in the ears and vertigo are two symptoms that may indicate dysfunction of the eighth cranial nerve. Ototoxicity is a toxic effect of therapy with aminoglycosides and could result in permanent hearing loss. The nurse should hold the dose and notify the physician. Options 1, 2, and 4 are incorrect nursing actions.

Test-Taking Strategy: Focus on the client's complaints and recall that ototoxicity can occur with this medication. Recalling that the physician is notified if toxicity is suspected will direct you to option 3. Review the toxic effects of this medication if you had difficulty with this question.

Level of Cognitive Ability: Application
Client Needs: Safe, Effective Care Environment
Integrated Process: Nursing Process/Implementation
Content Area: Pharmacology

Reference:
Hodgson, B., & Kizior, R. (2004). *Saunders nursing drug handbook 2004.* Philadelphia: Saunders, p. 992.

---

37. A nurse is preparing to administer amiodarone (Cordarone) intravenously. To provide a safe environment, the nurse ensures that which specific item is in place for the client before administering the medication?
    1 Noninvasive blood pressure cuff
    2 Oxygen saturation monitor
    3 Oxygen therapy
    4 Continuous cardiac monitoring

Answer: 4
Rationale: Amiodarone is an antidysrhythmic used to treat life-threatening ventricular dysrhythmias. The client should have continuous cardiac monitoring in place, and the medication should be infused by intravenous pump. Although options 1, 2, and 3 may be in place for the client, they are not specific items needed for the administration of this medication.

Test-Taking Strategy: Focus on the name of the medication. Recalling that this medication is an antidysrhythmic will direct you to option 4. Review the classification of this medication and the nursing considerations when administering this medication if you had difficulty with this question.

Level of Cognitive Ability: Application
Client Needs: Safe, Effective Care Environment
Integrated Process: Nursing Process/Implementation
Content Area: Pharmacology

Reference:
Hodgson, B., & Kizior, R. (2004). *Saunders nursing drug handbook 2004.* Philadelphia: Saunders, p. 48.

---

38. A client is admitted to the hospital for a bowel resection following a diagnosis of a bowel tumor. During the admission assessment, the client tells the nurse that a living will was prepared 3 years ago. The client asks the nurse if this document is still effective. The nurse makes which response to the client?

1   "Yes it is."
2   "You will have to ask your lawyer."
3   "It should be reviewed yearly with your physician."
4   "I have no idea."

Answer: 3

Rationale: The client should discuss the living will with the physician, and it should be reviewed annually to ensure that it contains the client's present wishes and desires. Option 1 is incorrect. Option 4 is not at all helpful to the client and is in fact a communication block. Although a lawyer would need to be consulted if the living will needed to be changed, the accurate nursing response would be to inform the client that the living will should be reviewed annually.

Test-Taking Strategy: Use the process of elimination. Eliminate options 1 and 4 first because they are nontherapeutic and close-ended statements and place the client's question on hold. From the remaining options, it is necessary to know that the document is reviewed annually. Review the concepts related to living wills if you had difficulty with this question.

Level of Cognitive Ability: Application
Client Needs: Safe, Effective Care Environment
Integrated Process: Communication and Documentation
Content Area: Fundamental Skills

Reference:
Brent, N. (2001). *Nurses and the law* (2nd ed.). Philadelphia: Saunders, pp. 216-217.

---

39. A nurse is told that an assigned client has acquired multidrug-resistant *Staphylococcus aureus* (MRSA). In addition to standard precautions, the nurse places the client on which type of transmission-based precautions?

1   Airborne precautions
2   Droplet precautions
3   Enteric precautions
4   Contact precautions

Answer: 4

Rationale: Contact precautions include standard precautions and the use of barrier precautions such as gloves and impermeable gowns. Contact precautions are used for clients with diarrhea, draining wounds not contained by a sterile dressing, or who have acquired antibiotic-resistant infections. The goal of these precautions is to eliminate disease transmission resulting either from direct contact with the client or from indirect contact through an intermediary infected object or surface that has been in contact with the client, such as instruments, linens, or dressing materials. Enteric precautions are initiated if the organism is transmitted via the gastrointestinal tract. Airborne and droplet precautions are used if the organism is transmitted via the respiratory tract.

Test-Taking Strategy: Focus on the client's diagnosis and think about the method of transmission of the infection to others. Eliminate options 1 and 2 first because they are similar. From the remaining options, recalling that MRSA can be transmitted by contact with the infecting organism will assist in answering the question. Review contact precautions if you had difficulty with this question.

Level of Cognitive Ability: Application
Client Needs: Safe, Effective Care Environment
Integrated Process: Nursing Process/Implementation
Content Area: Fundamental Skills

Reference:
Potter, P., & Perry, A. (2005). *Fundamentals of nursing* (6th ed.). St. Louis: Mosby, p. 797.

---

40. A nurse is caring for a client immediately following a bronchoscopy. The client received intravenous sedation and a topical anesthetic for the procedure. In order to provide a safe environment for the client at this time, the nurse plans to:

1 Place a padded tongue blade at the bedside in case of a seizure
2 Check the bedside to ensure that no food or fluid is within the client's reach to prevent aspiration
3 Connect the client to a bedside ECG to monitor for dysrhythmias
4 Place a water-seal chest drainage set at the bedside in case of a pneumothorax

Answer: 2
Rationale: Following this procedure, the client remains NPO until the cough and swallow reflexes have returned, which is usually in 1 to 2 hours. Once the client can swallow, oral intake may begin with ice chips and small sips of water. No data in the question suggests that the client is at risk for a seizure. Even though the client is monitored for signs of any distress, seizures would not be anticipated, and therefore a padded tongue blade would not be placed at the bedside routinely. A pneumothorax is a possible complication of this procedure, and the nurse should monitor the client for signs of distress. However, a water-seal chest drainage set would not be placed routinely at the bedside. No data is given to support that the client is at increased risk for cardiac dysrhythmias.

Test-Taking Strategy: Note the key words "immediately following a bronchoscopy" and "topical anesthetic." Use the ABCs—airway, breathing, and circulation—to direct you to option 2. Review postprocedure care for this procedure if you had difficulty with this question.

Level of Cognitive Ability: Application
Client Needs: Safe, Effective Care Environment
Integrated Process: Nursing Process/Planning
Content Area: Adult Health/Respiratory

Reference:
Ignatavicius, D., & Workman, M. (2002). *Medical surgical nursing: Critical thinking for collaborative care* (4th ed.). Philadelphia: Saunders, p. 486.

---

41. A client with a history of silicosis is admitted to the hospital with respiratory distress and impending respiratory failure. To ensure a safe environment, the nurse plans to have which of the following items readily available at the client's bedside?

1 Chest tube and drainage system
2 Intubation tray
3 Thoracentesis tray
4 Code cart

Answer: 2
Rationale: The client with impending respiratory failure may need intubation and mechanical ventilation. The nurse ensures that an intubation tray is readily available. The other items are not needed at the client's bedside.

Test-Taking Strategy: Focus on the client's diagnosis. Use the ABCs—airway, breathing, and circulation—to direct you to option 2. Review care of the client with impending respiratory failure if you had difficulty with this question.

Level of Cognitive Ability: Application
Client Needs: Safe, Effective Care Environment
Integrated Process: Nursing Process/Planning
Content Area: Adult Health/Respiratory

Reference:
Ignatavicius, D., & Workman, M. (2002). *Medical surgical nursing: Critical thinking for collaborative care* (4th ed.). Philadelphia: Saunders, pp. 558; 599-601.

---

42. A nurse is preparing to administer a first dose of pentamidine (Pentam-300) intravenously to a client. Before administering the dose, the nurse should place the client:
1 On respiratory precautions
2 In a private room
3 In a supine position
4 In semi-Fowler's position

Answer: 3
Rationale: Pentamidine can cause severe and sudden hypotension, even with administration of a single dose. The client should be lying down during administration of this medication. The blood pressure is monitored frequently during administration. Options 1 and 2 are unnecessary. Option 4 is incorrect.

Test-Taking Strategy: Use the process of elimination. Note that both options 3 and 4 address a client position. This indicates that one of these options may be correct. Recalling that the medication causes hypotension will direct you to option 3. Review the nursing considerations related to this medication if you had difficulty with this question.

Level of Cognitive Ability: Application
Client Needs: Safe, Effective Care Environment
Integrated Process: Nursing Process/Implementation
Content Area: Pharmacology

Reference:
Hodgson, B., & Kizior, R. (2004). *Saunders nursing drug handbook 2004.* Philadelphia: Saunders, p. 794.

---

43. A nurse is administering a dose of intravenous hydralazine (Apresoline) to a client. To provide a safe environment, the nurse ensures that which item is in place before injecting the medication?
1 Central line
2 Foley catheter
3 Cardiac monitor
4 Noninvasive blood pressure cuff

Answer: 4
Rationale: Hydralazine is an antihypertensive medication used in the management of moderate to severe hypertension. The blood pressure and pulse should be monitored frequently after administration, so a noninvasive blood pressure cuff is the item to have in place. Options 1, 2, and 3 are not necessary.

Test-Taking Strategy: Focus on the name of the medication. The name of the medication "*Apres*oline" may provide you with the clue that the medication is used to lower the blood pressure. This will direct you to option 4. Review the action of this medication if you had difficulty with this question.

Level of Cognitive Ability: Application
Client Needs: Safe, Effective Care Environment
Integrated Process: Nursing Process/Implementation
Content Area: Pharmacology

Reference:
Hodgson, B., & Kizior, R. (2004). *Saunders nursing drug handbook 2004.* Philadelphia: Saunders, p. 498.

44. A nurse is preparing to care for a client who has undergone left pneumonectomy. The nurse plans to do which of the following immediately after transfer from the postanesthesia care unit?
  1 Place the client's intravenous (IV) fluid on a pump
  2 Assist the client to sit in the bedside chair
  3 Position the client supine
  4 Position the client on the left side

Answer: 1
Rationale: Following pneumonectomy, the fluid status of the client is monitored closely to prevent fluid overload, because the size of the pulmonary vascular bed has been reduced as a result of the pneumonectomy. Complete lateral turning and positioning is avoided. The head of the bed should be elevated to promote lung expansion. The client should remain on bed rest in the immediate postoperative period.

Test-Taking Strategy: Use the process of elimination. Eliminate options 3 and 4 first, because the client should not lie flat and because lateral positioning is avoided. Eliminate option 2 next, because the client should not be sitting in a chair immediately after a surgical procedure such as this. Review postoperative care following pneumonectomy if you had difficulty with this question.

Level of Cognitive Ability: Application
Client Needs: Safe, Effective Care Environment
Integrated Process: Nursing Process/Planning
Content Area: Adult Health/Respiratory

Reference:
Ignatavicius, D., & Workman, M. (2002). *Medical surgical nursing: Critical thinking for collaborative care* (4th ed.). Philadelphia: Saunders, pp. 568-569.

45. A client being seen in the emergency room is being evaluated for possible pleurisy. The nurse preparing the client for a chest X-ray plans to:
  1 Ask the client to remove a neck chain being worn
  2 Ask the client about the time of last food intake
  3 Scrub the chest with betadine
  4 Determine if the client has any metallic implants

Answer: 1
Rationale: If a chest X-ray is prescribed, jewelry or metal objects that might obstruct the X-ray need to be removed. The client does not need to have food or fluid restricted before a chest X-ray, and skin preparation is not required. Notation of metallic implants is required before a magnetic resonance imaging (MRI), but an MRI is not used to diagnose pleurisy.

Test-Taking Strategy: Use the process of elimination, noting the diagnostic test addressed in the question. Focus on the anatomic area of the X-ray and recall the principles related to client preparation to direct you to option 1. Review this diagnostic test if you had difficulty with this question.

Level of Cognitive Ability: Application
Client Needs: Safe, Effective Care Environment
Integrated Process: Nursing Process/Planning
Content Area: Adult Health/Respiratory

Reference:
Chernecky, C., & Berger, B. (2004). *Laboratory tests and diagnostic procedures* (4th ed.). Philadelphia: Saunders, p. 360.

46. A nurse has administered diazepam (Valium) 5 mg intravenously (IV) to a client. To ensure safety, the nurse plans to maintain the client on bed rest for at least:
1 Thirty minutes
2 One hour
3 Three hours
4 Eight hours

Answer: 3

Rationale: The client should remain in bed for at least 3 hours following a parenteral dose of diazepam. The medication is a centrally acting skeletal muscle relaxant and also has antianxiety, sedative-hypnotic, and anticonvulsant properties. Cardiopulmonary side effects include apnea, hypotension, bradycardia, or cardiac arrest. For this reason, resuscitative equipment is also kept nearby.

Test-Taking Strategy: Think about the effects of diazepam administered intravenously to answer this question. Options 1 and 2 can be eliminated first because of the short time frames. From the remaining options, eliminate option 4 because of the lengthy time frame. Review the nursing considerations related to the administration of this medication if you had difficulty with this question.

Level of Cognitive Ability: Application
Client Needs: Safe, Effective Care Environment
Integrated Process: Nursing Process/Planning
Content Area: Pharmacology

Reference:
Hodgson, B., & Kizior, R. (2004). *Saunders nursing drug handbook 2004.* Philadelphia: Saunders, p. 300.

47. A nurse is caring for a hospitalized client who is having a prescribed dosage of clonazepam (Klonopin) adjusted. Because of the adjustment in the medication that is being made, the nurse plans to:
1 Monitor blood glucose levels
2 Institute seizure precautions
3 Weigh the client daily
4 Observe for ecchymoses

Answer: 2

Rationale: Clonazepam is a benzodiazepine that is used as an anticonvulsant. During initial therapy and during periods of dosage adjustment, the nurse should initiate seizure precautions for the client. Options 1, 3, and 4 are unrelated to the use of this medication.

Test-Taking Strategy: Focus on the name of the medication. Recalling that this medication is an anticonvulsant will direct you to option 2. Review the nursing considerations related to this medication if you had difficulty with this question.

Level of Cognitive Ability: Application
Client Needs: Safe, Effective Care Environment
Integrated Process: Nursing Process/Planning
Content Area: Pharmacology

Reference:
Hodgson, B., & Kizior, R. (2004). *Saunders nursing drug handbook 2004.* Philadelphia: Saunders, p. 230.

48. A nurse is planning to obtain an arterial blood gas (ABG) from a client with chronic obstructive pulmonary disease (COPD). To prevent bleeding following the procedure, the nurse plans time for which activity after the arterial blood is drawn?

1 Holding a warm compress over the puncture site for 5 minutes
2 Applying pressure to the puncture site by applying a 2 × 2 gauze for 5 minutes
3 Encouraging the client to open and close the hand rapidly for 2 minutes
4 Having the client keep the radial pulse puncture site in a dependent position for 5 minutes

Answer: 2

Rationale: Applying pressure over the puncture site reduces the risk of hematoma formation and damage to the artery. A cold compress would aid in limiting blood flow; a warm compress would increase blood flow. Keeping the extremity still and out of a dependent position will aid in the formation of a clot at the puncture site.

Test-Taking Strategy: Use the process of elimination. Focus on the issue, preventing bleeding. Options 1, 3, and 4 promote bleeding. Option 2 aids in the prevention of bleeding into the surrounding tissues. Review nursing responsibilities following ABGs if you had difficulty with this question.

Level of Cognitive Ability: Application
Client Needs: Safe, Effective Care Environment
Integrated Process: Nursing Process/Planning
Content Area: Adult Health/Respiratory

Reference:
Chernecky, C., & Berger, B. (2004). *Laboratory tests and diagnostic procedures* (4th ed.). Philadelphia: Saunders, p. 249.

49. A nurse is admitting to the nursing unit a client who has an arteriovenous (AV) fistula in the right arm for hemodialysis. The nurse plans to best prevent injury to the site by:

1 Putting a large note about the access site on the front of the medical record
2 Applying an allergy bracelet to the right arm
3 Placing a sign at the bedside that says: "No blood pressure (BP) measurements or venipunctures in the right arm."
4 Telling the client to inform all caregivers who enter the room about the presence of the access site

Answer: 3

Rationale: There should be no venipunctures or blood pressure measurements in the extremity with a hemodialysis access device. This is commonly communicated to all caregivers by placing a sign at the client's bedside. Placing a note on the front of the medical record does not ensure that everyone caring for the client is aware of the access device. An allergy bracelet is placed on the client with an allergy. Some health care agencies, however, do have policies that require application of a wrist bracelet of some type to be placed on the client with a hemodialysis access device. The client should not be responsible for informing the caregivers.

Test-Taking Strategy: Use the process of elimination, noting the key word "best." Eliminate option 2 because an allergy bracelet is used for a client with an allergy. Eliminate option 4 next because this responsibility should not be placed on the client. From the remaining options, note that option 3 best informs those caring for the client of the presence of the fistula. Review care of the client with an AV fistula if you had difficulty with this question.

Level of Cognitive Ability: Application
Client Needs: Safe, Effective Care Environment
Integrated Process: Nursing Process/Planning
Content Area: Adult Health/Renal

Reference:
Ignatavicius, D., & Workman, M. (2002). *Medical surgical nursing: Critical thinking for collaborative care* (4th ed.). Philadelphia: Saunders, p. 1692.

50. Regular insulin by continuous intravenous (IV) infusion is prescribed for a client with a blood glucose level of 700 mg/dL. The nurse plans to:
1 Infuse the medication via an electronic infusion pump
2 Mix the solution in 5% dextrose
3 Change the solution every 6 hours
4 Titrate the infusion according to the client's urine glucose levels

Answer: 1
Rationale: Insulin is administered via an infusion pump to prevent inadvertent overdose and subsequent hypoglycemia. Dextrose is added to the IV infusion once the serum glucose level reaches 250 mg/dL to prevent the occurrence of hypoglycemia. Administering dextrose to a client with a serum glucose level of 700 mg/dL would counteract the beneficial effects of insulin in reducing the glucose level. Glycosuria is not a reliable indicator of the actual serum glucose levels because many factors affect the renal threshold for glucose loss in the urine. There is no reason to change the solution every 6 hours.

Test-Taking Strategy: Use the process of elimination. Eliminate option 4, knowing that urine glucose levels do not provide an accurate indication of the client's status. Next, eliminate option 2, knowing that dextrose would not be administered to a client with a blood glucose of 700 mg/dL. From the remaining options, recalling the complications associated with a continuous infusion of insulin will direct you to option 1. Review nursing care of a client with a continuous IV infusion of insulin if you had difficulty with this question.

Level of Cognitive Ability: Application
Client Needs: Safe, Effective Care Environment
Integrated Process: Nursing Process/Planning
Content Area: Adult Health/Endocrine

Reference:
Ignatavicius, D., & Workman, M. (2002). *Medical surgical nursing: Critical thinking for collaborative care* (4th ed.). Philadelphia: Saunders, p. 1460.

51. A nurse is developing a plan of care for a client with diabetic ketoacidosis (DKA). The nurse includes which intervention in the plan?
1 Maintain side rails in the upright position
2 Ambulate the client every 2 hours
3 Assess for fluid overload
4 Limit family visitation time

Answer: 1
Rationale: The client with DKA may experience a decrease in the level of consciousness (LOC) secondary to acidosis. Safety becomes a priority for any client with a decreased LOC, thus requiring the use of side rails to prevent fall injuries. The client may be too ill to ambulate and will experience fluid loss (dehydration) rather than overload. Family visitation is helpful for both the client and family to assist with psychosocial adaptation.

Test-Taking Strategy: Focus on the client's diagnosis to eliminate options 2 and 4. From the remaining options, recalling that dehydration is an issue in DKA and that mental status changes occur will direct you to option 1. Review care of the client with DKA if you had difficulty with this question.

Level of Cognitive Ability: Application
Client Needs: Safe, Effective Care Environment
Integrated Process: Nursing Process/Planning
Content Area: Adult Health/Endocrine

References:
Black, J., & Hawks, J. (2005). *Medical-surgical nursing: Clinical management for positive outcomes* (7th ed.). Philadelphia: Saunders, p. 1269.
Elkin, M., Perry, A., & Potter, P. (2004). *Nursing interventions & clinical skills* (3rd ed.). St. Louis: Mosby, p. 84.

52. A nurse practicing in a nurse-managed clinic wants to set up a diabetic teaching seminar. The nurse understands that to meet the clients' needs, the nurse must first:

1 Assess the clients' functional abilities
2 Ensure that insurance documentation is up-to-date
3 Discuss the focus of the seminar with the multidisciplinary team
4 Include everyone who comes into the clinic in the teaching sessions

Answer: 1

Rationale: Nurse-managed clinics focus on individualized disease prevention and health promotion and maintenance. Therefore, the nurse must first assess the clients and their needs in order to effectively plan the seminar. Options 2, 3, and 4 do not address the clients' needs.

Test-Taking Strategy: Use the process of elimination and the steps of the nursing process. Remember the first step is assessment. Option 1 reflects assessment. Review teaching/learning principles if you had difficulty with this question.

Level of Cognitive Ability: Application
Client Needs: Safe, Effective Care Environment
Integrated Process: Teaching/Learning
Content Area: Leadership/Management

Reference:
Potter, P., & Perry, A. (2005). *Fundamentals of nursing* (6th ed.). St. Louis: Mosby, pp. 451-454.

---

53. A nurse notes that a postoperative client has not been obtaining relief of pain with the prescribed narcotics, but only while a particular licensed practical nurse (LPN) is assigned to the client. The nurse:

1 Reviews the client's medication administration record and immediately discusses the situation with the nursing supervisor
2 Notifies the physician that the client needs an increase in narcotic dosage
3 Avoids assigning the LPN to the care of clients receiving narcotics
4 Confronts the LPN with the information about the client having pain control problems and asks if the LPN is using the narcotics personally

Answer: 1

Rationale: In this situation, the nurse has noted an unusual occurrence, but before deciding what action to take next, the nurse needs more data than just suspicion. This can be obtained by reviewing the client's record. State and Federal labor and narcotic regulations, as well as institutional policies and procedures, must be followed. It is therefore most appropriate that the nurse discuss the situation with the nursing supervisor before taking further action. The client does not need an increase in narcotics. To avoid assigning the LPN to clients receiving narcotics ignores the issue. A confrontation is not the most advisable action because the appropriate administrative authorities need to be consulted first.

Test-Taking Strategy: Use the process of elimination and knowledge regarding the roles and responsibilities of the nurse and the organizational channels of communication. Option 1 is the only option that includes consultation with an authority figure, the nursing supervisor. Review the nurse's role when substance abuse in another nurse is suspected if you had difficulty with this question.

Level of Cognitive Ability: Application
Client Needs: Safe, Effective Care Environment
Integrated Process: Nursing Process/Implementation
Content Area: Leadership/Management

Reference:
Stuart, G., & Laraia, M. (2005). *Principles and practice of psychiatric nursing* (8th ed.). St. Louis: Mosby, pp. 510-511.

54. A medication nurse is supervising a newly hired licensed practical nurse (LPN) during the administration of oral pyridostigmine (Mestinon) to a client with myasthenia gravis. Which observation by the medication nurse would indicate safe practice by the LPN?

1 Asking the client to lie down on his or her right side
2 Instructing the client to void before taking the medication
3 Asking the client to take sips of water
4 Asking the client to look up at the ceiling for 30 seconds

Answer: 3

Rationale: Myasthenia gravis can affect the client's ability to swallow. The primary assessment is to determine the client's ability to handle oral medications or any oral substance. Options 1 and 4 are not appropriate. Option 1 could result in aspiration and option 4 has no useful purpose. There is no specific reason for the client to void before taking this medication.

Test-Taking Strategy: Use the process of elimination. Recalling that myasthenia gravis affects the client's ability to swallow will direct you to option 3. Also, note the relation between the words "oral" in the question and "sips of water" in the correct option. Review nursing care of the client with myasthenia gravis if you had difficulty with this question.

Level of Cognitive Ability: Analysis
Client Needs: Safe, Effective Care Environment
Integrated Process: Nursing Process/Evaluation
Content Area: Leadership/Management

Reference:
Phipps, W., Monahan, F., Sands, J., Marek, J., & Neighbors, M. (2003). *Medical-surgical nursing: Health and illness perspectives* (7th ed.). St. Louis: Mosby, pp. 1398; 1400.

---

55. A client's vital signs have noticeably deteriorated over the past 4 hours following surgery. A nurse does not recognize the significance of these changes in vital signs and takes no action. The client later requires emergency surgery. The nurse could be prosecuted for inaction according to the definition of which of these terms?

1 Tort
2 Misdemeanor
3 Common law
4 Statutory law

Answer: 1

Rationale: A tort is a wrongful act intentionally or unintentionally committed against a person or his or her property. The nurse's inaction in the situation described is consistent with the definition of a tort offense. Option 2 is an offense under criminal law. Option 3 describes case law that has evolved over time via precedents. Option 4 describes laws that are enacted by State, Federal, or local governments.

Test-Taking Strategy: Focus on the data in the question and the definition of the terms in the options. Recalling that a tort is a wrongful act will direct you to option 1. Review the definitions related to the various types of laws if you had difficulty with this question.

Level of Cognitive Ability: Analysis
Client Needs: Safe, Effective Care Environment
Integrated Process: Nursing Process/Analysis
Content Area: Fundamental Skills

References:
Brent, N. (2001). *Nurses and the law* (2nd ed.). Philadelphia: Saunders, p. 54.
Potter, P., & Perry, A. (2005). *Fundamentals of nursing* (6th ed.). St. Louis: Mosby, pp. 413-414.

56. A well-known individual from the community is admitted to the hospital with a diagnosis of Parkinson's disease. The nurse
gives medical information regarding the
client's condition to a person who is
assumed to be a family member. Later, the
nurse discovers that this person is not a
family member and realizes that she has
violated which legal concept of the nurse-
client relationship?
  1 Client's right to privacy
  2 Nurse's lack of experience
  3 Teaching/learning principles
  4 Performing focused physical assess-
     ment

Answer: 1
Rationale: Discussing a client's condition without client permission violates a client's rights and places the nurse in legal jeopardy. This action by the nurse is both an invasion of privacy and
affects the confidentiality issue with client rights. Options 2, 3,
and 4 do not represent violation of the situation presented.

Test-Taking Strategy: Focus on the information in the question.
The issue of the question is related to sharing information, which
constitutes an invasion of privacy. Review client rights and the situations that involve invasion of privacy if you had difficulty with
this question.

Level of Cognitive Ability: Analysis
Client Need: Safe, Effective Care Environment
Integrated Process: Nursing Process/Analysis
Content Area: Adult Health/Neurological

Reference:
Potter, P., & Perry, A. (2005). *Fundamentals of nursing* (6th ed.). St. Louis: Mosby,
  pp. 413-414.

---

57. A clinic nurse is assessing a client for environmental risk factors related to neurological disorders. The nurse understands that
which of the following is least likely associated with neurological disorders?
  1 Exposure to fumes, such as paints or
     bonding agents (glue)
  2 Exposure to pesticides
  3 Ventilation in the work area
  4 Number of windows in the work area

Answer: 4
Rationale: The nurse would assess for the risk of exposure to neu-
rotoxic fumes and chemicals. These could include paint, bonding
agents, pesticides, and many more. The nurse also inquires about
the adequacy of ventilation in the home and work area. Many
work spaces (such as factories, insurance companies, and operating rooms) are adequately ventilated without the use of windows.

Test-Taking Strategy: Note the key words "least likely." Focusing
on the issue, environmental risk factors will direct you to option
4. Review environmental risk factors associated with neurological
disorders if you had difficulty with this question.

Level of Cognitive Ability: Analysis
Client Needs: Safe, Effective Care Environment
Integrated Process: Nursing Process/Assessment
Content Area: Adult Health/Neurological

Reference:
Black, J., & Hawks, J. (2005). *Medical-surgical nursing: Clinical management for positive outcomes* (7th ed.). Philadelphia: Saunders, pp. 2034; 2037.

---

58. A nurse performing an initial admission
assessment notes that a client has been
taking metoclopramide (Reglan) for a prolonged period. The nurse would immediately call the physician if which signs or
symptoms were then noted by the nurse?
  1 Anxiety or irritability
  2 Dry mouth relieved with the use of
     sugar-free hard candy
  3 Excessive drowsiness
  4 Uncontrolled rhythmic movements of
     the face or limbs

Answer: 4
Rationale: If the client experiences tardive dyskinesia (rhythmic
movements of the face or limbs), the nurse should call the physician because these side effects may be irreversible. The medication
would be discontinued, and no further doses should be given by
the nurse. Anxiety, irritability, and dry mouth are mild side effects
that do not harm the client.

Test-Taking Strategy: Note that the question contains the key word "immediately," which guides you to select the most harmful option. Recalling that this medication causes tardive dyskinesia will direct you to option 4. Review the side effects of this medication and the signs of tardive dyskinesia if you had difficulty with this question.

Level of Cognitive Ability: Analysis
Client Needs: Safe, Effective Care Environment
Integrated Process: Communication and Documentation
Content Area: Pharmacology

Reference:
McKenry, L., & Salerno, E. (2003). *Mosby's pharmacology in nursing* (21st ed.). St. Louis: Mosby, p. 761.

---

59. A nurse calls the physician of a client scheduled for a cardiac catheterization because the client has numerous questions regarding the procedure and has requested to speak to the physician. The physician is very upset with the nurse and arrives at the unit to visit the client after prompting by the nurse. The nurse is outside of the client's room and hears the physician tell the client in a derogatory manner that the nurse "doesn't know anything." Which legal tort has the physician violated?
1 Libel
2 Slander
3 Assault
4 Negligence

Answer: 2
Rationale: Defamation takes place when something untrue is said (slander) or written (libel) about a person, resulting in injury to that person's good name and reputation. An assault occurs when a person puts another person in fear of a harmful or an offensive contact. Negligence involves the actions of professionals that fall below the standard of care for a specific professional group.

Test-Taking Strategy: Use the process of elimination and eliminate options 3 and 4 first. From the remaining options, recalling that slander constitutes verbal defamation will direct you to option 2. Review the torts identified in each option if you had difficulty with this question.

Level of Cognitive Ability: Analysis
Client Needs: Safe, Effective Care Environment
Integrated Process: Nursing Process/Analysis
Content Area: Fundamental Skills

References:
Brent, N. (2001). *Nurses and the law* (2nd ed.). Philadelphia: Saunders, p. 121.
Potter, P., & Perry, A. (2005). *Fundamentals of nursing* (6th ed.). St. Louis: Mosby, p. 414.

---

60. A nurse enters a client's room and finds the client sitting on the floor. The nurse performs a thorough assessment and assists the client back into bed. The nurse completes an incident report and notifies the physician of the incident. Which of the following is the next appropriate nursing action regarding the incident?
1 Make a copy of the incident report for the physician
2 Place the incident report in the client's chart
3 Document a complete entry in the client's record concerning the incident
4 Document in the client's record that an incident report has been completed

Answer: 3
Rationale: The incident report is confidential and privileged information and should not be copied, placed in the chart, or have any reference made to it in the client's record. The incident report is not a substitute for a complete entry in the client's record concerning the incident.

Test-Taking Strategy: Use the process of elimination and eliminate options 2 and 4 first because they are similar. From the remaining options, recalling that incident reports should not be copied will direct you to option 3. Review nursing responsibilities related to incident reports if you had difficulty with this question.

Level of Cognitive Ability: Application
Client Needs: Safe, Effective Care Environment
Integrated Process: Communication and Documentation
Content Area: Fundamental Skills

Reference:
Potter, P., & Perry, A. (2005). *Fundamentals of nursing* (6th ed.). St. Louis: Mosby, pp. 419; 497.

---

61. A client had a colon resection. A nasogastric tube was in place when a regular diet was brought to the client's room. The client did not want to eat solid food and asked that the physician be called. The nurse insisted that the solid food was the correct diet. The client ate and subsequently had additional surgery as a result of complications. The determination of negligence in this situation is based on:
    1 A duty existed and it was breached
    2 Not calling the physician
    3 The dietary department sending the wrong food
    4 The nurse's persistence

Answer: 1
Rationale: For negligence to be proven, there must be a duty, and then a breach of duty; the breach of duty must cause the injury, and damages or injury must be experienced. Options 2, 3, and 4 do not fall under the criteria for negligence. Option 1 is the only option that fits the criteria of negligence.

Test-Taking Strategy: Use the process of elimination. Options 2, 3, and 4 do not directly support the issue of negligence because it would be difficult to determine that these elements caused injury. The focus relates to what the nurse is responsible for. Option 1 is an umbrella (global) response to the question. Review the legal elements of nursing practice and criteria for negligence if you had difficulty with this question.

Level of Cognitive Ability: Analysis
Client Needs: Safe, Effective Care Environment
Integrated Process: Nursing Process/Analysis
Content Area: Fundamental Skills

Reference:
Brent, N. (2001). *Nurses and the law* (2nd ed.). Philadelphia: Saunders, pp. 54-55.

---

62. A nurse is caring for a child with intussusception. During care, the child passes a normal brown stool. The appropriate nursing action is to:
    1 Report the passage of a normal brown stool to the physician
    2 Prepare the child and parents for the possibility of surgery
    3 Note the child's physical symptoms
    4 Prepare the child for hydrostatic reduction

Answer: 1
Rationale: Passage of a normal brown stool usually indicates that the intussusception has reduced itself. This is immediately reported to the physician, who may choose to alter the diagnostic or therapeutic plan of care. Hydrostatic reduction and surgery may not be necessary. Although the nurse would note the child's physical symptoms, based on the data in the question, option 1 is the appropriate action.

Test-Taking Strategy: Use the process of elimination. Note the similarity between the information in the question and the correct option. Also, recalling the physiology associated with intussusception will direct you to option 1. Review care of the child with intussusception if you had difficulty with this question.

Level of Cognitive Ability: Application
Client Needs: Safe, Effective Care Environment
Integrated Process: Nursing Process/Implementation
Content Area: Child Health

Reference:
Wong, D., & Hockenberry, M. (2003). *Wong's nursing care of infants and children* (7th ed.). St. Louis: Mosby, p. 1449.

63. A new nursing graduate is attending an agency orientation regarding the nursing model of practice implemented in the facility. The nurse is told that the nursing model is a primary nursing approach. The nurse understands that which of the following is a characteristic of this type of nursing model of practice?
  1 The nurse manager assigns tasks to the staff members.
  2 Critical paths are used in providing client care.
  3 A single registered nurse (RN) is responsible for planning and providing individualized nursing care.
  4 Nursing staff are led by an RN leader in providing care to a group of clients.

Answer: 3
Rationale: Primary nursing is concerned with keeping the nurse at the bedside actively involved in direct care while planning goal-directed, individualized client care. Option 1 identifies functional nursing. Option 2 identifies a component of case management. Option 4 identifies team nursing.

Test-Taking Strategy: Note that the issue of the question relates to primary nursing. Keep this issue in mind and use the process of elimination. Option 3 is the only option that identifies the concept of a primary approach. Review the various types of nursing delivery systems if you had difficulty with this question.

Level of Cognitive Ability: Comprehension
Client Needs: Safe, Effective Care Environment
Integrated Process: Nursing Process/Implementation
Content Area: Leadership/Management

Reference:
Potter, P., & Perry, A. (2005). *Fundamentals of nursing* (6th ed.). St. Louis: Mosby, p. 373.

64. A client asks the nurse how to become an organ donor. The nurse includes which statement in the response to the client?
  1 The donor must be 25 years of age or older.
  2 The donation is done by written consent.
  3 The family is responsible for making organ donor decisions at the time of death.
  4 A witness and a family member must be present to sign a form if an individual wants to donate his or her own organs for transplantation.

Answer: 2
Rationale: The client has the right to donate her or his own organs for transplantation. Any person 18 years of age or older may become an organ donor by written consent. In the absence of appropriate documentation, a family member or legal guardian may authorize donation of the decedent's organs.

Test-Taking Strategy: Use the process of elimination and focus on the issues related to client rights. This will direct you to option 2. Review the procedure for organ donation if you had difficulty with this question.

Level of Cognitive Ability: Application
Client Needs: Safe, Effective Care Environment
Integrated Process: Nursing Process/Evaluation
Content Area: Fundamental Skills

Reference:
Potter, P., & Perry, A. (2005). *Fundamentals of nursing* (6th ed.). St. Louis: Mosby, pp. 410; 589.

65. A registered nurse (RN) is observing a licensed practical nurse (LPN) caring for a deceased client whose eyes will be donated. The RN intervenes if the LPN performs which action?
  1 Elevates the head of the bed
  2 Closes the client's eyes
  3 Places wet saline gauze pads and an ice pack on the eyes
  4 Closes the client's eyes and places a dry sterile dressing over the eyes

Answer: 4
Rationale: When a corneal donor dies, the eyes are closed and gauze pads wet with saline are placed over them with a small ice pack. Within 2 to 4 hours, the eyes are enucleated. The cornea is usually transplanted within 24 to 48 hours. The head of the bed should also be elevated. There is no useful purpose to place dry sterile dressings over the eyes.

Test-Taking Strategy: Note that the issue relates to donation of the eyes. Also note the key word "intervenes" in the stem of the question. This key word indicates a false-response question and that you need to select the option that is an incorrect nursing action. Visualize each option and think about the issue of preserving the eyes. This will direct you to option 4. Review this procedure if you had difficulty with the question.

Level of Cognitive Ability: Application
Client Needs: Safe, Effective Care Environment
Integrated Process: Nursing Process/Implementation
Content Area: Leadership/Management

References:
Ignatavicius, D., & Workman, M. (2002). *Medical surgical nursing: Critical thinking for collaborative care* (4th ed.). Philadelphia: Saunders, p. 1031.
Phipps, W., Monahan, F., Sands, J., Marek, J., & Neighbors, M. (2003). *Medical-surgical nursing: Health and illness perspectives* (7th ed.). St. Louis: Mosby, p. 1703.

---

66. A clinical nurse manager conducts an inservice educational session for the staff nurses about case management. The clinical nurse manager determines that a review of the material needs to be done if a staff nurse stated that case management:
   1 Represents a primary health prevention focus managed by a single case manager
   2 Manages client care by managing the client care environment
   3 Is designed to promote appropriate use of hospital personnel and material resources
   4 Maximizes hospital revenues while providing for optimal outcome of client care

Answer: 1
Rationale: Case management represents an interdisciplinary health care delivery system to promote appropriate use of hospital personnel and material resources to maximize hospital revenues while providing for optimal outcome of care. It manages client care by managing the client care environment.

Test-Taking Strategy: Note the key words "a review of the material needs to be done." These key words indicate a false-response question and that you need to select the option that is an incorrect characteristic of case management. Noting the word "single" in option 1 will direct you to this option. Review the characteristics of case management if you had difficulty with this question.

Level of Cognitive Ability: Analysis
Client Needs: Safe, Effective Care Environment
Integrated Process: Teaching/Learning
Content Area: Leadership/Management

Reference:
Potter, P., & Perry, A. (2005). *Fundamentals of nursing* (6th ed.). St. Louis: Mosby, pp. 485; 487.

---

67. A registered nurse is delegating activities to the nursing staff. Which activity is least appropriate for the nursing assistant?
   1 Assisting a post-cardiac catheterization client who needs to lie flat to eat lunch
   2 Obtaining frequent oral temperatures on a client
   3 Accompanying a man being discharged to his transportation to home
   4 Collecting a urine specimen from a client

Answer: 1
Rationale: Work that is delegated to others must be done consistent with the individual's level of expertise and licensure or lack of licensure. Based on the options provided, the least appropriate activity for a nursing assistant would be assisting a post-cardiac catheterization client who needs to lie flat to eat lunch. Because the client needs to eat lying flat, the client is at risk for aspiration. The remaining three options do not include situations to indicate that these activities carry any risk.

Test-Taking Strategy: Note the key words "least appropriate." Use the ABCs—i.e., airway, breathing, and circulation—and recall the principles of delegation in answering the question. Review the principles of assignments and delegation if you had difficulty with this question.

Level of Cognitive Ability: Application
Client Needs: Safe, Effective Care Environment
Integrated Process: Nursing Process/Planning
Content Area: Delegating/Prioritizing

Reference:
Potter, P., & Perry, A. (2005). *Fundamentals of nursing* (6th ed.). St. Louis: Mosby, pp. 378; 418.

---

68. A clinical nurse manager is reviewing the critical paths of the clients on the nursing unit. The nurse manager collaborates with each nurse assigned to the clients and performs a variance analysis. Which of the following would indicate the need for further action and analysis?
 1 A client is performing his own colostomy care.
 2 A one-day postoperative client has a temperature of 98.8 degrees Fahrenheit.
 3 Purulent drainage is noted from a postoperative wound incision.
 4 A client newly diagnosed with diabetes mellitus is preparing his own insulin for injection.

Answer: 3
Rationale: Variances are actual deviations or detours from the critical paths. Variances can be either positive or negative, avoidable, or unavoidable and can be caused by a variety of things. Positive variance occurs when the client achieves maximum benefit and is discharged earlier than anticipated. Negative variance occurs when untoward events prevent a timely discharge. Variance analysis occurs continually in order to anticipate and recognize negative variance early so that appropriate action can be taken. Option 3 is the only option that identifies the need for further action.

Test-Taking Strategy: Use the process of elimination, identifying the negative variance. Options 1, 2, and 4 identify positive outcomes. Option 3 identifies a negative outcome. Review the purpose of variance analysis if you had difficulty with this question.

Level of Cognitive Ability: Analysis
Client Needs: Safe, Effective Care Environment
Integrated Process: Nursing Process/Evaluation
Content Area: Leadership/Management

Reference:
Potter, P., & Perry, A. (2005). *Fundamentals of nursing* (6th ed.). St. Louis: Mosby, p. 485.

---

69. A nurse manager is conducting a conference with the nursing staff regarding concerns and proposals for actions related to the nursing unit. The nurse manager presents his or her own analysis of the problem and proposals for actions to team members, and invites the team members to comment and provide input. Which style of leadership is the nurse manager specifically employing?
 1 Laissez faire
 2 Authoritarian
 3 Situational
 4 Participative

Answer: 4
Rationale: Participative leadership suggests a compromise between the authoritarian and the democratic style. In participative leadership, the manager presents his or her own analysis of problems and proposals for actions to team members, inviting critique and comments. The participative leader then analyzes the comments and makes the final decision. A laissez-faire leader abdicates leadership and responsibilities, allowing staff to work without assistance, direction, or supervision. The autocratic style of leadership is task oriented and directive. The situational leadership style utilizes a style depending on the situation and events.

Test-Taking Strategy: Focus on the data in the question. Noting the words "invites the team members to comment and provide input" will direct you to option 4. Review the various types of leadership styles if you had difficulty with this question.

Level of Cognitive Ability: Comprehension
Client Needs: Safe, Effective Care Environment
Integrated Process: Nursing Process/Implementation
Content Area: Leadership/Management

Reference:
Yoder-Wise, P. (2003). *Leading and managing in nursing* (3rd ed.). St. Louis: Mosby, p. 147.

---

70. A clinic nurse teaches a pregnant client with herpes genitalis about the measures that will be implemented during the pregnancy. Which statement by the client indicates that teaching was effective?
1 "I must continue to take my acyclovir (Zovirax)."
2 "I need to abstain from sexual intercourse during the entire pregnancy."
3 "I need to take sitz baths four times a day."
4 "I may need a cesarean section if the lesions are present at the time of labor."

Answer: 4
Rationale: For women with active lesions, either recurrent or primary, at the time of labor, delivery should be cesarean; therefore, option 4 is correct. Acyclovir is used with caution during pregnancy. Clients should be advised to abstain from sexual contact while the lesions are present. If it is an initial infection, they should continue to abstain until they become culture negative because prolonged viral shedding may occur in such cases. Option 3 is incorrect. Keeping the genital area clean and dry will promote healing.

Test-Taking Strategy: Use the process of elimination and eliminate option 1 first because of the absolute word "must." Next, eliminate option 2 because of the word "entire." Knowing that the genital area should remain clean and dry will assist in eliminating option 3. Review the health care measures related to herpes genitalis if you had difficulty with this question.

Level of Cognitive Ability: Analysis
Client Needs: Safe, Effective Care Environment
Integrated Process: Teaching/Learning
Content Area: Maternity/Antepartum

Reference:
Lowdermilk, D., & Perry, A. (2004). *Maternity & women's health care* (8th ed.). St. Louis: Mosby, p. 201.

---

71. A nurse has an order to test a client's stools using hemoccult slides. The nurse would question the order if the client was taking which medication that could cause a false-negative result?
1 Ascorbic acid (Vitamin C)
2 Colchicine
3 Iodine
4 Acetylsalicylic acid (Aspirin)

Answer: 1
Rationale: Ascorbic acid can interfere with the result of occult blood testing, causing false-negative findings. Colchicine and iodine can cause false-positive results. Acetylsalicylic acid would either have no effect on results or could cause a positive result, because aspirin is irritating to the stomach lining.

Test-Taking Strategy: Focus on the key words "false-negative results." Specific knowledge of the factors that interfere with occult blood testing is needed to answer this question accurately. Review the nursing considerations associated with this test if you had difficulty with this question.

Level of Cognitive Ability: Application
Client Needs: Safe, Effective Care Environment
Integrated Process: Communication and Documentation
Content Area: Adult Health/Gastrointestinal

Reference:
Chernecky, C., & Berger, B. (2004). *Laboratory tests and diagnostic procedures* (4th ed.). Philadelphia: Saunders, p. 819.

---

72. A community health nurse is providing instructions to a group of mothers regarding the safe use of car seats for toddlers. The nurse determines that the mother of a toddler understands the instructions if the mother states which of the following?
   1 "The car seat can be placed in a face-forward position when the height of the toddler is 27 inches."
   2 "The car seat should never be placed in a face-forward position."
   3 "The car seat can be placed in a face-forward position at any time."
   4 "The car seat is suitable for the toddler until the toddler reaches the weight of 40 pounds."

Answer: 4
Rationale: The transition point for switching to the forward-facing position is defined by the manufacturer of the safety seat but is generally at a body weight of 9 kg (20 pounds). The car safety seat should be used until the child weighs at least 40 pounds regardless of age. Options 1, 2, and 3 are incorrect.

Test-Taking Strategy: Use the process of elimination and focus on the issue of the question. Eliminate options 2 and 3 first because of the absolute words "never" and "any." From the remaining options, visualize each and use knowledge regarding car safety and the toddler to answer the question. Review these safety principles if you had difficulty with this question.

Level of Cognitive Ability: Analysis
Client Needs: Safe, Effective Care Environment
Integrated Process: Nursing Process/Evaluation
Content Area: Child Health

Reference:
Wong, D., & Hockenberry, M. (2003). *Wong's nursing care of infants and children* (7th ed.). St. Louis: Mosby, p. 1758.

---

73. A home care nurse is providing instructions to the mother of a toddler regarding safety measures in the home to prevent an accidental burn injury. Which statement by the mother indicates a need for further instruction?
   1 "I need to remain in the kitchen when I prepare meals."
   2 "I need to be sure to place my cup of coffee on the counter."
   3 "I need to use the back burners for cooking."
   4 "I need to turn pot handles inward and to the middle of the stove."

Answer: 2
Rationale: Toddlers, with their increased mobility and developing motor skills, can reach hot water or hot objects placed on counters and open fires or burners on stoves above their eye level. Parents should be encouraged to remain in the kitchen when preparing a meal, to use the back burners on the stove, and to turn pot handles inward and toward the middle of the stove. Hot liquids should never be left unattended, and the toddler should always be supervised. The mother's statement in option 2 does not indicate an adequate understanding of the principles of safety.

Test-Taking Strategy: Use the process of elimination and note the key words "a need for further instruction." These key words indicate a false-response question and that you need to select the option that identifies an incorrect statement by the mother. Options 1, 3, and 4 can be eliminated because they identify basic safety principles. Also recalling that the toddler is in the stage of developing motor skills will assist in directing you to option 2. Review these safety principles if you had difficulty with this question.

Level of Cognitive Ability: Analysis
Client Needs: Safe, Effective Care Environment
Integrated Process: Teaching/Learning
Content Area: Child Health

Reference:
Wong, D., & Hockenberry, M. (2003). *Wong's nursing care of infants and children* (7th ed.). St. Louis: Mosby, p. 10.

---

74. A client with a right pleural effusion noted on a chest X-ray is being prepared for a thoracentesis. The client experiences severe dizziness when sitting upright. To provide a safe environment, the nurse assists the client to which position for the procedure?
1 Prone with the head turned toward the side supported by a pillow
2 Sims' position with the head of the bed flat
3 Right side-lying with the head of the bed elevated 45 degrees
4 Left side-lying with the head of the bed elevated 45 degrees

Answer: 4
Rationale: To facilitate removal of fluid from the chest wall, the client is positioned sitting at the edge of the bed leaning over the bedside table with the feet supported on a stool. If the client is unable to sit up, the client is positioned lying in bed on the unaffected side with the head of the bed elevated 30 to 45 degrees. The prone and Sims' positions are inappropriate positions for this procedure.

Test-Taking Strategy: Use the process of elimination. Eliminate option 3 first because if the client was lying on the affected side, it would be difficult to perform the procedure. Option 2 can be eliminated next because the Sims' position is primarily used for rectal enemas or irrigations. Next, visualize the prone position. In the prone position, the client is lying on the abdomen, which is not an appropriate position for this procedure. Review the procedure for a thoracentesis if you had difficulty with this question.

Level of Cognitive Ability: Application
Client Needs: Safe, Effective Care Environment
Integrated Process: Nursing Process/Implementation
Content Area: Fundamental Skills

Reference:
Chernecky, C., & Berger, B. (2004). *Laboratory tests and diagnostic procedures* (4th ed.). Philadelphia: Saunders, p. 1043.

---

75. A physician has written an order to administer methylergonovine (Methergine) to a postpartum client with uterine atony. The nurse would contact the physician to verify the order if which of the following conditions were present in the mother?
1 Excessive lochia
2 Excessive bleeding and saturation of more than one peripad per hour
3 Hypertension
4 Difficulty locating the uterine fundus

Answer: 3
Rationale: Methergine is contraindicated for the hypertensive woman, individuals with severe hepatic or renal disease, and during the third stage of labor. A uterine fundus that is difficult to locate, excessive bleeding, and excessive lochia are clinical manifestations of uterine atony indicating the need for methylergonovine.

Test-Taking Strategy: Use the process of elimination. Eliminate options 1, 2, and 4 because they are similar in that they are clinical manifestations of uterine atony. Review this content if you had difficulty with this question or are unfamiliar with the use of this medication and its contraindications.

Level of Cognitive Ability: Application
Client Needs: Safe, Effective Care Environment
Integrated Process: Communication and Documentation
Content Area: Maternity/Postpartum

Reference:
Lowdermilk, D., & Perry, A. (2004). *Maternity & women's health care* (8th ed.). St. Louis: Mosby, p. 1040.

---

76. A client is scheduled for a colonoscopy and the physician has provided detailed information to the client regarding the procedure. The nurse brings the informed consent form to the client to obtain the client's signature and discovers that the client cannot write. What is the nurse's appropriate action?
1 Contact the physician
2 Send the client for the procedure without a signed informed consent
3 Explain the procedure to the client with another nurse present and send the client for the procedure without a signed informed consent
4 Obtain a second nurse to also act as a witness and ask the client to sign the form with an X

Answer: 4
Rationale: Clients who cannot write may sign an informed consent with an X. This is witnessed by two nurses. Nurses serve as a witness to the client's signature and not to the fact that the client is informed. It is the physician's responsibility to inform the client about a procedure. The nurse clarifies facts presented by the physician. There is no useful reason to contact the physician at this time. A client is not sent to a procedure without a signed informed consent if one is needed.

Test-Taking Strategy: Note that in this situation the physician has informed the client about the procedure. This will assist in eliminating option 1. Eliminate options 2 and 3 next because they are similar. Review the principles related to informed consent if you had difficulty with this question.

Level of Cognitive Ability: Application
Client Needs: Safe, Effective Care Environment
Integrated Process: Nursing Process/Implementation
Content Area: Fundamental Skills

Reference:
Ignatavicius, D., & Workman, M. (2002). *Medical surgical nursing: Critical thinking for collaborative care* (4th ed.). Philadelphia: Saunders, p. 248.

---

77. A child with a brain tumor is admitted to the hospital for removal of the tumor. To ensure a safe environment for the child, the nurse includes which of the following in the plan of care?
1 Assisting the child with ambulation at all times
2 Avoiding contact with other children on the nursing unit
3 Initiating seizure precautions
4 Using a wheelchair for out-of-bed activities

Answer: 3
Rationale: Seizure precautions should be implemented for any child with a brain tumor, both preoperatively and postoperatively. Options 1 and 4 are not required unless functional deficits exist. Based on the child's diagnosis, option 2 is not necessary.

Test-Taking Strategy: Note the key words "safe environment" in the stem of the question. Eliminate options 1 and 4 first because they are similar. Additionally, note the absolute word "all" in option 1. From the remaining options, eliminate option 2 because there is no reason for the child to avoid contact with other children. Review nursing interventions related to the child with a brain tumor if you had difficulty with this question.

Level of Cognitive Ability: Application
Client Needs: Safe, Effective Care Environment
Integrated Process: Nursing Process/Planning
Content Area: Child Health

Reference:
McKinney, E., James, S., Murray, S., & Ashwill, J. (2005). *Maternal-child nursing* (2nd ed.). St. Louis: Elsevier, p. 1347.

---

78. A home care nurse provides instructions to the mother of a child with croup. The mother expresses concern regarding the occurrence of an acute spasmodic episode, and the nurse instructs the mother regarding management if an acute episode occurs. Which statement by the mother indicates a need for further instructions?
1 "I will place a steam vaporizer in my child's room."
2 "I will place my child in a closed bathroom and allow my child to inhale steam from warm running water."
3 "I will place a cool mist humidifier in my child's room."
4 "I will take my child outside to breathe the cool humid night air."

Answer: 1
Rationale: Steam from warm running water in a closed bathroom and cool mist from a bedside humidifier are effective in reducing mucosal edema. Cool mist humidifiers are recommended over steam vaporizers, which present a danger of scald burns. Taking the child outside to breathe the cool humid night air may also relieve mucosal swelling.

Test-Taking Strategy: Focus on the issue of the question: to reduce mucosal edema and to provide a safe environment. Also note the key words "need for further instructions." These key words indicate a false-response question and that you need to select the incorrect statement or unsafe action. Option 1 would provide an unsafe environment for the child. Review management of acute spasmodic croup if you had difficulty with this question.

Level of Cognitive Ability: Analysis
Client Needs: Safe, Effective Care Environment
Integrated Process: Teaching/Learning
Content Area: Child Health

Reference:
Wong, D., & Hockenberry, M. (2003). *Wong's nursing care of infants and children* (7th ed.). St. Louis: Mosby, p. 1364.

---

79. A nurse is reviewing the results of the rubella screening (titer) with a pregnant 24-year-old client. The test results are positive, and the mother asks if it is safe for her toddler to receive the vaccine. The appropriate nursing response is:
1 "You are still susceptible to rubella, so your toddler should receive the vaccine."
2 "Most children do not receive the vaccine until they are 5 years of age."
3 "It is not advised for children of pregnant women to be vaccinated during their mother's pregnancy."
4 "Your titer supports your immunity to rubella, and it is safe for your toddler to receive the vaccine at this time."

Answer: 4
Rationale: All pregnant women should be screened for prior rubella exposure during pregnancy. All children of pregnant women should receive their immunizations according to schedule. Additionally, no definitive evidence suggests that the rubella vaccine virus is transmitted from person to person. A positive maternal titer further indicates that a significant antibody titer has developed in response to a prior exposure to the rubivirus.

Test-Taking Strategy: Focus on the data in the question. Recalling that a positive titer indicates immunity will direct you to option 4. Review this important screening test if you had difficulty with this question.

Level of Cognitive Ability: Application
Client Needs: Safe, Effective Care Environment
Integrated Process: Nursing Process/Implementation
Content Area: Maternity/Antepartum

Reference:
Murray, S., McKinney, E., & Gorrie, T., (2002). *Foundations of maternal-newborn nursing* (3rd ed.). Philadelphia: Saunders, p. 145.

80. Following delivery, the postpartum nurse instructs the client with known cardiac disease to call for the nurse when she needs to get out of bed or when she plans to care for her newborn infant. The nurse informs the mother that this is necessary to:

1 Minimize the potential of postpartum hemorrhage

2 Help the mother assume the parenting role

3 Provide an opportunity for the nurse to teach newborn infant care techniques

4 Avoid maternal or infant injury caused by the potential for syncope or overexertion

Answer: 4

Rationale: The immediate postpartum period is associated with increased risks for the cardiac client. Hormonal changes and fluid shifts from extravascular tissues to the circulatory system cause additional stress on cardiac functioning. Although options 1, 2, and 3 are appropriate nursing concerns during the postpartum period, the primary concern for the cardiac client is to maintain a safe environment because of the potential for cardiac compromise.

Test-Taking Strategy: Focus on the issue of the question as it relates to safety, and use the process of elimination. Option 4 is the only option that relates directly to the issue of safety. Review the physiological manifestations that occur in a cardiac client following delivery and the need to implement safety precautions if you had difficulty with this question.

Level of Cognitive Ability: Application
Client Needs: Safe, Effective Care Environment
Integrated Process: Teaching/Learning
Content Area: Maternity/Postpartum

Reference:
Lowdermilk, D., & Perry, A. (2004). *Maternity & women's health care* (8th ed.). St. Louis: Mosby, p. 916.

81. A nurse is assessing a client who has just been measured and fitted for crutches. The nurse determines that the client's crutches are fitted correctly if:

1 The elbow is at a 30-degree angle when the hand is on the handgrip.

2 The elbow is straight when the hand is on the handgrip.

3 The client's axilla is resting on the crutch pad during ambulation.

4 The top of the crutch is even with the axilla.

Answer: 1

Rationale: For optimal upper extremity leverage, the elbow should be at approximately 30 degrees of flexion when the hand is resting on the handgrip. The top of the crutch needs to be two to three fingerwidths lower than the axilla. When crutch walking, all weight needs to be on the hands to prevent nerve palsy from pressure on the axilla.

Test-Taking Strategy: Use the process of elimination. Options 3 and 4 are similar and can be eliminated first. Visualize the mechanics of crutch walking to assist in selecting from the remaining options. If the weight should be resting on the hands, then there needs to be some flexion to push off from during ambulation. Review crutch walking and the safe and appropriate associated measures if you had difficulty with this question.

Level of Cognitive Ability: Analysis
Client Needs: Safe, Effective Care Environment
Integrated Process: Nursing Process/Evaluation
Content Area: Adult Health/Musculoskeletal

References:
Harkreader, H., & Hogan, M.A. (2004). *Fundamentals of nursing: Caring and clinical judgment* (2nd ed.). Philadelphia: Saunders, pp. 793-794.
Ignatavicius, D., & Workman, M. (2002). *Medical surgical nursing: Critical thinking for collaborative care* (4th ed.). Philadelphia: Saunders, p. 1140.

82. A physician has written an order for a vest restraint to be applied on a client from 10:00 PM to 7:00 AM because the client becomes disoriented during the night and is at risk for falls. At 11:00 PM, the charge nurse makes rounds on all of the clients in the unit. When assessing the client with the vest restraint, which observation by the charge nurse would indicate that the nurse who cared for this client performed an unsafe action in the use of the restraint?

1 A hitch knot was used to secure the restraint.

2 The client's record indicates that the restraint will be released every 2 hours.

3 The restraint was applied tightly.

4 The call light was placed within reach of the client.

Answer: 3

Rationale: Restraints should never be applied tightly because it could impair circulation. The restraint should be applied securely (not tightly) to prevent the client from slipping through the restraint and endangering him or herself. A hitch knot may be used on the client because it can easily be released in an emergency. Restraints, especially limb restraints, must be released every 2 hours (or per agency policy) to inspect the skin for abnormalities. The call light must always be within the client's reach in case the client needs assistance.

Test-Taking Strategy: Note the key word "unsafe" in the stem of the question. This key word indicates a false-response question and that you need to select the option that indicates an unsafe action. Noting the word "tightly" in option 3 will direct you to this option. Review the principles regarding the safe use of restraints if you had difficulty with this question.

Level of Cognitive Ability: Analysis
Client Needs: Safe, Effective Care Environment
Integrated Process: Nursing Process/Evaluation
Content Area: Leadership/Management

References:
Harkreader, H., & Hogan, M.A. (2004). *Fundamentals of nursing: Caring and clinical judgment* (2nd ed.). Philadelphia: Saunders, pp. 510-511.
Ignatavicius, D., & Workman, M. (2002). *Medical surgical nursing: Critical thinking for collaborative care* (4th ed.). Philadelphia: Saunders, pp. 40-41.

83. A nurse has documented an entry regarding client care in the client's medical record. When checking the entry, the nurse realizes that incorrect information was documented. How does the nurse correct the error?

1 Covers up the incorrect information completely using a black pen and writes in the correct information

2 Uses correction fluid to cover up the incorrect information and writes in the correct information

3 Erases the error and writes in the correct information

4 Draws one line to cross out the incorrect information and then initials the change

Answer: 4

Rationale: To correct an error documented in a medical record, the nurse draws one line through the incorrect information and then initials the error. An error is never erased and correction fluid is never used in a medical record.

Test-Taking Strategy: Focus on the issue: correcting an error documented in a medical record. Note that options 1, 2, and 3 are similar in that they all indicate complete covering up or eliminating the correct information. Review the principles of documentation if you are unfamiliar with them.

Level of Cognitive Ability: Application
Client Needs: Safe, Effective Care Environment
Integrated Process: Communication and Documentation
Content Area: Fundamental Skills

Reference:
Ignatavicius, D., & Workman, M. (2002). *Medical surgical nursing: Critical thinking for collaborative care* (4th ed.). Philadelphia: Saunders, p. 16.

84. A nurse is preparing to suction a client through a tracheostomy tube. Which protective items would the nurse wear to perform this procedure?
1 Gown, mask, and sterile gloves
2 Goggles, mask, and sterile gloves
3 Mask, gown, and a cap
4 Mask, sterile gloves, and a cap

Answer: 2

Rationale: The nurse should wear a mask and goggles when suctioning the client. Sterile gloves are also worn. A mask would offer full protection of the nurse's nose and mouth. Goggles would protect the nurse's eyes from getting splashed with sputum. A gown would protect the nurse's uniform, and a cap would protect the nurse's hair, but these items are not required for suctioning a client.

Test-Taking Strategy: Use the process of elimination. Visualize the suctioning procedure and the potential exposure of body fluids that this procedure could cause. This should direct you to option 2. Review standard precautions if you had difficulty with this question.

Level of Cognitive Ability: Application
Client Needs: Safe, Effective Care Environment
Integrated Process: Nursing Process/Implementation
Content Area: Fundamental Skills

References:
Harkreader, H., & Hogan, M.A. (2004). *Fundamentals of nursing: Caring and clinical judgment* (2nd ed.). Philadelphia: Saunders. p. 468.
Potter, P., & Perry, A. (2005). *Fundamentals of nursing* (6th ed.). St. Louis: Mosby, p. 797.

85. A nurse is instructing a client how to safely use crutches for ambulating at home. Which measure would the nurse recommend to minimize the risk of falls while ambulating with the crutches?
1 Use grab bars in the bath tub or shower
2 Remove scatter rugs in the home
3 Keep all pets out of the house
4 Use soft-soled slippers when walking with the crutches

Answer: 2

Rationale: To reduce the risk of falls, all obstacles should be removed from the home. Not all pets are trip hazards (e.g., fish, birds, guinea pigs). Grab bars in the bath tub or shower will not necessarily assist the client while walking with crutches. Shoes with nonslip soles should be worn.

Test-Taking Strategy: Focus on the issue "minimize the risk of falls." Use the process of elimination and principles related to safety measures. Eliminate option 3 first because of the word "all." Visualize the items identified in the remaining options to assist in directing you to option 2. Review home care measures related to safety and ambulation if you had difficulty with this question.

Level of Cognitive Ability: Application
Client Needs: Safe, Effective Care Environment
Integrated Process: Teaching/Learning
Content Area: Fundamental Skills

Reference:
Potter, P., & Perry, A. (2005). *Fundamentals of nursing* (6th ed.). St. Louis: Mosby, pp. 949; 979-980.

86. The nurse has observed that an older post-operative client has episodes of extreme agitation. Which nursing measure would be appropriate for the nurse to implement to avoid episodes of agitation?
1 Walk up behind the client and gently put a hand on the client's shoulder while speaking
2 Speak to the client at the entrance of the room to avoid any episodes of violence
3 Speak and move slowly toward the client while assessing the client's needs
4 Wait until the client's agitation has subsided before approaching the client

Answer: 3
Rationale: Speaking and moving slowly toward the client will prevent the client from becoming further agitated. Any sudden moves or speaking too quickly may cause the client to have a violent episode. Walking up behind the client may cause the client to become startled and react violently. Remaining at the entrance of the room may make the client feel alienated. If the client's agitation is not addressed, it will only increase. Therefore, waiting for the agitation to subside is not an appropriate option.

Test-Taking Strategy: Remember that one of the most basic principles in preventing episodes of agitation or violent episodes is to avoid further agitation. Remember to be empathetic to the client while avoiding actions that would startle the client. These principles will direct you to option 3. Review nursing interventions for the client who is agitated if you had difficulty with this question.

Level of Cognitive Ability: Application
Client Needs: Safe, Effective Care Environment
Integrated Process: Nursing Process/Implementation
Content Area: Fundamental Skills

Reference:
Lewis, S., Heitkemper, M., & Dirksen, S. (2004). *Medical-surgical nursing: Assessment and management of clinical problems* (6th ed.). St. Louis: Mosby, p. 1836.

87. A 17-year-old client is about to be discharged to home with her newborn baby, and the nurse provides information to the client about home safety for children. Which statement by the client would alert the nurse that further teaching is required regarding home safety?
1 "I have locks on all my cabinets that contain my cleaning supplies."
2 "I have a car seat that I will put in the front seat to keep my baby safe."
3 "I will not use the microwave oven to heat my baby's formula."
4 "I keep all my pots and pans in my lower cabinets."

Answer: 2
Rationale: A baby car seat should never be placed in the front seat because of the potential for injury on impact. Any cabinets that contain dangerous items that a baby or child could swallow should be locked. Microwave ovens should never be used to heat formula because the formula heats unevenly, and it could burn and even scald the baby's mouth. Even though the bottle may feel warm, it could contain hot spots that could severely damage the baby's mouth. It is perfectly safe to leave pots and pans in the lower cabinets for a child to investigate, as long as they are not made of glass, which would harm the baby if broken.

Test-Taking Strategy: Note the key words "further teaching is required." These key words indicate a false-response question and that you need to select the incorrect client statement. Remember that a baby car seat should never be placed in the front seat because of the potential for injury on impact. Review these safety principles if you had difficulty with this question.

Level of Cognitive Ability: Analysis
Client Needs: Safe, Effective Care Environment
Integrated Process: Teaching/Learning
Content Area: Child Health

Reference:
Wong, D., & Hockenberry, M. (2003). *Wong's nursing care of infants and children* (7th ed.). St. Louis: Mosby, p. 288.

88. A nurse has administered an injection to a client. After the injection, the nurse accidentally drops the syringe on the floor. Which nursing action is appropriate in this situation?
1 Carefully pick up the syringe from the floor and gently recap the needle
2 Carefully pick up the syringe from the floor and dispose of it in a sharps container
3 Obtain a dust pan and mop to sweep up the syringe
4 Call the housekeeping department to pick up the syringe

Answer: 2

Rationale: Syringes should never be recapped in any circumstances because of the risk of getting pricked with a contaminated needle. Used syringes should always be placed in a sharps container immediately after use to avoid individuals from getting injured. A syringe should not be swept up because this action poses an additional risk for getting pricked. It is not the responsibility of the housekeeping department to pick up the syringe.

Test-Taking Strategy: Use the process of elimination and basic principles related to the safe disposal of syringes to answer the question. Remember that a needle is never recapped and is always disposed of in a sharps container. Review these safety principles if you had difficulty with this question.

Level of Cognitive Ability: Application
Client Needs: Safe, Effective Care Environment
Integrated Process: Nursing Process/Implementation
Content Area: Fundamental Skills

Reference:
Potter, P., & Perry, A. (2005). *Fundamentals of nursing* (6th ed.). St. Louis: Mosby, p. 891.

---

89. A nurse is assigned to care for a client who is in traction. The nurse ensures a safe environment for the client by:
1 Monitoring the weights to be sure that they are resting on a firm surface
2 Checking the weights to be sure that they are off the floor
3 Making sure that the knots are at the pulleys
4 Making sure that the head of the bed is kept at a 90-degree angle

Answer: 2

Rationale: To achieve proper traction, weights need to be free-hanging with knots kept away from the pulleys. Weights are not to be kept resting on a firm surface. The head of the bed is usually kept low to provide countertraction.

Test-Taking Strategy: Use the process of elimination. Visualize the traction, recalling that there must be weight to exert the pull from the traction setup. This concept will assist in eliminating options 1 and 3. Recalling that countertraction is needed will assist in eliminating option 4. Review care of the client in traction if you had difficulty with this question.

Level of Cognitive Ability: Application
Client Needs: Safe, Effective Care Environment
Integrated Process: Nursing Process/Implementation
Content Area: Adult Health/Musculoskeletal

References:
Lewis, S., Heitkemper, M., & Dirksen, S. (2004). *Medical-surgical nursing: Assessment and management of clinical problems* (6th ed.). St. Louis: Mosby, pp. 1659-1661.
Phipps, W., Monahan, F., Sands, J., Marek, J., & Neighbors, M. (2003). *Medical-surgical nursing: Health and illness perspectives* (7th ed.). St. Louis: Mosby, p. 1480.

90. A nurse is observing a client using a walker. The nurse determines that the client is using the walker correctly if the client:
1 Puts all four points of the walker flat on the floor, puts weight on the hand pieces, and then walks into it
2 Puts weight on the hand pieces, moves the walker forward, and then walks into it
3 Puts weight on the hand pieces, slides the walker forward, and then walks into it
4 Walks into the walker, puts weight on the hand pieces, and then puts all four points of the walker flat on the floor

Answer: 1
Rationale: When the client uses a walker, the nurse stands adjacent to the affected side. The client is instructed to put all four points of the walker 2 feet forward flat on the floor before putting weight on the hand pieces. This will ensure client safety and prevent stress cracks in the walker. The client is then instructed to move the walker forward and walk into it.

Test-Taking Strategy: Visualize each of the options. Options 2 and 3 can be eliminated because putting weight on the hand pieces initially would cause an unsafe situation. From the remaining options, recalling that the walker is placed on all four points first will direct you to option 1. Review this procedure if you had difficulty with this question.

Level of Cognitive Ability: Analysis
Client Needs: Safe, Effective Care Environment
Integrated Process: Nursing Process/Evaluation
Content Area: Fundamental Skills

References:
Harkreader, H., & Hogan, M.A. (2004). *Fundamentals of nursing: Caring and clinical judgment* (2nd ed.). Philadelphia: Saunders, p. 792.
Ignatavicius, D., & Workman, M. (2002). *Medical surgical nursing: Critical thinking for collaborative care* (4th ed.). Philadelphia: Saunders, p. 1440.
Lewis, S., Heitkemper, M., & Dirksen, S. (2004). *Medical-surgical nursing: Assessment and management of clinical problems* (6th ed.). St. Louis: Mosby, p. 1670.

91. A client is fitted for crutches, and the nurse observes the client to evaluate for the correct height of the crutches. The nurse expects to note which of the following?
1 The client is able to rest the axillae on the axillary bars.
2 The nurse is able to place two fingers comfortably between the axillae and the axillary bars.
3 The client is able to maintain the arms in a straight position when standing with the crutches.
4 The nurse is able to place four fingers comfortably between the axillae and the axillary bars.

Answer: 2
Rationale: With the client's elbows flexed 20 to 30 degrees, the shoulders in a relaxed position, and the crutches placed approximately 15 cm (6 inches) anterolateral from the toes, the nurse should be able to place two fingers comfortably between the axillae and the axillary bars. The crutches are adjusted if there is too much or too little space at the axillary area. The client is advised never to rest the axillae on the axillary bars because this could injure the brachial plexus (the nerves in the axillae that supply the arm and shoulder area). The nurse should terminate ambulation and recheck the crutch height if the client complains of numbness or tingling in the hands or arms.

Test-Taking Strategy: Focus on the issue: correct height of crutches, and visualize each of the options. This will direct you to option 2, because the incorrect options are not reasonable and would not provide safety. Review this procedure if you had difficulty with this question.

Level of Cognitive Ability: Analysis
Client Needs: Safe, Effective Care Environment
Integrated Process: Nursing Process/Evaluation
Content Area: Fundamental Skills

Reference:
Potter, P., & Perry, A. (2005). *Fundamentals of nursing* (6th ed.). St. Louis: Mosby, pp. 949-950.

92. A nurse is caring for an adolescent client with conjunctivitis. The nurse provides instructions to the client and tells the adolescent to:
1 Avoid using all eye makeup to prevent possible reinfection
2 Apply warm compresses to decrease pain and lessen irritation
3 Obtain a new set of contact lenses for use after the infection clears
4 Stay home for 3 days after starting antibiotic eye drops to avoid the spread of infection

Answer: 3
Rationale: Eye makeup should be replaced but can still be worn. Cool compresses decrease pain and irritation. Isolation for 24 hours after antibiotics are initiated is necessary. A new set of contact lenses should be obtained.

Test-Taking Strategy: Use the process of elimination. Eliminate option 1 because of the absolute word "all." Recalling the principles related to the effectiveness of antibiotics will assist in eliminating option 4. From the remaining options, recalling the effects related to cool and warm compresses will direct you to option 3. Review home care instructions for the client with conjunctivitis if you had difficulty with this question.

Level of Cognitive Ability: Application
Client Needs: Safe, Effective Care Environment
Integrated Process: Teaching/Learning
Content Area: Child Health

Reference:
James, S., Ashwill, J., & Droske, S. (2002). *Nursing care of children: Principles & practice* (2nd ed.). Philadelphia: Saunders, p. 1048.

---

93. A client who has experienced a cerebrovascular accident has partial hemiplegia of the left leg. The straight-leg cane formerly used by the client is not sufficient to provide support. The nurse interprets that the client could benefit from the somewhat greater support and stability provided by a:
1 Quad-cane
2 Wooden crutch
3 Lofstrand crutch
4 Wheelchair

Answer: 1
Rationale: A quad-cane may be prescribed for the client who requires greater support and stability than is provided by a straight-leg cane. The quad-cane provides a four-point base of support and is indicated for use by clients with partial or complete hemiplegia. Neither crutches nor a wheelchair are indicated for use with a client such as described in this question. A Lofstrand crutch is useful for clients with bilateral weakness.

Test-Taking Strategy: Use the process of elimination. Providing a wheelchair to a client with partial hemiplegia is excessive and is eliminated first. Wooden crutches are not indicated, because there is no restriction in weight bearing. From the remaining options, recalling that a Lofstrand crutch is useful for bilateral weakness will direct you to option 1. Review the use of assistive devices for ambulation if you had difficulty with this question.

Level of Cognitive Ability: Analysis
Client Needs: Safe, Effective Care Environment
Integrated Process: Nursing Process/Assessment
Content Area: Adult Health/Neurological

Reference:
Potter, P., & Perry, A. (2005). *Fundamentals of nursing* (6th ed.). St. Louis: Mosby, p. 949.

94. A postoperative client begins to drain small amounts of bright red blood from the tracheostomy tube 24 hours after a laryngectomy. The best nursing action is to:
1 Notify the surgeon
2 Increase the frequency of suctioning
3 Add moisture to the oxygen delivery system
4 Document the character and amount of drainage

Answer: 1

Rationale: Immediately following laryngectomy, a small amount of bleeding occurs from the tracheostomy that resolves within the first few hours. Otherwise, bleeding that is bright red may be a sign of impending rupture of a vessel. The bleeding in this instance represents a potential life-threatening situation, and the surgeon is notified to further evaluate the client and suture or repair the bleed. The other options do not address the urgency of the problem. Failure to notify the surgeon places the client at risk.

Test-Taking Strategy: Note the key words "bright red blood" and "24 hours after." This should indicate that a potential complication exists and direct you to option 1. Review the complications following laryngectomy if you had difficulty with this question.

Level of Cognitive Ability: Application
Client Needs: Safe, Effective Care Environment
Integrated Process: Nursing Process/Implementation
Content Area: Adult Health/Respiratory

References:

Ignatavicius, D., & Workman, M. (2002). *Medical surgical nursing: Critical thinking for collaborative care* (4th ed.). Philadelphia: Saunders, p. 1668.
Lewis, S., Heitkemper, M., & Dirksen, S. (2004). *Medical-surgical nursing: Assessment and management of clinical problems* (6th ed.). St. Louis: Mosby, p. 586.
Potter, P., & Perry, A. (2005). *Fundamentals of nursing* (6th ed.). St. Louis: Mosby, p. 1116.

95. A client has a risk for infection following radical vulvectomy. The nurse avoids which of the following when giving perineal care to this client?
1 Cleanses using warm tap water
2 Intermittently exposes the wound to air
3 Provides perineal care after each voiding and bowel movement (BM)
4 Provides prescribed sitz baths after the sutures are removed

Answer: 1

Rationale: A sterile solution such as normal saline should be used for perineal care using an aseptic syringe or a water pick. This should be done regularly at least twice a day and after each voiding and BM. The wound is intermittently exposed to air to permit drying and prevent maceration. Once sutures are removed, sitz baths may be prescribed to stimulate healing and for the soothing effect.

Test-Taking Strategy: Note the key word "avoids." This key word indicates a false-response question and that you need to select the incorrect action. Focusing on the issue: risk for infection, using principles of asepsis, and noting the words "tap water" in option 1 will direct you to this option. Review these principles if you had difficulty with this question.

Level of Cognitive Ability: Application
Client Needs: Safe, Effective Care Environment
Integrated Process: Nursing Process/Implementation
Content Area: Fundamental Skills

References:

Ignatavicius, D., & Workman, M. (2002). *Medical surgical nursing: Critical thinking for collaborative care* (4th ed.). Philadelphia: Saunders, p. 1779.
Phipps, W., Monahan, F., Sands, J., Marek, J., & Neighbors, M. (2003). *Medical-surgical nursing: Health and illness perspectives* (7th ed.). St. Louis: Mosby, p. 1783.

96. A nurse prepares to assist a postoperative client to progress from a lying to a sitting position to prepare for ambulation. Which nursing action is appropriate to maintain the safety of the client?
1 Assist the client to move quickly from the lying position to the sitting position
2 Assess the client for signs of dizziness and hypotension
3 Elevate the head of the bed quickly to assist the client to a sitting position
4 Allow the client to rise from the bed to a standing position unassisted

Answer: 2
Rationale: Early ambulation should not exceed the client's tolerance. The client should be assessed before sitting. The client is assisted to rise from the lying position to the sitting position gradually until any evidence of dizziness, if present, has subsided. This position can be achieved by raising the head of the bed slowly. After sitting, the client may be assisted to a standing position. The nurse should be at the client's side to provide physical support and encouragement.

Test-Taking Strategy: Use the process of elimination. Eliminate options 1 and 3 because of the word "quickly" and option 4 because of the word "unassisted." Additionally, option 2 is the only option that reflects assessment, the first step of the nursing process. Review safety measures for ambulation if you had difficulty with this question.

Level of Cognitive Ability: Application
Client Needs: Safe, Effective Care Environment
Integrated Process: Nursing Process/Implementation
Content Area: Fundamental Skills

Reference:
Phipps, W., Monahan, F., Sands, J., Marek, J., & Neighbors, M. (2003). *Medical-surgical nursing: Health and illness perspectives* (7th ed.). St. Louis: Mosby, p. 446.

97. A client has an order for a stool culture. The nurse avoids doing which of the following when carrying out this order?
1 Wearing sterile gloves
2 Using a sterile container
3 Refrigerating the specimen
4 Sending the specimen directly to the laboratory

Answer: 3
Rationale: Storing a stool specimen for culture in a refrigerator is contraindicated because it can retard the growth of organisms. A stool specimen is obtained using sterile gloves and a sterile container. After obtaining the specimen, the stool is sent immediately to the laboratory.

Test-Taking Strategy: Note the key word "avoids." This key word indicates a false-response question and that you need to select the action that is incorrect. Recalling that a culture is done to identify organisms will assist you in determining that options 1, 2, and 4 must be carried out to ensure accuracy of results. Review this procedure if you had difficulty with this question.

Level of Cognitive Ability: Application
Client Needs: Safe, Effective Care Environment
Integrated Process: Nursing Process/Implementation
Content Area: Adult Health/Gastrointestinal

References:
Black, J., & Hawks, J. (2005). *Medical-surgical nursing: Clinical management for positive outcomes* (7th ed.). Philadelphia: Saunders, p. 783.
Chernecky, C., & Berger, B. (2004). *Laboratory tests and diagnostic procedures* (4th ed.). Philadelphia: Saunders, p. 1023.

98. A client is being transferred to the nursing unit from the postanesthesia care unit following spinal fusion with rod insertion. The nurse prepares to transfer the client from the stretcher to the bed by using:

1 A bath blanket and the assistance of three people
2 A bath blanket and the assistance of four people
3 A transfer board and the assistance of two people
4 A transfer board and the assistance of four people

Answer: 4

Rationale: Following spinal fusion, with or without instrumentation, the client is transferred from the stretcher to the bed using a transfer board and the assistance of four people. This permits optimal stabilization and support of the spine, while allowing the client to be moved smoothly and gently.

Test-Taking Strategy: Use the process of elimination. Think about the level of comfort and stability provided to the client's spine with the amounts of assistance given in each option. Using this approach will assist in eliminating options 1, 2, and 3. Review care of the client following spinal fusion with rod insertion if you had difficulty with this question.

Level of Cognitive Ability: Application
Client Needs: Safe, Effective Care Environment
Integrated Process: Nursing Process/Planning
Content Area: Adult Health/Neurological

References:
Black, J., & Hawks, J. (2005). *Medical-surgical nursing: Clinical management for positive outcomes* (7th ed.). Philadelphia: Saunders, pp. 2144; 2146-2147.
Potter, P., & Perry, A. (2005). *Fundamentals of nursing* (6th ed.). St. Louis: Mosby, pp. 1472; 1475.

---

99. A nurse is preparing to nasotracheally suction a client with acquired immunodeficiency syndrome (AIDS) who has had blood-tinged sputum with previous suctioning. The nurse plans to use which of the following items as part of standard precautions for this client?

1 Gloves, mask, and protective eyewear
2 Gloves, gown, and mask
3 Gown, mask, and protective eyewear
4 Gloves, gown, and protective eyewear

Answer: 1

Rationale: Standard precautions include the use of gloves whenever there is actual or potential contact with blood or body fluids. During procedures that aerosolize blood, the nurse wears a mask and protective eyewear or a face shield. Impervious gowns are worn in those instances when it is anticipated that there will be contact with a large amount of blood.

Test-Taking Strategy: Focus on the data in the question. Note the issue, suctioning, so expect airborne secretions and possibly airborne particles of blood with this procedure. This will direct you to the option that includes a mask, protective eyewear, and gloves. Review standard precautions if you had difficulty this question.

Level of Cognitive Ability: Application
Client Needs: Safe, Effective Care Environment
Integrated Process: Nursing Process/Planning
Content Area: Adult Health/Immune

Reference:
Black, J., & Hawks, J. (2005). *Medical-surgical nursing: Clinical management for positive outcomes* (7th ed.). Philadelphia: Saunders, pp. 428-429.

100. A nurse is inserting an indwelling urinary catheter into a male client. As the catheter is inserted into the urethra, urine begins to flow into the tubing. At this point, the nurse:

1 Immediately inflates the balloon
2 Withdraws the catheter approximately 1 inch and inflates the balloon
3 Inserts the catheter until resistance is met and inflates the balloon
4 Inserts the catheter 2.5 to 5 cm and inflates the balloon

Answer: 4

Rationale: The catheter's balloon is behind the opening at the insertion tip. The catheter is inserted 2.5 to 5 cm after urine begins to flow in order to provide sufficient space to inflate the balloon. Inserting the catheter the extra distance will ensure that the balloon is inflated inside the bladder and not in the urethra. Inflating the balloon in the urethra could produce trauma. Options 1, 2, and 3 are incorrect actions.

Test-Taking Strategy: Visualize the procedure described in the question and the effects of each description in the options to direct you to option 4. Review the procedure for inserting a urinary catheter into a male if you had difficulty with this question.

Level of Cognitive Ability: Application
Client Needs: Safe, Effective Care Environment
Integrated Process: Nursing Process/Implementation
Content Area: Fundamental Skills

Reference:
Potter, P., & Perry, A. (2005). *Fundamentals of nursing* (6th ed.). St. Louis: Mosby, pp. 1356-1357.

---

101. A nurse is preparing to administer oxygen to a client who has chronic obstructive pulmonary disease (COPD) and is at risk for carbon dioxide narcosis. The nurse checks to see that the oxygen flow rate is prescribed at:

1 2 to 3 liters per minute
2 4 to 5 liters per minute
3 6 to 8 liters per minute
4 8 to 10 liters per minute

Answer: 1

Rationale: In carbon dioxide narcosis, the central chemoreceptors lose their sensitivity to increased levels of carbon dioxide and no longer respond by increasing the rate and depth of respiration. For these clients, the stimulus to breathe is a decreased arterial oxygen concentration. In the client with COPD, a low arterial oxygen level is the client's primary drive for breathing. If oxygen is given too freely, the client loses the respiratory drive, and respiratory failure results. Thus, the nurse checks the flow of oxygen to see that it does not exceed 2 to 3 liters per minute.

Test-Taking Strategy: Focus on the client's diagnosis. Recalling the pathophysiology that occurs in COPD and that a low arterial oxygen level is the client's primary drive for breathing will direct you to option 1, the lowest oxygen liter flow. Review the concerns related to the administration of oxygen to a client with COPD if you had difficulty with this question.

Level of Cognitive Ability: Application
Client Needs: Safe, Effective Care Environment
Integrated Process: Nursing Process/Implementation
Content Area: Adult Health/Respiratory

References:
Ignatavicius, D., & Workman, M. (2002). *Medical surgical nursing: Critical thinking for collaborative care* (4th ed.). Philadelphia: Saunders, pp. 490; 545.
Lewis, S., Heitkemper, M., & Dirksen, S. (2004). *Medical-surgical nursing: Assessment and management of clinical problems* (6th ed.). St. Louis: Mosby, pp. 670; 1833.

102. A client undergoes a subtotal thyroidectomy. The nurse ensures that which priority item is at the client's bedside upon arrival from the operating room?

1 An apnea monitor
2 A blood transfusion warmer
3 A suction unit and oxygen
4 An ampule of phytonadione (Vitamin K)

Answer: 3

Rationale: Following thyroidectomy, respiratory distress can occur from tetany, tissue swelling, or hemorrhage. It is important to have oxygen and suction equipment readily available and in working order if such an emergency were to arise. Apnea is not a problem associated with thyroidectomy, unless the client experienced a respiratory arrest. Blood transfusions can be administered without a warmer if necessary. Vitamin K would not be administered for a client who is hemorrhaging, unless deficiencies in clotting factors warrant its administration.

Test-Taking Strategy: Recall the anatomic location of the thyroid gland and its proximity to the trachea. Use the ABCs—airway, breathing, and circulation—to direct you to option 3. Review postoperative care following thyroidectomy if you had difficulty with this question.

Level of Cognitive Ability: Application
Client Needs: Safe, Effective Care Environment
Integrated Process: Nursing Process/Planning
Content Area: Adult Health/Endocrine

Reference:
Ignatavicius, D., & Workman, M. (2002). *Medical surgical nursing: Critical thinking for collaborative care* (4th ed.). Philadelphia: Saunders, p. 1429.

---

103. A nurse places a hospitalized client with active tuberculosis in a private, well-ventilated isolation room. In addition, which critical action(s) should the nurse take before entering the client's room?

1 Wash the hands
2 Wash the hands and place a high-efficiency particulate air (HEPA) respirator over the nose and mouth
3 The nurse needs no special precautions, but the client is instructed to cover his or her mouth and nose when coughing or sneezing.
4 Wash the hands and wear a gown and gloves

Answer: 2

Rationale: The nurse wears a HEPA respirator when caring for a client with active tuberculosis. Hands are always thoroughly washed before and after caring for the client. Option 1 is an incomplete action. Option 3 is an incorrect statement. Option 4 is also inaccurate and incomplete. Gowning is only indicated when there is a possibility of contaminating clothing.

Test-Taking Strategy: Use the process of elimination. Noting the client's diagnosis and recalling the need for respiratory precautions will direct you to option 2. Review these respiratory isolation precautions if you had difficulty with this question.

Level of Cognitive Ability: Application
Client Needs: Safe, Effective Care and Environment
Integrated Process: Nursing Process/Implementation
Content Area: Adult Health/Respiratory

Reference:
Ignatavicius, D., & Workman, M. (2002). *Medical surgical nursing: Critical thinking for collaborative care* (4th ed.). Philadelphia: Saunders, p. 588.

104. A nurse is assigned to care for a hospitalized toddler. The nurse plans care knowing that the highest priority should be directed toward:
1 Protecting the toddler from injury
2 Adapting the toddler to the hospital routine
3 Allowing the toddler to participate in play and divisional activities
4 Providing a consistent caregiver

Answer: 1

Rationale: The toddler is at high risk for injury as a result of developmental abilities and an unfamiliar environment. While adaptation, diversion, and consistency are important, protection from injury is the highest priority.

Test-Taking Strategy: Note the key words "highest priority." Use Maslow's hierarchy of needs theory. Physiological needs come first, followed by safety. Because no physiological needs are addressed, the safety option of preventing injury takes priority. Review care of the hospitalized toddler if you had difficulty with this question.

Level of Cognitive Ability: Application
Client Needs: Safe, Effective Care Environment
Integrated Process: Nursing Process/Planning
Content Area: Child Health

Reference:
James, S., Ashwill, J., & Droske, S. (2002). *Nursing care of children: Principles & practice* (2nd ed.). Philadelphia: Saunders, p. 315.

105. A client is to undergo pleural biopsy at the bedside. Knowing the potential complications of the procedure, the nurse plans to have which of the following items available at the bedside?
1 Chest tube and drainage system
2 Intubation tray
3 Portable chest X-ray machine
4 Morphine sulfate injection

Answer: 1

Rationale: Complications following pleural biopsy include hemothorax, pneumothorax, and temporary pain from intercostal nerve injury. The nurse has a chest tube and drainage system available at the bedside for use if hemothorax or pneumothorax develops. An intubation tray is not indicated. The client should be premedicated before the procedure, or a local anesthetic is used. A portable chest X-ray machine would be called for to verify placement of a chest tube if one was inserted, but it is unnecessary to have at the bedside before the procedure.

Test-Taking Strategy: Note that the client is having a pleural biopsy. Recalling the complications of this procedure and noting the relation of this procedure to option 1 will direct you to this option. Review this procedure and its complications if you had difficulty with this question.

Level of Cognitive Ability: Application
Client Needs: Safe, Effective Care Environment
Integrated Process: Nursing Process/Planning
Content Area: Adult Health/Respiratory

Reference:
Black, J., & Hawks, J. (2005). *Medical-surgical nursing: Clinical management for positive outcomes* (7th ed.). Philadelphia: Saunders, p. 1773.

106. A nurse manager of a hemodialysis unit is observing a new nurse preparing to begin hemodialysis on a client with renal failure. The nurse manager intervenes if the new nurse planned to:

1 Put on a mask and gives one to the client to wear during connection to the machine
2 Wears full protective clothing such as goggles, mask, apron, and gloves
3 Covers the connection site with a bath blanket to enhance extremity warmth
4 Uses sterile technique for needle insertion

Answer: 3

Rationale: Infection is a major concern with hemodialysis. For that reason, the use of sterile technique and the application of a face mask for both the nurse and client are extremely important. It is also imperative that standard precautions be followed, which includes the use of goggles, mask, gloves, and an apron. The connection site should not be covered and it should be visible so that the nurse can assess for bleeding, ischemia, and infection at the site during the hemodialysis procedure.

Test-Taking Strategy: Note the key word "intervenes." This key word indicates a false-response question and that you need to select the option that indicates an incorrect nursing action. Eliminate options 1, 2, and 4 because they are similar in that they relate to infection control and standard precautions. Review the basic procedure related to hemodialysis if you had difficulty with this question.

Level of Cognitive Ability: Application
Client Needs: Safe, Effective Care Environment
Integrated Process: Nursing Process/Implementation
Content Area: Adult Health/Renal

Reference:
Phipps, W., Monahan, F., Sands, J., Marek, J., & Neighbors, M. (2003). *Medical-surgical nursing: Health and illness perspectives* (7th ed.). St. Louis: Mosby, p. 1269.

107. A nurse is going to suction an adult client with a tracheostomy who has copious amounts of respiratory secretions. The nurse does which of the following to perform this procedure safely?

1 Hyperoxygenates the client using a manual resuscitation bag
2 Sets the suction pressure range between 160 to 180 mm Hg
3 Occludes the Y-port of the suction catheter while advancing it into the tracheostomy
4 Applies continuous suction in the airway for up to 20 seconds

Answer: 1

Rationale: To perform suctioning, the nurse hyperoxygenates the client using a manual resuscitation bag or the sigh mechanism if the client is on a mechanical ventilator. The safe suction range for an adult is 100 to 120 mm Hg. The nurse advances the suction catheter into the tracheostomy without occluding the Y-port; suction is never applied while introducing the catheter because it would traumatize mucosa and remove oxygen from the respiratory tract. The nurse uses intermittent suction in the airway for up to 10 to 15 seconds.

Test-Taking Strategy: Use the process of elimination and visualize this procedure. Recalling that suction is applied intermittently and on catheter withdrawal only eliminates options 3 and 4. From the remaining options, use the ABCs—airway, breathing, and circulation—to direct you to option 1. Review this procedure if you had difficulty with this question.

Level of Cognitive Ability: Application
Client Needs: Safe, Effective Care Environment
Integrated Process: Nursing Process/Implementation
Content Area: Adult Health/Respiratory

Reference:
Potter, P., & Perry, A. (2005). *Fundamentals of nursing* (6th ed.). St. Louis: Mosby, p. 1106.

108. A nurse is collecting a sputum specimen for culture and sensitivity testing from a client who has a productive cough. The nurse plans to implement which intervention to obtain the specimen?
1 Ask the client to expectorate a small amount of sputum into the emesis basin
2 Ask the client to obtain the specimen after breakfast
3 Use a sterile plastic container for obtaining the specimen
4 Provide tissues for expectoration and obtaining the specimen

Answer: 3

Rationale: Sputum specimens for culture and sensitivity testing need to be obtained using sterile techniques because the test is done to determine the presence of organisms. If the procedure for obtaining the specimen is not sterile, then the specimen would be contaminated and the results of the test would be invalid. A first morning specimen is preferred because it represents overnight secretions of the tracheobronchial tree.

Test-Taking Strategy: Note the key words "culture and sensitivity." This tells you that the test is being done to identify the presence of microorganisms. Recalling that microorganisms will multiply in the specimen and that accurate identification of organisms is needed to determine treatment will direct you to option 3. Also noting the word "sterile" in option 3 will direct you to this option. Review the procedure for sputum collection if you had difficulty with this question.

Level of Cognitive Ability: Application
Client Needs: Safe, Effective Care Environment
Integrated Process: Nursing Process/Planning
Content Area: Fundamental Skills

Reference:
Chernecky, C., & Berger, B. (2004). *Laboratory tests and diagnostic procedures* (4th ed.). Philadelphia: Saunders, p. 1019.

109. The postmyocardial infarction client is scheduled for a technetium 99m ventriculography (multigated acquisition [MUGA] scan). The nurse ensures that which item is in place before the procedure?
1 Signed informed consent
2 Notation of allergies to iodine or shellfish
3 A central venous pressure (CVP) line
4 A Foley catheter

Answer: 1

Rationale: MUGA is a radionuclide study used to detect myocardial infarction, decreased myocardial blood flow, and left ventricular function. A radioisotope is injected intravenously. Therefore, a signed informed consent is necessary. The procedure does not use radiopaque dye. Therefore, allergies to iodine and shellfish is not a concern. A Foley catheter and CVP line are not required.

Test-Taking Strategy: Focus on the procedure. Recalling that the procedure involves injection of a radioisotope will direct you to option 1. Review preparation for this procedure if you had difficulty with this question.

Level of Cognitive Ability: Application
Client Needs: Safe, Effective Care Environment
Integrated Process: Nursing Process/Implementation
Content Area: Adult Health/Cardiovascular

References:
Black, J., & Hawks, J. (2005). *Medical-surgical nursing: Clinical management for positive outcomes* (7th ed.). Philadelphia: Saunders, pp. 1591-1592.
Chernecky, C., & Berger, B. (2004). *Laboratory tests and diagnostic procedures* (4th ed.). Philadelphia: Saunders, p. 1137.

110. A nurse is developing a nursing care plan for a client with severe Alzheimer's disease. The nurse identifies which nursing diagnosis as the priority?
1 Impaired verbal communication
2 Ineffective role performance
3 Risk for injury
4 Social isolation

Answer: 3
Rationale: Clients who have Alzheimer's disease have significant cognitive impairment and are therefore at risk for injury. It is critical for the nurse to maintain a safe environment, particularly as the client's judgment becomes increasingly impaired. Options 1, 2, and 4 may be appropriate, but the highest priority is directed toward safety.

Test-Taking Strategy: Use Maslow's hierarchy of needs theory. When a physiological need is not addressed, safety needs receive priority. Review care of the client with Alzheimer's disease if you had difficulty with this question.

Level of Cognitive Ability: Analysis
Client Needs: Safe, Effective Care Environment
Integrated Process: Nursing Process/Analysis
Content Area: Adult Health/Neurological

Reference:
Black, J., & Hawks, J. (2005). *Medical-surgical nursing: Clinical management for positive outcomes* (7th ed.). Philadelphia: Saunders, pp. 2168-2169.

111. A client with a diagnosis of recurrent major depression who is exhibiting psychotic behaviors is admitted to the psychiatric unit. In creating a safe environment for the client, the nurse most importantly develops a plan of care that deals specifically with the client's:
1 Disturbed thought processes
2 Imbalanced nutrition: less than body requirements
3 Bathing/hygiene self-care deficit
4 Deficient knowledge

Answer: 1
Rationale: Major depression, recurrent, with psychotic behaviors alerts the nurse that in addition to the criteria that designate the diagnosis of major depression, one must also deal with a client's psychosis. *Psychosis* is defined as a state in which a person's mental capacity to recognize reality and communicate and relate to others is impaired, thus interfering with the person's capacity to deal with life's demands. Disturbed thought processes generally indicates a state of increased anxiety in which hallucinations and delusions prevail. Although options 2 and 3 are important, option 1 is specific to the client. Option 4 is not a priority at this time.

Test-Taking Strategy: Focus on the client's diagnosis and the key word "specifically." Recall that the client with psychotic behavior experiences disturbed thought processes, such as hallucinations and delusions, and that disturbed thought processes present a risk related to safety. Review care of the client with major depression and psychosis if you had difficulty with this question.

Level of Cognitive Ability: Analysis
Client Needs: Safe, Effective Care Environment
Integrated Process: Nursing Process/Analysis
Content Area: Mental Health

Reference:
Fortinash, K., & Holoday-Worret, P. (2004) *Psychiatric mental health nursing* (3rd ed.). St. Louis: Mosby, p. 458.

112. A client is being admitted to the hospital after receiving a radium implant for cervical cancer. The nurse takes which priority action in the care of this client?
1 Encourages the client to take frequent rest periods
2 Admits the client to a private room
3 Encourages the family to visit
4 Places the client on reverse isolation

Answer: 2

Rationale: The client who has a radiation implant is placed in a private room and has limited visitors. This reduces the exposure of others to the radiation. Frequent rest periods are a helpful general intervention but are not a priority for the client in this situation. Reverse isolation is unnecessary.

Test-Taking Strategy: Note the key word "priority" and focus on the issue: radiation implant. Recalling the concepts related to environmental safety and that other individuals should have limited exposure to clients with radium implants will direct you to option 2. Review care of the client with a radiation implant if you had difficulty with this question.

Level of Cognitive Ability: Application
Client Needs: Safe, Effective Care Environment
Integrated Process: Nursing Process/Implementation
Content Area: Adult Health/Oncology

Reference:
Black, J., & Hawks, J. (2005). *Medical-surgical nursing: Clinical management for positive outcomes* (7th ed.). Philadelphia: Saunders, p. 363.

---

113. A client is to undergo weekly intravesical chemotherapy for bladder cancer for the next 8 weeks. The nurse interprets that the client understands how to manage the urine as a biohazard if the client states to:
1 Disinfect the urine and toilet with bleach for 6 hours following a treatment
2 Have one bathroom strictly set aside for the client's use for the next 8 weeks
3 Purchase extra bottles of scented disinfectant for daily bathroom cleansing
4 Void into a bedpan and then empty the urine into the toilet

Answer: 1

Rationale: After intravesical chemotherapy, the client treats the urine as a biohazard. This involves disinfecting the urine and the toilet with household bleach for 6 hours following a treatment. Scented disinfectants are of no particular use. The client does not need to have a separate bathroom for personal use. There is no value in using a bedpan for voiding.

Test-Taking Strategy: Use the process of elimination. Option 4 makes no sense and is eliminated first. Because scented disinfectants have no value, option 3 is eliminated next. Knowing that the urine and toilet needs special treatment for 6 hours after each treatment directs you to option 1. Also, option 2 is unnecessary and may be unrealistic for many clients. Review care of the client receiving intravesical chemotherapy if you had difficulty with this question.

Level of Cognitive Ability: Analysis
Client Needs: Safe, Effective Care Environment
Integrated Process: Teaching/Learning
Content Area: Adult Health/Oncology

Reference:
Black, J., & Hawks, J. (2005). *Medical-surgical nursing: Clinical management for positive outcomes* (7th ed.). Philadelphia: Saunders, p. 871.

114. A male client who is admitted to the hospital for an unrelated medical problem is diagnosed with urethritis caused by chlamydial infection. The nursing assistant assigned to the client asks the nurse what measures are necessary to prevent contraction of the infection during care. The nurse tells the nursing assistant that:
  1 Enteric precautions should be instituted for the client.
  2 Contact isolation should be initiated, because the disease is highly contagious.
  3 Standard precautions are sufficient, because the disease is transmitted sexually.
  4 Gloves and mask should be used when in the client's room.

Answer: 3
Rationale: Chlamydia is a sexually transmitted disease and is frequently called nongonococcal urethritis in the male client. It requires no special precautions other than standard precautions. Caregivers cannot acquire the disease during administration of care, and standard precautions are the only measure that needs to be used.

Test-Taking Strategy: Use the process of elimination. Recall that this infection is sexually transmitted. Also, note that option 3 is the umbrella (global) option. Review transmission of this disorder and standard precautions if you had difficulty with this question.

Level of Cognitive Ability: Application
Client Needs: Safe, Effective Care Environment
Integrated Process: Teaching/Learning
Content Area: Leadership/Management

References:
Black, J., & Hawks, J. (2005). *Medical-surgical nursing: Clinical management for positive outcomes* (7th ed.). Philadelphia: Saunders, p. 1131.
Lewis, S., Heitkemper, M., & Dirksen, S. (2004). *Medical-surgical nursing: Assessment and management of clinical problems* (6th ed.). St. Louis: Mosby, pp. 222; 1390.
Potter, P., & Perry, A. (2005). *Fundamentals of nursing* (6th ed.). St. Louis: Mosby, p. 797.

115. A client is in extreme pain from scrotal swelling that is caused by epididymitis. The nurse administers a subcutaneous narcotic analgesic in the left arm to relieve the pain. After administering the subcutaneous injection, the nurse takes which action next?
  1 Tells the client to do range of motion (ROM) exercises with the left arm to absorb the medication into the bloodstream
  2 Checks the name bracelet of the client
  3 Puts the side rails up on the bed
  4 Dims the lights in the room

Answer: 3
Rationale: The client who receives a narcotic analgesic should immediately have the side rails raised on the bed to prevent injury once the medication has taken effect. Dimming the light in the room is the next most helpful action. The name bracelet should have been checked before administering the medication. It is unnecessary to do ROM exercises at the site of injection.

Test-Taking Strategy: Use the process of elimination. Eliminate option 2 first because this should have been done before administering the medication. Option 1 is not necessary and is eliminated next. From the remaining options, note the key word "next" to direct you to option 3. As part of protecting the client's safety after administration of a narcotic analgesic, you would put the side rails up. Review nursing interventions when administering a narcotic analgesic if you had difficulty with this question.

Level of Cognitive Ability: Application
Client Needs: Safe, Effective Care Environment
Integrated Process: Nursing Process/Implementation
Content Area: Pharmacology

References:
Kee, J., & Hayes, E. (2003). *Pharmacology: A nursing process approach* (4th ed.). Philadelphia: Saunders, p. 271.
McKenry, L., & Salerno, E. (2003). *Mosby's pharmacology in nursing* (21st ed.). St. Louis: Mosby, p. 363.

116. A nurse is preparing the client's morning NPH insulin dose and notices a clumpy precipitate inside the insulin vial. The nurse should:
1 Draw up and administer the dose
2 Shake the vial in an attempt to disperse the clumps
3 Draw the dose from a new vial
4 Warm the bottle under running water to dissolve the clump

Answer: 3
Rationale: The nurse should always inspect the vial of insulin before use for solution changes that may signify loss of potency. NPH insulin is normally uniformly cloudy. Clumping, frosting, and precipitates are signs of insulin damage. In this situation, because potency is questionable, it is safer to discard the vial and draw up the dose from a new vial.

Test-Taking Strategy: Remember that NPH insulin is cloudy but not clumpy. This will direct you to option 3, the safest action. Remember: when in doubt, throw it out. Review the characteristics of NPH insulin if you had difficulty with this question.

Level of Cognitive Ability: Application
Client Needs: Safe, Effective Care Environment
Integrated Process: Nursing Process/Implementation
Content Area: Pharmacology

Reference:
Lehne, R. (2004). *Pharmacology for nursing care* (5th ed.). Philadelphia: Saunders, pp. 604; 616.

---

117. A nurse is preparing the bedside for a postoperative parathyroidectomy client who is expected to return to the nursing unit from the recovery room in 1 hour. The nurse ensures that which piece of medical equipment is at the client's bedside?
1 Underwater seal chest drainage
2 Tracheotomy set
3 Intermittent gastric suction
4 Cardiac monitor

Answer: 2
Rationale: Respiratory distress caused by hemorrhage and swelling and compression of the trachea is a primary concern for the nurse managing the care of a postoperative parathyroidectomy client. An emergency tracheotomy set is always routinely placed at the bedside of the client with this type of surgery, in anticipation of this potential complication. Options 1, 3, and 4 are not specifically needed with the surgical procedure.

Test-Taking Strategy: Use the process of elimination. Think about the location of the surgical incision and what potential problems might occur from that location. This will direct you to option 2. Review postoperative care following parathyroidectomy if you had difficulty with this question.

Level of Cognitive Ability: Application
Client Needs: Safe, Effective Care Environment
Integrated Process: Nursing Process/Planning
Content Area: Adult Health/Endocrine

Reference:
Ignatavicius, D., & Workman, M. (2002). *Medical surgical nursing: Critical thinking for collaborative care* (4th ed.). Philadelphia: Saunders, p. 1438.

118. A nurse has an order to administer foscarnet (Foscavir) intravenously to a client with acquired immunodeficiency syndrome (AIDS). Before administering this medication, the nurse plans to:
1 Place the solution on a controlled infusion pump
2 Obtain folic acid (Folvite) as an antidote
3 Ensure that liver enzyme levels have been drawn as a baseline
4 Obtain a sputum culture

Answer: 1

Rationale: Foscarnet is an antiviral agent used to treat cytomegalovirus (CMV) retinitis in clients with AIDS. Because of the potential toxicity of the medication, it is administered with the use of a controlled infusion device. It is highly toxic to the kidneys, and serum creatinine levels are measured frequently during therapy. Folic acid is not an antidote. A sputum culture is not necessary.

Test-Taking Strategy: Use the process of elimination. Eliminate option 4 because the medication is usually indicated in the treatment of CMV retinitis, not respiratory infection. Additionally, no data in the question indicates the need for a sputum culture. Option 2 is eliminated next, because folic acid is not an antidote. From the remaining options, it is necessary to know that the medication can be toxic and cannot be infused too quickly. This will direct you to option 1. Also, recalling that the medication is toxic to the kidneys, not the liver, will direct you to the correct option. Review this medication if you had difficulty with this question.

Level of Cognitive Ability: Application
Client Needs: Safe, Effective Care Environment
Integrated Process: Nursing Process/Planning
Content Area: Adult Health/Immune

Reference:
McKenry, L., & Salerno, E. (2003). *Mosby's pharmacology in nursing* (21st ed.). St. Louis: Mosby, p. 1027.

---

119. A client who is scheduled for gallbladder surgery is mentally impaired and is unable to communicate. With regard to obtaining permission for the surgical procedure, which nursing intervention would be appropriate?
1 Ensure that the family has signed the informed consent
2 Ensure that the client has signed the informed consent
3 Inform the family about the advanced directive process
4 Inform the family about the process of a living will

Answer: 1

Rationale: A client must be alert, able to communicate, and competent to sign an informed consent. If the client is unable to, then the family can sign the consent. A living will lists the medical treatment a person chooses to omit or refuse if the person becomes unable to make decisions and is terminally ill. Advanced directives are forms of communication in which persons can give direction on how they would like to be treated when they cannot speak for themselves.

Test-Taking Strategy: Focus on the issue: obtaining permission for the surgical procedure. Recalling that an informed consent is required will eliminate options 3 and 4. From the remaining options, noting the words "mentally impaired" in the question will direct you to option 1. Review the process of informed consent if you had difficulty with this question.

Level of Cognitive Ability: Application
Client Needs: Safe, Effective Care Environment
Integrated Process: Nursing Process/Implementation
Content Area: Fundamental Skills

Reference:
Potter, P., & Perry, A. (2005). *Fundamentals of nursing* (6th ed.). St. Louis: Mosby, pp. 416-417.

120. A client diagnosed with tuberculosis (TB) is scheduled to go to the radiology department for a chest X-ray. Which nursing intervention would be appropriate when preparing to transport the client?
1 Apply a mask to the client
2 Apply a mask and gown to the client
3 Apply a mask, gown, and gloves to the client
4 Notify the X-ray department so that the personnel can be sure to wear a mask when the client arrives

Answer: 1
Rationale: Clients known or suspected of having TB should wear a mask when out of the hospital room to prevent the spread of the infection to others. A gown or gloves are not necessary.

Test-Taking Strategy: Use the process of elimination. Recalling that the route of transmission of TB is airborne will direct you to option 1. Review the transmission associated with TB if you had difficulty with this question.

Level of Cognitive Ability: Application
Client Needs: Safe, Effective Care Environment
Integrated Process: Nursing Process/Implementation
Content Area: Fundamental Skills

Reference:
Potter, P., & Perry, A. (2005). *Fundamentals of nursing* (6th ed.). St. Louis: Mosby, pp. 788; 797.

121. A registered nurse (RN) is planning the assignments for the day and has a licensed practical nurse (LPN) and a nursing assistant (NA) working on the team. The nurse assigns which client to the LPN?
1 Client with dementia
2 A one-day postoperative mastectomy client
3 A client who requires some assistance with bathing
4 A client who requires some assistance with ambulation

Answer: 2
Rationale: Assignment of tasks needs to be implemented based on the job description of the LPN and NA, the level of education and clinical competence, and state law. The one-day postoperative mastectomy client will need care that requires the skill of a licensed nurse. The nursing assistant has the skills to care for a client with dementia, a client who requires some assistance with bathing, and a client who requires some assistance with ambulation.

Test-Taking Strategy: Focus on the clients identified in the options and the job description and level of education of the LPN and NA. Think about the needs of each client to assist in determining the assignment. Remember that the LPN will be performing at a higher skill level than the NA. Review the principles associated with delegating and assignment making if you had difficulty with this question.

Level of Cognitive Ability: Application
Client Needs: Safe, Effective Care Environment
Integrated Process: Nursing Process/Planning
Content Area: Delegating/Prioritizing

Reference:
Potter, P., & Perry, A. (2005). *Fundamentals of nursing* (6th ed.). St. Louis: Mosby, pp. 42; 378-379; 418.

122. A client requests pain medication and the nurse administers an intramuscular injection. After administration of the injection, the nurse does which of the following first?
1 Massages the injection site
2 Removes the gloves
3 Washes the hands
4 Places the syringe in the puncture-resistant needle box container

Answer: 1
Rationale: Following administration of an intramuscular injection, the nurse would massage the site to assist in medication absorption. Then, the nurse assists the client to a comfortable position. The uncapped needle and syringe is discarded in a puncture-resistant container, gloves are removed, and the hands are washed. Of the options provided, the nurse would perform option 1 first.

Test-Taking Strategy: Note the key word "first." Visualize the procedure and read each option to identify the first action. Review this procedure if you had difficulty with this question.

Level of Cognitive Ability: Application
Client Needs: Safe, Effective Care Environment
Integrated Process: Nursing Process/Implementation
Content Area: Delegating/Prioritizing

Reference:
Potter, P., & Perry, A. (2005). *Fundamentals of nursing* (6th ed.). St. Louis: Mosby, pp. 891; 887.

---

123. A nurse is in the process of giving a client a bed bath. In the middle of the procedure, the unit secretary calls the nurse on the intercom to tell the nurse that there is an emergency phone call. The appropriate nursing action is to:
  1 Leave the client's door open so the client can be monitored and the nurse can answer the phone call
  2 Finish the bath before answering the phone call
  3 Immediately walk out of the client's room and answer the phone call
  4 Cover the client, place the call light within reach, and answer the phone call

Answer: 4
Rationale: Because the telephone call is an emergency, the nurse may need to answer it. The other appropriate action is to ask another nurse to accept the call. This, however, is not one of the options. To maintain privacy and safety, the nurse covers the client and places the call light within the client's reach. Additionally, the client's door should be closed or the room curtains pulled around the bathing area.

Test-Taking Strategy: Use the process of elimination. Noting the key words "emergency phone call" will assist in eliminating option 2. From the remaining options, recalling the rights of the client and the principles related to safety will direct you to option 4. Review these guidelines for care if you had difficulty with this question.

Level of Cognitive Ability: Application
Client Needs: Safe, Effective Care Environment
Integrated Process: Nursing Process/Implementation
Content Area: Fundamental Skills

Reference:
Potter, P., & Perry, A. (2005). *Fundamentals of nursing* (6th ed.). St. Louis: Mosby, p. 1030.

---

124. A nursing manager is reviewing the purpose for applying restraints to a client with the nursing staff. The nurse manager determines that further review is necessary if a nursing staff member states that which of the following is an indication for the use of a restraint?
  1 To be sure that the client remains in bed at nighttime
  2 To restrict movement of a limb
  3 To prevent the client from pulling out intravenous lines and catheters
  4 To prevent the violent client from injuring self and others

Answer: 1
Rationale: Restraints are devices used to restrict the client's movement in situations when it is necessary to immobilize a limb or other body part. They are applied to prevent the client from injuring self or others; from pulling out intravenous lines, catheters, or tubes; or from removing dressings. Restraints also may be used to keep children still and from injuring themselves during treatments and diagnostic procedures. Restraints are not applied to keep a client in bed at nighttime and should never be used as a form of punishment.

Test-Taking Strategy: Note the key words "further review is necessary." These words indicate a false-response question and that you need to select the option that identifies an inaccurate use for restraints. Eliminate options 2 and 3 first because they are similar. From the remaining options, read each option carefully. Recalling the guidelines for the use of restraints will direct you to option 1. Review these guidelines if you had difficulty with this question.

Level of Cognitive Ability: Application
Client Needs: Safe, Effective Care Environment
Integrated Process: Teaching/Learning
Content Area: Leadership/Management

Reference:
Potter, P., & Perry, A. (2005). *Fundamentals of nursing* (6th ed.). St. Louis: Mosby, pp. 411; 981.

---

125. A client has an order to receive valproic acid (Depakene) 250 mg once daily. To maximize the client's safety, the nurse schedules administration of the medication:
1 At bedtime
2 Before breakfast
3 With breakfast
4 With lunch

Answer: 1

Rationale: Valproic acid is an anticonvulsant that causes central nervous system (CNS) depression. For this reason, the side effects include sedation, dizziness, ataxia, and confusion. When the client is taking this medication as a single daily dose, administering it at bedtime negates the risk of injury from sedation and enhances client safety. Otherwise, it may be given after meals to avoid gastrointestinal upset.

Test-Taking Strategy: Note the key words "to maximize the client's safety." Recalling that this medication is an anticonvulsant with CNS depressant properties and that sedation is a side effect will direct you to option 1. Administration at bedtime allows the sedative effects of the medication to occur at a time when the client is sleeping. Also note that options 2, 3, and 4 are similar in that they indicate administering the medication with meals. Review the side effects of this medication if you had difficulty with this question.

Level of Cognitive Ability: Application
Client Needs: Safe, Effective Care Environment
Integrated Process: Nursing Process/Implementation
Content Area: Pharmacology

Reference:
McKenry, L., & Salerno, E. (2003). *Mosby's pharmacology in nursing* (21st ed.). St. Louis: Mosby, p. 375.

126. A client with an acute respiratory infection is admitted to the hospital with a diagnosis of sinus tachycardia. The nurse develops a plan of care for the client and includes which intervention?
  1 Providing the client with short, frequent walks
  2 Measuring the client's pulse once each shift
  3 Eliminating sources of caffeine from meal trays
  4 Limiting oral and intravenous fluids

Answer: 3

Rationale: Sinus tachycardia is often caused by fever, physical and emotional stress, heart failure, hypovolemia, certain medications, nicotine, caffeine, and exercise. Exercise and fluid restriction will not alleviate tachycardia. Measuring the client's pulse during each shift will not decrease the heart rate. Additionally, the pulse should be taken more frequently than once each shift.

Test-Taking Strategy: Use the process of elimination, focusing on the client's diagnosis. Recalling the causes of tachycardia will direct you to option 3. Remember that caffeine is a stimulant and will increase the heart rate. Review care of the client with tachycardia if you had difficulty with this question.

Level of Cognitive Ability: Application
Client Needs: Safe, Effective Care Environment
Integrated Process: Nursing Process/Planning
Content Area: Adult Health/Cardiovascular

Reference:
Black, J., & Hawks, J. (2005). *Medical-surgical nursing: Clinical management for positive outcomes* (7th ed.). Philadelphia: Saunders, pp. 1557; 1570.

---

127. A nurse has an order to obtain a urinalysis from a client with an indwelling urinary catheter. The nurse avoids which of the following, which could contaminate the specimen?
  1 Obtaining the specimen from the urinary drainage bag
  2 Clamping the tubing of the drainage bag
  3 Aspirating a sample from the port on the drainage bag
  4 Wiping the port with an alcohol swab before inserting the syringe

Answer: 1

Rationale: A urine specimen is not taken from the urinary drainage bag. Urine undergoes chemical changes while sitting in the bag and does not necessarily reflect the current client status. In addition, it may become contaminated with bacteria from opening the system.

Test-Taking Strategy: Use the process of elimination, focusing on the issue of preventing contamination. Also note the key word "avoids." This key word indicates a false-response question and that you need to select an option that indicates an incorrect nursing action. Recalling basic principles of asepsis will direct you to option 1. Review this procedure if you had difficulty with this question.

Level of Cognitive Ability: Application
Client Needs: Safe, Effective Care Environment
Integrated Process: Nursing Process/Implementation
Content Area: Fundamental Skills

Reference:
Harkreader, H., & Hogan, M.A. (2004). *Fundamentals of nursing: Caring and clinical judgment* (2nd ed.). Philadelphia: Saunders, pp. 702-703.

128. A nursing assistant is caring for an older client with cystitis who has an indwelling urinary catheter. The registered nurse provides directions regarding urinary catheter care and ensures that the nursing assistant:
1 Uses soap and water to cleanse the perineal area
2 Keeps the drainage bag above the level of the bladder
3 Loops the tubing under the client's leg
4 Lets the drainage tubing rest under the leg

Answer: 1

Rationale: Proper care of an indwelling urinary catheter is especially important to prevent prolonged infection or reinfection in the client with cystitis. The perineal area is cleansed thoroughly using mild soap and water at least twice a day and following a bowel movement. The drainage bag is kept below the level of the bladder to prevent urine from being trapped in the bladder, and for the same reason, the drainage tubing is not placed or looped under the client's leg. The tubing must drain freely at all times.

Test-Taking Strategy: Use the process of elimination. Eliminate options 3 and 4 first because they are similar. From the remaining options, noting the word "above" in option 2 will assist in eliminating this option. Also, note that option 1 relates to preventing infection. Review care of the client with an indwelling urinary catheter if you had difficulty with this question.

Level of Cognitive Ability: Application
Client Needs: Safe, Effective Care Environment
Integrated Process: Teaching/Learning
Content Area: Leadership/Management

Reference:
Potter, P., & Perry, A. (2005). *Fundamentals of nursing* (6th ed.). St. Louis: Mosby, p. 1349.

129. A nurse is assigned to care for a woman with preeclampsia. The nurse plans to initiate which action to provide a safe environment?
1 Turn off the room lights and draw the window shades
2 Maintain fluid and sodium restrictions
3 Take the woman's vital signs every 4 hours
4 Encourage visits from family and friends for psychosocial support

Answer: 1

Rationale: Clients with preeclampsia are at risk of developing eclampsia (seizures). Bright lights and sudden loud noises may initiate seizures in this client. A woman with preeclampsia should be placed in a dimly lighted, quiet, private room. Visitors should be limited to allow for rest and prevent overstimulation. Clients with preeclampsia have decreased plasma volume, and adequate fluid and sodium intake is necessary to maintain fluid volume and tissue perfusion. Vital signs need to be monitored more frequently than every 4 hours when preeclampsia is present.

Test-Taking Strategy: Use the process of elimination. Eliminate option 4 because it is not a physiological need. Eliminate option 3 next because vital signs need to be monitored more frequently than every 4 hours. From the remaining options, knowing that seizures may be precipitated by sudden loud noises and bright lights will assist in directing you to option 1. Review care of the client with preeclampsia if you had difficulty with this question.

Level of Cognitive Ability: Application
Client's Needs: Safe, Effective Care Environment
Integrated Process: Nursing Process/Planning
Content Area: Maternity/Antepartum

Reference:
Lowdermilk, D., & Perry, A. (2004). *Maternity & women's health care* (8th ed.). St. Louis: Mosby, p. 852.

130. A client is scheduled for a bronchoscopy. The nurse plans to implement which priority measure?
  1 Restricting the diet to clear liquids on the day of the test
  2 Asking the client about allergies to shellfish
  3 Obtaining informed consent for an invasive procedure
  4 Administration of preprocedure antibiotics prophylactically

Answer: 3

Rationale: Bronchoscopy requires that informed consent be obtained from the client before the procedure. The client is kept NPO for at least 6 hours before the procedure. It is unnecessary to inquire about allergies to shellfish before this procedure, because contrast dye is not injected. There is also no need for prophylactic antibiotics.

Test-Taking Strategy: Use the process of elimination. Recalling that bronchoscopy is an invasive procedure and requires an informed consent will direct you to option 3. Review preprocedure preparation for bronchoscopy if you had difficulty with this question.

Level of Cognitive Ability: Application
Client Needs: Safe, Effective Care Environment
Integrated Process: Nursing Process/Planning
Content Area: Adult Health/Respiratory

Reference:
Chernecky, C., & Berger, B. (2004). *Laboratory tests and diagnostic procedures* (4th ed.). Philadelphia: Saunders, p. 297.

---

131. A nurse has given a subcutaneous injection to a client with acquired immunodeficiency syndrome (AIDS). The nurse disposes of the used needle and syringe by:
  1 Placing the uncapped needle and syringe in a labeled, rigid plastic container
  2 Recapping the needle and discarding the syringe in a disposal unit
  3 Breaking the needle before discarding it
  4 Placing the uncapped needle and syringe in a labeled cardboard box

Answer: 1

Rationale: Standard precautions include specific guidelines for handling of needles. Needles should not be recapped, bent, broken, or cut after use. They should be disposed of in a labeled, impermeable container specific for this purpose. Needles should not be discarded in cardboard boxes, because these type of boxes are not impervious. Needles should never be left lying around after use.

Test-Taking Strategy: Use the process of elimination and focus on the guidelines related to standard precautions. Recalling that a needle should never be recapped or broken will eliminate option 2 and 3. From the remaining options, noting the key words "rigid plastic container" in option 1 will direct you to this option. Review the principles related to needle disposal if you had difficulty with this question.

Level of Cognitive Ability: Application
Client Needs: Safe, Effective Care Environment
Integrated Process: Nursing Process/Implementation
Content Area: Adult Health/Immune

Reference:
Harkreader, H., & Hogan, M.A. (2004). *Fundamentals of nursing: Caring and clinical judgment* (2nd ed.). Philadelphia: Saunders, p. 469.

132. A nurse is planning care for a client with acute glomerulonephritis. The nurse instructs the nursing assistant to do which of the following in the care of the client?

1 Monitor the temperature every 2 hours
2 Remove the water pitcher from the bedside
3 Ambulate the client frequently
4 Encourage a diet that is high in protein

Answer: 2

Rationale: A client with acute glomerulonephritis commonly experiences fluid volume excess and fatigue. Interventions include fluid restriction, as well as monitoring weight and intake and output. The client may be placed on bed rest or at least encouraged to rest, because a direct correlation exists between proteinuria, hematuria, edema, and increased activity levels. The diet is high in calories but low in protein. It is unnecessary to monitor the temperature as frequently as every 2 hours.

Test-Taking Strategy: Use the process of elimination. The question provides no information about the client's actual temperature, so option 1 is eliminated first. Knowing that the client needs rest eliminates option 3. From the remaining options, it is necessary to know either that fluid is restricted or that protein is limited. Review interventions related to this condition if you had difficulty with this question.

Level of Cognitive Ability: Application
Client Needs: Safe, Effective Care Environment
Integrated Process: Teaching/Learning
Content Area: Leadership/Management

Reference:
Ignatavicius, D., & Workman, M. (2002). *Medical surgical nursing: Critical thinking for collaborative care* (4th ed.). Philadelphia: Saunders, p. 1652.

---

133. A nurse is caring for a client with a C-6 spinal cord injury during the spinal shock phase. The nurse implements which of the following when preparing the client to sit in a chair?

1 Teaches the client to lock the knees during the pivoting stage of the transfer
2 Administers a vasodilator in order to improve circulation of the lower limbs
3 Raises the head of the bed slowly to decrease orthostatic hypotensive episodes
4 Applies knee splints to stabilize the joints during transfer

Answer: 3

Rationale: Spinal shock is often accompanied by vasodilation in the lower limbs, which results in a fall in blood pressure upon rising. The client can have dizziness and feel faint. The nurse should provide for a gradual progression in head elevation while monitoring the blood pressure. A vasodilator would exacerbate the problem. Clients with cervical cord injuries cannot lock their knees, and the use of splints would impair the transfer.

Test-Taking Strategy: Use the process of elimination. Focusing on the client's diagnosis will assist in eliminating options 1 and 4. From the remaining options, recalling that spinal shock is accompanied by vasodilation will direct you to option 3. Review care of the client with spinal shock if you had difficulty with this question.

Level of Cognitive Ability: Application
Client Needs: Safe, Effective Care Environment
Integrated Process: Nursing Process/Implementation
Content Area: Adult Health/Neurological

Reference:
Black, J., & Hawks, J. (2005). *Medical-surgical nursing: Clinical management for positive outcomes* (7th ed.). Philadelphia: Saunders, p. 2215.

134. A nurse notes that a client's lithium level is 3.9 mEq/L. The nurse implements which priority intervention?
1 Determining visual acuity
2 Monitoring intake and output
3 Assisting with ambulation
4 Instituting seizure precautions

Answer: 4

Rationale: A therapeutic regimen is designed to attain a serum lithium level of 1.0 to 1.5 mEq/L during acute mania, and levels of 0.6 to 1.4 mEq/L for maintenance treatment. A level of 3.9 mEq/L is within the toxic range, and seizures may occur at levels of 3.5 mEq/L and higher. Options 1, 2, and 3 are appropriate interventions but are not the priority.

Test-Taking Strategy: Use the process of elimination. Focusing on the word "priority" and recalling the manifestations that occur in a toxic level will direct you to option 4. Review toxicity related to lithium and the manifestations that occur as a result of toxicity if you had difficulty with this question.

Level of Cognitive Ability: Application
Client Needs: Safe, Effective Care Environment
Integrated Process: Nursing Process/Implementation
Content Area: Pharmacology

References:
Chernecky, C., & Berger, B. (2001). *Laboratory tests and diagnostic procedures* (3rd ed.). Philadelphia: Saunders, p. 683.
Hodgson, B., & Kizior, R. (2004). *Saunders nursing drug handbook 2004.* Philadelphia: Saunders, p. 608.

135. A hospitalized client with a diagnosis of anorexia nervosa and in a state of starvation is in a two-bed hospital room. A newly admitted client will be assigned to this client's room. Which client would be inappropriate to assign to this two-bed room?
1 A client with pneumonia
2 A client with a fractured leg that is casted
3 A client who can care for self
4 A client who is scheduled for a diagnostic test

Answer: 1

Rationale: The client in a state of starvation has a compromised immune system. Having a roommate with pneumonia would place the client at risk for infection. Options 2, 3, and 4 are appropriate roommates.

Test-Taking Strategy: Note the client's diagnosis and the key words "in a state of starvation." Also note the key word "inappropriate." This key word indicates a false-response question and that you need to select the client who should not be assigned to the room of the client with anorexia nervosa. Thinking about the physiological risks for this client will direct you to option 1. Review care of the client with anorexia nervosa if you had difficulty with this question.

Level of Cognitive Ability: Application
Client Needs: Safe, Effective Care Environment
Integrated Process: Nursing Process/Implementation
Content Area: Leadership/Management

Reference:
Stuart, G., & Laraia, M. (2005). *Principles and practice of psychiatric nursing* (8th ed.). St. Louis: Mosby, p. 522.

136. A hospitalized child develops exanthema (rash) that covers the trunk and the extremities. The nurse reviews the child's health history and notes that the child was exposed to varicella 2 weeks ago. The appropriate nursing intervention is to:
1 Allow the child to play in the playroom until the physician can be contacted
2 Place the child in a private room on strict isolation
3 Immediately admit the client to any available bed
4 Assess the progression of the exanthema and report it to the physician

Answer: 2
Rationale: The child with undiagnosed exanthema needs to be placed on strict isolation. Varicella causes a profuse rash on the trunk with a sparse rash on the extremities. The incubation period is 14 to 21 days. It is important to prevent the spread of this communicable disease by placing the child in isolation until further diagnosis and treatment is made. Options 1 and 3 are inaccurate, and option 4 is not the most appropriate intervention.

Test-Taking Strategy: Use the process of elimination. Noting the key words "exposed to varicella" will direct you to option 2. This action will prevent exposure of this communicable disease to others. Review care of the child with varicella if you had difficulty with this question.

Level of Cognitive Ability: Application
Client Needs: Safe, Effective Care Environment
Integrated Process: Nursing Process/Implementation
Content Area: Child Health

Reference:
Wong, D., & Hockenberry, M. (2003). *Wong's nursing care of infants and children* (7th ed.). St. Louis: Mosby, pp. 653; 1092.

137. A nurse is observing a second nurse who is performing hemodialysis on a client. The second nurse is drinking coffee and eating a doughnut next to the hemodialysis machine while talking with the client about the events of the client's week. The first nurse should:
1 Appreciate what a wonderful therapeutic relationship this second nurse and client have
2 Get a cup of coffee and join in on the conversation
3 Ask the client if he would also like a cup of coffee
4 Ask the second nurse to refrain from eating and drinking in the client area

Answer: 4
Rationale: A potential complication of hemodialysis is the acquisition of dialysis-associated hepatitis B. This is a concern for clients (who may carry the virus), client families (at risk from contact with the client and with environmental surfaces), and staff (who may acquire the virus from contact with the client's blood). This risk is minimized by the use of standard precautions, appropriate handwashing and sterilization procedures, and the prohibition of eating, drinking, or other hand-to-mouth activity in the hemodialysis unit. The first nurse should ask the second nurse to stop eating and drinking in the client area.

Test-Taking Strategy: Use the process of elimination and the principles related to standard precautions to direct you to option 4. Review infection control measures related to the client receiving hemodialysis if you had difficulty with this question.

Level of Cognitive Ability: Application
Client Needs: Safe, Effective Care Environment
Integrated Process: Nursing Process/Implementation
Content Area: Leadership/Management

Reference:
Black, J., & Hawks, J. (2005). *Medical-surgical nursing: Clinical management for positive outcomes* (7th ed.). Philadelphia: Saunders, p. 959.

138. A nurse is caring for a client who is going to have an arthrogram using a contrast medium. Which preprocedure assessment would be of highest priority?
1 Allergy to iodine or shellfish
2 Ability of the client to remain still during the procedure
3 Whether the client has any remaining questions about the procedure
4 Whether the client wishes to void before the procedure

Answer: 1

Rationale: Because of the risk of allergy to contrast medium, the nurse places highest priority on assessing whether the client has an allergy to iodine or shellfish. The nurse also reinforces information about the test, tells the client about the need to remain still during the procedure, and encourages the client to void before the procedure for comfort.

Test-Taking Strategy: Note the key words "highest priority." This tells you that more than one or all of the options are correct. Although options 2, 3, and 4 all compete for priority, only option 1 presents a life-threatening situation. Review priority assessments of a client receiving a contrast medium if you had difficulty with this question.

Level of Cognitive Ability: Analysis
Client Needs: Safe, Effective Care Environment
Integrated Process: Nursing Process/Assessment
Content Area: Delegating/Prioritizing

Reference:
Chernecky, C., & Berger, B. (2004). *Laboratory tests and diagnostic procedures* (3rd ed.). Philadelphia: Saunders, p. 202.

---

139. A client with a possible rib fracture has never had a chest X-ray. The nurse plans to tell the client which of the following about the procedure?
1 The X-ray stimulates a small amount of pain
2 It is necessary to remove jewelry and any other metal objects from the chest area
3 The client will be asked to breathe in and out during the X-ray
4 The X-ray technologist will stand next to the client during the X-ray

Answer: 2

Rationale: An X-ray is a photographic image of a part of the body on a special film, which is used to diagnose a wide variety of conditions. The X-ray is painless and any discomfort would arise from repositioning a painful part for filming. The nurse may premedicate a client, if prescribed, who is at risk for pain. Any radiopaque objects such as jewelry or other metal must be removed from the chest area because they will interfere with the interpretation of the results. The client is asked to breathe in deeply and then hold the breath while the chest X-ray is taken. To minimize the risk of radiation exposure, the X-ray technologist stands in a separate area protected by a lead wall. The client also wears a lead shield over the reproductive organs.

Test-Taking Strategy: Note the name of the diagnostic procedure and the relation between the procedure and option 2. Remember that any radiopaque objects such as jewelry or other metal must be removed from the chest area because they will interfere with the interpretation of the chest X-ray results. Review the procedure for a chest X-ray if you had difficulty with this question.

Level of Cognitive Ability: Application
Client Needs: Safe, Effective Care Environment
Integrated Process: Nursing Process/Implementation
Content Area: Adult Health/Musculoskeletal

Reference:
Chernecky, C., & Berger, B. (2004). *Laboratory tests and diagnostic procedures* (4th ed.). Philadelphia: Saunders, p. 360.

140. A nurse is planning a discharge teaching plan for a client with a spinal cord injury. To provide for a safe environment regarding home care, which of the following would be the priority in the discharge teaching plan?
1 What the physician has indicated needs to be taught
2 Follow-up laboratory and diagnostic tests that need to be done
3 Assisting the client to deal with long-term care placement
4 Including the client's significant others in the teaching session

Answer: 4

Rationale: Involving the client's significant others in discharge teaching is a priority in planning for the client with a spinal cord injury. The client will need the support of the significant others. Knowledge and understanding of what to expect will help both the client and significant others deal with the client's limitations. A physician's order is not necessary for discharge planning and teaching; this is an independent nursing action. Laboratory and diagnostic testing are not priority discharge instructions for this client. Long-term placement is not the only option for a client with spinal cord injury.

Test-Taking Strategy: Use the process of elimination. Eliminate option 3 first because long-term placement is not the only option for a client with a spinal cord injury. Eliminate option 1 next because although the physician's orders need to be addressed, teaching is an independent nursing action. From the remaining options, focusing on the client's diagnosis will direct you to option 4. Remember, home care and support will be needed. Review care of the client with a spinal cord injury if you had difficulty with this question.

Level of Cognitive Ability: Application
Client Needs: Safe, Effective Care Environment
Integrated Process: Teaching/Learning
Content Area: Adult Health/Neurological

Reference:
Ignatavicius, D., & Workman, M. (2002). *Medical surgical nursing: Critical thinking for collaborative care* (4th ed.). Philadelphia: Saunders, p. 941.

141. A nurse observes a client wringing her hands and looking frightened. The client reports to the nurse that she "feels out of control." Which approach by the nurse is most appropriate to maintain a safe environment?
1 Administer the prescribed prn antianxiety medication immediately
2 Move the client to a quiet room and talk about her feelings
3 Isolate the client in a "time-out" room
4 Observe the client in an ongoing manner but do not intervene

Answer: 2

Rationale: The anxiety symptoms demonstrated by this client require some form of intervention. Moving the client to a quiet room decreases environmental stimulus. Talking provides the nurse an opportunity to assess the cause of the client's feelings and to identify appropriate interventions. Isolation is appropriate if a client is a danger to self or others. Medication is used only when other noninvasive approaches have been unsuccessful.

Test-Taking Strategy: Use therapeutic communication techniques. Option 2 is the only option that addresses the client's feelings. Remember that a client's feelings are most important. Review therapeutic communication techniques if you had difficulty with this question.

Level of Cognitive Ability: Application
Client Needs: Safe, Effective Care Environment
Integrated Process: Nursing Process/Implementation
Content Area: Mental Health

Reference:
Varcarolis, E.M. (2002). *Foundations of psychiatric mental health nursing* (4th ed.). Philadelphia: Saunders, pp. 285-288.

142. A client with urolithiasis is scheduled for extracorporeal shock wave lithotripsy. The nurse ensures that the client understands the procedure and tells the client that:

1 The procedure involves breaking up the stone by a vibrating needle that is inserted into the urinary tract

2 He will be anesthetized and placed in a water bath

3 There is no pain at all involved with this procedure

4 There are no side effects or complications associated with this procedure

Answer: 2

Rationale: In extracorporeal shock wave lithotripsy, a noninvasive procedure, the client is anesthetized (spinal or general) and placed in a water bath. Anesthesia is necessary to keep the client very still during the procedure. Shock waves are administered that shatter the stone without damaging the surrounding tissues. The stone is broken into fine sand, which is secreted into the client's urine within a few days after the procedure. Hematuria is common after the procedure. The presence of clots in the urine needs to be reported to the physician. Clots could indicate a complication such as a hematoma.

Test-Taking Strategy: Use the process of elimination. Eliminate options 3 and 4 first because of the absolute word "no" in these options. From the remaining options, recalling that the procedure is noninvasive and is done via shock waves (not a vibrating needle) will direct you to option 2. Review this procedure if you had difficulty with this question.

Level of Cognitive Ability: Application
Client Needs: Safe, Effective Care Environment
Integrated Process: Nursing Process/Implementation
Content Area: Adult Health/Renal

Reference:
Lewis, S., Heitkemper, M., & Dirksen, S. (2004). *Medical-surgical nursing: Assessment and management of clinical problems* (6th ed.). St. Louis: Mosby, p. 1188.

143. A nurse is assisting at a code and the physician is going to defibrillate the client. Of the following items, which is the only one that the nurse does not need to remove from the client just before the client is defibrillated?

1 Back board

2 Oxygen

3 Nitroglycerin patch

4 Pulse oximetry machine plugged into an electrical socket

Answer: 1

Rationale: Flammable materials and metal devices or liquids (that are capable of carrying electricity) are removed from the client and bed before discharging the paddles of the defibrillator. The nitroglycerin patch has a metallic backing and should be removed.

Test-Taking Strategy: Use the process of elimination. Note the key words "does not need to remove." Eliminate options 2 and 4 because they are similar. From the remaining options, recall that the back board is needed to resume cardiopulmonary resuscitation immediately if defibrillation is unsuccessful. Review procedures for defibrillation if you had difficulty with this question.

Level of Cognitive Ability: Application
Client Needs: Safe, Effective Care Environment
Integrated Process: Nursing Process/Implementation
Content Area: Adult Health/Cardiovascular

References:
Black, J., & Hawks, J. (2005). *Medical-surgical nursing: Clinical management for positive outcomes* (7th ed.). Philadelphia: Saunders, p. 1689.
Ignatavicius, D., & Workman, M. (2002). *Medical surgical nursing: Critical thinking for collaborative care* (4th ed.). Philadelphia: Saunders, p. 691.

144. A nurse is planning the discharge instructions from the emergency department for an adult client who is a victim of family violence. The nurse understands that the discharge plans must include:

1 Instructions to call the police the next time the abuse occurs
2 Exploration of the pros and cons of remaining with the abusive family member
3 Specific information regarding "safe havens" or shelters in the client's neighborhood
4 Specific information about self-defense classes

Answer: 3

Rationale: Any of the options might be included in the discharge plan at some point if long-term therapy or a long-term relationship with the nurse is established. The question refers to an emergency department setting. It is most important to assist victims of abuse with identifying a plan for how to remove self from harmful situations should they arise again. An abused person is usually reluctant to call the police. Teaching the victim to fight back (as in the use of self-defense) is not the best action when dealing with a violent person.

Test-Taking Strategy: Use Maslow's hierarchy of needs theory. Remember that if a physiological need is not present, then safety is the priority. Review care of the victim of abuse if you had difficulty with this question.

Level of Cognitive Ability: Application
Client Needs: Safe, Effective Care Environment
Integrated Process: Nursing Process/Planning
Content Area: Mental Health

Reference:
Stuart, G., & Laraia, M. (2005). *Principles and practice of psychiatric nursing* (8th ed.). St. Louis: Mosby, pp. 806; 812.

---

145. A physician is about to defibrillate a client in ventricular fibrillation and says in a loud voice "CLEAR!" The nurse immediately:

1 Shuts off the intravenous infusion going into the client's arm
2 Shuts off the mechanical ventilator
3 Steps away from the bed and makes sure all others have done the same
4 Places the conductive gel pads for defibrillation on the client's chest

Answer: 3

Rationale: For the safety of all personnel, when the defibrillator paddles are being discharged, all personnel must stand back and be clear of all contact with the client or the client's bed. It is the primary responsibility of the person defibrillating to communicate the "clear" message loudly enough for all to hear and ensure their compliance. All personnel must immediately comply with this command. The gel pads should have been placed on the client's chest before the defibrillator paddles were applied. A ventilator is not in use during a code; rather an Ambu (resuscitation) bag is used. Shutting off the intravenous infusion has no useful purpose. Stepping back from the bed prevents the nurse or others from being defibrillated along with the client.

Test-Taking Strategy: Use the process of elimination, focusing on the issue: the procedure for defibrillation. Recalling the risks associated with this procedure and noting the word "CLEAR" in the question will direct you to option 3. Review the risks associated with this procedure if you had difficulty with this question.

Level of Cognitive Ability: Application
Client Needs: Safe, Effective Care Environment
Integrated Process: Nursing Process/Implementation
Content Area: Adult Health/Cardiovascular

Reference:
Black, J., & Hawks, J. (2005). *Medical-surgical nursing: Clinical management for positive outcomes* (7th ed.). Philadelphia: Saunders, p. 1689.

146. A client with chronic renal failure has an indwelling peritoneal catheter in the abdomen for peritoneal dialysis. While bathing, the client spills water on the abdominal dressing covering the abdomen. The nurse plans to immediately:

1 Reinforce the dressing
2 Change the dressing
3 Flush the peritoneal dialysis catheter
4 Scrub the catheter with povidone iodine

Answer: 2

Rationale: Clients with peritoneal dialysis catheters are at high risk for infection. A dressing that is wet is a conduit for bacteria to reach the catheter insertion site. The nurse ensures that the dressing is kept dry at all times. Reinforcing the dressing is not a safe practice to prevent infection in this circumstance. Flushing the catheter is not indicated. Scrubbing the catheter with povidone iodine is done at the time of connection or disconnection of peritoneal dialysis.

Test-Taking Strategy: Focus on the issue: that the dressing is wet. The correct option would focus on the dressing, not the catheter. Therefore, eliminate options 3 and 4. Knowing that it is better to change a wet dressing than reinforce it will direct you to option 2. Review care of the client with a peritoneal dialysis catheter if you had difficulty with this question.

Level of Cognitive Ability: Application
Client Needs: Safe, Effective Care Environment
Integrated Process: Nursing Process/Planning
Content Area: Adult Health/Renal

Reference:
Black, J., & Hawks, J. (2005). *Medical-surgical nursing: Clinical management for positive outcomes* (7th ed.). Philadelphia: Saunders, p. 958.

---

147. A client is scheduled for elective cardioversion to treat chronic high-rate atrial fibrillation. The nurse determines that the client is not yet ready for the procedure after noting that the:

1 Client's digoxin (Lanoxin) has been withheld for the last 48 hours
2 Client has received a dose of midazolam (Versed) intravenously
3 Client is wearing a nasal cannula delivering oxygen at 2 liters per minute
4 Defibrillator has the synchronizer turned on and is set at 50 joules

Answer: 3

Rationale: Digoxin may be withheld for up to 48 hours before cardioversion because it increases ventricular irritability and may cause ventricular dysrhythmias post countershock. The client typically receives a dose of an intravenous sedative or antianxiety agent. The defibrillator is switched to synchronizer mode to time the delivery of the electrical impulse to coincide with the QRS and avoid the T wave, which could cause ventricular fibrillation. Energy level is typically set at 50 to 100 joules. During the procedure, any oxygen is removed temporarily, because oxygen supports combustion, and a fire could result from electrical arcing.

Test-Taking Strategy: Use the process of elimination, noting the key words "not yet ready for the procedure." Think about the procedure and recall the concept related to oxygen combustion to direct you to option 3. Review this procedure if you had difficulty with this question.

Level of Cognitive Ability: Analysis
Client Needs: Safe, Effective Care Environment
Integrated Process: Nursing Process/Evaluation
Content Area: Adult Health/Cardiovascular

References:
Black, J., & Hawks, J. (2005). *Medical-surgical nursing: Clinical management for positive outcomes* (7th ed.). Philadelphia: Saunders, p. 1678.
Ignatavicius, D., & Workman, M. (2002). *Medical surgical nursing: Critical thinking for collaborative care* (4th ed.). Philadelphia: Saunders, p. 690.

148. A nurse is planning activities for a depressed client who was just admitted to the hospital. The nurse plans to:
 1 Provide an activity that is quiet and solitary in nature to avoid increased fatigue, such as working on a puzzle or reading a book
 2 Plan nothing until the client asks to participate in the milieu
 3 Offer the client a menu of daily activities and insist that the client participate in all of them
 4 Provide a structured daily program of activities and encourage the client to participate

Answer: 4
Rationale: A depressed person is often withdrawn. Also, the person experiences difficulty concentrating, loss of interest or pleasure, low energy and fatigue, and feelings of worthlessness and poor self-esteem. The plan of care needs to provide stimulation in a structured environment. Options 1 and 2 are restrictive and offer little or no structure and stimulation. The nurse should not insist that a client participate in all activities.

Test-Taking Strategy: Use the process of elimination, focusing on the client's diagnosis. Eliminate option 3 first because of the word "insist" and the absolute word "all." From the remaining options, noting the word "structured" in option 4 will direct you to this option. Review care of the client with depression if you had difficulty with this question.

Level of Cognitive Ability: Application
Client Needs: Safe, Effective Care Environment
Integrated Process: Nursing Process/Planning
Content Area: Mental Health

Reference:
Stuart, G., & Laraia, M. (2005). *Principles and practice of psychiatric nursing* (8th ed.). St. Louis: Mosby, p. 348.

149. A nurse is caring for an older client who had a hip pinning following a fracture. In planning care, the nurse avoids which of the following to minimize the chance for further injury?
 1 Side rails in the "up" position
 2 Use of the nightlight in hospital room and bathroom
 3 Call bell placed within the client's reach
 4 Delays in responding to the call light but telling the client via the intercom system that someone will attend to his or her needs

Answer: 4
Rationale: Safe nursing actions intended to prevent injury to the client include keeping the side rails up, the bed in low position, use of a nightlight, and providing a call bell that is within the client's reach. Responding promptly to the client's use of the call light minimizes the chance that the client will try to get up alone, which could result in a fall. Communicating with the client via an intercom does not meet the client's needs to prevent potential injury.

Test-Taking Strategy: Note the key word "avoids." This word tells you that you need to select the action that is incorrect. Focusing on the issue, preventing injury, will direct you to option 4. Delays will give the client a reason to try to get up unattended and risk a fall and possible injury. Review measures to prevent injury if you had difficulty with this question.

Level of Cognitive Ability: Application
Client Needs: Safe, Effective Care Environment
Integrated Process: Nursing Process/Planning
Content Area: Fundamental Skills

Reference:
Ebersole, P., & Hess, P. (2001). *Geriatric nursing & healthy aging.* St. Louis: Mosby, p. 467.

150. A nurse is assisting in the care of a client who is to be cardioverted. The nurse plans to set the defibrillator to which of the following starting energy range levels, depending on the specific physician order?

1 50 to 100 joules
2 150 to 200 joules
3 250 to 300 joules
4 350 to 400 joules

Answer: 1

Rationale: When a client is cardioverted, the defibrillator is charged to the energy level ordered by the physician. Cardioversion is usually started at 50 to 100 joules. Options 2, 3, and 4 are incorrect and identify energy levels that are too high for cardioversion.

Test-Taking Strategy: Use the process of elimination. Remember that in instances when cardioversion is used, an underlying cardiac rhythm needs to be converted to a better rhythm. So, lower voltages are used. Review this procedure if you had difficulty with this question.

Level of Cognitive Ability: Application
Client Needs: Safe, Effective Care Environment
Integrated Process: Nursing Process/Planning
Content Area: Adult Health/Cardiovascular

Reference:
Ignatavicius, D., & Workman, M. (2002). *Medical surgical nursing: Critical thinking for collaborative care* (4th ed.). Philadelphia: Saunders, p. 690.

151. A nurse has an order to get the client out of bed to a chair on the first postoperative day following total knee replacement. The nurse plans to do which of the following to protect the knee joint?

1 Apply a knee immobilizer before getting the client up and elevate the client's surgical leg while sitting
2 Apply a compression dressing and put ice on the knee while sitting
3 Lift the client to the bedside chair, leaving the continuous passive motion (CPM) machine in place
4 Obtain a walker to minimize weight-bearing by the client on the affected leg

Answer: 1

Rationale: The nurse assists the client to get out of bed on the first postoperative day after putting a knee immobilizer on the affected joint to provide stability. The surgeon orders the weight-bearing limits on the affected leg. The leg is elevated while the client is sitting in the chair to minimize edema. Ice is not used unless prescribed. A compression dressing should already be in place on the wound. A CPM machine is used only while the client is in bed.

Test-Taking Strategy: Use the process of elimination. Note the relation between the issue "protect the knee joint" and "knee immobilizer" in option 1. Review postoperative care following total knee replacement if you had difficulty with this question.

Level of Cognitive Ability: Application
Client Needs: Safe, Effective Care Environment
Integrated Process: Nursing Process/Planning
Content Area: Adult Health/Musculoskeletal

References:
Black, J., & Hawks, J. (2005). *Medical-surgical nursing: Clinical management for positive outcomes* (7th ed.). Philadelphia: Saunders, p. 596.
Phipps, W., Monahan, F., Sands, J., Marek, J., & Neighbors, M. (2003). *Medical-surgical nursing: health and illness perspectives* (7th ed.). St. Louis: Mosby, pp. 1531; 1537.

152. A client is admitted to the psychiatric unit following a suicide attempt by hanging. The nurse's most important aspect of care is to maintain client safety, and the nurse plans to:

1 Assign a staff member to the client who will remain with the client

2 Place the client in a seclusion room where all potentially dangerous articles are removed

3 Remove the client's clothing and place the client in a hospital gown

4 Request that a client's peer remain with the client at all times

Answer: 1

Rationale: Hanging is a serious suicide attempt. The plan of care must reflect the action that will promote the client's safety. Constant observation by a staff member is necessary. It is not a peer's responsibility to safeguard a client. Removing one's clothing does not maximize all possible safety strategies. Placing the client in seclusion further isolates the client.

Test-Taking Strategy: Use the process of elimination, focusing on the issue: suicide attempt. Recalling that one-to-one supervision is necessary will direct you to option 1. Review suicide precautions if you had difficulty with this question.

Level of Cognitive Ability: Application
Client Needs: Safe, Effective Care Environment
Integrated Process: Nursing Process/Planning
Content Area: Mental Health

Reference:
Stuart, G., & Laraia, M. (2005). *Principles and practice of psychiatric nursing* (8th ed.). St. Louis: Mosby, p. 379.

153. A nurse receives a telephone call from a male client who states that he wants to kill himself and has a loaded gun on the table. The best nursing intervention is to:

1 Insist that the client give you his name and address so that you can get the police there immediately

2 Keep the client talking and allow the client to ventilate feelings

3 Use therapeutic communication techniques, especially the reflection of feelings

4 Keep the client talking and signal to another staff member to trace the call so that appropriate help can be sent

Answer: 4

Rationale: In a crisis, the nurse must take an authoritative, active role to promote the client's safety. A loaded gun in the home of the client who verbalizes he wants to kill himself is a crisis. The client's safety is of prime concern. Keeping the client on the phone and getting help to the client is the best intervention. Insisting may anger the client and he might hang up. Option 2 lacks the authoritative action stance of securing the client's safety. Using therapeutic communication techniques is important, but overuse of reflection may sound uncaring or superficial and is lacking direction and a solution to the immediate problem of the client's safety.

Test-Taking Strategy: Use the process of elimination and focus on the crisis: a potential for suicide. The only option that will provide direct help is option 4. Review crisis intervention for a client contemplating suicide if you had difficulty with this question.

Level of Cognitive Ability: Application
Client Needs: Safe, Effective Care Environment
Integrated Process: Nursing Process/Implementation
Content Area: Mental Health

References:
Stuart, G., & Laraia, M. (2005). *Principles and practice of psychiatric nursing* (8th ed.). St. Louis: Mosby, p. 367.
Varcarolis, E.M. (2002). *Foundations of psychiatric mental health nursing* (4th ed.). Philadelphia: Saunders, p. 651.

154. Following a thorough assessment, the nurse determines the need to place a vest restraint on a client. The client tells the nurse that he does not want the vest restraint applied. The best nursing action is to:
1 Apply the restraint anyway
2 Contact the physician
3 Medicate the client with a sedative and then apply the restraint
4 Compromise with the client and use wrist restraints

Answer: 2

Rationale: The use of restraints needs to be avoided if possible. If the nurse determines that a restraint is necessary, this should be discussed with the family, and an order needs to be obtained from the physician. The nurse should explain carefully to the client and family about the reasons why the restraint is necessary, the type of restraint selected, and the anticipated duration of restraint. If the nurse applied the restraint on a client who was refusing such, the nurse could be charged with battery. Compromising with the client is unethical.

Test-Taking Strategy: Use the process of elimination and principles and concepts related to ethical and legal issues. Eliminate options 1 and 3 first because they are similar. From the remaining options, eliminate option 4 because it is unethical. Review the legal implications related to the use of restraints if you had difficulty with this question.

Level of Cognitive Ability: Application
Client Needs: Safe, Effective Care Environment
Integrated Process: Nursing Process/Implementation
Content Area: Fundamental Skills

References:
Brent, N. (2001). *Nurses and the law* (2nd ed.). Philadelphia: Saunders, p. 420.
Ignatavicius, D., & Workman, M. (2002). *Medical surgical nursing: Critical thinking for collaborative care* (4th ed.). Philadelphia: Saunders, pp. 40-41.

155. A client is being discharged from the hospital and will receive oxygen therapy at home. The nurse is teaching the client and family about oxygen safety measures. Which statement by the client indicates the need for further teaching?
1 "I realize that I should check the oxygen level of the portable tank on a consistent basis."
2 "It is all right to burn my scented candles as long as they are a few feet away from my oxygen tank."
3 "I will not sit in front of my wood-burning fireplace with my oxygen on."
4 "I will call the physician if I experience any shortness of breath."

Answer: 2

Rationale: Oxygen is a highly combustible gas, although it will not spontaneously burn or cause an explosion. It can easily cause a fire to ignite in a client's room if it contacts a spark from a cigarette, burning candle, or electrical equipment. Options 1, 3, and 4 are appropriate oxygen safety measures.

Test-Taking Strategy: Use the process of elimination, noting the key words "need for further teaching." These key words indicate a false-response question and that you need to select the option that is an incorrect client statement. Recalling that oxygen is a highly combustible gas will direct you to option 2. Review teaching points related to home care and oxygen if you had difficulty with this question.

Level of Cognitive Ability: Analysis
Client Needs: Safe, Effective Care Environment
Integrated Process: Teaching/Learning
Content Area: Fundamental Skills

Reference:
Perry, A., & Potter, P. (2004). *Clinical nursing skills and techniques* (5th ed.). St. Louis: Mosby, p. 1131.

156. A home care nurse visits a client who is to receive intravenous (IV) therapy via an IV pump. To ensure electrical safety, the nurse would:

1   Use an extension cord to allow the client freedom to move around and ambulate
2   Tape the electrical cord from the IV pump to the floor before plugging it in
3   Run the electrical cord from the IV pump under the carpet before plugging it in
4   Obtain a three-prong grounded plug adapter

Answer: 4

Rationale: Electrical equipment should be grounded. The third longer prong in an electrical plug is the ground. Theoretically, the ground prong carries any stray electrical current back to the ground, hence its name. The other two prongs carry the power to the piece of electrical equipment. In this situation, the nurse obtains a three-prong grounded plug adapter, attaches it to the cord, and plugs it into the wall. Options 1, 2, and 3 are unsafe actions.

Test-Taking Strategy: Use principles of basic electrical safety to direct you to the correct option. Remember that extension cords should not be used unless they are approved for use and that taping cords and running cords under carpets is unsafe. Review these safety principles, if you had difficulty with this question.

Level of Cognitive Ability: Application
Client Needs: Safe, Effective Care Environment
Integrated Process: Nursing Process/Implementation
Content Area: Fundamental Skills

Reference:
Potter, P., & Perry, A. (2005). *Fundamentals of nursing* (6th ed.). St. Louis: Mosby, p. 992.

---

157. On an initial home care visit, the home care nurse assesses the client's environment for potential hazards. Which observation is an indication that the client needs instruction about safety?

1   Skid-resistant small area rugs in the living room
2   Clothes hamper at the end of the hallway
3   Area rugs on the stairs
4   Carpeted stairs secured with carpet tacks

needs instruction = answer wrong one.

Answer: 3

Rationale: Area rugs and runners should not be used on stairs. Any carpeting on the stairs should be secured with carpet tacks. Injuries in the home frequently result from objects, including small rugs, on the stairs and floor, wet spots on the floor, and clutter on bedside tables, on closet shelves, on the top of the refrigerator, and on bookshelves. Care should also be taken to ensure that end tables are secure and have stable straight legs. Nonessential items should be placed in drawers to eliminate clutter.

Test-Taking Strategy: Focus on the key words "needs instruction about safety." These words indicate a false-response question and that you need to select the option that indicates an unsafe observation. Recalling that area rugs are not secured will direct you to option 3. Review these safety principles if you had difficulty with this question.

Level of Cognitive Ability: Analysis
Client Needs: Safe, Effective Care Environment
Integrated Process: Nursing Process/Assessment
Content Area: Fundamental Skills

Reference:
Potter, P., & Perry, A. (2005). *Fundamentals of nursing* (6th ed.). St. Louis: Mosby, p. 980.

158. A hospitalized client with a history of alcohol abuse says to the nurse, "I am leaving now. I have to go. I don't want any more treatment. I have things that I have to do right away." The client has not been discharged. In fact, the client is scheduled for an important diagnostic test to be performed in 1 hour. After discussing the client's concerns with the client, the client dresses and begins to walk out of the hospital room. The appropriate nursing action is to:

1 Restrain the client until the physician can be reached
2 Call security to block all exit areas
3 Tell the client that he cannot return to this hospital again if he leaves now
4 Call the nursing supervisor

Answer: 4
Rationale: A nurse can be charged with false imprisonment if clients are made to wrongfully believe that they cannot leave the hospital. Most health care facilities have documents for clients to sign that relate to the clients' responsibilities when they leave against medical advice (AMA). The client should be asked to sign this document before leaving. The nurse should request that the client wait to speak to the physician before leaving, but if the client refuses to do so, the nurse cannot hold the client against his or her will. Restraining the client and calling security to block exits constitutes false imprisonment. Any client has a right to health care and cannot be told otherwise.

Test-Taking Strategy: Use the process of elimination. Keeping the concept of false imprisonment in mind, eliminate options 1 and 2 because they are similar. Eliminate option 3 knowing that any client has a right to health care. Review the points related to false imprisonment if you had difficulty with this question.

Level of Cognitive Ability: Application
Client Needs: Safe, Effective Care Environment
Integrated Process: Nursing Process/Implementation
Content Area: Fundamental Skills

Reference:
Brent, N. (2001). *Nurses and the law* (2nd ed.). Philadelphia: Saunders, pp. 214-215.

159. Two nurses are in the cafeteria having lunch in a quiet, secluded area. A physical therapist from the physical therapy department joins the nurses. During lunch, the nurses discuss a client who was physically abused. After lunch, the physical therapist provides therapy as prescribed to this physically abused client and asks the client questions about the physical abuse. The client discovers that the nurses told the therapist about the abuse situation and is emotionally harmed. The ramifications associated with the nurses' discussion about the client are associated with which of the following?

1 None, because the discussion took place in a quiet, secluded area
2 They can be charged with slander.
3 They can be charged with libel.
4 None, because the physical therapist is involved in the client's care

Answer: 2
Rationale: Defamation occurs when information is communicated to a third party that causes damage to someone else's reputation either in writing (libel) or verbal (slander). Common examples are discussing information about a client in public areas or speaking negatively about coworkers. The situation identified in the question can cause emotional harm to the client, and the nurses could be charged with slander. This situation also violates the client's right to confidentiality.

Test-Taking Strategy: Use the process of elimination and focus on the issue: client's rights and confidentially. This will assist in eliminating options 1 and 4 first. From the remaining options, recall that slander constitutes verbal discussion regarding a client. Review this legal responsibility if you had difficulty with this question.

Level of Cognitive Ability: Analysis
Client Needs: Safe, Effective Care Environment
Integrated Process: Nursing Process/Analysis
Content Area: Fundamental Skills

Reference:
Brent, N. (2001). *Nurses and the law* (2nd ed.). Philadelphia: Saunders, pp. 121-122.

160. A nurse arrives at work and is told that the intensive care unit (ICU) is in need of assistance. The nurse is told by the supervisor that the assignment today is to work in the ICU. The nurse has never worked in the ICU and shares concerns with the supervisor regarding unfamiliarity with the technological equipment used in that unit. The nurse is again told to report to the ICU. The appropriate action by the nurse is to:

1   Refuse to go to the ICU
2   Go to the ICU and tell the charge nurse she is feeling ill and needs to go home
3   Call the hospital lawyer
4   Go to the ICU and inform the charge nurse of those tasks that cannot be performed

Answer: 4

Rationale: Legally, a nurse cannot refuse to float unless a union contract guarantees that nurses can only work in a specified area or the nurse can prove the lack of knowledge for the performance of assigned task. When encountered with this situation, the nurse should set priorities and identify potential areas of harm to the client. All pertinent facts related to client care problems and safety issues should be documented. The nurse should perform only those tasks in which training has been received. It is the nurse's responsibility to clearly describe these tasks.

Test-Taking Strategy: Use the process of elimination. Eliminate option 1 because if a nurse refuses to care for a client, the nurse can be charged with abandonment. Eliminate option 2 next because it is similar to option 1 and because it is ethically unsound. From the remaining options, focusing on the issue, the legalities surrounding floating, will direct you to option 4. Review the issues related to floating and abandonment of the client if you had difficulty with this question.

Level of Cognitive Ability: Application
Client Needs: Safe, Effective Care Environment
Integrated Process: Nursing Process/Implementation
Content Area: Fundamental Skills

Reference:
Potter, P., & Perry, A. (2005). *Fundamentals of nursing* (6th ed.). St. Louis: Mosby, pp. 418-419.

---

161. A registered nurse (RN) asks a licensed practical nurse (LPN) to change the colostomy bag on a client. The LPN tells the RN that although attendance at the hospital inservice was completed regarding this procedure, the procedure has never been performed on a client. The appropriate action by the RN is to:

1   Request that the LPN review the materials from the inservice before performing the procedure
2   Request that the LPN review the procedure in the hospital manual and bring the written procedure into the client's room for guidance during the procedure
3   Request that the LPN observe another LPN perform the procedure
4   Perform the procedure with the LPN

Answer: 4

Rationale: The RN must remember that even though a task may be delegated to someone, the nurse who delegates maintains accountability for the overall nursing care of the client. Only the task, not the ultimate accountability, may be delegated to another. The RN is responsible for ensuring that competent and accurate care is delivered to the client. Requesting that the LPN observe another LPN perform the procedure does not ensure that the procedure will be done correctly. Because this is a new procedure for this LPN, the RN should accompany the LPN, provide guidance, and answer questions following the procedure. Although it is appropriate to review the inservice materials and the hospital procedure manual, it is best for the RN to accompany the LPN to perform the procedure.

Test-Taking Strategy: Use the process of elimination and eliminate options 1 and 2 first. Although it may be important for the LPN to review inservice materials and the hospital procedure manual, these options are not complete. From the remaining options, select option 4 because option 3 does not ensure that the LPN will perform this procedure safely. Additionally, it is the RN's responsibility to educate. Review the principles related to delegating and accountability if you had difficulty with this question.

Level of Cognitive Ability: Application
Client Needs: Safe, Effective Care Environment
Integrated Process: Teaching/Learning
Content Area: Delegating/Prioritizing

Reference:
Potter, P., & Perry, A. (2005). *Fundamentals of nursing* (6th ed.). St. Louis: Mosby, pp. 19; 42; 375.

---

162. A nurse has applied the patch electrodes of an automatic external defibrillator (AED) to the chest of a client who is pulseless. The defibrillator has interpreted the rhythm to be ventricular fibrillation. The nurse then:
1 Orders any personnel away from the client, charges the machine, and defibrillates through the console
2 Performs cardiopulmonary resuscitation (CPR) for 1 minute before defibrillating
3 Charges the machine and immediately pushes the "discharge" buttons on the console
4 Administers rescue breathing during the defibrillation

Answer: 1
Rationale: If the AED advises to defibrillate, the nurse or rescuer orders all persons away from the client, charges the machine, and pushes both of the "discharge" buttons on the console at the same time. The charge is delivered through the patch electrodes, and this method is known as "hands-off" defibrillation, which is safest for the rescuer. The sequence of charges (up to three consecutive attempts at 200, 300, 360 joules) is similar to that of conventional defibrillation. Option 4 is contraindicated for the safety of any rescuer. Performing CPR delays the defibrillation attempt.

Test-Taking Strategy: Use the process of elimination and the guidelines related to defibrillation. Recalling the need to avoid contact with the client during this procedure will direct you to option 1. Review this procedure if you had difficulty with this question.

Level of Cognitive Ability: Application
Client Needs: Safe, Effective Care Environment
Integrated Process: Nursing Process/Implementation
Content Area: Adult Health/Cardiovascular

Reference:
Ignatavicius, D., & Workman, M. (2002). *Medical surgical nursing: Critical thinking for collaborative care* (4th ed.). Philadelphia: Saunders, p. 691.

---

163. A nurse is planning care for a client diagnosed with deep vein thrombosis (DVT) of the left leg. Which intervention would the nurse avoid in the care of this client?
1 Application of moist heat to the left leg
2 Administration of acetaminophen (Tylenol)
3 Elevation of the left leg
4 Ambulation in the hall three times per shift

Answer: 4
Rationale: Standard management of the client with DVT includes bed rest; limb elevation; relief of discomfort with warm moist heat and analgesics as needed; anticoagulant therapy; and monitoring for signs of pulmonary embolism. Ambulation increases the likelihood of dislodgment of the tail of the thrombus, which could travel to the lungs as a pulmonary embolism.

Test-Taking Strategy: Use the process of elimination, noting the key word "avoid." This key word indicates a false-response question and that you need to select the option that is an incorrect nursing action. Recalling that pulmonary embolism is a complication of DVT will direct you to option 4. Review care of the client with DVT if you had difficulty with this question.

Level of Cognitive Ability: Application
Client Needs: Safe, Effective Care Environment
Integrated Process: Nursing Process/Implementation
Content Area: Adult Health/Cardiovascular

Reference:
Ignatavicius, D., & Workman, M. (2002). *Medical surgical nursing: Critical thinking for collaborative care* (4th ed.). Philadelphia: Saunders, pp. 763-764.

---

164. A nurse is caring for a client with severe toxemia of pregnancy who is receiving an intravenous (IV) infusion of magnesium sulfate. To provide a safe environment, the nurse ensures that which priority item is at the bedside?
1 Percussion hammer
2 Tongue blade
3 Potassium chloride injection
4 Calcium gluconate injection

Answer: 4
Rationale: Toxic effects of magnesium sulfate may cause loss of deep tendon reflexes, heart block, respiratory paralysis, and cardiac arrest. The antidote for magnesium sulfate is calcium gluconate and should be available at the client's bedside. A percussion hammer may be important to assess reflexes, but is not the priority item. An airway rather than a tongue blade is also an appropriate item. Potassium chloride is not related to the administration of magnesium sulfate.

Test-Taking Strategy: Use the process of elimination. Note the key word "priority." This key word indicates that more than one or all of the options may be correct but that you need to identify the most important one. Remember, the percussion hammer would identify the decrease in deep tendon reflexes, but the calcium gluconate is required to treat the life-threatening condition that can occur. Review care of the client receiving IV magnesium sulfate if you had difficulty with this question.

Level of Cognitive Ability: Application
Client Needs: Safe, Effective Care Environment
Integrated Process: Nursing Process/Implementation
Content Area: Pharmacology

Reference:
McKenry, L., & Salerno, E. (2003). *Mosby's pharmacology in nursing* (21st ed.). St. Louis: Mosby, p. 372.

---

165. A nurse administers the morning dose of digoxin (Lanoxin) to the client. When the nurse charts the medication, the nurse discovers that a dose of 0.25 mg was administered rather than the prescribed dose of 0.125 mg. The nurse should take which appropriate action?
1 Administer the additional 0.125 mg
2 Tell the client that the dose administered was not the total amount and administer the additional dose
3 Tell the client that too much medication was administered and an error was made
4 Complete an incident report

Answer: 4
Rationale: In accord with the agency's policies, nurses are required to file incident reports when a situation arises that could or did cause a client harm. The nurse also contacts the physician. If a dose of 0.125 mg was prescribed, and a dose of 0.25 mg was administered, then the client received too much medication. Additional medication is not administered and in fact could be detrimental to the client. The client should be informed when an error has occurred, but in a professional manner so as not to cause fear and concern. In many situations, the physician will discuss this with the client.

Test-Taking Strategy: Use the process of elimination. Simple math calculation will assist in eliminating options 1 and 2. From the remaining options, noting the key word "appropriate" will direct you to option 4. Remember, the nurse completes an incident report when an error occurs. Review the principles related to incident reports if you had difficulty with this question.

Level of Cognitive Ability: Application
Client Needs: Safe, Effective Care Environment
Integrated Process: Nursing Process/Implementation
Content Area: Fundamental Skills

Reference:
Potter, P., & Perry, A. (2005). *Fundamentals of nursing* (6th ed.). St. Louis: Mosby, pp. 419; 497.

---

166. When planning the discharge of a client with chronic anxiety, the nurse develops goals to promote a safe environment at home. The appropriate maintenance goal for the client should focus on which of the following?
  1 Maintaining continued contact with a crisis counselor
  2 Identifying anxiety-producing situations
  3 Ignoring feelings of anxiety
  4 Eliminating all anxiety from daily situations

Answer: 2
Rationale: Recognizing situations that produce anxiety allows the client to prepare to cope with anxiety or avoid a specific stimulus. Counselors will not be available for all anxiety-producing situations. Additionally, this option does not encourage the development of internal strengths. Ignoring feelings will not resolve anxiety. It is impossible to eliminate all anxiety from life.

Test-Taking Strategy: Use the process of elimination. Eliminate option 4 first because of the absolute word "all." Eliminate option 3 next because feelings should not be ignored. From the remaining options, select option 2 because this option is more client-centered and provides the preparation for the client to deal with anxiety if it occurs. Review goals of care for the client with anxiety if you had difficulty with this question.

Level of Cognitive Ability: Application
Client Needs: Safe, Effective Care Environment
Integrated Process: Nursing Process/Planning
Content Area: Mental Health

References:
Stuart, G., & Laraia, M. (2005). *Principles and practice of psychiatric nursing* (8th ed.). St. Louis: Mosby, p. 268.
Varcarolis, E.M. (2002). *Foundations of psychiatric mental health nursing* (4th ed.). Philadelphia: Saunders, pp. 321-322.

---

167. A nurse is planning to instruct a client with chronic vertigo about safety measures to prevent exacerbation of symptoms or injury. The nurse plans to teach the client that it is important to:
  1 Drive at times when the client does not feel dizzy
  2 Go to the bedroom and lie down when vertigo is experienced
  3 Remove throw rugs and clutter in the home
  4 Turn the head slowly when spoken to

Answer: 3
Rationale: The client with chronic vertigo should avoid driving and using public transportation. The sudden movements involved in each could precipitate an attack. To further prevent vertigo attacks, the client should change position slowly, and should turn the entire body, not just the head, when spoken to. If vertigo does occur, the client should immediately sit down or grasp the nearest piece of furniture. The client should maintain the home in a clutter-free state and have throw rugs removed, because the effort of trying to regain balance after slipping could trigger the onset of vertigo.

Test-Taking Strategy: Use the process of elimination, focusing on the issue: chronic vertigo and preventing injury. Eliminate options 1 and 2 first, because they put the client at greatest risk of injury secondary to vertigo. From the remaining options, recalling that the client is taught to turn the entire body, not just the head, will direct you to option 3. Review safety measures for the client with chronic vertigo if you had difficulty with this question.

Level of Cognitive Ability: Application
Client Needs: Safe, Effective Care Environment
Integrated Process: Teaching/Learning
Content Area: Adult Health/Ear

References:

Black, J., & Hawks, J. (2005). *Medical-surgical nursing: Clinical management for positive outcomes* (7th ed.). Philadelphia: Saunders, pp. 1990-1991.

Ignatavicius, D., & Workman, M. (2002). *Medical surgical nursing: Critical thinking for collaborative care* (4th ed.). Philadelphia: Saunders, p. 1068.

---

168. A client receiving heparin therapy for acute myocardial infarction has an activated partial thromboplastin time (aPTT) value of 100 seconds. Before reporting the results to the physician, the nurse verifies that which of the following are available for use if prescribed?

1 Protamine sulfate
2 Phytonadione (vitamin K)
3 Cyanocobalamin (Vitamin B_{12})
4 Methylene blue (Urolene blue)

Answer: 1

Rationale: Therapeutic values of the aPTT for clients on heparin ranges between 60 and 70 seconds, depending on the control value. A value of 100 seconds indicates that the client has received too much heparin. The antidote for heparin overdosage is protamine sulfate. Vitamin K is the antidote for warfarin sodium (Coumadin) overdosage. Methylene blue is an antidote for cyanide poisoning. Vitamin B_{12} is used to treat clients with pernicious anemia.

Test-Taking Strategy: Focus on the issue: heparin therapy, and note the key words "available for use." Recalling that protamine sulfate is the antidote for heparin will direct you to option 1. Review the normal aPTT and the antidote for heparin if you had difficulty with this question.

Level of Cognitive Ability: Application
Client Needs: Safe, Effective Care Environment
Integrated Process: Nursing Process/Implementation
Content Area: Pharmacology

Reference:

Hodgson, B., & Kizior, R. (2004). *Saunders nursing drug handbook 2004.* Philadelphia: Saunders, p. 493.

---

169. A male suicidal client is being discharged home with his family. Which statement by a family member might constitute criteria for delaying discharge?

1 The client's wife asks, "Does he know that I've already moved out and filed for a divorce?"
2 The client's son states, "One of his friends visited last week to tell us Dad's union is out on strike."
3 The client's daughter states, "I've decided to postpone my wedding until Dad's feeling better."
4 The client's brother asks, "Will my brother be able to continue as executor of our parent's trust?"

Answer: 1

Rationale: Single, divorced, and widowed clients have suicide rates that are greater than those who are married. While the situation of the strike is stressful, the client will probably receive a portion of his wages and can derive hope and a sense of belonging from being a member of the union. While the client might feel responsible for his daughter's postponement of the wedding, if presented as an action to include him, the client will feel loved and cared for. While being suicidal may reduce the ability to concentrate, if the client perceives the executorship positively, taking the role away reinforces the client's low self-esteem and self-worth. This statement by the client's brother also indicates a need for the client's brother to be educated about depressive illness.

Test-Taking Strategy: Use the process of elimination and focus on the issue: delaying discharge. Recalling the risks associated with a suicide intent will direct you to option 1. Review these risks if you had difficulty with this question.

Level of Cognitive Ability: Analysis
Client Needs: Safe, Effective Care Environment
Integrated Process: Nursing Process/Analysis
Content Area: Mental Health

Reference:
Stuart, G., & Laraia, M. (2005). *Principles and practice of psychiatric nursing* (8th ed.). St. Louis: Mosby, p. 374.

---

170. A nurse is preparing to ambulate a client with Parkinson's disease who has recently been started on L-Dopa (Levadopa). The nurse assesses which most important item before performing this activity with the client?
  1 Assistive devices used by the client
  2 The degree of intention tremors exhibited by the client
  3 The client's history of falls
  4 The client's postural (orthostatic) vital signs

Answer: 4
Rationale: Clients with Parkinson's disease are at risk for postural (orthostatic) hypotension from the disease. This problem is exacerbated with the introduction of Levadopa, which can also cause postural hypotension and increase the client's risk for falls. Although knowledge of the client's use of assistive devices and history of falls is helpful, it is not the most important piece of assessment data based on the wording of this question. Clients with Parkinson's disease generally have resting, not intention, tremors.

Test-Taking Strategy: Focus on the key words "most important." Postural hypotension presents the greatest safety risk to the client. Also, use of the ABCs—airway, breathing, and circulation—will direct you to option 4. Checking postural vital signs is one way to assess circulation. Review the complications associated with Parkinson's disease and the effects of Levadopa if you had difficulty with this question.

Level of Cognitive Ability: Application
Client Needs: Safe, Effective Care Environment
Integrated Process: Nursing Process/Assessment
Content Area: Pharmacology

References:
Lehne, R. (2004). *Pharmacology for nursing care* (5th ed.). Philadelphia: Saunders, p. 184.
McKenry, L., & Salerno, E. (2003). *Mosby's pharmacology in nursing* (21st ed.). St. Louis: Mosby, p. 497.

---

171. A nurse is preparing to transfer an average-sized client with right-sided hemiplegia from the bed to the wheelchair. The client is able to support weight on the unaffected side. The nurse plans to use the hemiplegic transfer technique. The client is dangling on the side of the bed. For the safest transfer, the wheelchair should be positioned:
  1 Near the client's right leg
  2 Next to either leg
  3 As space in the room permits
  4 Near the client's left leg

Answer: 4
Rationale: Although space in the room is an important consideration for placement of the wheelchair for a transfer, when the client has an affected lower extremity, movement should always occur toward the client's unaffected (strong) side. For example, if the client's right leg is involved, and the client is sitting on the edge of the bed, position the wheelchair next to the client's left side. This wheelchair position allows the client to use the unaffected leg effectively and safely.

Test-Taking Strategy: Use the process of elimination, focusing on the issue: a safe transfer technique. Noting that the client has right-sided hemiplegia and visualizing each of the options will direct you to option 4. Positioning the wheelchair next to the client's unaffected leg allows the client to use the stronger leg more effectively for a safe transfer. Review transfer techniques if you had difficulty with this question.

Level of Cognitive Ability: Application
Client Needs: Safe, Effective Care Environment
Integrated Process: Nursing Process/Implementation
Content Area: Fundamental Skills

Reference:

Potter, P., & Perry, A. (2005). *Fundamentals of nursing* (6th ed.). St. Louis: Mosby, pp. 1469-1470.

---

172. A nurse is caring for a client with a serious condition who is a potential organ donor. Before approaching the family to discuss organ donation, the nurse reviews the client's medical record for contraindications to organ donation, which would include:

1 Allergy to penicillin-type antibiotics
2 Age of 38 years
3 Hepatitis B infection
4 Negative rapid plasma reagin (RPR) laboratory result

Answer: 3

Rationale: A potential organ donor must meet age eligibility requirements, which vary by organ. For example, age must not exceed 65 years for kidney donation, 55 years for pancreas or liver donation, and 40 years for heart donation. The client should be free of communicable disease, such as human immunodeficiency virus, hepatitis, or syphilis, and the involved organ must not be diseased. Another contraindication is malignancy, with the exception of noninvolved skin and cornea.

Test-Taking Strategy: Focus on the issue: contraindications to organ donations. Noting the word "infection" in option 3 will direct you to this option. Review these contraindications if you had difficulty with this question.

Level of Cognitive Ability: Analysis
Client Needs: Safe, Effective Care Environment
Integrated Process: Nursing Process/Assessment
Content Area: Fundamental Skills

References:

Black, J., & Hawks, J. (2005). *Medical-surgical nursing: Clinical management for positive outcomes* (7th ed.). Philadelphia: Saunders, p. 2430.
Lewis, S., Heitkemper, M., & Dirksen, S. (2004). *Medical-surgical nursing: Assessment and management of clinical problems* (6th ed.). St. Louis: Mosby, p. 1240.

---

173. A nurse is monitoring the ongoing care given to the potential organ donor who has been diagnosed with brain death. The nurse determines that the standard of care had been maintained if which of the following data is observed?

1 Urine output: 45 mL/hour
2 Capillary refill: 5 seconds
3 Serum pH: 7.32
4 Blood pressure: 90/48 mmHg

Answer: 1

Rationale: Adequate perfusion must be maintained to all vital organs in order for the client to remain viable as an organ donor. A urine output of 45 mL per hour indicates adequate renal perfusion. Low blood pressure and delayed capillary refill time are circulatory system indicators of inadequate perfusion. A serum pH of 7.32 is acidotic, which adversely affects all body tissues.

Test-Taking Strategy: Use the process of elimination and eliminate options 2, 3, and 4 because they are abnormal values. Review normal values for physical assessment measurements and the criteria related to organ donation if you had difficulty with this question.

Level of Cognitive Ability: Analysis
Client Needs: Safe, Effective Care Environment
Integrated Process: Nursing Process/Evaluation
Content Area: Fundamental Skills

References:
Black, J., & Hawks, J. (2005). *Medical-surgical nursing: Clinical management for positive outcomes* (7th ed.). Philadelphia: Saunders, p. 2430.
Lewis, S., Heitkemper, M., & Dirksen, S. (2004). *Medical-surgical nursing: Assessment and management of clinical problems* (6th ed.). St. Louis: Mosby, p. 1240.
Phipps, W., Monahan, F., Sands, J., Marek, J., & Neighbors, M. (2003). *Medical-surgical nursing: health and illness perspectives* (7th ed.). St. Louis: Mosby, p. 1688.

---

174. The client who suffered a severe head injury has had vigorous treatment to control cerebral edema. Brain death has now been determined. The nurse prepares to carry out which of the following that will maintain viability of the kidneys before organ donation?
1 Monitoring temperature
2 Administering intravenous (IV) fluids
3 Assessing lung sounds
4 Performing range of motion exercises to extremities

Answer: 2
Rationale: Perfusion to the kidney is affected by blood pressure, which is in turn affected by blood vessel tone and fluid volume. Therefore, the client who was previously dehydrated to control intracranial pressure is now in need of rehydration to maintain perfusion to the kidneys. Thus, the nurse prepares to infuse IV fluids as prescribed, and continues to monitor urine output. Options 1, 3, and 4 will not maintain viability of the kidneys.

Test-Taking Strategy: Focus on the issue: maintaining viability of the kidneys. Use the process of elimination, noting the relation between the issue and option 2. Review the concepts related to organ donation of the kidneys if you had difficulty with this question.

Level of Cognitive Ability: Application
Client Needs: Safe, Effective Care Environment
Integrated Process: Nursing Process/Planning
Content Area: Fundamental Skills

Reference:
Lewis, S., Heitkemper, M., & Dirksen, S. (2004). *Medical-surgical nursing: Assessment and management of clinical problems* (6th ed.). St. Louis: Mosby, p. 1241.

---

175. A nurse is working in the emergency room of a small local hospital when a client with multiple gunshot wounds arrives by ambulance. Which of the following actions by the nurse is contraindicated in the proper care of handling legal evidence?
1 Cut clothing along seams, avoiding bullet holes
2 Initiate a chain of custody log
3 Place personal belongings in a labeled, sealed paper bag
4 Give clothing and wallet to the family

Answer: 4
Rationale: Basic rules for handling evidence include limiting the number of people with access to the evidence; initiating a chain of custody log to track handling and movement of evidence; and careful removal of clothing to avoid destroying evidence. This usually includes cutting clothes along seams, while avoiding areas where there are obvious holes or tears. Potential evidence is never released to the family to take home.

Test-Taking Strategy: Focus on the client situation and note the key word "contraindicated." This key word indicates a false-response question and that you need to select the option that identifies an incorrect nursing action. Use knowledge of basic emergency care principles related to a potential crime to eliminate each of the incorrect options. Remember that giving the client's belongings to the family may be giving up evidence. Review the legal principles related to care of a client with a gunshot wound if you had difficulty with this question.

Level of Cognitive Ability: Application
Client Needs: Safe, Effective Care Environment
Integrated Process: Nursing Process/Implementation
Content Area: Leadership/Management

Reference:
Brent, N. (2001). *Nurses and the law* (2nd ed.). Philadelphia: Saunders, p. 289.

---

176. A nurse working on a medical nursing unit during an external disaster is called to assist with care for clients coming into the emergency room. Using principles of triage, the nurse initiates immediate care for a client with which of the following injuries?
1 Bright red bleeding from a neck wound
2 Penetrating abdominal injury
3 Fractured tibia
4 Open massive head injury in deep coma

Answer: 1
Rationale: The client with arterial bleeding from a neck wound is in "immediate" need of treatment to save the client's life. This client is classified as such and would wear a color tag of red from the triage process. The client with a penetrating abdominal injury would be tagged yellow and classified as "delayed," requiring intervention within 30 to 60 minutes. A green or "minimal" designation would be given to the client with a fractured tibia, who requires intervention but who can provide self-care if needed. A designation of "expectant" would be applied to the client with massive injuries and minimal chance of survival. This client would be color-coded "black" in the triage process. The client who is color-coded "black" is given supportive care and pain management, but is given definitive treatment last.

Test-Taking Strategy: Use the process of elimination and focus on the key words "initiates immediate care." Use the principles of triage and prioritize. Noting the words "bright red" in option 1 will direct you to this option. Review disaster planning and the principles of triage if you had difficulty with this question.

Level of Cognitive Ability: Application
Client Needs: Safe, Effective Care Environment
Integrated Process: Nursing Process/Implementation
Content Area: Delegating/Prioritizing

References:
Black, J., & Hawks, J. (2005). *Medical-surgical nursing: Clinical management for positive outcomes* (7th ed.). Philadelphia: Saunders, p. 2509.
Lewis, S., Heitkemper, M., & Dirksen, S. (2004). *Medical-surgical nursing: Assessment and management of clinical problems* (6th ed.). St. Louis: Mosby, pp. 1846-1847.
Phipps, W., Monahan, F., Sands, J., Marek, J., & Neighbors, M. (2003). *Medical-surgical nursing: health and illness perspectives* (7th ed.). St. Louis: Mosby, p. 119.

---

177. A nurse working on an adult nursing unit is told to review the client census to determine which clients could be discharged if there are a large number of admissions from a newly declared disaster. The nurse determines that the client with which of the following problems would need to remain hospitalized?
1 Laparoscopic cholecystectomy
2 Ongoing ventricular dysrhythmias while on procainamide (Procan)
3 Diabetes mellitus with blood glucose at 180 mg/dL
4 Fractured hip pinned 5 days ago

Answer: 2
Rationale: The client with ongoing ventricular dysrhythmias requires ongoing medical evaluation and treatment, because of potentially lethal complications of the problem. Each of the other problems listed may be managed at home with appropriate agency referrals for home care services and support from the family at home.

Test-Taking Strategy: Use the principles of triage. Severity of illness usually guides the determination of who requires ongoing monitoring and care. Use of the ABCs—airway, breathing, and circulation—will direct you to option 2. Review the principles of triage and prioritizing if you had difficulty with this question.

Level of Cognitive Ability: Analysis
Client Needs: Safe, Effective Care Environment
Integrated Process: Nursing Process/Analysis
Content Area: Delegating/Prioritizing

References:

Black, J., & Hawks, J. (2005). *Medical-surgical nursing: Clinical management for positive outcomes* (7th ed.). Philadelphia: Saunders, p. 2484.

Lewis, S., Heitkemper, M., & Dirksen, S. (2004). *Medical-surgical nursing: Assessment and management of clinical problems* (6th ed.). St. Louis: Mosby, pp. 1846-1847.

---

178. A registered nurse (RN) is orienting a nursing assistant to the clinical nursing unit. The RN would intervene if the nursing assistant did which of the following during a routine handwashing procedure?

1 Kept hands lower than elbows
2 Used 3 to 5 mL of soap from the dispenser
3 Washed continuously for 10 to 15 seconds
4 Dried from forearm down to fingers

Answer: 4

Rationale: Proper handwashing procedure involves wetting the hands and wrists and keeping the hands lower than the forearms so water flows toward the fingertips. The nurse uses 3 to 5 mL of soap and scrubs for 10 to 15 seconds using rubbing and circular motions. The hands are rinsed and then dried, moving from the fingers to the forearms. The paper towel is then discarded, and a second one is used to turn off the faucet to avoid hand contamination.

Test-Taking Strategy: Note the key word "intervene." This key word indicates a false-response question and that you need to select the option that identifies an incorrect action by the nursing assistant. Use basic principles of medical asepsis and visualize each of the actions in the options to assist in directing you to option 4. Review this fundamental nursing procedure if you had difficulty with this question.

Level of Cognitive Ability: Application
Client Needs: Safe, Effective Care Environment
Integrated Process: Nursing Process/Implementation
Content Area: Leadership/Management

Reference:

Potter, P., & Perry, A. (2005). *Fundamentals of nursing* (6th ed.). St. Louis: Mosby, pp. 790-793.

---

179. A nurse is developing a plan of care for a client being admitted to the hospital who is immunosuppressed and will be placed on neutropenic precautions. With regard to neutropenic precautions, which intervention is incorrect?

1 Placing a mask on the client if the client leaves the room
2 Removing a vase with fresh flowers left by a previous client
3 Admitting the client to a semi-private room
4 Placing a precaution sign on the door to the room

Answer: 3

Rationale: The client who is on neutropenic precautions is immunosuppressed and is admitted to a single (private) room on the nursing unit. A precaution sign should be placed on the door to the client's room. Standing water and fresh flowers should be removed to decrease the microorganism count. The client should wear a mask whenever leaving the room to be protected from exposure to microorganisms.

Test-Taking Strategy: Use the process of elimination, noting the key word "incorrect." This key word indicates a false-response question and that you need to select the option that identifies an incorrect action. Recalling that neutropenic precautions are instituted when the client is at risk for infection because of impaired immune function will direct you to option 3. Review this type of infection control precaution if you had difficulty with this question.

Level of Cognitive Ability: Application
Client Needs: Safe, Effective Care Environment
Integrated Process: Nursing Process/Planning
Content Area: Adult Health/Oncology

References:

Black, J., & Hawks, J. (2005). *Medical-surgical nursing: Clinical management for positive outcomes* (7th ed.). Philadelphia: Saunders, pp. 381-382.
Lewis, S., Heitkemper, M., & Dirksen, S. (2004). *Medical-surgical nursing: Assessment and management of clinical problems* (6th ed.). St. Louis: Mosby, p. 734.

---

180. A nurse is preparing to change the linens and clean a client who was incontinent of urine. The nurse wears which of the following protective items?
  1 Mask and gloves
  2 Gown and gloves
  3 Mask, gown, and gloves
  4 Gown, gloves, and eyewear

Answer: 2
Rationale: In caring for the incontinent client, the nurse should wear gloves and a gown to protect the hands and uniform from contamination.

Test-Taking Strategy: Note that the potential source of contamination in this situation is the client's urine. Because urine present on the hospital gown and bedclothes is not likely to splash, eliminate options 1, 3, and 4. Review standard precautions if you had difficulty with this question.

Level of Cognitive Ability: Application
Client Needs: Safe, Effective Care Environment
Integrated Process: Nursing Process/Implementation
Content Area: Adult Health/Oncology

Reference:

Potter, P., & Perry, A. (2005). *Fundamentals of nursing* (6th ed.). St. Louis: Mosby, p. 797.

---

181. A nurse receives a telephone call from the hospital admission office and is informed that a client is being admitted who will undergo implantation of a sealed internal radiation source. The nurse asks the admission office clerk if which of the following rooms is selected for the client?
  1 A single room at the distant end of the hall
  2 A single room near the nurse's station
  3 A semiprivate room between two isolation rooms
  4 A semiprivate room near the nurse's station

Answer: 1
Rationale: The client receiving an implantation of a sealed internal radiation source should be placed in a single room in an area that reduces the risk of exposure to others. For this reason, rooms are often used that are at the end of a hall or near a stairwell.

Test-Taking Strategy: Use of the principles of shielding related to radiation therapy will assist to eliminate options 2, 3, and 4 because they do not provide distance to protect other clients. Review the protective measures related to the care of a client with a sealed internal radiation source if you had difficulty with this question.

Level of Cognitive Ability: Application
Client Needs: Safe, Effective Care Environment
Integrated Process: Nursing Process/Planning
Content Area: Adult Health/Oncology

References:

Black, J., & Hawks, J. (2005). *Medical-surgical nursing: Clinical management for positive outcomes* (7th ed.). Philadelphia: Saunders, p. 363.
Ignatavicius, D., & Workman, M. (2002). *Medical surgical nursing: Critical thinking for collaborative care* (4th ed.). Philadelphia: Saunders, p. 429.

182. A nurse is assessing the corneal reflex on an unconscious client. The nurse would use which of the following as the safest stimulus to touch the client's cornea?
1 Wisp of cotton
2 Sterile tongue depressor
3 Sterile glove
4 Tip of a 1-mL syringe with the needle removed

Answer: 1
Rationale: The corneal reflex is tested in selected situations, such as with the unconscious client. The client who is unconscious is at great risk for corneal abrasion. For this reason, the safest way to test the corneal reflex is by touching the cornea lightly with cotton. The lids of both eyes blink when the cornea is touched. Use of the items in options 2, 3, and 4 can cause injury to the cornea.

Test-Taking Strategy: Use the process of elimination, noting the key words "unconscious" and "safest." Visualize each item in the options and eliminate options 2, 3, and 4 because they are blunt objects. Review care of an unconscious client if you had difficulty with this question.

Level of Cognitive Ability: Application
Client Needs: Safe, Effective Care Environment
Integrated Process: Nursing Process/Assessment
Content Area: Adult Health/Neurological

Reference:
Wilson, S., & Giddens, J. (2005). *Health assessment for nursing practice* (3rd ed.). St. Louis: Mosby, p. 310.

183. A nurse is preparing to assist the client from the bed to a chair using a hydraulic lift. The nurse would do which of the following to move the client safely with this device?
1 Have three people available to assist
2 Position the client in the center of the sling
3 Have the client grasp the chains attaching the sling to the lift
4 Lower the client rapidly once positioned over the chair

Answer: 2
Rationale: When using a hydraulic lift, the client is positioned in the center of the sling, which is then attached to chains or straps that attach the sling to the lift. The client's hands and arms are crossed over the chest, and the client is raised from the bed into a sitting position. The client is also raised off the mattress with the lift and is lowered slowly once the sling is positioned over the chair.

Test-Taking Strategy: Focus on the issue: moving the client safely. Visualize this procedure and each description in the options to direct you to option 2. Review this procedure if you had difficulty with this question.

Level of Cognitive Ability: Application
Client Needs: Safe, Effective Care Environment
Integrated Process: Nursing Process/Implementation
Content Area: Fundamental Skills

Reference:
Potter, P., & Perry, A. (2005). *Fundamentals of nursing* (6th ed.). St. Louis: Mosby, p. 1473.

184. An older client in a long-term care facility has a nursing diagnosis of Risk for Injury related to confusion. Because the client's gait is stable, the nurse uses which method of restraint to prevent injury to the client?
1 Vest restraint
2 Waist restraint
3 Chair with locking lap tray
4 Alarm-activating (Ambularm) bracelet

Answer: 4
Rationale: If the client is confused and has a stable gait, the least intrusive method of restraint is the use of an alarm-activating bracelet, or "wandering bracelet." This allows the client to move about the residence freely while preventing the client from leaving the premises. Options 1, 2, and 3 are restrictive devices and should not be used.

Test-Taking Strategy: Use the process of elimination and knowledge of the ethical and legal ramifications related to restraints. Noting the key words "gait is stable" will direct you to option 4. Review the guidelines related to the use of restraints if you had difficulty with this question.

Level of Cognitive Ability: Application
Client Needs: Safe, Effective Care Environment
Integrated Process: Nursing Process/Implementation
Content Area: Fundamental Skills

Reference:
Potter, P., & Perry, A. (2005). *Fundamentals of nursing* (6th ed.). St. Louis: Mosby, p. 990.

---

185. Furosemide (Lasix) 40 mg orally has been prescribed for the client. In error, the nurse administers furosemide 80 mg orally to the client at 10:00 AM. Following discovery of the error, the nurse completes an incident report. Which of the following would the nurse document on this report?
  1 "Furosemide 80 mg was given to the client instead of 40 mg."
  2 "The wrong dose of medication was given to the client at 10:00 AM."
  3 "I meant to give 40 mg of furosemide but I was rushed to get to another client who needed me and I gave the wrong dose."
  4 "Furosemide 80 mg administered at 10:00 AM."

Answer: 4
Rationale: When completing an incident report, the nurse should state the fact clearly. The nurse should not record assumptions, opinions, judgments, or conclusions about what occurred. The nurse should not point blame or suggest how to prevent an occurrence of a similar incident.

Test-Taking Strategy: Read the occurrence as stated in the question. Use the process of elimination and select the option that clearly and most directly states what has occurred. Options 1 and 2 are similar and point out that an error was made; therefore, eliminate these options. Option 3 provides a judgment. Option 4 clearly and simply states the occurrence. Review the principles associated with incident reports if you had difficulty with this question.

Level of Cognitive Ability: Application
Client Needs: Safe, Effective Care Environment
Integrated Process: Communication and Documentation
Content Area: Fundamental Skills

Reference:
Potter, P., & Perry, A. (2005). *Fundamentals of nursing* (6th ed.). St. Louis: Mosby, p. 419.

---

186. A registered nurse (RN) on the night shift assists a staff member in completing an incident report for a client who was found sitting on the floor. Following completion of the report, the RN intervenes if the staff member prepares to:
  1 Document in the nurses' notes that an incident report was filed
  2 Forward the incident report to the Continuous Quality Improvement Department
  3 Ask the unit secretary to call the physician
  4 Notify the nursing supervisor

Answer: 1
Rationale: Nurses are advised not to document the filing of an incident report in the nurses' notes for legal reasons. Incident reports inform the facility's administration of the incident so that risk management personnel can consider changes that might prevent similar occurrences in the future. Incident reports also alert the facility's insurance company to a potential claim and the need for further investigation. Options 2, 3, and 4 are accurate interventions.

Test-Taking Strategy: Note the key word "intervenes" in the stem of the question. This key word indicates a false-response question and that you need to select the option that identifies an incorrect action by the staff member. Note that options 2, 3, and 4 all relate to notification of key individuals or departments. Option 1 relates to documentation of filing an incident report. Review the concepts that relate to incident reports if you had difficulty with this question.

Level of Cognitive Ability: Application
Client Needs: Safe, Effective Care Environment
Integrated Process: Nursing Process/Implementation
Content Area: Leadership/Management

Reference:
Brent, N. (2001). *Nurses and the law* (2nd ed.). Philadelphia: Saunders, pp. 95-99.

---

187. A physician visits a client on the nursing unit. During the visit, the physician is paged and notified that the monthly physician's breakfast meeting is about to start. The physician states to the nurse: "I'm in a hurry. Can you write an order to decrease the atenolol (Tenormin) to 25 mg daily." Which of the following is the appropriate nursing action?
1 Write the order
2 Call the nursing supervisor to write the order
3 Ask the physician to return to the nursing unit to write the order
4 Inform the client of the change of medication

Answer: 3
Rationale: Nurses are encouraged not to accept verbal orders from the physician because of the risks of error. The only exception to this may be in an emergency situation, and then the agency policy and procedure must be adhered to. Although the client will be informed of the change in the treatment plan, this is not the appropriate action at this time. The physician needs to write the new order. It is inappropriate to ask another individual other than the physician to write the order.

Test-Taking Strategy: Use the process of elimination. Recall that verbal orders are not acceptable. Options 1 and 2 are similar, so therefore eliminate these options. Option 4 is appropriate, but not at this time. Option 3 clearly identifies the nurse's responsibility in this situation. Review these principles if you had difficulty with this question.

Level of Cognitive Ability: Application
Client Needs: Safe, Effective Care Environment
Integrated Process: Nursing Process/Implementation
Content Area: Leadership/Management

Reference:
Potter, P., & Perry, A. (2005). *Fundamentals of nursing* (6th ed.). St. Louis: Mosby, pp. 497; 838.

---

188. A nurse is caring for a hospitalized client who has an order for dextroamphetamine (Dexedrine) 25 mg orally daily. The nurse collaborates with the dietician to limit the amount of which of the following items on the client's dietary trays?
1 Starch
2 Caffeine
3 Protein
4 Fat

Answer: 2
Rationale: Dextroamphetamine is a central nervous system (CNS) stimulant. Caffeine is also a stimulant and should be limited in the client taking this medication. The client should be taught to limit caffeine intake as well. Options 1, 3, and 4 are acceptable dietary items.

Test-Taking Strategy: Use the process of elimination. Recalling that this medication is a CNS stimulant will direct you to option 2. Review this medication if you had difficulty with this question.

Level of Cognitive Ability: Application
Client Needs: Safe, Effective Care Environment
Integrated Process: Nursing Process/Implementation
Content Area: Pharmacology

References:
Lehne, R. (2004). *Pharmacology for nursing care* (5th ed.). Philadelphia: Saunders, p. 356.
McKenry, L., & Salerno, E. (2003). *Mosby's pharmacology in nursing* (21st ed.). St. Louis: Mosby, p. 383.

---

189. A nurse is planning preoperative care for a client scheduled for insertion of an inferior vena cava (IVC) filter. The nurse questions the physician about withholding which regularly scheduled medication on the day before surgery?
1 Furosemide (Lasix)
2 Potassium chloride (K-Dur)
3 Docusate (Colace)
4 Warfarin sodium (Coumadin)

Answer: 4
Rationale: In the preoperative period, the nurse consults with the physician about withholding warfarin sodium to avoid the occurrence of hemorrhage. Furosemide is a diuretic, potassium chloride is a supplement, and docusate is a stool softener.

Test-Taking Strategy: Note the issue: witholding a medication. Use the process of elimination, evaluating each medication in terms of its potential harm to the preoperative client. Review these medications if you had difficulty with this question.

Level of Cognitive Ability: Application
Client Needs: Safe, Effective Care Environment
Integrated Process: Nursing Process/Implementation
Content Area: Adult Health/Cardiovascular

Reference:
Ignatavicius, D., & Workman, M. (2002). *Medical surgical nursing: Critical thinking for collaborative care* (4th ed.). Philadelphia: Saunders, p. 765.

---

190. A hospitalized client with hypertension has been started on captopril (Capoten). The nurse ensures that the client does which of the following specific to this medication?
1 Eats foods that are high in potassium
2 Takes in sufficient amounts of high-fiber foods
3 Moves from a sitting to a standing position slowly
4 Drinks plenty of water

Answer: 3
Rationale: Orthostatic hypotension is a concern for clients taking antihypertensive medications. Clients are advised to avoid standing in one position for lengthy amounts of time, to change positions slowly, and to avoid extreme warmth (showers, bath, weather). Clients are also taught to recognize the symptoms of orthostatic hypotension, including dizziness, lightheadedness, weakness, and syncope. Options 1, 2, and 4 are not specific to this medication.

Test-Taking Strategy: Use the process of elimination. Recalling that captopril is an antihypertensive will direct you to option 3. Remember that the risk of orthostatic hypotension is present with all types of antihypertensives. Review the effects of this medication if you had difficulty with this question.

Level of Cognitive Ability: Application
Client Needs: Safe, Effective Care Environment
Integrated Process: Nursing Process/Implementation
Content Area: Adult Health/Cardiovascular

Reference:
McKenry, L., & Salerno, E. (2003). *Mosby's pharmacology in nursing* (21st ed.). St. Louis: Mosby, p. 586.

191. A nurse is preparing to ambulate a client. The best and safest position for the nurse in assisting the client is to stand:
1 Behind the client
2 In front of the client
3 On the unaffected side of the client
4 On the affected side of the client

Answer: 4
Rationale: When walking with clients, the nurse should stand on the affected side and grasp the security belt in the midspine area of the small of the back. The nurse should position the free hand at the shoulder area so that the client can be pulled toward the nurse in the event that there is a forward fall. The client is instructed to look up and outward rather than at his or her feet. Options 1, 2, and 3 are incorrect positions.

Test-Taking Strategy: Use the process of elimination. Recalling that support is needed on the affected side will assist in directing you to option 4. Review this procedure if you had difficulty with this question.

Level of Cognitive Ability: Application
Client Needs: Safe, Effective Care Environment
Integrated Process: Nursing Process/Implementation
Content Area: Fundamental Skills

Reference:
Potter, P., & Perry, A. (2005). *Fundamentals of nursing* (6th ed.). St. Louis: Mosby, pp. 947-948.

---

192. A client receiving lisinopril (Prinivil) has a white blood cell (WBC) count of 3,800 mm^3. The nurse plans to do which of the following in the care of this client?
1 Follow strict aseptic technique
2 Request prophylactic antibiotics from the physician
3 Place the client on respiratory isolation
4 Use antibacterial soap when bathing the client

Answer: 1
Rationale: The client taking angiotensin-converting enzyme (ACE) inhibitors, such as lisinopril, may be at risk of developing neutropenia. These clients require the use of strict aseptic technique by all who care for the client. The client should also be taught to report signs and symptoms of infection, such as sore throat and fever, to the physician. The WBC count with differential may be monitored monthly for up to 6 months in clients deemed at risk. Options 2, 3, and 4 are not appropriate interventions. No data in the question indicates the need for antibiotics, respiratory isolation, or the use of antibacterial soap.

Test-Taking Strategy: Use the process of elimination. This question can be correctly answered even without knowing that ACE inhibitors cause neutropenia, as long as you can recognize abnormally low WBC values. Recognizing that a WBC count of 3,800 mm^3 is a low count and that a low count places the client at risk for infection directs you to option 1. Review this medication if you had difficulty with this question.

Level of Cognitive Ability: Application
Client Needs: Safe, Effective Care Environment
Integrated Process: Nursing Process/Planning
Content Area: Pharmacology

Reference:
McKenry, L., & Salerno, E. (2003). *Mosby's pharmacology in nursing* (21st ed.). St. Louis: Mosby, p. 587.

193. A nurse is taking the temperature of a client using a glass thermometer. The nurse shakes down the thermometer and drops the thermometer on the floor. Which of the following actions should the nurse take?
 1 Carefully wipe up the spill, avoiding getting cut from the glass
 2 Use a mop and dust pan to clean up the spill, avoiding contact with the glass and mercury
 3 Notify the Environmental Services Department of the spill
 4 Call the Housekeeping Department to clean up the spill and broken glass

Answer: 3
Rationale: Mercury is a hazardous material. Accidental breakage of a mercury-in-glass thermometer is a health hazard to the client, nurse, and other health care workers. Mercury droplets are not to be touched. If a breakage or spill occurs, the Environmental Services Department is called and a mercury spill kit is used to clean up the spill.

Test-Taking Strategy: Use the process of elimination. Remembering that mercury is a hazardous material will direct you to option 3. Review the principles associated with mercury spills if you had difficulty with this question.

Level of Cognitive Ability: Application
Client Needs: Safe, Effective Care Environment
Integrated Process: Nursing Process/Implementation
Content Area: Fundamental Skills

Reference:
Potter, P., & Perry, A. (2005). *Fundamentals of nursing* (6th ed.). St. Louis: Mosby, p. 633.

---

194. A nurse is called to a client's room by another nurse. When the nurse arrives at the room, she discovers that a fire has occurred in the client's waste basket. The first nurse has removed the client from the room. What is the second nurse's next action?
 1 Evacuate the unit
 2 Extinguish the fire
 3 Confine the fire
 4 Activate the fire alarm

Answer: 4
Rationale: Remember the acronym RACE (i.e., rescue, alarm, confine, extinguish) to set priorities if a fire occurs. In this situation, the client has been rescued from the immediate vicinity of the fire. The next action is to activate the fire alarm.

Test-Taking Strategy: Use the RACE acronym to set priorities and answer the question. This will direct you to option 4. Review fire safety if you had difficulty with this question.

Level of Cognitive Ability: Application
Client Needs: Safe, Effective Care Environment
Integrated Process: Nursing Process/Implementation
Content Area: Delegating/Prioritizing

Reference:
Potter, P., & Perry, A. (2005). *Fundamentals of nursing* (6th ed.). St. Louis: Mosby, p. 991.

---

195. A nurse is caring for a client with cervical cancer who has an internal radiation implant. Which of the following required items would the nurse ensure is kept in the client's room during this treatment?
 1 A bedside commode
 2 A lead apron
 3 Long-handled forceps and a lead container (pig)
 4 A number 16 Foley catheter

Answer: 3
Rationale: In the case of dislodgment of an internal radiation implant, the radioactive source is never touched with the bare hands. It is retrieved with long-handled forceps and placed in the lead container (pig) kept in the client's room. In many situations, the client has a Foley catheter inserted and is on bed rest during treatment to prevent dislodgment. A lead apron, although one may be in the room, is not the required item. Nurses wear a dosimeter badge while in the client's room to measure the exposure to radiation and limit time spent in the room.

Test-Taking Strategy: Note the key word "required". Eliminate options 1 and 4 because they are similar and relate to urinary output. From the remaining options, select option 3 over option 2, keeping in mind that the risk of dislodgment can occur. Review these principles if you had difficulty with this question.

Level of Cognitive Ability: Application
Client Needs: Safe, Effective Care Environment
Integrated Process: Nursing Process/Implementation
Content Area: Fundamental Skills

References:

Black, J., & Hawks, J. (2005). *Medical-surgical nursing: Clinical management for positive outcomes* (7th ed.). Philadelphia: Saunders, p. 363.
Ignatavicius, D., & Workman, M. (2002). *Medical surgical nursing: Critical thinking for collaborative care* (4th ed.). Philadelphia: Saunders, p. 429.

196. A nurse enters the client's room and finds the client lying on the floor. Following assessment of the client, the nurse calls the nursing supervisor and the physician to inform them of the occurrence. The nursing supervisor instructs the nurse to complete an incident report. The nurse understands that incident reports allow the analysis of adverse client events by:

1 Evaluating quality care and the potential risks for injury to the client
2 Determining the effectiveness of nursing interventions in relation to outcomes
3 Providing a method of reporting injuries to local, state, and federal agencies
4 Providing clients with necessary stabilizing treatments

Answer: 1

Rationale: Proper documentation of unusual occurrences, incidents, and accidents, and the nursing actions taken as a result of the occurrence are internal to the institution or agency and allow the nurse and administration to review the quality of care and determine any potential risks present. Incident reports are not routinely filled out for interventions, nor are they used to report occurrences to other agencies.

Test-Taking Strategy: Use the process of elimination and knowledge regarding the purpose of incident reports. Eliminate option 2, recalling that incident reports are not routinely filled out for interventions. Eliminate option 3 because incident reports are not used to report occurrences to other agencies. Eliminate option 4 because it is unrelated to the purpose of an incident report. Review the purpose of incident reports if you had difficulty with this question.

Level of Cognitive Ability: Analysis
Client Needs: Safe, Effective Care Environment
Integrated Process: Nursing Process/Analysis
Content Area: Fundamental Skills

References:

Brent, N. (2001). *Nurses and the law* (2nd ed.). Philadelphia: Saunders, p. 95.
Potter, P., & Perry, A. (2005). *Fundamentals of nursing* (6th ed.). St. Louis: Mosby, p. 419.

197. A registered nurse suspects that a colleague is substance impaired and notes signs of alcohol intoxication in the colleague. The Nurse Practice Act requires that the registered nurse do which of the following?
1 Talk with the colleague
2 Report the information to a nursing supervisor
3 Call the impaired nurse organization
4 Ask the colleague to go to the nurses' lounge to sleep for a while

Answer: 2
Rationale: Nurse Practice Acts require reporting the suspicion of impaired nurses. The Board of Nursing has jurisdiction over the practice of nursing and may develop plans for treatment and supervision. This suspicion needs to be reported to the nursing supervisor, who will then report to the Board of Nursing. Confronting the colleague may cause conflict. Asking the colleague to go to the nurses' lounge to sleep for a while does not safeguard clients.

Test-Taking Strategy: Use the process of elimination and knowledge regarding the agency channels of communication when reporting an incident. Remember to report suspicions of substance abuse to the nursing supervisor. Review nursing responsibilities related to suspicion of an impaired nurse if you had difficulty with this question.

Level of Cognitive Ability: Application
Client Needs: Safe, Effective Care Environment
Integrated Process: Nursing Process/Implementation
Content Area: Leadership/Management

References:
Brent, N. (2001). *Nurses and the law* (2nd ed.). Philadelphia: Saunders, pp. 302-304.
Stuart, G., & Laraia, M. (2005). *Principles and practice of psychiatric nursing* (8th ed.). St. Louis: Mosby, pp. 510-511.

198. A nurse lawyer provides an education session to the nursing staff regarding client rights. A staff nurse asks the lawyer to describe an example that might relate to invasion of client privacy. Which of the following indicates a violation of this right?
1 Taking photographs of the client without consent
2 Telling the client that he or she cannot leave the hospital
3 Threatening to place a client in restraints
4 Performing a surgical procedure without consent

Answer: 1
Rationale: Invasion of privacy takes place when an individual's private affairs are unreasonably intruded into. Telling the client that he or she cannot leave the hospital constitutes false imprisonment. Threatening to place a client in restraints constitutes assault. Performing a surgical procedure without consent is an example of battery.

Test-Taking Strategy: Use the process of elimination, noting the key words "invasion of client privacy." Note the relation of these key words to option 1. Review those situations that include invasion of privacy if you had difficulty with this question.

Level of Cognitive Ability: Analysis
Client Needs: Safe, Effective Care Environment
Integrated Process: Nursing Process/Analysis
Content Area: Leadership/Management

Reference:
Brent, N. (2001). *Nurses and the law* (2nd ed.). Philadelphia: Saunders, pp. 122-123.

199. A nurse witnesses an automobile accident and provides care to the open wound of a young child at the scene of the accident. The family is extremely grateful and insists that the nurse accept monetary compensation for the care provided to the child. Because of the family's insistence, the nurse accepts the compensation to avoid offending the family. The child subsequently develops an infection and sepsis and is hospitalized, and the family files suit against the nurse who provided care to the child at the scene of the accident. Which of the following is accurate regarding the nurse's immunity from this suit?

1 The Good Samaritan Law will protect the nurse
2 The Good Samaritan Law will protect the nurse if the care given at the scene was not negligent
3 The Good Samaritan Law will not provide immunity from the suit if the nurse accepted compensation for the care provided
4 The Good Samaritan Law protects laypersons and not professional health care providers

Answer: 3
Rationale: A Good Samaritan Law is passed by a state legislature to encourage nurses and other health care providers to provide care to a person when an accident, emergency, or injury occurs, without fear of being sued for the care provided. Called "immunity from suit," this protection usually applies only if all of the conditions of the law are met, such as the heath care provider receives no compensation for the care provided and the care given is not willfully and wantonly negligent.

Test-Taking Strategy: Note the key words "accepts the compensation" in the question. Note the relation of these words to option 3. Also eliminate options 1, 2, and 4 because they are similar. Review the Good Samaritan Law if you had difficulty with this question.

Level of Cognitive Ability: Analysis
Client Needs: Safe, Effective Care Environment
Integrated Process: Nursing Process/Analysis
Content Area: Fundamental Skills

Reference:
Brent, N. (2001). *Nurses and the law* (2nd ed.). Philadelphia: Saunders, pp. 66; 407-408.

---

200. A client brought to the emergency room after a serious accident is unconscious and bleeding profusely. Surgery is required immediately in order to save the client's life. In regard to informed consent for the surgical procedure, which of the following is the best nursing action?

1 Try to obtain the spouse's telephone number and call the spouse to obtain telephone consent before the surgical procedure
2 Transport the client to the operating room immediately as required by the physician without obtaining an informed consent
3 Ask the friend who accompanied the client to the emergency room to sign the consent form
4 Call the nursing supervisor to initiate a court order for the surgical procedure

Answer: 2
Rationale: Generally, the informed consent of an adult client is not needed in two instances: (1) when an emergency is present and delaying treatment to obtain informed consent would result in injury or death to the client, and (2) when the client waives the right to give informed consent. Option 3 is inappropriate. Options 1 and 4 would delay treatment.

Test-Taking Strategy: Use the process of elimination. Option 3 can be eliminated first because it is inappropriate to ask a nonfamily member to sign a consent form. Next, note the key words "surgery is required immediately." Eliminate options 1 and 4 because these actions would delay treatment. Review the issues surrounding informed consent if you had difficulty with this question.

Level of Cognitive Ability: Application
Client Needs: Safe, Effective Care Environment
Integrated Process: Nursing Process/Implementation
Content Area: Fundamental Skills

References:
Brent, N. (2001). *Nurses and the law* (2nd ed.). Philadelphia: Saunders, p 210.
Potter, P., & Perry, A. (2005). *Fundamentals of nursing* (6th ed.). St. Louis: Mosby, pp. 416-417.

201. A home care nurse arrives at the client's home for the scheduled home visit. The client's lawyer is present and the client is preparing a living will. The living will requires that the client's signature be witnessed, and the client asks the nurse to witness the signature. The nurse should do which of the following?

1 Sign the will as a witness to signature only
2 Sign the will, clearly identifying credentials and employment agency
3 Decline to sign the will
4 Call the home health care office and notify the supervisor that the will is being witnessed

Answer: 3

Rationale: Living wills are required to be in writing and signed by the client. The client's signature either must be witnessed by specified individuals or notarized. Many states prohibit any employee, including a nurse of a facility where the declaring is receiving care, from being a witness. The nurse should decline to sign the will.

Test-Taking Strategy: Use the process of elimination. Eliminate options 1, 2, and 4 because they are similar and indicate that the nurse will sign as a witness. Review legal implications associated with wills if you had difficulty with this question.

Level of Cognitive Ability: Application
Client Needs: Safe, Effective Care Environment
Integrated Process: Nursing Process/Implementation
Content Area: Fundamental Skills

References:
Brent, N. (2001). *Nurses and the law* (2nd ed.). Philadelphia: Saunders, pp. 216-217.
Potter, P., & Perry, A. (2005). *Fundamentals of nursing* (6th ed.). St. Louis: Mosby, pp. 409-410.

202. An older woman is brought to the emergency room. On physical assessment, the nurse notes old and new ecchymotic areas on both arms and buttocks. The nurse asks the client how the bruises were sustained. The client, although reluctant, tells the nurse in confidence that her daughter frequently hits her if she gets in the way. Which of the following is the appropriate nursing response?

1 "I promise I will not tell anyone, but let's see what we can do about this."
2 "I have a legal obligation to report this type of abuse."
3 "Let's talk about ways that will prevent your daughter from hitting you."
4 "This should not be happening, and if it happens again, you must call the emergency department."

Answer: 2

Rationale: Confidential issues are not to be discussed with nonmedical personnel or the person's family or friends without the person's permission. Clients should be assured that information is kept confidential, unless it places the nurse under a legal obligation. The nurse must report situations related to child or elderly abuse, gunshot wounds, crimes, and certain infectious diseases.

Test-Taking Strategy: Use the process of elimination. Option 4 can be eliminated first because this action does not protect the client from injury. Options 1 and 3 are similar and should be eliminated next. Review the nursing responsibilities related to reporting obligations if you had difficulty with this question.

Level of Cognitive Ability: Application
Client Needs: Safe, Effective Care Environment
Integrated Process: Nursing Process/Implementation
Content Area: Fundamental Skills

Reference:
Brent, N. (2001). *Nurses and the law* (2nd ed.). Philadelphia: Saunders, pp. 283; 285.

203. A client is brought to the emergency room by the ambulance team following collapse at home. Cardiopulmonary resuscitation is attempted but is unsuccessful. The wife of the client tells the nurse that the client is an organ donor and that the eyes are to be donated. The nurse does which of the following?
1 Places the client in a supine position
2 Calls the National Donor Association to confirm that the client is a donor
3 Places wet saline gauze pads and an ice pack on the eyes
4 Asks the wife to obtain the legal documents regarding organ donation from the lawyer

Answer: 3

Rationale: When a corneal donor dies, the eyes are closed and gauze pads wet with saline are placed over them with a small ice pack. Within 2 to 4 hours, the eyes are enucleated. The cornea is usually transplanted within 24 to 48 hours. The head of the bed should also be elevated. There is no useful reason to call the National Donor Association or lawyer at this time.

Test-Taking Strategy: Note that the issue relates to donation of the eyes. This should assist in eliminating options 2 and 4. From the remaining options, recalling that the supine position will result in edema in the location of the eyes will assist in eliminating option 1. Review the procedure for caring for an eye donor if you had difficulty with the question.

Level of Cognitive Ability: Application
Client Needs: Safe, Effective Care Environment
Integrated Process: Nursing Process/Implementation
Content Area: Fundamental Skills

Reference:
Ignatavicius, D., & Workman, M. (2002). *Medical surgical nursing: Critical thinking for collaborative care* (4th ed.). Philadelphia: Saunders, p. 1031.

---

204. A client tells the home care nurse of his decision to refuse external cardiac massage. Which of the following is the most appropriate initial nursing action?
1 Notify the physician of the client's request
2 Document the client's request in the home care nursing care plan
3 Conduct a client conference with the home care staff to share the client's request
4 Discuss the client's request with the family

Answer: 1

Rationale: External cardiac massage is a life-saving treatment that a client can refuse. The most appropriate initial nursing action is to notify the physician, because a written Do Not Resuscitate (DNR) order from the physician is needed. The DNR order must be reviewed or renewed on a regular basis per agency policy. Although options 2, 3, and 4 may be appropriate, remember that first a written physician's order is necessary.

Test-Taking Strategy: Use the process of elimination and prioritize the options. Note the key words "most appropriate initial." These key words indicate that more than one option may be correct. Although options 2, 3, and 4 may be appropriate, remember that first a written physician's order is necessary. Review DNR procedures if you had difficulty with this question.

Level of Cognitive Ability: Application
Client Needs: Safe, Effective Care Environment
Integrated Process: Nursing Process/Implementation
Content Area: Delegating/Prioritizing

References:
Lewis, S., Heitkemper, M., & Dirksen, S. (2004). *Medical-surgical nursing: Assessment and management of clinical problems* (6th ed.). St. Louis: Mosby, pp. 164-165.
Potter, P., & Perry, A. (2005). *Fundamentals of nursing* (6th ed.). St. Louis: Mosby, p. 410.

205. A client is to be discharged to home and will continue with intermittent infusions of antibiotics via a peripherally inserted central catheter (PICC line). The nurse plans to include which instruction to be done on a daily basis in the discharge plan?

1 Keep the affected arm immobilized with an arm board or other splint
2 Assess the insertion site and length of the arm for signs of infection
3 Aspirate a small amount of blood from the catheter to determine patency
4 Maintain continuous infusion of fluids in between doses of antibiotics

Answer: 2

Rationale: A PICC is designed to be a long-term indwelling catheter and is usually inserted into the median cubital vein. The tip of the catheter should lie in the superior vena cava. A PICC does not require the affected arm to be immobilized (a major advantage of a PICC) and can be used for intermittent or continuous fluid infusion. Although the risk of infection is less with a PICC than with a subclavian or other central line, it is possible for phlebitis or infection to develop. Clients must be aware of the need for daily inspection and to report any discharge, redness, or pain immediately to the nurse or physician. Although a PICC can be used for obtaining blood specimens, it is not recommended to routinely aspirate blood to determine patency.

Test-Taking Strategy: Use the process of elimination. Eliminate option 1 because this action would be appropriate for a short-length peripheral intravenous catheter if placed in a mobile and vulnerable spot (such as the wrist). Option 3 is incorrect because aspiration of blood from the catheter is not recommended as a routine means of determining placement. Because the nature of a PICC allows for either continuous or intermittent infusions, option 4 is also incorrect. Basic principles of infection control could lead you to choose option 2 as the correct option. Additionally, option 2 addresses the first step of the nursing process: assessment. Review home care instructions for a client with a PICC if you had difficulty with this question.

Level of Cognitive Ability: Application
Client Needs: Safe, Effective Care Environment
Integrated Process: Nursing Process/Planning
Content Area: Fundamental Skills

References:
Perry, A., & Potter, P. (2004). *Clinical nursing skills & techniques* (5th ed.). St. Louis: Mosby, pp. 586-587.
Potter, P., & Perry, A. (2005). *Fundamentals of nursing* (6th ed.). St. Louis: Mosby, pp. 586-587.

206. A nursing instructor is discussing professional liability insurance with the senior class of nursing students. The instructor should most appropriately advise the students who will be graduating in 2 months:

1 To obtain their own malpractice insurance
2 That malpractice insurance is not required and is expensive
3 To discuss liability insurance with the employment agency
4 That most lawsuits are filed against physicians

Answer: 1

Rationale: Nurses need their own liability insurance for protection against malpractice lawsuits. Nurses erroneously assume that they are protected by an agency's professional liability policies. Usually when a nurse is sued, the employer is also sued for the nurse's actions or inaction's. Even though this is the norm, nurses are encouraged to have their own malpractice insurance.

Test-Taking Strategy: Note the key words "most appropriately" in the stem of the question. These key words tell you that one or more options may be correct. Although options 2, 3, and 4 may be accurate, the most appropriate advice is identified in option 1. Review liability related to malpractice insurance if you had difficulty with this question.

Level of Cognitive Ability: Application
Client Needs: Safe, Effective Care Environment
Integrated Process: Teaching/Learning
Content Area: Fundamental Skills

Reference:
Brent, N. (2001). *Nurses and the law* (2nd ed.). Philadelphia: Saunders, p. 56.

207. A charge nurse observes that a staff nurse is not able to meet client needs in a reasonable time frame, does not problem-solve situations, and does not prioritize nursing care. The charge nurse has the responsibility to:
  1 Supervise the staff nurse more closely so tasks are completed
  2 Provide support and identify the underlying cause of the staff nurse's problem
  3 Ask other staff members to help the staff nurse get the work done
  4 Report the staff nurse to the supervisor so something is done to resolve the problem

Answer: 2
Rationale: Option 2 empowers the charge nurse to assist the staff nurse while trying to identify and reduce the behaviors that make it difficult for the staff nurse to function. Options 1, 3, and 4 are punitive actions, shift the burden to other workers, and do not solve the problem.

Test-Taking Strategy: Remember that assessment is the first step of the nursing process. The charge nurse needs to gather information before making any decisions or deciding on a course of action. Identifying the underlying cause of the problem is a process of assessment. Review the leadership role of the nurse if you had difficulty with this question.

Level of Cognitive Ability: Application
Client Needs: Safe, Effective Care Environment
Integrated Process: Nursing Process/Implementation
Content Area: Leadership/Management

Reference:
Potter, P., & Perry, A. (2005). *Fundamentals of nursing* (6th ed.). St. Louis: Mosby, pp. 384-385.

208. A registered nurse is a preceptor for a new nursing graduate and is observing the new nursing graduate organize the client assignment and daily tasks. The registered nurse intervenes if the new nursing graduate does which of the following?
  1 Prioritizes client needs and daily tasks
  2 Provides time for unexpected tasks
  3 Lists the supplies needed for a task
  4 Plans to document task completion at the end of the day

Answer: 4
Rationale: The nurse should document task completion continuously throughout the day. Options 1, 2, and 3 identify accurate components of time management.

Test-Taking Strategy: Note the key word "intervenes" in the stem of the question. This key word indicates a false-response question and that you need to select the incorrect component of time management. Recalling that the nurse needs to document client data and task completion continuously throughout the day will direct you to option 4. Review time management principles and the principles related to documentation if you had difficulty with this question.

Level of Cognitive Ability: Application
Client Needs: Safe, Effective Care Environment
Integrated Process: Teaching/Learning
Content Area: Leadership/Management

Reference:
Potter, P., & Perry, A. (2005). *Fundamentals of nursing* (6th ed.). St. Louis: Mosby, pp. 480-483.

209. A registered nurse is a preceptor for a new nursing graduate and is describing critical paths and variance analysis to the new nursing graduate. The registered nurse instructs the new nursing graduate that a variance analysis is performed on all clients:
1   Daily during hospitalization
2   Every other day of hospitalization
3   Every third day of hospitalization
4   Continuously

Answer: 4
Rationale: Variance analysis occurs continually as the case manager and other caregivers monitor client outcomes against critical paths. The goal of critical paths is to anticipate and recognize negative variance early so that appropriate action can be taken. A negative variance occurs when untoward events preclude a timely discharge and the length of stay is longer than planned for a client on a specific critical path. Options 1, 2, and 3 are incorrect.

Test-Taking Strategy: Focus on the issue: critical paths and variance analysis. Recall that the goal of critical paths is to recognize negative variance early. This will direct you to option 4. Remember that it is best to monitor a client continuously rather than daily. Review the characteristics of critical paths and variance analysis if you had difficulty with this question.

Level of Cognitive Ability: Application
Client Needs: Safe, Effective Care Environment
Integrated Process: Teaching/Learning
Content Area: Leadership/Management

Reference:
Potter, P., & Perry, A. (2005). *Fundamentals of nursing* (6th ed.). St. Louis: Mosby, p. 485.

---

210. A nurse manager employs a leadership style in which decisions regarding the management of the nursing unit are made without input from the staff. The type of leadership style that is implemented by this nurse manager is:
1   Autocratic
2   Situational
3   Democratic
4   Laissez faire

Answer: 1
Rationale: The autocratic style of leadership is task oriented and directive. The leader uses his or her power and position in an authoritarian manner to set and implement organizational goals. Decisions are made without input from the staff. Democratic styles best empower staff toward excellence because this style of leadership allows nurses to provide input regarding the decision-making process and an opportunity to grow professionally. The situational leadership style utilizes a style depending on the situation and events. The laissez-faire style allows staff to work without assistance, direction, or supervision.

Test-Taking Strategy: Use the process of elimination. Noting the key words "made without input from the staff" will assist in directing you to option 1. Review the various leadership styles if you had difficulty with this question.

Level of Cognitive Ability: Application
Client Needs: Safe, Effective Care Environment
Integrated Process: Nursing Process/Implementation
Content Area: Leadership/Management

References:
Huber, D. (2000). *Leadership and nursing care management* (2nd ed.). Philadelphia: Saunders, pp. 59-61.
Yoder-Wise, P. (2003). *Leading and managing in nursing* (3rd ed.). St. Louis: Mosby, pp. 147; 374.

211. A hospital administration has implemented a change in the method of assignments of nurses to nursing units. Nurses will now be required to work in other nursing departments and will not be specifically assigned to a nursing unit. A group of registered nurses is resistant to the change, and nursing administration anticipates that the nurses will not facilitate the process of change. Which of the following would be the best approach on the part of administration in dealing with the resistance?

1 Ignore the resistance
2 Exert coercion with the nurses
3 Manipulate the nurses to participate in the change
4 Confront the nurses to encourage verbalization of feelings regarding the change

Answer: 4

Rationale: Confrontation is an important strategy to meet resistance head-on. Face-to-face meetings to confront the issue at hand will allow verbalization of feelings, identification of problems and issues, and the development of strategies to solve the problem. Option 1 will not address the problem. Option 2 may produce additional resistance. Option 3 may provide a temporary solution to the resistance, but will not specifically address the concern.

Test-Taking Strategy: Use the process of elimination. Options 1 and 2 can be easily eliminated first because these actions do not address the problem and may produce additional resistance. From the remaining options, select option 4 because this option specifically addresses the issue and would provide problem-solving measures. Review the strategies associated with dealing with resistance to change if you had difficulty with this question.

Level of Cognitive Ability: Application
Client Needs: Safe, Effective Care Environment
Integrated Process: Nursing Process/Implementation
Content Area: Leadership/Management

Reference:
Potter, P., & Perry, A. (2005). *Fundamentals of nursing* (6th ed.). St. Louis: Mosby, p. 440.

212. A registered nurse (RN) in charge of the nursing unit is preparing the assignments for the day. The RN assigns a nursing assistant to make beds and bathe one of the clients on the unit and assigns another nursing assistant to fill the water pitchers and serve juice to all of the clients. Another RN is assigned to administer all medications. Based on the assignments designed by the RN in charge, which type of nursing care is being implemented?

1 Functional nursing
2 Team nursing
3 Exemplary model of nursing
4 Primary nursing

Answer: 1

Rationale: The functional model of care involves an assembly-line approach to client care, with major tasks being delegated by the charge nurse to individual staff members. Team nursing is characterized by a high degree of communication and collaboration between members. The team is generally led by a registered nurse, who is responsible for assessing, developing nursing diagnoses, planning, and evaluating each client's plan of care. In an exemplary model of team nursing, each staff member works fully within the realm of his or her educational and clinical experience in an effort to provide comprehensive individualized client care. Each staff member is accountable for client care and outcomes of care. In primary nursing, concern is with keeping the nurse at the bedside actively involved in care, providing goal-directed and individualized client care.

Test-Taking Strategy: Focus on the information provided in the question to assist in directing you to the correct option. Noting that each staff member is assigned a specific task will direct you to option 1. Review the various nursing delivery systems if you had difficulty with this question.

Level of Cognitive Ability: Application
Client Needs: Safe, Effective Care Environment
Integrated Process: Nursing Process/Implementation
Content Area: Leadership/Management

Reference:
Potter, P., & Perry, A. (2005). *Fundamentals of nursing* (6th ed.). St. Louis: Mosby, p. 372.

213. A nurse is receiving a client in transfer from the postanesthesia care unit following a left above-the-knee amputation. The nurse should take which action to safely position the client at this time?
1 Put the bed in reverse Trendelenburg
2 Keep the stump flat with the client lying on the operative side
3 Position the stump flat on the bed
4 Elevate the foot of the bed

Answer: 4
Rationale: Edema of the stump is controlled by elevating the foot of the bed for the first 24 hours after surgery. Following the first 24 hours, the stump is usually placed flat on the bed to reduce hip contracture. Edema is also controlled by stump wrapping techniques.

Test-Taking Strategy: Use the process of elimination. Eliminate options 2 and 3 first because they are similar positions. To select from the remaining options, note that the client has just returned from surgery. Using basic principles related to immediate postoperative care and preventing postoperative edema will assist in directing you to option 4. Review postoperative positioning following amputation if you had difficulty with this question.

Level of Cognitive Ability: Application
Client Needs: Safe, Effective Care Environment
Integrated Process: Nursing Process/Implementation
Content Area: Adult Health/Cardiovascular

Reference:
Black, J., & Hawks, J. (2005). *Medical-surgical nursing: Clinical management for positive outcomes* (7th ed.). Philadelphia: Saunders, p. 1524.

---

214. A charge nurse knows that drug and alcohol use by nurses is a reason for the increasing numbers of disciplinary cases by the Board of Nursing. The charge nurse understands that when dealing with a nurse with such an illness, it is most important to assess the impaired nurse to determine the:
1 Physiological impact of the illness on practice
2 Types of illegal activities related to the abuse
3 If falsification of client records occurred
4 Magnitude of drug diversion over time

Answer: 1
Rationale: A nurse must be able to function at a level that does not affect the ability to provide safe, quality care. The highest priority is to determine how the illness affects the nurse's ability to practice. The other options will be addressed if an investigation is carried out.

Test-Taking Strategy: Use Maslow's hierarchy of needs theory. Option 1 addresses physiological integrity and also focuses on the client of the question: the impaired nurse. Review the concepts related to the impaired nurse if you had difficulty with this question.

Level of Cognitive Ability: Analysis
Client Needs: Safe, Effective Care Environment
Integrated Process: Nursing Process/Analysis
Content Area: Leadership/Management

References:
Potter, P., & Perry, A. (2005). *Fundamentals of nursing* (6th ed.). St. Louis: Mosby, pp. 66; 93.
Stuart, G., & Laraia, M. (2005). *Principles and practice of psychiatric nursing* (8th ed.). St. Louis: Mosby, pp. 510-511.

215. A pregnant client tests positive for the hepatitis B virus. The client asks the nurse if she will be able to breastfeed the baby as planned after delivery. The nurse makes which response to the client?
1 "You will not be able to breastfeed the baby until 6 months after delivery."
2 "Breastfeeding is not a problem, and you will be able to breastfeed immediately after delivery."
3 "Breastfeeding is allowed if the baby receives prophylaxis at birth and remains on the scheduled immunization."
4 "Breastfeeding is not advised, and you should seriously consider bottle-feeding the baby."

Answer: 3
Rationale: The pregnant client who tests positive for hepatitis B virus should be reassured that breastfeeding is not contraindicated if the infant receives prophylaxis at birth and remains on the schedule for immunizations. Options 1, 2, and 4 are incorrect.

Test-Taking Strategy: Use the process of elimination. Eliminate options 1, 2, and 4 because of the absolute word "not" in these options. Also use therapeutic communication techniques to direct you to option 3. Review the management of hepatitis B virus if you had difficulty with this question.

Level of Cognitive Ability: Application
Client Needs: Safe, Effective Care Environment
Integrated Process: Teaching/Learning
Content Area: Maternity/Antepartum

Reference:
Lowdermilk, D., & Perry, A. (2004). *Maternity & women's health care* (8th ed.). St. Louis: Mosby, p. 1065.

216. A nurse manager is planning to implement a change in the method of the documentation system in the nursing unit. Many problems have occurred as a result of the present documentation system, and the nurse manager determines that a change is required. The initial step in the process of change for the nurse manager is which of the following?
1 Plan strategies to implement the change
2 Identify potential solutions and strategies for the change process
3 Set goals and priorities regarding the change process
4 Identify the inefficiency that needs improvement or correction

Answer: 4
Rationale: When beginning the change process, the nurse should identify and define the problem that needs improvement or correction. This important first step can prevent many future problems, because if the problem is not correctly identified, a plan for change may be aimed at the wrong problem. This is followed by goal setting, prioritizing, and identifying potential solutions and strategies to implement the change.

Test-Taking Strategy: Use the steps of the nursing process and knowledge regarding the change process to answer this question. Option 4 is the only option that identifies an assessment step. Review the steps of the change process if you had difficulty with this question.

Level of Cognitive Ability: Application
Client Needs: Safe, Effective Care Environment
Integrated Process: Nursing Process/Planning
Content Area: Leadership/Management

Reference:
Potter, P., & Perry, A. (2005). *Fundamentals of nursing* (6th ed.). St. Louis: Mosby, pp. 266-267.

217. A delivery room nurse is preparing a client for a cesarean delivery. The client is placed on the delivery room table and the nurse positions the client:

1. In Trendelenburg position
2. In semi-Fowler's position
3. In the supine position with a wedge under the right hip
4. In the prone position

Answer: 3

Rationale: Vena cava and descending aorta compression by the pregnant uterus impedes blood return from the lower trunk and extremities, therefore decreasing cardiac return, cardiac output, and blood flow to the uterus and subsequently the fetus. The best position to prevent this would be side-lying with the uterus displaced off the abdominal vessels. Positioning for abdominal surgery necessitates a supine position, however, so a wedge placed under the right hip provides displacement of the uterus. Trendelenburg positioning places pressure from the pregnant uterus on the diaphragm and lungs, decreasing respiratory capacity and oxygenation. A semi-Fowler's or prone position is not practical for this type of abdominal surgery.

Test-Taking Strategy: Use the process of elimination and visualize each of the positions in the options. Recalling the concern in the pregnant client related to vena cava and descending aorta compression will direct you to option 3. Review positioning concepts if you had difficulty with this question.

Level of Cognitive Ability: Application
Client Needs: Safe, Effective Care Environment
Integrated Process: Nursing Process/Implementation
Content Area: Maternity/Intrapartum

Reference:
Lowdermilk, D., & Perry, A. (2004). *Maternity & women's health care* (8th ed.). St. Louis: Mosby, p. 1019.

218. A nurse in the day care center is told that a child with autism will be attending the center. The nurse collaborates with the staff of the day care center and plans activities that will meet the child's needs. The priority consideration in planning activities for the child is to ensure:

1. Social interactions with other children in the same age group
2. Safety with activities
3. Familiarity with all activities and providing orientation throughout the activities
4. That activities provide verbal stimulation

Answer: 2

Rationale: Safety with activities is a priority in planning activities with the child. The child with autism is unable to anticipate danger, has a tendency for self-mutilation, and has sensory perceptual deficits. Although social interactions, verbal communications, and providing familiarity and orientation are also appropriate interventions, the priority is safety.

Test-Taking Strategy: Use Maslow's hierarchy of needs theory to answer this question. Physiological needs take priority. When a physiological need does not exist, safety needs are the priority. None of the options addresses a physiological need. Option 2 addresses the safety need. Options 1, 3, and 4 address psychosocial needs. Review care of the child with autism if you had difficulty with this question.

Level of Cognitive Ability: Application
Client Needs: Safe, Effective Care Environment
Integrated Process: Nursing Process/Planning
Content Area: Child Health

Reference:
Wong, D., & Hockenberry, M. (2003). *Wong's nursing care of infants and children* (7th ed.). St. Louis: Mosby, p. 1010.

219. A registered nurse is reviewing a plan of care developed by a nursing student for a child who is being admitted to the pediatric unit with a diagnosis of seizures. The registered nurse determines that the student nurse needs to revise the plan of care if which incorrect intervention is documented?

1 Pad the side rails of the bed with blankets
2 Maintain the bed in a low position
3 Restrain the child if a seizure occurs
4 Place the child in a side-lying lateral position if a seizure occurs

Answer: 3

Rationale: Restraints are not to be applied to a child with a seizure because they could cause injury to the child. The side rails of the bed are padded with blankets, and the bed is maintained in low position to provide safety in the event that the child has a seizure. Positioning the child on his or her side will prevent aspiration as the saliva drains out of the child's mouth during the seizure.

Test-Taking Strategy: Note the key word "incorrect" in the stem of the question. This key word indicates a false-response question and that you need to select the incorrect intervention. Focus on safety to eliminate the incorrect options and recall that restraints are not to be used. Review safety measures related to the child with seizures if you had difficulty with this question.

Level of Cognitive Ability: Analysis
Client Needs: Safe, Effective Care Environment
Integrated Process: Teaching/Learning
Content Area: Child Health

Reference:
Wong, D., & Hockenberry, M. (2003). *Wong's nursing care of infants and children* (7th ed.). St. Louis: Mosby, p. 1697.

220. In the role as a caregiver, the nurse's primary responsibility is to assess the client's ability to:

1 Restore physical, emotional, and social well-being
2 Decide the best approach(s) for care
3 Take steps to prevent injury
4 Protect self

Answer: 1

Rationale: A primary role of the caregiver is to assess the client's ability to restore well-being. Options 2, 3, and 4 identify the nurse's role as a client advocate.

Test-Taking Strategy: Use the process of elimination. Focus on the key word "caregiver" to direct you to option 1. Options 2, 3, and 4 are similar and address the nurse's role as a client advocate. Review the roles and responsibilities of the nurse as a caregiver if you had difficulty with this question.

Level of Cognitive Ability: Application
Client Needs: Safe, Effective Care Environment
Integrated Process: Nursing Process/Implementation
Content Area: Leadership/Management

Reference:
Potter, P., & Perry, A. (2005). *Fundamentals of nursing* (6th ed.). St. Louis: Mosby, p. 19.

221. A cooling blanket is prescribed for a child with a fever. A nurse caring for the child has never used this type of equipment, and the charge nurse provides instructions and observes the nurse using the cooling blanket. The charge nurse intervenes if the nurse:
1 Places the cooling blanket on the bed and covers it with a sheet
2 Checks the skin condition of the child before, during, and after the use of the cooling blanket
3 Keeps the child uncovered to assist in reducing the fever
4 Keeps the child dry while on the cooling blanket to prevent the risk of frostbite

Answer: 3
Rationale: While on a cooling blanket, the child should be covered lightly to maintain privacy and reduce shivering. Options 1, 2, and 4 are important interventions to prevent shivering, frostbite, and skin breakdown.

Test-Taking Strategy: Note the key word "intervenes." This word indicates a false-response question and that you need to select the option that identifies an incorrect nursing action. Recalling the physiological response associated with fever and noting the word "uncovered" in option 3 will direct you to this option. Review the procedure associated with the use of a cooling blanket if you had difficulty with this question.

Level of Cognitive Ability: Analysis
Client Needs: Safe, Effective Care Environment
Integrated Process: Teaching/Learning
Content Area: Leadership/Management

Reference:
James, S., Ashwill, J., & Droske, S. (2002). *Nursing care of children: Principles & practice* (2nd ed.). Philadelphia: Saunders, p. 370.

222. A child with respiratory syncytial virus (RSV) who is in an oxygen tent is receiving ribavirin (Virazole). Which precaution will the nurse specifically take while caring for the child?
1 Wear head covering
2 Wear goggles and a mask
3 Wear a gown
4 Wear a gown and mask

Answer: 2
Rationale: Some caregivers experience headaches, burning nasal passages and eyes, and crystallization of soft contact lenses as a result of contact with ribavirin (Virazole). Therefore, goggles and a mask may be worn. A gown or head covering are not necessary.

Test-Taking Strategy: Note the key words "specifically take" in the question. Recalling the effects of this medication on contact with it will direct you to option 2. Review the procedures related to the administration of this medication if you had difficulty with this question.

Level of Cognitive Ability: Application
Client Needs: Safe, Effective Care Environment
Integrated Process: Nursing Process/Implementation
Content Area: Child Health

References:
McKinney, E., James, S., Murray, S., & Ashwill, J. (2005). *Maternal-child nursing* (2nd ed.). St. Louis: Elsevier, p. 1214.
McKenry, L., & Salerno, E. (2003). *Mosby's pharmacology in nursing* (21st ed.). St. Louis: Mosby, p. 1029.

223. A nurse receives a telephone call from the emergency room and is told that a child with a diagnosis of tonic-clonic seizures will be admitted to the pediatric unit. The nurse prepares for the admission of the child and instructs the nursing assistant to place which items at the bedside?
1 Suction apparatus and an airway
2 A tracheotomy set and oxygen
3 An emergency cart and padded side rails
4 An endotracheal tube and an airway

Answer: 1

Rationale: Tonic-clonic seizures cause tightening of all body muscles followed by tremors. Obstructed airway and increased oral secretions are the major complications during and following a seizure. Suction is helpful to prevent choking and cyanosis. Options 2 and 4 are incorrect because inserting an endotracheal tube or a tracheostomy is not done. It is not necessary to have an emergency cart at the bedside, but a cart should be available in the treatment room or on the nursing unit.

Test-Taking Strategy: Use the process of elimination. Recalling that tonic-clonic seizures produce excessive oral secretions and airway obstruction will assist in selecting the correct option. Review the plan of care associated with seizure precautions if you had difficulty with this question.

Level of Cognitive Ability: Application
Client Needs: Safe, Effective Care Environment
Integrated Process: Nursing Process/Planning
Content Area: Leadership/Management

Reference:
James, S., Ashwill, J., & Droske, S. (2002). *Nursing care of children: Principles & practice* (2nd ed.). Philadelphia: Saunders, pp. 976; 971.

---

224. The nurse in a well baby clinic is providing safety instructions to the mother of a 1-month-old infant. Which safety instruction is most appropriate at this age?
1 Cover electrical outlets
2 Remove hazardous objects from low places
3 Lock all poisons
4 Never shake the infant's head

Answer: 4

Rationale: The age-appropriate instruction that is most important is to instruct the mother not to shake or vigorously jiggle the baby's head. Options 1, 2, and 3 are most important instructions to provide to the mother as the child reaches the age of 6 months and begins to explore the environment.

Test-Taking Strategy: Focus on the age of the infant to direct you to the correct option. A 1-month-old is not at a developmental level to explore the environment, which will assist in eliminating options 1, 2, and 3. Review age-appropriate safety measures if you had difficulty with this question.

Level of Cognitive Ability: Application
Client Needs: Safe, Effective Care Environment
Integrated Process: Teaching/Learning
Content Area: Child Health

References:
James, S., Ashwill, J., & Droske, S. (2002). *Nursing care of children: Principles & practice* (2nd ed.). Philadelphia: Saunders, p. 1008.
Wong, D., & Hockenberry, M. (2003). *Wong's nursing care of infants and children* (7th ed.). St. Louis: Mosby, p. 687.

225. A nurse is caring for a 9-month-old child following cleft palate repair who has elbow restraints applied. The mother visits the child and asks the nurse to remove the restraints. The nurse takes which appropriate action?

1 Removes both restraints

2 Tells the mother that the restraints cannot be removed

3 Removes a restraint from one extremity

4 Loosens the restraints but tells the mother that they cannot be removed

Answer: 3

Rationale: Elbow restraints are used following cleft palate repair to prevent the child from touching the repair site, which could cause accidental rupture and tearing of the sutures. The restraints can be removed one at a time only if a parent or nurse is in constant attendance. Options 1, 2, and 4 are inaccurate nursing actions.

Test-Taking Strategy: Use the process of elimination. Eliminate options 2 and 4 first because they are similar. From the remaining options, recall the purpose of the restraints following this surgical procedure. This will assist in directing you to option 3, the safest nursing action. Review postoperative nursing interventions following cleft palate repair if you had difficulty with this question.

Level of Cognitive Ability: Application
Client Needs: Safe, Effective Care Environment
Integrated Process: Nursing Process/Implementation
Content Area: Child Health

Reference:
Wong, D., & Hockenberry, M. (2003). *Wong's nursing care of infants and children* (7th ed.). St. Louis: Mosby, p. 461.

CRITICAL THINKING: ALTERNATE FORMAT QUESTIONS

1. A home care nurse visits a client who has been recently discharged from the hospital following an acute myocardial infarction. The client tells the nurse that a living will was prepared and asks the nurse where a copy of the will can be kept. Select all areas where the client's living will is kept:

___ Lawyer's office
___ Physician's office
___ Medical record at the hospital
___ Hospital emergency room files
___ In the client's home
___ At the social security office

Answer:
Lawyer's office
Physician's office
Medical record at the hospital
In the client's home

Rationale: Copies of a living will should be kept with the medical record, at the physician's office, and in the client's home. A copy should also be maintained in the lawyer's office. The emergency room does not maintain these documents in its files. A copy of a client's living will is not sent to the social security office.

Test-Taking Strategy: Recall that a living will is a legal document and recall the issues surrounding confidentiality. Note that the question addresses a home care nurse. Therefore, it seems reasonable that the client should have a copy in the home because this document identifies the client's wishes. It would also seem reasonable that both a physician and lawyer would hold a copy of this document and that a copy would be maintained in the client's medical record to provide guidance to care providers if a situation arose during hospitalization requiring referral to this document. It is not realistic for an emergency room to maintain such documents in its files, especially if the client's medical record will contain this document anyway. Review the concepts related to living wills if you had difficulty with this question.

Level of Cognitive Ability: Application
Client Needs: Safe, Effective Care Environment
Integrated Process: Nursing Process/Implementation
Content Area: Fundamental Skills

Reference:
Phipps, W., Monahan, F., Sands, J., Marek, J., & Neighbors, M. (2003). *Medical-sur-gical nursing: Health and illness perspectives* (7th ed.). St. Louis: Mosby, p. 106.

2. A nurse is providing an educational session to a group of students who are enrolled in a nursing assistant program and prepares an instructional list for the students regarding the correct procedure for handwashing. Select in order of priority the correct procedure for performing handwashing. (Number 1 is the first step in the procedure)

___ Apply soap to the hands, keep the hands pointed downward, and rub them vigorously

___ Turn on the water

___ Allow the warm water to wet the hands

___ Dry the hands using a paper towel

___ Turn the water faucet off with the paper towel

___ Rinse the hands

Answer: 312564

Rationale: The nurse turns the water on first and then allows the warm water to wet the hands, applies soap to the hands, keeps the hands pointed downward, and rubs them vigorously. Warm water is used for handwashing because it increases the sudsing action of the soap. Hands should be kept downward to enable the unsanitary material to fall off the skin. The nurse then rinses the hands, dries the hands using a paper towel, and turns the water faucet off with the paper towel. The faucet is turned off by using a paper towel to prevent the hands from getting recontaminated.

Test-Taking Strategy: Visualize the procedure to answer the question. Recall that care must be taken to avoid recontamination of the hands during and after this procedure. This will assist in determining the order of action. Review the procedure for handwashing if you had difficulty with this question.

Level of Cognitive Ability: Application
Client Needs: Safe, Effective Care Environment
Integrated Process: Nursing Process/Implementation
Content Area: Delegating/Prioritizing

References:
Harkreader, H., & Hogan, M.A. (2004). *Fundamentals of nursing: Caring and clinical judgment* (2nd ed.). Philadelphia: Saunders. pp. 465-467.
Lewis, S., Heitkemper, M., & Dirksen, S. (2004). *Medical-surgical nursing: Assessment and management of clinical problems* (6th ed.). St. Louis: Mosby, p. 223.
Phipps, W., Monahan, F., Sands, J., Marek, J., & Neighbors, M. (2003). *Medical-surgical nursing: Health and illness perspectives* (7th ed.). St. Louis: Mosby, p. 199.

3. A nurse is taking care of a client on contact isolation. After nursing care has been performed and upon leaving the room, the nurse removes protective items in which order of priority? (Number 1 is the first action)

___ Unties the gown at the waist

___ Unties the gown at the neck, allows it to fall forward toward the shoulders, and removes it

___ Performs handwashing

___ Discards the gown in the appropriate receptacle

___ Removes the gloves

___ Removes the mask and eye wear (goggles)

Answer: 136425

Rationale: At the door of the room and next to an appropriate receptacle, the nurse unties the gown at the waist but does not remove it yet. The nurse then removes the gloves. The gown is then untied at the neck, allowed to fall forward from the shoulders, and removed. The gown is then discarded in the appropriate receptacle. The nurse then removes the mask and goggles and discards them. The hands are then washed.

Test-Taking Strategy: Use the principles of standard precautions and the methods of preventing contamination to answer the question. Visualize the correct process of removing contaminated clothing and items after caring for a client. Review this procedure if you had difficulty with this question.

Level of Cognitive Ability: Application
Client Needs: Safe, Effective Care Environment
Integrated Process: Nursing Process/Implementation
Content Area: Delegating/Prioritizing

Reference:
Harkreader, H., & Hogan, M.A. (2004). *Fundamentals of nursing: Caring and clinical judgment* (2nd ed.). Philadelphia: Saunders, pp. 472-473.

---

4. The registered nurse (RN) is observing a licensed practical nurse (LPN) prepare medications for a client. The physician's order reads: theophylline (Slo-bid) 100 mg orally every 6 hours. The medication label reads: theophylline 50-mg capsules. The RN determines that the LPN prepared the correct and safe dose if the LPN plans to administer how many capsule(s) to the client?

Answer: _____

Answer: 2
Rationale: Use the formula for calculating medication dosages.

Formula:

$$\frac{\text{Desired}}{\text{Available}} \times 1 \text{ Capsule} = \text{Capsule(s) per dose}$$

$$\frac{100 \text{ mg}}{50 \text{ mg}} \times 1 \text{ Capsule} = 2 \text{ Capsules}$$

Test-Taking Strategy: Identify the key components of the question and what the question is asking. In this case, the question asks for capsule(s) per dose. Set up the formula knowing that desired dose is 100 mg and available is 50 mg in one capsule. Use a calculator to verify your answer and make sure that the answer makes sense. Review medication calculations if you had difficulty with this question.

Level of Cognitive Ability: Analysis
Client Needs: Safe, Effective Care Environment
Integrated Process: Nursing Process/Evaluation
Content Area: Leadership/Management

Reference:
Kee, J., & Marshall, S. (2004). *Clinical calculations: With applications to general and specialty areas* (5th ed.). Philadelphia: Saunders, pp. 84-85.

---

5. The physician's order reads heparin sodium 25,000 units in 250 mL 5% dextrose in water to infuse intravenously continuously at a rate of 800 units per hour. To ensure that the solution infuses safely at the rate prescribed, the nurse sets the intravenous pump to how many mL per hr?

Answer: _____

Answer: 8
Rationale: Use the formula for calculating mL per hour with the use of an infusion pump.

Desired: 800 units per hour

Available: 25,000 units in 250 mL 5% dextrose in water

First, divide the 25,000 units by the 250 mL to yield a concentration of 100 units per mL.

Next, 800 units per hour is divided by 100 units per mL. The nurse would set the pump at 8 mL per hour.

Test-Taking Strategy: Think about what the question is asking. Determine units per mL and then use the standard "desired over available" formula. This will assist in determining that the pump should be set at 8 mL per hour. Review this formula if you had difficulty with this question.

Level of Cognitive Ability: Application
Client Needs: Safe, Effective Care Environment
Integrated Process: Nursing Process/Implementation
Content Area: Fundamental Skills

Reference:
Kee, J., & Marshall, S. (2004). *Clinical calculations: With applications to general and specialty areas* (5th ed.). Philadelphia: Saunders, p. 212.

REFERENCES

Black, J., & Hawks, J. (2005). *Medical-surgical nursing: Clinical management for positive outcomes* (7th ed.). Philadelphia: Saunders.

Brent, N. (2001). *Nurses and the law* (2nd ed.). Philadelphia: Saunders.

Chernecky, C., & Berger, B. (2004). *Laboratory tests and diagnostic procedures* (4th ed.). Philadelphia: Saunders.

Ebersole, P., & Hess, P. (2005). *Geriatric nursing & healthy aging* (2nd ed.). St. Louis: Mosby.

Elkin, M., Perry, A., & Potter, P. (2004). *Nursing interventions & clinical skills* (3rd ed.). St. Louis: Mosby.

Fortinash, K., & Holoday-Worret, P. (2004). *Psychiatric mental health nursing* (3rd ed.). St. Louis: Mosby.

Harkreader, H., & Hogan, M.A. (2004). *Fundamentals of nursing: Caring and clinical judgment* (2nd ed.). Philadelphia: Saunders.

Hodgson, B., & Kizior, R. (2004). *Saunders nursing drug handbook 2004.* Philadelphia: Saunders.

Huber, D. (2000). *Leadership and nursing care management* (2nd ed.). Philadelphia: Saunders.

Ignatavicius, D., & Workman, M. (2002). *Medical surgical nursing: Critical thinking for collaborative care* (4th ed.). Philadelphia: Saunders.

James, S., Ashwill, J., & Droske, S. (2002). *Nursing care of children: Principles & practice* (2nd ed.). Philadelphia: Saunders.

Kee, J., & Hayes, E. (2003). *Pharmacology: A nursing process approach* (4th ed.). Philadelphia: Saunders.

Kee, J., & Marshall, S. (2004). *Clinical calculations: With applications to general and specialty areas* (5th ed.). Philadelphia: Saunders.

Lehne, R. (2004). *Pharmacology for nursing care* (5th ed.). Philadelphia: Saunders.

Lewis, S., Heitkemper, M., & Dirksen, S. (2004). *Medical-surgical nursing: Assessment and management of clinical problems* (6th ed.). St. Louis: Mosby.

Lowdermilk, D., & Perry, A. (2004). *Maternity & women's health care* (8th ed.). St. Louis: Mosby.

McKenry, L., & Salerno, E. (2003). *Mosby's pharmacology in nursing* (21st ed.). St. Louis: Mosby.

McKinney, E., James, S., Murray, S., & Ashwill, J. (2005). *Maternal-child nursing* (2nd ed.). St. Louis: Elsevier.

Perry, A., & Potter, P. (2004). *Clinical nursing skills and techniques* (5th ed.). St. Louis: Mosby.

Phipps, W., Monahan, F., Sands, J., Marek, J., & Neighbors, M. (2003). *Medical-surgical nursing: Health and illness perspectives* (7th ed.). St. Louis: Mosby.

Potter, P., & Perry, A. (2005). *Fundamentals of nursing* (6th ed.). St. Louis: Mosby.

Stuart, G., & Laraia, M. (2005). *Principles and practice of psychiatric nursing* (8th ed.). St. Louis: Mosby.

Varcarolis, E.M. (2002). *Foundations of psychiatric mental health nursing* (4th ed.). Philadelphia: Saunders.

Wilson, S., & Giddens, J. (2005). *Health assessment for nursing practice* (3rd ed.). St. Louis: Mosby.

Wong, D., & Hockenberry, M. (2003). *Wong's nursing care of infants and children* (7th ed.). St. Louis: Mosby.

Yoder-Wise, P. (2003). *Leading and managing in nursing* (3rd ed.). St. Louis: Mosby.

Health Promotion and Maintenance

1. A mother of a teenage client with an anxiety disorder is concerned about her daughter's progress upon discharge. She states that her daughter "stashes food, eats all the wrong things that make her hyperactive," and "hangs out with the wrong crowd." To promote optimal health and to assist the mother in preparing for her daughter's discharge, the nurse advises the mother to:

1 Restrict the daughter's socializing time with her friends

2 Consider taking time off from work to help her daughter readjust to the home environment

3 Limit the amount of chocolate and caffeine products in the home

4 Keep her daughter out of school until she can adjust to the school environment

Answer: 3

Rationale: Clients with anxiety disorder are advised to limit their intake of caffeine, chocolate, and alcohol. These products have the potential of increasing anxiety. Options 1 and 4 are unreasonable and are an unhealthy approach. It may not be realistic for a family member to take time off from work.

Test-Taking Strategy: Note the daughter's diagnosis and focus on the issue: to promote health. Options 1, 2, and 4 are similar and are concerned with monitoring or curtailing the daughter's physical activities, whereas option 3 focuses on the issue. Review health promotion measures for the client with anxiety disorder if you had difficulty with this question.

Level of Cognitive Ability: Application
Client Needs: Health Promotion and Maintenance
Integrated Process: Teaching/Learning
Content Area: Mental Health

Reference:
Stuart, G., & Laraia, M. (2005). *Principles and practice of psychiatric nursing* (8th ed.). St. Louis: Mosby, p. 266.

---

2. A nurse is performing an assessment on a client with hepatic encephalopathy and assesses for asterixis. To appropriately test for asterixis, the nurse:

1 Asks the client to extend an arm, dorsiflex the wrist, and extend the fingers

2 Checks the stools for clay-colored pigmentation

3 Asks the client to sign his or her name on a piece of paper and looks for any deterioration in hand movements

4 Reviews laboratory serum levels of bilirubin and alkaline phosphatase for elevation

Answer: 1

Rationale: Asterixis is an abnormal muscle tremor often associated with hepatic encephalopathy. Asterixis is sometimes called "liver flap." Options 2, 3, and 4 are associated with hepatitis but are not signs of asterixis.

Test-Taking Strategy: Recalling the signs and symptoms of hepatic encephalopathy will direct you to option 1. Also, focus on the definition of asterixis to answer correctly. Review this technique if you are unfamiliar with assessment for asterixis.

Level of Cognitive Ability: Application
Client Needs: Health Promotion and Maintenance

Integrated Process: Nursing Process/Assessment
Content Area: Fundamental Skills

Reference:
Ignatavicius, D., & Workman, M. (2002). *Medical surgical nursing: Critical thinking for collaborative care* (4th ed.). Philadelphia: Saunders, pp. 1303; 1653.

---

3. A nurse assesses the 12th cranial nerve in the client who sustained a cerebrovascular accident (CVA). To assess this cranial nerve, the nurse asks the client to:
   1 Extend the arms
   2 Turn the head toward the nurse's arm
   3 Extend the tongue
   4 Focus the eyes on an object held by the nurse

Answer: 3
Rationale: To assess the function of the 12th cranial (hypoglossal) nerve, the nurse would assess the client's ability to extend the tongue. Impairment of the 12th cranial nerve can occur with a CVA. Options 1, 2, and 4 do not test the function of the 12th cranial nerve.

Test-Taking Strategy: Recalling that the 12th cranial nerve is the hypoglossal nerve will direct you to option 3. Review the cranial nerves and the method of testing these nerves if you had difficulty with this question.

Level of Cognitive Ability: Application
Client Needs: Health Promotion and Maintenance
Integrated Process: Nursing Process/Assessment
Content Area: Adult Health/Neurological

Reference:
Ignatavicius, D., & Workman, M. (2002). *Medical surgical nursing: Critical thinking for collaborative care* (4th ed.). Philadelphia: Saunders, p. 981.

---

4. A client with type 2 diabetes mellitus is being discharged from the hospital after an occurrence of hyperglycemic hyperosmolar nonketotic syndrome (HHNS). The nurse develops a discharge teaching plan for the client and identifies which of the following as the priority?
   1 Exercise routines
   2 Monitoring for signs of dehydration
   3 Keeping follow-up appointments
   4 Controlling dietary intake

Answer: 2
Rationale: Clients at risk for HHNS should immediately report signs and symptoms of dehydration to health care providers. Dehydration can be severe and may progress rapidly. Although options 1, 3, and 4 are a component of the teaching plan, in the client with HHNS, dehydration is the priority.

Test-Taking Strategy: Use the process of elimination, noting the key word "priority." Look at each option in terms of its seriousness and recall that dehydration can rapidly progress to HHNS. Review HHNS if you had difficulty with this question.

Level of Cognitive Ability: Application
Client Needs: Health Promotion and Maintenance
Integrated Process: Teaching/Learning
Content Area: Delegating/Prioritizing

References:
Black, J., & Hawks, J. (2005). *Medical-surgical nursing: Clinical management for positive outcomes* (7th ed.). Philadelphia: Saunders, p. 1273.
Ignatavicius, D., & Workman, M. (2002). *Medical surgical nursing: Critical thinking for collaborative care* (4th ed.). Philadelphia: Saunders, p. 1484.

5. A nurse develops a plan of care for an older client with diabetes mellitus. The nurse plans to first:

1 Teach with videotapes showing insulin administration to ensure competence
2 Assess the client's ability to read label markings on syringes and blood glucose monitoring equipment
3 Structure menus for adherence to diet
4 Encourage dependence on others to prepare the client for the chronicity of the disease

Answer: 2

Rationale: The nurse first assesses the client's ability to care for self. Allowing the client to have "hands-on" experience rather than teaching with videos is more effective. Independence should be encouraged. Structuring menus for the client promotes dependence.

Test-Taking Strategy: Use the steps of the nursing process. Option 2 reflects assessment, the first step of the nursing process. Review teaching/learning principles and the teaching/learning needs of the older client if you had difficulty with this question.

Level of Cognitive Ability: Application
Client Needs: Health Promotion and Maintenance
Integrated Process: Teaching/Learning
Content Area: Adult Health/Endocrine

Reference:
Black, J., & Hawks, J. (2005). *Medical-surgical nursing: Clinical management for positive outcomes* (7th ed.). Philadelphia: Saunders, pp. 154; 1265.

---

6. A nurse is conducting a health screening on a client with a family history of hypertension. Which assessment finding would alert the nurse to the need for teaching related to cerebrovascular accident (CVA) prevention?

1 Eats two bowls of high-fiber grain cereal with skim milk for breakfast
2 Works as the manager of a busy medical-surgical unit yet jogs two miles daily
3 Uses oral contraceptives and condoms for pregnancy and disease prevention
4 Has a blood pressure (BP) of 136/86 mmHg and has lost 10 pounds recently

Answer: 3

Rationale: Obesity, hypertension, hypercholesterolemia, smoking, and use of oral contraceptives are all modifiable risk factors for CVA. Oral contraceptive use is discouraged in some clients because of the side effect of clot formation. Low-fat diet and stress reduction methods are encouraged and identified in options 1 and 2. Although option 4 identifies a borderline BP, the client has made a change in eating habits as noted by the weight loss mentioned in this option.

Test-Taking Strategy: Note the key words "need for teaching." These key words indicate a false-response question and that you need to select the option that is a risk factor for CVA. Noting the words "oral contraceptives" in option 3 will direct you to this option. Review this content if you had difficulty with this question and are unfamiliar with the risk factors related to CVA.

Level of Cognitive Ability: Analysis
Client Needs: Health Promotion and Maintenance
Integrated Process: Nursing Process/Assessment
Content Area: Adult Health/Neurological

References:
Ignatavicius, D., & Workman, M. (2002). *Medical surgical nursing: Critical thinking for collaborative care* (4th ed.). Philadelphia: Saunders, pp. 734-735.
Lewis, S., Heitkemper, M., & Dirksen, S. (2004). *Medical-surgical nursing: Assessment and management of clinical problems* (6th ed.). St. Louis: Mosby, pp. 794-795.

7. A nurse is reviewing assessment data on a clinic client. Which finding would be most important for the client to modify to lessen the risk for coronary artery disease (CAD)?
  1 Elevated high-density lipoprotein (HDL) levels
  2 Elevated low-density lipoprotein (LDL) levels
  3 Elevated triglyceride levels
  4 Elevated serum lipase levels

Answer: 2
Rationale: LDL is more directly associated with CAD than other lipoproteins. LDL levels, along with cholesterol, have a higher predictive association for CAD than triglycerides. Additionally, HDL is inversely associated with the risk of CAD. Lipase is a digestive enzyme that breaks down ingested fats in the gastrointestinal tract.

Test-Taking Strategy: Focus on the issue: the risk factor related to cardiac disease. Recalling that LDL is the "bad" type of cholesterol will direct you to option 2. Review this content if you are unfamiliar with these risk factors.

Level of Cognitive Ability: Analysis
Client Needs: Health Promotion and Maintenance
Integrated Process: Nursing Process/Assessment
Content Area: Adult Health/Cardiovascular

Reference:
Lewis, S., Heitkemper, M., & Dirksen, S. (2004). *Medical-surgical nursing: Assessment and management of clinical problems* (6th ed.). St. Louis: Mosby, pp. 806-808.

---

8. A nurse is taking a history from a client suspected of having testicular cancer. Which of the following data will be most helpful in determining risk factors for this type of cancer?
  1 Number of sexual partners
  2 Age and race
  3 Number of children
  4 Marital status

Answer: 2
Rationale: Two basic but important risk factors for testicular cancer are age and race. The disease occurs most frequently in Caucasian males between the ages of 18 and 40 years. Other risk factors include a history of undescended testis and a family history of testicular cancer. Marital status and number of children do not pose a risk factor for males and testicular cancer.

Test-Taking Strategy: Use knowledge of the risk factors associated with this type of cancer to answer the question. Recalling that testicular cancer most often occurs between ages 18 and 40 will direct you to option 2. Review the risk factors related to testicular cancer if you had difficulty with this question.

Level of Cognitive Ability: Analysis
Client Needs: Health Promotion and Maintenance
Integrated Process: Nursing Process/Assessment
Content Area: Adult Health/Oncology

Reference:
Lewis, S., Heitkemper, M., & Dirksen, S. (2004). *Medical-surgical nursing: Assessment and management of clinical problems* (6th ed.). St. Louis: Mosby, p. 1454.

---

9. A client with a history of ear problems is going on vacation by aircraft. The nurse advises the client to avoid which of the following to prevent barotrauma during ascent and descent of the airplane?
  1 Sucking hard candy
  2 Swallowing
  3 Yawning
  4 Keeping the mouth motionless

Answer: 4
Rationale: Clients who are prone to barotrauma should perform any of a variety of mouth movements to equalize pressure in the ear, particularly during ascent and descent of an aircraft. These can include yawning, swallowing, drinking, chewing, or sucking on hard candy. Valsalva maneuver may also be helpful. The client should avoid sitting with the mouth motionless during this time, because this aggravates pressure build-up behind the tympanic membrane.

Test-Taking Strategy: Use the process of elimination, and note the key word "avoid." This key word indicates a false-response question and that you need to select the option that identifies an incorrect client action. Eliminate options 1, 2, and 3 because they are similar and involve movement of the mouth. Review the measures that will prevent barotrauma of the ear if you had difficulty with this question.

Level of Cognitive Ability: Application
Client Needs: Health Promotion and Maintenance
Integrated Process: Teaching/Learning
Content Area: Adult Health/Ear

References:

Black, J., & Hawks, J. (2005). *Medical-surgical nursing: Clinical management for positive outcomes* (7th ed.). Philadelphia: Saunders, p. 1981.
Ignatavicius, D., & Workman, M. (2002). *Medical surgical nursing: Critical thinking for collaborative care* (4th ed.). Philadelphia: Saunders, p. 1067.

---

10. A community health nurse is working with food services in a rural school setting. A goal for the school dietary program is to avoid nutritional deficiencies and enhance the children's nutritional status through healthy dietary practices. In implementing interventions by levels of prevention, which of the following would be a primary prevention intervention that the nurse could use?
1 Case finding in the school to identify dietary practices
2 School screening programs for early detection of children with poor eating habits
3 Providing educational programs, literature, and posters to promote awareness of healthy eating
4 Conduct a community-wide dietary screening activity to detect community dietary trends

Answer: 3
Rationale: Primary prevention interventions are those measures that keep illness, injury, or potential problems from occurring, therefore option 3 is correct. Options 1, 2, and 4 are secondary prevention measures that seek to detect existing health problems or trends.

Test-Taking Strategy: Note the issue of the question: primary prevention intervention. Knowledge that primary prevention interventions are those measures that keep illness from occurring will direct you to option 3. Review the levels of prevention if you had difficulty with this question.

Level of Cognitive Ability: Application
Client Needs: Health Promotion and Maintenance
Integrated Process: Nursing Process/Implementation
Content Area: Fundamental Skills

Reference:

Black, J., & Hawks, J. (2005). *Medical-surgical nursing: Clinical management for positive outcomes* (7th ed.). Philadelphia: Saunders, pp. 22; 668-669.

---

11. A nursing instructor asks a nursing student to identify situations that indicate a secondary level of prevention in health care. Which situation, if identified by the student, would indicate a need for further study of the levels of prevention?
1 Teaching a stroke client how to use a walker
2 Encouraging a client to take antihypertensive medications as prescribed
3 Screening for hypertension in a community
4 Encouraging a woman over age 40 to obtain periodic mammograms

Answer: 1
Rationale: Secondary prevention focuses on the early diagnosis and prompt treatment of disease. Tertiary prevention is represented by rehabilitation services. Options 3 and 4 identify screening procedures, and option 2 identifies a treatment of a disease. Option 1 identifies a rehabilitative service.

Test-Taking Strategy: Note the key words "indicate a need for further study." These key words indicate a false-response question and that you need to select the option that does not represent secondary level of prevention. Recalling that secondary prevention focuses on the early diagnosis and prompt treatment of disease will direct you to option 1. Review the levels of prevention if you had difficulty with this question.

Level of Cognitive Ability: Analysis
Client Needs: Health Promotion and Maintenance
Integrated Process: Teaching/Learning
Content Area: Leadership/Management

References:

Ignatavicius, D., & Workman, M. (2002). *Medical surgical nursing: Critical thinking for collaborative care* (4th ed.). Philadelphia: Saunders, p. 6.

Potter, P., & Perry, A. (2005). *Fundamentals of nursing* (6th ed.). St. Louis: Mosby, p. 97.

---

12. To promote health, a substance abuse clinic nurse is providing dietary instructions to clients. A client asks the nurse about foods that are high in thiamine. The nurse tells the client that which food is especially rich in this vitamin?

1 Chicken
2 Broccoli
3 Pork
4 Milk

Answer: 3

Rationale: Thiamine is present in a variety of foods of plant and animal origin. Pork products are especially rich in this vitamin. Other good sources include nuts, whole-grain cereals, and legumes. Chicken is high in protein. Broccoli is high in iron and vitamin K. Milk is high in calcium.

Test-Taking Strategy: Use the process of elimination and knowledge regarding food items high in thiamine to answer this question. Review this content if you are unfamiliar with foods high in thiamine.

Level of Cognitive Ability: Application
Client Needs: Health Promotion and Maintenance
Integrated Process: Teaching/Learning
Content Area: Fundamental Skills

Reference:

Peckenpaugh, N. (2003). *Nutrition essentials and diet therapy* (9th ed.). Philadelphia: Saunders, pp. 155-156.

---

13. A nurse provides home care instructions to a mother of an infant with a diagnosis of hydrocephalus. Which statement by the mother indicates an understanding of the care for the infant?

1 "I need to keep my infant's head in a pushed-back position during sleep."
2 "I need to feed my infant in a flat, side-lying position."
3 "I need to place my infant on its stomach with a towel under the neck for sleep."
4 "I need to support my infant's neck and head."

Answer: 4

Rationale: Hydrocephalus is a condition characterized by an enlargement of the cranium caused by an abnormal accumulation of cerebrospinal fluid within the cerebral ventricular system. This characteristic causes an increase in the weight of the infant's head. The infant's head becomes top heavy. Supporting the infant's head and neck when picking the infant up will prevent the hyperextension of the neck area and the infant from falling backward. Hyperextension of the infant's head can put pressure on the neck vertebrae, causing injury. Options 1 and 3 will cause hyperextension. The infant should be fed with the head elevated for proper motility of food processing.

Test-Taking Strategy: Note the key words "indicates an understanding." Use the process of elimination, and eliminate option 2 first because feeding any infant in this position is unsafe. Note the similarity between options 1 and 3. Both of these positions will cause hyperextension of the infant's neck. Review care of the infant with hydrocephalus if you had difficulty with this question.

Level of Cognitive Ability: Analysis
Client Needs: Health Promotion and Maintenance
Integrated Process: Teaching/Learning
Content Area: Child Health

Reference:
James, S., Ashwill, J., & Droske, S. (2002). *Nursing care of children: Principles & practice* (2nd ed.).Philadelphia: Saunders, p. 961.

---

14. A nurse is preparing a teaching plan for the parents of an infant with a ventricular peritoneal shunt who will be discharged from the hospital. The nurse plans to include which instruction in the plan of care?
 1 Call the physician if the infant is fussy
 2 Position the infant on the side of the shunt when the infant is put to bed
 3 Expect an increased urine output from the shunt
 4 Call the physician if the infant has a high-pitched cry

Answer: 4
Rationale: If the shunt is broken or malfunctioning, the fluid from the ventricle part of the brain will not be diverted to the peritoneal cavity. The cerebrospinal fluid will build up in the cranial area. The result is intracranial pressure, which then causes a high-pitched cry in the infant. The infant should not be positioned on the side of the shunt because this will cause pressure on the shunt and skin breakdown. This type of shunt affects the gastrointestinal system, not the genitourinary system, and an increased urinary output is not expected. Option 1 is only a concern if other signs indicative of a complication are occurring.

Test-Taking Strategy: Use the process of elimination. Remember that a high-pitched cry in an infant indicates a concern or problem. Review significant assessment findings and home care instructions for the parents of an infant with a ventricular peritoneal shunt if you had difficulty with this question.

Level of Cognitive Ability: Application
Client Needs: Health Promotion and Maintenance
Integrated Process: Teaching/Learning
Content Area: Child Health

Reference:
Wong, D., & Hockenberry, M. (2003). *Wong's nursing care of infants and children* (7th ed.). St. Louis: Mosby, p. 441.

---

15. A home care nurse visits a child with Reye's syndrome and plans to provide instructions to the mother regarding care of the child. The nurse instructs the mother to:
 1 Increase the stimuli in the environment
 2 Give the child frequent, small meals if vomiting occurs
 3 Avoid daytime naps so the child will sleep at night
 4 Check the child's skin and eyes every day for a yellow discoloration

Answer: 4
Rationale: Checking for jaundice will assist in identifying the presence of liver complications that are characteristic of Reye's syndrome. If vomiting occurs in Reye's syndrome, it is caused by cerebral edema, is a sign of increased intracranial pressure, and needs to be reported. Decreasing stimuli and providing rest decreases stress on the brain tissue. Options 1 and 3 do not promote a restful environment for the child.

Test-Taking Strategy: Read each option carefully and think about the manifestations and complications associated with Reye's syndrome. Recalling that increased intracranial pressure is a concern will assist in eliminating option 2. Eliminate options 1 and 3 next because they are similar in that they do not promote a restful environment for the child. Review care of the child with Reye's syndrome if you had difficulty with this question.

Level of Cognitive Ability: Application
Client Needs: Health Promotion and Maintenance
Integrated Process: Teaching/Learning
Content Area: Child Health

References:

James, S., Ashwill, J., & Droske, S. (2002). *Nursing care of children:Principles & practice* (2nd ed.).Philadelphia: Saunders, p. 458.

Wong, D., & Hockenberry, M. (2003). *Wong's nursing care of infants and children* (7th ed.). St. Louis: Mosby, p. 1683.

---

16. A nurse in the well baby clinic has provided instructions regarding dental care to the mother of a 10-month-old child. Which statement by the mother indicates a need for further instructions?

1 "I need to start dental hygiene as soon as the primary teeth erupt."
2 "I need to use fluoride supplements if the water is not fluoridated."
3 "I can coat a pacifier with honey during the day as long as I do not give my child a bottle at nap or bedtime."
4 "I need to limit the amount of concentrated sweets."

Answer: 3

Rationale: The practice of coating pacifiers with honey or using commercially available hard-candy pacifiers is discouraged. Besides being cariogenic, honey may also cause botulism, and parts of the candy pacifier may be aspirated. Additionally, a bottle at nap or bedtime that contains sweet milk or other fluids such as juice bathes the teeth, producing caries. Fluoride, an essential mineral for building caries-resistant teeth, is needed beginning at 6 months of age or as directed by the physician if the infant does not receive adequate fluoride content. A diet that is low in sweets and high in nutritious food promotes dental health.

Test-Taking Strategy: Note the key words "indicates a need for further instructions." These key words indicate a false-response question and that you need to select the option that indicates an incorrect statement by the mother. Focus on the issue as it relates to the prevention of dental caries and recall that honey is cariogenic and may also cause botulism. This will direct you to option 3. Review dental care measures if you had difficulty with this question.

Level of Cognitive Ability: Analysis
Client Needs: Health Promotion and Maintenance
Integrated Process: Teaching/Learning
Content Area: Child Health

Reference:

James, S., Ashwill, J., & Droske, S. (2002). *Nursing care of children: Principles & practice* (2nd ed.).Philadelphia: Saunders, p. 167.

---

17. A 7-year-old child is hospitalized with a fracture of the femur and is placed in traction. In meeting the growth and development needs of the child, the nurse most appropriately selects which of the following play activities for the child?

1 A coloring book with crayons
2 A finger-painting set
3 A large puzzle
4 A board game

Answer: 4

Rationale: The school-aged child becomes organized with more direction with play activities. Such activities include collections, drawing, construction, dolls, pets, guessing games, board games, riddles, hobbies, competitive games, and listening to the radio or television. Options 1 and 2 are most appropriate for a preschooler. Option 3 is most appropriate for a toddler.

Test-Taking Strategy: Note the age and the diagnosis of the child to answer this question. Recalling the specific types of age-related play activities that are appropriate for the school-aged child will direct you to option 4. Review age-appropriate activities for the school-aged child if you had difficulty with this question.

Level of Cognitive Ability: Application
Client Needs: Health Promotion and Maintenance
Integrated Process: Nursing Process/Implementation
Content Area: Child Health

References:
James, S., Ashwill, J., & Droske, S. (2002). *Nursing care of children: Principles & practice* (2nd ed.).Philadelphia: Saunders, p. 316.
Wong, D., & Hockenberry, M. (2003). *Wong's nursing care of infants and children* (7th ed.). St. Louis: Mosby, p. 1768.

---

18. A clinic nurse has provided information to the mother of a toddler regarding toilet-training. Which statement by the mother would indicate a need for further instructions?
   1   "I should wait until my child is between 18 and 24 months old."
   2   "I know that my child will develop bowel control before bladder control."
   3   "I should have my child sit on the potty until she urinates."
   4   "I know my child is ready to begin toilet training if my child is walking."

Answer: 3
Rationale: The child should not be forced to sit on the potty for long periods of time. The physical ability to control the anal and urethral sphincters is achieved some time after the child is walking, probably between ages 18 and 24 months. Bowel control is usually achieved before bladder control.

Test-Taking Strategy: Note the key words "a need for further instructions" in the stem of the question. These key words indicate a false-response question and that you need to select the option that is an incorrect statement by the mother. Recall that forcing a child to develop this behavior will result in a negative response. This will direct you to option 3. Review the task of toilet-training if you had difficulty with this question.

Level of Cognitive Ability: Analysis
Client Needs: Health Promotion and Maintenance
Integrated Process: Teaching/Learning
Content Area: Child Health

Reference:
Wong, D., & Hockenberry, M. (2003). *Wong's nursing care of infants and children* (7th ed.). St. Louis: Mosby, p. 603.

---

19. A clinic nurse is performing an assessment on a 12-month-old infant. The nurse determines that the infant is demonstrating the highest level of developmental achievement if the 12-month-old is able to:
   1   Produce cooing sounds
   2   Produce babbling sounds
   3   Obey simple commands
   4   Begin to use simple words

Answer: 4
Rationale: Simple words such as "mama" and the use of gestures to communicate begins between 9 and 12 months of age. A 1- to 3-month-old infant will produce cooing sounds. Babbling is common in a 3- to 4-month-old infant. Between 8 and 9 months, the infant begins to understand and obey simple commands such as "wave bye-bye." Using single-consonant babbling occurs between 6 and 8 months.

Test-Taking Strategy: Note that the infant is 12 months of age, and note the key words "highest level." Use the process of elimination and knowledge of language and communication developmental milestones to answer the question. Review these milestones if you had difficulty with this question.

Level of Cognitive Ability: Analysis
Client Needs: Health Promotion and Maintenance
Integrated Process: Nursing Process/Assessment
Content Area: Child Health

Reference:
Wong, D., & Hockenberry, M. (2003). *Wong's nursing care of infants and children* (7th ed.). St. Louis: Mosby, p. 515.

---

20. A nurse is assisting in conducting a session on relaxation techniques to a group of pregnant woman attending a childbirth class. The nurse informs the group that active relaxation techniques will assist with coping with the discomfort of contractions. The nurse determines teaching has been effective when a client says that active relaxation includes:

1 "Assuming a state of mind that is open to suggestions from a coach."

2 "Remembering that the contractions will be over after delivery."

3 "Relaxing uninvolved muscles while the uterus contracts."

4 "Understanding that the causes of contraction discomfort are more psychological than physical."

Answer: 3

Rationale: Active relaxation includes specific relaxation exercises and conditioned responses such as distraction from the discomfort of labor. The woman is an active participant in the use of the technique, which focuses on relaxing uninvolved muscles while the uterus contracts. Options 1, 2, and 4 are incorrect.

Test-Taking Strategy: Use the process of elimination, noting the key words "active relaxation." Option 3 contains an active verb and is different from the other options. Options 1, 2, and 4 are all similar in that the verb is passive. Review the purpose of active relaxation techniques during labor if you had difficulty with this question.

Level of Cognitive Ability: Analysis
Client Needs: Health Promotion and Maintenance
Integrated Concept/Process: Teaching/Learning
Content Area: Maternity/Antepartum

Reference:
McKinney, E., James, S., Murray, S., & Ashwill, J. (2005). *Maternal-child nursing* (2nd ed.). St. Louis: Elsevier, pp. 420-421.

---

21. A nurse is performing an assessment of a prenatal client being seen in the clinic for the first time. Following the assessment, the nurse determines that which piece of data places the client into the high-risk category for contracting human immunodeficiency virus (HIV)?

1 Living in an area where population rate of HIV infection is low

2 A history of intravenous (IV) drug use in the past year

3 A history of one sexual partner within the past 10 years

4 A spouse who is heterosexual and had only one sexual partner in the past 10 years

Answer: 2

Rationale: HIV is transmitted by intimate sexual contact and the exchange of body fluids, exposure of infected blood, and transmission from an infected woman to her fetus. Women who fall into the high-risk category for HIV infection include those with persistent and recurrent sexually transmitted diseases, those with a history of multiple sexual partners, and those who have used IV drugs. A heterosexual partner, particularly a partner who has had only one sexual partner in 10 years, is not a high-risk factor for developing HIV.

Test-Taking Strategy: Use the process of elimination, recalling that that exchange of blood and body fluids places the client at high risk for HIV infection. This will assist in directing you to the correct option. Review the risk factors for HIV if you had difficulty with this question.

Level of Cognitive Ability: Analysis
Client Needs: Health Promotion and Maintenance
Integrated Process: Nursing Process/Assessment
Content Area: Adult Health/Immune

References:
Murray, S., McKinney, E., & Gorrie, T. (2002). *Foundations of maternal-newborn nursing* (3rd ed.). Philadelphia: Saunders, p. 928.
Lewis, S., Heitkemper, M., & Dirksen, S. (2004). *Medical-surgical nursing: Assessment and management of clinical problems* (6th ed.). St. Louis: Mosby, p. 277.

22. A nurse instructs a perinatal client about measures to prevent urinary tract infections. Which statement by the client would indicate an understanding of these measures?
   1 "I can take a bubble bath as long as the soap doesn't contain any oils."
   2 "I should always use scented toilet paper."
   3 "I can wear my tight-fitting jeans."
   4 "I should choose underwear with a cotton panel liner."

Answer: 4
Rationale: Wearing items with a cotton panel liner allows for air movement in and around the genital area. Bubble bath or other bath oils should be avoided because these may be irritating to the urethra. Harsh, scented, or printed toilet paper may cause irritation. Wearing tight clothes irritates the genital area and does not allow for air circulation.

Test-Taking Strategy: Use the process of elimination, and note the key words "indicate an understanding." Eliminate option 2 because of the absolute word "always" and option 3 because of the words "tight-fitting." From the remaining options, recall that bubble baths need to be avoided. Review measures to prevent urinary tract infections if you had difficulty with this question.

Level of Cognitive Ability: Analysis
Client Need: Health Promotion and Maintenance
Integrated Process: Nursing Process/Evaluation
Content Area: Maternity/Antepartum

References:
Ignatavicius, D., & Workman, M. (2002). *Medical surgical nursing: Critical thinking for collaborative care* (4th ed.). Philadelphia: Saunders, p. 1621.
Lowdermilk, D., & Perry, A. (2004). *Maternity & women's health care* (8th ed.). St. Louis: Mosby, 422.

23. A nurse instructs a client with mild preeclampsia about home care measures. The nurse determines that the teaching has been effective concerning assessment of complications when the client states:
   1 "As long as the home care nurse is visiting me daily, I do not have to keep my next physician's appointment."
   2 "I need to take my blood pressure each morning and alternate arms each time."
   3 "I need to check my weight every day at different times during the day."
   4 "I need to check my urine with a dipstick every day for protein and call the physician if it is 2+ or more."

Answer: 4
Rationale: The client needs to be instructed to report any increases in blood pressure, +2 proteinuria, weight gain greater than one pound per week, presence of edema, and decreased fetal activity to the physician or health care provider immediately to prevent worsening of the preeclamptic condition. It is important to keep physician appointments even if the client is receiving visits from a home care nurse. Blood pressures need to be taken in the same arm, in a sitting position, every day in order to obtain a consistent and accurate reading. The weight needs to be checked at the same time each day, wearing the same clothes, after voiding, and before breakfast in order to obtain reliable weights.

Test-Taking Strategy: Use the process of elimination, noting the key words "teaching has been effective." Basic principles related to health care teaching and focusing on the specific issue of the question, mild preeclampsia, will assist in directing you to option 4. Review home care teaching points for the client with preeclampsia if you had difficulty with this question.

Level of Cognitive Ability: Analysis
Client Needs: Health Promotion and Maintenance
Integrated Process: Nursing Process/Evaluation
Content Area: Maternity/Antepartum

Reference:
Lowdermilk, D., & Perry, A. (2004). *Maternity & women's health care* (8th ed.). St. Louis: Mosby, p. 850.

24. The nurse is providing instructions to a client and family regarding home care following left eye cataract removal. The nurse tells the client and family which of the following about positioning in the postoperative period?

1 Lower the head between the knees three times a day
2 Bend below the waist as frequently as able
3 Sleep on the right side or back
4 Sleep only on the left side

Answer: 3

Rationale: Following cataract surgery, the client should not sleep on the side of the body that was operated on. The client should also avoid bending below the level of the waist or lowering the head because these actions will increase intraocular pressure.

Test-Taking Strategy: Use the process of elimination. Eliminate options 1 and 2 first because they are similar and indicate that lowering the head below waist level is acceptable. From the remaining options, remembering that the client needs to be instructed to remain off of the operative side will direct you to option 3. Review postoperative instructions for the client following cataract surgery if you had difficulty with this question.

Level of Cognitive Ability: Application
Client Needs: Health Promotion and Maintenance
Integrated Process: Teaching/Learning
Content Area: Adult Health/Eye

References:
Lewis, S., Heitkemper, M., & Dirksen, S. (2004). *Medical-surgical nursing: Assessment and management of clinical problems* (6th ed.). St. Louis: Mosby, p. 452.
Phipps, W., Monahan, F., Sands, J., Marek, J., & Neighbors, M. (2003). *Medical-surgical nursing: Health and illness perspectives* (7th ed.). St. Louis: Mosby, p. 1901.

25. A nurse has provided instructions to a new mother with a urinary tract infection regarding foods and fluids to consume that will acidify the urine. The nurse determines that further instructions are needed if the mother indicates that which fluid will acidify the urine?

1 Apricot juice
2 Carbonated drinks
3 Prune juice
4 Cranberry juice

Answer: 2

Rationale: Acidification of the urine inhibits multiplication of bacteria. Fluids that acidify the urine include apricot, plum, and prune, or cranberry juice. Carbonated drinks should be avoided because they increase urine alkalinity.

Test-Taking Strategy: Use the process of elimination, noting the key words "further instructions are needed." These key words indicate a false-response question and that you need to select the fluid item that will not acidify the urine. Note the similarity between options 1, 3, and 4 in that these items are fruit juices. This will assist in directing you to option 2. Review foods and fluids that cause urine acidification if you had difficulty with this question.

Level of Cognitive Ability: Analysis
Client Needs: Health Promotion and Maintenance
Integrated Process: Teaching/Learning
Content Area: Maternity/Postpartum

Reference:
Murray, S., McKinney, E., & Gorrie, T. (2002). *Foundations of maternal-newborn nursing* (3rd ed.). Philadelphia: Saunders, p. 792.

26. A postpartum nurse has instructed a new mother on how to bathe her newborn infant. The nurse demonstrates the procedure to the mother, and on the following day, asks the mother to perform the procedure. Which observation by the nurse indicates that the mother is performing the procedure correctly?

1 The mother cleans the ears and then moves to the eyes and the face.
2 The mother begins to wash the newborn infant by starting with the eyes and face.
3 The mother washes the arms, chest, and back followed by the neck, arms, and face.
4 The mother washes the entire newborn infant's body and then washes the eyes, face, and scalp.

Answer: 2
Rationale: Bathing should start at the eyes and face and with the cleanest area first. Next, the external ears and behind the ears are cleaned. The newborn infant's neck should be washed because formula, lint, or breast milk will often accumulate in the folds of the neck. Hands and arms are then washed. The newborn infant's legs are washed next, with the diaper area washed last.

Test-Taking Strategy: Use the process of elimination, and use the basic techniques and principles of bathing a client to answer this question. Remember to always start with the cleanest area of the body first and proceed to the dirtiest area. This principle will direct you to option 2. Review home care measures related to the care of the newborn infant if you had difficulty with this question.

Level of Cognitive Ability: Analysis
Client Needs: Health Promotion and Maintenance
Integrated Process: Nursing Process/Evaluation
Content Area: Maternity/Postpartum

Reference:
Murray, S., McKinney, E., & Gorrie, T. (2002). *Foundations of maternal-newborn nursing* (3rd ed.). Philadelphia: Saunders, p. 569.

27. A nurse is teaching umbilical cord care to a new mother. The nurse tells the mother that:

1 Cord care is done only at birth to control bleeding
2 Alcohol is the only agent to use to clean the cord
3 The process of keeping the cord clean and dry will decrease bacterial growth
4 It takes at least 21 days for the cord to dry up and fall off

Answer: 3
Rationale: The cord should be kept clean and dry to decrease bacterial growth. The cord should be cleansed two to three times a day using alcohol or other agents. Cord care is required until the cord dries up and falls off between 7 to 14 days after birth. Additionally, the diaper should be folded below the cord to keep urine away from the cord.

Test-Taking Strategy: Use the process of elimination. Eliminate options 1 and 2 first because of the absolute word "only." From the remaining options, recalling the purpose of cord care will direct you to option 3. Review concepts related to cord care if you had difficulty with this question.

Level of Cognitive Ability: Application
Client Needs: Health Promotion and Maintenance
Integrated Process: Teaching/Learning
Content Area: Maternity/Postpartum

Reference:
Murray, S., McKinney, E., & Gorrie, T. (2002). *Foundations of maternal-newborn nursing* (3rd ed.). Philadelphia: Saunders, pp. 559; 568.

28. The parents of a male newborn infant who is uncircumcised request information on how to clean the newborn's penis. The nurse tells the parents to:

1 "Retract the foreskin and cleanse the glans when bathing the infant."
2 "Avoid retraction of the foreskin to clean the penis because this may cause adhesions."
3 "Retract the foreskin no farther than it will easily go and replace it over the glans after cleaning."
4 "Retract the foreskin and cleanse with every diaper change."

Answer: 2

Rationale: In male newborn infants, prepuce is continuous with the epidermis of the gland and is not retractable. If retraction is forced, this may cause adhesions to develop. The mother should be told to allow separation to occur naturally, which usually occurs between 3 years old and puberty. Most foreskins are retractable by 3 years of age and should be pushed back gently at this time for cleaning once a week. Options 1, 3, and 4 identify an action that addresses retraction of the foreskin.

Test-Taking Strategy: Use the process of elimination. Note that options 1, 3, and 4 are similar in that they all identify retracting the foreskin. Option 2 is the option that is different. Review teaching points related to cleaning the penis of an uncircumcised newborn infant if you had difficulty with this question.

Level of Cognitive Ability: Application
Client Needs: Health Promotion and Maintenance
Integrated Process: Teaching/Learning
Content Area: Maternity/Postpartum

References:
Lowdermilk, D., & Perry, A. (2004). *Maternity & women's health care* (8th ed.). St. Louis: Mosby, p. 695.
Wong, D., & Hockenberry, M. (2003). *Wong's nursing care of infants and children* (7th ed.). St. Louis: Mosby, p. 254.

29. The nurse prepares a teaching plan about the administration of ear drops for the parents of a 6-year-old child. The nurse tells the parents that when administering the drops, they should:

1 Pull the ear up and back
2 Wear gloves
3 Hold the child in a sitting position
4 Position the child so that the affected ear is facing downward

Answer: 1

Rationale: To administer ear drops in a child older than 3 years of age, the ear is pulled upward and back. The ear is pulled down and back in children younger than 3 years of age. Gloves do not need to be worn by the parents, but handwashing before and after the procedure needs to be performed. The child needs to be in a side-lying position with the affected ear facing upward to facilitate the flow of medication down the ear canal by gravity.

Test-Taking Strategy: Visualizing this procedure will assist in eliminating options 2, 3, and 4. Also, recalling the anatomy of the child's ear canal and noting the age of the child will direct you to option 1. Review this procedure if you had difficulty with this question.

Level of Cognitive Ability: Application
Client Needs: Health Promotion and Maintenance
Integrated Process: Teaching/Learning
Content Area: Child Health

Reference:
Wong, D., & Hockenberry, M. (2003). *Wong's nursing care of infants and children* (7th ed.). St. Louis: Mosby, p. 1160.

30. A nurse is providing discharge instructions to the mother of an 8-year-old child who had a tonsillectomy. The mother tells the nurse that the child loves tacos and asks when the child can safely eat one. The most appropriate response to the mother is:
1 "In 1 week"
2 "In 3 weeks"
3 "Six days following surgery"
4 "When the physician says it's okay"

Answer: 2
Rationale: Rough or scratchy foods or spicy foods are to be avoided for 3 weeks following a tonsillectomy. Citrus juices that irritate the throat need to be avoided for 10 days. Red liquids are avoided because they will give the appearance of blood if the child vomits. The mother is instructed to add full liquids on the second day and soft foods as the child tolerates them.

Test-Taking Strategy: Use the process of elimination. Eliminate options 1 and 3 first because they identify similar time frames. From the remaining options, focus on the key words "most appropriate" and eliminate option 4 because it places the mother's question on hold. Review these dietary instructions if you had difficulty with this question.

Level of Cognitive Ability: Application
Client Needs: Health Promotion and Maintenance
Integrated Process: Teaching/Learning
Content Area: Child Health

References:
James, S., Ashwill, J., & Droske, S. (2002). *Nursing care of children: Principles & practice* (2nd ed.).Philadelphia: Saunders, p. 637.
Wong, D., & Hockenberry, M. (2003). *Wong's nursing care of infants and children* (7th ed.). St. Louis: Mosby, p. 1354.

31. Following a cleft lip repair, the nurse instructs the parents about cleaning of the lip repair site. The nurse uses which solution in demonstrating this procedure to the parents?
1 Tap water
2 Sterile water
3 Full-strength hydrogen peroxide
4 Half-strength hydrogen peroxide

Answer: 2
Rationale: The lip repair site is cleansed with sterile water using a cotton swab after feeding and as prescribed. The parents should be instructed to use a rolling motion starting at the suture line and rolling out. Tap water is not a sterile solution. Hydrogen peroxide may disrupt the integrity of the site.

Test-Taking Strategy: Use the process of elimination. Eliminate options 3 and 4 first because they are similar. From the remaining options, recall the importance of asepsis in treating a surgical site to direct you to option 2. Review this procedure if you had difficulty with this question.

Level of Cognitive Ability: Application
Client Needs: Health Promotion and Maintenance
Integrated Process: Teaching/Learning
Content Area: Child Health

Reference:
James, S., Ashwill, J., & Droske, S. (2002). *Nursing care of children: Principles & practice* (2nd ed.).Philadelphia: Saunders, p. 538.

32. A child with a diagnosis of umbilical hernia has been scheduled for surgical repair in 2 weeks. The clinic nurse instructs the parents about the signs of possible hernial strangulation. The nurse tells the parents that which sign would require physician notification?

1 Fever
2 Diarrhea
3 Constipation
4 Vomiting

Answer: 4

Rationale: The parents of a child with an umbilical hernia need to be instructed in the signs of strangulation, which include vomiting, pain, and irreducible mass at the umbilicus. The parents should be instructed to contact the physician immediately if strangulation is suspected.

Test-Taking Strategy: Use the process of elimination and the definition of the word "strangulation" to assist in eliminating options 1 and 2. From the remaining options, think about the anatomy of the body and the expected occurrence if strangulation developed to direct you to option 4. Review the signs of strangulation if you had difficulty with this question.

Level of Cognitive Ability: Application
Client Needs: Health Promotion and Maintenance
Integrated Process: Teaching/Learning
Content Area: Child Health

Reference:
James, S., Ashwill, J., & Droske, S. (2002). *Nursing care of children: Principles & practice* (2nd ed.).Philadelphia: Saunders, p. 547.

33. A client with a compound (open) fracture of the radius has a plaster of Paris cast applied in the emergency room. The nurse provides home care instructions and tells the client to seek medical attention if which of the following occurs?

1 The cast feels heavy and damp after 24 hours of application.
2 Numbness and tingling are felt in the fingers.
3 Bloody drainage is noted on the cast during the first 6 hours after application.
4 The entire cast feels warm in the first 24 hours after application.

Answer: 2

Rationale: A limb encased in a cast is at risk for nerve damage and diminished circulation from increased pressure caused by edema. Signs of increased pressure from the cast include numbness, tingling, and increased pain. A plaster of Paris cast can take up to 48 hours to dry and generates heat while drying. Some drainage may occur initially with a compound (open) fracture.

Test-Taking Strategy: Note the key words "compound (open)" in the question. These key words and use of the ABCs—airway, breathing, and circulation—will direct you to option 2. Review teaching points for the client with a plaster cast if you had difficulty with this question.

Level of Cognitive Ability: Application
Client Needs: Health Promotion and Maintenance
Integrated Process: Teaching/Learning
Content Area: Adult Health/Musculoskeletal

Reference:
Phipps, W., Monahan, F., Sands, J., Marek, J., & Neighbors, M. (2003). *Medical-surgical nursing: Health and illness perspectives* (7th ed.). St. Louis: Mosby, p. 1481.

34. A mother of a child with celiac disease asks the nurse how long a special diet is necessary. The nurse tells the mother that:
    1 A gluten-free diet will need to be followed for life
    2 Adequate nutritional status will help prevent celiac crisis
    3 Supplemental vitamins, iron, and folate will prevent complications
    4 A lactose-free diet will need to be followed temporarily

Answer: 1
Rationale: The main nursing consideration with celiac disease is helping the child adhere to dietary management. Treatment of celiac disease consists primarily of dietary management with a gluten-free diet. Options 2, 3, and 4 are all true statements but do not answer the question the client is asking. Children with untreated celiac disease may have lactose intolerance, which usually improves with gluten withdrawal. Nutritional deficiencies resulting from malabsorption are treated with appropriate supplements.

Test-Taking Strategy: Focus on the issue of the question: "the length of time a special diet is necessary." Option 1 directly relates to this issue. Review dietary requirements for celiac disease if you had difficulty with this question.

Level of Cognitive Ability: Application
Client Needs: Health Promotion and Maintenance
Integrated Process: Teaching/Learning
Content Area: Child Health

Reference:
Wong, D., & Hockenberry, M. (2003). *Wong's nursing care of infants and children* (7th ed.). St. Louis: Mosby, pp. 1450-1451.

---

35. A nurse teaches a mother of a newly circumcised infant about post-circumcision care. Which statement by the mother indicates an understanding of the care required?
    1 "I need to check for bleeding every hour for the first 12 hours."
    2 "I need to clean the penis every hour with baby wipes."
    3 "I need to wrap the penis completely in dry sterile gauze, making sure it is dry when I change his diaper."
    4 "My baby will not urinate for the next 24 hours because of swelling."

Answer: 1
Rationale: The mother needs to be taught to observe for bleeding and to assess the site hourly for 8 to 12 hours following the circumcision. Voiding needs to be assessed. The mother should call the physician if the baby has not urinated within 24 hours because swelling or damage may obstruct urine output. When the diaper is changed, Vaseline gauze should be reapplied. Frequent diaper changing prevents contamination of the site. Water is used for cleaning because soap or baby wipes may irritate the area and cause discomfort.

Test-Taking Strategy: Use the process of elimination. Eliminate option 2 because baby wipes will cause stinging in the newly circumcised penis. Eliminate option 3 because gauze will stick to the penis if it is completely dry. Eliminate option 4 because penile swelling that prevents voiding needs to be reported to the physician. Review post-circumcision care if you had difficulty answering the question.

Level of Cognitive Ability: Analysis
Client Needs: Health Promotion and Maintenance
Integrated Process: Nursing Process/Evaluation
Content Area: Maternity/Postpartum

Reference:
Lowdermilk, D., & Perry, A. (2004). *Maternity & women's health care* (8th ed.). St. Louis: Mosby, pp. 749; 793.

36. A nurse is developing a teaching plan for a client who will be receiving phenelzine sulfate (Nardil). The nurse plans to tell the client to avoid:
1 Aged cheeses
2 Cherries and blueberries
3 Digitalis preparations
4 Vasodilators

Answer: 1
Rationale: Phenelzine sulfate is in the monoamine oxidase inhibitor (MAOI) class of antidepressant medications. An individual on an MAOI must avoid aged cheeses, alcoholic beverages, avocados, bananas, and caffeine drinks. There are also other food items to avoid, including chocolate, meat tenderizers, pickled herring, raisins, sour cream, yogurt, and soy sauce. Medications that should be avoided include amphetamines, antiasthmatics, and certain antidepressants. The client should also avoid antihistamines, antihypertensive medications, levodopa (L-Dopa), and meperidine (Demerol).

Test-Taking Strategy: Note the key word "avoid." This key word indicates a false-response question and that you need to select the food item that the client is not allowed to consume. Recalling that phenelzine sulfate is an MAOI and recalling the foods that need to be avoided will direct you to option 1. Review this medication if you had difficulty with this question.

Level of Cognitive Ability: Application
Client Needs: Health Promotion and Maintenance
Integrated Process: Teaching/Learning
Content Area: Pharmacology

Reference:
Hodgson, B., & Kizior, R. (2004). *Saunders nursing drug handbook 2004.* Philadelphia: Saunders, p. 799.

37. A nurse is providing home care instructions to the parents of an infant who had surgical repair of an inguinal hernia. The nurse instructs the parents to do which of the following to prevent infection at the surgical site?
1 Change the diapers as soon as they become damp
2 Report a fever immediately
3 Soak the infant in a tub bath twice a day for the next 5 days
4 Restrict the infant's physical activity

Answer: 1
Rationale: Changing diapers as soon as they become damp helps prevent infection at the surgical site. Parents are instructed to change diapers more frequently than usual during the day and once or twice during the night. Parents are also instructed to give the infant sponge baths instead of tub baths for 2 to 5 days postoperatively. There are no restrictions placed on the infant's activity. A fever could indicate the presence of an infection.

Test-Taking Strategy: Focus on the issue: to prevent infection. This will assist in eliminating options 2 and 3. From the remaining options, thinking about the anatomical location of an inguinal hernia will direct you to option 1. Review measures to prevent infection following inguinal hernia repair if you had difficulty with this question.

Level of Cognitive Ability: Application
Client Needs: Health Promotion and Maintenance
Integrated Process: Teaching/Learning
Content Area: Child Health

Reference:
Wong, D., & Hockenberry, M. (2003). *Wong's nursing care of infants and children* (7th ed.). St. Louis: Mosby, p. 478.

38. A client is experiencing difficulty using an incentive spirometer. The nurse teaches the client that which of the following may interfere with effective use of the device?
  1 Breathing through the nose
  2 Forming a tight seal around the mouthpiece with the lips
  3 Inhaling slowly
  4 Removing the mouthpiece to exhale

Answer: 1

Rationale: Incentive spirometry is not effective if the client breathes through the nose. The client should exhale, form a tight seal around the mouthpiece, inhale slowly, hold to the count of three, and remove the mouthpiece to exhale. The client should repeat the exercise approximately 10 times every hour for best results.

Test-Taking Strategy: Note the key words "may interfere with effective use." These key words indicate a false-response question and that you need to select the option that identifies an incorrect client action. Visualizing the use of this device will direct you to option 1. Review this procedure if you had difficulty with this question.

Level of Cognitive Ability: Application
Client Needs: Health Promotion and Maintenance
Integrated Process: Teaching/Learning
Content Area: Adult Health/Respiratory

Reference:
Phipps, W., Monahan, F., Sands, J., Marek, J., & Neighbors, M. (2003). *Medical-surgical nursing: Health and illness perspectives* (7th ed.). St. Louis: Mosby, p. 383.

---

39. A client with chronic obstructive pulmonary disease (COPD) has a knowledge deficit related to positions used to breathe more easily. The nurse teaches the client to:
  1 Lie on the side with the head of the bed at a 45-degree angle
  2 Sit bolt upright in bed with the arms crossed over the chest
  3 Sit on the edge of the bed with the arms leaning on an overbed table
  4 Sit in a reclining chair tilted slightly back with the feet elevated

Answer: 3

Rationale: Proper positioning can decrease episodes of dyspnea in a client. These include sitting upright while leaning on an overbed table, sitting upright in a chair with the arms resting on the knees, and leaning against a wall while standing. Option 1 restricts expansion of the lateral wall of the lung. Option 2 restricts movement of the anterior and posterior walls. Option 4 restricts posterior lung expansion.

Test-Taking Strategy: Use the process of elimination. Visualize each of the positions described in the options. Think about how each position affects lung expansion to direct you to option 3. Review positions that relieve dyspnea in the client with COPD if you had difficulty with this question.

Level of Cognitive Ability: Application
Client Needs: Health Promotion and Maintenance
Integrated Process: Teaching/Learning
Content Area: Adult Health/Respiratory

References:
Ignatavicius, D., & Workman, M. (2002). *Medical surgical nursing: Critical thinking for collaborative care* (4th ed.). Philadelphia: Saunders, pp. 547-548.
Phipps, W., Monahan, F., Sands, J., Marek, J., & Neighbors, M. (2003). *Medical-surgical nursing: health and illness perspectives* (7th ed.). St. Louis: Mosby, p. 576.

40. A nurse has taught the client with pleurisy about measures to promote comfort during recuperation. The nurse determines that the client has understood the instructions if the client states to:
1 Try to take only small, shallow breaths
2 Splint the chest wall during coughing and deep breathing
3 Lie as much as possible on the unaffected side
4 Take as much pain medication as possible

Answer: 2
Rationale: The client with pleurisy should splint the chest wall during coughing and deep breathing. The client may also lie on the affected side to minimize movement of the affected chest wall. Taking small, shallow breaths promotes atelectasis. The client should take medication cautiously so that adequate coughing and deep breathing is performed and an adequate level of comfort is maintained.

Test-Taking Strategy: Focus on the issue: to promote comfort. Eliminate option 1 because of the absolute word "only." From the remaining options, noting the word "splint" in option 2 will direct you to this option. Review the measures that will promote comfort in a client with pleurisy if you had difficulty with this question.

Level of Cognitive Ability: Analysis
Client Needs: Health Promotion and Maintenance
Integrated Process: Nursing Process/Evaluation
Content Area: Adult Health/Respiratory

Reference:
Lewis, S., Heitkemper, M., & Dirksen, S. (2004). *Medical-surgical nursing: Assessment and management of clinical problems* (6th ed.). St. Louis: Mosby, p. 630.

41. A client with a diagnosis of trigeminal neuralgia is started on a regimen of carbamazepine (Tegretol). The nurse provides instructions to the client about the medication and determines that the client understands the instructions if the client states:
1 "I will report a fever or sore throat to my doctor."
2 "My urine may turn red in color, but this is nothing to be concerned about."
3 "I must brush my teeth frequently to avoid damage to my gums."
4 "Some joint pain is expected and is nothing to worry about."

Answer: 1
Rationale: Agranulocytosis is an adverse effect of carbamazepine and places the client at risk for infection. If the client develops a fever or a sore throat, the physician should be notified. Unusual bruising or bleeding are also adverse effects of the medication and need to be reported to the physician if they occur.

Test-Taking Strategy: Use the process of elimination. Eliminate option 3 because of the absolute word "must." Next eliminate options 2 and 4 because both indicate that development of an adverse effect is "nothing to be concerned about." Also recalling that agranulocytosis is an adverse effect will direct you to option 1. Review the adverse effects of this medication and the laboratory tests that need monitoring if you had difficulty with this question.

Level of Cognitive Ability: Analysis
Client Needs: Health Promotion and Maintenance
Integrated Process: Nursing Process/Evaluation
Content Area: Pharmacology

Reference:
Hodgson, B., & Kizior, R. (2004). *Saunders nursing drug handbook 2004.* Philadelphia: Saunders, p. 149.

42. A nurse teaches a preoperative client about the nasogastric (NG) tube that will be inserted in preparation for surgery. The nurse determines that the client understands when the tube will be removed in the postoperative period when the client states:

1   "When my gastrointestinal (GI) system is healed."
2   "When I can tolerate food without vomiting."
3   "When my bowels begin to function again, and I begin to pass gas."
4   "When the doctor says so."

Answer: 3

Rationale: NG tubes are discontinued when normal function returns to the GI tract. The tube will be removed before GI healing. Food would not be administered unless bowel function returns. Although the physician determines when the NG tube will be removed, option 4 does not determine effectiveness of teaching.

Test-Taking Strategy: Use the process of elimination. Option 4 can be easily eliminated first. Eliminate option 1 next, considering the time factor associated with healing of the GI tract. From the remaining options, recalling that food would not be administered unless bowel function returns will assist in eliminating option 2. Review the use and care of the NG tube if you had difficulty with this question.

Level of Cognitive Ability: Analysis
Client Needs: Health Promotion and Maintenance
Integrated Process: Nursing Process/Evaluation
Content Area: Adult Health/Gastrointestinal

Reference:
Potter, P., & Perry, A. (2005). *Fundamentals of nursing* (6th ed.). St. Louis: Mosby, p. 1408.

---

43. A client is receiving intralipids (fat emulsion) intravenously at home, and the client's spouse manages the infusion. The health care nurse makes a visit and discusses potential adverse reactions and side effects of the therapy with the client and the spouse. Following the discussion, the nurse expects the spouse to verbalize that in case of a suspected adverse reaction, the priority action is to:

1   Take a blood pressure
2   Stop the infusion
3   Contact the nurse
4   Contact the local area emergency response team

Answer: 2

Rationale: Fat emulsion therapy can cause overloading syndrome (focal seizures, fever, shock) and adverse effects, including chest pain, chills, and shock. The priority action is to stop the infusion and limit the adverse response before obtaining additional assistance. Although options 1, 2, and 4 are correct interventions, the priority is to stop the infusion.

Test-Taking Strategy: Note the key words "suspected adverse reactions" and "priority." Remembering that the priority action when an adverse reaction occurs is to stop the infusion will direct you to the correct option. Review the adverse reactions of fat emulsion therapy and the priority actions if an adverse reaction occurs if you had difficulty with this question.

Level of Cognitive Ability: Analysis
Client Needs: Health Promotion and Maintenance
Integrated Process: Teaching/Learning
Content Area: Delegating/Prioritizing

References:
Black, J., & Hawks, J. (2005). *Medical-surgical nursing: Clinical management for positive outcomes* (7th ed.). Philadelphia: Saunders, p. 708.
Ignatavicius, D., & Workman, M. (2002). *Medical surgical nursing: Critical thinking for collaborative care* (4th ed.). Philadelphia: Saunders, p. 1129.

44. A home care nurse suspects that a client's spouse is experiencing caregiver strain. The nurse assesses for this occurrence by:

1 Obtaining feedback from the client about the coping abilities of the caregiver

2 Gathering subjective and objective assessment from the caregiver and client

3 Waiting until the caregiver expresses concern about the significant responsibility in caring for the client

4 Making a referral to the home care agency social worker to perform an assessment

Answer: 2

Rationale: Caregiver strain can occur when a client is significantly dependent on someone for personal and health care needs. Option 1 is not appropriate. The nurse should not expect the client to assess the coping abilities of the caregiver. Although a social worker may be helpful, the nurse needs to assess the situation before making a referral. Waiting for the caregiver to express concern is not appropriate. The caregiver may be exhausted or incapable of caring for the client by this time.

Test-Taking Strategy: Use the steps of the nursing process to eliminate options 3 and 4. From the remaining options, select option 2 because it addresses both the client and the caregiver. Review the concepts of caregiver strain if you had difficulty with this question.

Level of Cognitive Ability: Application
Client Needs: Health Promotion and Maintenance
Integrated Process: Nursing Process/Assessment
Content Area: Fundamental Skills

Reference:
Potter, P., & Perry, A. (2005). *Fundamentals of nursing* (6th ed.). St. Louis: Mosby, pp. 609-610.

---

45. A client being discharged from the hospital will be taking warfarin (Coumadin) at home on a daily basis. The nurse has provided instructions to the client about the medication and determines that further teaching is needed if the client states:

1 "This medicine thins my blood and allows me to clot slower."

2 "I need to have a prothrombin time checked in 2 weeks."

3 "If I notice any increased bleeding or bruising, I need to call my doctor."

4 "I need to increase the intake of foods high in vitamin K in my diet."

Answer: 4

Rationale: Warfarin sodium (Coumadin) is an oral anticoagulant that is used mainly to prevent thromboembolitic events, such as thrombophlebitis, pulmonary embolism, and embolism formation caused by atrial fibrillation or other disorders. Oral anticoagulants prolong the clotting time and are monitored by the prothrombin time (PT) and the International Normalized Ratio (INR). Client education should include signs and symptoms of adverse effects and dietary restrictions such as limiting foods high in vitamin K (leafy green vegetables, liver, cheese, and egg yolk) because these increase clotting times.

Test-Taking Strategy: Note the key words "further teaching is needed." These key words indicate a false-response question and that you need to select the incorrect client statement. Recalling that warfarin sodium is an anticoagulant will assist in eliminating options 1, 2, and 3. Also, remembering the role vitamin K plays in the clotting mechanism will direct you to option 4. Review client teaching points related to this medication if you had difficulty with this question.

Level of Cognitive Ability: Analysis
Client Needs: Health Promotion and Maintenance
Integrated Process: Teaching/Learning
Content Area: Pharmacology

References:
Hodgson, B., & Kizior, R. (2004). *Saunders nursing drug handbook 2004.* Philadelphia: Saunders, p. 1063.
McKenry, L., & Salerno, E. (2003). *Mosby's pharmacology in nursing* (21st ed.). St. Louis: Mosby, pp. 631-632.

46. A teenager returns to the gynecological (GYN) clinic for a follow-up visit for a sexually transmitted disease (STD). Which statement by the teenager indicates the need for further teaching?
  1 "I always make sure my boyfriend uses a condom."
  2 "I know you won't tell my parents I'm sick."
  3 "My boyfriend doesn't have to come in for treatment, does he?"
  4 "I finished all of the antibiotics, just like you said."

Answer: 3
Rationale: In treating STDs, all sexual contacts must be contacted and treated with medication. Clients should always use a condom with any sexual contact. Treatment of a teenager at a GYN clinic is confidential and parents will not be contacted, even if the client is under 18 years of age. Any client should always finish the course of antibiotics prescribed by the health care provider.

Test-Taking Strategy: Note the key words "need for further teaching." These key words indicate a false-response question and that you need to select the incorrect client statement. Recalling the concepts related to "safe sex," the treatment of STDs in the teenager, and the principles related to antibiotic therapy will direct you to option 3. Review this content if you had difficulty with this question.

Level of Cognitive Ability: Analysis
Client Needs: Health Promotion and Maintenance
Integrated Process: Teaching/Learning
Content Area: Child Health

Reference:
Wong, D., & Hockenberry, M. (2003). *Wong's nursing care of infants and children* (7th ed.). St. Louis: Mosby, p. 862.

47. A nurse is teaching a client newly diagnosed with diabetes mellitus about blood glucose monitoring. The nurse teaches the client to report glucose levels that exceed:
  1 150 mg/dL
  2 200 mg/dL
  3 250 mg/dL
  4 350 mg/dL

Answer: 3
Rationale: The client should be taught to report blood glucose levels that exceed 250 mg/dL, unless otherwise instructed by the physician. Options 1 and 2 are low levels that do not require physician notification. Option 4 is a high value.

Test-Taking Strategy: Use the process of elimination. Recalling the basic principles related to diabetic home care instructions will direct you to option 3. Review this common area of teaching for clients with diabetes mellitus if you had difficulty with this question.

Level of Cognitive Ability: Application
Client Needs: Health Promotion and Maintenance
Integrated Process: Teaching/Learning
Content Area: Adult Health/Endocrine

References:
Chernecky, C., & Berger, B. (2004). *Laboratory tests and diagnostic procedures* (4th ed.). Philadelphia: Saunders, p. 599.
Ignatavicius, D., & Workman, M. (2002). *Medical surgical nursing: Critical thinking for collaborative care* (4th ed.). Philadelphia: Saunders, p. 1450.

48. A client with gastritis asks the nurse at a screening clinic about analgesics that will not cause epigastric distress. The nurse tells the client to take which of the following medications?
1 Bufferin
2 Tylenol
3 Ecotrin
4 Ascriptin

Answer: 2

Rationale: Aspirin is irritating to the gastrointestinal (GI) tract of the client with a history of gastritis. The client should be advised to take analgesics that do not contain aspirin, such as acetaminophen (Tylenol). The other medications listed have aspirin in them. Another category of medications that is irritating to the GI tract is the nonsteroidal antiinflammatory drugs (NSAIDs).

Test-Taking Strategy: Use the process of elimination. Note that options 1, 3 and 4 are similar and are aspirin-containing medications. Review these medications if you had difficulty with this question.

Level of Cognitive Ability: Application
Client Needs: Health Promotion and Maintenance
Integrated Process: Teaching/Learning
Content Area: Pharmacology

Reference:
McKenry, L., & Salerno, E. (2003). *Mosby's pharmacology in nursing* (21st ed.). St. Louis: Mosby, p. 208.

49. A client is diagnosed with thromboangiitis obliterans (Buerger's disease). The nurse places highest priority on teaching the client about modifications of which risk factor related to this disorder?
1 Exposure to heat
2 Excessive water intake
3 Diet low in vitamin C
4 Cigarette smoking

Answer: 4

Rationale: Buerger's disease occurs predominantly in men between 25 to 40 years of age who smoke cigarettes. A familial tendency is noted, but cigarette smoking is consistently a risk factor. Symptoms of the disease improve with smoking cessation. Options 1, 2, and 3 are not risk factors.

Test-Taking Strategy: Note the key words "highest priority" and "risk factor." Recalling the pathophysiology related to this disorder will direct you to option 4. Review the risk factors of this disorder if you had difficulty with this question.

Level of Cognitive Ability: Application
Client Needs: Health Promotion and Maintenance
Integrated Process: Teaching/Learning
Content Area: Adult Health/Cardiovascular

Reference:
Ignatavicius, D., & Workman, M. (2002). *Medical surgical nursing: Critical thinking for collaborative care* (4th ed.). Philadelphia: Saunders, p. 761.

50. A client has a new prescription for timolol (Betimol). The nurse determines that the client has misunderstood instructions given about the medication if the client stated to:
1 Report shortness of breath to the physician
2 Change positions slowly
3 Taper or discontinue the medication once the client feels well
4 Have enough medication on hand to last through weekends and vacations

Answer: 3

Rationale: Common client teaching points about beta-adrenergic blocking agents include to take the pulse daily and hold for a rate under 60 beats per minute (and notify physician) and to report shortness of breath. The client should not discontinue or change the medication dose. The client is also instructed to keep enough medication on hand so as not to run out, to change positions slowly, not to take over-the-counter medications (especially decongestants, cough, and cold preparations) without consulting the physician, and to carry medical identification stating a beta-blocker is being taken.

Test-Taking Strategy: Use the process of elimination, noting the key words "has misunderstood." These key words indicate a false-response question and that you need to select the incorrect client statement. Noting the word "discontinue" in option 3 will direct you to this option. Review client teaching points related to this medication if you had difficulty with this question.

Level of Cognitive Ability: Analysis
Client Needs: Health Promotion and Maintenance
Integrated Process: Teaching/Learning
Content Area: Pharmacology

Reference:
McKenry, L., & Salerno, E. (2003). *Mosby's pharmacology in nursing* (21st ed.). St. Louis: Mosby, p. 485.

---

51. A nurse has completed giving medication instructions to the client receiving benazepril (Lotensin) to treat hypertension. The nurse determines that the client needs further instruction if the client stated to:
1 Change positions slowly
2 Report signs and symptoms of infection to the physician
3 Monitor the blood pressure every week
4 Use salt moderately to taste in cooking and on foods

Answer: 4
Rationale: The client taking an angiotensen-converting enzyme (ACE) inhibitor is instructed to take the medication exactly as prescribed, monitor blood pressure weekly, and continue with other lifestyle changes to control hypertension. The client should change positions slowly to avoid orthostatic hypotension, report fever, mouth sores, and sore throat to the physician (neutropenia), and avoid the use of salt.

Test-Taking Strategy: Use the process of elimination, noting the key words "needs further instruction." These key words indicate a false-response question and that you need to select the incorrect client statement. Noting that the medication is prescribed to treat hypertension will assist in eliminating options 1, 2, and 3. Review this medication if you had difficulty with this question.

Level of Cognitive Ability: Analysis
Client Needs: Health Promotion and Maintenance
Integrated Process: Teaching/Learning
Content Area: Pharmacology

Reference:
Hodgson, B., & Kizior, R. (2004). *Saunders nursing drug handbook 2004*. Philadelphia: Saunders, p. 98.

---

52. A nurse has given medication instructions to a client receiving lovastatin (Mevacor). The nurse determines that the client understands the effects of the medication if the client stated the need to adhere to the periodic evaluation of serum:
1 Creatinine levels
2 Liver function studies
3 Blood glucose levels
4 Bleeding times

Answer: 2
Rationale: Lovastatin is a reductase inhibitor. It results in an increase in the high-density lipoprotein (HDL) cholesterol and a decrease in the triglycerides and low-density lipoprotein (LDL) cholesterol. This medication is converted by the liver to active metabolites, and therefore is not used in clients with active hepatic disease or elevated transaminase levels. For this reason, clients are recommended to have periodic liver function studies. Periodic cholesterol levels are also needed to monitor the effectiveness of therapy.

Test-Taking Strategy: Focus on the name of the medication. Recalling that medication names that contain the letters "statin" are cholesterol-lowering medications and that cholesterol is synthesized in the liver will direct you to option 2. Review this medication if you had difficulty with this question.

Level of Cognitive Ability: Analysis
Client Needs: Health Promotion and Maintenance
Integrated Process: Nursing Process/Evaluation
Content Area: Pharmacology

References:
Hodgson, B., & Kizior, R. (2004). *Saunders nursing drug handbook 2004.* Philadelphia: Saunders, p. 620.
McKenry, L., & Salerno, E. (2003). *Mosby's pharmacology in nursing* (21st ed.). St. Louis: Mosby, p. 661.

53. A home care nurse visits a client at home. Clonazepam (Klonopin) has been prescribed for the client, and the nurse teaches the client about the medication. Which statement by the client indicates that further teaching is necessary?
1 "I can take my medicine at bedtime if it tends to make me feel drowsy."
2 "My drowsiness will decrease over time with continued treatment."
3 "I should take my medicine with food to decrease stomach problems."
4 "If I experience slurred speech, it will disappear in about 8 weeks."

Answer: 4
Rationale: Clients who are experiencing signs and symptoms of toxicity with the administration of clonazepam exhibit slurred speech, sedation, confusion, respiratory depression, hypotension, and eventually coma. Some drowsiness may occur but will decrease with continued use. The medication may be taken with food to decrease gastrointestinal irritation. Options 1, 2, and 3 are correct and represent an accurate understanding of the medication.

Test-Taking Strategy: Use the process of elimination, noting the key words "further teaching is necessary." These key words indicate a false-response question and that you need to select the incorrect client statement. Recalling the toxic effects that can occur with the use of this medication will direct you to option 4. Review this medication if you had difficulty with this question.

Level of Cognitive Ability: Analysis
Client Needs: Health Promotion and Maintenance
Integrated Process: Teaching/Learning
Content Area: Pharmacology

Reference:
Hodgson, B., & Kizior, R. (2004). *Saunders nursing drug handbook 2004.* Philadelphia: Saunders, p. 230.

54. The home care nurse visits a client at home. Persantine (Dipyridamole) has been prescribed for the client, and the nurse teaches the client about the medication. Which statement by the client indicates that the client understands the medication instructions?
1 "If I take this medicine with my warfarin sodium (Coumadin), it will protect my artificial heart valve."
2 "This medication will prevent a heart attack."
3 "This medication will prevent a stroke."
4 "This medication will help me to keep my blood pressure down."

Answer: 1
Rationale: Persantine combined with warfarin sodium is prescribed to protect the client's artificial heart valves. Persantine does not prevent heart attacks or strokes. It is an antiplatelet medication, not an antihypertensive.

Test-Taking Strategy: Use the process of elimination. Recalling that this medication is an antiplalelet not an antihypertensive will assist in eliminating option 4. Noting the word "prevent" in options 2 and 3 will assist in eliminating these options. Review the use of this medication if you had difficulty with this question.

Level of Cognitive Ability: Analysis
Client Needs: Health Promotion and Maintenance
Integrated Process: Nursing Process/Evaluation
Content Area: Pharmacology

References:
Hodgson, B., & Kizior, R. (2004). *Saunders nursing drug handbook 2004.* Philadelphia: Saunders, p. 320.
McKenry, L., & Salerno, E. (2003). *Mosby's pharmacology in nursing* (21st ed.). St. Louis: Mosby, p. 636.

---

55. A nurse is preparing to care for the mother of a preterm infant. The nurse plans to begin discharge planning:
1 When the discharge date is set
2 When the parents feel comfortable with and can demonstrate adequate care of their infant
3 When the mother is in labor
4 After stabilization of the infant in the early stages of hospitalization

Answer: 4
Rationale: Discharge planning begins upon admission. Determination of the services, needs, supplies, and equipment requirements should not be made on the day of discharge. Options 1 and 2 are incorrect because it is much too late to make the plans that need to be made. Option 3 is incorrect because during labor, the outcome of the delivery in not known.

Test-Taking Strategy: Use the process of elimination, remembering that discharge planning always begins upon admission to the hospital. Noting the key words "early stages of hospitalization" will direct you to option 4. Review the guidelines related to discharge planning if you had difficulty with this question.

Level of Cognitive Ability: Application
Client Needs: Health Promotion and Maintenance
Integrated Process: Nursing Process/Planning
Content Area: Maternity/Postpartum

Reference:
Wong, D., & Hockenberry, M. (2003). *Wong's nursing care of infants and children* (7th ed.). St. Louis: Mosby, p. 368.

56. A nurse is providing home care instructions to a client recovering from an acute inferior myocardial infarction (MI) with recurrent angina. The nurse teaches the client to:

1 Avoid sexual intercourse for at least 4 months
2 Replace sublingual nitroglycerin tablets yearly
3 Recognize the adverse effects of acetylsalicylic acid (aspirin), which include tinnitus and hearing loss
4 Participate in an exercise program that includes overhead lifting and reaching

Answer: 3

Rationale: After an acute MI, many clients are instructed to take one aspirin daily. Adverse effects include tinnitus, hearing loss, epigastric distress, gastrointestinal bleeding, and nausea. Following an acute MI, sexual intercourse usually can be resumed in 4 to 8 weeks if the physician agrees. Clients should be advised to purchase a new supply of nitroglycerin tablets every 6 to 9 months. Expiration dates on the medication bottle should also be checked. Activities that include lifting and reaching over the head should be avoided because they reduce cardiac output.

Test-Taking Strategy: Use the process of elimination and focus on the client's diagnosis. Noting the time limits in options 1 and 2, "4 months" and "yearly," will assist in eliminating these options. From the remaining options, "overhead lifting and reaching" in option 4 should indicate that this is incorrect. Review client teaching points following an MI if you had difficulty with this question.

Level of Cognitive Ability: Application
Client Needs: Health Promotion and Maintenance
Integrated Process: Teaching/Learning
Content Area: Adult Health/Cardiovascular

Reference:
Phipps, W., Monahan, F., Sands, J., Marek, J., & Neighbors, M. (2003). *Medical-surgical nursing: health and illness perspectives* (7th ed.). St. Louis: Mosby, p. 655.

---

57. A nurse is reviewing home care instructions with an older client who has type 1 diabetes mellitus and a history of diabetic ketoacidosis (DKA). The client's spouse is present when the instructions are given. Which statement by the spouse indicates that further teaching is necessary?

1 "If the grandchildren are sick, they probably shouldn't come to visit."
2 "I should call the doctor if he has nausea or abdominal pain lasting for more than one or two days."
3 "If he is vomiting, I shouldn't give him any insulin."
4 "I should bring him to the physician's office if he develops a fever."

Answer: 3

Rationale: Infection and stopping insulin are precipitating factors for DKA. Nausea and abdominal pain that lasts more than one or two days need to be reported, because these signs may be indicative of DKA.

Test-Taking Strategy: Note the key words "further teaching is necessary." These key words indicate a false-response question and that you need to select the incorrect client statement. Eliminate options 1 and 4 first because both relate to infection. From the remaining options, recalling the causes of DKA will direct you to option 3. Review the precipitating factors associated with DKA if you had difficulty with this question.

Level of Cognitive Ability: Analysis
Client Needs: Health Promotion and Maintenance
Integrated Process: Teaching/Learning
Content Area: Adult Health/Endocrine

Reference:
Black, J., & Hawks, J. (2005). *Medical-surgical nursing: Clinical management for positive outcomes* (7th ed.). Philadelphia: Saunders, p. 1269.

58. A home care nurse provides self-care instructions to a client with chronic venous insufficiency caused by deep vein thrombosis. Which statement by the client indicates a need for further instructions?

1 "I can cross the legs at the knee, but not the ankle."
2 "I need to elevate the foot of the bed during sleep."
3 "I need to avoid prolonged standing or sitting."
4 "I should continue to wear elastic hose for at least 6 to 8 weeks."

Answer: 1

Rationale: Clients with chronic venous insufficiency are advised to avoid crossing the legs, sitting in chairs where the feet don't touch the floor, and wearing garters or sources of pressure above the legs (such as girdles). The client should wear elastic hose for 6 to 8 weeks, and in some situations for life. The client should sleep with the foot of the bed elevated to promote venous return during sleep. Venous problems are characterized by insufficient drainage of blood from the legs returning to the heart. Thus, interventions need to be aimed at promoting flow of blood out of the legs and back to the heart.

Test-Taking Strategy: Note the key words "need for further instructions." These key words indicate a false-response question and that you need to select the incorrect client statement. Use the concept of gravity when answering questions that relate to peripheral vascular problems. Option 1 is the only action that does not promote venous drainage. Review home care instructions for the client with chronic venous insufficiency if you had difficulty with this question.

Level of Cognitive Ability: Analysis
Client Needs: Health Promotion and Maintenance
Integrated Process: Teaching/Learning
Content Area: Adult Health/Cardiovascular

References:
Black, J., & Hawks, J. (2005). *Medical-surgical nursing: Clinical management for positive outcomes* (7th ed.). Philadelphia: Saunders, p. 1540.
Lewis, S., Heitkemper, M., & Dirksen, S. (2004). *Medical-surgical nursing: Assessment and management of clinical problems* (6th ed.). St. Louis: Mosby, pp. 929; 934.

59. A nurse is providing home care instructions to a client who had varicose vein stripping and ligation and is being discharged from the ambulatory care unit. The nurse tells the client to:

1 Maintain bed rest for the first 3 days
2 Ambulate for 5 to 10 minutes twice a day beginning the day after surgery
3 Elevate the foot of the bed while in bed
4 Remove elastic hose after 24 hours

Answer: 3

Rationale: Standard postoperative care following vein ligation and stripping consists of bed rest for 24 hours, with ambulation for 5 to 10 minutes every 2 hours thereafter. Continuous elastic compression of the leg is maintained usually for one week following the procedure, followed by long-term use of elastic hose. The foot of the bed should be elevated to promote venous drainage.

Test-Taking Strategy: Use knowledge of the concepts related to blood flow and immobility to answer this question. Options 1 and 4 will promote venous stasis, so they are eliminated first. From the remaining options, noting the words "twice a day" in option 2 will eliminate this option. Review postoperative teaching points following varicose vein stripping and ligation if you had difficulty with this question.

Level of Cognitive Ability: Application
Client Needs: Health Promotion and Maintenance
Integrated Process: Teaching/Learning
Content Area: Adult Health/Cardiovascular

Reference:
Ignatavicius, D., & Workman, M. (2002). *Medical surgical nursing: Critical thinking for collaborative care* (4th ed.). Philadelphia: Saunders, p. 769.

60. A nurse is developing a teaching plan for the client with Raynaud's disease. The nurse plans to tell the client that the symptoms may improve with:

1 A high-protein diet, which will minimize tissue malnutrition
2 Vitamin K administration, which will prevent tendencies toward bleeding
3 Keeping the hands and feet warm and dry, which will prevent vasoconstriction
4 Daily cool baths, which will provide an analgesic effect

Answer: 3

Rationale: Use of measures to prevent vasoconstriction are helpful in managing Raynaud's disease. The hands and feet should be kept dry. Gloves and warm fabrics should be worn in cold weather, and the client should avoid exposure to nicotine and caffeine. Avoidance of situations that trigger stress is also helpful. Options 1, 2, and 4 are not components of the treatment for this disorder.

Test-Taking Strategy: Use the process of elimination. Recalling the pathophysiology of the disorder and the need to promote vasodilation will direct you to option 3. Review teaching points related to Raynaud's disease if you had difficulty with this question.

Level of Cognitive Ability: Application
Client Needs: Health Promotion and Maintenance
Integrated Process: Teaching/Learning
Content Area: Adult Health/Cardiovascular

Reference:
Ignatavicius, D., & Workman, M. (2002). *Medical surgical nursing: Critical thinking for collaborative care* (4th ed.). Philadelphia: Saunders, p. 762.

61. A client with peripheral arterial disease has received instructions from the nurse about how to limit progression of the disease. The nurse determines that the client needs further instructions if which statement was made by the client?

1 "I should walk daily to increase the circulation to my legs."
2 "A heating pad on my leg will help soothe the leg pain."
3 "I need to take special care of my feet to prevent injury."
4 "I need to eat a balanced diet."

Answer: 2

Rationale: Long-term management of peripheral arterial disease consists of measures that increase peripheral circulation (exercise), promote vasodilation (warmth), relieve pain, and maintain tissue integrity (foot care and nutrition). Application of heat directly to the extremity is contraindicated. The limb may have decreased sensitivity and be more at risk for burns. Additionally, direct application of heat raises oxygen and nutritional requirements of the tissue even further.

Test-Taking Strategy: Focus on the client's diagnosis and note the key words "needs further instructions." These key words indicate a false-response question and that you need to select the incorrect client statement. Noting the key word "heating" in option 2 will direct you to the correct option. Review the teaching points related to peripheral arterial disease if you had difficulty with this question.

Level of Cognitive Ability: Analysis
Client Needs: Health Promotion and Maintenance
Integrated Process: Teaching/Learning
Content Area: Adult Health/Cardiovascular

Reference:
Ignatavicius, D., & Workman, M. (2002). *Medical surgical nursing: Critical thinking for collaborative care* (4th ed.). Philadelphia: Saunders, p. 745; 750.

62. A nurse is teaching a client with hypertension about items that contain sodium and reviews a written list of items sent from the cardiac rehabilitation department. The nurse tells the client that which of the following items on the list is acceptable to use?
   1 Demineralized water
   2 Antacids
   3 Laxatives
   4 Toothpaste

Answer: 1
Rationale: Sodium intake can be increased by use of several types of products, including toothpaste and mouthwashes; over-the-counter (OTC) medications such as analgesics, antacids, cough remedies, laxatives, and sedatives; softened water, as well as some mineral waters. Water that is bottled, distilled, deionized, or demineralized may be used for drinking and cooking. Clients are advised to read labels for sodium content.

Test-Taking Strategy: Note the key words "acceptable to use" and focus on the issue: the item that is low in sodium. Noting the word "demineralized," which means having the minerals taken out of, will direct you to option 1. Review items that are low and high in sodium content if you had difficulty with this question.

Level of Cognitive Ability: Application
Client Needs: Health Promotion and Maintenance
Integrated Process: Teaching/Learning
Content Area: Adult Health/Cardiovascular

References:
Peckenpaugh, N. (2003). *Nutrition essentials and diet therapy* (9th ed.). Philadelphia: Saunders, pp. 156; 241-242.
Williams, S. (2001). *Basic nutrition & diet therapy* (11th ed.). St. Louis: Mosby, pp. 360-362.

63. A school nurse provides several teaching sessions to a group of high school students regarding the hazards of smoking. Which comment by a student indicates the need for further teaching?
   1 "Inhalation of tobacco smoke from active smoking, and passive smoke inhaled from other people smoking, are both public health issues."
   2 "Chewing tobacco is a safer method of tobacco use than is smoking the tobacco."
   3 "My health is at risk when my parents smoke."
   4 "Smoking during pregnancy increases the risk of stillbirth and miscarriages."

Answer: 2
Rationale: All forms of tobacco use are health hazards. Options 1, 3, and 4 are accurate regarding the health hazards of tobacco use.

Test-Taking Strategy: Note the key words "need for further teaching." These key words indicate a false-response question and that you need to select the incorrect student statement. This should direct you to option 2. Review the hazards of tobacco use if you had difficulty with this question.

Level of Cognitive Ability: Analysis
Client Needs: Health Promotion and Maintenance.
Integrated Process: Teaching/Learning
Content Area: Fundamental Skills

Reference:
Potter, P., & Perry, A. (2005). *Fundamentals of nursing* (6th ed.). St. Louis: Mosby, p. 212.

64. A nurse is developing goals for the postpartum client who is at risk for uterine infection. Which goal would be most appropriate for this client?

1 The client will verbalize a reduction of pain.

2 The client will no longer have a positive Homan's sign.

3 The client will report how to treat an infection.

4 The client will be able to identify measures to prevent infection.

Answer: 4

Rationale: The uterus is theoretically sterile during pregnancy until the membranes rupture. It is capable of being invaded by pathogens after membrane rupture. Options 1 and 2 are unrelated to the issue of infection. Option 3 indicates that an infection is present. Option 4 is a goal for the client "at risk" for infection.

Test-Taking Strategy: Focus on the key words "at risk for infection." Noting the word "prevent" in option 4 will direct you to this option. Option 3 implies that an infection has been diagnosed. Options 1 and 2 are unrelated to the issue of the question. Review the goals for a client at risk for infection if you had difficulty with this question.

Level of Cognitive Ability: Analysis
Client Needs: Health Promotion and Maintenance
Integrated Process: Nursing Process/Planning
Content Area: Maternity/Postpartum

Reference:
Lowdermilk, D., & Perry, A. (2004). *Maternity & women's health care* (8th ed.). St. Louis: Mosby, pp. 1046-1048.

---

65. A neonatal intensive care unit (NICU) nurse teaches handwashing techniques to the parents of an infant who is receiving antibiotic treatment for a neonatal infection. The nurse determines that the parents understand the purpose of handwashing if they state that this is primarily done to:

1 Reduce their fears

2 Minimize the spread of infection to other siblings

3 Reduce the possibility of transmitting an environmental infection to their infant

4 Allow them an opportunity to communicate with each other and staff

Answer: 3

Rationale: Appropriate handwashing by staff and parents has been effective in the prevention of nosocomial infections in nursery units. This action also promotes parents taking an active part in the care of their infant. Options 1 and 4 are not the primary reason to perform handwashing. Because the infant has the infection and is in the NICU, option 2 is incorrect.

Test-Taking Strategy: Note the key word "primarily" to assist in eliminating options 1 and 4. Noting that the infant is in the NICU will assist in eliminating option 2. Review the purposes of handwashing if you had difficulty with this question.

Level of Cognitive Ability: Analysis
Clients Needs: Health Promotion and Maintenance
Integrated Process: Teaching/Learning
Content Area: Maternity/Postpartum

Reference:
Lowdermilk, D., & Perry, A. (2004). *Maternity & women's health care* (8th ed.). St. Louis: Mosby, p. 46.

66. Following shoulder arthroplasty, a nurse monitors the client for brachial plexus compromise and is checking the status of the ulnar nerve. Which technique would the nurse use to assess the status of this nerve?

1   Have the client grasp the nurse's hand and note the strength of the client's first and second fingers
2   Ask the client to move the thumb toward the palm and back to the neutral position
3   Have the client spread all the fingers wide and resist pressure
4   Ask the client to raise the forearm above the head

Answer: 3

Rationale: To assess the ulnar nerve status, the client is asked to spread all of the fingers wide and resist pressure. Weakness against pressure may indicate compromise of the ulnar nerve. Option 1 describes assessment of the status of the medial nerve. Option 2 describes assessment of the status of the radial nerve. Option 4 assesses the flexion of the biceps and determines the status of the cutaneous nerve.

Test-Taking Strategy: Focus on the issue: the status of the ulnar nerve. Recalling the location and the function of this nerve will direct you to option 3. Review this assessment technique if you are unfamiliar with this procedure.

Level of Cognitive Ability: Application
Client Needs: Health Promotion and Maintenance
Integrated Process: Nursing Process/Assessment
Content Area: Adult Health/Musculoskeletal

Reference:
Black, J., & Hawks, J. (2005). *Medical-surgical nursing: Clinical management for positive outcomes* (7th ed.). Philadelphia: Saunders, pp. 1250-1251.

---

67. A hospitalized client with active pulmonary tuberculosis has been receiving multidrug therapy for the past month and is being prepared for discharge to home. The nurse determines that respiratory isolation is no longer required and that medication therapy has been effective when:

1   Nausea and vomiting has stopped
2   The Mantoux Test (PPD) is negative
3   Sputum cultures are negative
4   Stools are clay-colored

Answer: 3

Rationale: The primary diagnostic tool for pulmonary tuberculosis is a sputum culture. A negative culture indicates effectiveness of treatment. Nausea and vomiting and clay-colored stools are side effects of the medication used to treat tuberculosis. Their presence or absence does not measure the therapeutic effectiveness of the medication. The Mantoux test is a screening tool, not a diagnostic test for tuberculosis. Because the Mantoux test indicates exposure to the organism but not active disease, the test results will remain positive.

Test-Taking Strategy: Use the process of elimination, noting the key words "therapy has been effective." Remember that the absence of infectious organisms is a desired outcome in communicable diseases. The sputum is the only diagnostic test that will determine the absence of infectious organisms. Review the measures that present the spread of this communicable disease if you had difficulty with this question.

Level of Cognitive Ability: Analysis
Client Needs: Health Promotion and Maintenance
Integrated Process: Nursing Process/Evaluation
Content Area: Adult Health/Respiratory

Reference:
Ignatavicius, D., & Workman, M. (2002). *Medical surgical nursing: Critical thinking for collaborative care* (4th ed.). Philadelphia: Saunders, pp. 585; 587.

68. A nurse has conducted a class for pregnant clients with diabetes mellitus on signs and symptoms of potential complications. The nurse determines that the teaching was effective if a client made which of the following statements?

1 "I'm glad I don't have to worry about developing hypoglycemia while I am pregnant."

2 "I need to watch my weight for any sudden gains because I am prone to pregnancy-induced hypertension."

3 "My insulin needs should decrease in the last two months because I will be using some of the baby's insulin supply."

4 "I should not have ultrasounds done because I am diabetic."

Answer: 2

Rationale: Hypoglycemia is a problem during pregnancy and needs to be assessed. A diabetic pregnant client has a higher incidence of developing pregnancy-induced hypertension than the nondiabetic pregnant client. Insulin needs will increase during the last trimester because of increased placenta degradation. Ultrasounds are done frequently during a diabetic pregnancy to check for congenital anomalies and determine appropriate growth patterns.

Test-Taking Strategy: Use the process of elimination, focusing on the issue: a pregnant client with diabetes mellitus. Options 1 and 4 can be easily eliminated, recalling that hypoglycemia is a concern and that ultrasounds need to be done. From the remaining options, remember that insulin needs will increase during the last trimester of pregnancy. This will assist in eliminating option 3. Review the complications associated with diabetes and pregnancy if you had difficulty with this question.

Level of Cognitive Ability: Analysis
Client Needs: Health Promotion and Maintenance
Integrated Process: Nursing Process/Evaluation
Content Area: Maternity/Antepartum

Reference:
Lowdermilk, D., & Perry, A. (2004). *Maternity & women's health care* (8th ed.). St. Louis: Mosby, p. 887.

---

69. A postpartum client recovering from disseminated intravascular coagulopathy (DIC) is to be discharged on low dosages of an anticoagulant medication. The nurse provides home care instructions and tells the client to avoid which of the following?

1 All activities because bruising injuries can occur

2 Walking long distances and climbing stairs

3 Taking acetylsalicylic acid (aspirin)

4 Brushing her teeth

Answer: 3

Rationale: Aspirin can interact with the anticoagulant medication and increase clotting time beyond therapeutic ranges. Avoiding aspirin is a priority. Not *all activities* need to be avoided. Walking and climbing stairs are acceptable activities. The client does not need to avoid brushing the teeth; however, the client should be instructed to use a soft toothbrush.

Test-Taking Strategy: Note the key word "avoid" in the question. Recalling that bleeding is an adverse effect of anticoagulants will direct you to the correct option. Review teaching points related to anticoagulants if you had difficulty with this question.

Level of Cognitive Ability: Application
Client Needs: Health Promotion and Maintenance
Integrated Process: Teaching/Learning
Content Area: Pharmacology

Reference:
McKenry, L., & Salerno, E. (2003). *Mosby's pharmacology in nursing* (21st ed.). St. Louis: Mosby, p. 211.

70. A client with a diagnosis of depression admits that one reason for her depression is that too many demands drain her energy. The client also admits that one reason the situation is bad is because the word "no" is not part of her vocabulary when it comes to the requests and needs of others. After 7 days of hospitalization, another client asks for assistance in cleaning the unit immediately. The client with depression says, "No, I can't help you now. I am enjoying watching this movie." The nurse interprets this response as:
1 A shirking of responsibility
2 Withdrawal from peers
3 Increased control over decisions
4 Decreased cooperation with others

Answer: 3
Rationale: The client has been unable to refuse requests in the past. Saying "no" now indicates that the client is trying to meet her own needs. "No" is being said now without guilt and apology. During the treatment process, the client has learned how to meet her own needs, and this can help to maintain health upon discharge. Options 1, 2, and 4 are incorrect interpretations.

Test-Taking Strategy: Use the process of elimination. Focusing on the data in the question will direct you to option 3. Review measures that assist in increasing control in the client with depression if you had difficulty with this question.

Level of Cognitive Ability: Analysis
Client Needs: Health Promotion and Maintenance
Integrated Process: Nursing Process/Analysis
Content Area: Mental Health

Reference:
Keltner, N., Schwecke, L., & Bostrom, C. (2003). *Psychiatric nursing* (4th ed.). St. Louis: Mosby, pp. 354-355.

71. A client with depression who was admitted to the mental health unit approximately 7 days ago is preparing for discharge to home, and the nurse is evaluating the client's understanding of depression and coping strategies learned during hospitalization. The nurse determines that further teaching needs to occur if the client makes which of the following statements?
1 "This hospital experience and the therapy has been a positive experience in my life."
2 "I know I must continue to take my medications just as prescribed."
3 "I now know that I can't be all things to all people."
4 "I know that I probably won't have depression in the future."

Answer: 4
Rationale: Depression may be a recurring illness for some people. The client needs to understand the symptoms of depression and recognize when or if treatment needs to begin again. The other statements indicate that the client has learned some coping skills, such as setting limits, taking medications, and reframing an a potentially unpleasant experience into a more positive one.

Test-Taking Strategy: Note the key words "further teaching needs to occur." These key words indicate a false-response question and that you need to select the option that indicates a lack of client understanding about depression. Recalling that depression may reoccur will direct you to option 4. Review the characteristics of depression if you had difficulty with this question.

Level of Cognitive Ability: Analysis
Client Needs: Health Promotion and Maintenance
Integrated Process: Teaching/Learning
Content Area: Mental Health

References:
Keltner, N., Schwecke, L., & Bostrom, C. (2003). *Psychiatric nursing* (4th ed.). St. Louis: Mosby, p. 355.
Stuart, G., & Laraia, M. (2005). *Principles and practice of psychiatric nursing* (8th ed.). St. Louis: Mosby, p. 358.

72. A nurse demonstrates to a mother how to correctly take an axillary temperature to determine if the child has a fever. Which action by the mother would indicate a need for further teaching?

1 She selects a thermometer with a slender tip.
2 She holds the thermometer in the axilla for one minute.
3 She records the actual temperature reading and route.
4 She places the thermometer in the center of the axilla.

Answer: 2

Rationale: Taking an axillary temperature for at least 5 minutes is most accurate. Options 1, 3, and 4 are correct steps for taking axillary temperature.

Test-Taking Strategy: Note the key words "a need for further teaching." These key words indicate a false-response question and that you need to select the option that identifies an incorrect action by the mother. Visualizing the procedure and noting the words "one minute" in option 2 will direct you to this option. Review the procedure for obtaining an axillary temperature if you had difficulty with this question.

Level of Cognitive Ability: Analysis
Client Needs: Health Promotion and Maintenance
Integrated Process: Teaching/Learning
Content Area: Child Health

Reference:
Wong, D., & Hockenberry, M. (2003). *Wong's nursing care of infants and children* (7th ed.). St. Louis: Mosby, pp. 178; 180.

---

73. A school nurse is teaching an athletic coach how to prevent dehydration in athletes during football practice. Which action by the coach during football practice indicates that the teaching was ineffective?

1 Schedules fluid breaks every 30 minutes throughout practice
2 Weighs athletes before, during, and after football practice
3 Asks the athletes to take a salt tablet before football practice
4 Tells the athletes to drink 16 ounces of fluid per pound lost during practice

Answer: 3

Rationale: Salt tablets should not be taken because they can contribute to dehydration. Frequent fluid breaks should be taken to prevent dehydration. Early detection of decreased body weight alerts an individual to drink fluids before becoming dehydrated. Sixteen ounces of fluid should be consumed for every pound lost to prevent dehydration.

Test-Taking Strategy: Note the key words "teaching was ineffective." These key words indicate a false-response question and that you need to select the option that identifies an incorrect action by the coach. Recalling the principles of fluid and electrolyte balance and the causes of dehydration will direct you to option 3. Options 1, 2, and 4 are measures that prevent the occurrence of dehydration in athletes. Review these measures if you had difficulty with this question.

Level of Cognitive Ability: Analysis
Client Needs: Health Promotion and Maintenance
Integrated Process: Teaching/Learning
Content Area: Fundamental Skills

References:
Black, J., & Hawks, J. (2005). *Medical-surgical nursing: Clinical management for positive outcomes* (7th ed.). Philadelphia: Saunders, pp. 208-209.
Ignatavicius, D., & Workman, M. (2002). *Medical surgical nursing: Critical thinking for collaborative care* (4th ed.). Philadelphia: Saunders, p. 165.

74. A nurse instructs a hospitalized client in a low-fat diet. The client indicates understanding of this diet by choosing which of the following from the dietary menu?
1 Liver, potato salad, sherbet
2 Shrimp and bacon salad
3 Turkey breast, boiled rice, and angel food cake
4 Lean hamburger steak, macaroni and cheese

Answer: 3
Rationale: Major sources of fats include meats, salad dressings, eggs, butter, cheese, and bacon. Options 1, 2, and 4 contain high-fat foods.

Test-Taking Strategy: Use the process of elimination. Eliminate options 2 and 4 first because both a hamburger steak and bacon are high in fat. From the remaining options, look at the foods closely. Option 3 does not contain any high-fat foods. Potato salad (option 1) will contain mayonnaise, which is high in fat. Review those foods that contain fat if you had difficulty with this question.

Level of Cognitive Ability: Analysis
Client Needs: Health Promotion and Maintenance
Integrated Process: Nursing Process/Evaluation
Content Area: Fundamental Skills

Reference:
Peckenpaugh, N. (2003). *Nutrition essentials and diet therapy* (9th ed.). Philadelphia: Saunders, pp. 217; 234.

75. A nurse has provided discharge instructions regarding nitroglycerin therapy to the client with angina. Which statement by the client indicates an understanding of home use of the nitroglycerin?
1 "When I have chest pain, I should put a tablet under my tongue. If I have a burning sensation, I should call my doctor immediately."
2 "When I experience chest pain, I can continue what I'm doing. If it doesn't go away in 10 minutes, I should use a nitroglycerin tablet."
3 "When I have pain, I should lie down and place a tablet under my tongue. If unrelieved in 5 minutes, I should take another tablet."
4 "If I use a nitroglycerin, and the pain does not subside in 15 minutes, I should go to the hospital."

Answer: 3
Rationale: The client taking sublingual nitroglycerin should lie down upon taking the medication because lightheadedness and dizziness may occur as a result of postural hypotension. The client should use up to three tablets at 5-minute intervals before seeking medical attention. Options 1, 2, and 4 are incorrect regarding the use of nitroglycerin. A burning sensation is a common side effect of nitroglycerin. Nitroglycerin should be taken with the onset of anginal pain. The client should repeat nitroglycerin if relief is not obtained with the first or second dose.

Test-Taking Strategy: Use the process of elimination. Recalling that nitroglycerin may be taken at 5-minute intervals times three will direct you to option 3. Review client teaching related to nitroglycerin if you had difficulty with this question.

Level of Cognitive Ability: Analysis
Client Needs: Health Promotion and Maintenance
Integrated Process: Nursing Process/Evaluation
Content Area: Adult Health/Cardiovascular

References:
Hodgson, B., & Kizior, R. (2004). *Saunders nursing drug handbook 2004.* Philadelphia: Saunders, p. 735.
Lehne, R. (2004). *Pharmacology for nursing care* (5th ed.). Philadelphia: Saunders, p. 534.
McKenry, L., & Salerno, E. (2003). *Mosby's pharmacology in nursing* (21st ed.). St. Louis: Mosby, pp. 89-90.

76. A client has urinary calculi that are composed of uric acid, and the nurse teaches the client dietary measures to prevent further development of the calculi. The nurse determines that the client understands the dietary measures if the client states that it is necessary to avoid consuming:
  1 Milk
  2 Foods such as spinach, chocolate, and tea
  3 Foods such as fish with fine bones and organ meats
  4 Dairy products

Answer: 3
Rationale: With a uric acid stone, the client should limit intake of foods high in purines. Organ meats, sardines, herring, and other high-purine foods are eliminated from the diet. Foods with moderate levels of purines, such as red and white meats and some seafood, are also limited. Options 1, 2, and 4 are recommended dietary changes for calculi composed of calcium phosphate or calcium oxalate.

Test-Taking Strategy: Note the key words "uric acid." Remembering that organ meats are high in purines will direct you to the correct option. Also note that options 1, 2, and 4 are similar in that they are foods that are avoided if the client has calcium phosphate or calcium oxalate calculi. Review the foods to avoid with uric acid calculi if you had difficulty with this question.

Level of Cognitive Ability: Analysis
Client Needs: Health Promotion and Maintenance
Integrated Process: Nursing Process/Evaluation
Content Area: Adult Health/Renal

Reference:
Ignatavicius, D., & Workman, M. (2002). *Medical surgical nursing: Critical thinking for collaborative care* (4th ed.). Philadelphia: Saunders, p. 1637.

77. A nurse is teaching a mother with diabetes mellitus who delivered a large for gestational age (LGA) male infant about care of the infant. The nurse tells the mother that LGA infants appear to be more mature because of their large size, and in reality, these infants frequently need to be aroused to facilitate nutritional intake and attachment. Which statement by the mother indicates the need for additional information about care of the infant?
  1 "I will talk to my baby when he is in a quiet alert state."
  2 "I will watch my baby closely because I know he may not be as mature in motor development."
  3 "I will breast feed my baby every 2 1/2 to 3 hours and will use arousing techniques."
  4 "I will allow my baby to sleep through the night because he needs his rest."

Answer: 4
Rationale: LGA infants tend to be more difficult to arouse and therefore will need to be aroused to facilitate nutritional intake and attachment opportunities. These infants also have problems maintaining a quiet alert state. It is beneficial for the mother to interact with the infant during this time to enhance and lengthen the quiet alert state. Even though the infant is large, motor function is not usually as mature as in the term infant. LGA infants need to be aroused for feedings, usually every 2 1/2 to 3 hours for breast feeding.

Test-Taking Strategy: Note the key words "need for additional information." These key words indicate a false-response question and that you need to select the option that identifies an incorrect statement by the mother. Focusing on the words "frequently need to be aroused" in the question will direct you to option 4. Options 1, 2, and 3 address observation and arousal, whereas option 4 does not. Review care of the LGA infant if you had difficulty with this question.

Level of Cognitive Ability: Analysis
Client Needs: Health Promotion and Maintenance
Integrated Process: Teaching/Learning
Content Area: Maternity/Postpartum

Reference:
Murray, S., McKinney, E., & Gorrie, T. (2002). *Foundations of maternal-newborn nursing* (3rd ed.). Philadelphia: Saunders, p. 542.

78. A client has been experiencing muscle weakness over a period of several months. The physician suspects polymyositis, and the client asks the nurse about the disorder. The nurse tells the client that in this disorder:
1 Muscle fibers are thickened
2 There is a decrease in elastic tissue
3 Muscle fibers are inflamed
4 There are increased fibers and tissue

Answer: 3
Rationale: In polymyositis, necrosis and inflammation are seen in muscle fibers and myocardial fibers. Option 1 is an opposite of what is noted in this disorder. Option 2 is incorrect, however, decreased elastic tissue in the aorta would be noted in a condition known as Marfan's syndrome. Option 4 refers to increased fibrous tissue seen in ankylosis.

Test-Taking Strategy: Note the issue of the question: polymyositis. "Itis" indicates inflammation. The only option that addresses inflammation is option 3. Review the description of polymyositis if you had difficulty with this question.

Level of Cognitive Ability: Application
Client Needs: Health Promotion and Maintenance
Integrated Process: Nursing Process/Implementation
Content Area: Adult Health/Musculoskeletal

Reference:
Ignatavicius, D., & Workman, M. (2002). *Medical surgical nursing: Critical thinking for collaborative care* (4th ed.). Philadelphia: Saunders, p. 359.

---

79. A client has two chest tubes inserted into the right pleural space following thoracic surgery, which are attached to Pleur-Evac drainage systems. To promote optimal respiratory functioning, the nurse plans to:
1 Milk and strip the chest tubes once a shift
2 Maintain the client on bed rest until the chest tubes are removed
3 Position the client only on the back and on the right side
4 Encourage the client to cough and deep breathe every hour

Answer: 4
Rationale: The client who has chest tubes following thoracic surgery should be encouraged to cough and deep breathe every 1 to 2 hours after surgery. This helps facilitate drainage of fluid from the pleural space, as well as facilitate the clearance of secretions from the respiratory tract. Milking and stripping of the chest tube may be done when there is an occlusion, such as with a small clot. Even then, it is done only with a physician's order or when allowed by agency policy. The client is maintained in semi-Fowler's position and may lie on the back or on the nonoperative side. The client may be allowed to lie on the operative side according to surgeon preference, but care must be taken not to compress the chest tube or attached drainage tubing. Ambulation is generally allowed and also facilitates optimal respiratory function.

Test-Taking Strategy: Focus on the issue: to promote optimal respiratory functioning. Option 1 is eliminated first because milking and stripping a chest tube is done only with a physician's order or when allowed by agency policy. Bed rest (option 2) does not promote respiratory function and is eliminated next. From the remaining options, recalling that positioning is done according to surgeon preference directs you to option 4. Review the measures that promote optimal respiratory function in the client with a chest tube if you had difficulty with this question.

Level of Cognitive Ability: Application
Client Needs: Health Promotion and Maintenance
Integrated Process: Nursing Process/Planning
Content Area: Adult Health/Respiratory

Reference:
Black, J., & Hawks, J. (2005). *Medical-surgical nursing: Clinical management for positive outcomes* (7th ed.). Philadelphia: Saunders, pp. 1857-1859.

80. A nurse in an ambulatory clinic administers a Mantoux skin test to a client on a Monday. The nurse plans to have the client return to the clinic to have the results read on:
1 Tuesday or Wednesday
2 Wednesday or Thursday
3 Thursday or Friday
4 The following Monday

Answer: 2
Rationale: The Mantoux skin test for tuberculosis is read in 48 to 72 hours. The client should return to the clinic on Wednesday or Thursday.

Test-Taking Strategy: Use the process of elimination. Recalling that this test is read within 48 to 72 hours will direct you to option 2. Review the procedure for this test if you had difficulty with this question.

Level of Cognitive Ability: Application
Client Needs: Health Promotion and Maintenance
Integrated Process: Nursing Process/Planning
Content Area: Adult Health/Respiratory

Reference:
Chernecky, C., & Berger, B. (2004). *Laboratory tests and diagnostic procedures* (4th ed.). Philadelphia: Saunders, p. 766.

---

81. A client with chronic airflow limitation (CAL) is admitted to the hospital with exacerbation and has a nursing diagnosis of Ineffective Airway Clearance. The nurse assesses the client to determine the extent that which of the following prehospitalization factors could have contributed most to this nursing diagnosis?
1 Anxiety level
2 Amount of sleep
3 Fat intake
4 Fluid intake

Answer: 4
Rationale: The client with Ineffective Airway Clearance has ineffective coughing and excess sputum in the airways. The nurse assesses for knowledge of contributing factors, such as dehydration and lack of knowledge of proper coughing techniques. Reduction of these factors helps limit exacerbations of the disease. Options 1, 2, and 3 are not directly associated with this nursing diagnosis.

Test-Taking Strategy: Note the nursing diagnosis: Ineffective Airway Clearance. This calls to mind the concept of sputum production and clearance. Evaluate each of the options in terms of their potential ability to inhibit sputum production or clearance. The fluid intake is the only factor that could affect the viscosity of secretions, thus affecting airway clearance. Review the defining characteristics of Ineffective Airway Clearance if you had difficulty with this question.

Level of Cognitive Ability: Analysis
Client Needs: Health Promotion and Maintenance
Integrated Process: Nursing Process/Assessment
Content Area: Adult Health/Respiratory

Reference:
Gulanick, M., Myers, J., Klopp, A., Gradishar, D., Galanes, S., & Puzas, M. (2003). *Nursing care plans: Nursing diagnosis and intervention* (5th ed.). St. Louis: Mosby, pp. 10-11.

82. A client with acquired immunodeficiency syndrome (AIDS) gets recurrent *Candida* infections (thrush) of the mouth. The nurse has given instructions to the client to minimize the occurrence of thrush and determines that the client understands the instructions if which statement is made by the client?

1 "I should brush my teeth and rinse my mouth once a day."
2 "I should use a strong mouthwash at least once a week."
3 "Increasing red meat in my diet will keep this from recurring."
4 "I should use warm saline or water to rinse my mouth."

Answer: 4

Rationale: When a client is in a state of immunosuppression or has decreased levels of some normal oral flora, an overgrowth of the normal flora *Candida* can occur. Careful routine mouth care is helpful in preventing recurrence of *Candida* infections. The client should use a mouthwash consisting of warm saline (or water). Red meat will not prevent thrush. The timeframes for oral hygiene in options 1 and 2 are too infrequent.

Test-Taking Strategy: Use the process of elimination. Eliminate options 1 and 2 because they are similar and the timeframes are too infrequent. From the remaining options, recalling that red meat is not likely to minimize the occurrence of thrush will direct you to option 4. Review teaching points related to the prevention of *Candida* infections if you had difficulty with this question.

Level of Cognitive Ability: Analysis
Client Needs: Health Promotion and Maintenance
Integrated Process: Nursing Process/Evaluation
Content Area: Adult Health/Immune

Reference:
Black, J., & Hawks, J. (2005). *Medical-surgical nursing: Clinical management for positive outcomes* (7th ed.). Philadelphia: Saunders, p. 2391.

83. A nurse is teaching a client with acquired immunodeficiency syndrome (AIDS) how to avoid food-borne illnesses. The nurse instructs the client to prevent acquiring infection from food by avoiding which of the following items?

1 Raw oysters
2 Pasteurized milk
3 Products with sorbitol
4 Bottled water

Answer: 1

Rationale: The client is taught to avoid raw or undercooked seafood, meat, poultry, and eggs. The client should also avoid unpasteurized milk and dairy products. Fruits that can be peeled are safe, as are bottled beverages. The client may be taught to avoid sorbitol, but this is to diminish diarrhea and has nothing to do with food-borne infections.

Test-Taking Strategy: Use the process of elimination focusing on the issue, food-borne illness. Sorbitol can cause diarrhea but is unrelated to food-borne illness, so option 3 is eliminated first. Eliminate option 2 next because products that are pasteurized are free of microbes. From the remaining options, noting the key word "raw" in option 1 will direct you to this option. Review dietary teaching for the client with AIDS if you had difficulty with this question.

Level of Cognitive Ability: Application
Client Needs: Health Promotion and Maintenance
Integrated Process: Teaching/Learning
Content Area: Adult Health/Immune

Reference:
Black, J., & Hawks, J. (2005). *Medical-surgical nursing: Clinical management for positive outcomes* (7th ed.). Philadelphia: Saunders, p. 2396.

84. A client with histoplasmosis has an order for ketoconazole (Nizoral). The nurse teaches the client to do which of the following while taking this medication?
1 Take the medication on an empty stomach
2 Take the medication with an antacid
3 Avoid exposure to sunlight
4 Limit alcohol to 2 ounces per day

Answer: 3
Rationale: The client should be taught that ketoconazole is an antifungal medication. It should be taken with food or milk. Antacids should be avoided for 2 hours after it is taken because gastric acid is needed to activate the medication. The client should avoid concurrent use of alcohol, because the medication is hepatotoxic. The client should also avoid exposure to sunlight, because the medication increases photosensitivity.

Test-Taking Strategy: Use the process of elimination and general guidelines related to medication administration to eliminate options 2 and 4. From the remaining options, it is necessary to know that the medication causes photosensitivity reaction and should be taken with food or milk. Review this medication if you had difficulty with this question.

Level of Cognitive Ability: Application
Client Needs: Health Promotion and Maintenance
Integrated Process: Teaching/Learning
Content Area: Pharmacology

Reference:
McKenry, L., & Salerno, E. (2003). *Mosby's pharmacology in nursing* (21st ed.). St. Louis: Mosby, p. 1018.

85. A nurse is planning to teach a teenage client about sexuality. The nurse would begin the instruction by:
1 Establishing a relationship and determining prior knowledge
2 Providing written information about sexually transmitted diseases
3 Informing the teenager of the dangers of pregnancy
4 Advising the teenager to maintain sexual abstinence until marriage

Answer: 1
Rationale: The first step in effective communication is establishing a relationship. By exploring the client's interest and prior knowledge, rapport is established and learning needs are assessed. The other options may or may not be later steps depending on the data obtained.

Test-Taking Strategy: Use the steps of the nursing process and select an assessment option. This will direct you to option 1. When teaching, assessing motivation, interest, and level of knowledge is done before providing information. Review the principles of teaching and learning if you had difficulty with this question.

Level of Cognitive Ability: Application
Client Needs: Health Promotion and Maintenance
Integrated Process: Teaching/Learning
Content Area: Child Health

Reference:
Wong, D., & Hockenberry, M. (2003). *Wong's nursing care of infants and children* (7th ed.). St. Louis: Mosby, pp. 710;815.

86. A nurse provides home care instructions to a client with Cushing's syndrome. The nurse determines that the client understands the hospital discharge instructions if the client makes which statement?
  1 "I need to eat foods low in potassium."
  2 "I need to take aspirin rather than Tylenol for a headache."
  3 "I need to check the color of my stools."
  4 "I need to check the temperature of my legs twice a day."

Answer: 3
Rationale: Cushing's syndrome results in an increased secretion of cortisol. Cortisol stimulates the secretion of gastric acid, and this can result in the development of peptic ulcers and gastrointestinal bleeding. The client should be encouraged to eat potassium-rich foods to correct hypokalemia that occurs in this disorder. Aspirin can increase the risk for gastric bleeding and skin bruising. Cushing's syndrome does not affect temperature changes in lower extremities.

Test-Taking Strategy: Note the key words "understands the hospital discharge instructions." Recalling the pathophysiology in this disorder and that cortisol stimulates the secretion of gastric acid will direct you to option 3. Review Cushing's syndrome if you had difficulty with this question.

Level of Cognitive Ability: Analysis
Client Needs: Health Promotion and Maintenance
Integrated Process: Nursing Process/Evaluation
Content Area: Adult Health/Endocrine

References:
Black, J., & Hawks, J. (2005). *Medical-surgical nursing: Clinical management for positive outcomes* (7th ed.). Philadelphia: Saunders, p. 1156.
Ignatavicius, D., & Workman, M. (2002). *Medical surgical nursing: Critical thinking for collaborative care* (4th ed.). Philadelphia: Saunders, p. 1419.

---

87. A client with congestive heart failure and secondary hyperaldosteronism is started on spironolactone (Aldactone) to manage this disorder. The nurse anticipates the need for dosage adjustment of which of the following medications, if it is also being taken by the client?
  1 Warfarin sodium (Coumadin)
  2 Alprazolam (Xanax)
  3 Verapamil hydrochloride (Calan)
  4 Potassium chloride

Answer: 4
Rationale: Spironolactone (Aldactone) is a potassium-sparing diuretic. If the client was taking potassium chloride or another potassium supplement, the risk for hyperkalemia exists. Potassium doses would need to be adjusted while on this medication. A dosage adjustment would not be necessary if the client was taking the medications identified in options 1, 2, or 3.

Test-Taking Strategy: Focus on the issue: a dosage adjustment. Recalling that spironolactone is a potassium-sparing diuretic will direct you to option 4. Review potassium-sparing diuretics if you had difficulty with this question.

Level of Cognitive Ability: Analysis
Client Needs: Health Promotion and Maintenance
Integrated Process: Nursing Process/Analysis
Content Area: Adult Health/Cardiovascular

References:
Hodgson, B., & Kizior, R. (2004). *Saunders nursing drug handbook 2004.* Philadelphia: Saunders, p. 931.
Ignatavicius, D., & Workman, M. (2002). *Medical surgical nursing: Critical thinking for collaborative care* (4th ed.). Philadelphia: Saunders, p. 739.

88. A nurse is teaching health education classes to a group of expectant parents, and the topic is preventing mental retardation caused by congenital hypothyroidism. The nurse tells the parents that the most effective means of preventing this disorder is by:

1 Adequate protein intake
2 Limiting alcohol consumption
3 Vitamin intake
4 Neonatal screening

Answer: 4

Rationale: Congenital hypothyroidism is the most common preventable cause of mental retardation. Neonatal screening is the only means of early diagnosis and subsequent prevention of mental retardation. Newborn infants are screened for congenital hypothyroidism before discharge from the nursery and before 7 days of life. Treatment is begun immediately if necessary. Adequate protein and vitamin intake will not specifically prevent this disorder. Alcohol consumption during pregnancy needs to be restricted, not limited.

Test-Taking Strategy: Focus on the issue: preventing mental retardation caused by congenital hypothyroidism. Options 1, 2, and 3 are measures to prevent all birth defects. Also note that neonatal screening is the umbrella (global) option. Review congenital hypothyroidism and its complications if you had difficulty with this question.

Level of Cognitive Ability: Application
Client Needs: Health Promotion and Maintenance
Integrated Process: Teaching/Learning
Content Area: Maternity/Antepartum

Reference:
Lowdermilk, D., & Perry, A. (2004). *Maternity & women's health care* (8th ed.). St. Louis: Mosby, p. 902.

89. A nurse in an outpatient diabetes clinic is monitoring a client with type 1 diabetes mellitus. Today's blood work reveals a glycosylated hemoglobin (HbA1c) of 10%. The nurse interprets this blood work as indicating which of the following?

1 A normal value indicating that the client is managing blood glucose control well
2 A low value indicating that the client is not managing blood glucose control very well
3 A high value indicating that the client is not managing blood glucose control very well
4 The value does not offer information regarding client management of their disease

Answer: 3

Rationale: Glycosylated hemoglobin is a measure of glucose control during the past 6 to 8 weeks before the test. It is a reliable measure to determine the degree of glucose control in diabetic clients over a period of time and is not influenced by good glucose or dietary management a day or two before the test is done. The HbA1c should be 7.5% or less, with elevated levels indicating poor glucose control.

Test-Taking Strategy: Specific knowledge regarding the normal values for this test will direct you to option 3. Review this test if you had difficulty with this question.

Level of Cognitive Ability: Analysis
Client Needs: Health Promotion and Maintenance
Integrated Process: Nursing Process/Analysis
Content Area: Adult Health/Endocrine

Reference:
Chernecky, C., & Berger, B. (2004). *Laboratory tests and diagnostic procedures* (4th ed.). Philadelphia: Saunders, p. 615.

90. A nurse is instructing a client with type 1 diabetes mellitus about management of hypoglycemic reactions. The nurse instructs the client that hypoglycemia most likely occurs during what time interval after insulin administration?
  1 Onset
  2 Peak
  3 Duration
  4 Anytime

Answer: 2
Rationale: Insulin reactions are most likely to occur during the peak time of the insulin, when the medication is at its maximum action. Peak action depends on type of insulin, amount administered, injection site, and other factors.

Test-Taking Strategy: Remember that insulin is a hypoglycemic agent. The word "peak" means the "highest point." Remembering this should assist in directing you to the correct option. Review the occurrence of hypoglycemia when a client is taking insulin if you had difficulty with this question.

Level of Cognitive Ability: Application
Client Needs: Health Promotion and Maintenance
Integrated Process: Teaching/Learning
Content Area: Adult Health/Endocrine

Reference:
Phipps, W., Monahan, F., Sands, J., Marek, J., & Neighbors, M. (2003). *Medical-surgical nursing: Health and illness perspectives* (7th ed.). St. Louis: Mosby, pp. 946-947.

91. A nurse is caring for a client who is scheduled to have a thyroidectomy and provides instructions to the client about the surgical procedure. Which statement by the client would indicate an understanding of the nurse's instructions?
  1 "I will definitely have to continue taking antithyroid medications after this surgery."
  2 "I need to place my hands behind my neck when I have to cough or change positions."
  3 "I need to turn my head and neck front, back, and side to side every hour for the first 12 hours after surgery."
  4 "I expect to experience some tingling of my toes, fingers, and lips after surgery."

Answer: 2
Rationale: The client is taught that tension needs to be avoided on the suture line; otherwise, hemorrhage may develop. One way of reducing incisional tension is to teach the client how to support the neck when coughing or being repositioned. Likewise, during the postoperative period, the client should avoid any unnecessary movement of the neck. That is why sandbags and pillows are frequently used to support the head and neck. Removal of the thyroid does not mean that the client will be taking antithyroid medications postoperatively. If a client experiences tingling in the fingers, toes, and lips, it is probably a result of injury to the parathyroid gland during surgery resulting in hypocalcemia. These signs and symptoms need to be reported immediately.

Test-Taking Strategy: Use the process of elimination. Focusing on the type of surgery and the anatomical location of the surgical procedure will assist in eliminating options 1, 3, and 4. Review postoperative care following thyroidectomy if you had difficulty with this question.

Level of Cognitive Ability: Analysis
Client Needs: Health Promotion and Maintenance
Integrated Process: Nursing Process/Evaluation
Content Area: Adult Health/Endocrine

Reference:
Ignatavicius, D., & Workman, M. (2002). *Medical surgical nursing: Critical thinking for collaborative care* (4th ed.). Philadelphia: Saunders, p. 1429.

92. A nurse has been preparing a client with chronic obstructive pulmonary disease (COPD) for discharge to home. Which statement by the client indicates a need for further teaching in relation to nutrition?
1 "I will certainly try to drink 3 liters of fluid every day."
2 "It's best to eat three large meals a day so I will get all my nutrients."
3 "I will not eat as much cabbage as I once did."
4 "I will rest a few minutes before I eat."

Answer: 2
Rationale: Adequate fluid intake helps liquefy pulmonary secretions. Large meals distend the abdomen and elevate the diaphragm, which may interfere with breathing. Gas-forming foods may cause bloating, which interferes with normal diaphragmatic breathing. Resting before eating may decrease the fatigue that is often associated with COPD.

Test-Taking Strategy: Use the process of elimination, noting the key words "need for further teaching." These key words indicate a false-response question and that you need to select the option that identifies an incorrect client statement. Focusing on the client's diagnosis and recalling the activities that produce dyspnea will direct you to option 2. Review nutrition and the client with a chronic respiratory disorder if you had difficulty with this question.

Level of Cognitive Ability: Analysis
Client Needs: Health Promotion and Maintenance
Integrated Process: Teaching/Learning
Content Area: Adult Health/Respiratory

Reference:
Ignatavicius, D., & Workman, M. (2002). *Medical surgical nursing: Critical thinking for collaborative care* (4th ed.). Philadelphia: Saunders, p. 550.

---

93. A nurse is preparing a client with pneumonia for discharge to home. Which statement by the client would alert the nurse to the fact that the client is in need of further discharge teaching?
1 "I will take all of my antibiotics even if I do feel 100% better."
2 "I understand that it may be weeks before my usual sense of well-being returns."
3 "It is a good idea for me to take a nap every afternoon for the next couple of weeks."
4 "You can toss out that incentive spirometer as soon as I leave for home."

Answer: 4
Rationale: Deep breathing and coughing exercises and use of incentive spirometry should be practiced for 6 to 8 weeks after the client is discharged from the hospital in order to keep the alveoli expanded and promote the removal of lung secretions. If the entire regimen of antibiotics is not taken, the client may suffer a relapse. Adequate rest is needed to maintain progress toward recovery. The period of convalescence with pneumonia is often lengthy, and it may be weeks before the client feels a sense of well being.

Test-Taking Strategy: Note the key words "in need of further discharge teaching." These key words indicate a false-response question and that you need to select the option that identifies an incorrect client statement. Focusing on the client's diagnosis and recalling the need to promote removal of lung secretions will direct you to option 4. Review teaching points for the client with pneumonia if you had difficulty with this question.

Level of Cognitive Ability: Analysis
Client Needs: Health Promotion and Maintenance
Integrated Process: Teaching/Learning
Content Area: Adult Health/Respiratory

References:
Ignatavicius, D., & Workman, M. (2002). *Medical surgical nursing: Critical thinking for collaborative care* (4th ed.). Philadelphia: Saunders, p. 581.
Lewis, S., Heitkemper, M., & Dirksen, S. (2004). *Medical-surgical nursing: Assessment and management of clinical problems* (6th ed.). St. Louis: Mosby, p. 599.

94. A community health nurse provides an educational session to members of the local community regarding breast self-examination (BSE). Which statement by a member indicates a need for further education?

1 "I should perform BSE when I have my period."
2 "It is easiest to perform BSE when I am in the shower when my hands are soapy."
3 "I need to perform BSE every month."
4 "I'll use the finger pads of my three middle fingers to feel for lumps and thickening."

Answer: 1

Rationale: The best time to perform BSE is after (not during) the monthly period, when the breasts are not tender and swollen. Options 2, 3 and 4 identify accurate information regarding this self-examination.

Test-Taking Strategy: Note the key words "need for further education." These key words indicate a false-response question and that you need to select the option that identifies an incorrect member statement. Focusing on the issue, BSE, and visualizing this procedure will direct you to option 1. Review this procedure if you had difficulty with this question.

Level of Cognitive Ability: Analysis
Client Needs: Health Promotion and Maintenance
Integrated Process: Teaching/Learning
Content Area: Adult Health/Oncology

Reference:
Potter, P., & Perry, A. (2005). *Fundamentals of nursing* (6th ed.). St. Louis: Mosby, pp. 736-737.

---

95. A nurse makes a home care visit to a client with Bell's palsy. Which statement by the client requires clarification by the nurse?

1 "I have been gently massaging my face."
2 "I wear dark glasses when I go out."
3 "I wear an eye patch at night."
4 "I am staying on a liquid diet."

Answer: 4

Rationale: It is not necessary for a client with Bell's palsy to stay on a liquid diet. The client should be encouraged to chew on the unaffected side. Options 1, 2, and 3 identify accurate statements related to managing Bell's palsy.

Test-Taking Strategy: Note the key words "requires clarification by the nurse." These key words indicate a false-response question and that you need to select the option that identifies an incorrect client statement. Recalling that Bell's palsy relates to the face will assist in eliminating options 1, 2, and 3. Review interventions associated with this disorder if you had difficulty with this question.

Level of Cognitive Ability: Analysis
Client Needs: Health Promotion and Maintenance
Integrated Process: Nursing Process/Evaluation
Content Area: Adult Health/Neurological

References:
Black, J., & Hawks, J. (2005). *Medical-surgical nursing: Clinical management for positive outcomes* (7th ed.). Philadelphia: Saunders, p. 2154.
Lewis, S., Heitkemper, M., & Dirksen, S. (2004). *Medical-surgical nursing: Assessment and management of clinical problems* (6th ed.). St. Louis: Mosby, p. 1606.

96. A home care nurse is evaluating a client's understanding of self-management of trigeminal neuralgia. Which client statement indicates that teaching is necessary?
1 "An analgesic will help relieve my pain."
2 "I should chew on my good side."
3 "I should use warm mouthwash for oral hygiene."
4 "Taking my carbamazepine (Tegretol) will help control my pain."

Answer: 1
Rationale: Chronic irritation of the fifth cranial nerve results in trigeminal neuralgia and is characterized by intermittent episodes of intense pain of sudden onset on the affected side of the face. The pain is rarely relieved by analgesics. It is recommended that clients chew on the unaffected side and use warm mouthwash for oral hygiene. Medications such as carbamazepine (Tegretol) help control the pain of trigeminal neuralgia.

Test-Taking Strategy: Use the process of elimination, noting the key words "indicates that teaching is necessary." These key words indicate a false-response question and that you need to select the option that identifies an incorrect client statement. Recalling that trigeminal neuralgia is characterized by intense pain will direct you to option 1. Review this disorder if you had difficulty with this question.

Level of Cognitive Ability: Analysis
Client Needs: Health Promotion and Maintenance
Integrated Process: Teaching/Learning
Content Area: Adult Health/Neurological

Reference:
Black, J., & Hawks, J. (2005). *Medical-surgical nursing: Clinical management for positive outcomes* (7th ed.). Philadelphia: Saunders, pp. 2153-2154

97. A nurse is caring for a client with type 1 diabetes mellitus. Because the client is at risk for hypoglycemia, the nurse teaches the client to:
1 Omit the evening dose of NPH insulin if the client is exercising
2 Monitor the urine for acetone
3 Assess for signs of drowsiness and coma
4 Keep glucose tablets and subcutaneous glucagon available

Answer: 4
Rationale: Glucose tablets are taken if a hypoglycemic reaction occurs. Glucagon is administered subcutaneously or intramuscularly if the client loses consciousness and is unable to take glucose by mouth. Glucagon releases glycogen stores and raises blood glucose levels in hypoglycemia. Family members can be taught to administer this medication and possibly prevent an emergency room visit. The nurse would not instruct a client to omit insulin. Acetone in the urine may indicate hyperglycemia. Although signs of hypoglycemia need to be taught to the client, drowsiness and coma are not the initial and key signs of this complication.

Test-Taking Strategy: Use the process of elimination. Eliminate option 1 first because the nurse would not instruct a client to omit insulin doses. Options 2 and 3 can be eliminated next because they are not related to the issue of hypoglycemia. Review the signs of hypoglycemia and the appropriate interventions if you had difficulty with this question.

Level of Cognitive Ability: Application
Client Needs: Health Promotion and Maintenance
Integrated Process: Teaching/Learning
Content Area: Adult Health/Endocrine

Reference:
Hodgson, B., & Kizior, R. (2004). *Saunders nursing drug handbook 2004.* Philadelphia: Saunders, p. 477.

98. A nurse is caring for a client with a precipitate labor. The nurse tells the client that in this type of labor:
1 The labor will last less than 3 hours
2 A lengthy period of pushing may be necessary
3 The onset of contractions is gradual
4 Induction may be necessary

Answer: 1
Rationale: Precipitate labor is defined as that which lasts 3 or fewer hours for the entire labor and delivery. It usually has an abrupt, not a gradual onset. Induction, particularly with an oxytocic agent, is contraindicated because of the enhanced stimulatory effects on the uterine muscle and an increased risk for fetal hypoxia.

Test-Taking Strategy: Use the process of elimination. The word "precipitate" should assist in defining this condition. Note the relationship between this word and "less than 3 hours" in option 1. Review information related to precipitate labor if you had difficulty answering this question.

Level of Cognitive Ability: Application
Client Needs: Health Promotion and Maintenance
Integrated Process: Nursing Process/Implementation
Content Area: Maternity/Intrapartum

Reference:
Lowdermilk, D., & Perry, A. (2004). *Maternity & women's health care* (8th ed.). St. Louis: Mosby, p. 1003.

---

99. A nurse is instructing a pregnant client on measures to prevent a recurrent episode of preterm labor. Which statement by the client indicates a need for further teaching?
1 "I will report any feeling of pelvic pressure."
2 "I will adhere to the limitations in activity and stay off my feet."
3 "I will avoid sexual intercourse at this time."
4 "I will limit my fluid intake to three 8-ounce glasses of fluid a day."

Answer: 4
Rationale: Risks for preterm labor include dehydration. A client should not restrict fluids (except for those containing alcohol and caffeine). A sign of preterm labor may be pelvic pressure, without the perception of a contraction. A decrease in activity and bed rest is often prescribed in an attempt to decrease pressure on the cervix and increase uterine blood flow. Mechanical stimulation of the cervix during intercourse can stimulate contractions.

Test-Taking Strategy: Note the key words "need for further teaching." These key words indicate a false-response question and that you need to select the option that identifies an incorrect client statement. Focusing on the issue, preventing preterm labor, will direct you to option 4. Remember, generally it is not a good practice for the client to limit fluid intake to three 8-ounce glasses of fluid a day. Review this content if you had difficulty answering the question.

Level of Cognitive Ability: Analysis
Client Needs: Health Promotion and Maintenance
Integrated Process: Teaching/Learning
Content Area: Maternity/Antepartum

Reference:
Lowdermilk, D., & Perry, A. (2004). *Maternity & women's health care* (8th ed.). St. Louis: Mosby, p. 436.

100. A nurse has completed discharge teaching with the parents of a child with glomerulonephritis. Which statement by the parents indicates that further teaching is necessary?

1 "We'll check our child's blood pressure every day."

2 "We'll be sure that our child eats a lot of vegetables and does not add extra salt to food."

3 "It'll be so good to have my child back in tap dancing classes next week."

4 "We'll test our child's urine for albumin every week."

Answer: 3

Rationale: After discharge, parents should allow the child to return to his or her normal routine and activities, with adequate periods allowed for rest. Tap dancing classes one week after discharge would be a too rapid increase in activity and unrealistic. Options 1, 2, and 4 are correct home care measures.

Test-Taking Strategy: Use the process of elimination, noting the key words "further teaching is necessary." These key words indicate a false-response question and that you need to select the option that identifies an incorrect statement by the parents. Select option 3 because tap dancing is an aggressive exercise. Review home care measures for glomerulonephritis if you had difficulty with this question.

Level of Cognitive Ability: Analysis
Client Needs: Health Promotion and Maintenance
Integrated Process: Teaching/Learning
Content Area: Child Health

Reference:
Wong, D., & Hockenberry, M. (2003). *Wong's nursing care of infants and children* (7th ed.). St. Louis: Mosby, p. 1274.

---

101. A nurse is planning discharge teaching for parents of a child who had sustained a head injury and is now on tapering doses of dexamethasone sodium phosphate (Decadron). The nurse plans to make which statement to the parents?

1 "This medication decreases chances of infections."

2 "This medication will be discontinued after two doses."

3 "If your child's face becomes puffy, the medication dose needs to be increased."

4 "This medication is tapered to decrease the chance of recurring swelling in the brain."

Answer: 4

Rationale: Rebounding of cerebral edema is a side effect of dexamethasone sodium phosphate (Decadron) withdrawal if done abruptly. Dexamethasone sodium phosphate decreases inflammation not infection. Facial edema is a common side effect that disappears when the medication is discontinued.

Test-Taking Strategy: Focus on the name of the medication and recall that it is a corticosteroid. Remember that tapering is required with corticosteroids to prevent a rebound effect as a result of adrenal insufficiency. Review this medication if you had difficulty with this question.

Level of Cognitive Ability: Application
Client Needs: Health Promotion and Maintenance
Integrated Process: Teaching/Learning
Content Area: Pharmacology

Reference:
McKenry, L., & Salerno, E. (2003). *Mosby's pharmacology in nursing* (21st ed.). St. Louis: Mosby, p. 959.

102. A nurse has implemented a plan of care for a client with a C-5 spinal cord injury to promote health maintenance. Which client outcome would indicate effectiveness of the interventions?
1 Regains bladder and bowel control
2 Performs activities of daily living independently
3 Maintains intact skin
4 Independently transfers self to and from the wheelchair

Answer: 3

Rationale: A client with a C-5 spinal cord injury results in quadriplegia with no sensation below the clavicle, including most of the arms and hands. The client maintains partial movement of the shoulders and elbows. Maintaining intact skin is an outcome for spinal cord injury clients. The remaining options are inappropriate for this client.

Test-Taking Strategy: Focus on the key words "C-5 spinal cord injury." Eliminate options 2 and 4 first because they are similar. From the remaining options, recalling the effects of a C-5 spinal cord injury will assist in eliminating option 1 because it is unrealistic. If you are unfamiliar with this type of injury, review this content.

Level of Cognitive Ability: Analysis
Client Needs: Health Promotion and Maintenance
Integrated Process: Nursing Process/Evaluation
Content Area: Adult Health/Neurological

Reference:
Ignatavicius, D., & Workman, M. (2002). *Medical surgical nursing: Critical thinking for collaborative care* (4th ed.). Philadelphia: Saunders, p. 939.

103. A home care nurse visits a child who is being treated with penicillin G potassium (Pfizerpen) for scarlet fever. The mother tells the nurse that the child has only voided a small amount of tea-colored urine since the previous day. The mother also reports that the child's appetite has decreased and the child's face was swollen this morning. The nurse interprets that these new symptoms are:
1 Signs of the normal progression of scarlet fever
2 Nothing to be concerned about
3 The symptoms of acute glomerulonephritis
4 Symptoms of an allergic reaction to penicillin

Answer: 3

Rationale: The symptoms identified in the question indicate acute glomerulonephritis. Although the child is on penicillin, these are not symptoms of an allergic reaction. These symptoms are not normal and should not be ignored.

Test-Taking Strategy: Use the process of elimination. Eliminate options 1 and 2 because they are similar. From the remaining options, recalling the complications of scarlet fever and the symptoms of a medication reaction will direct you to option 3. Review the complications of scarlet fever and the symptoms of acute glomerulonephritis if you had difficulty with this question.

Level of Cognitive Ability: Analysis
Client Needs: Health Promotion and Maintenance
Integrated Process: Nursing Process/Analysis
Content Area: Child Health

Reference:
Wong, D., & Hockenberry, M. (2003). *Wong's nursing care of infants and children* (7th ed.). St. Louis: Mosby, p. 1271.

104. A client who sustained a thoracic cord injury a year ago returns to the clinic for a follow-up visit, and the nurse notes a small reddened area on the coccyx. The client is not aware of the reddened area. After counseling the client to relieve pressure on the area according to a turning schedule, which action by the nurse is most appropriate?

1 Ask a family member to assess the skin daily
2 Schedule the client to return to the clinic daily for a skin check
3 Teach the client to feel for reddened areas
4 Teach the client to use a mirror for skin assessment

Answer: 4

Rationale: The client should be encouraged to be as independent as possible. The most effective way of skin self-assessment for this client is with the use of a mirror. Asking a family member to assess the skin daily does not promote independence. It is unnecessary and unrealistic for the client to return to the clinic daily for a skin check. Redness cannot be felt.

Test-Taking Strategy: Use the process of elimination, recalling that independence is the key in rehabilitation of clients. Options 1 and 2 involve others in performing a task that the client can do independently. Option 3 is an inaccurate assessment technique, because redness cannot be felt. Option 4 is the only option that addresses client self-assessment. Review home care measures for the client with a thoracic cord injury if you had difficulty with this question.

Level of Cognitive Ability: Application
Client Needs: Health Promotion and Maintenance
Integrated Process: Nursing Process/Implementation
Content Area: Adult Health/Neurological

References:
Black, J., & Hawks, J. (2005). *Medical-surgical nursing: Clinical management for positive outcomes* (7th ed.). Philadelphia: Saunders, pp. 2234; 2228.
Phipps, W., Monahan, F., Sands, J., Marek, J., & Neighbors, M. (2003). *Medical-surgical nursing: health and illness perspectives* (7th ed.). St. Louis: Mosby, p. 775.

105. A nurse has given instructions to a client returning home following an arthroscopy of the knee. The nurse determines that the client understands the home care instructions if the client stated to:

1 Stay off the leg entirely for the rest of the day
2 Resume strenuous exercise the following day
3 Refrain from eating food for the remainder of the day
4 Report fever or site inflammation to the physician

Answer: 4

Rationale: After arthroscopy, the client can usually walk carefully on the leg once sensation has returned. The client is instructed to avoid strenuous exercise for at least a few days. The client may resume the usual diet. Signs and symptoms of infection should be reported to the physician.

Test-Taking Strategy: Use the process of elimination, focusing on the procedure: arthroscopy. Recalling that the procedure is invasive will direct you to option 4. Additionally, the client is always taught the signs and symptoms of infection to report to the physician. Review home care instructions for the client following arthroscopy if you had difficulty with this question.

Level of Cognitive Ability: Analysis
Client Needs: Health Promotion and Maintenance
Integrated Process: Nursing Process/Evaluation
Content Area: Adult Health/Musculoskeletal

References:
Ignatavicius, D., & Workman, M. (2002). *Medical surgical nursing: Critical thinking for collaborative care* (4th ed.). Philadelphia: Saunders, p. 1091.

106. Allopurinol (Zyloprim) has been prescribed for a client to treat gouty arthritis. The nurse teaches the client to anticipate which of the following prescriptions if an acute attack occurs?
1 Adding colchicine or a nonsteroidal antiinflammatory drug (NSAID) to the treatment plan
2 Doubling the dose of the allopurinol
3 Stopping the allopurinol and taking an NSAID
4 Stopping the allopurinol and taking acetylsalicylic acid (aspirin)

Answer: 1
Rationale: Allopurinol helps prevent an attack of gouty arthritis, but it does not relieve the pain. Therefore, another medication such as colchicine or an NSAID must be added if an acute attack occurs. Because acute attacks may occur more frequently early in the course of therapy with allopurinol, some physicians recommend taking the two products concurrently during the first 3 to 6 months.

Test-Taking Strategy: Use the process of elimination. Eliminate options 3 and 4 first because it is unlikely that medication will be stopped. From the remaining options, recalling that an acute attack of gouty arthritis is painful will assist in selecting option 1, because of the antiinflammatory action of the NSAID. Review interventions for an acute attack of gouty arthritis if you had difficulty with this question.

Level of Cognitive Ability: Application
Client Needs: Health Promotion and Maintenance
Integrated Process: Teaching/Learning
Content Area: Pharmacology

Reference:
Lehne, R. (2004). *Pharmacology for nursing care* (5th ed.). Philadelphia: Saunders, p. 776.

107. A nursing instructor asks a nursing student to describe live or attenuated vaccines. The student tells the instructor that these types of vaccines are:
1 Vaccines that have their virulence (potency) diminished so as to not produce a full-blown clinical illness
2 Vaccines that contain pathogens made inactive by either chemicals or heat
3 Bacterial toxins that have been made inactive by either chemicals or heat
4 Vaccines that have been obtained from the pooled blood of many people and provide antibodies to a variety of diseases

Answer: 1
Rationale: Live or attenuated vaccines have their virulence (potency) diminished so as to not produce a full-blown clinical illness. In response to vaccination, the body produces antibodies and causes immunity to be established. Option 2 identifies killed or inactivated vaccines. Option 3 identifies toxoids. Option 4 identifies human immune globulin.

Test-Taking Strategy: Use the process of elimination, focusing on the issue of the question. Noting the key word "live" in the question will assist in eliminating options 2, 3, and 4. If you are unfamiliar with the types of vaccines, review this content.

Level of Cognitive Ability: Comprehension
Client Needs: Health Promotion and Maintenance
Integrated Process: Teaching/Learning
Content Area: Child Health

Reference:
Lehne, R. (2004). *Pharmacology for nursing care* (5th ed.). Philadelphia: Saunders, p. 714.

108. A client has received a prescription for lisinopril (Prinivil). The nurse teaches the client that which of the following frequent side effects may occur?
1 Hypertension
2 Polyuria
3 Hypothermia
4 Cough

Answer: 4

Rationale: Cough is a frequent side effect of therapy with any of the angiotensin-converting enzyme (ACE) inhibitors. Hypertension is the reason to administer the medication, not a side effect. Fever is an occasional side effect. Proteinuria is another common side effect, but not polyuria.

Test-Taking Strategy: Note the name of the medication. Recalling that most ACE inhibitor medication names end in "pril" and that an ACE inhibitor is used to treat hypertension will assist in eliminating option 1. From the remaining options, it is necessary to know that cough is a frequent side effect of these medications. Review the side effects of this medication if you had difficulty with this question.

Level of Cognitive Ability: Application
Client Needs: Health Promotion and Maintenance
Integrated Process: Teaching/Learning
Content Area: Pharmacology

Reference:
McKenry, L., & Salerno, E. (2003). *Mosby's pharmacology in nursing* (21st ed.). St. Louis: Mosby, pp. 586-587.

109. A nurse has provided home care instructions to a client taking lithium carbonate (Eskalith). Which client statement indicates that the client understands the prescribed regimen?
1 "I make sure that my diet contains salt."
2 "I keep my medication next to the milk in the refrigerator so that I can remember to take it every day."
3 "It is not difficult to restrict my water intake."
4 "I am careful to avoid eating foods high in potassium."

Answer: 1

Rationale: Lithium replaces sodium ions in the cells and induces excretion of sodium and potassium from the body. Client teaching includes maintenance of sodium intake in the daily diet and increased fluid intake (at least 1 to 1 1/2 liters per day) during maintenance therapy. Lithium is stored at room temperature and protected from light and moisture.

Test-Taking Strategy: Note the key word "understands the prescribed regimen." Recalling that lithium is a salt that replaces sodium ions and induces excretion of sodium will direct you to the correct option. Review this medication if you had difficulty with this question.

Level of Cognitive Ability: Analysis
Client Needs: Health Promotion and Maintenance
Integrated Process: Nursing Process/Evaluation
Content Area: Pharmacology

References:
Hodgson, B., & Kizior, R. (2004). *Saunders nursing drug handbook 2004.* Philadelphia: Saunders, p. 606.
Lehne, R. (2004). *Pharmacology for nursing care* (5th ed.). Philadelphia: Saunders, p. 328.

110. An older client is given a prescription for haloperidol (Haldol). The nurse instructs the client and family to report any signs of pseudoparkinsonism and tells the family to monitor for:
  1 Stooped posture and a shuffling gait
  2 Muscle weakness and decreased salivation
  3 Tremors and hyperpyrexia
  4 Motor restlessness and aphasia

Answer: 1
Rationale: Pseudoparkinsonism is a common extrapyramidal side effect of antipsychotic medications. This condition is characterized by a stooped posture, shuffling gait, masklike facial appearance, drooling, tremors, and pill-rolling motions of the fingers. Hyperpyrexia is characteristic of another extrapyramidal side effect, neuroleptic malignant syndrome (NMS). Aphasia is not characteristic of pseudoparkinsonism.

Test-Taking Strategy: Focus on the word pseudo*parkinsonism*. Recalling the characteristics of Parkinson's disease will direct you to option 1. Review the characteristics and the effects of antipsychotic medications if you had difficulty with this question.

Level of Cognitive Ability: Application
Client Needs: Health Promotion and Maintenance
Integrated Process: Teaching/Learning
Content Area: Pharmacology

References:
Hodgson, B., & Kizior, R. (2004). *Saunders nursing drug handbook 2004.* Philadelphia: Saunders, p. 491.
McKenry, L., & Salerno, E. (2003). *Mosby's pharmacology in nursing* (21st ed.). St. Louis: Mosby, p. 402.

111. A client on tranylcypromine (Parnate) requests information on foods that are acceptable to eat while taking the medication. The nurse tells the client that it is safe to eat:
  1 Raisins
  2 Smoked fish
  3 Yogurt
  4 Oranges

Answer: 4
Rationale: Tranylcypromine is classified as a monoamine oxidase inhibitor (MAOI) and, as such, tyramine-containing food should be avoided. Types of food to be avoided include, but are not limited to, those items identified in options 1, 2, and 3. Additionally, beer, wine, caffeinated beverages, pickled meats, yeast preparations, avocados, bananas, and plums are to be avoided. Oranges are permissible.

Test-Taking Strategy: Use the process of elimination. Note the similarity in the food items in options 1, 2, and 3. These are food items that are either processed or contain some type of additive. The only natural food is option 4. Remember, however, that although bananas, avocados, or plums are natural foods, they are not permitted while taking an MAOI. Review foods that are high in tyramine if you had difficulty with this question.

Level of Cognitive Ability: Application
Client Needs: Health Promotion and Maintenance
Integrated Process: Teaching/Learning
Content Area: Pharmacology

Reference:
Hodgson, B., & Kizior, R. (2004). *Saunders nursing drug handbook 2004.* Philadelphia: Saunders, p. 1010.

112. A nurse is performing an assessment on a 3-year-old child with chickenpox. The child's mother tells the nurse that the child keeps scratching at night, and the nurse teaches the mother about measures that will prevent an alteration in skin integrity. Which statement by the mother indicates that teaching was effective?

1 "I will apply generous amounts of a cortisone cream to prevent itching."
2 "I need to place white gloves on my child's hands at night."
3 "I need to keep my child in a warm room at night so the covers will not cause my child to scratch."
4 "I will give my child a glass of warm milk at bedtime to help my child sleep."

Answer: 2

Rationale: Gloves will keep the child from preventing an alteration in skin integrity from scratching. Generous amounts of any topical cream can lead to medication toxicity. A warm room will increase the child's skin temperature and make the itching worse. Warm milk will have no effect on itching.

Test-Taking Strategy: Use the process of elimination. Note the key words "prevent an alteration in skin integrity." Eliminate option 3 first because this action will promote itching. Option 4 is eliminated next because it is unrelated to skin integrity. From the remaining options, the words "generous amounts" in option 1 should provide you with the clue that this option is incorrect. Review measures related to the child with chickenpox if you had difficulty with this question.

Level of Cognitive Ability: Analysis
Client Needs: Health Promotion and Maintenance
Integrated Process: Teaching/Learning
Content Area: Child Health

Reference:
Wong, D., & Hockenberry, M. (2003). *Wong's nursing care of infants and children* (7th ed.). St. Louis: Mosby, p. 653.

---

113. A nurse is providing instructions about foot care to a client with chronic arterial insufficiency. The nurse tells the client to:

1 Wear shoes that fit snugly
2 Clean the feet daily, drying them well
3 Cross the legs at the ankles only
4 Cut the toenails very short to prevent scratching

Answer: 2

Rationale: Foot care for the client with vascular disease is the same as for clients who have diabetes mellitus. This includes daily cleansing of the feet; drying well especially between the toes; applying lotion to dry areas; wearing shoes that fit well without pressure areas; and keeping the toenails trimmed short. The client is also instructed to avoid crossing the legs at the knees or ankles to prevent vasoconstriction.

Test-Taking Strategy: Recall that diabetes mellitus and vascular disease both result in impairment of the tissues of the feet and use the principles involved in diabetic foot care to answer this question. Eliminate option 1 because of the word "snugly," option 3 because of the absolute word "only," and option 4 because of the words "very short." Review foot care for the client with vascular disease if you had difficulty with this question.

Level of Cognitive Ability: Application
Client Needs: Health Promotion and Maintenance
Integrated Process: Teaching/Learning
Content Area: Adult Health/Cardiovascular

Reference:
Phipps, W., Monahan, F., Sands, J., Marek, J., & Neighbors, M. (2003). *Medical-surgical nursing: health and illness perspectives* (7th ed.). St. Louis: Mosby, p. 775.

114. A nurse is giving instructions to a client with peptic ulcer disease about symptom management. The nurse tells the client to:
1 Eat slowly and chew food thoroughly
2 Eat large meals to absorb gastric acid
3 Limit the intake of water
4 Use acetylsalicylic acid (aspirin) to relieve gastric pain

Answer: 1

Rationale: The client with a peptic ulcer is taught to eat smaller, more frequent meals to help keep the gastric secretions neutralized. The client should eat slowly and chew thoroughly to prevent excess gastric acid secretion. The client should consume fluids of 6 to 8 glasses of water per day to dilute gastric acid. The use of aspirin is avoided, because it is irritating to gastric mucosa.

Test-Taking Strategy: Use the process of elimination. Recalling the concepts related to digestion and knowledge of substances that are known gastric irritants will direct you to option 1. Review teaching points related to the client with peptic ulcer disease if you had difficulty with this question.

Level of Cognitive Ability: Application
Client Needs: Health Promotion and Maintenance
Integrated Process: Teaching/Learning
Content Area: Adult Health/Gastrointestinal

Reference:
Phipps, W., Monahan, F., Sands, J., Marek, J., & Neighbors, M. (2003). *Medical-surgical nursing: Health and illness perspectives* (7th ed.). St. Louis: Mosby, p. 1035.

115. A client with a hiatal hernia asks the nurse about fluids that are safe to drink and that will not irritate the gastric mucosa. The nurse tells the client to drink:
1 Tomato juice
2 Orange juice
3 Grapefruit juice
4 Apple juice

Answer: 4

Rationale: Substances that are irritating to the client with hiatal hernia include tomato products and citrus fruits, which should be avoided. Because caffeine stimulates gastric acid secretion, beverages that contain caffeine, such as coffee, tea, cola, and cocoa, are also eliminated from the diet.

Test-Taking Strategy: Use the process of elimination. Eliminate options 1, 2, and 3 because they are similar and are citrus products. Additionally, option 4 is the least irritating to the stomach. Review dietary measures for the client with hiatal hernia if you had difficulty with this question.

Level of Cognitive Ability: Application
Client Needs: Health Promotion and Maintenance
Integrated Process: Nursing Process/Implementation
Content Area: Adult Health/Gastrointestinal

Reference:
Phipps, W., Monahan, F., Sands, J., Marek, J., & Neighbors, M. (2003). *Medical-surgical nursing: Health and illness perspectives* (7th ed.). St. Louis: Mosby, p. 1015.

116. A client with a spinal cord injury experiences bladder spasms and reflex incontinence. In preparing for discharge to home, the nurse instructs the client to:

1 Limit fluid intake to 1000 mL in 24 hours
2 Take own temperature every day
3 Catheterize self every 2 hours prn to prevent spasm
4 Avoid caffeine in the diet

Answer: 4

Rationale: Caffeine in the diet can contribute to bladder spasms and reflex incontinence. This should be eliminated in the diet of the client with a spinal cord injury. Limiting fluid intake does not prevent spasm and could place the client at further risk of urinary tract infection. Self-monitoring of temperature would be useful in detecting infection, but does nothing to alleviate bladder spasm. Self-catheterization every 2 hours is too frequent and serves no useful purpose.

Test-Taking Strategy: Focus on the issue: preventive measures for bladder spasm and reflex incontinence. Eliminate options 1 and 3 first because they place the client at increased risk of urinary tract infection and are therefore not appropriate. From the remaining options, eliminate option 2 because this action would detect infection but does not deal with spasm and incontinence. Review measures to prevent bladder spasm and reflex incontinence if you had difficulty with this question.

Level of Cognitive Ability: Application
Client Needs: Health Promotion and Maintenance
Integrated Process: Teaching/Learning
Content Area: Adult Health/Neurological

References:
Black, J., & Hawks, J. (2005). *Medical-surgical nursing: Clinical management for positive outcomes* (7th ed.). Philadelphia: Saunders, pp. 209; 2227.
Lewis, S., Heitkemper, M., & Dirksen, S. (2004). *Medical-surgical nursing: Assessment and management of clinical problems* (6th ed.). St. Louis: Mosby, pp. 1620-1621; 1628.
Phipps, W., Monahan, F., Sands, J., Marek, J., & Neighbors, M. (2003). *Medical-surgical nursing: Health and illness perspectives* (7th ed.). St. Louis: Mosby, p. 1422.

117. A client seeks treatment in an ambulatory care center for symptoms of Raynaud's disease. The nurse instructs the client to:

1 Wear protective items, such as gloves and warm socks, as necessary
2 Alternate exposures to both heat and cold
3 Decrease cigarette smoking by one-half
4 Continue activity during vasospasm for quicker relief of symptoms

Answer: 1

Rationale: Treatment for Raynaud's disease includes avoidance of precipitating factors such as cold or damp weather, stress, and cigarettes. The client should get sufficient rest and sleep, protect the extremities by wearing protective clothing, and stop activity during vasospasm.

Test-Taking Strategy: Use the process of elimination. Recall that the symptoms of Raynaud's disease are caused by vasospasm. Eliminate options 2, 3, and 4 because they will cause vasospasm. Review client teaching points related to Raynaud's disease if you had difficulty with this question.

Level of Cognitive Ability: Application
Client Needs: Health Promotion and Maintenance
Integrated Process: Teaching/Learning
Content Area: Adult Health/Cardiovascular

Reference:
Phipps, W., Monahan, F., Sands, J., Marek, J., & Neighbors, M. (2003). *Medical-surgical nursing: Health and illness perspectives* (7th ed.). St. Louis: Mosby, pp. 777-778

118. A client with atherosclerosis asks the nurse about dietary modifications to lower the risk of heart disease. The nurse instructs the client to eat which of the following foods?
  1 Roast beef
  2 Fresh cantaloupe
  3 Broiled cheeseburger
  4 Mashed potato with gravy

Answer: 2

Rationale: To lower the risk of heart disease, the diet should be low in saturated fat with the appropriate number of total calories. The diet should include fewer red meats and more white meat, with the skin removed. Dairy products used should be low in fat, and foods with high amounts of empty calories should be avoided.

Test-Taking Strategy: Focus on the issue: lower the risk of heart disease. Use fat content of the foods in the options as a guide to answering this question. Eliminate options 1 and 3 first because of the fat content of the described meats. From the remaining options, eliminate option 4 because fresh fruits and vegetables are naturally low in fat. Review dietary measures that will lower the risk of heart disease if you had difficulty with this question.

Level of Cognitive Ability: Application
Client Needs: Health Promotion and Maintenance
Integrated Process: Teaching/Learning
Content Area: Adult Health/Cardiovascular

Reference:
Phipps, W., Monahan, F., Sands, J., Marek, J., & Neighbors, M. (2003). *Medical-surgical nursing: Health and illness perspectives* (7th ed.). St. Louis: Mosby, pp. 666-668.

119. A client is being discharged to home after angioplasty using the right femoral area as the catheter insertion site. The nurse instructs the client that which of the following signs and symptoms may be expected after the procedure?
  1 Coolness or discoloration of the right foot
  2 Temperature as high as 101°F
  3 Large area of bruising at the right groin
  4 Mild discomfort in the right groin

Answer: 4

Rationale: The client may feel some mild discomfort at the catheter insertion site following angioplasty. This is usually relieved by analgesics such as acetaminophen (Tylenol). The client is taught to report to the physician any neurovascular changes to the affected leg, bleeding or bruising at the insertion site, and signs of local infection, such as drainage at the site or increased temperature.

Test-Taking Strategy: Use the process of elimination, noting the key word "expected." Knowing that bleeding and infection are complications of the procedure guides you to eliminate options 2 and 3. From the remaining options, eliminate option 1, knowing that neurovascular status should not be impaired by the procedure, or by knowing that the area may be mildly uncomfortable. Review the complications associated with angioplasty if you had difficulty with this question.

Level of Cognitive Ability: Application
Client Needs: Health Promotion and Maintenance
Integrated Process: Teaching/Learning
Content Area: Adult Health/Cardiovascular

Reference:
Phipps, W., Monahan, F., Sands, J., Marek, J., & Neighbors, M. (2003). *Medical-surgical nursing: Health and illness perspectives* (7th ed.). St. Louis: Mosby, p. 661.

120. A nurse is teaching dietary modifications to the client with hypertension. The nurse instructs the client to eat which of the following snack foods?

1 Cheese and crackers
2 Raw carrots
3 Frozen pizza
4 Canned tomato soup

Answer: 2

Rationale: Sodium should be avoided by the client with hypertension. Fresh fruits and vegetables are naturally low in sodium. Hypertensive clients are also advised to keep fat intake to less than 30% of total calories as part of prudent heart living. Each of the incorrect options contains increased amounts of sodium, and options 1 and 3 are likely to be also higher in fat.

Test-Taking Strategy: Focus on the issue, the dietary modifications needed with hypertension. Eliminate options 1, 3, and 4 because they are similar and are all processed food items. Review dietary measures for the client with hypertension if you had difficulty with this question.

Level of Cognitive Ability: Application
Client Needs: Health Promotion and Maintenance
Integrated Process: Teaching/Learning
Content Area: Adult Health/Cardiovascular

Reference:
Phipps, W., Monahan, F., Sands, J., Marek, J., & Neighbors, M. (2003). *Medical-surgical nursing: Health and illness perspectives* (7th ed.). St. Louis: Mosby, p. 767.

121. A nurse teaches a client with hypertension to recognize the signs and symptoms that may occur during periods of an elevated blood pressure. The nurse determines that the client needs additional teaching if the client states that which sign or symptom is associated with an elevated blood pressure?

1 Dizziness
2 Epistaxis
3 Feeling of fullness in the head
4 Blurred vision

Answer: 3

Rationale: Cerebrovascular symptoms of hypertension include early morning headaches, occipital headaches, blurred vision, lightheadedness and vertigo, dizziness, and epistaxis. The client should be aware of these symptoms and report them if they occur. The client should also be taught self-monitoring of blood pressure. Feelings of fullness in the head is more likely associated with a sinus condition.

Test-Taking Strategy: Note the key words "needs additional teaching." These key words indicate a false-response question and that you need to select the option that identifies the incorrect client response. Focus on the issue: signs of an elevated blood pressure. Option 3 is the vague option, whereas options 1, 2, and 4 are specific and related to hypertension. Review the signs and symptoms of hypertension if you had difficulty with this question.

Level of Cognitive Ability: Application
Client Needs: Health Promotion and Maintenance
Integrated Process: Teaching/Learning
Content Area: Adult Health/Cardiovascular

Reference:
Phipps, W., Monahan, F., Sands, J., Marek, J., & Neighbors, M. (2003). *Medical-surgical nursing: Health and illness perspectives* (7th ed.). St. Louis: Mosby, p. 762.

122. A client is taking iron supplements to correct an iron-deficiency anemia. The nurse teaches the client which special consideration while on iron therapy?
1 Avoid taking iron with milk or antacids
2 Limit intake of meat, fish, and poultry
3 Eat a low-fiber diet
4 Limit intake of fluids

Answer: 1

Rationale: The client should avoid taking iron with milk or antacids, because these items decrease absorption of iron. The client should also avoid taking iron with food if possible. The client should increase natural sources of iron, such as meats, fish, and poultry. Finally, the client should take in sufficient fiber and fluids to prevent constipation as a side effect of iron therapy.

Test-Taking Strategy: Use the process of elimination. Begin to answer this question by eliminating options 3 and 4, knowing that constipation is a common side effect of iron therapy. Recalling that meat products contain iron would guide you to eliminate option 2 next. Remember that several medications have impaired absorption with milk products or antacids. Review home care measures for the client with iron-deficiency anemia if you had difficulty with this question.

Level of Cognitive Ability: Application
Client Needs: Health Promotion and Maintenance
Integrated Process: Teaching/Learning
Content Area: Pharmacology

Reference:
McKenry, L., & Salerno, E. (2003). *Mosby's pharmacology in nursing* (21st ed.). St. Louis: Mosby, pp. 62; 1165.

123. A client with a colostomy complains to the nurse of appliance odor. The nurse recommends that the client take in which of the following deodorizing foods?
1 Yogurt
2 Mushrooms
3 Cucumbers
4 Eggs

Answer: 1

Rationale: Foods that help eliminate odor with a colostomy include yogurt, buttermilk, spinach, beet greens, and parsley. Foods that cause odor are many, and include alcohol, beans, turnips, radishes, asparagus, onions, cucumbers, mushrooms, cabbage, asparagus, eggs, and fish.

Test-Taking Strategy: Use the process of elimination. Remember that foods that cause gas in the client with normal gastrointestinal (GI) function also form gas in the GI tract of the client with a colostomy. Use basic nutritional knowledge to eliminate options 2, 3, and 4. Review foods that are gas forming if you had difficulty with this question.

Level of Cognitive Ability: Application
Client Needs: Health Promotion and Maintenance
Integrated Process: Teaching/Learning
Content Area: Adult Health/Gastrointestinal

References:
Ignatavicius, D., & Workman, M. (2002). *Medical surgical nursing: Critical thinking for collaborative care* (4th ed.). Philadelphia: Saunders, p. 1254.
Lewis, S., Heitkemper, M., & Dirksen, S. (2004). *Medical-surgical nursing: Assessment and management of clinical problems* (6th ed.). St. Louis: Mosby, pp. 1090-1091.

124. A nurse is demonstrating colostomy care to a client with a newly created colostomy. The nurse demonstrates correct cutting of the appliance by making the circle how much larger than the client's stoma?

1 1/16 inch
2 1/8 inch
3 1/4 inch
4 1/2 inch

Answer: 2

Rationale: The size of the opening for the appliance is generally cut 1/8 inch larger than the size of the client's stoma. This minimizes the amount of exposed skin, but does not cause pressure on the stoma. Option 1 is an extremely small size that would cause irritation to the stoma. Options 3 and 4 leave too much skin area exposed for possible irritation by gastrointestinal contents.

Test-Taking Strategy: Use the process of elimination, and remember that the goal is to prevent stoma and skin irritation. Visualizing each of the appliance sizes in the options will direct you to option 2. Review home care instructions for a client with a colostomy if you had difficulty with this question.

Level of Cognitive Ability: Application
Client Needs: Health Promotion and Maintenance
Integrated Process: Teaching/Learning
Content Area: Adult Health/Gastrointestinal

Reference:
Ignatavicius, D., & Workman, M. (2002). *Medical surgical nursing: Critical thinking for collaborative care* (4th ed.). Philadelphia: Saunders, p. 1252.

125. A nurse teaches a client with a spinal cord injury about measures to prevent autonomic dysreflexia (hyperreflexia). Which statement by the client would indicate the need for additional teaching?

1 "I need to pay close attention to how frequently my bowels move."
2 "It is best if I avoid tight clothing and lumpy bed clothes."
3 "I should watch for headache, congestion, and flushed skin."
4 "Symptoms I should watch for include fever and chest pain."

Answer: 4

Rationale: Symptoms of autonomic dysreflexia include headache, congestion, flushed skin above the injury and cold skin below it, diaphoresis, nausea, and anxiety. Fever and chest pain are not associated with this condition.

Test-Taking Strategy: Use the process of elimination, noting the key words "need for additional teaching." These key words indicate a false-response question and that you need to select the option that identifies the incorrect client statement. Recalling the signs and symptoms and causes of autonomic dysreflexia will direct you to option 4. Review this content if you are unfamiliar with this syndrome.

Level of Cognitive Ability: Analysis
Client Needs: Health Promotion and Maintenance
Integrated Process: Teaching/Learning
Content Area: Adult Health/Neurological

References:
Black, J., & Hawks, J. (2005). *Medical-surgical nursing: Clinical management for positive outcomes* (7th ed.). Philadelphia: Saunders, p. 2229.
Ignatavicius, D., & Workman, M. (2002). *Medical surgical nursing: Critical thinking for collaborative care* (4th ed.). Philadelphia: Saunders, p. 931.

126. A nurse is discharging a female client from the hospital who has a diagnosis of T-11 fracture with cord transaction and has reinforced home care instructions with the client. Which of the following would indicate the need for further discharge teaching?

1 The client states she will have to be careful not to eat as many dairy products.

2 The client states she will wash her hands, perineum, and catheter with soap and water before performing self-catheterization.

3 The client jokes about no longer needing to worry about birth control.

4 The client verbalizes the need to eat her meals close to the same time every day.

Answer: 3

Rationale: Female spinal cord trauma clients remain fertile in their reproductive years. Contraception is necessary for these clients who are sexually active. Oral contraceptives may increase the risk for thrombophlebitis. Clients with paralysis should avoid dairy products to control the formation of urinary calculi. Clients who lack bladder control are taught to self-catheterize using clean technique. Meals should be eaten at the same time every day and include fiber and warm solid and liquid foods to promote and maintain regular evacuation of the bowel.

Test-Taking Strategy: Note the key words, "need for further discharge teaching." These key words indicate a false-response question and that you need to select the option that identifies the incorrect client statement. Remember that key aspects of dealing with a spinal cord injury client are nutrition and elimination. Options 1, 2 and 4 address these key areas. Review teaching points for a client with transection of the cord if you had difficulty with this question.

Level of Cognitive Ability: Analysis
Client Needs: Health Promotion and Maintenance
Integrated Process: Teaching/Learning
Content Area: Adult Health/Neurological

References:
Ignatavicius, D., & Workman, M. (2002). *Medical surgical nursing: Critical thinking for collaborative care* (4th ed.). Philadelphia: Saunders, p. 941.
Lewis, S., Heitkemper, M., & Dirksen, S. (2004). *Medical-surgical nursing: Assessment and management of clinical problems* (6th ed.). St. Louis: Mosby, pp. 1629-1630.

---

127. A client has been started on a monoamine oxidase inhibitor (MAOI). Which of the following should the nurse include when teaching the client about the medication?

1 The medication will begin to alleviate symptoms of depression almost immediately.

2 The medication is associated with a high rate of abuse.

3 This medication can cause severe drowsiness.

4 The client must avoid foods containing tyramine.

Answer: 4

Rationale: Although MAOIs usually produce hypotension as a side effect, potentially lethal hypertension can occur if the client eats foods that contain tyramine. Such foods include aged cheeses, hot dogs, and beer, among others. Option 1, 2, and 3 are incorrect statements.

Test-Taking Strategy: Note the key words "monoamine oxidase inhibitor (MAOI)." Recalling that MAOIs are associated with a food-medication interaction will direct you to option 4. Review these interactions if you had difficulty with this question.

Level of Cognitive Ability: Application
Client Needs: Health Promotion and Maintenance
Integrated Process: Teaching/Learning
Content Area: Pharmacology

Reference:
McKenry, L., & Salerno, E. (2003). *Mosby's pharmacology in nursing* (21st ed.). St. Louis: Mosby, pp. 62; 423.

128. A nurse is developing a plan of care for an older client with dementia and formulates a nursing diagnosis of self-care deficit. The nurse develops which realistic outcome for the client?
1 The client will be admitted to a nursing home to have activities of daily living (ADL) needs met.
2 The client will function at the highest level of independence possible.
3 The client will complete all ADLs independently within a 1- to 1 1/2-hour time frame.
4 The nursing staff will attend to all of the client's ADL needs during the hospital stay.

Answer: 2
Rationale: All clients, regardless of age, need to be encouraged to perform at the highest level of independence possible. This contributes to the client's sense of control and well-being. Options 1 and 4 are not client-centered goals. A 1- to 1 1/2-hour time frame may not be realistic for an older client with dementia.

Test-Taking Strategy: Use the process of elimination, focusing on the key words "realistic outcome for the client." Eliminate options 1 and 4 first because they are not client-centered. From the remaining options, eliminate option 3 because of the unrealistic time frame. Review care of the client with dementia if you had difficulty with this question.

Level of Cognitive Ability: Analysis
Client Needs: Health Promotion and Maintenance
Integrated Process: Nursing Process/Planning
Content Area: Mental Health

References:
Gulanick, M., Myers, J., Klopp, A., Gradishar, D., Galanes, S., & Puzas, M. (2003). *Nursing care plans: Nursing diagnosis and intervention* (5th ed.). St. Louis: Mosby, p. 132.
Lueckenotte, A. (2000). *Gerontologic nursing* (2nd ed.). St. Louis: Mosby, p. 631.

129. A client who is on haloperidol (Haldol) at bedtime also receives benztropine (Cogentin) at the same time. The nurse instructs the client that the benztropine is given to:
1 Combat extrapyramidal side effects (EPS)
2 Enhance sleep
3 Enhance the effects of haloperidol
4 Enhance the anticholinergic effects of the medications

Answer: 1
Rationale: Haloperidol is a neuroleptic medication that may cause the client to experience EPS. Antiparkinsonian medications such as benztropine may be administered concurrently to decrease the symptoms of EPS. Options 2, 3, and 4 are incorrect.

Test-Taking Strategy: Focus on the name of the medication and recall that haloperidol is a neuroleptic medication. Recalling that EPS is a concern with the use of neuroleptic medications will direct you to option 1. Review the purposes of these medications if you had difficulty with this question.

Level of Cognitive Ability: Application
Client Needs: Health Promotion and Maintenance
Integrated Process: Teaching/Learning
Content Area: Pharmacology

References:
Lehne, R. (2004). *Pharmacology for nursing care* (5th ed.). Philadelphia: Saunders, p. 297.
McKenry, L., & Salerno, E. (2003). *Mosby's pharmacology in nursing* (21st ed.). St. Louis: Mosby, p. 493.

130. A client is newly diagnosed with chronic obstructive pulmonary disease (COPD). The client returns home after a short hospitalization. The home care nurse visits the client and most importantly plans teaching strategies that are designed to:

1 Encourage the client to become a more active person
2 Improve oxygenation and minimize carbon dioxide retention
3 Identify irritants in the home that interfere with breathing
4 Promote membership in support groups

Answer: 2
Rationale: Improving oxygenation and minimizing carbon dioxide retention is the primary goal. The other options are interventions that will help achieve this primary goal.

Test-Taking Strategy: Note the key words "most importantly." Use the ABCs—airway, breathing, and circulation—to direct you to option 2. Review care of the client with COPD if you had difficulty with this question.

Level of Cognitive Ability: Application
Client Needs: Health Promotion and Maintenance
Integrated Process: Nursing Process/Planning
Content Area: Adult Health/Respiratory

References:
Lewis, S., Heitkemper, M., & Dirksen, S. (2004). *Medical-surgical nursing: Assessment and management of clinical problems* (6th ed.). St. Louis: Mosby, p. 677.
Phipps, W., Monahan, F., Sands, J., Marek, J., & Neighbors, M. (2003). *Medical-surgical nursing: Health and illness perspectives* (7th ed.). St. Louis: Mosby, p. 579.

131. A client is being discharged from the hospital following a bronchoscopy that was performed yesterday. Following discharge teaching, the client makes all of the following statements to the nurse. Which statement would the nurse identify as indicating a need for further teaching?

1 "I can expect to cough up bright red blood."
2 "I will stop smoking my cigarettes."
3 "I will get help immediately if I start having trouble breathing."
4 "I will use the throat lozenges as directed by the physician until my sore throat goes away."

Answer: 1
Rationale: After the procedure, the client should be observed for signs of respiratory distress, including dyspnea, changes in respiratory rate, use of accessory muscles, and changes in/or absent lung sounds. Expectorated secretions are inspected for hemoptysis, and if the client expectorates bright red blood the physician is notified. The client needs to avoid smoking. A sore throat is common, and lozenges would be helpful to alleviate the sore throat.

Test-Taking Strategy: Note the key words "need for further teaching." These key words indicate a false-response question and that you need to select the option that identifies the incorrect client statement. Note the words "bright red" in option 1. Remember bright red blood indicates active bleeding and needs to be reported to the physician. Review care of the client following bronchoscopy if you had difficulty with this question.

Level of Cognitive Ability: Analysis
Client Needs: Health Promotion and Maintenance
Integrated Process: Teaching/Learning
Content Area: Adult Health/Respiratory

Reference:
Chernecky, C., & Berger, B. (2004). *Laboratory tests and diagnostic procedures* (4th ed.). Philadelphia: Saunders, p. 297.

132. A client who is on chlorpromazine (Thorazine) is preparing for discharge. In developing a health promotion plan for the client, the nurse instructs the client:
1 To adhere to a strict tyramine-restricted diet
2 On the signs and symptoms of relapse of depression
3 To avoid prolonged exposure to the sun
4 To have the therapeutic blood levels drawn because there is a narrow range between the therapeutic and toxic levels of the medication

Answer: 3

Rationale: Chlorpromazine is an antipsychotic medication often used in the treatment of psychosis. Photosensitivity is sometimes a side effect of the phenothiazine class of antipsychotic medications to which chlorpromazine (Thorazine) belongs. Options 1, 2, and 4 are unrelated to the administration of this medication.

Test-Taking Strategy: Focus on the name of the medication. Because chlorpromazine is an antipsychotic medication, option 2 can be eliminated. Eliminate option 1 because this option relates to medications that are monoamine oxidase inhibitors. There is not a narrow range between therapeutic and toxic levels such as with lithium (Eskalith), therefore eliminate option 4. Review this medication if you had difficulty with this question.

Level of Cognitive Ability: Application
Client Needs: Health Promotion and Maintenance
Integrated Process: Teaching/Learning
Content Area: Pharmacology

Reference:
Lehne, R. (2004). *Pharmacology for nursing care* (5th ed.). Philadelphia: Saunders, p. 298.

---

133. A nurse instructs a client with hepatitis about measures to control fatigue. The nurse determines that the client needs additional instructions if the client states to:
1 Plan rest periods after meals
2 Rest between activities
3 Perform personal hygiene if not fatigued
4 Complete all daily activities in the morning when the client is most rested

Answer: 4

Rationale: A client with hepatitis has tremendous metabolic demands that lead to fatigue and interfere with activities of daily living (ADLs). The nurse encourages ADLs unless they cause excessive fatigue. The client is advised to plan rest periods after activities, such as meals. Activities should be spaced throughout the day with frequent planned rest periods. Clients who engage in excessive activity too early in the recovery stage may experience a relapse.

Test-Taking Strategy: Note the key word "needs additional instructions." These words indicate a false-response question and that you need to select the incorrect client statement. Use the basic principles associated with a balance of rest and activities to answer the question. By the process of elimination, the only option that does not provide this balance is option 4. Review measures to alleviate fatigue in the client with hepatitis if you had difficulty with this question.

Level of Cognitive Ability: Analysis
Client Needs: Health Promotion and Maintenance
Integrated Process: Teaching/Learning
Content Area: Adult Health/Gastrointestinal

Reference:
Black, J., & Hawks, J. (2005). *Medical-surgical nursing: Clinical management for positive outcomes* (7th ed.). Philadelphia: Saunders, p. 1329.

134. A nurse provides home care instructions to a client with multiple sclerosis. The nurse tells the client to:
  1 Avoid becoming pregnant
  2 Restrict fluid intake to 1000 mL daily
  3 Maintain a low-fiber diet
  4 Avoid taking hot baths or showers

Answer: 4
Rationale: Because fatigue can be precipitated by warm temperatures, the client is instructed to take cool baths and maintain a cool environmental temperature. A high-fiber diet and an adequate fluid intake of 2000 mL daily is encouraged to prevent alterations in elimination and bowel patterns. The client should not be told to avoid pregnancy, but the nurse should assist the client to make informed decisions regarding pregnancy.

Test-Taking Strategy: Use the process of elimination and knowledge regarding the effects of multiple sclerosis in answering the question. Eliminate option 1 first because it is inappropriate to tell a client to avoid pregnancy. Eliminate options 2 and 3 next because these measures are unhealthy in this client and would promote alterations in elimination patterns. Review teaching points related to the client with multiple sclerosis if you had difficulty with this question.

Level of Cognitive Ability: Application
Client Needs: Health Promotion and Maintenance
Integrated Process: Teaching/Learning
Content Area: Adult Health/Musculoskeletal

Reference:
Black, J., & Hawks, J. (2005). *Medical-surgical nursing: Clinical management for positive outcomes* (7th ed.). Philadelphia: Saunders, p. 2180.

---

135. A home care nurse provides instructions to the client with a halo vest. The nurse tells the client to:
  1 Have the spouse use the metal frame to assist the client to sit up
  2 Perform pin care three times a week using hydrogen peroxide or alcohol
  3 Loosen the bolts once a day for bathing
  4 Carry the correct size wrench to loosen the bolts in an emergency

Answer: 4
Rationale: The metal frame is never used or pulled on for turning or lifting. Pin care should be performed at least once a day using soap and water with cotton-tipped swabs or with alcohol swabs. The bolts should never be loosened except in an emergency. In fact, the physician should be notified if the bolts loosen. The client is instructed to carry the correct size wrench in case of an emergency requiring cardiopulmonary resuscitation (CPR). In such a situation, the anterior portion of the vest, including the anterior bolts, will need to be loosened, and the posterior portion should remain in place to provide stability for the spine during CPR.

Test-Taking Strategy: Try to visualize the appearance of a halo vest. Recall that the purpose of this vest is to stabilize a cervical fracture. Eliminate option 2 first because pin care should be done at least once a day. Eliminate option 1 because pulling on the frame will disrupt the stabilization of the fracture and possibly lead to serious complications. Remember that bolts should never be loosened except in an emergency situation. Review home care instructions for a client with a halo vest if you had difficulty with this question.

Level of Cognitive Ability: Application
Client Needs: Health Promotion and Maintenance
Integrated Process: Teaching/Learning
Content Area: Adult Health/Neurological

References:

Black, J., & Hawks, J. (2005). *Medical-surgical nursing: Clinical management for positive outcomes* (7th ed.). Philadelphia: Saunders, p. 636.

Lewis, S., Heitkemper, M., & Dirksen, S. (2004). *Medical-surgical nursing: Assessment and management of clinical problems* (6th ed.). St. Louis: Mosby, p. 1629.

Phipps, W., Monahan, F., Sands, J., Marek, J., & Neighbors, M. (2003). *Medical-surgical nursing: Health and illness perspectives* (7th ed.). St. Louis: Mosby, pp. 1470; 1480.

---

136. Haloperidol (Haldol) has been prescribed for a client with Tourette's syndrome, and the nurse instructs the client about the medication. Which statement by the client indicates the need for further instructions?

1 "It may take 6 weeks before the medication works."

2 "The drowsiness will probably go away as I continue the medication."

3 "I should stop the medication immediately if my vision becomes blurred."

4 "I need to avoid alcohol while taking this medication."

Answer: 3

Rationale: The client needs to be instructed not to abruptly stop the medication therapy. The client is informed that if visual disturbances occur, the physician should be notified. Options 1, 2, and 4 are accurate statements regarding the medication.

Test-Taking Strategy: Use the process of elimination, focusing on the key words "need for further instructions." These words indicate a false-response question and that you need to select the incorrect client statement. Eliminate option 4 first because this is a general principle with most medications. Knowledge that this medication is an antipsychotic will assist in eliminating options 1 and 2. Additionally, knowing that the medication should not be abruptly stopped will assist in directing you to option 3. Review this medication if you had difficulty with this question.

Level of Cognitive Ability: Analysis
Client Needs: Health Promotion and Maintenance
Integrated Process: Teaching/Learning
Content Area: Pharmacology

Reference:

Hodgson, B., & Kizior, R. (2004). *Saunders nursing drug handbook 2004.* Philadelphia: Saunders, p. 491.

---

137. A client with diabetes mellitus has received instructions about foot care. Which statement by the client would indicate that the client needs further instructions?

1 "The best time to cut my nails is after bathing."

2 "Cotton stockings should be worn to absorb excess moisture."

3 "The cuticles of my nails must be cut to prevent overgrowth."

4 "My feet should be inspected daily using a mirror."

Answer: 3

Rationale: Trimming or cutting the cuticles of the nails can lead to injury to the foot by scratching the skin. Even small injuries can be dangerous to the client with diabetes mellitus who has decreased peripheral vascular circulation. A manicure stick can be used to gently push the cuticle back under the nail. Nails can be cut straight across, and after a bath is the best time because the nails are softest. White, cotton stockings are best, and the client needs to inspect the feet daily.

Test-Taking Strategy: Use the process of elimination, noting the key words "needs further instructions." These words indicate a false-response question and that you need to select the incorrect client statement. Look for the option that could result in altered skin integrity. Using this principle, eliminate options 1, 2, and 4. Review diabetic foot care if you had difficulty with this question.

Level of Cognitive Ability: Analysis
Client Needs: Health Promotion and Maintenance

Integrated Process: Teaching/Learning
Content Area: Adult Health/Endocrine

Reference:
Ignatavicius, D., & Workman, M. (2002). *Medical surgical nursing: Critical thinking for collaborative care* (4th ed.). Philadelphia: Saunders, p. 1473.

---

138. A nurse has taught a client about the signs and symptoms and treatment of hyperglycemia. Which statement by the client reflects an accurate understanding?
1 "I may become diaphoretic and faint."
2 "I need to take an extra diabetic pill if my blood glucose is greater than 300."
3 "I may notice signs of fatigue, dry skin, and increased urination and thirst."
4 "I should restrict my fluid intake if my blood glucose is greater than 250 mg."

Answer: 3
Rationale: Fatigue, dry skin, polyuria, and polydipsia are classic symptoms of hyperglycemia. Fatigue occurs because of lack of energy from inability of the body to utilize glucose. Dry skin occurs secondary to dehydration related to the polyuria. Polydipsia occurs secondary to fluid loss. Diaphoresis is associated with hypoglycemia. Clients should not take extraoral hypoglycemic agents to reduce an elevated blood glucose level. A client with hyperglycemia becomes dehydrated secondary to the osmotic effect of elevated glucose; therefore, the client must increase fluid intake.

Test-Taking Strategy: Note the key words "reflects an understanding" and focus on the issue: hyperglycemia. Recalling that polyuria and polydipsia are signs of hyperglycemia will direct you to option 3. Review these signs if you had difficulty with this question.

Level of Cognitive Ability: Analysis
Client Needs: Health Promotion and Maintenance
Integrated Process: Nursing Process/Evaluation
Content Area: Adult Health/Endocrine

Reference:
Ignatavicius, D., & Workman, M. (2002). *Medical surgical nursing: Critical thinking for collaborative care* (4th ed.). Philadelphia: Saunders, p. 188.

---

139. A client taking famotidine (Pepcid) asks the home care nurse what would be the best medication to take for a headache. The nurse tells the client that it would be best to take:
1 Aspirin (acetylsalicylic acid, ASA)
2 Ibuprofen (Motrin)
3 Acetaminophen (Tylenol)
4 Naproxen (Naprosyn)

Answer: 3
Rationale: The client is taking famotidine, a histamine receptor antagonist. This implies that the client has a disorder characterized by gastrointestinal (GI) irritation. The only medication of the ones listed in the options that is not irritating to the GI tract is acetaminophen. The other medications could aggravate an already existing GI problem.

Test-Taking Strategy: Note the medication that the client is taking. Recalling that this medication is used for GI irritation will direct you to option 3. Also note that options 1, 2, and 4 are similar and are antiinflammatory medications. Review these medications if you had difficulty with this question.

Level of Cognitive Ability: Application
Client Needs: Health Promotion and Maintenance
Integrated Process: Teaching/Learning
Content Area: Pharmacology

References:
Hodgson, B., & Kizior, R. (2004). *Saunders nursing drug handbook 2004.* Philadelphia: Saunders, pp. 7-9;397.
McKenry, L., & Salerno, E. (2003). *Mosby's pharmacology in nursing* (21st ed.). St. Louis: Mosby, pp. 772-773.

140. A nurse is teaching the client taking cyclosporine (Sandimmune) after renal transplant about the medication. The nurse tells the client to be especially alert for:
1 Signs of infection
2 Hypotension
3 Weight loss
4 Hair loss

Answer: 1
Rationale: Cyclosporine is an immunosuppressant medication used to prevent transplant rejection. The client should be especially alert for signs and symptoms of infection while taking this medication, and report them to the physician if experienced. The client is also taught about other side effects of the medication, including hypertension, increased facial hair, tremors, gingival hyperplasia, and gastrointestinal complaints.

Test-Taking Strategy: Recalling that cyclosporine is an immunosuppressant, and that the client is at risk for infection while taking this medication, will direct you to option 1. Review this information if you had difficulty with this question because this is a major concern with transplant medication therapy.

Level of Cognitive Ability: Application
Client Needs: Health Promotion and Maintenance
Integrated Process: Teaching/Learning
Content Area: Pharmacology

Reference:
Hodgson, B., & Kizior, R. (2004). *Saunders nursing drug handbook 2004.* Philadelphia: Saunders, p. 259.

141. A client has undergone surgery for glaucoma. The nurse provides which discharge instruction to the client?
1 Wound healing usually takes 12 weeks
2 Expect that vision will be permanently impaired
3 A shield or eye patch should be worn to protect the eye
4 The sutures are removed after one week

Answer: 3
Rationale: After ocular surgery, the client should wear an eye patch or eyeglasses for protection of the eye. Healing takes place in about 6 weeks. Once the postoperative inflammation subsides, the client's vision should return to the preoperative level of acuity. Sutures are usually absorbable.

Test-Taking Strategy: Use the process of elimination, focusing on the issue: ocular surgery. Recalling that the eye requires protection after surgery will direct you to option 3. Review postoperative teaching points following eye surgery if you had difficulty with this question.

Level of Cognitive Ability: Application
Client Needs: Health Promotion and Maintenance
Integrated Process: Teaching/Learning
Content Area: Adult Health/Eye

Reference:
Phipps, W., Monahan, F., Sands, J., Marek, J., & Neighbors, M. (2003). *Medical-surgical nursing: health and illness perspectives* (7th ed.). St. Louis: Mosby, p. 1896.

142. A client has undergone surgery for cataracts. The nurse instructs the client to call the physician for which of the following complaints?
1 A sudden decrease in vision
2 Eye pain relieved by acetaminophen (Tylenol)
3 Small amounts of dried matter on the eyelashes after sleep
4 Gradual resolution of eye redness

Answer: 1

Rationale: The client should report a noticeable or sudden decrease in vision to the physician. The client is taught to take acetaminophen, which is usually effective in relieving discomfort. The eye may be slightly reddened postoperatively, but this should gradually resolve. Small amounts of dried material may be present on the lashes after sleep. This is expected and should be removed with a warm facecloth.

Test-Taking Strategy: Use the process of elimination, noting the key words "call the physician." Noting the words "sudden decrease" in option 1 will direct you to this option. Review home care instructions following eye surgery if you had difficulty with this question.

Level of Cognitive Ability: Application
Client Needs: Health Promotion and Maintenance
Integrated Process: Teaching/Learning
Content Area: Adult Health/Eye

Reference:
Phipps, W., Monahan, F., Sands, J., Marek, J., & Neighbors, M. (2003). *Medical-surgical nursing: Health and illness perspectives* (7th ed.). St. Louis: Mosby, p. 1897.

143. A home care nurse visits a client with a diagnosis of cirrhosis and ascites. The nurse provides dietary instructions and tells the client to:
1 Maintain a low-calorie diet
2 Decrease carbohydrate intake
3 Restrict calories to 1500 daily
4 Restrict sodium intake

Answer: 4

Rationale: If the client has ascites, sodium and possibly fluids should be restricted in the diet. Total daily calories should range between 2000 and 3000. The diet should supply sufficient carbohydrates to maintain weight and spare protein. The diet should provide ample protein to rebuild tissue but not enough protein to precipitate hepatic encephalopathy.

Test-Taking Strategy: Focus on the client's diagnosis: cirrhosis and ascites. Recalling that ascites indicates the accumulation of fluid will direct you to option 4. Review dietary measures for the client with cirrhosis and ascites if you had difficulty with this question.

Level of Cognitive Ability: Analysis
Client Needs: Health Promotion and Maintenance
Integrated Process: Teaching/Learning
Content Area: Adult Health/Gastrointestinal

Reference:
Phipps, W., Monahan, F., Sands, J., Marek, J., & Neighbors, M. (2003). *Medical-surgical nursing: Health and illness perspectives* (7th ed.). St. Louis: Mosby, pp. 1168; 1171.

144. A nurse is preparing a client with a diagnosis of multiple myeloma for discharge. The nurse tells the client to:

1 Restrict fluid intake to 1500 mL daily
2 Maintain bed rest
3 Maintain a high-calorie, low-fiber diet
4 Notify the physician if anorexia and nausea occurs and persists

Answer: 4

Rationale: Clients with multiple myeloma need to be taught to monitor for signs of hypercalcemia and to report them immediately to the physician. Anorexia, nausea, vomiting, polyuria, weakness and fatigue, constipation, and signs of dehydration are signs of moderate hypercalcemia. A fluid intake of 3000 mL daily is required to dilute the calcium overload and prevent protein from precipitating in the renal tubules. Activity is encouraged. Although a high-calorie diet is encouraged, a low-fiber diet can lead to constipation.

Test-Taking Strategy: Recall that hypercalcemia is a concern in multiple myeloma. Eliminate option 2 because bed rest will promote hypercalcemia. Next eliminate option 1 because this amount of fluid is rather low. Finally, eliminate option 3 because a low-fiber diet can lead to constipation. Review the signs of hypercalcemia if you had difficulty in selecting the correct option.

Level of Cognitive Ability: Analysis
Client Needs: Health Promotion and Maintenance
Integrated Process: Nursing Process/Implementation
Content Area: Adult Health/Oncology

Reference:
Phipps, W., Monahan, F., Sands, J., Marek, J., & Neighbors, M. (2003). *Medical-surgical nursing: Health and illness perspectives* (7th ed.). St. Louis: Mosby, pp. 1629-1632.

145. A nurse provides discharge instructions to the client who had a mastectomy and axillary lymph node dissection. The nurse tells the client to:

1 Avoid the use of insect repellent
2 Cut cuticles on the nails carefully using clean cuticle scissors
3 Wear protective gloves when doing the dishes
4 Avoid the use of lanolin hand cream on the affected arm

Answer: 3

Rationale: Following axillary node dissection, the affected arm may swell and is less able to fight infection. The client needs to be instructed in the several measures required to prevent complications. The client should use insect repellent to avoid bites and stings. Picking at or cutting cuticles should not be done because this could cause an alteration in skin integrity resulting in infection. Lanolin hand cream should be applied a few times daily. Protective gloves should be worn while doing dishes and cleaning.

Test-Taking Strategy: Note the client's diagnosis and focus on the issue: preventing altered skin integrity and thus infection. Keeping this in mind will assist in eliminating options 1, 2, and 4, which could potentially lead to a skin alteration. Review the client teaching points related to mastectomy and lymph node dissection if you had difficulty with this question.

Level of Cognitive Ability: Application
Client Needs: Health Promotion and Maintenance
Integrated Process: Teaching/Learning
Content Area: Adult Health/Oncology

References:
Black, J., & Hawks, J. (2005). *Medical-surgical nursing: Clinical management for positive outcomes* (7th ed.). Philadelphia: Saunders, p. 1106.
Ignatavicius, D., & Workman, M. (2002). *Medical surgical nursing: Critical thinking for collaborative care* (4th ed.). Philadelphia: Saunders, p. 1745.

146. A camp nurse provides instructions regarding skin protection from the sun to the parents who are preparing their children for a camping adventure. The nurse determines that further instructions are needed if a parent states:
1 To obtain sunscreen for use
2 That sunscreen will not be required on cloudy days
3 To pack a hat, long-sleeved shirt, and long pants for the child
4 To select tightly woven materials for greater protection from sun rays

Answer: 2
Rationale: The sun's rays are as damaging to the skin on cloudy, hazy days as they are on sunny days. Sunscreens are recommended and should be applied before exposure to the sun and reapplied frequently and liberally at least every 2 hours. A hat, long-sleeved shirt, and long pants should be worn when out in the sun. Tightly woven materials provide greater protection from the sun's rays.

Test-Taking Strategy: Note the key words "further instructions are needed." These words indicate a false-response question and that you need to select the incorrect parent statement. Recalling the concept that ultraviolet rays can be damaging regardless of cloudiness or haziness will assist in directing you to option 2. Also, eliminate options 1, 3, and 4 because these measures provide the greatest protection from the sun. Review guidelines that protect the skin from the damaging rays of the sun if you had difficulty with this question.

Level of Cognitive Ability: Application
Client Needs: Health Promotion and Maintenance
Integrated Process: Teaching/Learning
Content Area: Fundamental Skills

References:
Black, J., & Hawks, J. (2005). *Medical-surgical nursing: Clinical management for positive outcomes* (7th ed.). Philadelphia: Saunders, pp. 21; 1413.
Lewis, S., Heitkemper, M., & Dirksen, S. (2004). *Medical-surgical nursing: Assessment and management of clinical problems* (6th ed.). St. Louis: Mosby, pp. 487-488.

147. A client is receiving a course of chemotherapy on an outpatient basis for the diagnosis of lung cancer. Which home care instruction would the nurse provide to the client?
1 A bathroom can be shared with any member of the family.
2 Urinary and bowel excreta is not considered contaminated.
3 Disposable plates and plastic utensils must be used during the entire course of chemotherapy.
4 Contaminated linens should be washed separately and then washed a second time if necessary.

Answer: 4
Rationale: The client may excrete the chemotherapeutic agent for 48 hours or more after administration, depending on the medication administered. Blood, emesis, and excreta may be considered contaminated during this time. The client should not share a bathroom with children or pregnant women during this time. Any contaminated linens or clothing should be washed separately and then washed a second time if necessary. All contaminated disposable items should be sealed in plastic bags and disposed of as hazardous waste.

Test-Taking Strategy: Use the process of elimination. Eliminate options 1 and 2 first because they are similar. Eliminate option 3 next because it would seem unreasonable to have to use disposable utensils for the "entire" course of therapy. Also note the absolute word "must" in this option. Review client teaching points related to chemotherapy if you had difficulty with this question.

Level of Cognitive Ability: Application
Client Needs: Health Promotion and Maintenance
Integrated Process: Teaching/Learning
Content Area: Adult Health/Oncology

References:
Black, J., & Hawks, J. (2005). *Medical-surgical nursing: Clinical management for positive outcomes* (7th ed.). Philadelphia: Saunders, pp. 374-375.
Phipps, W., Monahan, F., Sands, J., Marek, J., & Neighbors, M. (2003). *Medical-surgical nursing: Health and illness perspectives* (7th ed.). St. Louis: Mosby, pp. 346; 350-351.

---

148. A home care nurse visits a client with bowel cancer who recently received a course of chemotherapy. The client has developed stomatitis, and the nurse provides instructions to the client about care of the mouth. The nurse determines that the client needs further instructions if the client states to:

1 Drink foods and liquids that are cold
2 Eat foods without spices
3 Maintain a diet of soft foods
4 Drink juices that are not citrus

Answer: 1

Rationale: Stomatitis is a term used to describe inflammation and ulceration of the mucosal lining of the mouth. Dietary modifications for this condition include avoiding extremely hot or cold foods, spices, and citrus fruits and juices. The client should be instructed to eat soft foods and take nutritional supplements as prescribed.

Test-Taking Strategy: Note the word "needs further instructions" in the stem of the question. These words indicate a false-response question and that you need to select the incorrect client statement. Recalling that stomatitis is an inflammation of the mucosal lining of the mouth will assist in eliminating options 2, 3, and 4, because these measures will alleviate further irritation and prevent discomfort. Review client teaching points for stomatitis if you had difficulty with this question.

Level of Cognitive Ability: Application
Client Needs: Health Promotion and Maintenance
Integrated Process: Teaching/Learning
Content Area: Adult Health/Oncology

References:
Black, J., & Hawks, J. (2005). *Medical-surgical nursing: Clinical management for positive outcomes* (7th ed.). Philadelphia: Saunders, p. 386.
Phipps, W., Monahan, F., Sands, J., Marek, J., & Neighbors, M. (2003). *Medical-surgical nursing: Health and illness perspectives* (7th ed.). St. Louis: Mosby, pp. 353; 1806.

---

149. A home care nurse provides instructions to a breast-feeding postpartum client who has developed breast engorgement. The nurse tells the mother to:

1 Feed the infant less frequently, every 4 to 6 hours, using bottle feeding in between
2 Apply cool packs to both breasts 20 minutes before a feeding
3 Avoid the use of a bra during engorgement
4 Gently massage the breast from the outer areas to the nipple during feeding

Answer: 4

Rationale: The client with breast engorgement should be advised to feed frequently, at least every 2 1/2 hours for 15 to 20 minutes per side. Moist heat should be applied to both breasts for about 20 minutes before a feeding. Between feedings, the mother should wear a supportive bra. During a feeding, it is helpful to gently massage the breast from the outer areas to the nipple to stimulate the letdown and flow of milk.

Test-Taking Strategy: Note the client's diagnosis. Think about the manifestations that occur with engorgement and recall that measures are initiated to facilitate the flow of milk. With this concept in mind, eliminate options 1, 2, and 3 because they will not facilitate the flow of milk. Review the measures used for breast engorgement if you had difficulty with this question.

Level of Cognitive Ability: Application
Client Needs: Health Promotion and Maintenance

Integrated Process: Teaching/Learning
Content Area: Maternity/Postpartum

Reference:
Lowdermilk, D., & Perry, A. (2004). *Maternity & women's health care* (8th ed.). St. Louis: Mosby, p. 777.

---

150. A client in the third trimester of pregnancy arrives at the clinic and tells the nurse that she frequently has a backache. Which instruction would the nurse provide to the client to alleviate the backache?
1 Sleep in a supine position and on a firm mattress
2 Perform pelvic rock exercises
3 Eat small meals frequently
4 Elevate the legs when sitting

Answer: 2
Rationale: To provide relief from backache, the nurse would advise the client to use good posture and body mechanics, perform pelvic rock exercises, and to wear flat supportive shoes. The client may also be advised to wear a maternity girdle, avoid overexertion, and sleep in the lateral position on a firm mattress. Back massage is also helpful. Eating small meals would more specifically assist in the relief of dyspnea. Leg elevation assists the client with varicosities.

Test-Taking Strategy: Use the process of elimination, keeping in mind that the issue of the question is backache. This should assist in eliminating options 3 and 4 because they are unrelated to the relief of backache. From the remaining options, recalling that the lateral position is most appropriate for the pregnant client will assist in directing you to option 2. Review relief measures for backache if you had difficulty with this question.

Level of Cognitive Ability: Application
Client Needs: Health Promotion and Maintenance
Integrated Process: Teaching/Learning
Content Area: Maternity/Antepartum

Reference:
Lowdermilk, D., & Perry, A. (2004). *Maternity & women's health care* (8th ed.). St. Louis: Mosby, pp. 425; 427; 428.

---

151. A nurse provides dietary instructions to the client receiving spironolactone (Aldactone). Which food item would the nurse instruct the client to avoid while taking this medication?
1 Crackers
2 Shrimp
3 Apricots
4 Popcorn

Answer: 3
Rationale: Spironolactone is a potassium-sparing diuretic, and the client needs to avoid foods high in potassium, such as whole-grain cereals, legumes, meat, bananas, apricots, orange juice, potatoes, and raisins. Option 3 provides the highest source of potassium and should be avoided.

Test-Taking Strategy: Use the process of elimination and note the key word "avoid." Recall that this medication is a potassium-sparing diuretic. Eliminate options 1 and 4 because they are food items that are similar. Remembering that fruits, vegetables, and fresh meats are high in potassium will direct you to option 3 as the food to avoid. Review this medication if you had difficulty with this question.

Level of Cognitive Ability: Application
Client Needs: Health Promotion and Maintenance
Integrated Process: Teaching/Learning
Content Area: Pharmacology

References:
Hodgson, B., & Kizior, R. (2004). *Saunders nursing drug handbook 2004.* Philadelphia: Saunders, p. 931.
McKenry, L., & Salerno, E. (2003). *Mosby's pharmacology in nursing* (21st ed.). St. Louis: Mosby, pp. 678-679.

---

152. Oral lactulose (Chronulac) is prescribed for a client with a hepatic disorder, and the home care nurse provides instructions to the client regarding the medication. The nurse determines that the client needs additional instructions if the client states to:

1 Take the medication with water
2 Increase fluid intake
3 Increase fiber in the diet
4 Notify the physician immediately if nausea occurs

Answer: 4

Rationale: Lactulose retains ammonia in the colon and promotes increased peristalsis and bowel evacuation, expelling ammonia from the colon. It should be taken with water or juice to aid in softening the stool. An increased fluid intake and a high-fiber diet will promote defecation. If nausea occurs, the client should be instructed to drink cola or eat unsalted crackers or dry toast. Notifying the physician immediately is not necessary.

Test-Taking Strategy: Use the process of elimination, noting the key word "needs additional instructions." These words indicate a false-response question and that you need to select the incorrect client statement. Eliminate options 1, 2, and 3 because they are similar in that they will promote defecation. Also recall that measures can be provided to the client to relieve nausea before notifying the physician. Review client teaching points related to this medication if you had difficulty with question.

Level of Cognitive Ability: Application
Client Needs: Health Promotion and Maintenance
Integrated Process: Teaching/Learning
Content Area: Pharmacology

Reference:
McKenry, L., & Salerno, E. (2003). *Mosby's pharmacology in nursing* (21st ed.). St. Louis: Mosby, p. 780.

---

153. A client with leukemia receives a course of chemotherapy. The home care nurse scheduled to visit the client receives a telephone call from the client's physician. The physician informs the nurse that the neutrophil count is 600/mm^3. Based on this laboratory value, the home care nurse tells the client to avoid doing which of the following?

1 Eating any raw fruits or vegetables
2 Taking aspirin or medications containing aspirin
3 Straining at bowel movements
4 Using a straight razor for shaving

Answer: 1

Rationale: Neutrophil counts should range between 3000 to 5800/mm^3. A low neutrophil count places the client at risk for infection. When the client is at risk for infection, the client should avoid exposure to individuals with colds or infections. All live plants, flowers, or objects that may harbor bacteria should be removed from the client's environment. The client should be on a low-bacteria diet and avoid eating any raw fruits and vegetables. Options 2, 3, and 4 are measures that would be implemented if the client was at risk for bleeding.

Test-Taking Strategy: Use the process of elimination. Recalling that a low neutrophil count places the client at risk for infection will direct you to option 1. Also, bearing in mind that the issue of the question relates to infection will assist in eliminating options 2, 3, and 4, because these options identify measures that reduce the risk of bleeding. Review care of the client with a low neutrophil count if you had difficulty with this question.

Level of Cognitive Ability: Application
Client Needs: Health Promotion and Maintenance

Integrated Process: Teaching/Learning
Content Area: Adult Health/Oncology

Reference:
Phipps, W., Monahan, F., Sands, J., Marek, J., & Neighbors, M. (2003). *Medical-surgical nursing: health and illness perspectives* (7th ed.). St. Louis: Mosby, p. 846.

---

154. A nurse provides instructions to the client who received cryosurgery for a local stage 0 cervical tumor. The nurse tells the client:
1 To call the physician if a watery discharge occurs
2 To call the physician if the discharge remains odorous after 1 week
3 To avoid tub baths
4 That pain indicates a complication of the procedure

Answer: 3
Rationale: Mild pain may occur and continue for several days following this procedure. A clear, watery discharge is expected. For about 14 days, this is followed by discharge containing debris, which may be odorous. If the discharge continues longer than 8 weeks, an infection is suspected. Healing takes about 10 weeks. Showers or sponge baths should be taken during this time. Tub baths and sitz baths need to be avoided.

Test-Taking Strategy: Use the process of elimination. Think about the anatomical area of the body in terms of where this procedure is performed. It would seem likely that the client would be instructed to avoid tub baths following this procedure. Review teaching points related to this procedure if you had difficulty with this question.

Level of Cognitive Ability: Application
Client Needs: Health Promotion and Maintenance
Integrated Process: Teaching/Learning
Content Area: Adult Health/Oncology

Reference:
Black, J., & Hawks, J. (2005). *Medical-surgical nursing: Clinical management for positive outcomes* (7th ed.). Philadelphia: Saunders, p. 1076.

---

155. A home care nurse provides instructions to the client taking digoxin (Lanoxin) 0.25 mg daily. Which client statement would indicate a need for further instructions?
1 "I will take my prescribed antacid if I become nauseated."
2 "It is important to have my blood drawn when prescribed."
3 "I will check my pulse before I take my medication."
4 "I will carry a medication identification (ID) card with me."

Answer: 1
Rationale: Digoxin is an antidysrhythmic. The most common early manifestations of toxicity are gastrointestinal (GI) disturbances, such as anorexia, nausea, and vomiting. Digoxin blood levels need to be obtained as prescribed to monitor for therapeutic plasma levels (0.5 to 2.0 ng/mL). The client is instructed to take the pulse, hold the medication if the pulse is below 60 beats per minute, and notify the physician. The client is instructed to wear or carry an ID bracelet or card.

Test-Taking Strategy: Use the process of elimination, recalling that toxicity can occur with the use of this medication. Also, note the key words, "a need for further instructions." These words indicate a false-response question and that you need to select the incorrect client statement. Remembering that GI disturbances are the earliest signs of digoxin toxicity will assist in directing you to option 1. Review this medication if you had difficulty with this question.

Level of Cognitive Ability: Analysis
Client Needs: Health Promotion and Maintenance

Integrated Process: Teaching/Learning
Content Area: Pharmacology

Reference:

Hodgson, B., & Kizior, R. (2004). *Saunders nursing drug handbook 2004.* Philadelphia: Saunders, p. 310-311.

---

156. A nurse is providing immediate postprocedure care to a client who had a thoracentesis to relieve a tension pneumothorax that resulted from rib fractures. The goal is that the client will exhibit normal respiratory functioning. The nurse provides instructions to assist the client toward this goal. Which statement by the client indicates that further instructions are needed?

1 "I will let you know at once if I have trouble breathing."

2 "I will lie on the affected side for an hour."

3 "I can expect a chest x-ray to be done shortly."

4 "I will notify you if I feel a crackling sensation on my chest."

Answer: 2

Rationale: After the procedure, the client is usually turned onto the unaffected side for 1 hour to facilitate lung expansion. Tachypnea, dyspnea, cyanosis, retractions, or diminished breath sounds, which may indicate pneumothorax, should be reported to the physician. A chest x-ray may be performed to evaluate the degree of lung reexpansion or pneumothorax. Subcutaneous emphysema may follow this procedure, because air in the pleural cavity leaks into subcutaneous tissues. The tissues feel like lumpy paper and crackle when palpated (crepitus). Usually subcutaneous emphysema causes no problems unless it is increasing and constricting vital organs, such as the trachea.

Test-Taking Strategy: Note the key words "further instructions are needed." These words indicate a false-response question and that you need to select the incorrect client statement. Focus on the issue, postprocedure care following thoracentesis, and recall that facilitating lung expansion is important. Noting the words "affected side" in option 2 will direct you to this option. Review postprocedure care for a thoracentesis if you had difficulty with this question.

Level of Cognitive Ability: Analysis
Client Needs: Health Promotion and Maintenance
Integrated Process: Teaching/Learning
Content Area: Adult Health/Respiratory

Reference:

Chernecky, C., & Berger, B. (2004). *Laboratory tests and diagnostic procedures* (4th ed.). Philadelphia: Saunders, p. 1043.

---

157. An older client with coronary artery disease is scheduled for hospital discharge and lives alone. The client states "I don't know how I'll be able to remember all these instructions and take care of myself once I get home." The nurse plans which of the following actions to assist the client?

1 Ask an out-of-town relative to stay with the client for a day or so

2 Ask the physician to delay the discharge until the client is better able to manage self-care

3 Ask the social worker to follow up with a telephone call after discharge to ensure the client is progressing

4 Ask the physician for a referral to a home health agency for nursing and home health aide support

Answer: 4

Rationale: With earlier hospital discharge, clients may require support from a home health agency until they are independent in functioning. Option 1 does not ensure that the client will receive continued care until able to be independent in managing own care. Option 3 does nothing to actively assist the client, and option 2 is not realistic in the current health care environment. Option 4 is the method of ensuring that the client has necessary assistance for as long as required.

Test-Taking Strategy: Use the process of elimination, focusing on the key words "lives alone." Note that option 4 is the umbrella (global) option and ensures client assistance at home. Review home care resources following hospital discharge if you had difficulty with this question.

Level of Cognitive Ability: Application
Client Needs: Health Promotion and Maintenance

Integrated Process: Nursing Process/Planning
Content Area: Fundamental Skills

References:
Black, J., & Hawks, J. (2005). *Medical-surgical nursing: Clinical management for positive outcomes* (7th ed.). Philadelphia: Saunders, pp. 170; 173.
Potter, P., & Perry, A. (2005). *Fundamentals of nursing* (6th ed.). St. Louis: Mosby, p. 36.

---

158. A client who has been newly diagnosed with angina pectoris asks the nurse how to prevent future angina attacks. The nurse plans to incorporate which instruction in a teaching session?
1 Eat fewer, larger meals for more efficient digestion
2 Plan all activities for early in the morning, when the client is most rested
3 Adjust medication doses freely until symptoms do not recur
4 Dress appropriately in very cold or very hot weather

Answer: 4
Rationale: Anginal episodes are triggered by events such as eating heavy meals, straining during bowel movements, smoking, overexertion, and experiencing emotional upset, or temperature extremes. Medication therapy is monitored and regulated by the physician.

Test-Taking Strategy: Use the process of elimination, focusing on the issue: preventing angina attacks. Recalling the causes of chest pain and principles of medication therapy will direct you to option 4. Review teaching points for the client with angina if you had difficulty with this question.

Level of Cognitive Ability: Application
Client Needs: Health Promotion and Maintenance
Integrated Process: Teaching/Learning
Content Area: Adult Health/Cardiovascular

References:
Black, J., & Hawks, J. (2005). *Medical-surgical nursing: Clinical management for positive outcomes* (7th ed.). Philadelphia: Saunders, p. 1706.
Lewis, S., Heitkemper, M., & Dirksen, S. (2004). *Medical-surgical nursing: Assessment and management of clinical problems* (6th ed.). St. Louis: Mosby, p. 828.

---

159. A nurse has performed a nutritional assessment on a client with cystitis. The nurse tells the client to consume which of the following beverages to minimize recurrence of cystitis?
1 Coffee
2 Tea
3 Water
4 White wine

Answer: 3
Rationale: Caffeine and alcohol can irritate the bladder. Therefore, alcohol and caffeine-containing beverages such as coffee, tea, and cocoa are avoided to minimize risk. Water helps flush bacteria out of the bladder, and an intake of 6 to 8 glasses per day is encouraged.

Test-Taking Strategy: Use the process of elimination. Option 4 is eliminated first, because alcohol intake is not encouraged for any disorder. Options 1 and 2 are similar in that they both contain caffeine. Thus, it is unlikely that either of these are correct options. Review client teaching points related to preventing cystitis if you had difficulty with this question.

Level of Cognitive Ability: Application
Client Needs: Health Promotion and Maintenance
Integrated Process: Teaching/Learning
Content Area: Adult Health/Renal

References:

Black, J., & Hawks, J. (2005). *Medical-surgical nursing: Clinical management for positive outcomes* (7th ed.). Philadelphia: Saunders, p. 792.

Lewis, S., Heitkemper, M., & Dirksen, S. (2004). *Medical-surgical nursing: Assessment and management of clinical problems* (6th ed.). St. Louis: Mosby, p. 1175.

---

160. A home care nurse has given instructions to a female client with cystitis about measures to prevent recurrence. The nurse determines that the client needs further instructions if the client verbalizes to:

1 Take bubble baths for more effective hygiene

2 Wear underwear made of cotton or with cotton panels

3 Drink a glass of water and void after intercourse

4 Avoid wearing pantyhose while wearing slacks

Answer: 1

Rationale: Measures to prevent cystitis include increasing fluid intake to 3 liters per day; eating an acid-ash diet; wiping front to back after urination; taking showers instead of tub baths; drinking water and voiding after intercourse; avoiding bubble baths, feminine hygiene sprays, or perfumed toilet tissue or sanitary pads; and wearing clothes that "breathe" (cotton pants, no tight jeans, no pantyhose under slacks). Other measures include teaching pregnant women to void every 2 hours and teaching menopausal women to use estrogen vaginal creams to restore vaginal pH.

Test-Taking Strategy: Note the key words "needs further instructions." These words indicate a false-response question and that you need to select the incorrect client statement. Eliminate option 3 first, knowing that drinking water is a basic measure to prevent cystitis. Next, eliminate options 2 and 4 because they are similar. Review teaching measures to prevent cystitis if you had difficulty with this question.

Level of Cognitive Ability: Analysis
Client Needs: Health Promotion and Maintenance
Integrated Process: Teaching/Learning
Content Area: Adult Health/Renal

Reference:

Lewis, S., Heitkemper, M., & Dirksen, S. (2004). *Medical-surgical nursing: Assessment and management of clinical problems* (6th ed.). St. Louis: Mosby, p. 1177.

---

161. A client with pyelonephritis is being discharged from the hospital. The nurse provides the client with discharge instructions to prevent recurrence. The nurse determines that the client understands the information that was given if the client states an intention to:

1 Report signs and symptoms of urinary tract infection (UTI) if they persist for more than one week

2 Take the prescribed antibiotics until all symptoms subside

3 Return to the physician's office for scheduled follow-up urine cultures

4 Modify fluid intake for the day based on the previous day's output

Answer: 3

Rationale: The client with pyelonephritis should take the full course of antibiotic therapy that has been prescribed and return to the physician's office for follow-up urine cultures if so instructed. The client should learn the signs and symptoms of UTI, and report them immediately if they occur. The client should use all measures that are used to prevent cystitis, which includes consuming fluids up to 3 liters per day.

Test-Taking Strategy: Use the process of elimination. Eliminate option 1 because UTI symptoms should never go unreported for a week. Option 2 is eliminated next because antibiotics should be taken for the full course of treatment for adequate elimination of the infection. From the remaining options, recalling the importance of increased fluids will direct you to option 3. Review client teaching points related to pyelonephritis if you had difficulty with this question.

Level of Cognitive Ability: Analysis
Client Needs: Health Promotion and Maintenance
Integrated Process: Nursing Process/Evaluation
Content Area: Adult Health/Renal

Reference:
Black, J., & Hawks, J. (2005). *Medical-surgical nursing: Clinical management for positive outcomes* (7th ed.). Philadelphia: Saunders, p. 920.

---

162. A client with nephrotic syndrome needs dietary teaching about how diet can help counteract the effects of altered renal function. The nurse plans to include which of the following statements in instructions to the client?
1 "Plan to drink at least 12 glasses of water a day."
2 "Add salt during cooking to replace sodium lost in the urine."
3 "Increase your intake of fish, meat, and eggs."
4 "Increase your intake of fatty foods to prevent protein loss."

Answer: 3
Rationale: The diet in nephrotic syndrome is limited in sodium. This is done to help control edema, which is a predominant part of the clinical picture. Fluids are not limited unless hyponatremia is present. On the other hand, the client is not encouraged to force fluids. Protein is increased, unless the glomerular filtration rate is impaired. This helps replace protein lost in the urine and ultimately also helps in controlling edema. A part of the clinical picture in nephrotic syndrome is hyperlipidemia, which results from the liver's synthesis of lipoproteins in response to hypoalbuminemia. Increasing fatty food intake would not be helpful in this circumstance.

Test-Taking Strategy: Use the process of elimination. Recalling that nephrotic syndrome is characterized by fluid retention and hypoalbuminemia will eliminate options 1 and 2. From the remaining options, knowing that hyperlipidemia accompanies this disorder will direct you to option 3. Review home care instructions for the client with nephrotic syndrome if you had difficulty with this question.

Level of Cognitive Ability: Application
Client Needs: Health Promotion and Maintenance
Integrated Process: Teaching/Learning
Content Area: Adult Health/Renal

Reference:
Black, J., & Hawks, J. (2005). *Medical-surgical nursing: Clinical management for positive outcomes* (7th ed.). Philadelphia: Saunders, p. 926.

---

163. A nurse is giving the client with polycystic kidney disease instructions in replacing elements lost in the urine as a result of impaired kidney function. The nurse instructs the client to increase intake of which of the following in the diet?
1 Sodium and potassium
2 Sodium and water
3 Water and phosphorus
4 Calcium and phosphorus

Answer: 2
Rationale: Clients with polycystic kidney disease waste sodium rather than retain it, and therefore need an increase in sodium and water in the diet. Potassium, calcium, and phosphorus need no special attention.

Test-Taking Strategy: Use the process of elimination. Recalling that this disorder causes sodium (not phosphorus) to be wasted will assist you in eliminating options 3 and 4. From the remaining options, recall that when the kidney excretes sodium, water is carried with it. This will direct you to option 2. Review care of the client with polycystic kidney disease if you had difficulty with this question.

Level of Cognitive Ability: Application
Client Needs: Health Promotion and Maintenance
Integrated Process: Teaching/Learning
Content Area: Adult Health/Renal

Reference:

Black, J., & Hawks, J. (2005). *Medical-surgical nursing: Clinical management for positive outcomes* (7th ed.). Philadelphia: Saunders, p. 938.

---

164. A client with acquired immunodeficiency syndrome (AIDS) is being treated for tuberculosis with isoniazid (INH). The nurse plans to teach the client which of the following regarding the administration of the medication?

1 Administer with an antacid to prevent gastrointestinal (GI) distress

2 Administer at least 1 hour before administering an aluminum-containing antacid to prevent a medication interaction

3 Administer with food to prevent rapid absorption of INH

4 Administer with a corticosteroid to potentiate the effects of INH

Answer: 2

Rationale: Aluminum hydroxide, a common ingredient in antacids, significantly decreases INH absorption. INH should be administered at least 1 hour before aluminum-containing antacids. Food affects the rate of absorption of rifampin (Rifadin), not INH. INH administration with a corticosteroid decreases INH's effects and increases the corticosteroids effects.

Test-Taking Strategy: Recall the general principles related to medication administration. In general, you would not usually administer a medication with an antacid because it would decrease absorption of the medication. Remembering this principle will direct you to the correct option. Review this medication to treat tuberculosis if you had difficulty with this question.

Level of Cognitive Ability: Application
Client Needs: Health Promotion and Maintenance
Integrated Process: Teaching/Learning
Content Area: Adult Health/Immune

Reference:

Hodgson, B., & Kizior, R. (2004). *Saunders nursing drug handbook 2004.* Philadelphia: Saunders, p. 560.

---

165. A nurse has provided dietary instructions to a client to minimize the risk of osteoporosis. The nurse determines that the client understands the recommended changes if the client verbalized to increase intake of which foods?

1 Rice

2 Yogurt

3 Sardines

4 Chicken

Answer: 2

Rationale: Calcium intake is encouraged to minimize the risk of osteoporosis. The major dietary source of calcium is from dairy foods, including milk, yogurt, and a variety of cheeses. Calcium may also be added to certain products, such as orange juice, which are then advertised as being fortified with calcium. Calcium supplements are available and recommended for those with typically low calcium intake. Rice, sardines, and chicken are not high-calcium foods.

Test-Taking Strategy: Note the client's diagnosis and recall that calcium intake is encouraged to minimize the risk of osteoporosis. Recalling that dairy products are high in calcium and that yogurt is a dairy product will direct you to option 2. Review osteoporosis and foods high in calcium if you had difficulty with this question.

Level of Cognitive Ability: Analysis
Client Needs: Health Promotion and Maintenance
Integrated Process: Teaching/Learning
Content Area: Adult Health/Musculoskeletal

References:
Black, J., & Hawks, J. (2005). *Medical-surgical nursing: Clinical management for positive outcomes* (7th ed.). Philadelphia: Saunders, p. 601.
Ignatavicius, D., & Workman, M. (2002). *Medical surgical nursing: Critical thinking for collaborative care* (4th ed.). Philadelphia: Saunders, p. 1101.

---

166. A nurse is conducting a health screening clinic for osteoporosis. The nurse determines that which client seen in the clinic is at greatest risk of developing this disorder?
1 A 36-year-old male who has asthma
2 A 25-year-old female who jogs
3 A sedentary 65-year-old female who smokes cigarettes
4 A 70-year-old male who consumes excess alcohol

Answer: 3
Rationale: Risk factors for osteoporosis include being female, postmenopausal, of advanced age, low-calcium diet, excessive alcohol intake, being sedentary, and smoking cigarettes. Long-term use of corticosteroids, anticonvulsants, and furosemide (Lasix) also increase the risk.

Test-Taking Strategy: Use the process of elimination, thinking about the risk factors associated with osteoporosis. Option 2 is eliminated first. The 25-year-old female who jogs (exercise using the long bones) has negligible risk. The 36-year-old male with asthma is eliminated next because the only risk factor may be long-term corticosteroid use prescribed for asthma. From the remaining options, the 65-year-old female is at higher risk (age, gender, postmenopausal, sedentary, smoking) than the 70-year-old male (age, alcohol consumption). Review the risk factors associated with osteoporosis if you had difficulty with this question.

Level of Cognitive Ability: Analysis
Client Needs: Health Promotion and Maintenance
Integrated Process: Nursing Process/Assessment
Content Area: Adult Health/Musculoskeletal

Reference:
Ignatavicius, D., & Workman, M. (2002). *Medical surgical nursing: Critical thinking for collaborative care* (4th ed.). Philadelphia: Saunders, p. 1095.

---

167. A client with right-sided weakness needs to learn how to use a cane for home maintenance of mobility. The nurse plans to teach the client to position the cane by holding it with the:
1 Left hand, and placing the cane in front of the left foot
2 Right hand, and placing the cane in front of the right foot
3 Left hand, and 6 inches lateral to the left foot
4 Right hand, and 6 inches lateral to the right foot

Answer: 3
Rationale: The client is taught to hold the cane on the opposite side of the weakness. This is because, with normal walking, the opposite arm and leg move together (called reciprocal motion). The cane is placed 6 inches lateral to the fifth toe.

Test-Taking Strategy: Use the process of elimination and visualize this procedure. Knowing that the cane is held at the client's side, not in front, helps eliminate options 1 and 2. Recalling that the preferred method is to have the cane positioned on the stronger side helps you choose option 3 over option 4. Review client teaching points related to the use of a cane if you had difficulty with this question.

Level of Cognitive Ability: Application
Client Needs: Health Promotion and Maintenance
Integrated Process: Teaching/Learning
Content Area: Adult Health/Musculoskeletal

Reference:
Potter, P., & Perry, A. (2005). *Fundamentals of nursing* (6th ed.). St. Louis: Mosby, pp. 948-949.

168. A nurse has taught a client with a below-the-knee amputation about prosthesis and stump care. The nurse determines that the client has understood the instructions if the client stated to:

1 Wear a clean nylon stump sock every day
2 Toughen the skin of the stump by rubbing it with alcohol
3 Prevent cracking of the skin of the stump by applying lotion daily
4 Use a mirror to inspect all areas of the stump each day

Answer: 4

Rationale: The client should wear a clean woolen stump sock each day. The stump is cleansed daily with a gentle soap and water, and is dried carefully. Alcohol is avoided because it could cause drying or cracking of the skin. Oils and creams are also avoided because they are too softening to the skin for safe prosthesis use. The client should inspect all surfaces of the stump daily for irritation, blisters, or breakdown.

Test-Taking Strategy: Use the process of elimination. Recall that nylon is a synthetic material that does not allow the best air circulation and holds in moisture. For this reason, option 1 is incorrect. Either alcohol or lotion can interfere with the natural condition of the skin, increasing the likelihood of breakdown either from drying or from excess moisture. For these reasons, eliminate options 2 and 3. Review client teaching points related to stump care following amputation if you had difficulty with this question.

Level of Cognitive Ability: Analysis
Client Needs: Health Promotion and Maintenance
Integrated Process: Teaching/Learning
Content Area: Adult Health/Musculoskeletal

References:
Black, J., & Hawks, J. (2005). *Medical-surgical nursing: Clinical management for positive outcomes* (7th ed.). Philadelphia: Saunders, pp. 1524-1525.
Lewis, S., Heitkemper, M., & Dirksen, S. (2004). *Medical-surgical nursing: Assessment and management of clinical problems* (6th ed.). St. Louis: Mosby, p. 1684.
Phipps, W., Monahan, F., Sands, J., Marek, J., & Neighbors, M. (2003). *Medical-surgical nursing: Health and illness perspectives* (7th ed.). St. Louis: Mosby, p. 781.

169. A nurse is ambulating a client with a right leg fracture who has an order for partial weight-bearing status. The nurse determines that the client demonstrates compliance with this restriction if the client:

1 Does not bear weight on the right leg
2 Allows the right leg to touch the floor only
3 Puts 30% to 50% of the weight on the right leg
4 Puts 60% to 80% of the weight on the right leg

Answer: 3

Rationale: The client who has partial weight-bearing status places 30% to 50% of the body weight on the affected limb. Full weight-bearing status is placing full weight on the limb. Non-weight-bearing status does not allow the client to let the limb touch the floor. Touch-down weight-bearing allows the client to let the limb touch the floor, but not bear weight. There is no classification for 60% to 80% weight-bearing status.

Test-Taking Strategy: Use the process of elimination, focusing on the key words "partial weight-bearing status." Option 3 is the only option that fits the description of partial weight-bearing. Review the categories related to weight-bearing if you had difficulty with this question.

Level of Cognitive Ability: Analysis
Client Needs: Health Promotion and Maintenance
Integrated Process: Teaching/Learning
Content Area: Adult Health/Musculoskeletal

Reference:
Black, J., & Hawks, J. (2005). *Medical-surgical nursing: Clinical management for positive outcomes* (7th ed.). Philadelphia: Saunders, p. 643.

170. A nurse is planning to teach a client in skeletal leg traction about measures to increase bed mobility. Which item would be most helpful for this client?
1 Television
2 Reading materials
3 Overhead trapeze
4 Fracture bedpan

Answer: 3
Rationale: The use of an overhead trapeze is extremely helpful in assisting a client to move about in bed and to get on and off the bedpan. This device has the greatest value in increasing overall bed mobility. A fracture bedpan is useful in reducing discomfort with elimination. Television and reading materials are helpful in reducing boredom and providing distraction.

Test-Taking Strategy: Note the key words "most helpful" and focus on the issue: increase bed mobility. Although all options are useful to the client in skeletal traction, the only one that helps with bed mobility is the trapeze. Review care of the client in traction if you had difficulty with this question.

Level of Cognitive Ability: Analysis
Client Needs: Health Promotion and Maintenance
Integrated Process: Nursing Process/Planning
Content Area: Adult Health/Musculoskeletal

Reference:
Phipps, W., Monahan, F., Sands, J., Marek, J., & Neighbors, M. (2003). *Medical-surgical nursing: Health and illness perspectives* (7th ed.). St. Louis: Mosby, p. 1480.

171. A nurse has given medication instructions to the client beginning anticonvulsant therapy with carbamazepine (Tegretol). The nurse determines that the client understands the use of the medication if the client stated to:
1 Drive as long as it is not at night
2 Use sunscreen when out of doors
3 Keep tissues handy because of excess salivation
4 Discontinue the medication if fever or a sore throat occur

Answer: 2
Rationale: Carbamazepine acts by depressing synaptic transmission in the central nervous system (CNS). Because of this, the client should avoid driving or doing other activities that require mental alertness until the effect on the client is known. The client should use protective clothing and sunscreen to avoid photosensitivity reactions. The medication may cause dry mouth, and the client should be instructed to provide good oral hygiene and use sugarless candy or gum as needed. The medication should not be abruptly discontinued, because it could cause the return of seizures. Fever and sore throat should be reported to the physician (leukopenia).

Test-Taking Strategy: Use the process of elimination. Recalling that this is an anticonvulsant medication with CNS depressant properties will assist in eliminating option 1 first. Option 4 is eliminated next because an anticonvulsant is not discontinued just because side effects or infection occur, rather, the physician should be called. From the remaining options, remembering that carbamazepine causes dry mouth will assist in eliminating option 3. Review client teaching points related to this medication if you had difficulty with this question.

Level of Cognitive Ability: Analysis
Client Needs: Health Promotion and Maintenance
Integrated Process: Teaching/Learning
Content Area: Pharmacology

References:
Kee, J., & Hayes, E. (2003). *Pharmacology: A nursing process approach* (4th ed.). Philadelphia: Saunders, p. 285.
Lehne, R. (2004). *Pharmacology for nursing care* (5th ed.). Philadelphia: Saunders, pp. 328-329.
McKenry, L., & Salerno, E. (2003). *Mosby's pharmacology in nursing* (21st ed.). St. Louis: Mosby, p. 369.

172. A nurse provides discharge instructions to a client with rheumatoid arthritis. The instructions focus on measures to lessen discomfort and provide joint protection, and the nurse tells the client to:

1 Change positions every hour
2 Lift items rather than sliding them
3 Perform prescribed exercises even if the joints are inflamed
4 Avoid stooping, bending, or overreaching

Answer: 4

Rationale: The client with rheumatoid arthritis should avoid remaining in one position and should change positions or stretch every 20 minutes. To reduce efforts by joints, the client should slide objects rather than lift them. The client should avoid exercises and activities other than gentle range of motion when the joints are inflamed. The client is instructed to avoid stooping, bending, or overreaching.

Test-Taking Strategy: Use the process of elimination. Eliminate option 1 because with rheumatoid arthritis, remaining in one position for 1 hour is rather lengthy. Eliminate option 3 based on the basic principle that joints should be rested if inflamed. From the remaining options, use the principles related to body mechanics to direct you to option 4. Review principles for joint protection in rheumatoid arthritis if you had difficulty with this question.

Level of Cognitive Ability: Application
Client Needs: Health Promotion and Maintenance
Integrated Process: Teaching/Learning
Content Area: Adult Health/Musculoskeletal

Reference:
Black, J., & Hawks, J. (2005). *Medical-surgical nursing: Clinical management for positive outcomes* (7th ed.). Philadelphia: Saunders, p. 2344.

173. A home care nurse visits an older client with arthritis. The client complains of difficulty instilling glaucoma eye drops because of shaking hands caused by the arthritis. Which instruction would the nurse provide to the client to alleviate this problem?

1 Keep the drops in the refrigerator so they will thicken and be easier to instill
2 Lie down on a bed or sofa to instill the eye drops
3 Tilt the head back to instill the eye drops
4 That a family member will have to instill the eye drops

Answer: 2

Rationale: Older clients with arthritis or shaking hands have difficulty instilling their own eye drops. The older client is instructed to lie down on a bed or sofa to instill the eye drops. Tilting the head back can lead to loss of balance. Placing eye drops in a refrigerator should not be done unless specifically prescribed. Eye drop regimen for glaucoma requires accurate timing, and it is unreasonable to expect a family member to instill the drops. Additionally, this discourages client independence.

Test-Taking Strategy: Use the process of elimination. Eliminate option 1 first because eye medication should not be refrigerated unless specifically prescribed. Considering the issue of promoting client independence, and the fact that the question does not provide data regarding family, eliminate option 4. From the remaining options, select option 2 because it provides greater safety for the older client. Review procedures for instilling eye drops if you had difficulty with this question.

Level of Cognitive Ability: Application
Client Needs: Health Promotion and Maintenance
Integrated Process: Teaching/Learning
Content Area: Adult Health/Eye

Reference:
Black, J., & Hawks, J. (2005). *Medical-surgical nursing: Clinical management for positive outcomes* (7th ed.). Philadelphia: Saunders, p. 1948.

---

174. A scleral buckling procedure is performed on a client with retinal detachment, and the nurse provides home care instructions to the client. Which statement by the client indicates a need for further instructions?

1 "I need to clean the eye daily with sterile water and a clean washcloth."

2 "I need to wear an eye shield during naps and at night."

3 "I need to avoid vigorous activity."

4 "I need to avoid heavy lifting."

Answer: 1

Rationale: In a scleral buckling procedure, the sclera is compressed from the outside by Silastic sponges or silicone bands that are sutured in place permanently. In addition, an intraocular injection of air or a gas bubble, or both, may be used to apply pressure on the retina from the inside of the eye to hold the retina in place. If an air or gas bubble has been injected, it may take several weeks to absorb. Vigorous activities and heavy lifting are avoided. An eye shield or glasses should be worn during the day, and a shield should be worn during naps and at night. The client is instructed to clean the eye with warm tap water using a clean washcloth.

Test-Taking Strategy: Use the process of elimination, noting the key words "need for further instructions." These words indicate a false-response question and that you need to select the incorrect client statement. It is not necessary to use sterile water to clean the eye. In fact, it does not make sense to use a sterile solution with a clean washcloth. Review client teaching points following scleral buckling if you had difficulty with this question.

Level of Cognitive Ability: Analysis
Client Needs: Health Promotion and Maintenance
Integrated Process: Teaching/Learning
Content Area: Adult Health/Eye

Reference:
Black, J., & Hawks, J. (2005). *Medical-surgical nursing: Clinical management for positive outcomes* (7th ed.). Philadelphia: Saunders, p. 1953.

---

175. A nurse provides dietary instruction to the parents of a child with a diagnosis of cystic fibrosis. The nurse tells the parents that the diet should be:

1 Low in protein

2 Fat free

3 High in calories

4 Low in sodium

Answer: 3

Rationale: Children with cystic fibrosis are managed with a high-calorie, high-protein diet, pancreatic enzyme replacement therapy, fat-soluble vitamin supplements, and if nutritional problems are severe, nighttime gastrostomy feedings or total parental nutrition. Fats are not restricted unless steatorrhea cannot be controlled by increased pancreatic enzymes. Sodium intake is unrelated to this disorder.

Test-Taking Strategy: Think about the pathophysiology associated with cystic fibrosis and use the process of elimination. Select option 3 because children require calories for growth and development and because this option is the umbrella (global) one. Review dietary measures for the child with cystic fibrosis if you had difficulty with this question.

Level of Cognitive Ability: Application
Client Needs: Health Promotion and Maintenance
Integrated Process: Teaching/Learning
Content Area: Child Health

Reference:
James, S., Ashwill, J., & Droske, S. (2002). *Nursing care of children: Principles & practice* (2nd ed.).Philadelphia: Saunders, p. 679.

---

176. A clinic nurse instructs an adolescent with iron-deficiency anemia about the administration of oral iron preparations. The nurse tells the adolescent that it is best to take the iron with:
1 Water
2 Soda
3 Tomato juice
4 Cola

Answer: 3
Rationale: Iron should be administered with vitamin C–rich fluids because vitamin C enhances the absorption of the iron preparation. Tomato juice contains a high content of ascorbic acid (vitamin C). Water, soda, and cola do not contain vitamin C.

Test-Taking Strategy: Use the process of elimination. Eliminate options 2 and 4 first because they are similar. From the remaining options, recall that vitamin C increases the absorption of iron to direct you to option 3. Review the administration of oral iron if you had difficulty with this question.

Level of Cognitive Ability: Application
Client Needs: Health Promotion and Maintenance
Integrated Process: Teaching/Learning
Content Area: Child Health

Reference:
James, S., Ashwill, J., & Droske, S. (2002). *Nursing care of children: Principles & practice* (2nd ed.).Philadelphia: Saunders, p. 746.

---

177. A nurse is conducting a home visit for the client who started taking a sustained-release preparation of procainamide hydrochloride (Pronestyl SR). The nurse plans on teaching the client which of the following items about this medication?
1 Not to crush, chew, or break the sustained-release preparations
2 The presence of a tablet wax matrix in the stool indicates poor medication absorption.
3 A double dose may be taken if the first daily dose is missed.
4 Monitoring the pulse rate is not necessary once this medication is begun.

Answer: 1
Rationale: Procainamide (Pronestyl) is an antidysrhythmic that is available in a sustained-release (SR) form. The SR preparations should not be broken, chewed, or crushed. The SR form has a wax matrix that may be noted in the stool, and if this occurs, it is not significant. If a dose is missed, an SR tablet may be taken if remembered within 4 hours (2 hours for regular-acting form); otherwise the dose should be omitted. The client or a family member should be taught to monitor the client's pulse and report any change in rate or rhythm.

Test-Taking Strategy: Use the process of elimination. Note the relation between the medication "Pronestyl SR" and option 1. Remember, SR preparations should not be broken, chewed, or crushed. Review the administration of this type of medication if you had difficulty with this question.

Level of Cognitive Ability: Application
Client Needs: Health Promotion and Maintenance
Integrated Process: Teaching/Learning
Content Area: Pharmacology

Reference:
Hodgson, B., & Kizior, R. (2004). *Saunders nursing drug handbook 2004.* Philadelphia: Saunders, p. 835.

178. A nurse has given the client with a nephrostomy tube instructions to follow after hospital discharge. The nurse determines that the client understands the instructions if the client verbalizes to drink at least how many glasses of water per day?

1 2 to 4
2 6 to 8
3 10 to 12
4 14 to 16

Answer: 2

Rationale: The client with a nephrostomy tube needs to have adequate fluid intake to dilute urinary particles that could cause calculus and to provide good mechanical flushing of the kidney and tube. The nurse encourages the client to take in at least 2000 mL of fluid per day, which is roughly equivalent to 6 to 8 glasses of water. Option 1 is an inadequate amount. Options 3 and 4 are amounts that could distend the renal pelvis.

Test-Taking Strategy: Use the process of elimination, noting that the client has a nephrostomy tube. Recall that the client needs at least 2 liters of fluid per day. This will direct you to option 2. Also, avoid options in the much higher range because these are unnecessary and could possibly place undue distention on the renal pelvis. Review care of the client with a nephrostomy tube if you had difficulty with this question.

Level of Cognitive Ability: Analysis
Client Needs: Health Promotion and Maintenance
Integrated Process: Nursing Process/Evaluation
Content Area: Adult Health/Renal

Reference:
Phipps, W., Monahan, F., Sands, J., Marek, J., & Neighbors, M. (2003). *Medical-surgical nursing: Health and illness perspectives* (7th ed.). St. Louis: Mosby, pp. 1223-1224.

179. A clinic nurse has provided home care instructions to a female client who has been diagnosed with recurrent trichomoniasis. Which statement by the client indicates a need for further instructions?

1 "I need to perform good perineal hygiene."
2 "I need to refrain from sexual intercourse."
3 "I need to discontinue treatment if my menstrual cycle begins."
4 "I need to take metronidazole (Flagyl) for seven days."

Answer: 3

Rationale: Treatment for a recurrent infection should be continued through the menstrual period because the vagina is more alkaline during this time and a flare-up is likely to occur. The client should refrain from sexual intercourse while the infection remains active. If this is not possible, a condom is recommended. Options 1, 2, and 4 are correct.

Test-Taking Strategy: Note the key words "need for further instructions." These words indicate a false-response question and that you need to select the incorrect client statement. Recalling basic principles related to taking prescribed medications will direct you to option 3. Review the treatment for this infection if you had difficulty with this question.

Level of Cognitive Ability: Analysis
Client Needs: Health Promotion and Maintenance
Integrated Process: Teaching/Learning
Content Area: Fundamental Skills

Reference:
Hodgson, B., & Kizior, R. (2004). *Saunders nursing drug handbook 2004.* Philadelphia: Saunders, p. 1055.

180. A nurse has provided home care instructions to a client recovering from a radical vulvectomy. Which statement by the client indicates a need for further instructions?
  1 "I need to take showers rather than tub baths."
  2 "I need to wipe from front to back after a bowel movement."
  3 "I need to monitor for foul-smelling perineal discharge."
  4 "I need to notify the physician if swelling of the groin or genital area persists for longer than 1 week."

Answer: 4
Rationale: The physician needs to be notified if any swelling of the groin or genital area occurs. The client should not wait 1 week before notifying the physician. Options 1, 2, and 3 are accurate instructions. Additionally, the client should monitor for pain, redness, or tenderness in the calves and for any signs of infection.

Test-Taking Strategy: Use the process of elimination, noting the key words "need for further instructions." These words indicate a false-response question and that you need to select the incorrect client statement. Basic hygiene principles will assist in eliminating options 1 and 2. From the remaining options, select option 4, noting the time frame in this option. Review client teaching points related to a radical vulvectomy if you had difficulty with this question.

Level of Cognitive Ability: Analysis
Client Needs: Health Promotion and Maintenance
Integrated Process: Teaching/Learning
Content Area: Adult Health/Oncology

Reference:
Black, J., & Hawks, J. (2005). *Medical-surgical nursing: Clinical management for positive outcomes* (7th ed.). Philadelphia: Saunders, pp. 1806-1807.

---

181. A client with a history of depression will be participating in cognitive therapy for health maintenance. The client says to the nurse, "How does this treatment work?" The nurse makes which statement to the client?
  1 "This type of treatment helps you examine how your thoughts and feelings contribute to your difficulties."
  2 "This type of treatment helps you examine how your past life has contributed to your problems."
  3 "This type of treatment helps you confront your fears by gradually exposing you to them."
  4 "This type of treatment will help you relax and develop new coping skills."

Answer: 1
Rationale: Cognitive therapy is frequently used with clients who have depression. This type of therapy is based on exploring the client's subjective experience. It includes examining the client's thoughts and feelings about situations as well as how these thoughts and feelings contribute to and perpetuate the client's difficulties and mood. Options 2, 3, and 4 are not characteristics of cognitive therapy.

Test-Taking Strategy: Note the key word "cognitive" and note the relation between this word and option 1. Option 1 uses the word "thoughts" in describing the treatment. Review this form of therapy if you had difficulty with this question.

Level of Cognitive Ability: Application
Client Needs: Health Promotion and Maintenance
Integrated Process: Nursing Process/Implementation
Content Area: Mental Health

Reference:
Keltner, N., Schwecke, L., & Bostrom, C. (2003). *Psychiatric nursing* (4th ed.). St. Louis: Mosby, p. 349.

182. A client with acquired immunodeficiency syndrome (AIDS) has a nursing diagnosis of Imbalanced Nutrition: Less Than Body Requirements. The nurse has instructed the client about methods to maintain and increase weight. The nurse determines that the client would benefit from further instruction if the client stated to:

1 Eat low-calorie snacks between meals
2 Eat small, frequent meals throughout the day
3 Consume nutrient-dense foods and beverages
4 Keep easy-to-prepare foods available in the home

Answer: 1
Rationale: The client should eat small, frequent meals throughout the day. The client also should take in nutrient-dense and high-calorie meals and snacks. The client is encouraged to eat favorite foods to keep intake up and plan meals that are easy to prepare. The client can also avoid taking fluids with meals to increase food intake before satiety sets in.

Test-Taking Strategy: Note the key words "would benefit from further instruction." These words indicate a false-response question and that you need to select the incorrect client statement. Also note the nursing diagnosis, Imbalanced Nutrition: Less Than Body Requirements. Recalling that the client should choose snacks that are high in calories (not low in calories) will direct you to option 1. Review care of the client with imbalanced nutrition if you had difficulty with this question.

Level of Cognitive Ability: Analysis
Client Needs: Health Promotion and Maintenance
Integrated Process: Teaching/Learning
Content Area: Adult Health/Immune

Reference:
Black, J., & Hawks, J. (2005). *Medical-surgical nursing: Clinical management for positive outcomes* (7th ed.). Philadelphia: Saunders, p. 2396.

---

183. A nurse has given a postoperative thoracotomy client instructions about how to perform arm and shoulder exercises after discharge from the hospital. The nurse determines that the client needs further instructions about effective techniques if the client is observed doing which movement on the affected side?

1 Moving the arm up over the head and back down
2 Holding the hands crossed in front and raising them over the head
3 Holding the upper arm straight out while moving the forearm up and down
4 Making circles with the wrist

Answer: 4
Rationale: A variety of exercises that involve moving the shoulder and elbow joints are indicated after thoracotomy. These include shrugging the shoulders and moving them back and forth; moving the arms up and down, forward, and backward; holding the hands crossed in front of the waist and then raising them over the head; and holding the upper arm straight out while moving the lower arm up and down. Exercises that move only the wrist joint are of no use after this surgery.

Test-Taking Strategy: Use the process of elimination, noting the key words "needs further instructions about effective techniques." These words indicate a false-response question and that you need to select the incorrect client action. Also focus on the issue: arm and shoulder exercises. Note that options 1 and 2 move the shoulder joint. Option 3 moves the shoulder and elbow joint. Option 4 moves only the wrist joint. Review arm and shoulder exercises after thoracotomy if you had difficulty with this question.

Level of Cognitive Ability: Analysis
Client Needs: Health Promotion and Maintenance
Integrated Process: Teaching/Learning
Content Area: Adult Health/Respiratory

Reference:
Lewis, S., Heitkemper, M., & Dirksen, S. (2004). *Medical-surgical nursing: Assessment and management of clinical problems* (6th ed.). St. Louis: Mosby, p. 404.

184. A nurse is teaching a client with histo-plasmosis infection about prevention of future exposure to infectious sources. The nurse determines that the client needs further instructions if the client states that potential infectious sources include:

1 Grape arbors
2 Mushroom cellars
3 Floors of chicken houses
4 Bird droppings

Answer: 1

Rationale: The client with histoplasmosis is taught to avoid exposure to potential sources of the fungus, which includes bird droppings (especially starlings and blackbirds), floors of chicken houses and bat caves, and mushroom cellars.

Test-Taking Strategy: Note the key words "needs further instructions." These words indicate a false-response question and that you need to select the incorrect client statement. Eliminate options 3 and 4 first because they are similar. Because histoplasmosis is a fungus, recall that there is increased exposure to areas where the fungus thrives. Therefore, the least likely option is the grape arbor, which is above ground and is not in a dark and damp area. Review the source and causes of histoplasmosis infection if you had difficulty with this question.

Level of Cognitive Ability: Analysis
Client Needs: Health Promotion and Maintenance
Integrated Process: Teaching/Learning
Content Area: Adult Health/Respiratory

References:
Black, J., & Hawks, J. (2005). *Medical-surgical nursing: Clinical management for positive outcomes* (7th ed.). Philadelphia: Saunders, pp. 420; 2391.
Lewis, S., Heitkemper, M., & Dirksen, S. (2004). *Medical-surgical nursing: Assessment and management of clinical problems* (6th ed.). St. Louis: Mosby, p. 608.

185. A nurse is teaching a client with pulmonary sarcoidosis about long-term ongoing management. The nurse plans to include which of the following in the instructions?

1 Need for daily corticosteroids
2 Usefulness of home oxygen
3 Need for follow-up chest X-rays every 6 months
4 Importance of using incentive spirometer daily

Answer: 3

Rationale: The client with pulmonary sarcoidosis needs to have follow-up chest X-rays every 6 months to monitor disease progression. If an exacerbation occurs, treatment is initiated with systemic corticosteroids, but corticosteroids are not a part of long-term ongoing management. Home oxygen and ongoing use of incentive spirometer are not indicated.

Test-Taking Strategy: Note the key words "long-term ongoing management" and focus on the client's diagnosis. Eliminate option 2 first because there is no specific information in the question to indicate a need for its use. Recalling that corticosteroids are used for exacerbation helps you eliminate this option as well. From the remaining options, it is necessary to know that serial monitoring with X-ray is needed to track progression of the disease. Review the treatment for pulmonary sarcoidosis if you had difficulty with this question.

Level of Cognitive Ability: Application
Client Needs: Health Promotion and Maintenance
Integrated Process: Teaching/Learning
Content Area: Adult Health/Respiratory

Reference:
Black, J., & Hawks, J. (2005). *Medical-surgical nursing: Clinical management for positive outcomes* (7th ed.). Philadelphia: Saunders, p. 1871.

186. A nurse has taught a client with silicosis about situations to avoid to prevent self-exposure to silica dust. The nurse determines that the client understands the instructions if the client verbalizes to give up or wear a mask for which of the following hobbies?
1 Pottery making
2 Woodworking
3 Painting
4 Gardening

Answer: 1
Rationale: Exposure to silica dust occurs with activities such as pottery making and doing stone masonry. Exposure to the finely ground silica, such as is used with soaps, polishes, and filters, is also dangerous. Silica is not a pesticide and is not found in the average soil. Silica is not inhaled in fumes, such as with woodworking or painting.

Test-Taking Strategy: Use the process of elimination, focusing on the issue: silica dust. Think about materials that could give off silica dust. Recalling that pottery is made from clay, which is dug from the earth, will direct you to option 1. Review the sources of silica dust if you had difficulty with this question.

Level of Cognitive Ability: Analysis
Client Needs: Health Promotion and Maintenance
Integrated Process: Nursing Process/Evaluation
Content Area: Adult Health/Respiratory

Reference:
Lewis, S., Heitkemper, M., & Dirksen, S. (2004). *Medical-surgical nursing: Assessment and management of clinical problems* (6th ed.). St. Louis: Mosby, p. 612.

187. A nurse is conducting dietary teaching with a client who is hypocalcemic. The nurse encourages the client to increase intake of which of the following foods?
1 Apples
2 Chicken breast
3 Cheese
4 Cooked pasta

Answer: 3
Rationale: Products that are naturally high in calcium are dairy products, including milk, cheese, ice cream, and yogurt. High-calcium foods generally have greater than 100 mg of calcium per serving. The other options are foods that are low in calcium, which means they have less than 25 mg of calcium per serving.

Test-Taking Strategy: Use the process of elimination, focusing on the client's diagnosis. Recalling that dairy products are naturally high in calcium will direct you to option 3. Review foods high in calcium if you had difficulty with this question.

Level of Cognitive Ability: Application
Client Needs: Health Promotion and Maintenance
Integrated Process: Teaching/Learning
Content Area: Fundamental Skills

Reference:
Ignatavicius, D., & Workman, M. (2002). *Medical surgical nursing: Critical thinking for collaborative care* (4th ed.). Philadelphia: Saunders, p. 186.

188. A client is diagnosed with hyperphosphatemia. The nurse encourages the client to limit intake of which item that will aggravate the condition?
1 Bananas
2 Grapes
3 Coffee
4 Carbonated beverages

Answer: 4
Rationale: Food items and liquids that are naturally high in phosphates should be avoided by the client with hyperphosphatemia. These include fish, eggs, milk products, vegetables, whole grains, and carbonated beverages. The food items in options 1, 2, and 3 are acceptable to consume.

Test-Taking Strategy: Focus on the client's diagnosis and the issue: the item to limit because it will aggravate the condition. Recalling the phosphate content of foods and fluids will direct you to option 4. Review dietary measures for the client with hyperphosphatemia if you had difficulty with this question.

Level of Cognitive Ability: Application
Client Needs: Health Promotion and Maintenance
Integrated Process: Teaching/Learning
Content Area: Fundamental Skills

Reference:

Lewis, S., Heitkemper, M., & Dirksen, S. (2004). *Medical-surgical nursing: Assessment and management of clinical problems* (6th ed.). St. Louis: Mosby, p. 348.

---

189. A nurse is caring for a client with a burn injury who has sustained thoracic burns and smoke inhalation and is at risk for Impaired Gas Exchange. The nurse avoids which least helpful action in caring for this client?

1 Repositioning the client from side to side every 2 hours
2 Positioning the client on the back with the head of the bed at a 45-degree angle only
3 Suctioning the airway on a prn basis
4 Providing humidified oxygen and incentive spirometry

Answer: 2

Rationale: Aggressive pulmonary measures are used to prevent respiratory complications in the client who has Impaired Gas Exchange as a result of a burn injury. These include turning and repositioning, positioning for comfort, using humidified oxygen, providing incentive spirometry, and suctioning the client on an as-needed basis. The least helpful measure is to keep the client in one single position. This will ultimately lead to atelectasis and possible pneumonia.

Test-Taking Strategy: Note the key words "avoids" and "least helpful." These words indicate a false-response question and that you need to select the incorrect nursing action. Use basic nursing knowledge of respiratory support measures to eliminate each of the incorrect options. Also, note the absolute word "only" in option 2. Review care of the client with Impaired Gas Exchange if you had difficulty with this question.

Level of Cognitive Ability: Application
Client Needs: Health Promotion and Maintenance
Integrated Process: Nursing Process/Implementation
Content Area: Adult Health/Integumentary

Reference:

Black, J., & Hawks, J. (2005). *Medical-surgical nursing: Clinical management for positive outcomes* (7th ed.). Philadelphia: Saunders, pp. 1447-1448.

---

190. A community health nurse provides an educational session on the risk factors of cervical cancer to women in a local community. The nurse determines that further teaching is needed if a woman attending the session identifies which of the following as a risk factor for this type of cancer?

1 Occurs most frequently in Caucasian women
2 Early age of first intercourse
3 Smoking tobacco
4 Low socioeconomic class

Answer: 1

Rationale: Risk factors for cervical cancer include African and Native American individuals, having multiple sexual partners or a partner who had multiple sexual partners, early age of first intercourse, smoking tobacco, low socioeconomic status, untreated chronic cervicitis, sexually transmitted diseases, and having a partner with a history of penile or prostate cancer.

Test-Taking Strategy: Note the key words "further teaching is needed." These words indicate a false-response question and that you need to select the incorrect client statement. Recalling the risk factors for cervical cancer will direct you to option 1. Review these risk factors if you had difficulty with this question.

Level of Cognitive Ability: Analysis
Client Needs: Health Promotion and Maintenance
Integrated Process: Teaching/Learning
Content Area: Adult Health/Oncology

Reference:
Black, J., & Hawks, J. (2005). *Medical-surgical nursing: Clinical management for positive outcomes* (7th ed.). Philadelphia: Saunders, p. 1072.

191. A high school nurse teaches the female students how to prevent pelvic inflammatory disease. The nurse tells the students:
  1 To avoid single sexual partners
  2 To consult with a gynecologist regarding placement of an intrauterine device (IUD)
  3 To douche monthly
  4 To avoid unprotected intercourse

Answer: 4
Rationale: Primary prevention for pelvic inflammatory disease includes avoiding unprotected intercourse, multiple sexual partners, the use of an IUD, and douching.

Test-Taking Strategy: Use the process of elimination and the principle of exposure of the pelvic area to factors that cause infection. With this concept in mind, eliminate options 1, 2, and 3. Review preventive measures for pelvic inflammatory disease if you had difficulty with this question.

Level of Cognitive Ability: Application
Client Needs: Health Promotion and Maintenance
Integrated Process: Teaching/Learning
Content Area: Fundamental Skills

Reference:
Black, J., & Hawks, J. (2005). *Medical-surgical nursing: Clinical management for positive outcomes* (7th ed.). Philadelphia: Saunders, p. 1063.

192. A nurse provides discharge teaching to a client following a vasectomy. Which statement by the client would indicate a need for further teaching?
  1 "If I have pain or swelling, I can use an ice bag and take Tylenol."
  2 "I can use a scrotal support if I need to."
  3 "I can resume sexual intercourse whenever I want."
  4 "I don't need to practice birth control any longer."

Answer: 4
Rationale: Following vasectomy, the client must continue to practice a method of birth control until the follow-up semen analysis shows azoospermia. Live sperm may be present in the ampulla of vas following this procedure. Options 1, 2, and 3 are appropriate client statements.

Test-Taking Strategy: Note the key words "need for further teaching." These words indicate a false-response question and that you need to select the incorrect client statement. Options 1 and 2 can be eliminated because these measures assist in alleviating discomfort or swelling following the procedure. Option 3 can be eliminated because there would be no reason to avoid sexual intercourse unless the client was experiencing discomfort. Also, thinking about the purpose of a vasectomy will direct you to option 4. Review client teaching following a vasectomy if you had difficulty with this question.

Level of Cognitive Ability: Analysis
Client Needs: Health Promotion and Maintenance
Integrated Process: Teaching/Learning
Content Area: Fundamental Skills

Reference:
Black, J., & Hawks, J. (2005). *Medical-surgical nursing: Clinical management for positive outcomes* (7th ed.). Philadelphia: Saunders, p. 1040.

193. A physician in a community clinic diagnoses a client with prostatitis, and a nurse provides home care instructions to the client. Which statement by the client would indicate a need for further instructions?

1 "I need to take the anti-inflammatory medications as prescribed."
2 "The warm sitz baths will help my condition."
3 "I need to avoid sexual activity for 2 weeks."
4 "There are no restrictions in my diet."

Answer: 3

Rationale: Interventions for prostatitis include anti-inflammatory agents or short-term antimicrobial medication. Warm sitz baths and normal sexual activity are recommended. Dietary restrictions are not necessary unless the person finds that certain foods are associated with manifestations.

Test-Taking Strategy: Note the key words "need for further instructions." These words indicate a false-response question and that you need to select the incorrect client statement. Eliminate option 1 first using the general principles associated with medication prescriptions. Option 4 can be eliminated next because there is no specific relationship of diet to this disorder. From the remaining options, eliminate option 2 because it would seem reasonable that sitz baths would provide comfort. Review home care instructions for the client with prostatitis if you had difficulty with this question.

Level of Cognitive Ability: Analysis
Client Needs: Health Promotion and Maintenance
Integrated Process: Teaching/Learning
Content Area: Fundamental Skills

Reference:
Black, J., & Hawks, J. (2005). *Medical-surgical nursing: Clinical management for positive outcomes* (7th ed.). Philadelphia: Saunders, p. 1036.

194. A nursing instructor asks a student to identify the risk factors and methods of preventing prostate cancer. Which statement by the student indicates a need to review this information?

1 Men older than 50 years of age should be monitored with a yearly digital rectal exam.
2 Men older than 50 years of age should be monitored with a prostate-specific antigen (PSA) assay.
3 A high-fat diet will assist in preventing this type of cancer.
4 Employment in fertilizer, textile, or rubber industries increase the risk of prostate cancer.

Answer: 3

Rationale: A high intake of dietary fat is a risk factor for prostate cancer. Options 1, 2, and 4 are accurate statements regarding the risks and prevention measures related to this type of cancer.

Test-Taking Strategy: Note the key words "a need to review this information." These words indicate a false-response question and that you need to select the incorrect student statement. Recalling the general principles related to cancer prevention will direct you to option 3. Review these measures if you had difficulty with this question.

Level of Cognitive Ability: Analysis
Client Needs: Health Promotion and Maintenance
Integrated Process: Teaching/Learning
Content Area: Fundamental Skills

Reference:
Black, J., & Hawks, J. (2005). *Medical-surgical nursing: Clinical management for positive outcomes* (7th ed.). Philadelphia: Saunders, p. 1028.

195. A clinic nurse provides information to a married couple regarding measures to prevent infertility. Which statement made by the husband indicates a need for providing further information?
  1 "We need to avoid excessive intake of alcohol."
  2 "We need to decrease exposure to environmental hazards."
  3 "We need to eat a nutritious diet."
  4 "I need to maintain warmth to my scrotum by taking hot baths frequently."

Answer: 4
Rationale: Keeping the testes cool by avoiding hot baths and tight clothing appears to improve the sperm count. Avoiding factors that depress spermatogenesis, such as the use of drugs, alcohol, marijuana, and exposure to occupational or environmental hazards, and maintaining good nutrition are key components to prevent infertility.

Test-Taking Strategy: Note the key words "need for providing further information." These words indicate a false-response question and that you need to select the incorrect client statement. Eliminate option 3 first because maintenance of a nutritious diet is important in all situations. From the remaining options, recalling that heat decreases motility of sperm will assist in directing you to the correct option. Review the measures that prevent infertility if you have difficulty with this question.

Level of Cognitive Ability: Analysis
Client Needs: Health Promotion and Maintenance
Integrated Process: Teaching/Learning
Content Area: Fundamental Skills

Reference:
Black, J., & Hawks, J. (2005). *Medical-surgical nursing: Clinical management for positive outcomes* (7th ed.). Philadelphia: Saunders, p. 1043.

196. A nurse teaches a client preparing for discharge from the hospital following a total hip replacement. Which statement by the client would indicate a need for further instructions?
  1 "I need to place a pillow between my knees when I lie down."
  2 "I need to wear a support stocking on my unaffected leg."
  3 "I should not sit in one position for longer than 4 hours."
  4 "I cannot drive a car for probably 6 weeks."

Answer: 3
Rationale: The client needs to be instructed not to sit continuously for longer than 1 hour. The client should be instructed to stand, stretch, and take a few steps periodically. The client cannot drive a car for 6 weeks after surgery unless allowed to do so by a physician. A support stocking should be worn on the unaffected leg and an Ace bandage usually is prescribed to be placed on the affected leg until there is no swelling in the legs and feet, and until full activities are resumed. The legs are abducted by placing a pillow between them when the client lies down.

Test-Taking Strategy: Note the key words "need for further instructions." These words indicate a false-response question and that you need to select the incorrect client statement. Recalling standard measures related to the postoperative period will assist in eliminating option 4. Knowing that leg abduction is maintained postoperatively during hospitalization will assist in eliminating option 1. From the remaining options, note the time frame of 4 hours in option 3. This is a lengthy time period for the client to remain in one position. Review teaching points following total hip replacement if you had difficulty with this question.

Level of Cognitive Ability: Analysis
Client Needs: Health Promotion and Maintenance
Integrated Process: Teaching/Learning
Content Area: Adult Health/Musculoskeletal

Reference:
Black, J., & Hawks, J. (2005). *Medical-surgical nursing: Clinical management for positive outcomes* (7th ed.). Philadelphia: Saunders, p. 593.

197. A client is diagnosed with hypothyroidism and is to begin on thyroid supplements, and the nurse instructs the client about the medication. Which statement by the client would indicate the need for further instructions?
1 "I need to take my daily dose every night at bedtime."
2 "I need to call my physician if I develop any chest pain."
3 "I need to speak to my physician when I begin to plan for parenthood."
4 "I may experience some gastrointestinal problems such as diarrhea."

Answer: 1
Rationale: The client is instructed to take the medication in the morning to prevent insomnia. If the client experiences any chest pain, it may indicate overdose, and the physician needs to be notified. The dose needs to be adjusted if the client is pregnant or plans to get pregnant. Gastrointestinal complaints from thyroid supplements include increased appetite, nausea, and diarrhea.

Test-Taking Strategy: Use the process of elimination, noting the key words "need for further instructions." Eliminate options 2 and 3 based on general principles related to medication therapy. Chest pain warrants follow-up, and pregnancy would require a review of the medication dosage. From the remaining options, think about the disorder: hypothyroidism. You would expect that thyroid hormone would have an effect on increasing body metabolism. This will assist in directing you to option 1. Review client teaching points related to thyroid supplements if you had difficulty with this question.

Level of Cognitive Ability: Analysis
Client Needs: Health Promotion and Maintenance
Integrated Process: Teaching/Learning
Content Area: Adult Health/Endocrine

Reference:
Lehne, R. (2004). *Pharmacology for nursing care* (5th ed.). Philadelphia: Saunders, p. 624.

198. A clinic nurse instructs a client with diabetes mellitus about how to prevent diabetic ketoacidosis (DKA) on days when the client is feeling ill. Which statement by the client indicates a need for further instructions?
1 "I need to stop my insulin if I am vomiting."
2 "I need to call my physician if I am ill for more than 24 hours."
3 "I need to eat 10 to 15 g of carbohydrates every 1 to 2 hours."
4 "I need to drink small quantities of fluid every 15 to 30 minutes."

Answer: 1
Rationale: The client needs to be instructed to take insulin even if he or she is vomiting and unable to eat. It is important to self-monitor blood glucose more frequently during illness (every 2 to 4 hours). If the premeal blood glucose is greater than 250 mg/dL, the client should test for urine ketones and contact the physician. Options 2, 3, and 4 are accurate interventions.

Test-Taking Strategy: Note the key words "need for further instructions." These words indicate a false-response question and that you need to select the incorrect client statement. Recalling that insulin needs to be taken every day will assist in directing you to option 1. Review sick day rules for the client with diabetes mellitus if you had difficulty with this question.

Level of Cognitive Ability: Analysis
Client Needs: Health Promotion and Maintenance
Integrated Process: Teaching/Learning
Content Area: Adult Health/Endocrine

Reference:
Black, J., & Hawks, J. (2005). *Medical-surgical nursing: Clinical management for positive outcomes* (7th ed.). Philadelphia: Saunders, p. 1286.

199. A nurse is instructing a client with diabetes mellitus regarding hypoglycemia. Which statement by the client indicates a need for further instructions?

1 "Hypoglycemia can occur at anytime of the day or night."
2 "If hypoglycemia occurs, I need to take my regular insulin as prescribed."
3 "If I feel sweaty or shaky, I might be experiencing hypoglycemia."
4 "I can drink 6 to 8 ounces of milk if hypoglycemia occurs."

Answer: 2

Rationale: If a hypoglycemic reaction occurs, the client will need to consume 10 to 15 g of carbohydrate. Six to eight ounces of milk contains this amount of carbohydrate. Tremors and diaphoresis are signs of mild hypoglycemia. Insulin is not taken as a treatment for hypoglycemia because the insulin will lower the blood glucose. Hypoglycemic reactions can occur at any time of the day or night.

Test-Taking Strategy: Note the key words "need for further instructions." Remember that in hypoglycemia the blood glucose is lowered. Insulin also lowers blood glucose, therefore it would seem reasonable that insulin is not a treatment for this condition. Review the signs of hypoglycemia and the appropriate interventions if you had difficulty with this question.

Level of Cognitive Ability: Analysis
Client Needs: Health Promotion and Maintenance
Integrated Process: Teaching/Learning
Content Area: Adult Health/Endocrine

Reference:
Black, J., & Hawks, J. (2005). *Medical-surgical nursing: Clinical management for positive outcomes* (7th ed.). Philadelphia: Saunders, p. 1277.

200. A client with nephrolithiasis arrives at the clinic for a follow-up visit. The laboratory analysis of the stone that the client passed one week ago indicates that the stone is composed of calcium oxalate. Based on this analysis, the nurse tells the client to avoid:

1 Lentils
2 Spinach
3 Lettuce
4 Pasta

Answer: 2

Rationale: Many kidney stones are composed of calcium oxalate. Foods that raise urinary oxalate excretion include spinach, rhubarb, strawberries, chocolate, wheat bran, nuts, beets, and tea.

Test-Taking Strategy: Note the key word "avoid" and focus on the type of stone. Recalling the foods, such as spinach, that raise urinary oxalate excretion will direct you to option 2. Review the foods that raise urinary oxalate excretion if you had difficulty with this question.

Level of Cognitive Ability: Application
Client Needs: Health Promotion and Maintenance
Integrated Process: Teaching/Learning
Content Area: Adult Health/Renal

Reference:
Black, J., & Hawks, J. (2005). *Medical-surgical nursing: Clinical management for positive outcomes* (7th ed.). Philadelphia: Saunders, pp. 883-885.

201. A nurse provides instructions to a new mother who is about to breastfeed her newborn infant. The nurse observes the new mother as she breastfeeds for the first time and intervenes if the new mother:

1 Turns the newborn infant on his side facing the mother
2 Draws the newborn the rest of the way onto the breast when the newborn opens his mouth
3 Tilts up the nipple or squeezes the areola, pushing it into the newborn's mouth
4 Places a clean finger in the side of the newborn's mouth to break the suction before removing the newborn from the breast

Answer: 3

Rationale: The mother is instructed to avoid tilting up the nipple or squeezing the areola and pushing it into the newborn's mouth. This action does not facilitate the breastfeeding process or flow of milk. Options 1, 2, and 4 are correct procedures for breastfeeding.

Test-Taking Strategy: Note the key word "intervenes." Visualize the descriptions in each of the options. This will eliminate options 1, 2, and 4. Also, careful reading of option 3 and noting the word "pushing," which suggests force or resistance, should assist in directing you to this option. Review the procedure for breastfeeding if you had difficulty with this question.

Level of Cognitive Ability: Analysis
Client Needs: Health Promotion and Maintenance
Integrated Process: Teaching/Learning
Content Area: Maternity/Postpartum

Reference:
Lowdermilk, D., & Perry, A. (2004). *Maternity & women's health care* (8th ed.). St. Louis: Mosby, p. 781.

---

202. A clinic nurse provides instructions to a mother regarding the care of her child who is diagnosed with croup. Which statement by the mother indicates a need for further instructions?

1 "I will place a cool mist humidifier next to my child's bed."
2 "Sips of warm fluids during a croup attack will help."
3 "I will give Tylenol for the fever."
4 "I will give cough syrup every night at bedtime."

Answer: 4

Rationale: The mother needs to be instructed that cough syrup and cold medicines are not to be administered because they may dry and thicken secretions. Sips of warm fluid will relax the vocal cords and thin mucus. A cool mist humidifier rather than a steam vaporizer is recommended because of the danger of the child pulling the machine over and causing a burn. Acetaminophen (Tylenol) will reduce the fever.

Test-Taking Strategy: Note the key words "need for further instructions." These words indicate a false-response question and that you need to select the incorrect client statement. Option 3 can be eliminated first, recalling that acetaminophen (Tylenol) is normally prescribed to reduce a fever. Recalling that warm fluids will thin secretions will assist you in eliminating option 2. From the remaining options, recalling that cough syrup will dry secretions will assist in directing you to option 4. Review home care instructions for the child with croup if you had difficulty with this question.

Level of Cognitive Ability: Analysis
Client Needs: Health Promotion and Maintenance
Integrated Process: Teaching/Learning
Content Area: Child Health

Reference:
Wong, D., & Hockenberry, M. (2003). *Wong's nursing care of infants and children* (7th ed.). St. Louis: Mosby, p. 364.

203. A client with anxiety disorder is taking buspirone (BuSpar) orally. The client tells the nurse that it is difficult to swallow the tablets. The nurse provides which instruction to the client?

1 To purchase the liquid preparation with the next refill

2 To crush the tablets before taking them

3 To call the physician for a change in medication

4 To mix the tablet uncrushed in apple sauce

Answer: 2

Rationale: Buspirone (BuSpar) may be administered without regard to meals, and the tablets may be crushed. This medication is not available in liquid form. It is premature to advise the client to call the physician for a change in medication without first trying alternative interventions. Mixing the tablet uncrushed in apple sauce will not ensure ease in swallowing.

Test-Taking Strategy: Use the process of elimination. Eliminate option 3 first because in most situations a nursing intervention can be instituted before calling the physician. Next, eliminate option 4 because this instruction will not ensure ease in swallowing. From the remaining options, it is necessary to know that this medication is not available in liquid form. Additionally, many tablets can be crushed. Review client instructions for administering this medication if you had difficulty with this question.

Level of Cognitive Ability: Application
Client Needs: Health Promotion and Maintenance
Integrated Process: Nursing Process/Implementation
Content Area: Pharmacology

Reference:
Hodgson, B., & Kizior, R. (2004). *Saunders nursing drug handbook 2004.* Philadelphia: Saunders, p. 130.

---

204. A nurse caring for a child with congestive heart failure provides instructions to the parents regarding the administration of digoxin (Lanoxin). Which statement by the mother indicates a need for further instructions?

1 "If my child vomits after I give the medication, I will not repeat the dose."

2 "I will check my child's pulse before giving the medication."

3 "I will check the dose of the medication with my husband before I give the medication."

4 "I will mix the medication with food."

Answer: 4

Rationale: The medication should not be mixed with food or formula because this method would not ensure that the child receives the entire dose of medication. Options 1, 2, and 3 are correct. Additionally, if a dosage is missed and is not identified until 4 or more hours later, the dose is not administered. If more than one consecutive dose is skipped, the physician needs to be notified.

Test-Taking Strategy: Note the key words "need for further instructions." General principles regarding medication administration to children should assist in directing you to the correct option. Mixing medications with formula or food may alter the effectiveness of the medication and, more important, if the child does not consume the entire formula or food, the total dosage would not be administered. Review parental instructions regarding administering digoxin if you had difficulty with this question.

Level of Cognitive Ability: Analysis
Client Needs: Health Promotion and Maintenance
Integrated Process: Teaching/Learning
Content Area: Pharmacology

References:
McKenry, L., & Salerno, E. (2003). *Mosby's pharmacology in nursing* (21st ed.). St. Louis: Mosby, 541.
Wong, D., & Hockenberry, M. (2003). *Wong's nursing care of infants and children* (7th ed.). St. Louis: Mosby, p. 1482.

205. A nurse provides discharge instructions to the mother of a child who was hospitalized for heart surgery. The nurse tells the mother that:

1 The child may return to school one week after hospital discharge
2 After bathing, rub lotion and sprinkle powder on the incision
3 The child can play outside for short periods of time
4 The physician is to be notified if the child develops a fever greater than 100.5° F

Answer: 4

Rationale: Following heart surgery, the child should not return to school until 3 weeks after hospital discharge, at which time the child should go to school for half days for the first few days. No creams, lotions, or powders should be placed on the incision until it is completely healed and without scabs. The mother is instructed to omit play outside for several weeks. The physician needs to be notified if the child develops a fever greater than 100.5° F.

Test-Taking Strategy: Use the process of elimination, bearing in mind the potential for infection in this child. Eliminate option 1 because of the time frame of 1 week. Eliminate option 3 because outside play can expose the child to infection and the risk of injury. Basic principles related to incision care should assist in eliminating option 2. Review home care instructions for the child following heart surgery if you had difficulty with this question.

Level of Cognitive Ability: Application
Client Needs: Health Promotion and Maintenance
Integrated Process: Teaching/Learning
Content Area: Child Health

Reference:
Wong, D., & Hockenberry, M. (2003). *Wong's nursing care of infants and children* (7th ed.). St. Louis: Mosby, p. 1509.

206. A clinic nurse provides instructions to a client who will begin on oral contraceptives. Which statement by the client indicates the need for further instructions?

1 "I will take one pill daily at the same time every day."
2 "I will not need to use an additional birth control method once I start these pills."
3 "If I miss a pill, I need to take it as soon as I remember."
4 "If I miss two pills, I will take them both as soon as I remember and I will take two pills the next day also."

Answer: 2

Rationale: The client needs to be instructed to use a second birth control method during the first pill cycle. Options 1, 3, and 4 are correct. Additionally, the client needs to be instructed that if she misses three pills, she will need to discontinue use for that cycle and use another birth control method.

Test-Taking Strategy: Note the key words "need for further instructions." These words indicate a false-response question and that you need to select the incorrect client statement. It would seem reasonable that during the first pill cycle, a second birth control method would need to be used to prevent conception. Review these guidelines if you had difficulty with this question.

Level of Cognitive Ability: Analysis
Client Needs: Health Promotion and Maintenance
Integrated Process: Teaching/Learning
Content Area: Pharmacology

References:
Lowdermilk, D., & Perry, A. (2004). *Maternity & women's health care* (8th ed.). St. Louis: Mosby, p. 233.
McKenry, L., & Salerno, E. (2003). *Mosby's pharmacology in nursing* (21st ed.). St. Louis: Mosby, p. 903.

207. A nurse is providing dietary instructions to the client hospitalized for pancreatitis. Which of the following foods would the nurse instruct the client to avoid?
1 Lentil soup
2 Bagel
3 Chili
4 Watermelon

Answer: 3
Rationale: The client needs to avoid alcohol, coffee and tea, spicy foods, and heavy meals, which stimulate pancreatic secretions and produce attacks of pancreatitis. The client is instructed in the benefit of eating small frequent meals that are high in protein, low in fat, and moderate to high in carbohydrates.

Test-Taking Strategy: Use the process of elimination, noting that options 1, 2, and 4 are foods that are moderately bland. Option 3 is different in that chili is a spicy food. Review dietary measures for the client with pancreatitis if you had difficulty with this question.

Level of Cognitive Ability: Application
Client Needs: Health Promotion and Maintenance
Integrated Process: Teaching/Learning
Content Area: Adult Health/Gastrointestinal

Reference:
Black, J., & Hawks, J. (2005). *Medical-surgical nursing: Clinical management for positive outcomes* (7th ed.). Philadelphia: Saunders, p. 1297.

208. A home care nurse visits a client who was recently diagnosed with cirrhosis. The nurse provides home care management instructions to the client. Which statement by the client indicates a need for further instructions?
1 "I will take acetaminophen (Tylenol) if I get a headache."
2 "I will obtain adequate rest."
3 "I should include sufficient carbohydrates in my diet."
4 "I should monitor my weight regularly."

Answer: 1
Rationale: Acetaminophen (Tylenol) is avoided because it can cause fatal liver damage in the client with cirrhosis. Adequate rest and nutrition is important. The diet should supply sufficient carbohydrates with a total daily calorie intake of 2000 to 3000. The client's weight should be monitored regularly.

Test-Taking Strategy: Note the key words "need for further instructions." These words indicate a false-response question and that you need to select the incorrect client statement. Recalling that acetaminophen (Tylenol) is a hepatotoxic agent will assist in directing you to the correct option. Review medications that are restricted or are avoided in clients with cirrhosis if you had difficulty with this question.

Level of Cognitive Ability: Analysis
Client Needs: Health Promotion and Maintenance
Integrated Process: Teaching/Learning
Content Area: Adult Health/Gastrointestinal

Reference:
Black, J., & Hawks, J. (2005). *Medical-surgical nursing: Clinical management for positive outcomes* (7th ed.). Philadelphia: Saunders, p. 1339.

209. A client who has a history of gout is also diagnosed with urolithiasis. The stones are determined to be of uric acid type. The nurse gives the client instructions in foods to limit, which includes:

1 Liver
2 Apples
3 Carrots
4 Milk

Answer: 1

Rationale: Foods containing high amounts of purines should be avoided in the client with uric acid stones. This includes limiting or avoiding organ meats, such as liver, brain, heart, and kidney. Other foods to avoid include sweetbreads, herring, sardines, anchovies, meat extracts, consommés, and gravies. Foods that are low in purines include all fruits, many vegetables, milk, cheese, eggs, refined cereals, coffee, tea, chocolate, and carbonated beverages.

Test-Taking Strategy: Use the process of elimination, focusing on the client's diagnosis and noting the key word "limit." Because purines are end-products of protein metabolism, eliminate options 2 and 3 first. From the remaining options, recall that organ meats such as liver provide a greater quantity of protein than milk does. Review dietary instructions for the client with uric acid stones if you had difficulty with this question.

Level of Cognitive Ability: Application
Client Needs: Health Promotion and Maintenance
Integrated Process: Teaching/Learning
Content Area: Fundamental Skills

Reference:
Black, J., & Hawks, J. (2005). *Medical-surgical nursing: Clinical management for positive outcomes* (7th ed.). Philadelphia: Saunders, pp. 885-886.

---

210. A client tells the nurse that he gets dizzy and lightheaded with each use of the incentive spirometer. The nurse asks the client to demonstrate use of the device, expecting that the client is:

1 Not forming a tight seal around the mouthpiece
2 Inhaling too slowly
3 Not resting adequately between breaths
4 Exhaling too slowly

Answer: 3

Rationale: If the client does not breathe normally between incentive spirometer breaths, hyperventilation and fatigue can result. Hyperventilation is the most common cause of respiratory alkalosis, which is characterized by lightheadedness and dizziness. Options 1, 2, and 4 would not be a cause of lightheadedness and dizziness.

Test-Taking Strategy: Focus on the issue: the cause of lightheadedness and dizziness. Think about each of the actions in the options to direct you to option 3. Options 1, 2, and 4 would result in ineffective use but would not cause dizziness and lightheadedness. Review the procedure for the use of the incentive spirometer if you had difficulty with this question.

Level of Cognitive Ability: Analysis
Client Needs: Health Promotion and Maintenance
Integrated Process: Nursing Process/Evaluation
Content Area: Adult Health/Respiratory

Reference:
Ignatavicius, D., & Workman, M. (2002). *Medical surgical nursing: Critical thinking for collaborative care* (4th ed.). Philadelphia: Saunders, p. 581.

211. A nurse is conducting a health screening clinic. The nurse interprets that which client participating in the screening has the greatest need for instruction to lower the risk of developing respiratory disease?
  1 A 50-year-old smoker with cracked asbestos lining on basement pipes in the home
  2 A 40-year-old smoker who works in a hospital
  3 A 36-year-old who works with pesticides
  4 A 25-year-old who does woodworking as a hobby

Answer: 1
Rationale: Smoking greatly enhances the client's risk of developing some form of respiratory disease. Other risk factors include exposure to harmful chemicals, airborne toxins, and dust or fumes. The client at greatest risk has two identified risk factors, one of which is smoking.

Test-Taking Strategy: Use the process of elimination. Eliminate options 3 and 4 first because the most harmful risk factor for the respiratory system is smoking. From the remaining options, select option 1 because asbestos is toxic to the lungs, if particles are inhaled. Also, two risk factors are identified in option 1, which makes this client at greater risk than the others who have one factor identified. Review the risk factors associated with respiratory disease if you had difficulty with this question.

Level of Cognitive Ability: Analysis
Client Needs: Health Promotion and Maintenance
Integrated Process: Nursing Process/Assessment
Content Area: Adult Health/Respiratory

References:
Ignatavicius, D., & Workman, M. (2002). *Medical surgical nursing: Critical thinking for collaborative care* (4th ed.). Philadelphia: Saunders, p. 557.
Lewis, S., Heitkemper, M., & Dirksen, S. (2004). *Medical-surgical nursing: Assessment and management of clinical problems* (6th ed.). St. Louis: Mosby, p. 659.

212. A nurse has conducted teaching with a client who has experienced pulmonary embolism about methods to prevent reoccurrence after discharge from the hospital. The nurse determines that the instructions have been effective if the client states an intention to:
  1 Continue to wear supportive hose
  2 Limit intake of fluids
  3 Cross the legs only at the ankle, but not at the knees
  4 Sit down whenever possible

Answer: 1
Rationale: Reoccurrence of pulmonary embolism can be minimized by wearing elastic or supportive hose. Elastic or supportive hose enhances venous return. The client also enhances venous return by avoiding crossing the legs at the knees or ankles, interspersing periods of sitting with walking, and doing active foot and ankle exercises. The client should also take in sufficient fluids to prevent hemoconcentration and hypercoagulability.

Test-Taking Strategy: Use the process of elimination, noting the key words "instructions have been effective." Recalling that promoting venous return will prevent pulmonary embolism will direct you to option 1. Review the measures that will prevent reoccurrence of pulmonary embolism if you had difficulty with this question.

Level of Cognitive Ability: Analysis
Client Needs: Health Promotion and Maintenance
Integrated Process: Nursing Process/Evaluation
Content Area: Adult Health/Respiratory

Reference:
Black, J., & Hawks, J. (2005). *Medical-surgical nursing: Clinical management for positive outcomes* (7th ed.). Philadelphia: Saunders, pp. 1539-1540.

213. A female client is being discharged from the hospital to home with an indwelling urinary catheter following surgical repair of the bladder following trauma. The nurse determines that the client understands the principles of catheter management if the client states to:

1 Cleanse the perineal area with soap and water once a day
2 Keep the drainage bag lower than the level of the bladder
3 Limit fluid intake so the bag won't become full so quickly
4 Coil the tubing and place it under the thigh when sitting to avoid tugging on the bladder

Answer: 2

Rationale: The perineal area should be cleansed twice daily and following each bowel movement with soap and water. The drainage bag should be lower than the level of the bladder, and the tubing should be free of kinks and compression. Coiling the tubing and placing it under the thigh can compress the tube. Adequate fluid intake is necessary to prevent infection and to provide natural irrigation of the catheter from increased urine flow.

Test-Taking Strategy: Note the key words "understands the principles." Option 4 is eliminated first because sitting on coiled tubing could cause compression and obstruct drainage. Option 3 is eliminated next, knowing that increased fluids are important. From the remaining options, noting the words "once a day" in option 1 will assist in eliminating this option. Review the principles related to catheter care if you had difficulty with this question.

Level of Cognitive Ability: Analysis
Client Needs: Health Promotion and Maintenance
Integrated Process: Nursing Process/Evaluation
Content Area: Adult Health/Renal

Reference:
Black, J., & Hawks, J. (2005). *Medical-surgical nursing: Clinical management for positive outcomes* (7th ed.). Philadelphia: Saunders, p. 906.

214. A 24-year-old female with a familial history of heart disease presents to the physician's office asking to begin oral contraceptive therapy for birth control. The nurse would next inquire whether the client:

1 Has taken oral contraceptives before
2 Exercises regularly
3 Eats a low-cholesterol diet
4 Is currently a smoker

Answer: 4

Rationale: Oral contraceptive use is a risk factor for heart disease, particularly when it is combined with cigarette smoking. Regular exercise and keeping total cholesterol levels under 200 mg/dL are general measures to decrease cardiovascular risk.

Test-Taking Strategy: Use the process of elimination, noting the key words "familial history of heart disease." Remember that smoking is the item that is linked to oral contraceptive use to make it a risk factor for cardiovascular disease. This will direct you to option 4. Review the risks associated with the use of oral contraceptives if you had difficulty with this question.

Level of Cognitive Ability: Analysis
Client Needs: Health Promotion and Maintenance
Integrated Process: Nursing Process/Assessment
Content Area: Adult Health/Cardiovascular

References:
Ignatavicius, D., & Workman, M. (2002). *Medical surgical nursing: Critical thinking for collaborative care* (4th ed.). Philadelphia: Saunders, p. 627.
Lewis, S., Heitkemper, M., & Dirksen, S. (2004). *Medical-surgical nursing: Assessment and management of clinical problems* (6th ed.). St. Louis: Mosby, p. 761.

215. A nurse is implementing measures to maintain adequate peripheral tissue perfusion in the post-cardiac surgery client. The nurse avoids which of the following in giving care to this client?
1 Range of motion (ROM) exercises to the feet
2 Application of compression stockings
3 Leg elevation while sitting in chair
4 Use of the knee gatch on the bed and placing pillows under the knees

Answer: 4

Rationale: After surgery, measures are taken to prevent venous stasis. They include applying elastic stockings or leg wraps, use of pneumatic compression boots, discouraging leg crossing, avoiding the use of the knee gatch, performing passive and active ROM, and avoiding the use of pillows in the popliteal space. Leg elevation while sitting will promote venous drainage and help prevent postoperative edema.

Test-Taking Strategy: Focus on the issue: post-cardiac surgery, and note the key word "avoids." Select the option that will impede venous return. The use of the knee gatch and placing pillows in the popliteal space puts pressure on blood vessels in the popliteal area, impeding venous return. Review care of the client following cardiac surgery if you had difficulty with this question.

Level of Cognitive Ability: Application
Client Needs: Health Promotion and Maintenance
Integrated Process: Nursing Process/Implementation
Content Area: Adult Health/Cardiovascular

Reference:
Black, J., & Hawks, J. (2005). *Medical-surgical nursing: Clinical management for positive outcomes* (7th ed.). Philadelphia: Saunders, pp. 1536-1537; 1655-1656.

216. A nurse is planning to teach a client with atrial fibrillation about the need to begin long-term anticoagulant therapy. Which explanation would the nurse use to best describe the reasoning for this therapy?
1 "Because of this dysrhythmia, blood backs up in the legs and puts you at risk for blood clots, also called deep vein thrombosis."
2 "The antidysrhythmic medications you are taking cause blood clots as a side effect, so you need this medication to prevent them."
3 "Because the atria are quivering, blood flows sluggishly through them, and clots can form along the heart wall, which could then loosen and travel to the lungs or brain."
4 "This dysrhythmia decreases the amount of blood flow coming from the heart, which can lead to blood clots forming in the brain."

Answer: 3

Rationale: A severe complication of atrial fibrillation is the development of mural thrombi. The blood stagnates in the "quivering" atria, because of the loss of organized atrial muscle contraction and "atrial kick." The blood that pools in the atria can then clot, which increases the risk of pulmonary and cerebral emboli.

Test-Taking Strategy: Use the process of elimination. Note the relationship between the client's diagnosis "atrial fibrillation" and the words "atria are quivering" in option 3. Review the pathophysiology of atrial fibrillation if you had difficulty with this question.

Level of Cognitive Ability: Application
Client Needs: Health Promotion and Maintenance
Integrated Process: Nursing Process/Implementation
Content Area: Adult Health/Cardiovascular

Reference:
Black, J., & Hawks, J. (2005). *Medical-surgical nursing: Clinical management for positive outcomes* (7th ed.). Philadelphia: Saunders, p. 1602.

217. A clinic nurse is providing instructions to a client in the third trimester of pregnancy regarding relief measures related to heartburn. Which instruction would the nurse provide to the client?
1 Eat fatty foods once a day in the morning only
2 Eat three large meals a day rather than small, frequent meals
3 Sip on milk or tea
4 Use antacids that contain sodium

Answer: 3
Rationale: Measures to provide relief of heartburn include eating small, frequent meals and avoiding fatty fried foods, coffee, and cigarettes. Mild antacids can be used if they do not contain aspirin or sodium. Frequent sips of milk or hot tea is helpful.

Test-Taking Strategy: Use the process of elimination. Eliminate option 4 first, because sodium will lead to edema and edema should be avoided. Eliminate option 1 next based on basic nutritional principles that fatty and fried foods should be avoided. From the remaining options, recalling that milk and hot tea can be soothing to the gastrointestinal tract will assist in eliminating option 2. Review the measures that relieve heartburn if you had difficulty with this question.

Level of Cognitive Ability: Application
Client Needs: Health Promotion and Maintenance
Integrated Process: Nursing Process/Implementation
Content Area: Maternity/Antepartum

Reference:
Lowdermilk, D., & Perry, A. (2004). *Maternity & women's health care* (8th ed.). St. Louis: Mosby, pp. 390; 432.

---

218. A nurse provides instructions regarding home care to a parent of a 3-year old child hospitalized with hemophilia. Which statement by the parent indicates a need for further instructions?
1 "I should not leave my child unattended."
2 "I need to pad table corners in my home."
3 "I need to remove household items that can tip over."
4 "My child should not have any immunizations."

Answer: 4
Rationale: The nurse needs to stress the importance of immunizations, dental hygiene, and routine well-child care. Options 1, 2, and 3 are appropriate. The parents are also instructed in measures to implement if blunt trauma occurs, especially trauma involving the joints, and how to apply prolonged pressure to superficial wounds until the bleeding has stopped.

Test-Taking Strategy: Note the key words "need for further instructions." These words indicate a false-response question and that you need to select the incorrect parent statement. Recalling that bleeding is a concern in this disorder will assist in eliminating options 1, 2, and 3, which include measures of protection and safety for the child. Also, recalling the importance of immunizations will direct you to option 4. If you had difficulty with this question, review care of the child with hemophilia.

Level of Cognitive Ability: Analysis
Client Needs: Health Promotion and Maintenance
Integrated Process: Teaching/Learning
Content Area: Child Health

References:
James, S., Ashwill, J., & Droske, S. (2002). *Nursing care of children: Principles & practice* (2nd ed.).Philadelphia: Saunders, pp. 756; 759.
Wong, D., & Hockenberry, M. (2003). *Wong's nursing care of infants and children* (7th ed.). St. Louis: Mosby, p. 1565.

219. A nurse provides instructions to the client taking clorazepate (Tranxene) for management of an anxiety disorder. The nurse tells the client that:

1 Drowsiness is a side effect that usually disappears with continued therapy
2 If dizziness occurs, call the physician
3 Smoking increases the effectiveness of the medication
4 If gastrointestinal (GI) disturbances occur, discontinue the medication

Answer: 1

Rationale: Dizziness is a common side effect of this medication and usually disappears with continued use. The client should be instructed that if dizziness occurs, to change positions slowly from lying, to sitting, to standing. Smoking reduces medication effectiveness. GI disturbance is an occasional side effect, and the medication can be given with food if this occurs.

Test-Taking Strategy: Use the process of elimination. Eliminate option 4 first because the client should not be instructed to discontinue medication. Eliminate option 2 next because episodes of dizziness commonly occur with antianxiety medications, and interventions to alleviate the dizziness should be implemented. From the remaining options, recall that drowsiness is commonly associated with antianxiety medications and normally disappears with continued therapy. Review client teaching points related to this medication if you had difficulty with this question.

Level of Cognitive Ability: Application
Client Needs: Health Promotion and Maintenance
Integrated Process: Teaching/Learning
Content Area: Mental Health

Reference:
Hodgson, B., & Kizior, R. (2004). *Saunders nursing drug handbook 2004.* Philadelphia: Saunders, p. 234.

220. A client with chlamydia infection has received instructions on self-care and prevention of further infection. The nurse determines that the client needs reinforcement of the instructions if the client states to:

1 Reduce the chance of reinfection by limiting the number of sexual partners
2 Use latex condoms to prevent disease transmission
3 Return to the clinic as requested for follow-up culture in 1 week
4 Use antibiotics prophylactically to prevent symptoms of chlamydia

Answer: 4

Rationale: Antibiotics are not taken prophylactically to prevent chlamydia. The risk of reinfection can be reduced by limiting the number of sexual partners and by the use of condoms. In some instances, follow-up culture is requested in 4 to 7 days to confirm a cure.

Test-Taking Strategy: Note the key words "needs reinforcement of the instructions." These words indicate a false-response question and that you need to select the incorrect client statement. Recalling the basic principles of antibiotic therapy will direct you to option 4, because antibiotics are not used intermittently for prophylaxis of infection. Review the treatment measures for chlamydia infection if you had difficulty with this question.

Level of Cognitive Ability: Analysis
Client Needs: Health Promotion and Maintenance
Integrated Process: Teaching/Learning
Content Area: Fundamental Skills

Reference:
Black, J., & Hawks, J. (2005). *Medical-surgical nursing: Clinical management for positive outcomes* (7th ed.). Philadelphia: Saunders, p. 1132.

221. The client with prostatitis asks the nurse, "Why do I need to take a stool softener? The problem is with my urine, not my bowels!" The nurse makes which response to the client?

1 "Being constipated puts you at more risk for developing complications of prostatitis."

2 "This is a standard medication order for anyone with an abdominal problem."

3 "This will keep the bowel free of feces, which will help decrease the swelling inside."

4 "This will help you prevent constipation, because straining is painful with prostatitis."

Answer: 4

Rationale: Stool softeners are ordered for the client with prostatitis to prevent constipation, which can be painful. It has no direct effect on decreasing swelling. Constipation does not cause complications of prostatitis. Stool softeners are not a standard prescription for "anyone with an abdominal problem."

Test-Taking Strategy: Use the process of elimination. Recalling the purpose and use of stool softeners, to prevent constipation, will direct you to option 4. Review care of the client with prostatitis if you had difficulty with this question.

Level of Cognitive Ability: Application
Client Needs: Health Promotion and Maintenance
Integrated Process: Teaching/Learning
Content Area: Adult Health/Renal

Reference:
Ignatavicius, D., & Workman, M. (2002). *Medical surgical nursing: Critical thinking for collaborative care* (4th ed.). Philadelphia: Saunders, p. 1803.

---

222. A client with Parkinson's disease has begun therapy with levodopa (L-dopa). The nurse determines that the client understands the action of the medication if the client verbalizes that results may not be apparent for:

1 24 hours
2 5 to 7 days
3 1 week
4 2 to 3 weeks

Answer: 4

Rationale: Signs and symptoms of Parkinson's disease usually begin to resolve within 2 to 3 weeks of starting therapy, although in some clients marked improvement may not be seen for up to 6 months. Clients need to understand this concept to aid in compliance with medication therapy.

Test-Taking Strategy: Use the process of elimination and knowledge regarding this medication. Eliminate options 2 and 3 because they are similar time frames. From the remaining options, eliminate option 1 because it is unlikely that results would be noted in 24 hours. Review this medication if you had difficulty with this question.

Level of Cognitive Ability: Analysis
Client Needs: Health Promotion and Maintenance
Integrated Process: Nursing Process/Evaluation
Content Area: Pharmacology

Reference:
McKenry, L., & Salerno, E. (2003). *Mosby's pharmacology in nursing* (21st ed.). St. Louis: Mosby, pp. 495-496.

---

223. A nurse in the physician's office is reviewing the results of a client's phenytoin (Dilantin) level drawn that morning. The nurse determines that the client had a therapeutic drug level if the client's result was:

1 3 mcg/mL
2 8 mcg/mL
3 15 mcg/mL
4 24 mcg/mL

Answer: 3

Rationale: The therapeutic range for serum phenytoin levels is 10 to 20 mcg/mL in clients with normal serum albumin levels and renal function. A level below this range indicates that the client is not receiving sufficient medication and is at risk for seizure activity. In this case, the medication dose should be adjusted upward. A level above the therapeutic range indicates that the client is entering the toxic range and is at risk for toxic side effects of the medication. In this case, the dose should be adjusted downward.

Test-Taking Strategy: Recalling that the therapeutic drug serum level for phenytoin is 10 to 20 mcg/mL will direct you to option 3. Review this level if you had difficulty with this question.

Level of Cognitive Ability: Analysis
Client Needs: Health Promotion and Maintenance
Integrated Process: Nursing Process/Evaluation
Content Area: Pharmacology

Reference:
Hodgson, B., & Kizior, R. (2004). *Saunders nursing drug handbook 2004.* Philadelphia: Saunders, p. 806.

---

224. A nurse is conducting a prostate screening clinic and is discussing prevention and risk factors for prostate cancer. The nurse determines that a client understands the educational information that was shared if the nurse overhears the client tell another participant that:

1 Green and yellow vegetables should be limited in the diet to prevent prostate cancer
2 A low-fiber diet should be followed to prevent prostate cancer
3 An annual prostate exam and a prostate-specific antigen (PSA) test should be done beginning at the age of 50
4 Eating foods high in fat is not a risk factor for prostate cancer

Answer: 3
Rationale: An annual prostate exam and a PSA test should be done beginning at the age of 50 and beginning at the age of 45 if the client is at high risk for this type of cancer. Increased intake of green or yellow vegetables or lycopenes contained in tomatoes may be helpful in reducing risk. A low-fat, high-fiber diet diminishes prostate cancer risk.

Test-Taking Strategy: Use the process of elimination and focus on the issue: prostate screening and prevention and risk factors for prostate cancer. Using general health principles will direct you to option 3. Review the screening measures for prostate cancer if you had difficulty with this question.

Level of Cognitive Ability: Analysis
Client Needs: Health Promotion and Maintenance
Integrated Process: Nursing Process/Evaluation
Content Area: Adult Health/Renal

References:
Black, J., & Hawks, J. (2005). *Medical-surgical nursing: Clinical management for positive outcomes* (7th ed.). Philadelphia: Saunders, p. 1028.
Lewis, S., Heitkemper, M., & Dirksen, S. (2004). *Medical-surgical nursing: Assessment and management of clinical problems* (6th ed.). St. Louis: Mosby, p. 300.

---

225. A client is being discharged to home without an indwelling urinary catheter following prostatectomy. The nurse plans to teach the client which of the following points as part of discharge teaching?

1 Drink at least 15 glasses of water a day to minimize clot formation
2 Mowing the lawn is allowed after 1 week
3 Notify the physician if fever, increased pain, or inability to void occurs
4 Avoid lifting more than 50 pounds for 4 to 6 weeks after surgery

Answer: 3
Rationale: The client should notify the physician if there are any signs of infection, bleeding, increased pain, or urinary obstruction. Lifting more than 20 pounds is prohibited for 4 to 6 weeks after surgery. Other strenuous activities that could increase intraabdominal tension are also restricted, such as mowing the lawn. The client should take in 6 to 8 glasses of water or nonalcoholic beverages per day to minimize the risk of clot formation.

Test-Taking Strategy: Use the process of elimination and focus on the client's diagnosis. Eliminate option 1 first as an excessive fluid intake. Noting that the activities identified in options 2 and 4 are excessive assists in eliminating these options. Review home care measures following prostatectomy if you had difficulty with this question.

Level of Cognitive Ability: Application
Client Needs: Health Promotion and Maintenance
Integrated Process: Teaching/Learning
Content Area: Adult Health/Renal

Reference:
Black, J., & Hawks, J. (2005). *Medical-surgical nursing: Clinical management for positive outcomes* (7th ed.). Philadelphia: Saunders, pp. 1025-1027.

---

226. A nurse is teaching a client with acute renal failure to include proteins in the diet that are considered high quality. Which food item would the nurse discourage because it is a low-quality protein source?

1 Eggs
2 Broccoli
3 Chicken
4 Fish

Answer: 2

Rationale: High-quality proteins come from animal sources and include such foods as eggs, chicken, meat, and fish. Low-quality proteins derive from plant sources and include vegetables and foods made from grains. Because the renal diet is limited in protein, it is important that the proteins ingested are of high quality.

Test-Taking Strategy: Use the process of elimination, noting the key words "low quality protein source." In comparing the options, note that option 2 (broccoli) is the only item that does not derive from a living source. Chicken, eggs, and fish derive from animal sources, whereas broccoli is a plant. Review food items that are high and low protein quality if you had difficulty with this question.

Level of Cognitive Ability: Application
Client Needs: Health Promotion and Maintenance
Integrated Process: Nursing Process/Implementation
Content Area: Adult Health/Renal

References:
Black, J., & Hawks, J. (2005). *Medical-surgical nursing: Clinical management for positive outcomes* (7th ed.). Philadelphia: Saunders, pp. 946-948.
Lewis, S., Heitkemper, M., & Dirksen, S. (2004). *Medical-surgical nursing: Assessment and management of clinical problems* (6th ed.). St. Louis: Mosby, p. 1215.
Phipps, W., Monahan, F., Sands, J., Marek, J., & Neighbors, M. (2003). *Medical-surgical nursing: Health and illness perspectives* (7th ed.). St. Louis: Mosby, p. 1258.

---

227. A home care nurse visits a client who had a cerebrovascular accident (CVA) with resultant unilateral neglect who was recently discharged from the hospital. The nurse provides instructions to the family regarding care and tells the family to:

1 Place personal items directly in front of the client
2 Assist the client from the affected side
3 Assist the client to groom the unaffected side first
4 Discourage the client from scanning the environment

Answer: 2

Rationale: Unilateral neglect is a pattern of lack of awareness of body parts such as paralyzed arms or legs. Initially, the environment is adapted to the deficit by focusing on the client's unaffected side, and the client's personal items are placed on the unaffected side. Gradually, the client's attention is focused to the affected side. The client is assisted from the affected side, and the client grooms the affected side first. The client needs to scan the entire environment.

Test-Taking Strategy: Note the client's diagnosis, unilateral neglect, and note the issue, home care instructions. Recalling the physiological alteration that occurs in unilateral neglect and that it involves a pattern of lack of awareness of body parts will direct you to option 2. Review interventions associated with unilateral neglect if you had difficulty with this question.

Level of Cognitive Ability: Application
Client Needs: Health Promotion and Maintenance
Integrated Process: Teaching/Learning
Content Area: Adult Health/Neurological

Reference:
Black, J., & Hawks, J. (2005). *Medical-surgical nursing: Clinical management for positive outcomes* (7th ed.). Philadelphia: Saunders, p. 2131.

---

228. A nurse has completed discharge teaching with a client who has had surgery for lung cancer. The nurse determines that the client has misunderstood essential elements of home management if the client verbalizes to:

1 Sit up and lean forward to breathe more easily
2 Deal with any increases in pain independently
3 Avoid exposure to crowds
4 Call the physician for increased temperature or shortness of breath

Answer: 2
Rationale: Health teaching includes using positions that facilitate respiration, such as sitting up and leaning forward. Health teaching also includes avoiding exposure to crowds or persons with respiratory infections and reporting signs and symptoms of respiratory infection or increases in pain. The client should not be expected to deal with increases in pain independently.

Test-Taking Strategy: Note the key words "has misunderstood." These words indicate a false-response question and that you need to select the incorrect client statement. Focusing on the client's diagnosis, lung cancer, will direct you to option 2. Review home care measures for the client who has had surgery for lung cancer if you had difficulty with this question.

Level of Cognitive Ability: Analysis
Client Needs: Health Promotion and Maintenance
Integrated Process: Nursing Process/Evaluation
Content Area: Adult Health/Oncology

Reference:
Black, J., & Hawks, J. (2005). *Medical-surgical nursing: Clinical management for positive outcomes* (7th ed.). Philadelphia: Saunders, p. 1862.

---

229. A nurse is evaluating the nutritional status of a client after radical neck dissection. The nurse determines that the client has maintained adequate nutritional status if the client maintains body weight or loses less than:

1 5 pounds
2 8 pounds
3 10 pounds
4 12 pounds

Answer: 1
Rationale: The nurse determines that the client has maintained adequate nutritional status if the client maintains baseline body weight or loses less than 5 pounds.

Test-Taking Strategy: Focus on the issue: maintaining adequate nutritional status. In this situation it is best to select the option that identifies the least amount of weight loss. This will direct you to option 1. Review nutritional principles if you had difficulty with this question.

Level of Cognitive Ability: Analysis
Client Needs: Health Promotion and Maintenance
Integrated Process: Nursing Process/Evaluation
Content Area: Fundamental Skills

Reference:
Black, J., & Hawks, J. (2005). *Medical-surgical nursing: Clinical management for positive outcomes* (7th ed.). Philadelphia: Saunders, p. 1791.

230. A nurse has given the client with a non-plaster (fiberglass) leg cast instructions on cast care at home. The nurse determines that the client needs further instructions if the client makes which statement?
1 "I should avoid walking on wet, slippery floors."
2 "It's all right to wipe dirt off the top of the cast with a damp cloth."
3 "I'm not supposed to scratch the skin underneath the cast."
4 "If the cast gets wet, I can dry it with a hair dryer turned to the warmest setting."

Answer: 4
Rationale: The client is instructed to avoid walking on wet, slippery floors to prevent falls. Surface soil on a cast may be removed with a damp cloth. If the cast gets wet, it can be dried with a hair dryer set to a cool setting. If the skin under the cast itches, cool air from a hair dryer may be used to relieve it. The client should never scratch under a cast because of the risk of skin breakdown and infection.

Test-Taking Strategy: Note the key words "needs further instructions." These words indicate a false-response question and that you need to select the incorrect client statement. Noting the words "warmest setting" in option 4 will direct you to this option. Review home care instructions for a client with a cast if you had difficulty with this question.

Level of Cognitive Ability: Analysis
Client Needs: Health Promotion and Maintenance
Integrated Process: Teaching/Learning
Content Area: Adult Health/Musculoskeletal

References:
Black, J., & Hawks, J. (2005). *Medical-surgical nursing: Clinical management for positive outcomes* (7th ed.). Philadelphia: Saunders, pp. 631-632.
Ignatavicius, D., & Workman, M. (2002). *Medical surgical nursing: Critical thinking for collaborative care* (4th ed.). Philadelphia: Saunders, pp. 1134-1135.

231. A child is seen in the health care clinic, and initial testing for human immunodeficiency virus (HIV) is performed because of the child's exposure to HIV infection. Which home care instruction would the nurse provide to the parents of the child?
1 Avoid all immunizations until the diagnosis is established
2 Avoid sharing toothbrushes
3 Wipe up any blood spills with soap and water and allow to air dry
4 Wash hands with half-strength bleach if they come in contact with the child's blood

Answer: 2
Rationale: Immunizations must be kept up to date. Blood spills are wiped up with a paper towel. The area is then washed with soap and water, rinsed with bleach and water, and allowed to air dry. Hands are washed with soap and water if they come in contact with blood. Parents are instructed that toothbrushes are not to be shared.

Test-Taking Strategy: Use the process of elimination. Eliminate option 1 first because of the absolute word "all." Eliminate option 3 next based on the knowledge that blood spills need to be cleaned with a bleach solution. Eliminate option 4 because bleach would be irritating and caustic to the skin. Review home care instructions for the child exposed to HIV infection if you had difficulty with this question.

Level of Cognitive Ability: Application
Client Needs: Health Promotion and Maintenance
Integrated Process: Teaching/Learning
Content Area: Child Health

References:
James, S., Ashwill, J., & Droske, S. (2002). *Nursing care of children: Principles & practice* (2nd ed.).Philadelphia: Saunders, p. 489.
Wong, D., & Hockenberry, M. (2003). *Wong's nursing care of infants and children* (7th ed.). St. Louis: Mosby, p. 1577.

232. A client is ready to be discharged to home health care for continued intravenous (IV) therapy in the home. Home care instructions regarding care of the IV have been given to the client. The best way to evaluate the client's ability to care for the IV site is to:

1 Ask the client to verbalize IV site care
2 Ask the client to change the IV dressing
3 Review the entire discharge plan with the client again
4 Demonstrate the dressing change again for the client one last time before discharge

Answer: 2

Rationale: Acquisition of psychomotor skills is best evaluated by observing how a client can carry out a procedure. The client may be able to verbalize how to do the procedure but may not be able to actually perform the psychomotor function. Reviewing the entire discharge plan again and demonstrating the procedure again will not evaluate the client's ability. Actively demonstrating is always the best method of evaluating a psychomotor skill.

Test -Taking Strategy: Use teaching/learning principles to answer the question and note the key word "best." The correct option needs to identify some type of active client participation. This concept will direct you to option 2. Review teaching/learning principles if you had difficulty with this question.

Level of Cognitive Ability: Analysis
Client Needs: Health Promotion and Maintenance
Integrated Process: Teaching/Learning
Content Area: Fundamental Skills

Reference:
Potter, P., & Perry, A. (2005). *Fundamentals of nursing* (6th ed.). St. Louis: Mosby, pp. 451-454; 1194.

233. A nurse provides home care instructions to a client with an implanted vascular access port. Which statement by the client indicates a need for further instructions?

1 "If the site becomes red, I will notify my physician."
2 "I should keep the site clean and dry."
3 "I should pump the port daily to maintain patency."
4 "The port will need to be flushed with saline to maintain patency."

Answer: 3

Rationale: An implanted vascular port does not need to be pumped in order to maintain patency. The site will need to be kept clean and dry, and the physician would need to be notified of signs and symptoms of infection. Saline is used to flush the site to maintain patency.

Test-Taking Strategy: Note the key words "need for further instructions." These words indicate a false-response question and that you need to select the incorrect client statement. Using principles related to vascular access ports and IV care will direct you to option 3. Review these principles if you had difficulty with this question.

Level of Cognitive Ability: Analysis
Client Needs: Health Promotion and Maintenance
Integrated Process: Teaching/Learning
Content Area: Fundamental Skills

Reference:
Perry, A., & Potter, P. (2004). *Clinical nursing skills and techniques* (5th ed.). St. Louis: Mosby, p. 610.

234. A nurse is planning to teach a client with below-the-knee amputation about skin care to prevent breakdown. Which of the following points would the nurse include in the teaching plan?
1 A stump sock must be worn at all times and changed twice a week.
2 The residual limb (stump) is washed gently and dried every other day.
3 The socket of the prosthesis needs to be washed with a strong bactericidal agent daily.
4 The socket of the prosthesis must be dried carefully before using it.

Answer: 4
Rationale: A stump sock must be worn at all times to absorb perspiration and is changed daily. The residual limb (stump) is washed, dried, and inspected for breakdown twice each day. The socket of the prosthesis is cleansed with a mild detergent, and rinsed and dried carefully each day. A strong bactericidal agent would not be used.

Test-Taking Strategy: Use the process of elimination. Recalling that the residual limb is cared for twice a day will assist in eliminating options 1 and 2. From the remaining options, noting the key word "strong" in option 3 will assist in eliminating this option. Review home care instructions following amputation if you had difficulty with this question.

Level of Cognitive Ability: Application
Client Needs: Health Promotion and Maintenance
Integrated Process: Teaching/Learning
Content Area: Adult Health/Musculoskeletal

Reference:
Phipps, W., Monahan, F., Sands, J., Marek, J., & Neighbors, M. (2003). *Medical-surgical nursing: Health and illness perspectives* (7th ed.). St. Louis: Mosby, p. 781.

235. A nurse has completed instructions on diet and fluid restriction for the client with chronic renal failure. The nurse determines that the client understands the information presented if the client selected which dessert from the dietary menu?
1 Angel food cake
2 Ice cream
3 Sherbet
4 Jello

Answer: 1
Rationale: Dietary fluid includes anything that is liquid at room temperature. This includes items such as ice cream, sherbet, and Jell-O. With clients on a fluid-restricted diet, it is helpful to avoid "hidden" fluids to whatever extent is possible. This allows the client more fluid for drinking, which can help alleviate thirst.

Test-Taking Strategy: Use the process of elimination, noting the key words "fluid restriction." Recalling that dietary fluid includes anything at room temperature will direct you to option 1. Review this type of dietary restriction if you had difficulty with this question.

Level of Cognitive Ability: Analysis
Client Needs: Health Promotion and Maintenance
Integrated Process: Nursing Process/Evaluation
Content Area: Adult Health/Renal

Reference:
Lewis, S., Heitkemper, M., & Dirksen, S. (2004). *Medical-surgical nursing: Assessment and management of clinical problems* (6th ed.). St. Louis: Mosby, p. 1223.

236. A nurse has given instructions to the client with chronic renal failure about reducing pruritis from uremia. The nurse determines that the client needs further instructions if the client states to use which item for skin care?
1 Mild soap
2 Oil in the bath water
3 Alcohol cleansing pads
4 Lanolin-based lotion

Answer: 3

Rationale: The client with chronic renal failure often has dry skin, accompanied by itching (pruritis) from uremia. The client should use mild soaps, lotions, and bath water oils to reduce dryness without increasing skin irritation. Products that contain perfumes or alcohol increase dryness and pruritis and should be avoided.

Test-Taking Strategy: Focus on the issue, reducing pruritis, and note the key words "needs further instructions." These words indicate a false-response question and that you need to select the incorrect client statement. Eliminate options 2 and 4 first because they are similar. From the remaining options, eliminate option 1, knowing that the client should avoid irritating products on the skin. Review measures to treat pruritis if you had difficulty with this question.

Level of Cognitive Ability: Analysis
Client Needs: Health Promotion and Maintenance
Integrated Process: Nursing Process/Evaluation
Content Area: Adult Health/Renal

Reference:
Ignatavicius, D., & Workman, M. (2002). *Medical surgical nursing: Critical thinking for collaborative care* (4th ed.). Philadelphia: Saunders, p. 1515.

237. A client who is scheduled for implantation of an automatic internal defibrillator-cardioverter (AICD) asks the nurse why there is a need to keep a diary and what to put in it. In formulating a reply, the nurse understands that the primary purpose of the diary is to:
1 Provide a count of the number of shocks delivered
2 Document events that precipitate a countershock
3 Record a variety of data useful for the physician in medical management
4 Analyze which activities to avoid

Answer: 3

Rationale: The client with an AICD maintains a log or diary of a variety of data. This includes recording date, time, activity before the shock and any symptoms experienced, number of shocks delivered, and how the client felt after the shock. The information is used by the physician to adjust the medical regimen, especially medication therapy, which must be maintained after AICD insertion.

Test-Taking Strategy: Use the process of elimination, noting the key words "primary purpose." Each of the incorrect options lists one of the items that should be logged in the diary, but the correct option is the only one that could be considered a "primary" purpose. Option 3 is the umbrella (global) option. Review home care instructions for the client with an AICD if you had difficulty with this question.

Level of Cognitive Ability: Application
Client Needs: Health Promotion and Maintenance
Integrated Process: Nursing Process/Implementation
Content Area: Adult Health/Cardiovascular

Reference:
Phipps, W., Monahan, F., Sands, J., Marek, J., & Neighbors, M. (2003). *Medical-surgical nursing: Health and illness perspectives* (7th ed.). St. Louis: Mosby, p. 701.

238. A nurse is evaluating a hypertensive client's understanding of dietary modifications to control the disease process. The nurse determines that the client's understanding is satisfactory if the client made which of the following meal selections?
1 Scallops, French fries, salad with bleu cheese dressing
2 Corned beef, fresh carrots, boiled potato
3 Hot dog in a bun, sauerkraut, baked beans
4 Turkey, baked potato, salad with oil and vinegar

Answer: 4
Rationale: The client with hypertension should avoid foods high in sodium. Foods from the meat group that are higher in sodium include bacon, hot dogs, luncheon meat, chipped or corned beef, Kosher meat, smoked or salted meat or fish, peanut butter, and a variety of shellfish.

Test-Taking Strategy: Use the process of elimination, focusing on the client's diagnosis. Eliminate options 2 and 3 because they are highly processed meats, which would be high in sodium. From the remaining options, recalling that shellfish and commercial salad dressing is high in sodium will assist in eliminating option 1. Review foods high in sodium if you had difficulty with this question.

Level of Cognitive Ability: Analysis
Client Needs: Health Promotion and Maintenance
Integrated Process: Nursing Process/Evaluation
Content Area: Adult Health/Cardiovascular

Reference:
Peckenpaugh, N. (2003). *Nutrition essentials and diet therapy* (9th ed.). Philadelphia: Saunders, p. 241.

239. A nurse has taught a client who will be taking warfarin sodium (Coumadin) indefinitely. Which statement by the client indicates a need for further teaching?
1 "I need to use a soft toothbrush."
2 "I need to avoid drinking alcohol while taking this medication."
3 "I need to carry identification about the medication being taken."
4 "I need to use a straight razor for shaving."

Answer: 4
Rationale: Client instructions for oral anticoagulant therapy include taking the medication only as prescribed and at the same time each day; avoiding other medications (including over-the-counter medications) without physician approval; avoiding alcohol; notifying all caregivers about the medication; carrying a Medic-Alert bracelet or card; reporting any signs of bleeding and implementing measures to prevent bleeding; and adhering to the schedule for follow-up blood work.

Test-Taking Strategy: Note the key words "need for further teaching." These words indicate a false-response question and that you need to select the incorrect client statement. Recalling that warfarin sodium is an anticoagulant and that the client is at risk for bleeding will direct you to option 4. Review home care instructions for the client on an anticoagulant if you had difficulty with this question.

Level of Cognitive Ability: Analysis
Client Needs: Health Promotion and Maintenance
Integrated Process: Teaching/Learning
Content Area: Pharmacology

Reference:
Hodgson, B., & Kizior, R. (2004). *Saunders nursing drug handbook 2004.* Philadelphia: Saunders, p. 1065.

240. A home care nurse has given instructions to a client recently discharged from the hospital about care to an arterial ischemic leg ulcer. The nurse determines that further instruction is needed if the client made which of the following statements?

1 "I should wear shoes and socks."
2 "I should cut my toenails straight across."
3 "I should raise my legs above the level of my heart periodically."
4 "I should inspect my feet daily."

Answer: 3

Rationale: Foot care instructions for the client with peripheral arterial ischemia are the same instructions given to the client with diabetic mellitus. The client with arterial disease, however, should avoid raising the legs above heart level, unless instructed to do so as part of an exercise program (such as Buerger-Allen exercises) or unless venous stasis is also present. Options 1, 2, and 4 are accurate client statements.

Test-Taking Strategy: Note the key words "further instruction is needed." These words indicate a false-response question and that you need to select the incorrect client statement. Also, note that the client has an arterial disorder. Recalling the anatomy of the blood vessels and the pattern of blood flow in the arteries will direct you to option 3. Review home care instructions for the client with an arterial disorder if you had difficulty with this question.

Level of Cognitive Ability: Analysis
Client Needs: Health Promotion and Maintenance
Integrated Process: Teaching/Learning
Content Area: Adult Health/Cardiovascular

Reference:
Lewis, S., Heitkemper, M., & Dirksen, S. (2004). *Medical-surgical nursing: Assessment and management of clinical problems* (6th ed.). St. Louis: Mosby, p. 921.

241. A client with chronic renal failure is about to begin hemodialysis therapy. The client asks the nurse about the frequency and scheduling of hemodialysis treatments. The nurse's response is based on an understanding that the typical schedule is:

1 5 hours of treatment 2 days per week
2 3 to 4 hours of treatment 3 days per week
3 2 to 3 hours of treatment 5 days per week
4 2 hours of treatment 6 days per week

Answer: 2

Rationale: The typical schedule for hemodialysis is 3 to 4 hours of treatment 3 days per week. Individual adjustments may be made according to variables, such as the size of the client, type of dialyzer, the rate of blood flow, personal client preferences, and others.

Test-Taking Strategy: Focus on the issue: the "typical" dialysis schedule. Recalling that the client receives dialysis 3 days per week will direct you to option 2. Review the typical dialysis schedule if you had difficulty with this question.

Level of Cognitive Ability: Application
Client Needs: Health Promotion and Maintenance
Integrated Process: Nursing Process/Implementation
Content Area: Adult Health/Renal

Reference:
Black, J., & Hawks, J. (2005). *Medical-surgical nursing: Clinical management for positive outcomes* (7th ed.). Philadelphia: Saunders, p. 957.

242. A client is being discharged from the hospital with a peripheral intravenous (IV) site for continued home IV therapy. In planning for the discharge, the nurse teaches the client which of the following to help prevent phlebitis and infiltration?

1 Gently massage the area around the site daily
2 Cleanse the site daily with alcohol
3 Keep the cannula stabilized or anchored properly with tape
4 Immobilize the extremity until the IV is discontinued

Answer: 3

Rationale: The principles of maintaining IV therapy at home are the same as in the hospital. It is extremely important to ensure that the IV site is anchored properly in order to reduce the risk of phlebitis and infiltration. Massaging the site may actually contribute to catheter movement and tissue damage. Dressings surrounding peripheral IV sites are changed and cleansed at various times (usually every 2 to 5 days) depending on facility protocols. Most dressings are to remain intact unless the dressing becomes wet, soiled, or loose. Alcohol is not normally used to cleanse the IV site. Immobilizing the extremity is not routinely necessary for peripheral IV sites. Arm boards are only used if a site is near a joint and the IV flow rate is positional.

Test-Taking Strategy: Use the process of elimination, focusing on the issue: preventing phlebitis and infiltration. Eliminate options 1, 2, and 4 because of the words "massage," "alcohol," and "immobilize," respectively. Review interventions related to the prevention of phlebitis and infiltration if you had difficulty with this question.

Level of Cognitive Ability: Application
Client Needs: Health Promotion and Maintenance
Integrated Process: Teaching/Learning
Content Area: Fundamental Skills

Reference:
Potter, P., & Perry, A. (2005). *Fundamentals of nursing* (6th ed.). St. Louis: Mosby, p. 1194.

---

243. A nurse is teaching a client how to stand on crutches. The nurse tells the client to place the crutches:

1 3 inches to the front and side of the toes
2 8 inches to the front and side of the toes
3 15 inches to the front and side of the toes
4 20 inches to the front and side of the toes

Answer: 2

Rationale: The classic tripod position is taught to the client before giving instructions on gait. The crutches are placed anywhere from 6 to 10 inches in front and to the side of the client's toes, depending on the client's body size. This provides a wide enough base of support to the client and improves balance.

Test-Taking Strategy: Use the process of elimination. Three inches (option 1) and 20 inches (option 4) seem excessively short and long, respectively, and these options should be eliminated first. From the remaining options, visualize this procedure. Eight inches seems more in keeping with the normal length of a stride than 15 inches. Review this procedure if you had difficulty with this question.

Level of Cognitive Ability: Application
Client Needs: Health Promotion and Maintenance
Integrated Process: Teaching/Learning
Content Area: Adult Health/Musculoskeletal

Reference:
Potter, P., & Perry, A. (2005). *Fundamentals of nursing* (6th ed.). St. Louis: Mosby, pp. 950-951.

244. A nurse is giving instructions to a client who is beginning therapy with digoxin (Lanoxin). The nurse teaches the client to:
1 Monitor the blood pressure once a week
2 Measure weight each morning before breakfast
3 Take the pulse daily
4 Have electrolyte levels drawn weekly

Answer: 3
Rationale: Clients taking digoxin should take the pulse each day and notify the physician if the heart rate is below 60 beats per minute or above 100 beats per minute. Options 1, 2, and 4 are not necessary interventions for the client taking digoxin.

Test-Taking Strategy: Use the process of elimination, focusing on the medication identified in the question. Recalling that digoxin is a cardiac medication will direct you to option 3. Review client instructions regarding this medication if you had difficulty with this question.

Level of Cognitive Ability: Application
Client Needs: Health Promotion and Maintenance
Integrated Process: Teaching/Learning
Content Area: Pharmacology

Reference:
Hodgson, B., & Kizior, R. (2004). *Saunders nursing drug handbook 2004.* Philadelphia: Saunders, p. 310.

245. A nurse has completed client teaching with a hemodialysis client about self-monitoring of fluid status between hemodialysis treatments. The nurse determines that the client understands the information given if the client states to record which of the following on a daily basis?
1 Pulse and respiratory rate
2 Intake and output and weight
3 Blood urea nitrogen and creatinine levels
4 Activity log

Answer: 2
Rationale: The client on hemodialysis should monitor fluid status between hemodialysis treatments. This can be done by recording intake and output and measuring weight on a daily basis. Ideally, the hemodialysis client should not gain more than 0.5 kg of weight per day. Options 1, 3, and 4 are not necessary.

Test-Taking Strategy: Use the process of elimination, and note the key words "daily basis." Focusing on these key words and the issue, fluid status, will direct you to option 2. Review self-care instructions for the hemodialysis client if you had difficulty with this question.

Level of Cognitive Ability: Analysis
Client Needs: Health Promotion and Maintenance
Integrated Process: Nursing Process/Evaluation
Content Area: Adult Health/Renal

Reference:
Ignatavicius, D., & Workman, M. (2002). *Medical surgical nursing: Critical thinking for collaborative care* (4th ed.). Philadelphia: Saunders, p. 1701.

246. Diltiazem hydrochloride (Cardizem) is prescribed for the client with Prinzmetal's angina. A nurse provides instructions to the client regarding this medication. Which statement by the client indicates a need for further instructions?
1 "I will call the physician if shortness of breath occurs."
2 "I will rise slowly when getting out of bed in the morning."
3 "I will take the medication after meals."
4 "I will avoid activities that require alertness until my body gets use to the medication."

Answer: 3
Rationale: Diltiazem hydrochloride (Cardizem) is a calcium-channel blocker. It is administered before meals and at bedtime as prescribed. Hypotension can occur, and the client is instructed to rise slowly. The client should avoid tasks that require alertness until a response to the medication is established. The client should call the physician if an irregular heartbeat, shortness of breath, pronounced dizziness, nausea, or constipation occurs.

Test-Taking Strategy: Note the key words "need for further instructions." These words indicate a false-response question and that you need to select the incorrect client statement. Focusing on the client's diagnosis will assist in eliminating options 1, 2, and 4.

Review home care instructions regarding this medication if you had difficulty with this question.

Level Cognitive Ability: Analysis
Client Needs: Health Promotion and Maintenance
Integrated Process: Teaching/Learning
Content Area: Pharmacology

Reference:
Hodgson, B., & Kizior, R. (2004). *Saunders nursing drug handbook 2004*. Philadelphia: Saunders, p. 314.

---

247. A nurse has provided instructions to a client being discharged from the hospital to home after an abdominal aortic aneurysm (AAA) resection. The nurse determines that the client understands the instructions if the client stated that an appropriate activity would be to:
  1 Lift objects up to 30 pounds
  2 Walk as tolerated, including stairs and out of doors
  3 Mow the lawn
  4 Play a game of 18-hole golf

Answer: 2
Rationale: The client can walk as tolerated after repair or resection of an AAA, including climbing stairs and walking outdoors. The client should not lift objects that weight more than 15 to 20 pounds for 6 to 12 weeks or engage in any activities that involve pushing, pulling, or straining. Driving is also prohibited for several weeks.

Test-Taking Strategy: Use the process of elimination, noting the key words "understands the instructions." Evaluate each option in terms of the strain it could put on the sutured graft. This will direct you to option 2. Review discharge instructions following AAA if you had difficulty with this question.

Level of Cognitive Ability: Analysis
Client Needs: Health Promotion and Maintenance
Integrated Process: Teaching/Learning
Content Area: Adult Health/Cardiovascular

Reference:
Black, J., & Hawks, J. (2005). *Medical-surgical nursing: Clinical management for positive outcomes* (7th ed.). Philadelphia: Saunders, p. 1531.

---

248. A nurse is planning dietary counseling for the client taking triamterene (Dyrenium). The nurse plans to include which of the following in a list of foods that are acceptable?
  1 Baked potato
  2 Bananas
  3 Oranges
  4 Pears canned in water

Answer: 4
Rationale: Triamterene is a potassium-sparing diuretic, and clients taking this medication should be cautioned against eating foods that are high in potassium, including many vegetables, fruits, and fresh meats. Because potassium is very water-soluble, foods that are prepared in water are often lower in potassium.

Test-Taking Strategy: Focus on the medication, noting the key words "foods that are acceptable." Recall that triamterene is a potassium-sparing diuretic. Next, review the options, identifying the food item lowest in potassium. Review high-potassium foods and this medication if you had difficulty with this question.

Level of Cognitive Ability: Application
Client Needs: Health Promotion and Maintenance
Integrated Process: Nursing Process/Planning
Content Area: Pharmacology

References:
Hodgson, B., & Kizior, R. (2004). *Saunders nursing drug handbook 2004.* Philadelphia: Saunders, pp. 1019-1020.
McKenry, L., & Salerno, E. (2003). *Mosby's pharmacology in nursing* (21st ed.). St. Louis: Mosby, 678.

---

249. Cyclophosphamide (Cytoxan) is prescribed for the client with breast cancer, and the nurse provides instructions to the client regarding the medication. Which statement by the client indicates a need for further instructions?
1 "I need to avoid contact with anyone who recently received a live virus vaccine."
2 "If I lose my hair, it will grow back."
3 "If I develop a sore throat, I should notify the physician."
4 "I need to limit my fluid intake while taking this medication."

Answer: 4
Rationale: Hemorrhagic cystitis is an adverse reaction associated with this medication. The client needs to be instructed to consume copious amounts of fluid during therapy. Avoiding contact with anyone who recently received a live virus vaccine is important because cyclophosphamide produces immunosuppression, placing the client at risk for infection. Hair will grow back, although it may have a different color and texture. A sore throat may be an indication of an infection and needs to be reported to the physician.

Test-Taking Strategy: Note the key words "need for further instructions." These words indicate a false-response question and that you need to select the incorrect client statement. Eliminate options 1 and 3 because they are similar in that they both relate to the risk of infection. From the remaining options, recalling that hemorrhagic cystitis is an adverse effect of this medication will direct you to option 4. Review the adverse effects of this medication if you had difficulty with this question.

Level of Cognitive Ability: Analysis
Client Needs: Health Promotion and Maintenance
Integrated Process: Teaching/Learning
Content Area: Pharmacology

Reference:
Hodgson, B., & Kizior, R. (2004). *Saunders nursing drug handbook 2004.* Philadelphia: Saunders, p. 258.

---

250. A community health nurse has reviewed information on the population in a local community and determines that there are groups in the population that are at high risk for infection with tuberculosis (TB). The nurse targets which high-risk group for screening?
1 White, Anglo-Saxon Americans
2 Adolescents ages 13 to 17
3 French Canadians
4 Older clients in long-term care facilities

Answer: 4
Rationale: Older clients, particularly those in long-term care facilities, are at high risk for infection with TB. Other people at risk include children ages 5 and younger, the malnourished, the immunosuppressed, the economically disadvantaged, foreign-born persons, and persons of a minority race who formerly lived in a place where TB is common, such as Asia and the Pacific Islands.

Test-Taking Strategy: Recalling the risk factors associated with TB will direct you to option 4. Remember that the very young and the very old often fall into a high-risk category. Review the risk factors associated with TB if you had difficulty with this question.

Level of Cognitive Ability: Analysis
Client Needs: Health Promotion and Maintenance
Integrated Process: Nursing Process/Assessment
Content Area: Adult Health/Respiratory

Reference:
Black, J., & Hawks, J. (2005). *Medical-surgical nursing: Clinical management for positive outcomes* (7th ed.). Philadelphia: Saunders, p. 1844.

CRITICAL THINKING: ALTERNATE FORMAT QUESTIONS

1. A nurse working at a health screening clinic gathers data from a client to identify the client's risk factors associated with coronary heart disease. The nurse is specifically interested in modifiable risk factors so that a health promotion and maintenance plan of care can be developed for the client. Select all risk factors that are modifiable.

___ Has a family history of heart disease
___ Has a personal history of diabetes mellitus
___ Is physically inactive
___ Is an African American
___ Is a cigarette smoker
___ Is female age 45 years
___ Has a blood pressure of 158/102 mmHg
___ Has an elevated serum cholesterol level
___ Is obese

Answer:
Has a personal history of diabetes mellitus
Is physically inactive
Is a cigarette smoker
Has a blood pressure of 158/102 mmHg
Has an elevated serum cholesterol level
Is obese

Rationale: Modifiable risk factors for coronary artery disease are those that can be modified or reduced by treatment. These include cigarette smoking, hypertension, elevated serum cholesterol level, diabetes mellitus, physical inactivity, and obesity. Nonmodifiable risk factors are those that cannot be modified or reduced by treatment and include such factors as heredity including race, age, and gender. Those whose parents had coronary heart disease are at higher risk. Increasing age influences both the risk and severity of the disease. Although men are at higher risk for heart attacks at a younger age, the risk for women increases significantly at menopause. The incidence of coronary heart disease is more prevalent in African-American women.

Test-Taking Strategy: Focus on the issue: modifiable risk factors. Recalling that modifiable risk factors are those that can be modified or reduced by treatment will assist in answering this question. Look at each risk factor listed and select the risk factors that can be changed. Review the modifiable and nonmodifiable risk factors for coronary heart disease if you had difficulty with this question.

Level of Cognitive Ability: Analysis
Client Needs: Health Promotion and Maintenance
Integrated Process: Nursing Process/Assessment
Content Area: Adult Health/Cardiovascular

Reference:
Black, J., & Hawks, J. (2005). *Medical-surgical nursing: Clinical management for positive outcomes* (7th ed.). Philadelphia: Saunders, p. 1628.

2. A client at risk for urinary tract infections is told to drink 3000 mL of fluid every day to decrease the risk. The nurse explains to the client that she needs to drink how many 10-ounce glasses of fluid per day to consume the prescribed 3000 mL?

Answer: _____

Answer: 10
Rationale: Each 10-ounce glass of fluid contains 300 mL (1 oz = 30 mL; therefore 10 oz = 300 mL). Therefore, the client will need to drink ten 10-ounce glasses of fluid daily (3000 mL divided by 300 mL = 10).

Test-Taking Strategy: Focus on the issue: the number of 10-ounce glasses of fluid that will equal 3000 mL. First change ounces to mL to determine the amount of mL in each 10-ounce glass of fluid. Next, divide the amount of fluid prescribed by the amount of mL in each 10-ounce glass of fluid. Review the formula for converting ounces to mL if you had difficulty with this question.

Level of Cognitive Ability: Application
Client Needs: Health Promotion and Maintenance
Integrated Process: Teaching/Learning
Content Area: Fundamental Skills

Reference:
Harkreader, H. & Hogan, M.A. (2004) *Fundamentals of nursing: Caring and clinical judgment.* (2nd ed.).Philadelphia: Saunders. pp. 406-407.

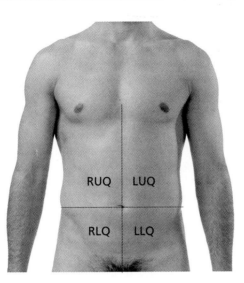

3. The nurse is performing a physical assessment on an adult client and is preparing to palpate the liver to assess for the location of the liver's lower border. The nurse plans to palpate in which abdominal quadrant.
1. Right upper quadrant (RUQ)
2. Left upper quadrant (LUQ)
3. Right lower quadrant (RLQ)
4. Left lower quadrant (LLQ)

Answer: _____

Answer: 1
Rationale: The liver is the largest organ in the body, weighing about 3.5 pounds (1.6 kg). It lies under the right diaphragm, spanning the upper quadrant of the abdomen from the fifth intercostal space to slightly below the costal margin. The rib cage covers a substantial portion of the liver; only the lower margin is exposed beneath it.

Teat-Taking Strategy: Use knowledge of anatomy of the body. Recalling that the liver is located on the right side of the body in the upper quadrant will direct you to the correct answer. Review the anatomical location of the liver and the technique for palpation if you had difficulty with this question.

Level of Cognitive Ability: Application
Client Needs: Health Promotion and Maintenance
Integrated Process: Nursing Process/Assessment
Content Area: Adult Health/Gastrointestinal

Reference:
Wilson, S., & Giddens, J. (2005). *Health assessment for nursing practice* (3rd ed.). St. Louis: Mosby, pp. 432; 443.

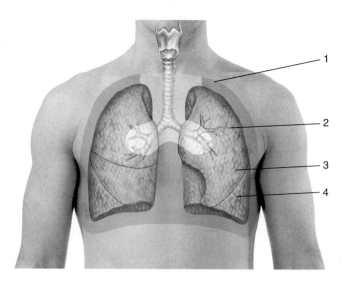

4. The nurse is performing a physical assessment on a client and is preparing to auscultate breath sounds. The nurse places the stethoscope in which area to assess bronchovesicular sounds?
1.
2.
3.
4.

Answer: 2
Rationale: Bronchovesicular breath sounds are heard over the main bronchi. Specifically, their normal location is between the first and second intercostal spaces at the sternal border anteriorly, and posteriorly at T4 medial to the scapula. These sounds are moderate in pitch, medium in intensity, and the duration of inspiration and expiration is equal. Bronchial breath sounds are heard over the trachea. Vesicular breath sounds are heard over the lesser bronchi, bronchioles, and lobes.

Test-Taking Strategy: Focus on the locations identified. Eliminate options 3 and 4 because they identify similar locations (peripheral lung fields). From the remaining options, recall that bronchial breath sounds are heard over the trachea. Review respiratory assessment techniques if you had difficulty with this question.

Level of Cognitive Ability: Application
Client Needs: Health Promotion and Maintenance
Integrated Process: Nursing Process/Assessment
Content Area: Adult Health/Respiratory

Reference:
Wilson, S., & Giddens, J. (2005). *Health assessment for nursing practice* (3rd ed.). St. Louis: Mosby, pp. 347-348.

5. The nurse prepares a discharge plan of care for a postoperative client who had a cystectomy and a urinary diversion (vesicostomy) created to treat bladder cancer. List in order of priority the nursing diagnoses identified in the plan of care. (Number 1 is the first priority.)

___ Risk for disturbed body image related to the presence of a pouch

___ Impaired urinary elimination related to urinary diversion and loss of ability to void normally

___ Risk for toileting self-care deficit related to poor hand-eye coordination

___ Risk for infection related to direct opening into the bladder

Answer: 4132

Rationale: A urinary diversion is a surgical diversion of urinary flow from its usual path through the urinary tract. As a result, the client has impaired urinary elimination. The nursing diagnosis, impaired urinary elimination, is the first priority because it is identified as an actual problem and directly relates to the client's surgical procedure. The client is also at risk for infection because of the direct opening into the bladder. Because infection can be life-threatening if it occurs, the nursing diagnosis risk for infection is the second priority. Because risk for toileting self-care deficit is a physiological need, it takes priority over risk for disturbed body image, which is a psychosocial need. Therefore, risk for toileting self-care deficit is the third priority, followed by risk for disturbed body image as the fourth priority.

Test-Taking Strategy: When presented with nursing diagnoses and asked to prioritize them, remember that in most situations an actual nursing diagnosis is the priority. This guideline assists you in selecting impaired urinary elimination as the first priority. From the remaining options, use Maslow's hierarchy of needs theory, and remember that physiological needs are the priority. This theory assists in determining that risk for disturbed body image is the fourth priority. When determining the second and third priority nursing diagnosis, recall that risk for infection can be life-threatening, whereas risk for toileting self-care deficit is not. Review care of the client with a urinary diversion if you had difficulty with this question.

Level of Cognitive Ability: Analysis
Client Needs: Health Promotion and Maintenance
Integrated Process: Nursing Process/Planning
Content Area: Adult Health/Renal

Reference:
Gulanick, M., Myers, J., Klopp, A., Gradishar, D., Galanes, S., & Puzas, M. (2003). *Nursing care plans: Nursing diagnosis and intervention* (5th ed.). St. Louis: Mosby, pp. 884-893.

REFERENCES

Black, J., & Hawks, J. (2005). *Medical-surgical nursing: Clinical management for positive outcomes* (7th ed.). Philadelphia: Saunders.

Chernecky, C., & Berger, B. (2004). *Laboratory tests and diagnostic procedures* (4th ed.). Philadelphia: Saunders.

Gulanick, M., Myers, J., Klopp, A., Gradishar, D., Galanes, S., & Puzas, M. (2003). *Nursing care plans: Nursing diagnosis and intervention* (5th ed.). St. Louis: Mosby.

Hodgson, B., & Kizior, R. (2004). *Saunders nursing drug handbook 2004.* Philadelphia: Saunders.

Ignatavicius, D., & Workman, M. (2005). *Medical surgical nursing: Critical thinking for collaborative care* (5th ed.). Philadelphia: Saunders.

James, S., Ashwill, J., & Droske, S. (2002). *Nursing care of children: Principles & practice* (2nd ed.). Philadelphia: Saunders.

Kee, J., & Hayes, E. (2003). *Pharmacology: A nursing process approach* (4th ed.). Philadelphia: Saunders.

Keltner, N., Schwecke, L., & Bostrom, C. (2003). *Psychiatric nursing* (4th ed.). St. Louis: Mosby.

Lehne, R. (2004). *Pharmacology for nursing care* (5th ed.). Philadelphia: Saunders.

Lewis, S., Heitkemper, M., & Dirksen, S. (2004). *Medical-surgical nursing: Assessment and management of clinical problems* (6th ed.). St. Louis: Mosby.

Lowdermilk, D., & Perry, A. (2004). *Maternity & women's health care* (8th ed.). St. Louis: Mosby.

Lueckenotte, A. (2000). *Gerontologic nursing* (2nd ed.). St. Louis: Mosby.

McKenry, L., & Salerno, E. (2003). *Mosby's pharmacology in nursing* (21st ed.). St. Louis: Mosby.

McKinney, E., James, S., Murray, S., & Ashwill, J. (2005). *Maternal-child nursing* (2nd ed.). St. Louis: Elsevier.

Murray, S., McKinney, E., & Gorrie, T. (2002). *Foundations of maternal-newborn nursing* (3rd ed.). Philadelphia: Saunders.

Peckenpaugh, N. (2003). *Nutrition essentials and diet therapy* (9th ed.). Philadelphia: Saunders.

Perry, A., & Potter, P. (2004). *Clinical nursing skills and techniques* (5th ed.). St. Louis: Mosby.

Phipps, W., Monahan, F., Sands, J., Marek, J., & Neighbors, M. (2003). *Medical-surgical nursing: Health and illness perspectives* (7th ed.). St. Louis: Mosby.

Potter, P., & Perry, A. (2005). *Fundamentals of nursing* (6th ed.). St. Louis: Mosby.

Stuart, G., & Laraia, M. (2005). *Principles and practice of psychiatric nursing* (8th ed.). St. Louis: Mosby.

Williams, S. (2001). *Basic nutrition & diet therapy* (11th ed.). St. Louis: Mosby.

Wong, D., & Hockenberry, M. (2003). *Wong's nursing care of infants and children* (7th ed.). St. Louis: Mosby.

Psychosocial Integrity

1. A mother comes to the pediatric clinic because her previously continent 6-year-old son has resumed bedwetting. After discovering that there is a new baby in the home, the nurse explains to the mother that the son is most likely using the defense mechanism of:
   1 Identification
   2 Regression
   3 Rationalization
   4 Repression

Answer: 2
Rationale: The defense mechanism of regression is characterized by returning to an earlier form of expressing an impulse. Option 1 occurs when a person models behavior after someone else. Option 3 occurs when a person unconsciously falsifies an experience by giving a "rational" explanation. Option 4 is characterized by blocking a wish or desire from conscious expression.

Test-Taking Strategy: Focus on the data in the question. Noting the key words "resumed bedwetting" will direct you to option 2. Review defense mechanisms if you had difficulty with this question.

Level of Cognitive Ability: Application
Client Needs: Psychosocial Integrity
Integrated Process: Nursing Process/Implementation
Content Area: Child Health

Reference:
Wong, D., & Hockenberry, M. (2003). *Wong's nursing care of infants and children* (7th ed.). St. Louis: Mosby, p. 609.

---

2. A nurse is obtaining a health history on an adolescent. Which statement by the adolescent indicates a need for follow-up assessment and intervention?
   1 "I find myself very moody—happy one minute and crying the next."
   2 "I can't seem to wake up in the morning. I would sleep until noon if I could."
   3 "I don't eat anything with fat in it and I've lost 8 pounds in 2 weeks."
   4 "When I get stressed out about school, I just like to be alone."

Answer: 3
Rationale: During the adolescent period, there is a heightened awareness of body image and peer pressure to go on excessively restrictive diets. The extreme limitation of omitting all fat in the diet and weight loss during a time of growth suggests inadequate nutrition and a possible eating disorder. Options 1, 2, and 4 are common and normal behaviors or feelings during adolescence.

Test-Taking Strategy: Note the key words "need for follow-up." These words indicate a false-response question and that you need to select the option that identifies a statement by the adolescent that is a concern. Options 1, 2, and 4 are common and normal behaviors or feelings during adolescence. Option 3 indicates a problem or abnormality. Review the developmental stage of the adolescent if you had difficulty with this question.

Level of Cognitive Ability: Analysis
Client Needs: Psychosocial Integrity
Integrated Process: Nursing Process/Analysis
Content Area: Child Health

Reference:
Wong, D., & Hockenberry, M. (2003). *Wong's nursing care of infants and children* (7th ed.). St. Louis: Mosby, p. 814.

---

3. A nurse is caring for a client who has bipolar disorder and is in a manic state. The nurse determines that which menu choice would be best for this client?
1 Scrambled eggs, orange juice, coffee with cream and sugar
2 Cheeseburger, banana, milk
3 Beef stew, fruit salad, tea
4 Macaroni and cheese, apple, milk

Answer: 2
Rationale: The client in a manic state often has inadequate food and fluid intake as a result of physical agitation. Foods that the client can eat "on the run" are best because the client is too active to sit at meals and use utensils. Additionally, clients in a manic state should not have caffeine-containing products.

Test-Taking Strategy: Use the process of elimination, focusing on the key words "manic state." Note the similarity between options 1, 3, and 4 in that the client needs to sit to eat some of these food items. Remember the concept of "finger foods" with the client with mania. Review care of the client with mania if you had difficulty with this question.

Level of Cognitive Ability: Application
Client Needs: Psychosocial Integrity
Integrated Process: Nursing Process/Planning
Content Area: Mental Health

Reference:
Stuart, G., & Laraia, M. (2005). *Principles and practice of psychiatric nursing* (8th ed.). St. Louis: Mosby, pp. 266; 336; 487.

---

4. A nurse is caring for a child who is a victim of child abuse and has determined that the child uses repression to cope with past life experiences. The nurse implements a plan of care that includes:
1 Placing the child on medications that will help forget the incidents
2 Having the child talk about the abuse in detail during the first therapy session
3 Encouraging the child to use play therapy to act out past experiences
4 Telling the child to let the past go and concentrate on the present and future

Answer: 3
Rationale: Play therapy is a nonthreatening avenue through which the child can use artwork, dolls, or puppets to act out frightening life experiences. Options 1 and 4 devalue the child and force the child to further repress harmful past experiences rather than facing them and moving on. Option 2 would be extremely threatening to the child and nontherapeutic.

Test-Taking Strategy: Use therapeutic communication techniques to eliminate options 2 and 4. From the remaining options, note the relationship of "past life experiences" in the question and "past experiences" in the correct option. Review care of the child who is a victim of abuse if you had difficulty with this question.

Level of Cognitive Ability: Application
Client Needs: Psychosocial Integrity
Integrated Process: Nursing Process/Implementation
Content Area: Child Health

Reference:
Wong, D., & Hockenberry, M. (2003). *Wong's nursing care of infants and children* (7th ed.). St. Louis: Mosby, p. 695.

5. An older female client is brought to the emergency room by a family member with whom she lives. The nurse notes that the client has poor hygiene, contractures, and decubiti ulcers on the sacrum, scapula, and heels. The client is suspected of which form of victimization?

1 Emotional abuse
2 Physical abuse
3 Psychological abuse
4 Sexual abuse

Answer: 2

Rationale: Victimization in a family can take many forms. When analyzing a specific client situation, it is important to understand which form of abuse is being considered. Physical abuse can take the form of battering (hitting, slapping, striking) or can be more subtle, such as neglect (failure to meet basic needs). Emotional and psychological abuse can involve inflicting verbal statements that cause mental anguish or alienation of the victim. Sexual abuse can involve unwanted sexual remarks, sexual advances, and physical sexual acts.

Test-Taking Strategy: Focus on the data in the question. This question identifies only physical signs of victimization. Option 2 is the only option that fits the description in the question. Review the signs of physical abuse in the older client if you had difficulty with this question.

Level of Cognitive Ability: Analysis
Client Needs: Psychosocial Integrity
Integrated Process: Nursing Process/Analysis
Content Area: Mental Health

Reference:
Stuart, G., & Laraia, M. (2005). *Principles and practice of psychiatric nursing* (8th ed.). St. Louis: Mosby, p. 811.

---

6. A female client is admitted to the inpatient mental health unit. When asked her name, she responds, "I am Elizabeth, the Queen of England." The nurse recognizes this response as a(n):

1 Visual illusion
2 Auditory hallucination
3 Grandiose delusion
4 Loose association

Answer: 3

Rationale: A delusion is an important personal belief that is almost certainly not true and resists modification. An illusion is a misperception or misinterpretation of externally real stimuli. A hallucination is a false perception. Loose association is thinking characterized by speech in which ideas that are unrelated shift from one subject to another.

Test-Taking Strategy: Use the process of elimination and focus on the information in the question. Eliminate options 1 and 2 because the client is not having any visual or auditory disturbances. Option 4 is eliminated next because there is no indication that the client is shifting from one subject to another. Making a reference to being a "queen" is a grandiose assumption. Review the description of grandiose delusions if you had difficulty with this question.

Level of Cognitive Ability: Analysis
Client Needs: Psychosocial Integrity
Integrated Process: Nursing Process/Assessment
Content Area: Mental Health

Reference:
Stuart, G., & Laraia, M. (2005). *Principles and practice of psychiatric nursing* (8th ed.). St. Louis: Mosby, p. 112.

7. A client newly admitted to the mental health unit with a diagnosis of bipolar disorder is trying to organize a dance with the other clients on the unit and is planning an on-unit supper. To decrease stimulation, the nurse should encourage the client to:
   1 Engage the help of other clients on the unit to accomplish the task
   2 Seek assistance from other staff members
   3 Postpone the dance and engage in a writing activity
   4 Firmly tell the client that this task is inappropriate

Answer: 3
Rationale: Because the client with bipolar disorder is easily stimulated by the environment, sedentary activities are the best outlets for energy release. Most bipolar clients enjoy writing, so the writing task is appropriate. An activity such as planning a dance or supper might be appropriate at some point, but not for the newly admitted client who is likely to have impaired judgment and a short attention span. Options 1 and 2 encourage planning the activity and therefore increase client stimulation. Option 4 could result in an angry outburst by the client.

Test-Taking Strategy: Use the process of elimination. Note the key words "to decrease stimulation." Options 1 and 2 encourage activity and should be eliminated. Option 4 tells the client that the activity is inappropriate, and this could result in an angry outburst by the client. Option 3 is the only option that limits activity. Review the appropriate activities for the bipolar client if you had difficulty with this question.

Level of Cognitive Ability: Application
Client Needs: Psychosocial Integrity
Integrated Process: Nursing Process/Implementation
Content Area: Mental Health

Reference:
Stuart, G., & Laraia, M. (2005). *Principles and practice of psychiatric nursing* (8th ed.). St. Louis: Mosby, pp. 355-356.

8. A client with obsessive compulsive disorder spends many hours during the day and night washing her hands. When initially planning for a safe environment, the nurse allows the client to continue this behavior because it:
   1 Relieves the client's anxiety
   2 Decreases the chance of infection
   3 Gives the client a feeling of self-control
   4 Increases self-esteem

Answer: 1
Rationale: The compulsive act provides immediate relief from anxiety and is used to cope with stress, conflict, or pain. Although the client may feel the need to increase self-esteem, that is not the primary goal of this behavior. Options 2 and 3 are also incorrect interpretations of the client's need to perform this behavior.

Test-Taking Strategy: Use the process of elimination. Focusing on the key word "initially" and recalling the effect of compulsive acts will direct you to option 1. Review this disorder if you are unfamiliar with this content.

Level of Cognitive Ability: Application
Client Needs: Psychosocial Integrity
Integrated Process: Nursing Process/Implementation
Content Area: Mental Health

Reference:
Varcarolis, E.M. (2002). *Foundations of psychiatric mental health nursing* (4th ed.). Philadelphia: Saunders, p. 313.

9. An adolescent is preparing to return home after psychiatric hospitalization following a suicide attempt. Which of the following would be least effective in preparing the client to return home?

1 Identify the family's strengths and weaknesses

2 Suggest that the mother's boyfriend move out of the home

3 Provide and offer the family options and resources

4 Encourage sharing of feelings among the family

Answer: 2

Rationale: Option 2 is clearly the least effective option because there is no information in the question that indicates that the boyfriend's involvement has anything to do with the suicide attempt. Options 1, 2, and 4 offer helpful ways to enhance the family processes.

Test-Taking Strategy: Note the key words "least effective." These words indicate a false-response question and indicate that you need to select the option that would be least helpful. Focus on the data in the question and note that options 1, 3, and 4 are similar and identify positive measures. Review the psychosocial issues related to preparing a client for discharge if you had difficulty with this question.

Level of Cognitive Ability: Application
Client Needs: Psychosocial Integrity
Integrated Process: Nursing Process/Implementation
Content Area: Mental Health

Reference:
Stuart, G., & Laraia, M. (2005). *Principles and practice of psychiatric nursing* (8th ed.). St. Louis: Mosby, pp. 271; 273-274.

10. An 11-year-old child scheduled for a diagnostic procedure will have an intravenous (IV) line inserted and will receive an intramuscular injection. The nurse most appropriately prepares the child for the procedure by:

1 Teaching the parents so they can explain everything to their child

2 Using pictures, concrete words, and demonstrations to describe what will happen

3 Telling the child not to worry because the doctors take care of everything

4 Reassuring the child that he or she will not feel any pain

Answer: 2

Rationale: The school-aged child understands best with visual aids and concrete language. Option 1 inappropriately delegates the responsibility for teaching to the parents. Option 3 is not therapeutic. Option 4 is inaccurate information because the injection will cause some discomfort.

Test-Taking Strategy: Use the process of elimination and therapeutic communication techniques. In option 1, a nursing responsibility is inappropriately delegated to parents. Option 3 is nontherapeutic, and option 4 is inaccurate information. Review care of the school-aged child if you had difficulty with this question.

Level of Cognitive Ability: Application
Client Needs: Psychosocial Integrity
Integrated Process: Nursing Process/Implementation
Content Area: Child Health

Reference:
Wong, D., & Hockenberry, M. (2003). *Wong's nursing care of infants and children* (7th ed.). St. Louis: Mosby, p. 152.

11. A nurse observes an anxious client blocking the hallway, walking three steps forward and then steps backward. Other clients are agitated trying to get past. The nurse intervenes by:

1 Standing alongside the client and saying, "You're very anxious today."
2 Stopping the behavior and saying, "You're going to get exhausted."
3 Taking the client to the TV lounge and saying, "Relax and watch television now."
4 Walking alongside the client and saying, "You're not going anywhere very fast doing this."

Answer: 1

Rationale: An important consideration in alleviating the anxiety is to assist the client to recognize their behavior. Options 2 and 3 do not address the increased anxiety and the need to control the underlying behavior, and may even escalate the behavior. Option 4 does not raise the client to a functioning level.

Test-Taking Strategy: Use the process of elimination. Note the relationship between "anxious" in the question and in the correct option. Remember, it is important to assist the client in recognizing their behavior. Review measures related to the care of an anxious client if you had difficulty with this question.

Level of Cognitive Ability: Application
Client Needs: Psychosocial Integrity
Integrated Process: Nursing Process/Implementation
Content Area: Mental Health

References:
Stuart, G., & Laraia, M. (2005). *Principles and practice of psychiatric nursing* (8th ed.). St. Louis: Mosby, p. 268.
Varcarolis, E.M. (2002). *Foundations of psychiatric mental health nursing* (4th ed.). Philadelphia: Saunders, pp. 286-289.

---

12. A nurse is assisting in providing a form of psychotherapy in which the client acts out situations that are of emotional significance. The nurse understands that this form of therapy is known as:

1 Reality therapy
2 Short-term dynamic psychotherapy
3 Psychoanalytic therapy
4 Psychodrama

Answer: 4

Rationale: Psychodrama involves enactment of emotionally charged situations. Reality therapy is used for individuals with cognitive impairment. Both short-term dynamic psychotherapy and psychoanalytic therapy depend on techniques drawn from psychoanalysis.

Test-Taking Strategy: Note the key words "the client acts out situations." This will assist in providing you with the definition of psychodrama. Review these types of therapy if you had difficulty with this question.

Level of Cognitive Ability: Analysis
Client Needs: Psychosocial Integrity
Integrated Process: Nursing Process/Analysis
Content Area: Mental Health

References:
Fortinash, K., & Holoday-Worret, P. (2004). *Psychiatric mental health nursing* (3rd ed.). St. Louis: Mosby, p. 451.
Varcarolis, E.M. (2002). *Foundations of psychiatric mental health nursing* (4th ed.). Philadelphia: Saunders, p. 878.

13. A manic client is placed in a seclusion room after an outburst of violent behavior that involved a physical assault on another client. As the client is secluded, the nurse:
1 Remains silent because verbal interaction would be too stimulating
2 Tells the client that she will be allowed to rejoin the others when she can behave
3 Asks the client if she understands why the seclusion is necessary
4 Informs the client that she is being secluded to help regain self-control

Answer: 4
Rationale: The client is removed to a nonstimulating environment as a result of behavior. Options 1, 2, and 3 are nontherapeutic actions. Additionally, option 2 implies punishment. It is best to directly inform the client of the purpose of the seclusion.

Test-Taking Strategy: Use therapeutic communication techniques. Select the option that presents reality most clearly to the client. Option 4 is the only option that provides a clear and direct purpose of the seclusion. Review care of the client requiring seclusion if you had difficulty with this question.

Level of Cognitive Ability: Application
Client Needs: Psychosocial Integrity
Integrated Process: Nursing Process/Implementation
Content Area: Mental Health

References:
Keltner, N., Schwecke, L., & Bostrom, C. (2003). *Psychiatric nursing* (4th ed.). St. Louis: Mosby, p. 139.
Stuart, G., & Laraia, M. (2005). *Principles and practice of psychiatric nursing* (8th ed.). St. Louis: Mosby, p. 646.

14. A client with angina pectoris is extremely anxious after being hospitalized for the first time. The nurse plans to do which of the following to minimize the client's anxiety?
1 Admit the client to a room as far as possible from the nursing station
2 Provide care choices to the client
3 Encourage the client to limit visitors to as few as possible
4 Keep the door open and hallway lights on at night

Answer: 2
Rationale: General interventions to minimize anxiety in the hospitalized client include providing information, social support, control over choices related to care, and acknowledging the client's feelings. Being far from the nursing station is unlikely to reduce anxiety for this client. Limiting visitors reduces social support, and leaving the door open with hallway lights on may keep the client oriented, but may interfere with sleep and increase anxiety.

Test-Taking Strategy: Use the process of elimination, focusing on the issue: minimizing anxiety. Thinking about each option and how it may either increase or minimize anxiety will direct you to option 2. Review interventions to minimize anxiety in the hospitalized client if you had difficulty with this question.

Level of Cognitive Ability: Application
Client Needs: Psychosocial Integrity
Integrated Process: Nursing Process/Planning
Content Area: Adult Health/Cardiovascular

References:
Lewis, S., Heitkemper, M., & Dirksen, S. (2004). *Medical-surgical nursing: Assessment and management of clinical problems* (6th ed.). St. Louis: Mosby, p. 1760.
Phipps, W., Monahan, F., Sands, J., Marek, J., & Neighbors, M. (2003). *Medical-surgical nursing: Health and illness perspectives* (7th ed.). St. Louis: Mosby, p. 672.

15. A male client diagnosed with catatonic stupor demonstrates severe withdrawal by lying on the bed with the body pulled into a fetal position. The nurse plans to:
1 Leave the client alone and intermittently check on him
2 Take the client into the dayroom with other clients so they can help watch him
3 Sit beside the client in silence and occasionally ask open-ended questions
4 Ask direct questions to encourage talking

Answer: 3
Rationale: Clients who are withdrawn may be immobile and mute, and require consistent, repeated approaches. Intervention includes establishment of interpersonal contact. The nurse facilitates communication with the client by sitting in silence, asking open-ended questions, and pausing to provide opportunities for the client to respond. The client is not left alone. Asking direct questions to this client is not therapeutic.

Test-Taking Strategy: Use the process of elimination. Eliminate option 1 because the nurse does not leave the client alone. Option 2 relies on other clients to care for this client, is inappropriate, and is eliminated next. From the remaining options, recall that asking direct questions to this client would not be therapeutic. Review care of the client with catatonic stupor if you had difficulty with this question.

Level of Cognitive Ability: Application
Client Needs: Psychosocial Integrity
Integrated Process: Nursing Process/Planning
Content Area: Mental Health

References:
Fortinash, K., & Holoday-Worret, P. (2004). *Psychiatric mental health nursing* (3rd ed.). St. Louis: Mosby, p. 250.
Keltner, N., Schwecke, L., & Bostrom, C. (2003). *Psychiatric nursing* (4th ed.). St. Louis: Mosby, p. 344.

16. A nurse is interviewing a client on admission to the mental health inpatient unit who was involved in a fire two months ago. The client is complaining of insomnia, difficulty concentrating, nervousness, hypervigilance, and is frequently thinking about fires. The nurse assesses these symptoms to be indicative of:
1 Obsessive compulsive disorder (OCD)
2 Phobia
3 Post-traumatic stress disorder (PTSD)
4 Dissociative disorder

Answer: 3
Rationale: PTSD is precipitated by events that are overwhelming, unpredictable, and sometimes life-threatening. Typical symptoms of PTSD include difficulty concentrating, sleep disturbances, intrusive recollections of the traumatic event, hypervigilance, and anxiety.

Test-Taking Strategy: Focus on the data in the question regarding the client's complaints. Recalling that flashbacks of traumatic events is a common symptom of PTSD will direct you to option 3. Review the clinical manifestations of PTSD if you are unfamiliar with this disorder.

Level of Cognitive Ability: Analysis
Client Needs: Psychosocial Integrity
Integrated Process: Nursing Process/Assessment
Content Area: Mental Health

Reference:
Stuart, G., & Laraia, M. (2005). *Principles and practice of psychiatric nursing* (8th ed.). St. Louis: Mosby, pp. 271; 273.

17. A 16-year-old client is hospitalized. Which statement by the client would alert the nurse to a potential developmental problem?

  1 "Is it okay if I have a couple of friends in to visit me this evening?"

  2 "When my friends get here, I would like to play some computer games with them."

  3 "Please tell my friends not to visit since I'll see them back at school next week."

  4 "I'd like my hair washed before my friends get here."

Answer: 3

Rationale: Adolescents who withdraw from peers into isolation struggle with developing identity, so option 3 should cause the nurse to be concerned. Option 1 indicates that the client is eager for companionship. Adolescents often develop special interests within their groups, which may help maximize certain skills, such as with computers. It is appropriate for the client to ask for hygiene measures to be attended to before the peer group arrives.

Test-Taking Strategy: Use the process of elimination. Options 1, 2, and 4 indicate that the client is anticipating the arrival of a peer group, which is appropriate. Option 3 indicates that the client may be withdrawing from appropriate relationships. Review the concepts of growth and development related to an adolescent if you had difficulty answering this question.

Level of Cognitive Ability: Analysis
Client Needs: Psychosocial Integrity
Integrated Process: Nursing Process/Assessment
Content Area: Child Health

Reference:
Wong, D., & Hockenberry, M. (2003). *Wong's nursing care of infants and children* (7th ed.). St. Louis: Mosby, pp.706-707.

---

18. A nurse obtains an electrocardiogram (ECG) rhythm strip on a client who is anxious about the result. The ECG shows that the rate is 90 beats per minute. To relieve anxiety, the nurse tells the client that:

  1 The rate is normal

  2 There is no need to worry

  3 Medication specific to the problem will be prescribed

  4 A slower heart rate is preferred

Answer: 1

Rationale: A normal adult resting pulse rate ranges between 60 and 100 beats per minute; therefore, the rate is normal. The nurse would not tell a client "not to worry." Options 3 and 4 indicate that the ECG is abnormal.

Test-Taking Strategy: Use the process of elimination and knowledge of the basic range of pulse rates for an adult. Eliminate option 2 because telling the client "not to worry" is an inappropriate action. Eliminate options 3 and 4 because they are similar and indicate that a problem exists. Review normal adult vital signs if you had difficulty with this question.

Level of Cognitive Ability: Application
Client Needs: Psychosocial Integrity
Integrated Process: Nursing Process/Implementation
Content Area: Adult Health/Cardiovascular

Reference:
Potter, P., & Perry, A. (2005). *Fundamentals of nursing* (6th ed.). St. Louis: Mosby, p. 619.

19. A nurse determines that a client recovering from a myocardial infarction is exhibiting signs of depression when the client:
  1 Reports insomnia at night
  2 Consumes 25% of meals and shows little interest when doing client teaching
  3 Ignores activity restrictions and does not report the experience of chest pain with activity
  4 Expresses apprehension about leaving the hospital and requests someone to stay at night

Answer: 2
Rationale: Signs of depression include withdrawal, lack of interest, crying, anorexia, and apathy. Insomnia may be a sign of anxiety or fear. Ignoring symptoms and activity restrictions are signs of denial. Apprehension is a sign of anxiety.

Test-Taking Strategy: Use the process of elimination, focusing on the issue: signs of depression. Recalling that anorexia and a lack of interest are associated with depression will direct you to option 2. Review the signs of depression if you had difficulty with this question.

Level of Cognitive Ability: Analysis
Client Needs: Psychosocial Integrity
Integrated Process: Nursing Process/Analysis
Content Area: Adult Health/Cardiovascular

References:
Ignatavicius, D., & Workman, M. (2002). *Medical surgical nursing: Critical thinking for collaborative care* (4th ed.). Philadelphia: Saunders, pp. 43; 794.
Lewis, S., Heitkemper, M., & Dirksen, S. (2004). *Medical-surgical nursing: Assessment and management of clinical problems* (6th ed.). St. Louis: Mosby, p. 829.

20. A client who recently had a gastrostomy feeding tube inserted refuses to participate in the plan of care, will not make eye contact, and does not speak to the family or visitors. The nurse assesses that the client is using which type of coping mechanism?
  1 Self-control
  2 Problem solving
  3 Accepting responsibility
  4 Distancing

Answer: 4
Rationale: Distancing is an unwillingness or inability to discuss events. Self-control is demonstrated by stoicism and hiding feelings. Problem solving involves making plans and verbalizing what will be done. Accepting responsibility places the responsibility for a situation on one's self.

Test-Taking Strategy: Focus on the data in the question. Noting the client's behavior will direct you to option 4, the least effective coping strategy. Review coping mechanisms if you had difficulty with this question.

Level of Cognitive Ability: Analysis
Client Needs: Psychosocial Integrity
Integrated Process: Nursing Process/Assessment
Content Area: Adult Health/Gastrointestinal

Reference:
Lewis, S., Heitkemper, M., & Dirksen, S. (2004). *Medical-surgical nursing: Assessment and management of clinical problems* (6th ed.). St. Louis: Mosby, pp. 244; 802.

21. A nurse reviews the preoperative teaching plan for a client scheduled for a radical neck dissection. When implementing the plan, the nurse initially focuses on:
  1 Postoperative communication techniques
  2 The financial status of the client
  3 The client's support systems and coping behaviors
  4 Information given to the client by the surgeon

Answer: 4
Rationale: The first step in client teaching is establishing what the client already knows. This allows the nurse to not only correct any misinformation but also to determine the starting point for teaching and to implement the education at the client's level. Although options 1, 2, and 3 may be a component of the plan, they are not the initial focus.

Test-Taking Strategy: Note the key word "initially." Remember that determining what the client already knows provides a starting point for teaching. Review the teaching/learning process if you had difficulty with this question.

Level of Cognitive Ability: Application
Client Needs: Psychosocial Integrity
Integrated Process: Teaching/Learning
Content Area: Delegating/Prioritizing

Reference:
Potter, P., & Perry, A. (2005). *Fundamentals of nursing* (6th ed.). St. Louis: Mosby, pp. 451-454.

---

22. A nurse is monitoring a client for signs of alcohol withdrawal. Which assessment data indicates early signs of withdrawal?
   1 Anxiety, tremor, irritability
   2 Disorientation, and sleepiness
   3 Dizziness, vomiting, headache
   4 Clouding of consciousness, tiredness, fatigue

Answer: 1
Rationale: The signs of alcohol withdrawal develop within a few hours after cessation or reduction of alcohol and peak after 24 to 48 hours. Early signs include anxiety, anorexia, insomnia, tremor, irritability, an elevation in pulse and blood pressure, nausea, vomiting, and poorly formed hallucinations or illusions.

Test-Taking Strategy: Use the process of elimination and eliminate options 2 and 4 first because they are similar. From the remaining options, focus on the key word "early" and remember that the client will become irritable and anxious. Review this content if you are unfamiliar with the signs and symptoms of alcohol withdrawal.

Level of Cognitive Ability: Analysis
Client Needs: Psychosocial Integrity
Integrated Process: Nursing Process/Assessment
Content Area: Mental Health

Reference:
Stuart, G., & Laraia, M. (2005). *Principles and practice of psychiatric nursing* (8th ed.). St. Louis: Mosby, p. 491.

---

23. A preschool child is placed in traction for treatment of a femur fracture. The child, who has reportedly been toilet-trained for at least one year, begins bedwetting. The nurse recognizes this as:
   1 Attention-seeking behavior requiring intervention by the child psychologist
   2 Loss of developmental milestones caused by prolonged immobilization
   3 Regressing to earlier developmental behavior, which is a normal psychological effect of immobilization
   4 A body image disturbance

Answer: 3
Rationale: The monotony of immobilization can lead to sluggish intellectual and psychomotor responses. Regressive behaviors are not uncommon in immobilized children and usually do not require professional intervention. Although "loss of developmental milestones" may seem like an appropriate option, "regressing to earlier developmental behavior" is a more accurate description of the psychological effects of immobilization. Body image may or may not be affected by long-term immobilization and does not relate to the information in the question.

Test-Taking Strategy: Use the process of elimination. Eliminate option 4 first because it is unrelated to the question. Eliminate option 1 because bedwetting by an immobilized child is not unusual, and a child psychologist is not needed. From the remaining options, recall that regression is a normal psychological response to immobilization to direct you to option 3. Review the psychological effects of immobilization if you had difficulty with this question.

Level of Cognitive Ability: Analysis
Client Needs: Psychosocial Integrity

Integrated Process: Nursing Process/Assessment
Content Area: Child Health

Reference:
Wong, D., & Hockenberry, M. (2003). *Wong's nursing care of infants and children* (7th ed.). St. Louis: Mosby, p. 1766.

---

24. A nurse is assessing a client to determine adjustment to presbycusis. Which of the following indicates successful adaptation to this problem?
1   Denial of a hearing impairment
2   Proper use of a hearing aid
3   Withdrawal from social activities
4   Reluctance to answer the telephone

Answer: 2

Rationale: Presbycusis occurs as part of the aging process and is a progressive sensorineural hearing loss. Some clients may not adapt well to the impairment, denying its presence. Others withdraw from social interactions and contact with others, embarrassed by the problem and the need to wear a hearing aid. Clients show adequate adaptation by obtaining and regularly using a hearing aid.

Test-Taking Strategy: The key words in the question are "successful adaptation." A review of each of the options shows that the only option with positive wording is option 2. The incorrect options indicate a need for further adaptation. Review the psychosocial issues related to the care of the client with a hearing aid if you had difficulty with this question.

Level of Cognitive Ability: Analysis
Client Needs: Psychosocial Integrity
Integrated Process: Nursing Process/Evaluation
Content Area: Adult Health/Ear

Reference:
Phipps, W., Monahan, F., Sands, J., Marek, J., & Neighbors, M. (2003). *Medical-surgical nursing: Health and illness perspectives* (7th ed.). St. Louis: Mosby, p. 1921.

---

25. A nurse is performing an admission assessment on a child and notes the presence of old and new bruises on the child's back and legs. The nurse suspects physical abuse and would:
1   File charges against the mother and father of the child
2   Report the case to legal authorities
3   Ask the mother to identify the individual who is physically abusing the child
4   Tell the child that she will need to go to a foster home until the situation is straightened out

Answer: 2

Rationale: The primary legal nursing responsibility when child abuse is suspected is to report the case. All 50 states require health care professionals to report all cases of suspected abuse. It is not appropriate for the nurse to file charges against the father or mother. It is also inappropriate to ask the mother to identify the abuser, because the abuser may be the mother. If so, the possibility exists that the mother may become defensive and leave the emergency room with the child. Option 4 is clearly inappropriate and will produce fear in the child.

Test-Taking Strategy: Use the process of elimination. In addition to the many implications associated with child abuse, abuse is a crime. With this in mind, option 2, reporting the case of abuse, is the primary responsibility of the nurse. Review the responsibilities of the nurse when child abuse is suspected if you had difficulty with this question.

Level of Cognitive Ability: Application
Client Needs: Psychosocial Integrity
Integrated Process: Nursing Process/Implementation
Content Area: Child Health

Reference:
Wong, D., & Hockenberry, M. (2003). *Wong's nursing care of infants and children* (7th ed.). St. Louis: Mosby, p. 692.

26. The emergency room nurse is performing an assessment on a 7-year-old child with a fractured arm. The child is hesitant to answer questions that the nurse is asking and consistently looks at the parents in a fearful manner. The nurse suspects physical abuse and continues with the assessment procedures. Which assessment finding would most likely assist in verifying the suspicion?

1 Poor hygiene
2 Bald spots on the scalp
3 Lacerations in the anal area
4 Swelling of the genitals

Answer: 2

Rationale: Bald spots on the scalp are most likely associated with physical abuse. The most likely assessment findings in sexual abuse include difficulty walking or sitting; torn, stained, or bloody underclothing; pain, swelling, or itching of the genitals; and bruises, bleeding, or lacerations in the genital or anal area. Poor hygiene may be indicative of physical neglect.

Test-Taking Strategy: Read the question carefully, noting the key words "physical abuse." The only option that specifically addresses an assessment finding related to physical abuse is option 2. Review the assessment findings in a child suspected of abuse if you had difficulty with this question.

Level of Cognitive Ability: Analysis
Client Needs: Psychosocial Integrity
Integrated Process: Nursing Process/Assessment
Content Area: Child Health

References:
James, S., Ashwill, J., & Droske, S. (2002). *Nursing care of children: Principles & practice* (2nd ed.). Philadelphia: Saunders, p. 233.
Wong, D., & Hockenberry, M. (2003). *Wong's nursing care of infants and children* (7th ed.). St. Louis: Mosby, p. 688.

27. A 4-year-old child who was recently hospitalized is brought to the clinic by his mother for a follow-up visit. The mother tells the nurse that the child has begun to wet the bed ever since the child was brought home from the hospital. The mother is concerned and asks the nurse what to do. The appropriate nursing response is which of the following?

1 "You need to discipline the child."
2 "This is a normal occurrence following hospitalization."
3 "We will need to discuss this behavior with the physician."
4 "The child probably has developed a urinary tract infection."

Answer: 2

Rationale: Regression can occur in a preschooler and is most often a result of the stress of the hospitalization. It is best to accept the regression if it occurs. Parents may be overly concerned about the regressive behavior and should be told that regression is normal following hospitalization. It is premature to discuss the situation with the physician. Options 1 and 4 are inappropriate responses to the mother.

Test-Taking Strategy: Note the key word "appropriate" in the stem of the question and use the process of elimination. Eliminate option 4 first because there is no data in the question to support this statement. Knowledge regarding the behavior patterns of a preschooler following hospitalization and the use of therapeutic communication techniques will assist in eliminating options 1 and 3. Review the psychosocial issues related to the hospitalized preschool child if you had difficulty with this question.

Level of Cognitive Ability: Application
Client Needs: Psychosocial Integrity
Integrated Process: Communication and Documentation
Content Area: Child Health

Reference:
Wong, D., & Hockenberry, M. (2003). *Wong's nursing care of infants and children* (7th ed.). St. Louis: Mosby, p. 1039.

28. During an office visit, a prenatal client with mitral stenosis states that she has been under a lot of stress lately. During the examination, the client questions everything the nurse does and behaves anxiously. The appropriate nursing action at this time would be to:

1 Tell her not to worry

2 Ignore her unfounded concerns and continue with the assessment

3 Explain the purpose of the nurse's actions and answer all questions

4 Refer her to a counselor

Answer: 3

Rationale: In the prenatal cardiac client, stress should be reduced as much as possible. The client should be provided with honest informed answers to questions to help alleviate unnecessary fears and emotional stress. Explaining the purpose of nursing actions will assist in decreasing the stress level of the client. Options 1, 2, and 4 are nontherapeutic methods of communication at this time.

Test-Taking Strategy: Use the process of elimination and therapeutic communication techniques to answer the question. Always address the client's concerns and feelings. Option 3 is the only option that addresses the client's concerns. Review therapeutic communication techniques if you had difficulty with this question.

Level of Cognitive Ability: Application
Client Needs: Psychosocial Integrity
Integrated Process: Nursing Process/Implementation
Content Area: Maternity/Antepartum

Reference:
Murray, S., McKinney, E., & Gorrie, T. (2002). *Foundations of maternal-newborn nursing* (3rd ed.). Philadelphia: Saunders, pp. 25-26.

29. A postpartum client with gestational diabetes is scheduled for discharge. During the discharge teaching, the client asks the nurse, "Do I have to worry about this diabetes anymore?" The appropriate response by the nurse is which of the following?

1 "Your blood glucose level is within normal limits now, so you will be all right."

2 "You will only have to worry about the diabetes if you become pregnant again."

3 "You will be at risk for developing gestational diabetes with your next pregnancy and developing diabetes mellitus."

4 "Once you have gestational diabetes you have diabetes forever and must be treated with medication for the rest of your life."

Answer: 3

Rationale: The client is at risk for developing gestational diabetes with each pregnancy. The client also has an increased risk of developing diabetes mellitus and needs to comply with follow-up assessments. She also needs to be taught techniques to lower her risk for developing diabetes mellitus, such as weight control. The diagnosis of gestational diabetes mellitus indicates that this client has an increased risk for developing diabetes mellitus; however, with proper care it may not develop.

Test-Taking Strategy: Identify the issue of the question, which is the long-term effect of gestational diabetes. Also use therapeutic communication techniques to answer the question and direct you to option 3. Review the long-term effects of gestational diabetes if you had difficulty with this question.

Level of Cognitive Ability: Application
Client Needs: Psychosocial Integrity
Integrated Process: Communication and Documentation
Content Area: Maternity/Postpartum

Reference:
Lowdermilk, D., & Perry, A. (2004). *Maternity & women's health care* (8th ed.). St. Louis: Mosby, p. 898.

30. A nurse is performing an assessment on a 16-year-old female client who has been diagnosed with anorexia nervosa. Which statement by the client would the nurse identify as a priority requiring further assessment?
1 "I exercise 3 to 4 hours every day to keep my slim figure."
2 "My best friend was in the hospital with this disease a year ago."
3 "I've been told that I am 10% below ideal body weight."
4 "I check my weight every day without fail."

Answer: 1

Rationale: Exercising 3 to 4 hours every day is excessive physical activity and unrealistic for a 16-year-old. The nurse needs to further assess this statement immediately to find out why the client feels the need to exercise this much to maintain her figure. Although it's unfortunate that her best friend had this disease, this is not considered a major threat to this client's physical well-being. A weight that exceeds 15% below the ideal weight is significant with anorexia nervosa. It is not considered abnormal to check weight every day. Many clients with anorexia nervosa check their weight close to 20 times a day.

Test-Taking Strategy: Note the key words "requiring further assessment" in the stem of the question. These words indicate a false-response question and that you need to select the option that identifies a concern. Eliminate options 3 and 4 first because these client statements are not significant or abnormal. From the remaining options, knowledge regarding the manifestations associated with anorexia nervosa will direct you to option 1. Review these significant manifestations if you had difficulty with this question.

Level of Cognitive Ability: Analysis
Client Needs: Psychosocial Integrity
Integrated Process: Nursing Process/Analysis
Content Area: Mental Health

Reference:
Stuart, G., & Laraia, M. (2005). *Principles and practice of psychiatric nursing* (8th ed.). St. Louis: Mosby, pp. 527; 530.

31. A physician has written an order to start progressive ambulation as tolerated on a hospitalized client who is experiencing periods of confusion as a result of bed rest and prolonged confinement to the hospital room. Which nursing intervention would be most appropriate when planning to implement the physician's order and in addressing the needs of the client?
1 Ambulate the client in the room for short distances frequently
2 Ambulate the client to the bathroom in the client's room three times a day
3 Progressively ambulate the client in the hall three times a day
4 Assist with range of motion exercises three times a day to increase strength

Answer: 3

Rationale: The cause of the confusion in this situation is bed rest and decreased sensory stimulation from prolonged confinement. Therefore, it is best to ambulate the client in the hall. This will increase sensory stimulation and may decrease confusion. Options 1 and 2 will not address the client's need for sensory stimulation. Option 4 is an action that should have been performed in preparation for ambulation while the client was on bed rest.

Test-Taking Strategy: Focus on the issue of "confusion as a result of bed rest and prolonged confinement." Eliminate option 4 first because this action should have been performed in preparation for ambulation while the client was on bed rest. Next eliminate options 1 and 2 because they are similar in that they both address ambulating the client in the hospital room. Review interventions related to promoting sensory stimulation if you had difficulty with this question.

Level of Cognitive Ability: Application
Client Needs: Psychosocial Integrity
Integrated Process: Nursing Process/Planning
Content Area: Fundamental Skills

Reference:
Potter, P., & Perry, A. (2005). *Fundamentals of nursing* (6th ed.). St. Louis: Mosby, p. 1477.

32. The nurse is caring for an older client who has been placed in Buck's extension traction following a hip fracture. On assessment of the client, the nurse notes that the client is disoriented. The most appropriate nursing intervention is to:

1 Ask the family to stay with the client
2 Apply restraints to the client
3 Ask the laboratory to perform electrolyte studies
4 Reorient the client frequently and place a clock and a calendar in the client's room

Answer: 4

Rationale: An inactive older person may become disoriented due to lack of sensory stimulation. The most appropriate nursing intervention would be to frequently reorient the client and to place objects such as a clock and a calendar in the client's room to maintain orientation. The family can assist with orientation of the client, but it is not appropriate to ask the family to stay with the client. It is not the within the scope of nursing practice to prescribe laboratory studies. Restraints may cause further disorientation and should not be applied unless specifically prescribed. Agency policies and procedures should be followed before application of restraints.

Test-Taking Strategy: Note the key words "most appropriate." Eliminate option 3 first because it is not within the realm of nursing practice to prescribe laboratory studies. Next, eliminate option 2 because restraints may add to the disorientation that the client is experiencing. It is not appropriate to place the responsibility of the client on the family, therefore eliminate option 1. Also, note the relationship between the words "disoriented" in the question and "reorient" in the correct option. Review the measures related to caring for a client who is disoriented if you had difficulty with this question.

Level of Cognitive Ability: Application
Client Needs: Psychosocial Integrity
Integrated Process: Nursing Process/Implementation
Content Area: Adult Health/Musculoskeletal

Reference:
Phipps, W., Monahan, F., Sands, J., Marek, J., & Neighbors, M. (2003). *Medical-surgical nursing: Health and illness perspectives* (7th ed.). St. Louis: Mosby, p. 1326.

33. An 8-year-old child is admitted to the hospital. The child was sexually abused by an adult family member and is withdrawn and appears frightened. Which of the following describes the best plan for the initial nursing encounter to convey concern and support?

1 Introduce self, explain role, and ask the child to act out the sexual encounter with the abuser using art therapy
2 Introduce self, then ask the child to express how he feels about the events leading up to this hospital admission
3 Introduce self and explain to the child that he is safe, now that he is in the hospital
4 Introduce self and tell the child that the nurse would like to sit with him for a little while

Answer: 4

Rationale: Victims of sexual abuse may exhibit fear and anxiety over what has just occurred. In addition, they may fear that the abuse could be repeated. On initiating contact with a child victim of sexual abuse who demonstrates fear of others, it is best to convey a willingness to spend time, and move slowly to initiate activities that may be perceived as threatening. Once rapport is established, the nurse may explore the child's feelings or use various therapeutic modalities to encourage recounting the sexual encounter. Option 4 conveys a plan for an initial encounter that establishes trust by sitting with the child in a nonthreatening atmosphere. Options 1 and 2 may be implemented once trust and rapport is established. Option 3 does not convey concern and support by the nurse.

Test-Taking Strategy: Use the process of elimination, focusing on the child's experience and that the child is frightened. This will assist in eliminating options 1 and 2. From the remaining options, recalling that rapport needs to be established first will direct you to option 4. Review care of the abused child if you had difficulty with this question.

Level of Cognitive Ability: Application
Client Needs: Psychosocial Integrity
Integrated Process: Caring
Content Area: Child Health

References:
James, S., Ashwill, J., & Droske, S. (2002). *Nursing care of children: Principles & practice* (2nd ed.). Philadelphia:Saunders, p. 1009.
Wong, D., & Hockenberry, M. (2003). *Wong's nursing care of infants and children* (7th ed.). St. Louis: Mosby, p. 697.

---

34. A female victim of a sexual assault is being seen in the crisis center for a third visit. She states that although the rape occurred nearly 2 months ago, she still feels "as though the rape just happened yesterday." The nurse would respond by stating:

1 "What can you do to alleviate some of your fears about being assaulted again?"
2 "Tell me more about those aspects of the rape that cause you to feel like the rape just occurred."
3 "In time, our goal will be to help you move on from these strong feelings about your rape."
4 "In reality, the rape did not just occur. It has been over 2 months now."

Answer: 2
Rationale: Option 2 allows for the client to express her ideas and feelings more fully, and portrays a nonhurried, nonjudgmental, supportive attitude. Clients need to be reassured that their feelings are normal and that they may freely express their concerns in a safe care environment. Option 1 places the problem solving totally on the client. Option 3 places the client's feelings on hold. Although option 4 is true, it immediately blocks communication.

Test-Taking Strategy: Use therapeutic communication techniques. Option 2 specifically addresses the client's feelings and concerns. Remember to always address the client's feelings first. Review therapeutic communication techniques if you had difficulty with this question.

Level of Cognitive Ability: Application
Client Needs: Psychosocial Integrity
Integrated Process: Communication and Documentation
Content Area: Mental Health

Reference:
Stuart, G., & Laraia, M. (2005). *Principles and practice of psychiatric nursing* (8th ed.). St. Louis: Mosby, pp. 30-34; 235.

---

35. A client is admitted to the mental health unit with a diagnosis of schizophrenia. A nursing diagnosis formulated for the client is Disturbed Thought Processes, secondary to paranoia. In formulating the plan of care with the health care team, the nurse includes instruction to the staff to:

1 Avoid laughing or whispering in front of the client
2 Increase socialization of the client with peers
3 Have the client sign a release of information to appropriate parties so that adequate data can be obtained for assessment purposes
4 Begin to educate the client about social supports in the community

Answer: 1
Rationale: A client experiencing paranoia is distrustful and suspicious of others. The health care team needs to establish rapport and trust with the client. Laughing or whispering in front of the client would increase the client's paranoia. Options 2, 3, and 4 ask the client to trust on a multitude of levels. These options are too intrusive for a client who is paranoid.

Test-Taking Strategy: Focus on the client's problem: paranoia. Recalling that the client with paranoia is distrustful and suspicious of others will direct you to option 1. Review this disorder if you had difficulty with this question.

Level of Cognitive Ability: Application
Client Needs: Psychosocial Integrity
Integrated Process: Nursing Process/Implementation
Content Area: Mental Health

Reference:
Stuart, G., & Laraia, M. (2005). *Principles and practice of psychiatric nursing* (8th ed.). St. Louis: Mosby, p. 786.

---

36. A nurse is assessing a client who has a nursing diagnosis of risk for self-directed violence. The client says, "You won't have to worry about me much longer." The nurse interprets this statement as:
1 An expression of hopelessness
2 An expression of depression
3 The intention for self-mutilation
4 The intention of suicide

Answer: 4
Rationale: A client with a risk for self-directed violence who says that he or she will not be around much longer is making an expression of a suicidal intent. Although hopelessness, depression, and self-mutilation may relate to self-directed violence, the statement that he or she will not be around is a direct comment about the act of suicide.

Test-Taking Strategy: Use the process of elimination. Focus on the client's statement to direct you to option 4. Review the characteristics related to risk for self-directed violence if you had difficulty with this question.

Level of Cognitive Ability: Analysis
Client Needs: Psychosocial Integrity
Integrated Process: Nursing Process/Analysis
Content Area: Mental Health

Reference:
Stuart, G., & Laraia, M. (2005). *Principles and practice of psychiatric nursing* (8th ed.). St. Louis: Mosby, pp. 308-309.

---

37. A nurse notes that an assigned client is lying tense in bed staring at the cardiac monitor. The client states, "There sure are a lot of wires around there. I sure hope we don't get hit by lightning." The appropriate nursing response is which of the following?
1 "Would you like a mild sedative to help you relax?"
2 "Oh, don't worry, the weather is suppose to be sunny and clear today."
3 "Yes, all those wires must be a little scary. Did someone explain what the cardiac monitor was for?"
4 "Your family can stay tonight if they wish."

Answer: 3
Rationale: The nurse should initially validate the client's concern and then assess the client's knowledge regarding the cardiac monitor. This gives the nurse an opportunity to provide client education if necessary. Options 1, 2, and 4 do not address the client's concern. Additionally, pharmacological interventions should be considered only if necessary.

Test-Taking Strategy: Use therapeutic communication techniques. Remember to address the client's feelings first. Option 3 is the only option that addresses the client's feelings. Review therapeutic communication techniques if you had difficulty with this question.

Level of Cognitive Ability: Application
Client Needs: Psychosocial Integrity
Integrated Process: Communication and Documentation
Content Area: Adult Health/Cardiovascular

Reference:
Potter, P., & Perry, A. (2005). *Fundamentals of nursing* (6th ed.). St. Louis: Mosby, p. 437.

38. A young adult male client with a spinal cord injury tells the nurse, "It's so depressing that I'll never get to have sex again." The nurse replies in a realistic way by making which of the following statements to the client?

1 "You're young, so you'll adapt to this more easily than if you were older."

2 "It must feel horrible to know you can never have sex again."

3 "It is still possible to have a sexual relationship, but it is different."

4 "Because of body reflexes, sexual functioning will be no different than before."

Answer: 3

Rationale: It is possible to have a sexual relationship after a spinal cord injury, but it is different than what the client experienced before the injury. Males may experience reflex erections, although they may not ejaculate. Females can have adductor spasm. Sexual counseling may help the client adapt to changes in sexuality after spinal cord injury.

Test-Taking Strategy: Use the process of elimination, knowledge regarding the effects of a spinal cord injury, and therapeutic communication techniques. Option 3 addresses the issue, is accurate, and a therapeutic response. Review the effects of a spinal cord injury if you had difficulty with this question.

Level of Cognitive Ability: Application
Client Needs: Psychosocial Integrity
Integrated Process: Communication and Documentation
Content Area: Adult Health/Neurological

Reference:
Phipps, W., Monahan, F., Sands, J., Marek, J., & Neighbors, M. (2003). *Medical-surgical nursing: Health and illness perspectives* (7th ed.). St. Louis: Mosby, pp. 1422-1423.

39. A family member of a client with a brain tumor states that he is distraught and feeling guilty for not encouraging the client to seek medical evaluation earlier. The nurse would incorporate which of the following items in formulating a response to the family member's statement?

1 It is true that brain tumors are easily recognizable.

2 The symptoms of a brain tumor may be easily attributed to another cause.

3 Brain tumors are never detected until very late in their course.

4 There are no symptoms of a brain tumor.

Answer: 2

Rationale: Signs and symptoms of a brain tumor vary depending on location and may easily be attributed to another cause. Symptoms include headache, vomiting, visual disturbances, and change in intellectual abilities or personality. Seizures occur in some clients. These symptoms can be easily attributed to other causes. The family requires support to assist them in the normal grieving process. Options 1, 3, and 4 are inaccurate.

Test-Taking Strategy: Use the process of elimination. Eliminate options 3 and 4 first because they contain the absolute words "never" and "no," respectively. From the remaining options, recall that the symptoms of a brain tumor may be easily attributed to another cause. Also, note the word "may" in the correct option. Review the symptoms of a brain tumor if you had difficulty with his question.

Level of Cognitive Ability: Application
Client Needs: Psychosocial Integrity
Integrated Process: Caring
Content Area: Adult Health/Neurological

Reference:
Phipps, W., Monahan, F., Sands, J., Marek, J., & Neighbors, M. (2003). *Medical-surgical nursing: Health and illness perspectives* (7th ed.). St. Louis: Mosby, p. 1344.

40. A male client is in a hip spica cast as a result of a hip fracture. On the day after the cast has been applied, the nurse finds the client surrounded by papers from his brief case and planning a phone meeting. The nurse's interaction with the client about the client's activities should be based on the knowledge that:

1 Setting limits on a client's behavior is a mandated nursing role.
2 Not keeping up with his job will increase his stress level.
3 Immediate involvement in his job will keep him from becoming bored while on bed rest.
4 Rest is an essential component in bone healing.

Answer: 4
Rationale: Rest is an essential component of bone healing. Nurses can help clients understand the importance of rest and find ways to balance work demands to promote healing. Nurses cannot demand these changes but need to encourage clients to choose them. It may be stress relieving to do work; however, in the immediate post-cast period, it may not be therapeutic. Stress should be kept at a minimum to promote bone healing. Setting limits on a client's behavior is not a mandated nursing role.

Test-Taking Strategy: Use the process of elimination. Eliminate options 2 and 3 because they are similar. From the remaining options, note that option 4 is the umbrella (global) option and addresses the issue of rest. Review the physiological and psychosocial needs of the client in a hip spica cast if you had difficulty with this question.

Level of Cognitive Ability: Analysis
Client Needs: Psychosocial Integrity
Integrated Process: Caring
Content Area: Adult Health/Musculoskeletal

Reference:
Black, J., & Hawks, J. (2005). *Medical-surgical nursing: Clinical management for positive outcomes* (7th ed.). Philadelphia: Saunders, p. 636.

41. A charge nurse observes a nursing assistant talking in an unusually loud voice to a client with delirium. The charge nurse takes which action?

1 Speaks to the nursing assistant immediately while in the client's room to solve the problem
2 Informs the client that everything is all right
3 Ascertains the client's safety, calmly asks the nursing assistant to join the nurse outside the room, and informs the nursing assistant that her voice was unusually loud
4 Explains to the nursing assistant that yelling in the client's room is tolerated only if the client is talking loudly

Answer: 3
Rationale: The nurse must ascertain that the client is safe, and then discuss the matter with the nursing assistant in an area away from the hearing of the client. If the client heard the conversation, the client may become more confused or agitated. Options 1, 2, and 4 are incorrect actions.

Test-Taking Strategy: Use Maslow's hierarchy of needs theory. Remember when a physiological need is not present, then safety needs are the priority. Review appropriate and therapeutic communication techniques and care of the client with delirium if you had difficulty with this question.

Level of Cognitive Ability: Application
Client Needs: Psychosocial Integrity
Integrated Process: Nursing Process/Implementation
Content Area: Leadership/Management

Reference:
Stuart, G., & Laraia, M. (2005). *Principles and practice of psychiatric nursing* (8th ed.). St. Louis: Mosby, p. 464.

42. A teenager who has celiac disease arrives at the emergency room complaining of profuse, watery diarrhea following a pizza party last night. The client states, "I don't want to be different from my friends." The nursing diagnosis that is most appropriate for this client is:
1 Deficient knowledge
2 Deficient fluid volume
3 Risk for situational low self-esteem
4 Celiac crisis

Answer: 3
Rationale: The client expresses concern over being different from friends. Although the question identifies that the client has profuse, watery diarrhea, no data identifies an actual deficient fluid volume. Also, the assessment data provided does not support a diagnosis of deficient knowledge. Celiac crisis is a medical diagnosis.

Test-Taking Strategy: Use the process of elimination, focusing on the data in the question. Eliminate option 4 because it is a medical diagnosis. Next, focus on the client's feelings of "being different." This will direct you to option 3. Review the defining characteristics of risk for situational low self-esteem if you had difficulty with this question.

Level of Cognitive Ability: Analysis
Client Needs: Psychosocial Integrity
Integrated Process: Nursing Process/Analysis
Content Area: Child Health

Reference:
Wong, D., & Hockenberry, M. (2003). *Wong's nursing care of infants and children* (7th ed.). St. Louis: Mosby, p. 804.

43. A nurse develops a plan of care for a one-month-old infant hospitalized for intussusception. Which nursing measure would be most effective to provide psychosocial support for the parent-child relationship?
1 Encourage the parents to go home and get some sleep
2 Encourage the parents to room-in with their infant
3 Provide educational materials
4 Initiate home nutritional support as early as possible

Answer: 2
Rationale: Rooming-in is effective in reducing separation anxiety and preserving the parent-child relationship. Parents are under stress when a child is ill and hospitalized. Telling a parent to go home and sleep will not relieve this stress. Educational materials may be beneficial but will not provide psychosocial support of the parent-child relationship. Home nutritional support is not usually necessary.

Test-Taking Strategy: Focus on the key words "parent-child relationship." Use the process of elimination, focusing on this concept. The only option that addresses a parent-child relationship is option 2. Review the measures that promote this relationship in a hospitalized infant if you had difficulty with this question.

Level of Cognitive Ability: Application
Client Needs: Psychosocial Integrity
Integrated Process: Caring
Content Area: Child Health

Reference:
James, S., Ashwill, J., & Droske, S. (2002). *Nursing care of children: Principles & practice* (2nd ed.). Philadelphia:Saunders, p. 310.

44. The parents of a male infant who will have a surgical repair of a hernia make the following comments. Which comment would require follow-up assessment by a nurse?
1 "I understand surgery will repair the hernia."
2 "The day nurse told me to give him sponge baths for a few days after surgery."
3 "I'll need to buy extra diapers because we need to change them more frequently now."
4 "I don't know if he will be able to father a child when he grows up."

Answer: 4
Rationale: The anatomical location of a hernia frequently causes more psychological concern to the parents than does the actual condition or treatment. Options 1, 2, and 3 all indicate accurate understanding. Option 4 is an incorrect comment.

Test-Taking Strategy: Focus on the key words "would require follow-up." Options 1, 2, and 3 do not require follow-up, whereas option 4 reflects parental fear and identifies a need for further assistance. Review parental instructions regarding the effects of a hernia repair if you had difficulty with this question.

Level of Cognitive Ability: Analysis
Client Needs: Psychosocial Integrity
Integrated Process: Nursing Process/Analysis
Content Area: Child Health

Reference:
Wong, D., & Hockenberry, M. (2003). *Wong's nursing care of infants and children* (7th ed.). St. Louis: Mosby, p. 478.

---

45. A nurse is leading a crisis intervention group. The clients are high school students who have experienced a recent death of a classmate. The classmate committed suicide at the school, and the clients are experiencing disbelief. The clients reviewed the details about finding the classmate dead in a bathroom. Initially, the nurse would:
1 Inquire how the clients recovered from death in the past
2 Reinforce the clients' sense of growth through this death experience
3 Reinforce the clients' ability to work through this death event
4 Inquire about the clients' perception of their classmate's suicide problem

Answer: 4
Rationale: It is essential to determine the clients' views. Inquiring about the clients' perception of the suicide will identify specifically the appraisal of the suicide and the meaning of the perception. Options 2 and 3 are similar in terms of attempts to foster clients' self-esteem. Such an approach is premature at this point. Although option 1 is exploratory, it does not address the "here and now" appraisal in terms of their classmate's suicide. Although the nurse is interested in how clients have coped in the past, this inquiry is not the most immediate assessment.

Test-Taking Strategy: Use the steps of the nursing process to eliminate options 2 and 3. From the remaining options, consider the issue of the question and select the option that deals with the "here and now." The nurse must first determine the clients' perception or appraisal of the stressful event. Review the phases of crisis if you had difficulty with this question.

Level of Cognitive Ability: Analysis
Client Needs: Psychosocial Integrity
Integrated Process: Nursing Process/Assessment
Content Area: Mental Health

Reference:
Stuart, G., & Laraia, M. (2005). *Principles and practice of psychiatric nursing* (8th ed.). St. Louis: Mosby, pp. 222-225.

46. A hospitalized client has participated in substance abuse therapy group sessions. The nurse is monitoring the client's response to the substance abuse sessions. Which statement by the client would best indicate that the client has assimilated session topics, coping response styles, and has processed information effectively for self-use?

1 "I know I'm ready to be discharged; I feel like I can say no and leave a group of friends if they are drinking . . . no problem."

2 "This group has really helped a lot. I know it will be different when I go home. But I'm sure that my family and friends will all help me, like the people in this group have. They'll all help me . . . I know they will . . . They won't let me go back to old ways."

3 "I'm looking forward to leaving here; I know that I will miss all of you. So, I'm happy and I'm sad. I'm excited and I'm scared. I know that I have to work hard to be strong and that everyone isn't going to be as helpful as you people. I know it isn't going to be easy. But, I'm going to try as hard as I can."

4 "I'll keep all my appointments; I'll do everything I'm supposed to . . . Nothing will go wrong that way."

Answer: 3

Rationale: In the defense mechanism of denial, the person denies reality. There can be varying degrees of this denial. In option 3, the client is expressing real concern and ambivalence about discharge from the hospital. The client is real in the appraisal about the changes the client will have to initiate in lifestyle as well as the fact that the client has to work hard and develop new friends and meeting places. Option 1 identifies denial. In option 2, the client is relying heavily on others, and the client's locus of control is external. In option 4, the client is concrete and procedure-oriented; again, the client verbalizes denial.

Test-Taking Strategy: Note the key words "has processed information effectively." Select the option that identifies the most realistic client verbalization. Recalling that in denial a person is unable to face reality will assist you in eliminating options 1, 2, and 4. Review the defense mechanism of denial if you had difficulty with this question.

Level of Cognitive Ability: Analysis
Client Needs: Psychosocial Integrity
Integrated Process: Nursing Process/Analysis
Content Area: Mental Health

References:
Stuart, G., & Laraia, M. (2005). *Principles and practice of psychiatric nursing* (8th ed.). St. Louis: Mosby, p. 492.
Varcarolis, E.M. (2002). *Foundations of psychiatric mental health nursing* (4th ed.). Philadelphia: Saunders, p. 292.

---

47. A client recovering from a head injury becomes agitated at times. Which action will most likely calm this client?

1 Turn on the television to a musical program

2 Talk to the client about the familiar objects, such as family pictures, that are kept in the client's room

3 Assign the client a new task to master

4 Make the client aware that the behavior is undesirable

Answer: 2

Rationale: Decreasing environmental stimuli aids in reducing agitation for the head-injured client. Option 1 increases stimuli. Option 3 does not simplify the environment because a new task may be frustrating. In option 4, the nurse uses negative reinforcement to help the client adjust. Providing familiar objects will decrease anxiety.

Test-Taking Strategy: Use the process of elimination, identifying those options that may increase stimuli, agitation, and frustration. This will assist in eliminating options 1, 3, and 4. Review measures that will relieve agitation if you had difficulty with this question.

Level of Cognitive Ability: Application
Client Needs: Psychosocial Integrity
Integrated Process: Caring
Content Area: Adult Health/Neurological

Reference:
Ignatavicius, D., & Workman, M. (2002). *Medical surgical nursing: Critical thinking for collaborative care* (4th ed.). Philadelphia: Saunders, p. 997.

48. A client recovering from a cerebrovascular accident (CVA) has become irritable and angry regarding limitations. Which of the following is the best nursing approach to help the client regain motivation to succeed?
  1 Allow longer and more frequent visitation by the spouse
  2 Use supportive statements to correct the client's behavior
  3 Tell the client that the nurses are experienced and know how the client feels
  4 Ignore the behavior, knowing that the client is grieving

Answer: 2
Rationale: Clients who have experienced a CVA have many and varied needs. The client may need his or her behavior pointed out so that correction can take place. It is also important to support and praise the client for accomplishments. Spouses of a CVA client are often grieving; therefore, more visitation may not be helpful. Additionally, short visits are often encouraged. Stating that the nurse knows how the client feels is inappropriate. The client's behavior should not be ignored.

Test-Taking Strategy: Use therapeutic communication techniques to eliminate options 3 and 4. From the remaining options, option 2 is the only option that addresses the client's behavior described in the question. Review the psychosocial aspects related to a CVA if you had difficulty with this question.

Level of Cognitive Ability: Application
Client Needs: Psychosocial Integrity
Integrated Process: Caring
Content Area: Adult Health/Neurological

Reference:
Ignatavicius, D., & Workman, M. (2002). *Medical surgical nursing: Critical thinking for collaborative care* (4th ed.). Philadelphia: Saunders, p. 982.

49. A client is admitted to the hospital with a fractured hip and is experiencing periods of confusion. The nurse formulates a nursing diagnosis of disturbed thought processes and identifies which priority psychosocial outcome?
  1 Improved sleep patterns
  2 Increased ability to concentrate and make decisions
  3 Meets self-care needs independently
  4 Reduced family fears and anxiety

Answer: 2
Rationale: The client needs to be able to concentrate and make decisions. Once the client is able to do that, the nurse can work with the client to achieve the other outcomes. The client is the center of the nurse's concern. Options 1 and 3 address physiological needs, not psychosocial outcomes. Option 4 is a secondary need.

Test-Taking Strategy: Use the process of elimination and note the key words "psychosocial outcome." Select the option that will have the greatest impact on the client's ability to function psychosocially. Option 4 can be eliminated because it does not address the client of the question. Options 1 and 3 address physiological not psychosocial needs. Review expected outcomes for the client with disturbed thought process if you had difficulty with this question.

Level of Cognitive Ability: Analysis
Client Needs: Psychosocial Integrity
Integrated Process: Nursing Process/Planning
Content Area: Adult Health/Musculoskeletal

References:
Black, J., & Hawks, J. (2005). *Medical-surgical nursing: Clinical management for positive outcomes* (7th ed.). Philadelphia: Saunders, p. 641.
Phipps, W., Monahan, F., Sands, J., Marek, J., & Neighbors, M. (2003). *Medical-surgical nursing: Health and illness perspectives* (7th ed.). St. Louis: Mosby, p. 1318.

50. A nurse is caring for a young woman dying from breast cancer. The nurse determines that a defining characteristic of anticipatory grieving is present when the woman:

1 Verbalizes unrealistic goals and plans for the future
2 Discusses thoughts and feelings related to loss
3 Has prolonged emotional reactions and outbursts
4 Ignores untreated medical conditions that requires treatment

Answer: 2
Rationale: The nurse can determine the client's stage of grief by observing the client's behavior. This is extremely important because the appropriate nursing diagnoses need to be developed so that the plan of care is appropriate. Options 1, 3, and 4 are examples of dysfunctional grieving.

Test-Taking Strategy: Focus on the issue: anticipatory grieving. Note the similarity in options 1, 3, and 4 in that they indicate dysfunctional grieving. Also noting the words "unrealistic," "prolonged," and ignores" in these options will assist in eliminating them. Review the stages of grief and anticipatory grieving if you had difficulty with this question.

Level of Cognitive Ability: Analysis
Client Needs: Psychosocial Integrity
Integrated Process: Nursing Process/Analysis
Content Area: Adult Health/Neurological

Reference:
Phipps, W., Monahan, F., Sands, J., Marek, J., & Neighbors, M. (2003). *Medical-surgical nursing: Health and illness perspectives* (7th ed.). St. Louis: Mosby, p. 97.

---

51. A nurse determines that a client is beginning to experience shock and hemorrhage secondary to a partial inversion of the uterus. The nurse pages the obstetrician STAT and calls for assistance. The client asks in an apprehensive voice, "What is happening to me? I feel so funny and I know I am bleeding. Am I dying?" The nurse responds to the client, knowing that the client is feeling:

1 Panic secondary to shock
2 Fear and anxiety related to unexpected and ambiguous sensations
3 Anticipatory grieving related to the fear of dying
4 Depression related to postpartum hormonal changes

Answer: 2
Rationale: Feelings of loss of control are common causes of anxiety. The unknown is the most common cause of fear. Apprehension and feelings of impending doom are also associated with shock, but the information in the question does not suggest panic at this point. Anticipatory grieving occurs when there is knowledge of the impending loss, but is not associated with a sudden situational crisis such as this one. It is far too early for the onset of postpartum depression.

Test-Taking Strategy: Focus on the data and the client's statement. Note the relationship between "I feel so funny" in the question and "unexpected and ambiguous sensations" in the correct option. Review client responses when a sudden situational crisis occurs if you had difficulty with this question.

Level of Cognitive Ability: Analysis
Client Needs: Psychosocial Integrity
Integrated Process: Nursing Process/Analysis
Content Area: Maternity/Postpartum

Reference:
Lowdermilk, D., & Perry, A. (2004). *Maternity & women's health care* (8th ed.). St. Louis: Mosby, p. 962.

52. A perinatal home care nurse has just assessed the fetal status of a client with a diagnosis of partial placental abruption of 20 weeks' gestation. The client is experiencing new bleeding and reports less fetal movement. The nurse informs the client that the physician will be contacted for possible hospital admission. The client begins to cry quietly while holding her abdomen with her hands. She murmurs, "No, no, you can't go, my little man." The nurse recognizes the client's behavior as an indication of:

1 Pain related to abdominal tetany
2 Cognitive confusion secondary to shock
3 Grieving, anticipatory related to perceived potential loss
4 Situational crisis, death of fetus related to fear and loss

Answer: 3
Rationale: Anticipatory grieving occurs when a client has knowledge of an impending loss. Anticipatory grieving is appropriate when signs of fetal distress accelerate. The first stages of anticipatory grieving may be characterized by shock, emotional numbness, disbelief, and strong emotions such as tears, screaming, or anger. There is no data that indicates the presence of pain, confusion, or fetal death.

Test-Taking Strategy: Use the process of elimination, focusing on the data in the question. Options 1 and 2 can be eliminated because there is no indication of pain or confusion. Note that in this situation, there is a situational crisis with feelings of grief, but no fetal loss has occurred at this point. Therefore, eliminate option 4. Review the defining characteristics of anticipatory grieving if you had difficulty with this question.

Level of Cognitive Ability: Analysis
Client Needs: Psychosocial Integrity
Integrated Process: Nursing Process/Analysis
Content Area: Maternity/Antepartum

Reference:
Lowdermilk, D., & Perry, A. (2004). *Maternity & women's health care* (8th ed.). St. Louis: Mosby, pp. 1151; 1155.

---

53. A postoperative client has been vomiting, has absent bowel sounds, and paralytic ileus has been diagnosed. The physician orders insertion of a nasogastric tube. The nurse explains the purpose of the tube and the insertion procedure to the client. The client says to the nurse, "I'm not sure I can take any more of this treatment." The nurse makes which statement to the client?

1 "It is your right to refuse any treatment. I'll notify the physician."
2 "You are feeling tired and frustrated with your recovery from surgery?"
3 "If you don't have this tube put down, you will just continue to vomit."
4 "Let's just put the tube down so you can get well."

Answer: 2
Rationale: In option 2, the nurse uses empathy. Empathy, comprehending, and sharing a client's frame of reference is an important component in a nurse-client relationship. It assists clients to express and explore feelings, which can lead to problem solving. The other options are examples of barriers to effective communication, including defensiveness (option 1), showing disapproval (option 3), and stereotyping (option 4).

Test-Taking Strategy: Use therapeutic communication techniques. Option 2 is an open-ended question and is a communication tool. It also focuses on the client feelings. Review these therapeutic techniques if you had difficulty with this question.

Level of Cognitive Ability: Application
Client Needs: Psychosocial Integrity
Integrated Process: Communication and Documentation
Content Area: Adult Health/Gastrointestinal

Reference:
Potter, P., & Perry, A. (2005). *Fundamentals of nursing* (6th ed.). St. Louis: Mosby, p. 437.

54. A client is admitted to the hospital with a bowel obstruction secondary to a recurrent malignancy, and the physician inserts a Miller-Abbott tube. After the procedure, the client asks the nurse, "Do you think this is worth all this trouble?" The most appropriate action or response by the nurse is:

1 To stay with the client and be silent
2 "Are you wondering whether you are going to get better?"
3 "Let's give this tube a chance."
4 "I remember a case similar to yours and the tube relieved the obstruction."

Answer: 2

Rationale: The nurse uses therapeutic communication tools to assist a client with a chronic terminal illness to express feelings. The nurse listens attentively to the client and uses clarifying and focusing to assist the client in expressing feelings. Responding with inappropriate silence (option 1), changing the subject (option 3), and offering false reassurance (option 4) are nontherapeutic communication techniques.

Test-Taking Strategy: Use therapeutic communications techniques. Option 2 encourages the client to verbalize. Review these techniques if you had difficulty with this question.

Level of Cognitive Ability: Application
Client Needs: Psychosocial Integrity
Integrated Process: Communication and Documentation
Content Area: Adult Health/Oncology

Reference:
Potter, P., & Perry, A. (2005). *Fundamentals of nursing* (6th ed.). St. Louis: Mosby, p. 437.

55. A nurse explains to a client receiving total parenteral nutrition (TPN) that intralipids, an intravenous fat emulsion, will also be administered. The client states to the nurse, "I was always overweight until I had this illness. I'm not sure I want to get that fat. The other IVs are probably enough." The nurse makes which initial response to the client?

1 "Fatty acids are essential for life. You'll develop deficiencies without the fats."
2 "I think you need to discuss this decision with the physician."
3 "Tell me how being ill has affected the way you think of yourself."
4 "I understand what you mean. I've dieted most of my life."

Answer: 3

Rationale: Clients receiving TPN are at risk for development of essential fatty acid deficiency. However, the client's comment requires more than an informational response initially. Option 3 assists the client to express feelings and deal with aspects of illness and treatment. Option 1 provides an opinion. Option 2 places the client's feelings on hold. Option 4 devalues the client's feelings.

Test-Taking Strategy: Note the key words "initial response." Use therapeutic communication techniques and focus on the client's feelings. Option 3 is the only option that addresses the client's feelings. Review therapeutic communication techniques if you had difficulty with this question.

Level of Cognitive Ability: Analysis
Client Needs: Psychosocial Integrity
Integrated Process: Communication and Documentation
Content Area: Fundamental Skills

Reference:
Potter, P., & Perry, A. (2005). *Fundamentals of nursing* (6th ed.). St. Louis: Mosby, p. 437.

56. A client has terminal cancer and is using narcotic analgesics for pain relief. The client is concerned about becoming addicted to the pain medication. The home care nurse allays the client's anxiety by:
1 Explaining to the client that his fears are justified but should be of no concern in the final stages of care
2 Encouraging the client to hold off as long as possible between doses of pain medication
3 Telling the client to take lower doses of medications even though the pain is not well controlled
4 Explaining to the client that addiction rarely occurs in individuals who are taking medication to relieve pain

Answer: 4
Rationale: Clients who are on narcotics often have well-founded fears about addiction, even in the face of pain. The nurse has a responsibility to provide correct information about the likelihood of addiction while still maintaining adequate pain control. Addiction is rare for individuals who are taking medication to relieve pain. Allowing the client to be in pain, as in options 2 and 3, is not acceptable nursing practice. Option 1 is only partially correct in that it acknowledges the client's fear.

Test-Taking Strategy: Use the process of elimination. Eliminate options 2 and 3 because these are not acceptable nursing practices. From the remaining options, eliminate option 1 because it is only partially correct. Review pain management if you had difficulty with this question.

Level of Cognitive Ability: Application
Client Needs: Psychosocial Integrity
Integrated Process: Caring
Content Area: Adult Health/Oncology

Reference:
Black, J., & Hawks, J. (2005). *Medical-surgical nursing: Clinical management for positive outcomes* (7th ed.). Philadelphia: Saunders, p. 450.

57. A client is very anxious about receiving chest physical therapy (CPT) for the first time at home. In planning for the client's care, the home care nurse proceeds in reassuring the client that:
1 There are no risks associated with this procedure.
2 CPT will resolve all of the client's respiratory symptoms.
3 CPT will assist in mobilizing secretions to enhance more effective breathing.
4 CPT will assist the client to cough more effectively.

Answer: 3
Rationale: There are risks associated with CPT, and these include cardiac, gastrointestinal, neurological, and pulmonary effects. CPT is an intervention to assist in mobilizing and clearing secretions and enhance more effective breathing. It will not resolve all respiratory symptoms. CPT will assist the client to cough, if the secretions have been mobilized and the cough stimulus is present.

Test-Taking Strategy: Use the process of elimination. Eliminate options 1 and 2 because they contain the absolute words "no" and "all." From the remaining options, focus on the purpose of CPT and recall that coughing will be stimulated once secretions are mobilized. Review the purpose of CPT if you had difficulty with this question.

Level of Cognitive Ability: Application
Client Needs: Psychosocial Integrity
Integrated Process: Teaching/Learning
Content Area: Adult Health/Respiratory

References:
Lewis, S., Heitkemper, M., & Dirksen, S. (2004). *Medical-surgical nursing: Assessment and management of clinical problems* (6th ed.). St. Louis: Mosby, pp. 672-673.
Ignatavicius, D., & Workman, M. (2002). *Medical surgical nursing: Critical thinking for collaborative care* (4th ed.). Philadelphia: Saunders, pp. 548-549.

58. A client with cardiomyopathy stops eating, takes long naps, and turns away from the nurse when the nurse talks to the client. The nurse interprets that this client is most likely experiencing:
1 Activity intolerance
2 Intractable pain
3 Noncompliance
4 Depression

Answer: 4
Rationale: Depression is a common problem related to clients who have long-term and debilitating illness. Options 1, 2, and 3 are not related to the symptoms present in the question and therefore are not appropriate interpretations.

Test-Taking Strategy: When a question asks for an interpretation of a client's symptoms, focus on the information in the question. Based on the data presented, the only appropriate interpretation is depression. Review the characteristics of depression if you had difficulty with this question.

Level of Cognitive Ability: Analysis
Client Needs: Psychosocial Integrity
Integrated Process: Nursing Process/Analysis
Content Area: Adult Health/Cardiovascular

References:
Black, J., & Hawks, J. (2005). *Medical-surgical nursing: Clinical management for positive outcomes* (7th ed.). Philadelphia: Saunders, pp. 532; 1607.
Phipps, W., Monahan, F., Sands, J., Marek, J., & Neighbors, M. (2003). *Medical-surgical nursing: Health and illness perspectives* (7th ed.). St. Louis: Mosby, pp. 81-82.

59. A nurse is caring for a pregnant client hospitalized for stabilization of diabetes mellitus. The client tells the nurse that her husband is caring for their 2-year-old daughter. The nurse develops which short-term psychosocial outcome for the client?
1 Teach the client and family about diabetes and its implications
2 Provide emotional support and education about interrupted family processes related to the pregnant woman's hospitalization
3 Protect from risk of injury secondary to convulsions
4 Be alert to the risks of early labor and birth

Answer: 2
Rationale: The short-term psychosocial well-being of the family is at risk as a result of the hospitalization of a client. Teaching about diabetes mellitus is a long-term goal related to diabetes. Options 3 and 4 are unrelated to diabetes mellitus and are more related to pregnancy-induced hypertension.

Test-Taking Strategy: Use the process of elimination. Eliminate options 3 and 4 because they are unrelated to diabetes mellitus. From the remaining options, note the words "short-term psychosocial outcome" and focus on the data in the question to direct you to option 2. Review outcomes for interrupted family processes if you had difficulty with this question.

Level of Cognitive Ability: Analysis
Client Needs: Psychosocial Integrity
Integrated Process: Nursing Process/Planning
Content Area: Maternity/Antepartum

References:
Lowdermilk, D., & Perry, A. (2004). *Maternity & women's health care* (8th ed.). St. Louis: Mosby, p. 22.
Murray, S., McKinney, E., & Gorrie, T. (2002). *Foundations of maternal-newborn nursing* (3rd ed.). Philadelphia: Saunders, p. 15.

60. A new parent is trying to make the decision whether to have her baby boy circumcised. The nurse makes which statement to assist the mother in making a decision?

1 "I had my son circumcised and I am so glad!"

2 "Circumcision is a difficult decision, but your physician is the best and you know it's better to get it done now than later!"

3 "Circumcision is a difficult decision. There are various controversies surrounding circumcision. Here, read this pamphlet that discusses the pros and cons, and we will talk after you read, to answer any questions that you have."

4 "You know they say it prevents cancer and sexually transmitted diseases, so I would definitely have my son circumcised!"

Answer: 3

Rationale: Informed decision making is the key point in answering this question. The nurse should provide educational material and answer questions pertaining to the education of the mother. Providing written information to the mother will give her the information she needs to make an educated and informed decision. The nurse's personal thoughts and feelings should not be part of the educational process.

Test-Taking Strategy: Use therapeutic communication techniques and the process of elimination. Options 1, 2, and 4 are communication blocks because the nurse is providing a personal opinion to the client. Review therapeutic communication techniques if you had difficulty with this question.

Level of Cognitive Ability: Application
Client Needs: Psychosocial Integrity
Integrated Process: Communication and Documentation
Content Area: Maternity/Postpartum

Reference:
Murray, S., McKinney, E., & Gorrie, T. (2002). *Foundations of maternal-newborn nursing* (3rd ed.). Philadelphia: Saunders, pp. 24-26.

---

61. A nurse is planning care for a client who is experiencing anxiety following a myocardial infarction. Which nursing intervention should be included in the plan of care?

1 Provide detailed explanations of all procedures

2 Administer an antianxiety medication to promote relaxation

3 Limit family involvement during the acute phase

4 Answer questions with factual information

Answer: 4

Rationale: Accurate information reduces fear, strengthens the nurse-client relationship, and assists the client to deal realistically with the situation. Providing detailed information may increase the client's anxiety. Information should be provided simply and clearly. Medication should not be used unless necessary. Limiting family involvement may or may not be helpful. The client's family may be a source of support for the client.

Test-Taking Strategy: Note that the client is experiencing anxiety. Eliminate option 1 because of the word "detailed." Eliminate option 2 because medication should not be the first intervention to alleviate anxiety. From the remaining options, eliminate option 3 because limiting family involvement is not anxiety-reducing in all situations. Review measures to reduce anxiety if you had difficulty with this question.

Level of Cognitive Ability: Application
Client Needs: Psychosocial Integrity
Integrated Process: Nursing Process/Implementation
Content Area: Adult Health/Cardiovascular

Reference:
Black, J., & Hawks, J. (2005). *Medical-surgical nursing: Clinical management for positive outcomes* (7th ed.). Philadelphia: Saunders, p. 1723.

62. A client recovering from an acute myocardial infarction will be discharged in one day. Which client action on the evening before discharge suggests that the client is in the denial phase?

1 Requests a sedative for sleep at 10:00 pm
2 Expresses hesitancy to leave the hospital
3 Walks up and down three flights of stairs unsupervised
4 Consumes 25% of foods and fluids for supper

Answer: 3

Rationale: Ignoring activity limitations and avoidance of lifestyle changes are signs of the denial stage. Walking three flights of stairs should be a supervised activity during this phase of the recovery process. Option 1 is an appropriate client action on the evening before discharge. Option 2, expressing hesitancy to leave, may be a manifestation of anxiety or fear, not of denial. Option 4, anorexia, is a manifestation of depression, not denial.

Test-Taking Strategy: Note the key word "denial." Focus on this key word and use the process of elimination. Option 1 is an appropriate client request. Option 2 identifies anxiety or fear. Option 4 identifies depression. Option 3 is the only option that identifies denial. Review the manifestations associated with denial if you had difficulty with this question.

Level of Cognitive Ability: Analysis
Client Needs: Psychosocial Integrity
Integrated Process: Nursing Process/Analysis
Content Area: Adult Health/Cardiovascular

Reference:
Black, J., & Hawks, J. (2005). *Medical-surgical nursing: Clinical management for positive outcomes* (7th ed.). Philadelphia: Saunders, pp. 525-526; 1719.

63. A nurse is caring for a client with Hodgkin's disease who will be receiving radiation and chemotherapy. Which statement by the client indicates a positive coping mechanism to be used during these treatments?

1 "I have selected a wig even though I will miss my own hair."
2 "I know losing my hair won't bother me."
3 "I will not leave the house bald."
4 "I will be one of the few who doesn't lose hair."

Answer: 1

Rationale: A combination of radiation and chemotherapy often causes alopecia. In order to use positive coping mechanisms, the client must identify personal feelings and positive interventions to deal with side effects. Options 2, 3, and 4 are not positive coping mechanisms.

Test-Taking Strategy: Focus on the issue: a positive coping mechanism. Options 2, 3, and 4 involve avoidance and denial. Option 1 is the only option that addresses a positive coping mechanism. Review coping mechanisms if you had difficulty with this question.

Level of Cognitive Ability: Analysis
Client Needs: Psychosocial Integrity
Integrated Process: Nursing Process/Analysis
Content Area: Adult Health/Oncology

Reference:
Black, J., & Hawks, J. (2005). *Medical-surgical nursing: Clinical management for positive outcomes* (7th ed.). Philadelphia: Saunders, pp. 1410-1411.

64. A male client is admitted to the hospital with diabetic ketoacidosis (DKA). The client's daughter says to the nurse, "My mother died last month, and now this. I've been trying to follow all of the instructions from the doctor, but what have I done wrong?" The nurse makes which response to the client's daughter?
 1 "Maybe we can keep your father in the hospital for a while longer to give you a rest."
 2 "An emotional stress, such as your mother's death, can trigger DKA in a diabetic client even though you are following the prescribed regimen."
 3 "You should talk to the social worker about getting you someone at home who is more capable in managing a diabetic's care."
 4 "Tell me what you think you did wrong."

Answer: 2
Rationale: Environment, infection, or an emotional stressor can initiate the physiological mechanism of DKA. Option 1 is not a cost-effective intervention. Options 3 and 4 substantiate the daughters' feelings of guilt and incompetence.

Test-Taking Strategy: Use the process of elimination. Eliminate option 1 first because this option is not cost effective. Options 3 and 4 devalue the client (the daughter) and block therapeutic communication and are eliminated next. Review therapeutic communication techniques if you had difficulty with this question.

Level of Cognitive Ability: Application
Client Needs: Psychosocial Integrity
Integrated Process: Caring
Content Area: Adult Health/Endocrine

References:
Black, J., & Hawks, J. (2005). *Medical-surgical nursing: Clinical management for positive outcomes* (7th ed.). Philadelphia: Saunders, p. 1627.
Potter, P., & Perry, A. (2005). *Fundamentals of nursing* (6th ed.). St. Louis: Mosby, p. 437.

---

65. A nurse has been working with a victim of rape in an outpatient setting for the past 4 weeks. The nurse identifies which client goal as an unrealistic short-term one?
 1 The client will resolve feelings of fear and anxiety related to the rape trauma.
 2 The client will experience physical healing of the wounds that were incurred at the time of the rape.
 3 The client will verbalize feelings about the rape event.
 4 The client will participate in the treatment plan by keeping appointments and following through with treatment options.

Answer: 1
Rationale: Short-term goals will include the beginning stages of dealing with the rape trauma. Clients will be expected initially to keep appointments, participate in care, begin to explore feelings, and begin to heal physical wounds that were inflicted at the time of the rape. Resolution of feelings of anxiety and fear is a long-term goal.

Test-Taking Strategy: Focus on the issue: an unrealistic short-term goal. Use the process of elimination, considering each option and the reality of the option statement being achieved short term. Note the word "resolve" in option 1. This word should provide you with the clue that this option is a long-term goal. Review appropriate goals for the client who is a victim of rape if you had difficulty with this question.

Level of Cognitive Ability: Analysis
Client Needs: Psychosocial Integrity
Integrated Process: Nursing Process/Analysis
Content Area: Mental Health

Reference:
Stuart, G., & Laraia, M. (2005). *Principles and practice of psychiatric nursing* (8th ed.). St. Louis: Mosby, p. 235.

66. A client is admitted to a surgical unit with a diagnosis of cancer. The client is scheduled for surgery in the morning. When the nurse enters the room and begins the surgical preparation, the client states, "I'm not having surgery. You must have the wrong person! My test results were negative. I'll be going home tomorrow." The nurse recognizes that the ego defense mechanism that may be operating here is:

1 Psychosis
2 Denial
3 Delusions
4 Displacement

Answer: 2

Rationale: By definition, ego defense mechanisms are operations outside of a person's awareness that the ego calls into play to protect against anxiety. Denial is the defense mechanism that blocks out painful or anxiety-inducing events or feelings. In this case, the client cannot deal with the upcoming surgery for cancer and therefore denies the illness. Psychosis and delusions are not defense mechanisms. Displacement is the discharging of pent-up feelings on persons less dangerous than those who initially aroused the feelings.

Test-Taking Strategy: Focus on the issue: ego defense mechanism. Options 1 and 3 are eliminated first because these are not ego defense mechanisms. From the remaining options, focus on the client's statement to direct you to option 2. Review ego defense mechanisms if you had difficulty with this question.

Level of Cognitive Ability: Analysis
Client Needs: Psychosocial Integrity
Integrated Process: Nursing Process/Analysis
Content Area: Adult Health/Oncology

Reference:
Stuart, G., & Laraia, M. (2005). *Principles and practice of psychiatric nursing* (8th ed.). St. Louis: Mosby, pp. 296; 279.

67. A community health nurse working in an industrial setting has received a memo indicating that a large number of employees will be laid off in the next 2 weeks. An analysis of previous layoffs suggested that workers experienced role crises, indecision, and depression. Using this data, the nurse should begin to:

1 Help the workers acquire unemployment benefits to avoid a gap in income
2 Reduce the staff in the occupational health department of the industrial setting
3 Notify the insurance carriers of the upcoming event to assist with potential health alterations
4 Identify referral, counseling, and vocational rehabilitative services for the employees being laid off

Answer: 4

Rationale: In preparation for this crisis, the nurse should identify the services that are available to the employees. These resources will provide immediate avenues for the assistance when the layoff occurs. Additional information about the industrial setting is needed to determine if options 1, 2, or 3 were necessary or possible.

Test-Taking Strategy: Use the steps of the nursing process to direct you to option 4. This option refers to assessment of resources and services for employees. Additionally, review crisis interventions if you had difficulty with this question.

Level of Cognitive Ability: Analysis
Client Needs: Psychosocial Integrity
Integrated Process: Nursing Process/Planning
Content Area: Mental Health

Reference:
Stuart, G., & Laraia, M. (2005). *Principles and practice of psychiatric nursing* (8th ed.). St. Louis: Mosby, pp. 228-229.

68. A primigravida client comes to the clinic and has been diagnosed with a urinary tract infection. She has repeatedly verbalized concern regarding safety of the fetus. Which of the following nursing diagnoses is appropriate at this time?
1 Acute Pain
2 Impaired Tissue Integrity
3 Urinary Tract Infection
4 Fear

Answer: 4
Rationale: The primary concern for this client is safety of her fetus, not herself. The priority nursing diagnosis at this time is Fear. Option 3 is a medical diagnosis and outside the scope of nursing practice. Acute Pain and Impaired Tissue Integrity are commonly seen in clients experiencing urinary tract infections, but the question includes no data to support either of the options.

Test-Taking Strategy: Focus on the data in the question and note the key words "verbalized concern." Eliminate option 3 because it is a medical diagnosis. Also, note that options 1, 2, and 3 are similar in that they are all physiological. Option 4 addresses the psychosocial issue. Review the defining characteristics of fear if you had difficulty with this question.

Level of Cognitive Ability: Analysis
Client Needs: Psychosocial Integrity
Integrated Process: Nursing Process/Analysis
Content Area: Maternity/Antepartum

Reference:
Gulanick, M., Myers, J., Klopp, A., Gradishar, D., Galanes, S., & Puzas, M. (2003). *Nursing care plans: Nursing diagnosis and intervention* (5th ed.). St. Louis: Mosby, pp. 59; 121; 169; 893.

69. A nurse is planning interventions for counseling the maternal client newly diagnosed with sickle cell anemia. The important psychosocial intervention at this time would be which of the following?
1 Provide all information regarding the disease
2 Allow the client to be alone if she is crying
3 Provide emotional support
4 Avoid the topic of the disease at all costs

Answer: 3
Rationale: One of the most important nursing functions is providing emotional support to the client and family during the counseling process. Option 1 overwhelms the client with information while the client is trying to cope with the news of the disease. Option 2 is only appropriate if the client requests to be alone. If not requested, the nurse is abandoning the client in a time of need. Option 4 is similar to option 2 and is nontherapeutic.

Test-Taking Strategy: Use the process of elimination. Eliminate options 1 and 4 because of the absolute words "all" and "avoid." Additionally, these actions are nontherapeutic. From the remaining options, remember that the client's feelings are the priority, and an extremely important role of the nurse is to provide emotional support. Review interventions related to providing emotional support if you had difficulty with this question.

Level of Cognitive Ability: Application
Client Needs: Psychosocial Integrity
Integrated Process: Caring
Content Area: Maternity/Antepartum

References:
Matteson, P. (2001). *Women's health during the childbearing years: A community-based approach.* St. Louis: Mosby, p. 171.
Stuart, G., & Laraia, M. (2005). *Principles and practice of psychiatric nursing* (8th ed.). St. Louis: Mosby, p. 246.

70. A neonatal intensive care nurse is caring for a newborn infant immediately following delivery with a suspected diagnosis of erythroblastosis fetalis. The nurse would make which of the following statements to the parents at this time?

1 "You must have many concerns. Please ask me any questions so I explain your infant's care."
2 "This is a common neonatal problem, so you shouldn't be concerned."
3 "There is no need to worry. We have the most updated equipment in this hospital."
4 "Your infant is very sick. The next 24 hours are most crucial."

Answer: 1

Rationale: Parental anxiety is expected related to the care of the infant with erythroblastosis fetalis. This anxiety is caused by a lack of knowledge regarding the disease process, treatments, and expected outcomes. Parents need to be encouraged to verbalize concerns and participate in care as appropriate. The nurse would not tell the parents "not to worry" or "not to be concerned." Option 4 will produce anxiety in the parents.

Test-Taking Strategy: Use therapeutic communication techniques. Eliminate options 2 and 3 because they are similar. Additionally, they are blocks to communication. Eliminate option 4 because it will produce anxiety in the parents. Remember to address the clients' feelings and concerns. Option 1 is the only option that encourages communication. Review therapeutic communication techniques if you had difficulty with this question.

Level of Cognitive Ability: Application
Clients Needs: Psychosocial Integrity
Integrated Process: Caring
Content Area: Maternity/Postpartum

References:
Matteson, P. (2001). *Women's health during the childbearing years: A community-based approach.* St. Louis: Mosby, pp. 52; 701.
McKinney, E., James, S., Murray, S., & Ashwill, J. (2005). *Maternal-child nursing* (2nd ed.). St. Louis: Elsevier, pp. 30-31.

71. A school nurse is weighing all the high school students. One of the teenagers, who has type 1 diabetes mellitus, has gained 15 pounds since last year with no gain in height. The nurse also notices this student eating alone in the cafeteria at lunch time and avoiding any interaction with her peers. Based on this data, the nurse is most concerned that the student may have:

1 Bulimia nervosa
2 Self-destructive thoughts
3 An alcohol abuse problem
4 A drug abuse problem

Answer: 2

Rationale: Diabetic teenagers are at risk for depression and suicide (self-destructive thoughts), which is frequently manifested by changing insulin and eating patterns. Social isolation is another indicator. Bulimics may be of normal weight but control weight gain by purging. Alcohol use and drug abuse is more likely to be related to weight loss.

Test-Taking Strategy: Focus on the data in the question and use the process of elimination. Eliminate options 3 and 4 first because they are similar. From the remaining options, noting the social isolation issue and the age of the client should direct you to option 2. Review the manifestations associated with depression and self-destructive thoughts if you had difficulty with this question.

Level of Cognitive Ability: Analysis
Client Needs: Psychosocial Integrity
Integrated Process: Nursing Process/Analysis
Content Area: Child Health

References:
Stuart, G., & Laraia, M. (2005). *Principles and practice of psychiatric nursing* (8th ed.). St. Louis: Mosby, p. 308.
Wong, D., & Hockenberry, M. (2003). *Wong's nursing care of infants and children* (7th ed.). St. Louis: Mosby, p. 719.

72. A school nurse is teaching a class of high school students about the risk of sexually transmitted diseases (STDs). What opening statement will best encourage participation within the group?
1 "At the end of the class, condoms will be distributed to everyone in the class."
2 "The topic today is very personal. For this reason, anything shared with the group will remain confidential."
3 "Please feel free to share your personal experiences with the group."
4 "Our goal today is to describe ways to prevent acquiring a sexually transmitted disease."

Answer: 2
Rationale: Option 2 identifies the rules for confidentiality, which will help develop a trust in sharing sensitive issues with the group. Option 1 may be an incentive for those attending to stay, but participation is not required to get the reward. Option 3 provides no protection of confidentiality. Option 4 does not foster trust, especially with those who may already have a STD.

Test-Taking Strategy: Focus on the issues, confidentiality, trust building, and sharing. Option 2 is the only option that addresses the issue of confidentiality. Review the concepts related to group process if you had difficulty with this question.

Level of Cognitive Ability: Application
Client Needs: Psychosocial Integrity
Integrated Process: Communication and Documentation
Content Area: Child Health

Reference:
Wong, D., & Hockenberry, M. (2003). *Wong's nursing care of infants and children* (7th ed.). St. Louis: Mosby, pp. 824-825.

73. A nurse is planning care for the client with an intrauterine fetal demise. Which of the following is an inappropriate goal for this client?
1 The woman and her family will express their grief about the loss of their desired infant.
2 The woman and her family will discuss plans for going home without the infant.
3 The woman and her family will contact their pastor or grief counselor for support following discharge.
4 The woman will recognize that thoughts of worthlessness and suicide are normal following a loss.

Answer: 4
Rationale: It is important for the nurse to assess whether the client is undergoing the normal grieving process. Signs that are a cause for concern and are not part of the normal grieving process include thoughts of worthlessness and suicide. Options 1, 2, and 3 are appropriate goals.

Test-Taking Strategy: Use the process of elimination, noting the key words "inappropriate goal." These key words should direct you to option 4 because thoughts of worthlessness and suicide are cause for concern. Review care of the client experiencing intrauterine fetal demise if you had difficulty with this question.

Level of Cognitive Ability: Analysis
Client Needs: Psychosocial Integrity
Integrated Process: Caring
Content Area: Maternity/Postpartum

Reference:
Lowdermilk, D., & Perry, A. (2004). *Maternity & women's health care* (8th ed.). St. Louis: Mosby, p. 1161.

74. A client with severe preeclampsia is admitted to the hospital. She is a student at a local college and insists on continuing her studies while in the hospital despite being instructed to rest. The nurse notes she studies about 19 hours a day between numerous visits from fellow students, family, and friends. The nurse plans to:
  1 Instruct the client that the health of the baby is more important than her studies at this time
  2 Ask her why she is not complying with the order of bed rest
  3 Include a significant other in helping the client understand the need for bed rest
  4 Develop a routine with the client to balance studies and rest needs

Answer: 4

Rationale: In options 1 and 2, the nurse is judging the client's opinion and asking probing questions. This will cause a breakdown in communication. Option 3 persuades the client's significant other to disagree with the client's action. This could cause problems with the relationship between the client and significant other and also conflict in communication with the health care workers. Option 4 involves the client in the decision making.

Test-Taking Strategy: Use the process of elimination. Eliminate options 1, 2, and 3 because these are blocks to communication and a therapeutic nurse-client relationship. Option 4 is the most thorough nursing action because it addresses rest, studies, and involves the client in the decision-making process. Review care of the client with preeclampsia if you had difficulty with this question.

Level of Cognitive Ability: Application
Client Needs: Psychosocial Integrity
Integrated Process: Nursing Process/Implementation
Content Area: Maternity/Antepartum

References:
Lowdermilk, D., & Perry, A. (2004). *Maternity & women's health care* (8th ed.). St. Louis: Mosby, 850.
Potter, P., & Perry, A. (2005). *Fundamentals of nursing* (6th ed.). St. Louis: Mosby, p. 437.

75. A pregnant client is newly diagnosed as having gestational diabetes. She cries during the remaining interview and keeps repeating, "What have I done to cause this? If I could only live my life over." Which nursing diagnosis should direct nursing care at this time?
  1 Situational low self-esteem related to a complication of pregnancy
  2 Deficient knowledge related to diabetic self-care during pregnancy
  3 Disturbed body image related to complications of pregnancy
  4 Risk for injury to the fetus related to maternal distress

Answer: 1

Rationale: The client is putting the blame for the diabetes on herself, lowering her self-esteem. She is expressing fear and grief. Deficient knowledge is an important nursing diagnosis for this client, but not at this time. The client will not be able to comprehend information at this time. There is no data in the question to support the nursing diagnoses in options 3 and 4.

Test-Taking Strategy: Use the data presented in the question to direct you to the correct option. The words "what have I done" should assist in eliminating options 2, 3, and 4. Review the defining characteristics of the nursing diagnosis, situational low self-esteem if you had difficulty with this question.

Level of Cognitive Ability: Analysis
Client Needs: Psychosocial Integrity
Integrated Process: Nursing Process/Analysis
Content Area: Maternity/Antepartum

Reference:
Lowdermilk, D., & Perry, A. (2004). *Maternity & women's health care* (8th ed.). St. Louis: Mosby, pp. 438; 882.

76. A client says to the nurse, "I'm going to die and I wish my family would stop hoping for a cure! I get so angry when they carry on like this! After all, I'm the one who's dying." The nurse makes which therapeutic response to the client?
1 "You're feeling angry that your family continues to hope for you to be cured?"
2 "I think we should talk more about your anger at your family."
3 "Well, it sounds like you're being pretty pessimistic. After all, years ago people died of pneumonia."
4 "Have you shared your feelings with your family?"

Answer: 1
Rationale: Reflection is the therapeutic communication technique that redirects the client's feelings back in order to validate what the client is saying. Option 1 uses the therapeutic technique of reflection. In option 2, the nurse attempts to use focusing, but the attempt to discuss central issues seems premature. In option 3, the nurse makes a judgment and is nontherapeutic in the one-to-one relationship. In option 4, the nurse is attempting to assess the client's ability to openly discuss feelings with family members. Although this is an appropriate assessment for this client, the timing is somewhat premature and closes off facilitation of the client's feelings.

Test-Taking Strategy: Use therapeutic communication techniques to answer the question. Option 1 is the only option that uses a therapeutic technique. Also, note the word "angry" in the question and in the correct option. Review the technique of reflection if you had difficulty with this question.

Level of Cognitive Ability: Application
Client Needs: Psychosocial Integrity
Integrated Process: Caring
Content Area: Mental Health

Reference:
Stuart, G., & Laraia, M. (2005). *Principles and practice of psychiatric nursing* (8th ed.). St. Louis: Mosby, pp. 31-32; 34; 43.

---

77. A nurse is caring for an older adult client who says, "I don't want to talk with you. You're only a nurse. I'll wait for my doctor." The nurse makes which appropriate response to the client?
1 "I understand. I'll leave you now and call your physician."
2 "I'm assigned to work with you. Your doctor placed you in my hands."
3 "You would prefer to speak with your doctor?"
4 "I'm angry with the way you've dismissed me. I am your nurse, not your servant."

Answer: 3
Rationale: In the correct option, the nurse uses reflection to redirect the client's feelings back for validation and focuses on the client's desire to talk with the physician. Options 2 and 4 are nontherapeutic responses. Option 1 reinforces acceptance for the client to continue this behavior.

Test-Taking Strategy: Use therapeutic communication techniques. Option 3 is the only therapeutic response and uses the technique of reflection. Review therapeutic communication techniques if you had difficulty with this question.

Level of Cognitive Ability: Application
Client Needs: Psychosocial Integrity
Integrated Process: Communication and Documentation
Content Area: Fundamental Skills

Reference:
Potter, P., & Perry, A. (2005). *Fundamentals of nursing* (6th ed.). St. Louis: Mosby, p. 437.

78. A female client and her newborn infant have undergone testing for human immunodeficiency virus (HIV), and both clients were found to be positive. The news is devastating, and the mother is crying. Using crisis intervention techniques, the nurse determines that which intervention is appropriate at this time?

1 Calling an HIV counselor and making an appointment for them
2 Describing the progressive stages and treatments for HIV
3 Examining with the mother how she got HIV
4 Listening quietly while the mother talks and cries

Answer: 4

Rationale: This client has just received devastating news and needs to have someone present with her as she begins to cope with this issue. The nurse needs to sit and actively listen while the mother talks and cries. Calling an HIV counselor may be helpful, but it is not what the client needs at this time. The other options are not appropriate for this stage of coping with the news that both she and the baby are HIV positive.

Test-Taking Strategy: Use the process of elimination. Note the key words "at this time." Options 2 and 3 can be eliminated first because they are premature interventions. From the remaining options, remember to address the client's feelings and to support the client. This will direct you to the correct option. The nurse should sit and listen and provide support, because this is the most caring response. Review crisis intervention and the measures that provide support if you had difficulty with this question.

Level of Cognitive Ability: Analysis
Client Needs: Psychosocial Integrity
Integrated Process: Caring
Content Area: Maternity/Postpartum

References:
Potter, P., & Perry, A. (2005). *Fundamentals of nursing* (6th ed.). St. Louis: Mosby, p. 437.
Stuart, G., & Laraia, M. (2005). *Principles and practice of psychiatric nursing* (8th ed.). St. Louis: Mosby, pp. 228-229.

---

79. A community health nurse visits a recently widowed, retired military man who is estranged from his only child because he was discharged from the service for being "gay." When the nurse visits, the ordinarily immaculate house is in chaos and the client is disheveled and has an alcohol type of odor on his breath. The nurse makes which therapeutic statement to the client?

1 "You seem to be having a very troubling time."
2 "I can see this isn't a good time to visit."
3 "What are you doing? How much are you drinking and for how long?"
4 "Do you think your wife would want you to behave like this?"

Answer: 1

Rationale: The therapeutic statement is the one that facilitates the client to explore his situation and to express his feelings. Reflection, by verbalizing to the client that the nurse feels he is experiencing a troubled or difficult time, is empathic and will assist the client to begin to ventilate. As the client begins to ventilate, the nurse can assist the client to discuss the reasons behind alienation from his only child. Option 2 uses humor to avoid therapeutic intimacy and effective problem solving. Option 3 uses social communication. Option 4 uses admonishment and tries to shame the client, which is not therapeutic or professional. This social communication belittles the client, will cause anger, and may evoke "acting out" by the client.

Test-Taking Strategy: Use therapeutic communication techniques. Remember to focus on the client's behavior and feelings. This will direct you to option 1. Review these techniques if you had difficulty with this question.

Level of Cognitive Ability: Application
Client Needs: Psychosocial Integrity
Integrated Process: Communication and Documentation
Content Area: Mental Health

Reference:
Stuart, G., & Laraia, M. (2005). *Principles and practice of psychiatric nursing* (8th ed.). St. Louis: Mosby, pp. 30-34.

80. A client says to the nurse, "I don't do anything right. I'm such a loser." The nurse makes which therapeutic statement to the client?
1 "You do things right all the time."
2 "Everything will get better."
3 "You don't do anything right?"
4 "You are not a loser, you are sick."

Answer: 3
Rationale: Option 3 provides the client the opportunity to verbalize. With this statement, the nurse can learn more about what the client really means by the statement. Options 1, 2, and 4 are closed statements and do not encourage the client to explore further.

Test-Taking Strategy: Use the process of elimination and therapeutic communication techniques. Option 3 repeats the client's statement and encourages further communication. Review therapeutic communication techniques if you had difficulty with this question.

Level of Cognitive Ability: Application
Client Needs: Psychosocial Integrity
Integrated Process: Communication and Documentation
Content Area: Mental Health

Reference:
Stuart, G., & Laraia, M. (2005). *Principles and practice of psychiatric nursing* (8th ed.). St. Louis: Mosby, pp. 30-34.

81. A client who is experiencing suicidal thoughts greets the nurse with the following statement, "It just doesn't seem worth it anymore. Why not just end it all?" The nurse would further assess the client by making which of the following responses?
1 "I'm sure your family is worried about you."
2 "I know you have had a stressful night."
3 "Did you sleep at all last night?"
4 "Tell me what you mean by that?"

Answer: 4
Rationale: Option 4 allows the client the opportunity to tell the nurse more about what his or her current thoughts are. Option 1 is false reassurance and may block communication. While option 2 is offering empathy to the client, it does not further assess. Option 3 changes the subject and may block communication.

Test-Taking Strategy: Note the key words "further assess." Use the nursing process and therapeutic communication techniques to select the correct option. Options 1 and 2 can be eliminated first because they do not reflect assessment. Both options 3 and 4 relate to assessment, but option 4 is directly related to the issue of the question and is most therapeutic. Review therapeutic communication techniques if you had difficulty with this question.

Level of Cognitive Ability: Application
Client Needs: Psychosocial Integrity
Integrated Process: Communication and Documentation
Content Area: Mental Health

Reference:
Stuart, G., & Laraia, M. (2005). *Principles and practice of psychiatric nursing* (8th ed.). St. Louis: Mosby, pp. 30-34; 111.

82. A mother says to the nurse, "I am afraid that my child might have another febrile seizure." The nurse makes which therapeutic statement to the mother?
1 "Why worry about something that you cannot control?"
2 "Most children will never experience a second seizure."
3 "Tell me what frightens you the most about seizures."
4 "Tylenol can prevent another seizure from occurring."

Answer: 3
Rationale: Option 3 is the only response that is an open-ended statement and provides the mother with an opportunity to express feelings. Option 1 is incorrect because it blocks communication by giving a flippant response to an expressed fear. Options 2 and 4 are incorrect because the nurse is giving false assurance that a seizure will not reoccur or can be prevented in this child.

Test-Taking Strategy: Note the key word "therapeutic." Use the process of elimination, seeking the option that is an example of a therapeutic communication technique. Options 1, 2, and 4 violate the principles of therapeutic communication and actually block communication. Review therapeutic communication techniques if you had difficulty with this question.

Level of Cognitive Ability: Application
Client Needs: Psychosocial Integrity
Integrated Process: Communication and Documentation
Content Area: Child Health

Reference:
Wong, D., & Hockenberry, M. (2003). *Wong's nursing care of infants and children* (7th ed.). St. Louis: Mosby, p. 144.

---

83. A mother has just given birth to a baby who has a cleft lip and palate. When planning to talk to the mother, the nurse should recognize that this client needs to be allowed to work through which of these emotions before maternal bonding can occur?
  1 Anger
  2 Grief
  3 Guilt
  4 Depression

Answer: 2
Rationale: The mother must first be assisted to grieve for the anticipated child that she did not have. Once this is accomplished, the mother can begin to focus on bonding with the infant she gave birth to. Options 1, 3, and 4 are incorrect because they are only one component of the grief process.

Test-Taking Strategy: Use the process of elimination and knowledge of the grief process. Options 1, 3, and 4 are incorrect because they are only one component of the grief process. Option 2 is the umbrella (global) option. Review the grief process if you had difficulty with this question.

Level of Cognitive Ability: Analysis
Client Needs: Psychosocial Integrity
Integrated Process: Nursing Process/Planning
Content Area: Maternity/Postpartum

References:
James, S., Ashwill, J., & Droske, S. (2002). *Nursing care of children: Principles & practice* (2nd ed.). Philadelphia: Saunders, p. 335.
Wong, D., & Hockenberry, M. (2003). *Wong's nursing care of infants and children* (7th ed.). St. Louis: Mosby, p. 462.

---

84. An infant is admitted to the hospital who has been diagnosed with acute chalasia. During the nursing history, the mother tells the nurse, "I am concerned that I am somehow causing my infant to vomit after feeding her." Considering this statement, which nursing diagnosis is most appropriate?
  1 Anxiety related to hospitalization of the infant for chalasia
  2 Noncompliance related to denial that chalasia is a physiological defect
  3 Deficient knowledge related to the lack of exposure to feeding an infant with chalasia
  4 Impaired parenting related to an unrealistic expectation of self

Answer: 4
Rationale: The infant is vomiting because of a physiological problem that is not caused by the parent. The misconception that the mother is responsible for the problem is an unrealistic expectation of self and may result in a decreased perception of her ability to adequately parent the child. The nurse should assist the parent to understand that she is not responsible for the child's condition. The mother's statement does not reflect symptoms of anxiety regarding the child's hospitalization. The mother states a concern about her behavior. There is no data in the question to support that the mother is experiencing denial that chalasia is a physiological defect. Again, there is insufficient data to support that the mother has not been instructed on feeding techniques for a child with chalasia.

Test-Taking Strategy: Use the process of elimination. Note that the mother is blaming herself for the child's health problem. As a result, the mother is at risk for Impaired Parenting. Review the defining characteristics for Impaired Parenting if you had difficulty with this question.

Level of Cognitive Ability: Analysis
Client Needs: Psychosocial Integrity
Integrated Process: Nursing Process/Analysis
Content Area: Child Health

Reference:
Wong, D., & Hockenberry, M. (2003). *Wong's nursing care of infants and children* (7th ed.). St. Louis: Mosby, pp. 144-146.

---

85. According to standard coronary care unit (CCU) orders, the client with an uncomplicated myocardial infarction (MI) may begin progressive activity after 3 days. The client who experienced an infarction 4 days ago refuses to dangle at the bedside, saying, "If my doctor tells me to do it, I will. Otherwise I won't." The nurse determines that the client is likely displaying:
1 Anger
2 Denial
3 Dependency
4 Depression

Answer: 3
Rationale: Clients may experience numerous emotional and behavioral responses following an MI. Dependency is one response that may be manifested by the client's refusal to perform any tasks or activities unless specifically approved by the physician. There is no data in the question to support denial or depression. Although the client's statement may express anger to some degree, it most specifically addresses dependency.

Test-Taking Strategy: Focus on the data in the question to determine the correct option. Begin by eliminating options 2 and 4 first because the client is not exhibiting signs of denial or depression. From the remaining options, focus on the client's statement to direct you to option 3. Review the characteristics related to dependency if you had difficulty with this question.

Level of Cognitive Ability: Analysis
Client Needs: Psychosocial Integrity
Integrated Process: Nursing Process/Analysis
Content Area: Adult Health/Cardiovascular

Reference:
Lewis, S., Heitkemper, M., & Dirksen, S. (2004). *Medical-surgical nursing: Assessment and management of clinical problems* (6th ed.). St. Louis: Mosby, p. 829.

86. A nurse is assessing a 45-year-old client admitted to the hospital for urinary calculi. The client has received 4 mg of morphine sulfate approximately 2 hours previously. The client states to the nurse, "I'm scared to death that it'll come back. That was the worst pain I ever had. Like a knife going from my right side to my groin." Which nursing diagnoses would be appropriate for the nurse to make regarding this statement?

1 Pain, acute, related to the presence of the calculus in right ureter
2 Deficient knowledge, related to the lack of information about the disease process
3 Anxiety, related to anticipation of recurrent severe pain
4 Urinary retention, related to obstruction of the urinary tract by calculi

Answer: 3

Rationale: The client has stated, "I'm scared to death that it'll come back." The anticipation of the recurring pain produces anxiety and threatens the client's psychological integrity. There is no evidence that the client has a calculus in the right ureter. There is also no evidence that either urinary retention or deficient knowledge exists.

Test-Taking Strategy: Use the data presented in the question to assist in answering the question. Note the key words, "I'm scared to death that it'll come back," and the relation of these key words to option 3, anxiety related to anticipation of recurrent severe pain. Review the defining characteristics of anxiety if you had difficulty with this question.

Level of Cognitive Ability: Analysis
Client Needs: Psychosocial Integrity
Integrated Process: Nursing Process/Analysis
Content Area: Mental Health

References:
Stuart, G., & Laraia, M. (2005). *Principles and practice of psychiatric nursing* (8th ed.). St. Louis: Mosby, pp. 267; 260.
Varcarolis, E.M. (2002). *Foundations of psychiatric mental health nursing* (4th ed.). Philadelphia: Saunders, p. 808.

87. A nurse is observing parents at the bedside of their small for gestational age (SGA) female infant, who is 27 weeks' gestation. The infant's mother states, "She is so tiny and fragile. I'll never be able to hold her with all those tubes." The nurse interprets the mother's statement to indicate which of the following nursing diagnoses?

1 Impaired Adjustment
2 Risk for Caregiver Role Strain
3 Compromised Family Coping
4 Risk for Impaired Parenting

Answer: 4

Rationale: One of the nursing diagnoses for the parents of a high-risk neonate, such as a preterm SGA infant, is risk for impaired parenting. Parent-infant bonding is affected if the infant does not exhibit normal newborn characteristics. Option 1 involves nonacceptance of a health status change or an inability to problem solve or set a goal. Option 2 addresses the strain of a caregiver, which during the initial hospitalization is too early to apply. Option 3 involves identification of compromised coping. At this time, there is inadequate data for these diagnoses, although they may become relevant at a later time.

Test-Taking Strategy: Use the data presented in the question to assist in answering. Eliminate options 1 and 3 first because these are actual nursing diagnoses. From the remaining options, note the key words, "I'll never be able to hold her." This should assist in directing you to the key words, "impaired parenting," in the correct option. Review the defining characteristics of impaired parenting if you had difficulty with this question.

Level of Cognitive Ability: Analysis
Client Needs: Psychosocial Integrity
Integrated Process: Nursing Process/Analysis
Content Area: Maternity/Postpartum

Reference:
Wong, D., & Hockenberry, M. (2003). *Wong's nursing care of infants and children* (7th ed.). St. Louis: Mosby, pp. 144-146.

88. After vaginal delivery of a large for gestational age (LGA) male infant, the nurse wraps the infant in a warm blanket and hands him to his mother. The mother verbalizes concern over the infant's facial bruising. To enhance attachment, the nurse makes which therapeutic statement?
1 "Since the bruising is painful, it is advisable that you not touch the baby's face."
2 "The bruising is caused by polycythemia, which usually leads to jaundice."
3 "It is a normal finding in large babies and nothing to be concerned about."
4 "The bruising is temporary, and it is important to interact with your infant."

Answer: 4
Rationale: The mother of an LGA infant with facial bruising may be reluctant to interact with the infant because of concern about causing additional pain to the infant. The bruising is temporary. Option 1 advises the mother not to touch the baby's face because the bruising is painful. Touch is an important component of the attachment process. Touching the infant gently with fingertips should be encouraged. The LGA infant may have polycythemia, which can contribute to bruising, but the bruising is not actually caused by the polycythemia. Option 3 avoids the mother's verbalized concerns.

Test-Taking Strategy: Use the process of elimination and note the issue: to enhance attachment. Eliminate options 2 and 3 first because they do not specifically address the issue of attachment. From the remaining options, note the relationship of the word "attachment" in the question and the word "interact" in the correct option. Review the interventions that promote mother-infant bonding if you had difficulty with this question.

Level of Cognitive Ability: Application
Client Needs: Psychosocial Integrity
Integrated Process: Nursing Process/Implementation
Content Area: Maternity/Postpartum

Reference:
Lowdermilk, D., & Perry, A. (2004). *Maternity & women's health care* (8th ed.). St. Louis: Mosby, p. 648.

---

89. A client with myasthenia gravis is ready to return home. The client confides that she is concerned that her husband will no longer find her physically attractive. The nurse would include in the plan of care to:
1 Encourage the client to start a support group
2 Insist that the client reach out and face this fear
3 Tell the client not to dwell on the negative
4 Encourage the client to share her feelings with her husband

Answer: 4
Rationale: Sharing feelings with her husband directly addresses the issue of the question. Encouraging the client to start a support group will not address the client's immediate and individual concerns. Options 2 and 3 are blocks to communication and avoid the client's concern.

Test-Taking Strategy: Focus on the issue of the question and use therapeutic communication techniques. Option 4 is the only option that addresses the client's immediate concern. Remember to address the client's feelings and concerns first. Review therapeutic communication techniques if you had difficulty with this question.

Level of Cognitive Ability: Application
Client Needs: Psychosocial Integrity
Integrated Process: Caring
Content Area: Adult Health/Neurological

References:
Black, J., & Hawks, J. (2005). *Medical-surgical nursing: Clinical management for positive outcomes* (7th ed.). Philadelphia: Saunders, p. 2183.
Potter, P., & Perry, A. (2005). *Fundamentals of nursing* (6th ed.). St. Louis: Mosby, p. 437.

90. A 9-year-old child is hospitalized for 2 months following a car accident. The best way to promote psychosocial development of this child is to plan for:
1 Tutoring to keep the child up with school work
2 A phone to call family and friends
3 Computer games, TV, and videos at the bedside
4 A portable radio and tape player with headphones

Answer: 1

Rationale: The developmental task of the school-aged child is industry versus inferiority. The child achieves success by mastering skills and knowledge. Maintaining school work provides for accomplishment and prevents feelings of inferiority from lagging behind the class. The other options provide diversion and are of lesser importance for a child of this age.

Test-Taking Strategy: Note the key words "psychosocial development" in the stem of the question. Note the age of the child and determine the developmental task for this child. Options 2, 3, and 4 address social and diversional issues, whereas option 1 specifically addresses psychosocial development. Review growth and development related to the school-aged child if you had difficulty with this question.

Level of Cognitive Ability: Application
Client Needs: Psychosocial Integrity
Integrated Process: Nursing Process/Planning
Content Area: Child Health

Reference:
Wong, D., & Hockenberry, M. (2003). *Wong's nursing care of infants and children* (7th ed.). St. Louis: Mosby, p. 1068.

---

91. A client who is in halo traction says to the visiting nurse, "I can't get used to this contraption. I can't see properly on the side and I keep misjudging where everything is." The nurse makes which therapeutic response to the client?
1 "Halo traction involves many difficult adjustments. Practice scanning with your eyes after standing up and before you move around."
2 "No one ever gets used to that thing! It's horrible. Many of our sports people who are in it complain vigorously."
3 "Why do you feel like this when you could have died from a broken neck? This is the way it is for several months. You need to accept it more, don't you think?"
4 "If I were you, I would have had the surgery rather than suffer like this."

Answer: 1

Rationale: In option 1, the nurse employs empathy and reflection. The nurse then offers a strategy for problem solving for the client's problem, which helps to increase peripheral vision for the client in halo traction. In option 2, the nurse provides a social response that contains emotionally charged language that could increase the client's anxiety. In option 3, the nurse uses excessive questioning and gives advice, which is nontherapeutic. In option 4, the nurse undermines the client's faith in the medical treatment being employed by giving advice that is insensitive and unprofessional.

Test-Taking Strategy: Use the process of elimination, seeking the option that represents a therapeutic communication technique. Focus on the client's statement and note that option 1 is the only statement that addresses the client's concern. Review therapeutic communication techniques if you had difficulty with this question.

Level of Cognitive Ability: Application
Client Needs: Psychosocial Integrity
Integrated Process: Caring
Content Area: Adult Health/Neurological

References:
Phipps, W., Monahan, F., Sands, J., Marek, J., & Neighbors, M. (2003). *Medical-surgical nursing: Health and illness perspectives* (7th ed.). St. Louis: Mosby, pp. 1413-1414.
Potter, P., & Perry, A. (2005). *Fundamentals of nursing* (6th ed.). St. Louis: Mosby, p. 437.

92. An older client has been admitted to the hospital with a hip fracture. The nurse prepares a plan of care for the client and identifies desired outcomes related to the impaired physical mobility. Which statement by the client most appropriately supports a positive adjustment to the impairment in mobility?
  1 "I wish you nurses would leave me alone! You are all telling me what to do!"
  2 "What took you so long? I called for you 30 minutes ago."
  3 "Hurry up and go away. I want to be alone."
  4 "I find it difficult to concentrate since the doctor talked with me about the surgery tomorrow."

Answer: 4
Rationale: Option 1 demonstrates acting out by the client. Option 2 is a demanding response. Option 3 demonstrates withdrawal behavior. Demanding, acting out, and withdrawn clients have not coped or adjusted with the injury or disease. Option 4 is reflective of an individual with moderate anxiety caused by difficulty to concentrate. It most appropriately supports a positive adjustment.

Test-Taking Strategy: Focus on the issue "positive adjustment" and use the process of elimination. You should easily be able to eliminate options 1, 2, and 3. Remember that age and impaired mobility, combined with medications, often contribute to anxiety and confusion. Review the psychosocial issues related to an older client with a hip fracture if you had difficulty with this question.

Level of Cognitive Ability: Analysis
Client Needs: Psychosocial Integrity
Integrated Process: Nursing Process/Evaluation
Content Area: Adult Health/Musculoskeletal

Reference:
Black, J., & Hawks, J. (2005). *Medical-surgical nursing: Clinical management for positive outcomes* (7th ed.). Philadelphia: Saunders, pp. 644-645.

93. A client who has a spinal cord injury and is paralyzed from the neck down frequently makes lewd sexual suggestions and uses profanity. The nurse interprets that the client is inappropriately using the defense mechanism of displacement and determines that the appropriate nursing diagnosis for this client is:
  1 Ineffective Coping
  2 Risk for Disuse Syndrome
  3 Impaired Environmental Interpretation Syndrome
  4 Disturbed Body Image

Answer: 1
Rationale: The definition of Ineffective Coping is the "state in which an individual demonstrates impaired adaptive behaviors and problem-solving abilities in meeting life's demands and roles." By displacing feelings onto the environment instead of in a constructive fashion, this nursing diagnosis clearly applies in this situation. Options 2 and 3 have no relation to this situation. Option 4 may be appropriate, but it has nothing to do with the displacement that the client is currently using.

Test-Taking Strategy: Focus on the data in the question to identify the correct option. Note that the question addresses the defense mechanism of displacement. Focusing on this issue and the definition of displacement will assist in directing you to the correct option. Review this defense mechanism if you had difficulty with this question.

Level of Cognitive Ability: Analysis
Client Needs: Psychosocial Integrity
Integrated Process: Nursing Process/Analysis
Content Area: Mental Health

References:
Fortinash, K., & Holoday-Worret, P. (2004). *Psychiatric mental health nursing* (3rd ed.). St. Louis: Mosby, p. 9.
Stuart, G., & Laraia, M. (2005). *Principles and practice of psychiatric nursing* (8th ed.). St. Louis: Mosby, pp. 296; 314-315.

94. A nurse in the newborn nursery is caring for a premature infant. The best way to assist the parents to develop attachment behaviors is to:

1 Encourage the parents to touch and speak to their infant
2 Place family pictures in the infant's view
3 Report only positive qualities and progress to the parents
4 Provide information on infant development and stimulation

Answer: 1

Rationale: Parents' involvement through touch and voice establishes and initiates the bonding process in the parent-infant relationship. Their active participation builds their confidence and supports the parenting role. Providing information and emphasizing only positives are not incorrect, but do not relate to the attachment process. Family pictures are ineffective for an infant.

Test-Taking Strategy: Use the process of elimination and focus on the issue: attachment behaviors. The only option that addresses attachment behaviors is option 1. Review measures that promote parent-infant bonding if you had difficulty with this question.

Level of Cognitive Ability: Application
Client Needs: Psychosocial Integrity
Integrated Process: Nursing Process/Implementation
Content Area: Maternity/Postpartum

Reference:
Lowdermilk, D., & Perry, A. (2004). *Maternity & women's health care* (8th ed.). St. Louis: Mosby, p. 655.

95. A 16-year-old is admitted to the hospital with hyperglycemia from failure to follow the diet, insulin, and glucose monitoring regimen. The client states, "I'm fed up with having my life ruled by doctors' orders and machines!" A priority nursing diagnosis is:

1 Imbalanced nutrition, greater than body requirements related to high blood glucose
2 Interrupted family processes, related to chronic illness
3 Disturbed thought processes, related to a personal crisis
4 Ineffective health maintenance of the therapeutic regimen, related to feelings of loss of control

Answer: 4

Rationale: Adolescents strive for identity and independence, and the situation describes a common fear of loss of control. The correct nursing diagnosis relates to the issues of the question, which are not following the prescribed regimen and the feelings of powerlessness. There is no indication of interrupted family or disturbed thought processes in the question. Imbalanced nutrition is inaccurate and limited.

Test-Taking Strategy: Focus on the information in the question. Eliminate options 1 and 2 because there is no data to support these nursing diagnoses. Eliminate option 3 because although the client may be experiencing a personal crisis, there is no evidence of disturbed thought process. Review the defining characteristics of ineffective health maintenance if you had difficulty with this question.

Level of Cognitive Ability: Analysis
Client Needs: Psychosocial Integrity
Integrated Process: Nursing Process/Analysis
Content Area: Child Health

Reference:
Wong, D., & Hockenberry, M. (2003). *Wong's nursing care of infants and children* (7th ed.). St. Louis: Mosby, pp. 1750-1751.

96. A client angrily tells a nurse that the doctor purposefully provided wrong information. Which of the following responses would hinder therapeutic communication?
1   "I'm certain the doctor would not lie to you."
2   "Can you describe the information that you are referring to?"
3   "I'm not sure what information you are referring to."
4   "Do you think it would be helpful to talk to your doctor about this?"

Answer: 1

Rationale: Option 1 hinders communication by disagreeing with the client. This technique could make the client defensive and block further communication. Options 2 and 3 attempt to clarify what the client is referring to. Option 4 attempts to explore if the client is comfortable talking to the doctor about this issue and encourages direct confrontation.

Test-Taking Strategy: Use the process of elimination and therapeutic communication techniques, noting the key word "hinder." This key word indicates a false-response question and that you need to select the option that identifies an incorrect nursing statement. Disagreeing or challenging a client's response will hinder or block therapeutic communication. Review therapeutic communication techniques if you had difficulty with this question.

Level of Cognitive Ability: Application
Client Needs: Psychosocial Integrity
Integrated Process: Communication and Documentation
Content Area: Mental Health

References:
Fortinash, K., & Holoday-Worret, P. (2004). *Psychiatric mental health nursing* (3rd ed.). St. Louis: Mosby, pp. 122-123.
Stuart, G., & Laraia, M. (2005). *Principles and practice of psychiatric nursing* (8th ed.). St. Louis: Mosby, p. 34.

---

97. A client with a diagnosis of major depression says to the nurse, "I should have died. I've always been a failure." The nurse makes which therapeutic response to the nurse?
1   "I see a lot of positive things in you."
2   "Feeling like a failure is part of your illness."
3   "You've been feeling like a failure for some time now?"
4   "You still have a great deal to live for."

Answer: 3

Rationale: Responding to the feelings expressed by a client is an effective therapeutic communication technique. The correct option is an example of the use of restating. Options 1, 2, and 4 block communication because they minimize the client's experience and do not facilitate exploration of the client's expressed feelings.

Test-Taking Strategy: Use the techniques that facilitate therapeutic communication to answer this question. Remember to address the client's feelings and concerns. Option 3 is the only option that is stated in the form of a question and is open-ended, and thus will encourage the verbalization of feelings. Review therapeutic communication techniques if you had difficulty with this question.

Level of Cognitive Ability: Application
Client Needs: Psychosocial Integrity
Integrated Process: Communication and Documentation
Content Area: Mental Health

Reference:
Stuart, G., & Laraia, M. (2005). *Principles and practice of psychiatric nursing* (8th ed.). St. Louis: Mosby, pp. 30-34.

98. Two months after a right mastectomy for breast cancer, the client comes to the office for a follow-up appointment. After being diagnosed with cancer in the right breast, the client was told that the risk for cancer in the left breast existed. When asked about Breast Self-Examination (BSE) practices since the surgery, the client replies, "I don't need to do that anymore." The nurse interprets that this response may indicate:

1 Change in body image
2 Change in role pattern
3 Denial
4 Grief and mourning

Answer: 3

Rationale: The coping strategy of denying or minimizing a health problem is manifested as anxiety and can produce health situations that may be life-threatening. Denial can lead to avoidance of self-care measures, such as taking medications or performing BSE. Options 1, 2, and 4 are unrelated to the client's statement.

Test-Taking Strategy: Focus on the data in the question. Note the client's statement "I don't need to do that anymore." Eliminate options 1, 2, and 4 because they are not directly related to the client's statement. Review the indicators of denial if you had difficulty with this question.

Level of Cognitive Ability: Analysis
Client Needs: Psychosocial Integrity
Integrated Process: Nursing Process/Analysis
Content Area: Adult Health/Oncology

Reference:
Black, J., & Hawks, J. (2005). *Medical-surgical nursing: Clinical management for positive outcomes* (7th ed.). Philadelphia: Saunders, pp. 525-526.

---

99. In planning for care of the client dying of cancer, one of the goals was that the client would verbalize acceptance of impending death. Which client statement indicates to the nurse that this goal has been reached?

1 "I'll be ready to die when my children finish school."
2 "I just want to live until my 100th birthday."
3 "I want to go to my daughter's wedding. Then I'll be ready to die."
4 "I'd like to have my family here when I die."

Answer: 4

Rationale: Acceptance is often characterized by plans for death. Often the client wants loved ones nearby. Options 1, 2, and 3 all reflect the bargaining stage of coping wherein the client tries to negotiate with his or her God or fate.

Test-Taking Strategy: Use the process of elimination. Note the similarity in options 1, 2, and 3. These options all demonstrate negotiating for something else to happen before death occurs. Option 4 is different and the option that reflects acceptance. Review the stages of death and dying if you had difficulty with this question.

Level of Cognitive Ability: Analysis
Client Needs: Psychosocial Integrity
Integrated Process: Nursing Process/Evaluation
Content Area: Adult Health/Oncology

Reference:
Black, J., & Hawks, J. (2005). *Medical-surgical nursing: Clinical management for positive outcomes* (7th ed.). Philadelphia: Saunders, p. 500.

100. A nurse is caring for a client with cancer who has a nursing diagnosis of Disturbed Body Image related to alopecia. The nurse plans to teach the client about which of the following related to this nursing diagnosis?

1 Proper dental hygiene with the use of a foam toothbrush
2 The importance of rinsing the mouth after eating
3 The use of wigs, which are often covered by insurance
4 The use of cosmetics to hide drug-induced rashes

Answer: 3

Rationale: The temporary or permanent thinning or loss of hair, known as alopecia, is common in clients with cancer receiving chemotherapy. This often causes a body image disturbance that can be easily addressed by the use of wigs, hats, or scarves. Options 1, 2, and 4 are all unrelated to alopecia.

Test-Taking Strategy: Focus on the definition of alopecia. Recalling that alopecia refers to hair loss will direct you to option 3. Review interventions to treat alopecia if you had difficulty with this question.

Level of Cognitive ability: Application
Client Needs: Psychosocial Integrity
Integrated Process: Nursing Process/Implementation
Content Area: Adult Health/Oncology

References:
Black, J., & Hawks, J. (2005). *Medical-surgical nursing: Clinical management for positive outcomes* (7th ed.). Philadelphia: Saunders, p. 386.
Lewis, S., Heitkemper, M., & Dirksen, S. (2004). *Medical-surgical nursing: Assessment and management of clinical problems* (6th ed.). St. Louis: Mosby, pp. 480; 484.

---

101. A client with aldosteronism has developed renal failure and says to the nurse, "This means that I will die very soon." The nurse makes which appropriate response to the client?

1 "What are you thinking about?"
2 "You will do just fine."
3 "You sound discouraged today."
4 "I read that death is a beautiful experience."

Answer: 3

Rationale: Option 3 uses the therapeutic communication technique of reflection, and clarifies and encourages further expression of the client's feelings. Option 1 requests an explanation and does not encourage expression of feelings. Options 2 and 4 deny the client's concerns and provide false reassurance.

Test-Taking Strategy: Use the therapeutic communication techniques. Note that option 3 facilitates the client's expression of feelings. Remember to focus on the client's feelings. Review therapeutic communication techniques if you had difficulty with this question.

Level of Cognitive Ability: Application
Client Needs: Psychosocial Integrity
Integrated Process: Communication and Documentation
Content Area: Adult Health/Endocrine

Reference:
Potter, P., & Perry, A. (2005). *Fundamentals of nursing* (6th ed.). St. Louis: Mosby, p. 437.

102. A client with diabetes mellitus has expressed frustration in learning the diabetic regimen and insulin administration. The home care nurse would initially:
1 Identify the cause of the frustration
2 Continue with diabetic teaching, knowing that the client will overcome any frustrations
3 Call the physician to discuss termination from home care services
4 Offer to administer the insulin on a daily basis until the client is ready to learn

Answer: 1

Rationale: The home care nurse must determine what is causing the client's frustration. Continuing to teach may only further block the learning process. Terminating the client from home care services achieves nothing and is considered abandonment unless other follow-up care is arranged. Administering the insulin only provides a short-term solution.

Test-Taking Strategy: Use the steps of the nursing process. Assessment is the first step. Of the options presented, options 2, 3, and 4 represent implementation phases of the nursing process. The only assessment option is option 1. Review teaching/learning principles if you had difficulty with this question.

Level of Cognitive Ability: Application
Client Needs: Psychosocial Integrity
Integrated Process: Teaching/Learning
Content Area: Adult Health/Endocrine

Reference:
Potter, P., & Perry, A. (2005). *Fundamentals of nursing* (6th ed.). St. Louis: Mosby, pp. 451-454.

103. A client with cancer is placed on permanent total parenteral nutrition (TPN) as a means of providing nutrition. The nurse includes psychosocial support when planning care for this client because:
1 Death is imminent
2 TPN requires disfiguring surgery for permanent port implantation
3 The client will need to adjust to the idea of living without eating by the usual route
4 Nausea and vomiting occur regularly with this type of treatment and will prevent the client from participating in social activity

Answer: 3

Rationale: Permanent TPN is indicated for clients who can no longer absorb nutrients via the enteral route. These clients will no longer take nutrition orally. Options 1, 2, and 4 are inaccurate. There is no indication in the question that death is imminent. Permanent port implantation is not disfiguring. TPN does not cause nausea and vomiting.

Test-Taking Strategy: Note the key words "permanent" and "as a means of providing nutrition" in the question. Note the relationship between the key words and option 3. Option 3 states "living without eating." Also, knowledge regarding TPN therapy will assist in eliminating options 1, 2, and 4. Review care of the client receiving permanent TPN if you had difficulty with this question.

Level of Cognitive Ability: Application
Client Needs: Psychosocial Integrity
Integrated Process: Nursing Process/Planning
Content Area: Adult Health/Oncology

Reference:
Black, J., & Hawks, J. (2005). *Medical-surgical nursing: Clinical management for positive outcomes* (7th ed.). Philadelphia: Saunders, p. 709.

104. A client who is to be discharged to home with a temporary colostomy says to the nurse, "I know I've changed this thing once, but I just don't know how I'll do it by myself when I'm home alone. Can't I stay here until the doctor puts it back?" The nurse makes which therapeutic response to the client?

1 "So you're saying that while you've practiced changing your colostomy bag once, you don't feel comfortable on your own yet?"

2 "Well, your insurance will not pay for a longer stay just to practice changing your colostomy, so you'll have to fight it out with them."

3 "Going home to care for yourself still feels pretty overwhelming? I will schedule you for home visits until you're feeling more comfortable."

4 "This is only temporary, but you need to hire a nurse companion until your surgery."

Answer: 3

Rationale: The client is expressing feelings of fear and helplessness. Option 3 assists in meeting this need. Option 1 is restating, but this response could cause the client to feel more helpless because the client's fears are reflected back to the client. Option 2 provides what is probably accurate information, but the words "just to practice" can be interpreted by the client as belittling. Option 4 provides information that the client already knows and then problem solves by using a client-centered action, which would probably overwhelm the client.

Test-Taking Strategy: Use therapeutic communication techniques and focus on the issue of the question: fear and helplessness. This will eliminate options 2 and 4. From the remaining options, remember the issue of the question and address the client's feelings and concerns. Option 1 is restating, but this intervention could cause the client to feel more helpless. Option 3 addresses the client's fear and dependency (helplessness) needs. Review therapeutic communication techniques if you had difficulty with this question.

Level of Cognitive Ability: Application
Client Needs: Psychosocial Integrity
Integrated Process: Communication and Documentation
Content Area: Adult Health/Gastrointestinal

Reference:
Lewis, S., Heitkemper, M., & Dirksen, S. (2004). *Medical-surgical nursing: Assessment and management of clinical problems* (6th ed.). St. Louis: Mosby, p. 362.

---

105. The parents of a newborn infant with congenital hypothyroidism and Down syndrome tell the nurse how sad they are that their child was born with these problems. They had many plans for a normal child, and now these will need to be adjusted. Based on these statements, the nurse plans to address which nursing diagnosis?

1 Anticipatory grieving
2 Dysfunctional grieving
3 Impaired adjustment
4 Disabled family coping

Answer: 1

Rationale: Anticipatory grieving is the intellectual and emotional responses and behaviors by which individuals and families work through the process of modifying self-concept based on the perception of potential loss. Defining characteristics include expressions of sorrow and distress at potential loss. Dysfunctional grieving or impaired adjustment are abnormal responses to changes in health status. The nursing diagnosis of disabled family coping is used when a usually supportive person is providing insufficient, ineffective, or compromised support, comfort, assistance, or encouragement.

Test-Taking Strategy: Focus on the data in the question. Noting the key words "how sad they are" should lead you to one of the options related to grieving. Recalling the defining characteristics of anticipatory grieving will direct you to this option. Review these two forms of grieving if you had difficulty with this question.

Level of Cognitive Ability: Analysis
Client Needs: Psychosocial Integrity
Integrated Process: Nursing Process/Analysis
Content Area: Maternity/Postpartum

Reference:
Wong, D., & Hockenberry, M. (2003). *Wong's nursing care of infants and children* (7th ed.). St. Louis: Mosby, pp. 923; 925.

---

106. A nurse is caring for a client who is diagnosed as having schizophrenia. The client is unable to speak, although there is no known pathological dysfunction of the organs of communication. The nurse documents that the client is experiencing:
  1 Pressured speech
  2 Verbigeration
  3 Poverty of speech
  4 Mutism

Answer: 4
Rationale: Mutism is the absence of verbal speech. The client does not communicate verbally, despite an intact physical structural ability to speak. Pressured speech refers to rapidity of speech reflecting the client's racing thoughts. Verbigeration is the purposeless repetition of words or phrases. Poverty of speech means diminished amounts of speech or monotonic replies.

Test-Taking Strategy: Use the process of elimination. Focus on the issue "unable to speak." This should assist in eliminating options 1 and 2. From the remaining options, recalling that poverty of speech indicates a diminished amount of speech will assist in eliminating option 3. Review altered thought and speech patterns if you had difficulty with this question.

Level of Cognitive Ability: Analysis
Client Needs: Psychosocial Integrity
Integrated Process: Communication and Documentation
Content Area: Mental Health

Reference:
Keltner, N., Schwecke, L., & Bostrom, C. (2003). *Psychiatric nursing* (4th ed.). St. Louis: Mosby, pp. 311; 331.

---

107. A client tells the nurse, "I am a spy for the FBI. I am an eye, an eye in the sky." The nurse recognizes that this is an example of:
  1 Loosened associations
  2 Echolalia
  3 Clang associations
  4 Word salad

Answer: 3
Rationale: Repetition of words or phrases that are similar in sound and in no other way (rhyming) is one altered thought and language pattern seen in schizophrenia. Clang associations often take the form of rhyming. Loosened associations occur when the individual speaks with frequent changes of subject, and the content is only obliquely related. Echolalia is the involuntary parrot-like repetition of words spoken by others. Word salad is the use of words with no apparent meaning attached to them or to their relationship to one another.

Test-Taking Strategy: Use the process of elimination, focusing on the client's statement. Recalling that clang associations often take the form of rhyming will direct you to option 3. Review altered thought and language patterns if you had difficulty with this question.

Level of Cognitive Ability: Analysis
Client Needs: Psychosocial Integrity
Integrated Process: Nursing Process/Analysis
Content Area: Mental Health

Reference:
Stuart, G., & Laraia, M. (2005). *Principles and practice of psychiatric nursing* (8th ed.). St. Louis: Mosby, p. 391.

108. A nurse is planning the hospital discharge of a young, newly diagnosed client with type 1 diabetes mellitus. The client tells the nurse that she is concerned about self-administering insulin while in school with other students around. Which statement by the nurse best supports the client's need at this time?

1 "You could contact the school nurse, who could provide a private area for you to administer your insulin."

2 "You could leave school early and take your insulin at home."

3 "You shouldn't be embarrassed by your diabetes. Lots of people have this disease."

4 "Oh, don't worry about that! You'll do fine!"

Answer: 1

Rationale: In planning this client's role transition, the nurse functions in the role of a problem solver in assisting the client to adapt to his or her illness. In option 1, the nurse offers information that addresses the client's need and promotes or assists the client to reach a decision that optimizes a sense of well-being. Option 2 requires a change in lifestyle. Options 3 and 4 are inappropriate statements and are similar in that they are both blocks to communication.

Test-Taking Strategy: Use therapeutic communication techniques. Focus on the issue: a concern of self-administering insulin while in school. Eliminate options 3 and 4 first because they are nontherapeutic. From the remaining options, select option 1 because it promotes the client's ability to continue the present lifestyle, whereas option 2 changes the lifestyle. Review measures that will assist the client in making a role transition if you had difficulty with this question.

Level of Cognitive Ability: Application
Client Needs: Psychosocial Integrity
Integrated Process: Communication and Documentation
Content Area: Adult Health/Endocrine

References:
Black, J., & Hawks, J. (2005). *Medical-surgical nursing: Clinical management for positive outcomes* (7th ed.). Philadelphia: Saunders, p. 1265.
Potter, P., & Perry, A. (2005). *Fundamentals of nursing* (6th ed.). St. Louis: Mosby, pp. 102-103.

109. A nurse is preparing a client for a parathyroidectomy. The client states, "I guess I'll have to learn to love wearing a scarf after this surgery!" Which nursing diagnosis would be appropriate to identify in the plan of care that addresses this client's need?

1 Impaired Comfort, related to surgical interruption of body tissue

2 Disturbed Body Image, related to perceived negative effect of the surgical incision

3 Risk for Impaired Physical Mobility, related to limited movement secondary to neck surgery

4 Ineffective Denial, related to poor coping mechanisms

Answer: 2

Rationale: The client's statement reflects a psychosocial concern regarding his or her appearance after surgery. Therefore, Disturbed Body Image is the correct option. Options 1 and 3 identify physiological nursing diagnoses, and option 4 is inappropriate because the client is addressing a concern, rather than avoiding one.

Test-Taking Strategy: Note that the client is expressing a concern. Keeping that in mind, eliminate option 4 because denial is a way of avoiding concerns. From the remaining options, focus on the client's statement to direct you to option 2. Review the psychosocial concerns following parathyroidectomy if you had difficulty with this question.

Level of Cognitive Ability: Analysis
Client Needs: Psychosocial Integrity
Integrated Process: Nursing Process/Analysis
Content Area: Fundamental Skills

Reference:
Phipps, W., Monahan, F., Sands, J., Marek, J., & Neighbors, M. (2003). *Medical-surgical nursing: Health and illness perspectives* (7th ed.). St. Louis: Mosby, p. 912.

110. A husband of a client with Graves' disease expresses concern regarding his wife's health because during the past 3 months she has been experiencing bursts of temper, nervousness, and inability to concentrate, even on trivial tasks. Based on this information, which nursing diagnosis would be appropriate for the client?

1 Ineffective coping
2 Disturbed sensory perception
3 Social isolation
4 Grieving

hyperthyrodism

Answer: 1

Rationale: A client with Graves' disease may become irritable, nervous, or depressed. The signs and symptoms in the question support the nursing diagnosis of ineffective coping. The information in the question does not support options 2, 3, and 4.

Test-Taking Strategy: Use the process of elimination. Focusing on the data in the question will direct you to option 1. Review the defining characteristics related to ineffective coping if you had difficulty with this question.

Level of Cognitive Ability: Analysis
Client Needs: Psychosocial Integrity
Integrated Process: Nursing Process/Analysis
Content Area: Adult Health/Endocrine

Reference:
Black, J., & Hawks, J. (2005). *Medical-surgical nursing: Clinical management for positive outcomes* (7th ed.). Philadelphia: Saunders, p. 1203.

---

111. A client who was admitted to the hospital for treatment of thyroid storm (hyperthyroidism) is preparing for discharge. The client is anxious about his illness and at times emotionally labile. Which intervention would the nurse include in the discharge plan of care for this client?

1 Avoid teaching the client anything about the disease until he is emotionally stable
2 Assist the client in identifying coping skills, support systems, and potential stressors
3 Reassure the client that everything will be fine once he is in his home environment
4 Confront the client and explain that he must control his behavior if he wants to go home

Answer: 2

Rationale: It is normal for clients who experience thyroid storm (hyperthyroidism) to continue to be anxious and emotionally labile at the time of discharge. Confrontation in option 4 will only heighten anxiety. In addition, options 1 and 3 block communication by either avoiding the issue or providing false reassurance. The best intervention is to help the client cope with these changes in behavior and anticipate potential stressors so that symptoms will not be as severe.

Test-Taking Strategy: Use the process of elimination and therapeutic communication techniques. Eliminate options 3 and 4 because they are blocks to communication. From the remaining options, note the key words "anxious about his illness." Eliminate option 1 because it is unrelated to addressing the client's anxiety. When confronted with psychosocial issues, always select the option that addresses the client's feelings and concerns. Review therapeutic communication techniques if you had difficulty with this question.

Level of Cognitive Ability: Application
Client Needs: Psychosocial Integrity
Integrated Process: Nursing Process/Planning
Content Area: Adult Health/Endocrine

References:
Black, J., & Hawks, J. (2005). *Medical-surgical nursing: Clinical management for positive outcomes* (7th ed.). Philadelphia: Saunders, p. 1202.
Potter, P., & Perry, A. (2005). *Fundamentals of nursing* (6th ed.). St. Louis: Mosby, p. 437.

112. A nurse is caring for a client admitted to the hospital for subclavian central line placement. Which psychosocial area of assessment should the nurse address with the client?
1   Strict restrictions of neck mobility
2   Loss of ability to ambulate as tolerated
3   Possible body image disturbance
4   Continuous pain related to ongoing placement of the subclavian line

Answer: 3
Rationale: When a client has a central line placed in the subclavian area, the client is able to move as tolerated with no restriction of movement. The client may have pain when the catheter is placed, but the pain will not last continuously. The client may, however, be self-conscious about the intravenous line, disturbing body image.

Test-Taking Strategy: Use the process of elimination, noting the key words "psychosocial area." Pain, altered mobility, and restricted neck movements are physical concerns. Review the psychosocial effects of a subclavian line if you had difficulty with this question.

Level of Cognitive Ability: Analysis
Client Needs: Psychosocial Integrity
Integrated Process: Nursing Process/Assessment
Content Area: Fundamental Skills

References:
Lewis, S., Heitkemper, M., & Dirksen, S. (2004). *Medical-surgical nursing: Assessment and management of clinical problems* (6th ed.). St. Louis: Mosby, p. 988.
Potter, P., & Perry, A. (2005). *Fundamentals of nursing* (6th ed.). St. Louis: Mosby, pp. 506-507.

---

113. A 12-year-old child is seen in the health care clinic. During the assessment, which finding would suggest to the nurse that the child is experiencing a disruption in the development of self-concept?
1   The child has a part-time babysitting job.
2   The child enjoys playing chess and mastering new skills with this game.
3   The child has many friends.
4   The child has an intimate relationship with a significant other.

Answer: 4
Rationale: A sense of industry is appropriate for this age group and may be exhibited by having a part-time job. The increase in self-esteem associated with skill mastery is an important part of development for the school-aged child. Friends are also important and appropriate in this age group. The formation of an intimate relationship would not be expected until young adulthood.

Test-Taking Strategy: Not the key words "disruption in the development of self-concept." Use the process of elimination, focusing on normal growth and development. Noting the age of the child in the question will assist in eliminating options 1, 2, and 3. Review normal growth and development and developmental tasks associated with this age group if you had difficulty with this question.

Level of Cognitive Ability: Analysis
Client Needs: Psychosocial Integrity
Integrated Process: Nursing Process/Assessment
Content Area: Child Health

Reference:
Wong, D., & Hockenberry, M. (2003). *Wong's nursing care of infants and children* (7th ed.). St. Louis: Mosby, p. 816.

114. A client newly diagnosed with tuberculosis (TB) is hospitalized and will be on respiratory isolation for at least 2 weeks. Which of the following would be appropriate in preventing psychosocial distress in the client?
1 Removing the calendar and clock in the room so that the client will not obsess about time
2 Noting whether the client has visitors
3 Giving the client a roommate with TB who persistently tries to talk
4 Instructing all staff members not to touch the client

Answer: 2
Rationale: The nurse should note whether the client has visitors and social contacts, because the presence of others can offer positive stimulation. The calendar and clock are needed to promote orientation to time. A roommate who insists on talking could create sensory overload. Additionally, the client on respiratory isolation should be in a private room. Touch may be important in order to help the client feel socially acceptable.

Test-Taking Strategy: Use the process of elimination. Note the key words "preventing psychosocial distress." Eliminate option 3 first because the client should be in a private room. From the remaining options, noting that the client will be on respiratory isolation for at least 2 weeks and recalling the basic principles related to sensory overload will direct you to option 2. Review the psychosocial concerns related to isolation if you had difficulty with this question.

Level of Cognitive Ability: Application
Client Needs: Psychosocial Integrity
Integrated Process: Nursing Process/Assessment
Content Area: Adult Health/Respiratory

Reference:
Potter, P., & Perry, A. (2005). *Fundamentals of nursing* (6th ed.). St. Louis: Mosby, pp. 797-798.

115. A nurse is interviewing a client with chronic obstructive pulmonary disease (COPD) who has a respiratory rate of 35 breaths per minute and is experiencing extreme dyspnea. Which nursing diagnosis would be appropriate for the client?
1 Impaired verbal communication, related to a physical barrier
2 Ineffective coping, related to the client's inability to handle a situational crisis
3 Disturbed body image, related to neurological deficit
4 Deficient knowledge, related to COPD

Answer: 1
Rationale: A client may suffer physical or psychological alterations that impair communication. To speak spontaneously and clearly, a person must have an intact respiratory system. Extreme dyspnea is a physical alteration affecting speech. There is no data in the question that supports options 2, 3, and 4.

Test-Taking Strategy: Use the process of elimination, focusing on the data in the question. Option 1 clearly addresses the problem that the client is experiencing. Option 2 is judgmental and inappropriate. There is nothing to indicate that the client has a neurological deficit. Option 4 identifies a medical diagnosis. Review the defining characteristics associated with impaired verbal communication if you had difficulty with this question.

Level of Cognitive Ability: Analysis
Client Needs: Psychosocial Integrity
Integrated Process: Nursing Process/Analysis
Content Area: Adult Health/Respiratory

Reference:
Potter, P., & Perry, A. (2005). *Fundamentals of nursing* (6th ed.). St. Louis: Mosby, p. 436.

116. A client was injured as a result of passing out from drinking alcohol and falling into the coals of a fire. A fourth-degree circumferential burn wound to the left leg resulted from this accident. In report, the nurse is told that the client just signed an informed consent for amputation of the limb and the procedure is scheduled for tomorrow. During the nursing assessment, the client is upset and withdrawn. The nurse takes which appropriate action at this time?

1 Let the client have some time alone to grieve over the future loss of the limb
2 Teach the client that the injury was a result of alcohol abuse and refer him for counseling
3 Inform the physician of the client's behavior and request medication to assist the client in coping with the diagnosis
4 Reflect back to the client that he appears upset

Answer: 4
Rationale: Reflection statements tend to elicit deeper awareness of feelings. A well-timed reflection can reveal an emotion that has escaped the client's notice. Additionally, option 4 validates the perception that the client is upset. Option 2 is inappropriate and a block to communication. Options 1 and 3 address interventions before assessing the situation.

Test-Taking Strategy: Use therapeutic communication techniques. Focus on the client's feelings. Select the option that encourages the client to express his feelings and talk more. This will direct you to option 4. Review therapeutic communication techniques if you had difficulty with this question.

Level of Cognitive Ability: Application
Client Needs: Psychosocial Integrity
Integrated Process: Nursing Process/Implementation
Content Area: Mental Health

Reference:
Stuart, G., & Laraia, M. (2005). *Principles and practice of psychiatric nursing* (8th ed.). St. Louis: Mosby, pp. 30-32.

---

117. A nurse is caring for a client with left-sided Bell's palsy. Which statement by the client requires further exploration by the nurse?

1 "My left eye is tearing a lot."
2 "I have trouble closing my left eyelid."
3 "I can't taste anything on the left side."
4 "I don't know how I'll live with the effects of this stroke for the rest of my life."

Answer: 4
Rationale: Bell's palsy is an inflammatory condition involving the facial nerve (cranial nerve VII). Although it results in facial paralysis, it is not the same as a stroke or cerebrovascular accident (CVA). Many clients fear that they have had a CVA when the symptoms of Bell's palsy appear, and they commonly believe that the paralysis is permanent. Symptoms resolve, although it may take several weeks. Options 1, 2, and 3 are expected assessment findings in the client with Bell's palsy.

Test-Taking Strategy: Note the key words "requiring further exploration." These key words indicate a false-response question and that you need to select the option that identifies an incorrect client statement. Recalling that this disorder is a temporary condition will direct you to option 4, which identifies an inaccurate understanding of the disorder and requires further exploration. Review this disorder if you had difficulty with this question.

Level of Cognitive Ability: Analysis
Client Needs: Psychosocial Integrity
Integrated Process: Nursing Process/Evaluation
Content Area: Adult Health/Neurological

Reference:
Black, J., & Hawks, J. (2005). *Medical-surgical nursing: Clinical management for positive outcomes* (7th ed.). Philadelphia: Saunders, p. 2154.

118. A client newly diagnosed with diabetes mellitus has a nursing diagnosis of Ineffective Health Maintenance, related to anxiety regarding the self-administration of insulin. Initially, the nurse should plan to:
1 Teach the family member to give the client the insulin
2 Use an orange for the client to inject into until the client is less anxious
3 Insert the needle and have the client push in the plunger and remove the needle
4 Give the injection until the client feels confident enough to do so by him or herself

Answer: 3

Rationale: Some clients find it difficult to insert a needle into their own skin. For these clients, the nurse might assist by selecting the site and inserting the needle. Then, as a first step in self-injection, the client can push in the plunger and remove the needle. Options 1 and 4 place the client into a dependent role. Option 2 is not realistic considering the issue of the question.

Test-Taking Strategy: Use the process of elimination, focusing on the issue: anxiety regarding self-administration of insulin. Eliminate options 1 and 4 because they place the client in a dependent position. From the remaining options, select option 3 because it addresses the issue of self-administration. Review teaching/learning principles related to an anxious client if you had difficulty with this question.

Level of Cognitive Ability: Application
Client Needs: Psychosocial Integrity
Integrated Process: Teaching/Learning
Content Area: Adult Health/Endocrine

Reference:
Potter, P., & Perry, A. (2005). *Fundamentals of nursing* (6th ed.). St. Louis: Mosby, pp. 451-454.

119. A client in labor has human immunodeficiency virus (HIV) and says to the nurse, "I know I will have a sick-looking baby." The nurse makes which appropriate response?
1 "There is no reason to worry. Our neonatal unit offers the latest treatments available."
2 "You have concerns about how HIV will affect your baby?"
3 "You are very sick, but your baby may not be."
4 "All babies are beautiful. I am sure your baby will be too."

Answer: 2

Rationale: Option 2 is the most therapeutic response and will elicit the best information. It addresses the therapeutic communication technique of paraphrasing. Parents need to know that their baby will not look sick from HIV at birth and that there may be a period of uncertainty before it is known whether the baby has acquired the infection. The client should not be told "there is no reason to worry." Options 3 and 4 provide false reassurances. Option 2 is an open-ended response that will provide an opportunity to the client to verbalize concerns.

Test-Taking Strategy: Use therapeutic communication techniques. Remember to address the client's feelings and concerns. This will direct you to option 2. Review these techniques if you had difficulty with this question.

Level of Cognitive Ability: Analysis
Client Needs: Psychosocial Integrity
Integrated Process: Communication and Documentation
Content Area: Maternity/Intrapartum

References:
Murray, S., McKinney, E., & Gorrie, T. (2002). *Foundations of maternal-newborn nursing* (3rd ed.). Philadelphia: Saunders, p. 25.
Potter, P., & Perry, A. (2005). *Fundamentals of nursing* (6th ed.). St. Louis: Mosby, p. 437.

120. A client who is scheduled for an abdominal peritoneoscopy states to the home care nurse, "The doctor told me to restrict food and liquids for at least eight hours before this procedure and to use a Fleet's enema four hours before entering the hospital. Do people ever get into trouble after this procedure?" The nurse makes which appropriate response to the client?
  1 "Any invasive procedure brings risk with it. You need to report any shoulder pain immediately."
  2 "There are relatively few problems, especially if you are having local anesthesia, but vaginal bleeding should be reported immediately."
  3 "Trouble? There is never any trouble with this procedure. That's why the surgeon will use local anesthesia."
  4 "You seem to understand the preparation very well. Are you having any concerns about the procedure?"

Answer: 4
Rationale: Abdominal peritoneoscopy is performed to directly visualize the liver, gallbladder, spleen, and stomach after the insufflation of nitrous oxide. During the procedure, a rigid laparoscope is inserted through a small incision in the abdomen. A microscope in the endoscope allows visualization of the organs and provides a way to collect a specimen for biopsy or to remove small tumors. The appropriate response is the one that facilitates the client's expression of feelings. Option 1 may increase the client's anxiety. In option 3, the nurse states that no problems are associated with this procedure. This is an absolute and is incorrect. Although option 2 contains accurate information, the word "immediately" can increase the client's anxiety.

Test-Taking Strategy: Use the process of elimination. Remember to focus on the client's feelings and concerns. Option 4 is the appropriate response because it provides an opportunity for the client to verbalize concerns. Review therapeutic communication techniques if you had difficulty with this question.

Level of Cognitive Ability: Application
Client Needs: Psychosocial Integrity
Integrated Process: Communication and Documentation
Content Area: Adult Health/Gastrointestinal

Reference:
Potter, P., & Perry, A. (2005). *Fundamentals of nursing* (6th ed.). St. Louis: Mosby, p. 437.

121. A nurse is caring for a client during a precipitate labor. In assessing the client's emotional needs, the nurse can anticipate the client having:
  1 Less pain and anxiety than with a normal labor
  2 A need for support in maintaining a sense of control
  3 Fewer fears regarding the effect on the newborn infant
  4 A sense of satisfaction regarding her quick labor

Answer: 2
Rationale: The client experiencing a precipitate labor may have more difficulty maintaining control because of the abrupt onset and quick progression of the labor. This may be very different from previous labor experiences; therefore, the client needs support from the nurse in order to understand and adapt to the rapid progression. The contractions often increase in intensity quickly, adding to the pain, anxiety, and lack of control. The client may also have an increased amount of concern about the effect of the labor on the newborn infant. Lack of control over the situation combined with increased pain and anxiety can result in a decreased level of satisfaction with the labor and delivery experience.

Test-Taking Strategy: Use the process of elimination. Focus on the client's condition: a precipitate labor. Note the key words "emotional needs" in the question and the key words "a need for support" in the correct option. Review care of the client with a precipitate labor if you had difficulty with this question.

Level of Cognitive Ability: Analysis
Client Needs: Psychosocial Integrity
Integrated Process: Nursing Process/Assessment
Content Area: Maternity/Intrapartum

Reference:
Lowdermilk, D., & Perry, A. (2004). *Maternity & women's health care* (8th ed.). St. Louis: Mosby, p. 584.

122. A nurse is planning care for a client who presents in active labor with a history of a previous cesarean delivery. The client complains of a "tearing" sensation in the lower abdomen, is upset, and expresses concern for the safety of her baby. The nurse makes which response to the client?

1 "Don't worry, you are in good hands."
2 "I can understand that you are fearful. We are doing everything possible for your baby."
3 "You'll have to talk to your doctor about that."
4 "I don't have time to answer questions now. We'll talk later."

Answer: 2

Rationale: Clients have a concern for the safety of their baby during labor and delivery, especially when a problem arises. Empathy and a calm attitude with realistic reassurances are an important aspect of client care. Dismissing or ignoring the client's concerns can lead to increased fear and lack of cooperation. Option 1 uses a cliché and false reassurance. Options 3 and 4 place the client's feelings "on hold."

Test-Taking Strategy: Use therapeutic communication techniques. Eliminate options 3 and 4 because they place the client's feelings "on hold." Next eliminate option 1 because the client should not be told, "Don't worry." Review therapeutic communication techniques if you had difficulty with this question.

Level of Cognitive Ability: Application
Client Needs: Psychosocial Integrity
Integrated Process: Communication and Documentation
Content Area: Maternity/Intrapartum

Reference:
Murray, S., McKinney, E., & Gorrie, T. (2002). *Foundations of maternal-newborn nursing* (3rd ed.). Philadelphia: Saunders, pp. 413-414.

123. A newborn male infant is diagnosed with an undescended testicle (cryptorchidism), and these findings are shared with the parents. The parents ask questions about the condition. The nurse responds, knowing that which of the following could have a psychosocial impact if this condition is not corrected?

1 Infertility
2 Malignancy
3 Feminization
4 Atrophy

Answer: 1

Rationale: Infertility can occur in this condition because proper function of the testes depends on a temperature cooler than 98.6°F. The psychological effects of an "empty scrotum" could affect the client's perception of self and the ability to reproduce. Options 2 and 4 are possible physical consequences of failure to treat cryptorchidism, not psychosocial consequences. Because all hormones responsible for secondary sex characteristics continue to be secreted directly into the bloodstream, option 3 is not correct.

Test-Taking Strategy: Use the process of elimination. Focusing on the issue, psychosocial impact, will assist in eliminating options 2 and 4. From the remaining options, it is necessary to know that infertility can occur if the condition is uncorrected. Review this disorder if you had difficulty with this question.

Level of Cognitive Ability: Analysis
Client Needs: Psychosocial Integrity
Integrated Process: Nursing Process/Analysis
Content Area: Maternity/Postpartum

Reference:
Wong, D., & Hockenberry, M. (2003). *Wong's nursing care of infants and children* (7th ed.). St. Louis: Mosby, p. 481.

124. A mother of an infant with hydrocephalus is concerned about the complication of mental retardation. The mother states to the nurse, "I'm not sure if I can care for my baby at home." The nurse makes which therapeutic response to the mother?

1 "There is no reason to worry. You have a good pediatrician."

2 "Mothers instinctively know what is best for their babies."

3 "You have concerns about your baby's condition and care?"

4 "All babies have individual needs."

Answer: 3

Rationale: Paraphrasing is restating the mother's message in the nurse's own words. Option 3 addresses the therapeutic technique of paraphrasing. In options 1 and 2, the nurse is offering a false reassurance, and these types of responses will block communication. In option 4, the nurse is minimizing the social needs involved with the baby's diagnosis, which is harmful for the nurse-parent relationship.

Test-Taking Strategy: Use therapeutic communication techniques and the process of elimination to answer the question. Option 3 is the only therapeutic response and addresses paraphrasing. This is the only option that will provide the client an opportunity to verbalize concerns. Review therapeutic communication techniques if you had difficulty with this question.

Level of Cognitive Ability: Application
Client Needs: Psychosocial Integrity
Integrated Process: Communication and Documentation
Content Area: Maternity/Postpartum

Reference:
Potter, P., & Perry, A. (2005). *Fundamentals of nursing* (6th ed.). St. Louis: Mosby, p. 437.

125. A preschooler is just diagnosed with impetigo. The child's mother tells the nurse, "But my children take baths every day." The nurse makes which therapeutic response to the mother?

1 "You are concerned about how your child got impetigo?"

2 "There is no need to worry. We will not tell daycare why your child is absent."

3 "Not only do you have to do a better job in keeping the children clean, you must also wash your hands more frequently."

4 "You should have seen the doctor before the wound became infected, and then you would not have had to worry about the child having impetigo."

Answer: 1

Rationale: By paraphrasing what the parent tells the nurse, the nurse is addressing the parent's thoughts. Option 1 is the therapeutic technique of paraphrasing. Options 2, 3, and 4 are blocks to communication because they make the parent feel guilty for the child's illness.

Test-Taking Strategy: Use therapeutic communication techniques and the process of elimination to answer the question. Option 1 is the only therapeutic technique and addresses paraphrasing. This is the only option that will provide the client an opportunity to verbalize concerns. Options 2, 3, and 4 are blocks to communication. Review therapeutic communication techniques if you had difficulty with this question.

Level of Cognitive Ability: Application
Client Needs: Psychosocial Integrity
Integrated Process: Communication and Documentation
Content Area: Child Health

References:
McKinney, E., James, S., Murray, S., & Ashwill, J. (2005). *Maternal-child nursing* (2nd ed.). St. Louis: Elsevier, p. 1365.
Potter, P., & Perry, A. (2005). *Fundamentals of nursing* (6th ed.). St. Louis: Mosby, p. 437.

126. A nurse is preparing to care for a child from a culture different from the nurse's. What is the best way to address the cultural needs of the child and family when the child is admitted to the health care facility?

1 Ask questions and explain to the family why the questions are being asked

2 Explain to the family that while the child is being treated, they need to discontinue cultural practices because they may be harmful to the child

3 Ignore cultural needs because they are not important to health care professionals

4 Only address those issues that directly affect the nurse's care of the child

Answer: 1

Rationale: When caring for individuals from a different culture, it is important to ask questions about their specific cultural needs and means of treatment. An understanding of the family's beliefs and health practices is essential to successful interventions for that particular family. Options 2, 3, and 4 ignore the cultural beliefs and values of the client.

Test-Taking Strategy: Use the process of elimination, focusing on the issue: cultural needs. Options 2, 3, and 4 are judgmental. Additionally, these options are all similar in that they ignore the cultural practices and values of the client. Review nursing interventions related to cultural diversity if you had difficulty with this question.

Level of Cognitive Ability: Application
Client Needs: Psychosocial Integrity
Integrated Process: Caring
Content Area: Child Health

Reference:
Wong, D., & Hockenberry, M. (2003). *Wong's nursing care of infants and children* (7th ed.). St. Louis: Mosby, pp. 35;45.

---

127. A client with a T-1 spinal cord injury has just learned that the cord was completely severed. The client says, "I'm no good to anyone. I might as well be dead." The nurse makes which appropriate response to the client?

1 "It makes me uncomfortable when you talk this way."

2 "I'll ask the psychologist to see you about this."

3 "You're not a useless person at all."

4 "You are feeling pretty bad about things right now."

Answer: 4

Rationale: Restating and reflecting keeps the lines of communication open and encourages the client to expand on current feelings of unworthiness and loss that require exploration. The nurse can block communication by showing discomfort, disapproval, or by postponing discussion of issues. Grief is a common reaction to loss of function. The nurse facilitates grieving through open communication.

Test-Taking Strategy: Use therapeutic communication techniques and the process of elimination. Options 1, 2, and 3 block communication. Option 4 identifies the therapeutic communication technique of restating and reflecting. Review therapeutic communication techniques if you had difficulty with this question.

Level of Cognitive Ability: Application
Client Needs: Psychosocial Integrity
Integrated Process: Communication and Documentation
Content Area: Adult Health/Musculoskeletal

References:
Black, J., & Hawks, J. (2005). *Medical-surgical nursing: Clinical management for positive outcomes* (7th ed.). Philadelphia: Saunders, p. 2231.
Potter, P., & Perry, A. (2005). *Fundamentals of nursing* (6th ed.). St. Louis: Mosby, p. 437.

128. A nurse enters the room of a client with myocardial infarction (MI) and finds the client quietly crying. After determining that there is no physiological reason for the client's distress, the nurse replies:
1 "Do you want me to call your daughter?"
2 "Can you tell me a little about what has you so upset?"
3 "I understand how you feel. I'd cry too if I had a major heart attack."
4 "Try not to be so upset. Psychological stress is bad for your heart."

Answer: 2
Rationale: Clients with MI often have a nursing diagnosis of Anxiety or Fear. The nurse allows the client to express concerns by showing genuine interest and concern and by facilitating communication using therapeutic communication techniques. Option 2 provides the client an opportunity to express concerns. Options 1, 3, and 4 do not address the client's feelings or promote client verbalization.

Test-Taking Strategy: Use the process of elimination. Select the option that has an exploratory approach, because the question does not identify why the client is upset. This technique helps you eliminate each of the incorrect options. Review therapeutic communication techniques if you had difficulty with this question.

Level of Cognitive Ability: Application
Client Needs: Psychosocial Integrity
Integrated Process: Communication and Documentation
Content Area: Adult Health/Cardiovascular

Reference:
Black, J., & Hawks, J. (2005). *Medical-surgical nursing: Clinical management for positive outcomes* (7th ed.). Philadelphia: Saunders, p. 1723.

129. A client with a recent complete T-4 spinal cord transection tells the nurse that he will walk again as soon as the spinal shock resolves. Which of the following will provide the most accurate basis for planning a response to the client?
1 In order to speed acceptance, the client needs reinforcement that he will not walk again.
2 The client needs to move through the grieving process rapidly in order to benefit from rehabilitation.
3 The client is projecting by insisting that walking is the rehabilitation goal.
4 Denial can be protective while the client deals with the anxiety created by the new disability.

Answer: 4
Rationale: In the adjustment period during the first few weeks after spinal cord injury, clients may use denial as a defense mechanism. Denial may decrease anxiety temporarily and is a normal part of grieving. After the spinal shock resolves, prolonged or excessive use of denial may impair rehabilitation. However, rehabilitation programs include psychological counseling to deal with denial and grief.

Test-Taking Strategy: Use the process of elimination and knowledge of the physiological effects of a T-4 spinal injury. The words "speed acceptance," "move through the grieving process rapidly," and "walking is the rehabilitation goal" should be indicators that these are incorrect options. Focus on the client's statement, which is an indication of denial, to direct you to option 4. Review the defining characteristics of denial if you had difficulty with this question.

Level of Cognitive Ability: Analysis
Client Needs: Psychosocial Integrity
Integrated Process: Nursing Process/Planning
Content Area: Adult Health/Musculoskeletal

Reference:
Black, J., & Hawks, J. (2005). *Medical-surgical nursing: Clinical management for positive outcomes* (7th ed.). Philadelphia: Saunders, pp. 525-526.

130. A nurse is developing a plan of care for a client scheduled for an above-the-knee leg amputation. The nurse should include which action in the plan when addressing psychosocial needs of a client?

1 Explain to the client that open grieving is abnormal
2 Discourage sharing feelings with others who have had similar experiences
3 Encourage the client to express feelings about body changes
4 Advise the client to seek psychological treatment after surgery

Answer: 3
Rationale: Surgical incisions or loss of a body part can alter a client's body image. The onset of problems coping with these changes may occur in the immediate or extended postoperative stage. Nursing interventions primarily involve providing psychological support. The nurse should encourage the client to express how he or she feels these postoperative changes will affect his or her life. Option 1 is an incorrect statement because open grieving in normal. Option 2 indicates disapproval, and in option 4, the nurse is giving advice.

Test-Taking Strategy: Use therapeutic communication techniques. Remember to always focus on the client's feelings first. This will direct you to option 3. Review therapeutic communication techniques if you had difficulty with this question.

Level of Cognitive Ability: Application
Client Needs: Psychosocial Integrity
Integrated Process: Caring
Content Area: Mental Health

Reference:
Stuart, G., & Laraia, M. (2005). *Principles and practice of psychiatric nursing* (8th ed.). St. Louis: Mosby, pp. 30-34.

---

131. A client in pulmonary edema exhibits severe anxiety. The nurse is preparing to carry out the medically prescribed orders. Which intervention would the nurse use to meet the needs of the client in a holistic manner?

1 Leave the client alone while gathering required equipment and medications
2 Give the client the call bell, and encourage its use if the client feels worse
3 Ask a family member to stay with the client
4 Stay with the client, and ask another nurse to gather equipment and supplies not already in the room

Answer: 4
Rationale: Pulmonary edema is accompanied by extreme fear and anxiety. Because the client typically experiences a sense of impending doom, the nurse should remain with the client as much as possible. Options 1 and 2 do not provide for the psychological needs of the client in distress. Family members (option 3) can emotionally support the client, but they are not able to respond to physiological needs and symptoms. In fact, they are typically in psychological distress themselves.

Test-Taking Strategy: Use the process of elimination. The word "holistic" in the stem of the question guides you to consider both the physical and emotional well-being of the client. Option 4 is the only option that addresses both needs. Review the psychosocial aspects of care for the client in pulmonary edema if you had difficulty with this question.

Level of Cognitive Ability: Application
Client Needs: Psychosocial Integrity
Integrated Process: Nursing Process/Implementation
Content Area: Adult Health/Respiratory

References:
Black, J., & Hawks, J. (2005). *Medical-surgical nursing: Clinical management for positive outcomes* (7th ed.). Philadelphia: Saunders, pp. 1890-1891.
Lewis, S., Heitkemper, M., & Dirksen, S. (2004). *Medical-surgical nursing: Assessment and management of clinical problems* (6th ed.). St. Louis: Mosby, pp. 59-60; 680.

132. A family of a client with myocardial infarction complicated by cardiogenic shock is visibly anxious and upset about the client's condition. The nurse plans to do which of the following to provide support to the family?
1 Insist they go home to sleep at night to keep up their own strength
2 Provide flexibility with visiting times according to the client's condition and family needs
3 Offer them coffee and other beverages on a regular basis
4 Ask the hospital chaplain to sit with them until the client's condition stabilizes

Answer: 2

Rationale: The use of flexible visiting hours meets the needs of both the client and family in reducing the anxiety levels of both. Insisting that the family go home is nontherapeutic. Offering the family beverages does not provide support. Although the chaplain may provide support, it is unrealistic for the chaplain to stay until the client stabilizes.

Test-Taking Strategy: Note the issue: the method of providing support. Options 1 and 4 may or may not be helpful, depending on the client and family situation. Coffee and beverages, while probably helpful to many, do not provide support. Review measures to provide support to the family of a client with a critical disorder if you had difficulty with this question.

Level of Cognitive Ability: Application
Client Needs: Psychosocial Integrity
Integrated Process: Caring
Content Area: Adult Health/Cardiovascular

Reference:
Lewis, S., Heitkemper, M., & Dirksen, S. (2004). *Medical-surgical nursing: Assessment and management of clinical problems* (6th ed.). St. Louis: Mosby, pp. 1761-1762.

---

133. A client with premature ventricular contractions says to the nurse, "I'm so afraid something bad will happen." Which action by the nurse would provide the most immediate help to the client?
1 Giving reassurance that nothing will happen to the client
2 Telephoning the client's family
3 Having a staff member stay with the client
4 Using television to distract the client

Answer: 3

Rationale: When a client experiences fear, the nurse can provide a calm, safe environment by offering appropriate reassurance, using therapeutic touch, and by having someone remain with the client as much as possible. Option 1 provides false reassurance. Options 2 and 4 do not address the client's fear.

Test-Taking Strategy: Use the process of elimination. Noting the key words "most immediate help" will direct you to option 3. Review measures to reduce a client's fear if you had difficulty with this question.

Level of Cognitive Ability: Application
Client Needs: Psychosocial Integrity
Integrated Process: Caring
Content Area: Adult Health/Cardiovascular

References:
Black, J., & Hawks, J. (2005). *Medical-surgical nursing: Clinical management for positive outcomes* (7th ed.). Philadelphia: Saunders, p. 1668.
Potter, P., & Perry, A. (2005). *Fundamentals of nursing* (6th ed.). St. Louis: Mosby, pp. 437; 920-921.

134. A client with Raynaud's disease tells the nurse that he has a stressful job and does not handle stressful situations well. The nurse most appropriately guides the client to:
1 Change jobs
2 Consider a stress management program
3 Seek help from a psychologist
4 Use earplugs to minimize environmental noise

Answer: 2
Rationale: Stress can trigger the vasospasm that occurs with Raynaud's disease, so referral to stress management programs or the use of biofeedback training may be helpful. Option 1 is unrealistic. Option 3 is not necessarily required at this time. Option 4 does not specifically address the issue.

Test-Taking Strategy: Use the process of elimination, focusing on the issue: stress. Note the relationship between this issue and option 2. Review measures that reduce stress if you had difficulty with this question.

Level of Cognitive Ability: Application
Client Needs: Psychosocial Integrity
Integrated Process: Nursing Process/Implementation
Content Area: Adult Health/Cardiovascular

References:
Black, J., & Hawks, J. (2005). *Medical-surgical nursing: Clinical management for positive outcomes* (7th ed.). Philadelphia: Saunders, p. 1533.
Potter, P., & Perry, A. (2005). *Fundamentals of nursing* (6th ed.). St. Louis: Mosby, p. 611.

135. A client with a history of pulmonary emboli is scheduled for insertion of an inferior vena cava filter. The nurse checks on the client 1 hour after the physician has explained the procedure and obtained consent from the client. The client is lying in bed, wringing the hands, and says to the nurse, "I'm not sure about this. What if it doesn't work and I'm just as bad off as before?" The nurse formulates which nursing diagnosis for the client?
1 Fear, related to the potential risks and outcome of surgery
2 Anxiety, related to the fear of death
3 Ineffective coping, related to the treatment regimen
4 Deficient knowledge, related to the surgical procedure

Answer: 1
Rationale: The North American Nursing Diagnosis Association (NANDA) defines Fear as "a feeling of dread related to an identifiable source that the person validates." This client has indicated the surgical procedure and its outcome as the object of fear. Anxiety is used when the client cannot identify the source of the uneasy feelings. Ineffective Coping is appropriate when the client is not making needed adaptations to deal with daily life. Deficient Knowledge is characterized by a lack of appropriate information.

Test-Taking Strategy: Focus on the data in the question and on the client's statement. Note the relationship of the client's statement and option 1. Review the defining characteristics of Fear if you had difficulty with this question.

Level of Cognitive Ability: Analysis
Client Needs: Psychosocial Integrity
Integrated Process: Nursing Process/Analysis
Content Area: Adult Health/Respiratory

References:
Gulanick, M., Myers, J., Klopp, A., Gradishar, D., Galanes, S., & Puzas, M. (2003). *Nursing care plans: Nursing diagnosis and intervention* (5th ed.). St. Louis: Mosby, pp. 14; 59; 47; 103.
Potter, P., & Perry, A. (2005). *Fundamentals of nursing* (6th ed.). St. Louis: Mosby, p. 1601.

136. A client has an oral endotracheal tube attached to a mechanical ventilator and is about to begin the weaning process. The nurse interprets that which of the following items should now be limited, which were previously useful in minimizing the client's anxiety?

1 Radio
2 Television
3 Family visitors
4 Antianxiety medications

Answer: 4

Rationale: Antianxiety medications and narcotic analgesics are used cautiously in the client being weaned from a mechanical ventilator. These medications may interfere with the weaning process by suppressing the respiratory drive. The client may exhibit anxiety during the weaning process as well for a variety of reasons, and therefore distractions such as radio, television, and visitors are still very useful.

Test-Taking Strategy: Note the key words "items should now be limited." Think about the items that could interfere with the client's strength, endurance, and respiratory drive in maintaining independent ventilation. Using this as the guideline, the only possible option is option 4. The side effects of these medications could include sedation, which could interfere with optimal respiratory function. Review care of the client who is weaning from a mechanical ventilator if you had difficulty with this question.

Level of Cognitive Ability: Analysis
Client Needs: Psychosocial Integrity
Integrated Process: Nursing Process/Analysis
Content Area: Adult Health/Respiratory

Reference:
Black, J., & Hawks, J. (2005). *Medical-surgical nursing: Clinical management for positive outcomes* (7th ed.). Philadelphia: Saunders, pp. 1893-1894.

---

137. A client scheduled for pulmonary angiography is fearful about the procedure and asks the nurse if the procedure involves significant pain and radiation exposure. The nurse provides a response to the client that provides reassurance, based on the understanding that:

1 The procedure is somewhat painful, but there is minimal exposure to radiation
2 Discomfort may occur with needle insertion, and there is minimal exposure to radiation
3 There is absolutely no pain, although a moderate amount of radiation must be used to get accurate results
4 There is very mild pain throughout the procedure, and the exposure to radiation is negligible

Answer: 2

Rationale: Pulmonary angiography involves minimal exposure to radiation. The procedure is painless, although the client may feel discomfort with insertion of the needle for the catheter that is used for dye injection. Options 1, 3, and 4 are incorrect.

Test-Taking Strategy: Focus on the diagnostic procedure. Eliminate option 3 because of the absolute word "no." From the remaining options, recalling that discomfort occurs with needle insertion will direct you to option 2. Review this procedure if you had difficulty with this question.

Level of Cognitive Ability: Analysis
Client Needs: Psychosocial Integrity
Integrated Process: Nursing Process/Analysis
Content Area: Adult Health/Respiratory

Reference:
Chernecky, C., & Berger, B. (2004). *Laboratory tests and diagnostic procedures* (4th ed.). Philadelphia: Saunders, p. 929.

138. A nurse is caring for an anxious client who has an open pneumothorax and a sucking chest wound. An occlusive dressing has been applied to the site. Which intervention by the nurse would best relieve the client's anxiety?

1 Encouraging the client to cough and deep breathe
2 Staying with the client
3 Interpreting the arterial blood gas report
4 Distracting the client with television

Answer: 2

Rationale: Staying with the client has a two-fold benefit. First, it relieves the anxiety of the dyspneic client. In addition, the nurse must stay with the client to observe respiratory status after application of the occlusive dressing. It is possible that the dressing could convert the open pneumothorax to a closed (tension) pneumothorax, resulting in a sudden decline in respiratory status and mediastinal shift. If this occurs, the nurse is present and able to remove the dressing immediately. Interpreting the arterial blood gas report and coughing and deep breathing has no immediate benefit for the client who is in distress. Option 4 is nontherapeutic.

Test-Taking Strategy: Focus on the issue: relieving the client's anxiety. Eliminate option 4 first, because the client is in distress. From the remaining options, use therapeutic nursing measures to direct you to option 2. Review the measures to relieve anxiety if you had difficulty with this question.

Level of Cognitive Ability: Application
Client Needs: Psychosocial Integrity
Integrated Process: Nursing Process/Implementation
Content Area: Adult Health/Respiratory

References:
Ignatavicius, D., & Workman, M. (2002). *Medical surgical nursing: Critical thinking for collaborative care* (4th ed.). Philadelphia: Saunders, p. 1820.
Phipps, W., Monahan, F., Sands, J., Marek, J., & Neighbors, M. (2003). *Medical-surgical nursing: Health and illness perspectives* (7th ed.). St. Louis: Mosby, p. 565.

139. A client with acquired immunodeficiency syndrome (AIDS) shares with the nurse feelings of social isolation since the diagnosis was made. The nurse suggests which of the following strategies as the most useful way to decrease the client's stated loneliness?

1 Using the Internet on the computer to facilitate communication while maintaining isolation
2 Use of the television and newspapers to maintain a feeling of being "in touch" with the world
3 Contacting a support group available in the local region for clients with AIDS
4 Reinstituting contact with the client's family, who live in a distant city

Answer: 3

Rationale: The nurse encourages the client to maintain social contact and support and assists the client in reducing barriers to social contact. This can include educating the client's family about the disease and transmission, and suggesting utilization of community resources and support groups. Options 1 and 2 will not decrease the client's loneliness. Option 4, although feasible, is the less likely solution to address the client's current feelings of loneliness.

Test-Taking Strategy: Use the process of elimination. Eliminate options 1 and 2 first, because they do not actually decrease the client's isolation and loneliness. These options maintain a measure of distance between the client and others. From the remaining options, note that the wording of option 4 implies that contact has been lost over time, and the logistics of distance make this the less likely solution to the client's current feelings of isolation. Review the strategies related to reducing social isolation if you had difficulty with this question.

Level of Cognitive Ability: Application
Client Needs: Psychosocial Integrity
Integrated Process: Nursing Process/Implementation
Content Area: Adult Health/Immune

Reference:
Phipps, W., Monahan, F., Sands, J., Marek, J., & Neighbors, M. (2003). *Medical-surgical nursing: Health and illness perspectives* (7th ed.). St. Louis: Mosby, p. 83.

---

140. A client has an initial positive result of an enzyme-linked immunosorbent assay (ELISA) test for human immunodeficiency virus (HIV). The client begins to cry and asks the nurse what this means. The nurse is able to provide support to the client using knowledge that:

1 The client is HIV positive, but the disease has been detected early

2 The client is HIV positive, but the client's CD4 cell count is high

3 False positive results can occur and more testing is needed before diagnosing the client's status as HIV positive

4 There are occasional false-positive readings with this test, which can be cleared up by repeating it one more time

Answer: 3

Rationale: If the client tests positive with the ELISA, the test is repeated. If it is positive a second time, the Western blot (a more specific test) is done to confirm the finding. The client is not diagnosed as HIV positive unless the Western blot is positive. (Some laboratories also run the Western blot a second time with a new specimen before making a final determination.)

Test-Taking Strategy: Recall that HIV is not diagnosed with a single laboratory test. With this in mind, eliminate options 1 and 2 first. From the remaining options, knowing that the ELISA would be repeated and then a Western blot would be done to confirm these results will direct you to option 3. Review the methods of diagnosing HIV if you had difficulty with this question.

Level of Cognitive Ability: Analysis
Client Needs: Psychosocial Integrity
Integrated Process: Nursing Process/Implementation
Content Area: Adult Health/Immune

Reference:
Ignatavicius, D., & Workman, M. (2002). *Medical surgical nursing: Critical thinking for collaborative care* (4th ed.). Philadelphia: Saunders, p. 375.

---

141. In performing a lethality assessment with a suicidal client, the nurse most appropriately asks the client:

1 "Do you ever think about ending it all?"

2 "Do you have any thoughts of killing yourself?"

3 "Do you wish your life was over?"

4 "Do you have a death wish?"

Answer: 2

Rationale: A lethality assessment requires direct communication between the client and the nurse concerning the client's intent. It is important to provide a question that is directly related to lethality. Euphemisms should be avoided.

Test-Taking Strategy: Use the process of elimination. Note the relationship between "suicidal" in the question and "killing" in the correct option. Although options 1, 3, and 4 infer a suicide intent, option 2 is most direct. Review assessment for suicide risk if you had difficulty with this question.

Level of Cognitive Ability: Application
Client Needs: Psychosocial Integrity
Integrated Process: Nursing Process/Assessment
Content Area: Mental Health

References:
Stuart, G., & Laraia, M. (2005). *Principles and practice of psychiatric nursing* (8th ed.). St. Louis: Mosby, p. 367.
Varcarolis, E.M. (2002). *Foundations of psychiatric mental health nursing* (4th ed.). Philadelphia: Saunders, pp. 642-643.

142. A client diagnosed with cancer of the bladder has a nursing diagnosis of "Fear related to the uncertain outcome of the upcoming cystectomy and urinary diversion." The nurse assesses that this diagnosis still applies if the client makes which of the following statements?

1 "I'm so afraid I won't live through all this."
2 "What if I have no help at home after going through this awful surgery?"
3 "I'll never feel like myself if I can't go to the bathroom normally."
4 "I wish I'd never gone to the doctor at all."

Answer: 1

Rationale: In order for Fear to be an actual diagnosis, the client must be able to identify the object of fear. In this question, the client is expressing a fear of an uncertain outcome related to cancer. The statement in option 2 reflects risk for impaired home maintenance. Option 3 reflects a disturbed body image. Option 4 is vague and nonspecific. Further exploration would be required to associate this statement with a nursing diagnosis.

Test-Taking Strategy: Note that the diagnostic statement includes wording about the uncertain outcome of surgery. Because option 4 is a general statement, it should be eliminated first. Options 2 and 3 focus on self after surgery, but do not contain statements about an uncertain outcome. In option 1, the client expresses a fear of dying after enduring the ordeal of surgery. Review the defining characteristics of Fear if you had difficulty with this question.

Level of Cognitive Ability: Analysis
Client Needs: Psychosocial Integrity
Integrated Process: Nursing Process/Analysis
Content Area: Adult Health/Renal

Reference:
Phipps, W., Monahan, F., Sands, J., Marek, J., & Neighbors, M. (2003). *Medical-surgical nursing: Health and illness perspectives* (7th ed.). St. Louis: Mosby, p. 364.

143. A client with nephrotic syndrome asks the nurse, "Why should I even bother trying to control my diet and the edema? It doesn't really matter what I do, if I can never get rid of this kidney problem anyway!" The nurse selects which most appropriate nursing diagnosis for this client?

1 Powerlessness
2 Ineffective Coping
3 Anxiety
4 Disturbed Body Image

Answer: 1

Rationale: Powerlessness is used when the client believes that personal actions will not affect an outcome in any significant way. Ineffective coping is used when the client has impaired adaptive abilities or behaviors in meeting the demands or roles expected. Anxiety is used when the client has a feeling of unease with a vague or undefined source. Disturbed body image occurs when there is an alteration in the way the client perceives body image.

Test-Taking Strategy: Focus on the data in the question and the client's statement. Note the statement, "It doesn't really matter what I do." This implies that the client has a sense of lack of control over the situation. This will direct you to option 1. Review the defining characteristics of powerlessness if you had difficulty with this question.

Level of Cognitive Ability: Analysis
Client Needs: Psychosocial Integrity
Integrated Process: Nursing Process/Analysis
Content Area: Adult Health/Renal

Reference:
Phipps, W., Monahan, F., Sands, J., Marek, J., & Neighbors, M. (2003). *Medical-surgical nursing: Health and illness perspectives* (7th ed.). St. Louis: Mosby, p. 81.

144. A client with renal cell carcinoma of the left kidney is scheduled for nephrectomy. The right kidney appears normal at this time. The client is anxious about whether dialysis will ultimately be a necessity. The nurse would use which of the following information in discussions with the client?

1 There is absolutely no chance of needing dialysis because of the nature of the surgery.

2 Dialysis could become likely, but it depends on how well the client complies with fluid restriction after surgery.

3 One kidney is adequate to meet the needs of the body as long as it has normal function.

4 There is a strong likelihood that the client will need dialysis within 5 to 10 years.

Answer: 3

Rationale: Fears about having only one functioning kidney are common in clients who must undergo nephrectomy for renal cancer. These clients need emotional support and reassurance that the remaining kidney should be able to fully meet the body's metabolic needs, as long as it has normal function. Options 1, 2, and 3 are inaccurate.

Test-Taking Strategy: Use the process of elimination. Eliminate option 1 because of the words "absolutely no chance." Knowing that there is no need for fluid restriction with a functioning kidney guides you to eliminate option 2 next. From the remaining options, recalling that an individual can donate a kidney without adverse consequences or the need for dialysis will direct you to option 3. Review the psychosocial aspects related to nephrectomy if you had difficulty with this question.

Level of Cognitive Ability: Application
Client Needs: Psychosocial Integrity
Integrated Process: Nursing Process/Implementation
Content Area: Adult Health/Oncology

References:
Ignatavicius, D., & Workman, M. (2002). *Medical surgical nursing: Critical thinking for collaborative care* (4th ed.). Philadelphia: Saunders, p. 1659.
Phipps, W., Monahan, F., Sands, J., Marek, J., & Neighbors, M. (2003). *Medical-surgical nursing: Health and illness perspectives* (7th ed.). St. Louis: Mosby, p. 1225.

145. A charge nurse is supervising a new registered nurse (RN) providing care to a client with end-stage heart failure. The client is withdrawn, reluctant to talk, and shows little interest in participating in hygienic care or activities. Which statement made by the new RN to the client indicates that the new RN needs further teaching in the use of therapeutic communication techniques?

1 "Many clients with end-stage heart failure fear death."

2 "Why don't you feel like getting up for your bath?"

3 "What are your feelings right now?"

4 "These dreams you mentioned, what are they like?"

Answer: 2

Rationale: When the nurse asks a "why" question of the client, the nurse is requesting an explanation for feelings and behaviors when the client may not know the reason. Requesting an explanation is a nontherapeutic communication technique. In option 1, the nurse is using the therapeutic communication technique of giving information. Imparting the common fear of death of clients with end-stage heart failure may encourage the client to voice concerns. In option 3, the nurse is encouraging verbalization of emotions or feelings, which is a therapeutic communication technique. In option 4, the nurse is using the therapeutic communication technique of exploring. Exploring is asking the client to describe something in more detail or to discuss it more fully.

Test-Taking Strategy: Note the key words "needs further teaching in the use of therapeutic communication techniques." These words indicate a false-response question and that you need to select the option that identifies an incorrect statement by the new RN. Select the option that is a block to communication. The word "why" in option 2 should guide you to this option. Review therapeutic communication techniques if you had difficulty with this question.

Level of Cognitive Ability: Analysis
Client Needs: Psychosocial Integrity
Integrated Process: Teaching/Learning
Content Area: Leadership/Management

Reference:
Potter, P., & Perry, A. (2005). *Fundamentals of nursing* (6th ed.). St. Louis: Mosby, p. 437.

---

146. A nurse is caring for a client with acute pulmonary edema. The nurse should include strategies for which of the following in the care of the client?
  1 Decreasing cardiac output
  2 Increasing fluid volume
  3 Promoting a positive body image
  4 Reducing anxiety

Answer: 4
Rationale: When cardiac output falls as a result of acute pulmonary edema, the sympathetic nervous system is stimulated. Stimulation of the sympathetic nervous system results in the flight-or-fight reaction, which further impairs cardiac function. The goal of treatment is to increase cardiac output and decrease fluid volume. A disturbed body image is not a common problem experienced by clients with acute pulmonary edema.

Test-Taking Strategy: Use the process of elimination. Thinking about the physiological occurrences of this condition will assist in eliminating options 1, 2, and 3. Also recalling that severe dyspnea occurs should assist in directing you to the correct option. Review care of the client with pulmonary edema if you had difficulty with this question.

Level of Cognitive Ability: Application
Client Needs: Psychosocial Integrity
Integrated Process: Nursing Process/Implementation
Content Area: Adult Health/Cardiovascular

Reference:
Ignatavicius, D., & Workman, M. (2002). *Medical surgical nursing: Critical thinking for collaborative care* (4th ed.). Philadelphia: Saunders, p. 710.

---

147. A client with acute renal failure is having trouble remembering information and instructions as a result of altered laboratory values. The nurse avoids doing which of the following when communicating with this client?
  1 Giving simple, clear directions
  2 Explaining treatments using understandable language
  3 Including the family in discussions related to care
  4 Giving thorough, complete explanations of treatment options

Answer: 4
Rationale: The client with acute renal failure may have difficulty remembering information and instructions because of anxiety and altered laboratory values. Communications should be clear, simple, and understandable. The family is included whenever possible. It is the physician's responsibility to explain treatment options.

Test-Taking Strategy: Use the process of elimination and note the key word "avoids." This key word indicates a false-response question and that you need to select the option that identifies an incorrect nursing action. Recalling the basic principles of effective communication would lead you to recognize that options 1, 2, and 3 are helpful in maintaining effective communication. Review the basic principles of effective communication if you had difficulty with this question.

Level of Cognitive Ability: Application
Client Needs: Psychosocial Integrity
Integrated Process: Nursing Process/Implementation
Content Area: Adult Health/Renal

Reference:
Black, J., & Hawks, J. (2005). *Medical-surgical nursing: Clinical management for positive outcomes* (7th ed.). Philadelphia: Saunders, p. 948.

---

148. A rehabilitation nurse witnessed a postoperative coronary artery bypass graft client and spouse arguing after a rehabilitation session. The appropriate statement by the nurse in identifying the feelings of the client would be:
1 "You seem upset . . ."
2 "You shouldn't get upset. It'll affect your heart."
3 "Oh, don't let this get you down."
4 "It will seem better tomorrow, smile."

Answer: 1
Rationale: Acknowledging the client's feelings without inserting your own values or judgments is a method of therapeutic communication. Therapeutic communication techniques assist the flow of communication and always focus on the client. Option 1 is an open-ended statement that allows the client to verbalize, which gives the nurse a direction or clarification of the true feelings. Options 2, 3, and 4 do not encourage verbalization by the client.

Test-Taking Strategy: Use therapeutic communication techniques. Focusing on the issue, identifying the feelings of the client, will direct you to option 1. Review therapeutic communication techniques if you had difficulty with this question.

Level of Cognitive Ability: Application
Client Needs: Psychosocial Integrity
Integrated Process: Communication and Documentation
Content Area: Adult Health/Cardiovascular

Reference:
Potter, P., & Perry, A. (2005). *Fundamentals of nursing* (6th ed.). St. Louis: Mosby, p. 437.

---

149. An acutely psychotic client displays increased psychomotor activity. The nurse anticipates that the physician will prescribe which of the following for the client?
1 Sertraline hydrochloride (Zoloft)
2 Haloperidol (Haldol)
3 Chloral Hydrate (Noctec)
4 Isocarboxazid (Marplan)

Answer: 2
Rationale: Antipsychotics are used to treat acute and chronic psychosis, especially when the client has increased psychomotor activity. A fast-acting, injectable agent would be the medication of choice. Antidepressants (options 1 and 4) and hypnotics (option 3) are not indicated for the presenting condition.

Test-Taking Strategy: Use the process of elimination, focusing on the issue: increased psychomotor activity. Eliminate options 1 and 4 first because they are both antidepressants. From the remaining options, recalling that haloperidol is an antipsychotic will direct you to option 2. Review these medications if you had difficulty with this question.

Level of Cognitive Ability: Analysis
Client Needs: Psychosocial Integrity
Integrated Process: Nursing Process/Analysis
Content Area: Pharmacology

Reference:
McKenry, L., & Salerno, E. (2003). *Mosby's pharmacology in nursing* (21st ed.). St. Louis: Mosby, p. 400.

---

150. A client is admitted to the mental health unit with a diagnosis of panic disorder. The nurse anticipates that the physician will prescribe a benzodiazepine and checks the physician's order sheet for which medication order?
1 Imipramine (Tofranil)
2 Alprazolam (Xanax)
3 Buproprion (Wellbutrin)
4 Doxepin (Sinequan)

Answer: 2
Rationale: Options 1, 3, and 4 are classified as antidepressants and act by stimulating the central nervous system (CNS) to elevate mood. Alprazolam (Xanax), a benzodiazepine antianxiety agent, depresses the CNS and induces relaxation in panic disorders.

Test-Taking Strategy: Knowledge regarding panic disorders and the classification of the medications identified in the options is needed to answer this question. Eliminate options 1, 3, and 4 because they are similar and are antidepressants. Review these medications if you had difficulty with this question.

Level of Cognitive Ability: Analysis
Client Needs: Psychosocial Integrity
Integrated Process: Nursing Process/Analysis
Content Area: Pharmacology

References:
Lehne, R. (2004). *Pharmacology for nursing care* (5th ed.). Philadelphia: Saunders, p. 348.
McKenry, L., & Salerno, E. (2003). *Mosby's pharmacology in nursing* (21st ed.). St. Louis: Mosby, p. 337.

---

151. A client with empyema is to undergo decortication to remove the inflamed tissue, pus, and debris. The nurse offers emotional support to the client based on the understanding that:
1 The client is likely to be in excruciating pain after surgery
2 The client will probably have chronic dyspnea after the surgery
3 Chest tubes will be in place after surgery for some time, and the healing process is slow
4 This problem may decrease the client's life expectancy

Answer: 3
Rationale: The client undergoing decortication to treat empyema needs ongoing support by the nurse. This is especially true because the client will have chest tubes in place after surgery, which must remain until the former pus-filled space is completely obliterated. This may take some time and may be discouraging to the client. Progress is monitored by chest X-ray. Options 1, 2, and 4 are not accurate.

Test-Taking Strategy: Use the process of elimination. Option 4 is the least likely response and is eliminated first. Option 1 is eliminated next, because no client should be in "excruciating pain" postoperatively. From the remaining options, it is necessary to know that the client will need chest tubes and that it may take some time for full healing to occur. Recalling that the client has chest tubes after thoracic surgery may be sufficient to help you select between these last two options. Review the psychosocial aspects of care following decortication if you had difficulty with this question.

Level of Cognitive Ability: Analysis
Client Needs: Psychosocial Integrity
Integrated Process: Caring
Content Area: Adult Health/Respiratory

Reference:
Black, J., & Hawks, J. (2005). *Medical-surgical nursing: Clinical management for positive outcomes* (7th ed.). Philadelphia: Saunders, p. 1873.

152. A client who has never been hospitalized before is having trouble initiating the stream of urine. Knowing that there is no pathological reason for this difficulty, the nurse avoids which of the following because it is the least helpful method of assisting the client?

1 Running tap water in the sink
2 Instructing the client to pour warm water over the perineal area
3 Assisting the client to a commode behind a closed curtain
4 Closing the bathroom door and instructing the client to pull the call bell when done

Answer: 3

Rationale: Lack of privacy is a key issue that may inhibit the ability of the client to void in the absence of known pathology. Using a commode behind a curtain may inhibit voiding in some people. Use of a bathroom is preferable and may be supplemented with the use of running water or pouring water over the perineum as needed.

Test-Taking Strategy: Use the process of elimination and note the key words "least helpful." Think about the issue related to decreased privacy and its effects on elimination. Review measures to assist in promoting urinary elimination if you had difficulty with this question.

Level of Cognitive Ability: Application
Client Needs: Psychosocial Integrity
Integrated Process: Nursing Process/Implementation
Content Area: Adult Health/Renal

Reference:
Potter, P., & Perry, A. (2005). *Fundamentals of nursing* (6th ed.). St. Louis: Mosby, p. 1327.

---

153. A client tells the nurse, "My doctor says I can have the surgery and go home the same day but I'm afraid. My husband's dead and my son is 3,000 miles away. I'm alone and what happens if something goes wrong? I'm not supposed to be up walking unless absolutely necessary." The nurse makes which therapeutic response to the client?

1 "I know, I know. They say, Managed Care is no Care! Have you got an alarm system so if you fall, it will alert someone to come? If worse comes to worse, call me and I'll come immediately."
2 "Don't worry. This procedure is done all the time without any problems. You'll be fine!"
3 "Your concern is well voiced. I advise you to call your son and insist he come home immediately! You can't be too careful."
4 "You seem very concerned about going home without help. Have you discussed your concerns with your doctor?"

Answer: 4

Rationale: The client has verbalized concerns. In option 4, the nurse uses reflection to direct the client's feelings and concerns. In option 1, the nurse is ventilating the nurse's own anger, frustration, and powerlessness. In addition, the nurse is trying to problem solve for the client but is overly controlling and takes the decision making out of the client's hands. In option 2, the nurse provides false reassurance and then minimizes the client's concerns. In option 3, the nurse is projecting the client's own fears, and the problem solving suggested by the nurse will increase fear and anxiety in the client.

Test-Taking Strategy: Use therapeutic communication techniques. Remember that the priority is to address the client's feelings. Option 4 is the only option that addresses the feelings and concerns of the client. Review therapeutic communication techniques if you had difficulty with this question.

Level of Cognitive Ability: Application
Client Needs: Psychosocial Integrity
Integrated Process: Communication and Documentation
Content Area: Mental Health

References:
Stuart, G., & Laraia, M. (2005). *Principles and practice of psychiatric nursing* (8th ed.). St. Louis: Mosby, pp. 30-31.
Varcarolis, E.M. (2002). *Foundations of psychiatric mental health nursing* (4th ed.). Philadelphia: Saunders, p. 673.

154. During the nursing assessment, the client says, "My doctor just told me that my cancer has spread and that I have less than 6 months to live." Which of the following nursing responses would be therapeutic?

1 "I know it seems desperate, but there have been a lot of breakthroughs. Something might come along in a month or so to change your status drastically."

2 "I hope you'll focus on the fact that your doctor says you have 6 months to live and that you'll think of how you'd like to live."

3 "I am sorry. There are no easy answers in times like this, are there?"

4 "I am sorry. Would you like to discuss this with me some more?"

Answer: 4

Rationale: The client has received very distressing news. The client is most likely still in the stage of shock and denial. In the correct option, the nurse invites the client to ventilate. Option 1 provides a social communication and false hope. Option 2 is patronizing and stereotypical. Option 3 is social and expresses the nurse's feelings rather than the client's feelings.

Test-Taking Strategy: Use therapeutic communication techniques. Note that option 4 is providing the opportunity for the client to express feelings. Remember to focus on the client's feelings. Review therapeutic communication techniques if you had difficulty with this question.

Level of Cognitive Ability: Application
Client Needs: Psychosocial Integrity
Integrated Process: Communication and Documentation
Content Area: Adult Health/Oncology

Reference:
Potter, P., & Perry, A. (2005). *Fundamentals of nursing* (6th ed.). St. Louis: Mosby, p. 437.

155. A client with an endotracheal tube gets easily frustrated when trying to communicate personal needs to the nurse. The nurse determines that which of the following methods for communication may be the easiest for the client?

1 Have the family interpret needs

2 Use a picture or word board

3 Use a pad and paper

4 Devise a system of hand signals

Answer: 2

Rationale: The client with an endotracheal tube in place cannot speak. The nurse devises an alternative communication system with the client. Use of a picture or word board is the simplest method of communication, because it requires only pointing at the word or object. A pad and pencil is an acceptable alternative, but it requires more client effort and more time. The use of hand signals may not be a reliable method, because it may not meet all needs and is subject to misinterpretation. The family does not need to bear the burden of communicating the client's needs, and they may not understand them either.

Test-Taking Strategy: Note the key words "frustrated" and "easiest." Options 3 and 4 are not the "easiest" and are therefore eliminated first. Because the family may not necessarily know what the client is trying to communicate, this option could cause added frustration for the client. Review alternative methods of communication if you had difficulty with this question.

Level of Cognitive Ability: Analysis
Client Needs: Psychosocial Integrity
Integrated Process: Communication and Documentation
Content Area: Adult Health/Respiratory

Reference:
Black, J., & Hawks, J. (2005). *Medical-surgical nursing: Clinical management for positive outcomes* (7th ed.). Philadelphia: Saunders, p. 1893.

156. A home care nurse visits a client who is receiving total parenteral nutrition (TPN) in the home. The client states, "I really miss eating with my family at dinner." The nurse makes which therapeutic response to the client?
1 "It is normal to miss something as basic as eating."
2 "I think in a few weeks you will probably be allowed to eat a little."
3 "Tell me more about how you feel about dinner time."
4 "You could sit with your family at dinner time anyway even if you do not eat."

Answer: 3
Rationale: The nurse assists the client to express feelings and deal with the aspects of illness and treatment. In option 3, the nurse uses clarifying and focusing to encourage the client to explore concerns. Blocks to communication such as giving opinions and changing the subject will stop the client from verbalizing feelings.

Test-Taking Strategy: Use therapeutic communication techniques. Always focus on client feelings first. This will direct you to option 3. Review therapeutic communication techniques if you had difficulty with this question.

Level of Cognitive Ability: Application
Client Needs: Psychosocial Integrity
Integrated Process: Communication and Documentation
Content Area: Fundamental Skills

Reference:
Potter, P., & Perry, A. (2005). *Fundamentals of nursing* (6th ed.). St. Louis: Mosby, p. 437.

157. A client has been receiving maprotiline (Ludiomil). The nurse notifies the health care provider if which adverse client response to the medication is noted?
1 Increased sense of well-being
2 Reported decrease in anxiety
3 Increased drowsiness
4 Increased appetite

Answer: 3
Rationale: Maprotiline is a tricyclic antidepressant used to treat various forms of depression and anxiety. The client is also often in psychotherapy while on this medication. Expected effects of the medication include improved sense of well-being, appetite, and sleep, as well as a reduced sense of anxiety. Common side effects to report to the health care provider include drowsiness, lethargy, and fatigue.

Test-Taking Strategy: Focus on the issue: an adverse response. Recall that this medication is an antidepressant. It would seem reasonable to expect options 1, 2, and 4 to occur as a positive response to this medication. Review this medication if you had difficulty with this question.

Level of Cognitive Ability: Analysis
Client Needs: Psychosocial Integrity
Integrated Process: Nursing Process/Evaluation
Content Area: Pharmacology

Reference:
Hodgson, B., & Kizior, R. (2004). *Saunders nursing drug handbook 2004.* Philadelphia: Saunders, p. 627.

158. A client who is to undergo thoracentesis is afraid of not being able to tolerate the procedure. The nurse interprets that the client needs honest support and reassurance, which can best be accomplished by which of the following statements?

1 "The procedure only takes 1 to 2 minutes, so you might try to get through it by mentally counting up to 120."

2 "The needle is a little uncomfortable going in, but this is controlled by rhythmically breathing in and out. I'll be with you to coach your breathing."

3 "The needle hurts when it goes in and you must remain still. I'll stay with you throughout the entire procedure and help you hold your position."

4 "I'll be right by your side, but the procedure will be totally painless as long as you don't move."

Answer: 3

Rationale: The needle insertion for thoracentesis is painful for the client. The nurse tells the client how important it is to remain still during the procedure, so the needle doesn't injure visceral pleura or lung tissue. The nurse reassures the client during the procedure and helps the client hold the proper position. Options 1, 2, and 4 are inaccurate statements.

Test-Taking Strategy: Use the process of elimination and therapeutic communication techniques. Recalling that the client must remain still during the procedure helps you eliminate option 2 first. Knowing that the procedure may be painful for the client and takes longer than 1 to 2 minutes helps you eliminate options 1 and 4. Review this procedure if you had difficulty with this question.

Level of Cognitive Ability: Application
Client Needs: Psychosocial Integrity
Integrated Process: Communication and Documentation
Content Area: Adult Health/Respiratory

Reference:
Chernecky, C., & Berger, B. (2004). *Laboratory tests and diagnostic procedures* (4th ed.). Philadelphia: Saunders, p. 1043.

159. A client with chronic respiratory failure is dyspneic. The client becomes anxious, which worsens the feelings of dyspnea. The nurse teaches the client which of the following methods to best interrupt the dyspnea-anxiety-dyspnea cycle?

1 Relaxation and breathing techniques
2 Biofeedback and coughing techniques
3 Guided imagery and limiting fluids
4 Distraction and increased dietary carbohydrates

Answer: 1

Rationale: The anxious client with dyspnea should be taught interventions to decrease anxiety, which include relaxation, biofeedback, guided imagery, and distraction. This will stop the escalation of feelings of anxiety and dyspnea. The dyspnea can be further controlled by teaching the client breathing techniques, which include pursed lip and diaphragmatic breathing. Coughing techniques are useful, but breathing techniques are more effective. Limiting fluids will thicken secretions and increased dietary carbohydrates will increase production of CO_2 by the body.

Test-Taking Strategy: Focus on the issue, relieving anxiety and dyspnea, and note the key word "best." Limiting fluids and increasing carbohydrates are contraindicated and are therefore eliminated. From the remaining options, recall that breathing techniques are more effective than coughing techniques. This will direct you to option 1. Review measures to relieve anxiety and dyspnea in the client with respiratory failure if you had difficulty with this question.

Level of Cognitive Ability: Application
Client Needs: Psychosocial Integrity
Integrated Process: Teaching/Learning
Content Area: Adult Health/Respiratory

References:
Black, J., & Hawks, J. (2005). *Medical-surgical nursing: Clinical management for positive outcomes* (7th ed.). Philadelphia: Saunders, p. 1825.
Ignatavicius, D., & Workman, M. (2002). *Medical surgical nursing: Critical thinking for collaborative care* (4th ed.). Philadelphia: Saunders, p. 86.

160. A client who has had drainage of a pleural effusion is in pain. Which intervention is least helpful in providing support to this client?
1 Offering verbal support and reassurance
2 Assisting the client to find positions of comfort
3 Leaving the client alone for an extended rest period
4 Providing pain medication for the client

Answer: 3

Rationale: The pain associated with drainage of pleural effusion is minimized by positioning the client for comfort and administering analgesics for relief of pain. The nurse also offers verbal support and reassurance. All of these measures help the client cope with the pain and discomfort associated with this problem. It is least helpful to leave the client alone for extended periods, because the client may experience continued pain, which may be augmented by isolation.

Test-Taking Strategy: Use the process of elimination, noting the key words "least helpful" in the stem of the question. Noting the words "alone" and "extended" in option 3 will direct you to this option. Review the psychosocial measures that provide support to a client in pain if you had difficulty with this question.

Level of Cognitive Ability: Application
Client Needs: Psychosocial Integrity
Integrated Process: Caring
Content Area: Fundamental Skills

Reference:
Black, J., & Hawks, J. (2005). *Medical-surgical nursing: Clinical management for positive outcomes* (7th ed.). Philadelphia: Saunders, pp. 453-454; 1872-1873.

---

161. A nurse is caring for a client who has just experienced a pulmonary embolism. The client is restless and very anxious. The nurse uses which approach in communicating with this client?
1 Explaining each treatment in great detail
2 Having the family reinforce the nurse's directions
3 Giving simple, clear directions and explanations
4 Speaking very little to the client until the crisis is over

Answer: 3

Rationale: The client who has suffered pulmonary embolism is fearful and apprehensive. The nurse effectively communicates with this client by staying with the client, providing simple, clear, and accurate information, and displaying a calm, efficient manner. Options 1, 2, and 4 will produce more anxiety for the client and family.

Test-Taking Strategy: Use the process of elimination. Eliminate option 1 because of the words "great detail." Next eliminate option 4 because of the words "speaking very little." From the remaining options, having the family reinforce the directions may place stress on the family and provide too much sensory input for the client. This will direct you to option 3. Review communication strategies for the client who is restless and anxious if you had difficulty with this question.

Level of Cognitive Ability: Application
Client Needs: Psychosocial Integrity
Integrated Process: Communication and Documentation
Content Area: Adult Health/Respiratory

Reference:
Black, J., & Hawks, J. (2005). *Medical-surgical nursing: Clinical management for positive outcomes* (7th ed.). Philadelphia: Saunders, p. 529.

162. A nurse in the emergency room is admitting a client with carbon monoxide poisoning from a suicide attempt. The nurse ensures that which most needed service is put in place for the client?
1 Pulmonary rehabilitation
2 Occupational therapy
3 Psychiatric consult
4 Neurological consult

Answer: 3
Rationale: The client with carbon monoxide poisoning as a result of a suicide attempt should have a psychiatric consult. The necessity of a neurological consult would depend on the sequelae to the nervous system from the carbon monoxide poisoning, and there is no data in the question indicating this need. Occupational therapy and pulmonary rehabilitation are not indicated.

Test-Taking Strategy: Focus on the client's diagnosis and note the key words "most needed." Eliminate occupational therapy first, because there is no indication of the need for that service. The client will need respiratory therapy, but not pulmonary rehabilitation, so option 1 is eliminated next. A neurological consult could be beneficial, but only if the client suffers long-term central nervous system damage from this suicide attempt. Review care of the client who attempted suicide if you had difficulty with this question.

Level of Cognitive Ability: Application
Client Needs: Psychosocial Integrity
Integrated Process: Nursing Process/Implementation
Content Area: Mental Health

Reference:
Stuart, G., & Laraia, M. (2005). *Principles and practice of psychiatric nursing* (8th ed.). St. Louis: Mosby, pp. 370-371.

163. A nurse is caring for a young adult diagnosed with sarcoidiosis. The client is angry and tells the nurse there is no point in learning disease management, because there is no possibility of ever being cured. The nurse formulates which nursing diagnosis for this client?
1 Disturbed Thought Processes
2 Ineffective Health Maintenance
3 Anxiety
4 Powerlessness

Answer: 4
Rationale: The client with Powerlessness expresses feelings of having no control over a situation or outcome. Ineffective Health Maintenance involves the inability to seek out help that is needed to maintain health. Anxiety is a vague sense of unease. Disturbed Thought Processes involves disruption in cognitive abilities or thought.

Test-Taking Strategy: Use the process of elimination and note the data in the question. Focusing on the issue, anger over a situation in which the client has little control, will direct you to option 4. Review the definitions of these nursing diagnoses if you had difficulty with this question.

Level of Cognitive Ability: Analysis
Client Needs: Psychosocial Integrity
Integrated Process: Nursing Process/Analysis
Content Area: Adult Health/Respiratory

Reference:
Stuart, G., & Laraia, M. (2005). *Principles and practice of psychiatric nursing* (8th ed.). St. Louis: Mosby, p. 245.

164. A client immobilized in skeletal leg traction complains of being bored and restless. Based on these complaints, the nurse formulates which nursing diagnosis for this client?
1 Deficient Diversional Activity
2 Powerlessness
3 Self-Care Deficit
4 Impaired Physical Mobility

Answer: 1

Rationale: A major defining characteristic of Deficient Diversional Activity is expression of boredom by the client. The question does not identify difficulties with coordination, range of motion, or muscle strength, which would indicate Impaired Physical Mobility. The question also does not identify client feelings of inability to perform activities of daily living (Self-Care Deficit) or lack of control (Powerlessness).

Test-Taking Strategy: Use the process of elimination, focusing on the data in the question. Noting the key words "bored and restless" will direct you to option 1. Review the defining characteristics of Deficient Diversional Activity if you had difficulty with this question.

Level of Cognitive Ability: Analysis
Client Needs: Psychosocial Integrity
Integrated Process: Nursing Process/Analysis
Content Area: Adult Health/Musculoskeletal

Reference:
Black, J., & Hawks, J. (2005). *Medical-surgical nursing: Clinical management for positive outcomes* (7th ed.). Philadelphia: Saunders, p. 637.

---

165. A client being mechanically ventilated after experiencing a fat embolus is visibly anxious. The nurse would take which appropriate action?
1 Encourage the client to sleep until arterial blood gas results improve
2 Ask a family member to stay with the client at all times
3 Ask the physician for an order for succinylcholine (Anectine)
4 Provide reassurance to the client and give small doses of morphine sulfate intravenously as prescribed

Answer: 4

Rationale: The nurse always speaks to the client calmly and provides reassurance to the anxious client. Morphine sulfate is often prescribed for pain and anxiety for the client receiving mechanical ventilation. In option 1, the nurse does nothing to reassure or help the client. It is not beneficial to ask the family to take on the burden of remaining with the client at all times. Succinylcholine is a paralyzing agent, but has no antianxiety properties.

Test-Taking Strategy: Use the process of elimination. Note that the client is anxious. Option 4 is the only option in which the nurse interacts with the client. Also note the words "provide reassurance" in the correct option. Review measures to relieve anxiety if you had difficulty with this question.

Level of Cognitive Ability: Application
Client Needs: Psychosocial Integrity
Integrated Process: Nursing Process/Implementation
Content Area: Adult Health/Respiratory

Reference:
Black, J., & Hawks, J. (2005). *Medical-surgical nursing: Clinical management for positive outcomes* (7th ed.). Philadelphia: Saunders, p. 1891.

166. A nurse is assessing a confused older client admitted to the hospital with a hip fracture. Which of the following data obtained by the nurse would prevent the risk for Disturbed Thought Processes?
1   Stress induced by the fracture
2   Hearing aid available and in working order
3   Unfamiliar hospital setting
4   Eyeglasses left at home

Answer: 2
Rationale: Confusion in the older client with a hip fracture could result from the unfamiliar hospital setting, stress caused by the fracture, concurrent systemic diseases, cerebral ischemia, or side effects of medications. Use of eyeglasses and hearing aids enhance the client's interaction with the environment and can reduce disorientation.

Test-Taking Strategy: Note the key word "prevent." This key word indicates that you need to select an option that will keep the client at the highest possible level of functioning from a cognitive perspective. Stress from the fracture (option 1) and an unfamiliar setting (option 3) is not likely to help the client's functional level, and these options are eliminated. Eyeglasses and hearing aids are both useful adjuncts in communicating with a client. Because the eyeglasses were left at home, they are of no use at the current time. Review the factors that place a hospitalized client at risk for Disturbed Thought Processes if you had difficulty with this question.

Level of Cognitive Ability: Analysis
Client Needs: Psychosocial Integrity
Integrated Process: Nursing Process/Assessment
Content Area: Fundamental Skills

Reference:
Black, J., & Hawks, J. (2005). *Medical-surgical nursing: Clinical management for positive outcomes* (7th ed.). Philadelphia: Saunders, p. 641.

---

167. A client is admitted to the nursing unit after a left below-the-knee amputation following a crush injury to the foot and lower leg. The client tells the nurse, "I think I'm going crazy. I can feel my left foot itching." The nurse interprets the client's statement to be:
1   A normal response, and indicates the presence of phantom limb sensation
2   A normal response, and indicates the presence of phantom limb pain
3   An abnormal response, and indicates that the client needs more psychological support
4   An abnormal response, and indicates that the client is in denial about the limb loss

Answer: 1
Rationale: Phantom limb sensations are felt in the area of the amputated limb. These can include itching, warmth, and cold. The sensations are caused by intact peripheral nerves in the area amputated. Whenever possible, clients should be prepared that they may experience these sensations. The client may also feel painful sensations in the amputated limb, called phantom limb pain. The origin of the pain is less well understood, but the client should be prepared for this, too, whenever possible. This is not an abnormal response.

Test-Taking Strategy: Focus on the client's complaint: itching. Recalling that sensation and pain may be felt in the residual limb eliminates options 3 and 4 first, because these feelings are not abnormal responses. From the remaining options, select option 1 because the client has complained of an itching sensation, but has not complained of pain in the residual limb. Review the expected findings in a client who had an amputation if you had difficulty with this question.

Level of Cognitive Ability: Analysis
Client Needs: Psychosocial Integrity
Integrated Process: Nursing Process/Analysis
Content Area: Adult Health/Cardiovascular

Reference:
Black, J., & Hawks, J. (2005). *Medical-surgical nursing: Clinical management for positive outcomes* (7th ed.). Philadelphia: Saunders, p. 450.

---

168. A client who has had a spinal fusion with insertion of hardware is extremely concerned with the perceived lengthy rehabilitation period. The client expresses concerns about finances and the ability to return to prior employment. The nurse understands that the client's needs could best be addressed by referral to the:

1 Surgeon
2 Clinical nurse specialist
3 Social worker
4 Physical therapist

Answer: 3
Rationale: Following spinal surgery, concerns about finances and employment are best handled by referral to a social worker. This individual is able to provide information about resources available to the client. The physical therapist has the best knowledge of techniques for increasing mobility and endurance. The clinical nurse specialist and surgeon would not have the necessary information related to financial resources.

Test-Taking Strategy: Use the process of elimination. Focusing on the client's concern about finances, and thinking about the role of each health care worker identified in the options, will direct you to option 3. Review the roles of these health care workers if you had difficulty with this question.

Level of Cognitive Ability: Analysis
Client Needs: Psychosocial Integrity
Integrated Process: Nursing Process/Planning
Content Area: Fundamental Skills

Reference:
Harkreader, H., & Hogan, M.A. (2004). *Fundamentals of nursing: caring and clinical judgment.* (2nd ed.). Philadelphia: Saunders, pp. 60-1094.

---

169. A client is fearful about having an arm cast removed. Which action by the nurse would be helpful to alleviate the client's fear?

1 Telling the client that the saw makes a frightening noise
2 Reassuring the client that no one has had an arm lacerated yet
3 Stating that the hot cutting blades have rarely caused burns
4 Showing the client the cast cutter and explaining how it works

Answer: 4
Rationale: Clients may be fearful of having a cast removed because of the cast cutting blade. The nurse should show the cast cutter to the client before it is used, and explain that the client may feel heat, vibration, and pressure. The cast cutter resembles a small electric saw with a circular blade. The nurse should reassure the client that the blade does not cut like a saw, but instead cuts the cast by vibrating side to side. Options 1, 2, and 3 are inappropriate and may increase the client's fear.

Test-Taking Strategy: Use the process of elimination, noting the key word "helpful." Focusing on the issue, the client's fear, will direct you to option 4. Option 4 gives the client the most reassurance because it best prepares the client for what will occur when the cast is removed. Review measures to relieve fear in a client preparing for a procedure if you had difficulty with this question.

Level of Cognitive Ability: Application
Client Needs: Psychosocial Integrity
Integrated Process: Nursing Process/Implementation
Content Area: Adult Health/Musculoskeletal

References:
Ignatavicius, D., & Workman, M. (2002). *Medical surgical nursing: Critical thinking for collaborative care* (4th ed.). Philadelphia: Saunders, p. 1136.
Potter, P., & Perry, A. (2005). *Fundamentals of nursing* (6th ed.). St. Louis: Mosby, p. 1601.

170. A client has several fractures of the lower leg and has been placed in an external fixation device. The client is upset about the appearance of the leg, which is very edematous. The nurse formulates which nursing diagnosis for the client?
1 Disturbed Body Image
2 Activity Intolerance
3 Risk for Impaired Physical Mobility
4 Social Isolation

Answer: 1
Rationale: The client is at risk for Disturbed Body Image related to a change in the structure and function of the affected leg. There is no data in the question to support a diagnosis of (actual) Activity Intolerance or Social Isolation. The client has an actual (not a risk for) Impaired Mobility because of the fixation device.

Test-Taking Strategy: Use the process of elimination, focusing on the data in the question. Noting the key words "upset about the appearance of the leg" will direct you to option 1. Review the defining characteristics for Disturbed Body Image if you had difficulty with this question.

Level of Cognitive Ability: Analysis
Client Needs: Psychosocial Integrity
Integrated Process: Nursing Process/Analysis
Content Area: Adult Health/Musculoskeletal

Reference:
Black, J., & Hawks, J. (2005). *Medical-surgical nursing: Clinical management for positive outcomes* (7th ed.). Philadelphia: Saunders, p. 1423.

171. A client and her husband are being discharged from the hospital after giving birth to a fetal demise. They ask about the possibility of attending a bereavement support group in the community. The nurse is aware that this is an indication of:
1 Denial
2 Prolonged sadness
3 Normal grieving
4 Anger

Answer: 3
Rationale: A perinatal bereavement support group can help the parents work through their pain by nonjudgmental sharing of feelings. It is a necessary part of normal grieving. The parents' request is not indicative of denial, prolonged sadness, or anger.

Test-Taking Strategy: Use the process of elimination, focusing on the issue of the question. Focus on the parents' request to assist in directing you to option 3. Review the normal grieving process if you had difficulty with this question.

Level of Cognitive Ability: Comprehension
Client Needs: Psychosocial Integrity
Integrated Process: Nursing Process/Analysis
Content Area: Maternity/Postpartum

References:
Potter, P., & Perry, A. (2005). *Fundamentals of nursing* (6th ed.). St. Louis: Mosby, p. 437.
McKinney, E., James, S., Murray, S., & Ashwill, J. (2005). *Maternal-child nursing* (2nd ed.). St. Louis: Elsevier, pp. 1223-1224.

172. A client was just told by the primary care physician that she will have an exercise stress test to evaluate the client's status after recent episodes of more severe chest pain. As the nurse enters the examining room, the client states, "Maybe I shouldn't bother going. I wonder if I should just take more medication instead." The nurse makes which therapeutic response to the client?

1 "Can you tell me more about how you're feeling?"

2 "Don't worry. Emergency equipment is available if it should be needed."

3 "Most people tolerate the procedure well without any complications."

4 "Don't you really want to control your heart disease?"

Answer: 1

Rationale: Anxiety and fear are often present before stress testing. The nurse should explore a client's feelings if concerns are expressed. Options 2, 3, and 4 are inappropriate statements and limit communication. Option 1 is open-ended and is the only option that is phrased to engender trust and sharing of concerns by the client.

Test-Taking Strategy: Use therapeutic communication techniques and the process of elimination. Remember to focus on the client's feelings. This will direct you to option 1. Review therapeutic communication techniques if you had difficulty with this question.

Level of Cognitive Ability: Application
Client Needs: Psychosocial Integrity
Integrated Process: Communication and Documentation
Content Area: Adult Health/Cardiovascular

Reference:
Potter, P., & Perry, A. (2005). *Fundamentals of nursing* (6th ed.). St. Louis: Mosby, p. 437.

173. A nurse is giving a client with heart failure home care instructions for use after hospital discharge. The client interrupts, saying, "What's the use? I'll never remember all of this, and I'll probably die anyway!" The nurse interprets that the client's response is most likely due to:

1 The teaching strategies used by the nurse

2 Anger about the new medical regimen

3 Insufficient financial resources to pay for the medications

4 Anxiety about the ability to manage the disease process at home

Answer: 4

Rationale: Anxiety and fear often develops after heart failure and can further tax the failing heart. The client's statement is made in the middle of receiving self-care instructions. There is no evidence in the question to support options 1, 2, or 3.

Test-Taking Strategy: Use the process of elimination. Focus on the data in the question. Note that the client's comment is made when preparing for self-care at home, which implies anxiety about disease self-management. Review the psychosocial concerns for a client with heart failure if you had difficulty with this question.

Level of Cognitive Ability: Analysis
Client Needs: Psychosocial Integrity
Integrated Process: Nursing Process/Analysis
Content Area: Adult Health/Cardiovascular

Reference:
Ignatavicius, D., & Workman, M. (2002). *Medical surgical nursing: Critical thinking for collaborative care* (4th ed.). Philadelphia: Saunders, p. 711.

174. Prior to initiating intravenous (IV) therapy, the nurse notes nonverbal signs of anxiety in the client. In order to help relieve the anxiety, the nurse should explain the procedure of IV initiation to the client. Which statement would be appropriate for the nurse to say to the client?

1 "I'll be starting an IV that will add fluid directly to your blood stream."
2 "I will be starting an IV, and it should not hurt much."
3 "A number eighteen angiocatheter will be inserted into your arm so fluid can be administered."
4 "Try not to worry. This procedure won't take long and will be over with before you know it."

Answer: 1

Rationale: Option 1 explains what an IV is in simple terms. Option 2 is incorrect and gives the client unwarranted reassurance because initiating an IV can be painful. Eliminate option 3 because the terminology of an 18-gauge angiocatheter is medical and will not be understood by the client. Suggesting the client not worry is a cliché and blocks client communication about fears and feelings.

Test Taking Strategy: Use therapeutic communication techniques. Remembering to avoid the use of medical jargon and terminology that clients will not understand will eliminate option 3. Eliminate option 4 because the client should not be told "not to worry." Eliminate option 2 because inserting an IV is painful. Review this procedure and therapeutic communication techniques if you had difficulty with this question.

Level of Cognitive Ability: Application
Client Needs: Psychosocial Integrity
Integrated Process: Communication and Documentation
Content Area: Fundamental Skills

Reference:
Potter, P., & Perry, A. (2005). *Fundamentals of nursing* (6th ed.). St. Louis: Mosby, p. 437.

175. A client scheduled for the insertion of an implanted port for intermittent chemotherapy treatments says, "I'm not sure if I can handle having a tube coming out of me all the time. What will my friends think?" Based on the client's statements, the nurse plans to do which of the following first?

1 Show the client various central line tubes and catheters
2 Explain that an implanted port is placed under the skin and is not visible
3 Notify the physician of the client's concerns
4 Explain that the client's friends probably will not see the tube under the clothing

Answer: 2

Rationale: An implanted port is placed under the skin and is not visible. There is no tubing external to the body. Tubing is used only when the port is accessed intermittently and the IV line is connected. Showing the client various other tubes will not be beneficial because the client will not be using them. It is premature to notify the physician. Option 4 does not correct the client's confusion regarding the implanted port.

Test-Taking Strategy: Use the process of elimination. Note the key words "implanted port" in the question and the relation to option 2. Review the concepts related to implanted catheters and the teaching/learning process if you had difficulty with this question.

Level of Cognitive Ability: Application
Client Needs: Psychosocial Integrity
Integrated Process: Teaching/Learning
Content Area: Fundamental Skills

Reference:
Potter, P., & Perry, A. (2005). *Fundamentals of nursing* (6th ed.). St. Louis: Mosby, pp. 451-454.

176. A client displays signs of anxiety when the nurse explains that the IV will need to be discontinued due to an infiltration. The nurse makes which appropriate statement to the client?
  1 "This will be a totally painless experience. It is nothing to worry about."
  2 "I'm sure it will be a real relief for you just as soon as I discontinue this IV for good."
  3 "Just relax and take a deep breath. This procedure will not take long and will be over soon."
  4 "I can see that you're anxious. Removal of the IV shouldn't be painful, but the IV will need to be restarted in another location."

Answer: 4
Rationale: Although discontinuing an IV is a painless experience, it is not therapeutic to tell a client not to worry. Option 2 does not acknowledge the client's feelings and does not tell the client that an infiltrated IV may need to be restarted. Option 3 does not address the client's feelings. Option 4 addresses the client's anxiety and honestly informs the client that the IV may need to be restarted. This option uses the therapeutic technique of giving information as well as acknowledging the client's feelings.

Test-Taking Strategy: Use therapeutic communication techniques, recalling that an infiltrated IV may need to be restarted. This will direct you to option 4. Also note that the correct option acknowledges the client's feelings. Review therapeutic communication techniques if you had difficulty with this question.

Level of Cognitive Ability: Application
Client Needs: Psychosocial Integrity
Integrated Process: Communication and Documentation
Content Area: Fundamental Skills

Reference:
Potter, P., & Perry, A. (2005). *Fundamentals of nursing* (6th ed.). St. Louis: Mosby, p. 437.

177. A toddler with suspected conjunctivitis is crying and refuses to sit still during the eye examination. Which of the following is the most appropriate nursing statement to the child?
  1 "If you will sit still, the exam will be over soon."
  2 "Would you like to see my flashlight?"
  3 "I know you are upset. We can do this exam later."
  4 "Don't be scared, the light won't hurt you."

Answer: 2
Rationale: Fears in this age group can be decreased by getting the child actively involved in the examination. Option 1 ignores the toddler's feelings. Option 3, although acknowledging feelings, falsely puts off the inevitable. Option 4 tells the toddler how to feel.

Test-Taking Strategy: Use knowledge regarding the stages of growth and development, noting that the child is a toddler. Also, the use of therapeutic communication techniques will direct you to option 2. Review growth and development related to the toddler if you had difficulty with this question.

Level of Cognitive Ability: Application
Client Needs: Psychosocial Integrity
Integrated Process: Communication and Documentation
Content Area: Child Health

Reference:
Wong, D., & Hockenberry, M. (2003). *Wong's nursing care of infants and children* (7th ed.). St. Louis: Mosby, p. 173.

178. A client with acute pyelonephritis is scheduled for a voiding cystourethrogram. The client is very shy and modest. The nurse interprets that this client would benefit from increased support and teaching about the procedure because:
1 Radiopaque contrast is injected into the bloodstream
2 Radioactive material is inserted into the bladder
3 The client must lie on an X-ray table in a cold, barren room
4 The client must void while the voiding process is filmed

Answer: 4
Rationale: Having to void in the presence of others can be very embarrassing for clients and may actually interfere with the client's ability to void. The nurse teaches the client about the procedure to try to minimize stress from lack of preparation and gives the client encouragement and emotional support. Screens may be used in the radiology department to try to provide an element of privacy during this procedure. Options 1, 2, and 3 are incorrect and do not address the issue of support.

Test-Taking Strategy: Use the process of elimination and knowledge regarding this procedure. Noting the key words "shy" and "modest" will direct you to option 4. Review this procedure if you had difficulty with this question.

Level of Cognitive Ability: Analysis
Client Needs: Psychosocial Integrity
Integrated Process: Nursing Process/Analysis
Content Area: Adult Health/Renal

Reference:
Chernecky, C., & Berger, B. (2004). *Laboratory tests and diagnostic procedures* (4th ed.). Philadelphia: Saunders, pp. 450-451.

179. A female client who is in a manic state emerges from her room. She is topless and is making sexual remarks and gestures toward staff and peers. The best initial nursing action is to:
1 Quietly approach the client, escort her to her room, and assist her in getting dressed
2 Approach the client in the hallway and insist that she go to her room
3 Confront the client on the inappropriateness of her behavior and offer her a time-out
4 Ask the other clients to ignore her behavior; eventually she will return to her room

Answer: 1
Rationale: A person who is experiencing mania lacks insight and judgment, has poor impulse control, and is highly excitable. The nurse must take control without creating increased stress or anxiety to the client. "Insisting" the client go to her room may meet with a great deal of resistance. Confronting the client and offering her a consequence of "time-out" may be meaningless to her. Asking other clients to ignore her is inappropriate. A quiet, firm approach while distracting the client (walking her to her room and assisting her to get dressed) achieves the goal of having her dressed appropriately and preserving her psychosocial integrity.

Test-Taking Strategy: Use the process of elimination, noting that the client is in a "manic state." Recalling that the nurse must take control to protect the client will direct you to option 1. Review care of the client with mania if you had difficulty with this question.

Level of Cognitive Ability: Application
Client Needs: Psychosocial Integrity
Integrated Process: Nursing Process/Implementation
Content Area: Mental Health

Reference:
Stuart, G., & Laraia, M. (2005). *Principles and practice of psychiatric nursing* (8th ed.). St. Louis: Mosby, p. 336.

180. Both the client who had cardiac surgery and the client's family express anxiety about how to cope with the recuperative process once they are home alone after discharge. The nurse plans to tell the client and family about which available resource?
1 Local library
2 United Way
3 American Heart Association Mended Heart's Club
4 American Cancer Society Reach for Recovery

Answer: 3

Rationale: Most clients and families benefit from knowing there are available resources to help them cope with the stress of self-care management at home. These can include telephone contact with the surgeon, cardiologist, and nurse; post-cardiac surgery sponsored cardiac rehabilitation programs; and community support groups such as the American Heart Association Mended Heart's Club (a nationwide program with local chapters). The United Way provides a wide variety of services to people who might otherwise not afford them. The American Cancer Society Reach for Recovery helps women recover after mastectomy. The library does not normally provide resources to cope.

Test-Taking Strategy: Use the process of elimination. Note that the options identify three organizations and a library. Eliminate the library first because the client and family need resources to cope, implying the need for interactive processes. From the remaining options, noting that the client had cardiac surgery will direct you to option 3. Review the support services for clients who have had cardiac surgery if you had difficulty with this question.

Level of Cognitive Ability: Application
Client Needs: Psychosocial Integrity
Integrated Process: Nursing Process/Planning
Content Area: Adult Health/Cardiovascular

References:
Black, J., & Hawks, J. (2005). *Medical-surgical nursing: Clinical management for positive outcomes* (7th ed.). Philadelphia: Saunders, p. 1644.
Lewis, S., Heitkemper, M., & Dirksen, S. (2004). *Medical-surgical nursing: Assessment and management of clinical problems* (6th ed.). St. Louis: Mosby, p. 843.
Phipps, W., Monahan, F., Sands, J., Marek, J., & Neighbors, M. (2003). *Medical-surgical nursing: Health and illness perspectives* (7th ed.). St. Louis: Mosby, p. 88.

181. An older client who has never been hospitalized before is to have a 12-lead electrocardiogram (ECG). The nurse would alleviate the client's anxiety about the test by giving which of the following explanations?
1 "The ECG can give the doctor information about what might be wrong with your heart."
2 "It's important to lie still during the procedure."
3 "It should only take about 20 minutes to complete the ECG tracing."
4 "The ECG electrodes are painless and will record the electrical activity of the heart."

Answer: 4

Rationale: The ECG uses painless electrodes, which are applied to the chest and limbs. It takes less than 5 minutes to complete and requires the client to lie still. The ECG measures the heart's electrical activity to determine rate, rhythm, and a variety of abnormalities. Options 1 and 2 are factual statements but are not stated to reduce anxiety.

Test-Taking Strategy: Use the process of elimination and focus on the issue: alleviating the client's anxiety. Eliminate option 3 because it is inaccurate. Next, eliminate options 1 and 2 because they will not alleviate anxiety. Review this diagnostic test and measures to alleviate anxiety if you had difficulty with this question.

Level of Cognitive Ability: Application
Client Needs: Psychosocial Integrity
Integrated Process: Communication and Documentation
Content Area: Adult Health/Cardiovascular

References:
Black, J., & Hawks, J. (2005). *Medical-surgical nursing: Clinical management for positive outcomes* (7th ed.). Philadelphia: Saunders, pp.1582-1583.
Chernecky, C., & Berger, B. (2004). *Laboratory tests and diagnostic procedures* (4th ed.). Philadelphia: Saunders, pp. 488-489.
Ignatavicius, D., & Workman, M. (2002). *Medical surgical nursing: Critical thinking for collaborative care* (4th ed.). Philadelphia: Saunders, p. 645.

---

182. A spouse of a client scheduled for insertion of an automatic implantable cardioverter-defibrillator (AICD) expresses anxiety about what would happen if the device discharges during physical contact. The nurse tells the spouse that:
1 Physical contact should be avoided whenever possible
2 A warning device sounds before countershock, so there is time to move away
3 The spouse would not feel or be harmed by the countershock
4 The shock would be felt, but it would not cause the spouse any harm

Answer: 4
Rationale: Clients and families are often fearful about activation of the AICD. Their fears are about the device itself, and also the occurrence of life-threatening dysrhythmias that triggers its function. Family members need reassurance that even if the device activates while touching the client, the level of the charge is not high enough to harm the family member, although it will be felt. The AICD emits a warning beep when the client is near magnetic fields, which could possibly deactivate it, but does not beep before countershock.

Test-Taking Strategy: Focus on the issue, anxiety, and use knowledge of the function of the AICD to answer this question. This will direct you to option 4. Review the concepts related to this device if you had difficulty with this question.

Level of Cognitive Ability: Application
Client Needs: Psychosocial Integrity
Integrated Process: Nursing Process/Implementation
Content Area: Adult Health/Cardiovascular

Reference:
Ignatavicius, D., & Workman, M. (2002). *Medical surgical nursing: Critical thinking for collaborative care* (4th ed.). Philadelphia: Saunders, pp. 694-695.

---

183. A client who is scheduled for permanent transvenous pacemaker insertion says to the nurse, "I know I need it, but I'm not sure this surgery is the best idea." Which nursing response will best help the nurse assess the client's preoperative concerns?
1 "Has anyone taught you about the procedure yet?"
2 "You sound uncertain about the procedure. Can you tell me more about what has you concerned?"
3 "You sound unnecessarily worried. Has anyone told you that the technology is quite advanced now?"
4 "How does your family feel about the surgery?"

Answer: 2
Rationale: Anxiety is common in the client with the need for pacemaker insertion. This can be related to fear of life-threatening dysrhythmias or to the surgical procedure. Options 1 and 3 are closed-ended and not exploratory. Option 4 is not indicated because it asks about the family and deflects attention away from the client's concerns. Option 2 is open-ended and uses clarification as a communication technique to explore the client's concerns.

Test-Taking Strategy: Use therapeutic communication techniques, focusing on the issue: addressing the client's preoperative concerns. Option 4 can be eliminated first because it addresses the family, not the client. From the remaining options, the only option that addresses the client's concerns is option 2. Review therapeutic communication techniques if you had difficulty with this question.

Level of Cognitive Ability: Application
Client Needs: Psychosocial Integrity

Integrated Process: Communication and Documentation
Content Area: Adult Health/Cardiovascular

Reference:
Potter, P., & Perry, A. (2005). *Fundamentals of nursing* (6th ed.). St. Louis: Mosby, p. 437.

---

184. A client with superficial varicose veins says to the nurse, "I hate these things. They're so ugly; I wish I could get them to go away." The nurse makes which therapeutic response to the client?
  1 "You should try sclerotherapy. It's great."
  2 "What have you been told about varicose veins and their management?"
  3 "There's not much you can do once you get them."
  4 "I understand how you feel, but you know, they really don't look too bad."

Answer: 2
Rationale: The client is expressing distress about physical appearance and has a risk for Disturbed Body Image. The nurse assesses knowledge and self-management of the condition as a means of empowering the client and helping in adapting to the body change. Options 1, 3, and 4 are nontherapeutic.

Test-Taking Strategy: Use the process of elimination. With questions that deal with client's feelings, select the option that facilitates sharing of information and concerns by the client. Options 1, 3, and 4 cut off or limit further comments by the client. Additionally, option 2 addresses assessment, the first step of the nursing process. Review therapeutic communication techniques if you had difficulty with this question.

Level of Cognitive Ability: Application
Client Needs: Psychosocial Integrity
Integrated Process: Communication and Documentation
Content Area: Adult Health/Cardiovascular

References:
Black, J., & Hawks, J. (2005). *Medical-surgical nursing: Clinical management for positive outcomes* (7th ed.). Philadelphia: Saunders, p. 1539.
Potter, P., & Perry, A. (2005). *Fundamentals of nursing* (6th ed.). St. Louis: Mosby, p. 437.

---

185. A client who has been diagnosed with chronic renal failure has been told that hemodialysis will be required. The client becomes angry and withdrawn, and states, "I'll never be the same now." The nurse formulates which nursing diagnosis for the client?
  1 Disturbed Thought Processes
  2 Disturbed Body Image
  3 Anxiety
  4 Noncompliance

Answer: 2
Rationale: A client with a renal disorder, such as renal failure, may become angry and depressed in response to the permanence of the alteration. Because of the physical change and the change in lifestyle that may be required to manage a severe renal condition, the client may experience Disturbed Body Image. Anxiety is not appropriate because the client is able to identify the cause of concern. The client is not cognitively impaired (option 1) or stating refusal to undergo therapy (option 4).

Test-Taking Strategy: Use the process of elimination and focus on the client's statement. Note that the client's statement focuses on self, which is consistent with Disturbed Body Image. Review the defining characteristics of Disturbed Body Image if you had difficulty with this question.

Level of Cognitive Ability: Analysis
Client Needs: Psychosocial Integrity
Integrated Process: Nursing Process/Analysis
Content Area: Adult Health/Renal

Reference:
Black, J., & Hawks, J. (2005). *Medical-surgical nursing: Clinical management for positive outcomes* (7th ed.). Philadelphia: Saunders, p. 1423.

186. A client with the diagnosis of hyperparathyroidism says to the nurse, "I can't stay on this diet. It is too difficult for me." When intervening in this situation, the nurse should respond:

1 "It is very important that you stay on this diet to avoid forming renal calculi."
2 "It really isn't difficult to stick to this diet. Just avoid milk products."
3 "Why do you think you find this diet plan difficult to adhere to?"
4 "You are having a difficult time staying on this plan. Let's discuss this."

Answer: 4
Rationale: By paraphrasing the client's statement, the nurse can encourage the client to verbalize emotions. The nurse also sends feedback to the client that the message was understood. An open-ended statement or question such as this prompts a lengthy response from the client. Option 1 is giving advice, which blocks communication. Option 2 devalues the client's feelings. Option 3 is requesting information that the client may not be able to express.

Test-Taking Strategy: Use therapeutic communication techniques and focus on the client's statement. Note that option 4 paraphrases the client's statement. Review therapeutic communication techniques if you had difficulty with this question.

Level of Cognitive Ability: Application
Client Needs: Psychosocial Integrity
Integrated Process: Communication and Documentation
Content Area: Adult Health/Endocrine

References:
Black, J., & Hawks, J. (2005). *Medical-surgical nursing: Clinical management for positive outcomes* (7th ed.). Philadelphia: Saunders, p. 1201.
Potter, P., & Perry, A. (2005). *Fundamentals of nursing* (6th ed.). St. Louis: Mosby, p. 437.

187. A nurse is caring for a client with newly diagnosed type 1 diabetes mellitus. In order to develop an effective teaching plan, it would be most important for the nurse to assess the client for:

1 Knowledge of the diabetic diet
2 Expressions of denial of having diabetes
3 Fear of performing insulin administration
4 Feelings of depression about lifestyle changes

Answer: 2
Rationale: When diabetes mellitus is first diagnosed, the client may go through the phases of grief: denial, fear, anger, bargaining, depression, and acceptance. Denial is the most detrimental phase to the teaching/learning process. If the client is denying the fact that he or she has diabetes, the client probably will not listen to discussions about the disease or how to manage it. Denial must be identified before the nurse can develop a teaching plan.

Test-Taking Strategy: Use the process of elimination, noting the key words "most important." All of the options may be appropriate to assess, but note that options 1, 3, and 4 relate to specific components of the teaching. Option 2 is the umbrella (global) option, and considering the principles of teaching and learning, this aspect needs to be assessed before implementation of teaching. Review teaching/learning principles if you had difficulty with this question.

Level of Cognitive Ability: Application
Client Needs: Psychosocial Integrity
Integrated Process: Teaching/Learning
Content Area: Adult Health/Endocrine

References:

Black, J., & Hawks, J. (2005). *Medical-surgical nursing: Clinical management for positive outcomes* (7th ed.). Philadelphia: Saunders, pp. 525-526.

Ignatavicius, D., & Workman, M. (2002). *Medical surgical nursing: Critical thinking for collaborative care* (4th ed.). Philadelphia: Saunders, p. 1487.

---

188. A client with newly diagnosed type 1 diabetes mellitus has been seen for three consecutive days in the emergency department with hyperglycemia. During the assessment, the client says to the nurse, "I'm sorry to keep bothering you every day, but I just can't give myself those awful shots." The nurse makes which therapeutic response?
  1 "You must learn to give yourself the shots."
  2 "I couldn't give myself a shot either."
  3 "I'm sorry you are having trouble with your injections. Has someone given you instructions on them?"
  4 "Let me see if the doctor can change your medication."

Answer: 3

Rationale: It is important to determine and deal with a client's underlying fear of self-injection. The nurse should determine if a knowledge deficit exists. Demanding a behavior or skill is inappropriate (option 1). Positive reinforcement is necessary instead of focusing on negative behaviors (option 2). The nurse should not offer a change in regimen that can't be accomplished (option 4).

Test-Taking Strategy: Use therapeutic communication techniques. Options 1, 2, and 4 are nontherapeutic. Additionally, option 4 may provide false reassurance regarding a change in medications. Review therapeutic communication techniques if you had difficulty with this question.

Level of Cognitive Ability: Application
Client Needs: Psychosocial Integrity
Integrated Process: Communication and Documentation
Content Area: Adult Health/Endocrine

References:

Ignatavicius, D., & Workman, M. (2002). *Medical surgical nursing: Critical thinking for collaborative care* (4th ed.). Philadelphia: Saunders, p. 1463.

Potter, P., & Perry, A. (2005). *Fundamentals of nursing* (6th ed.). St. Louis: Mosby, p. 437.

---

189. A nurse requests that a client with diabetes mellitus ask his or her significant other(s) to attend an educational conference on self-administration of insulin. The client questions why significant others need to be included. The nurse's best response would be:
  1 "Clients and families often work together to develop strategies for the management of diabetes."
  2 "Family members can take you to the doctor."
  3 "Family members are at risk of developing diabetes."
  4 "Nurses need someone to call and check on a client's progress."

Answer: 1

Rationale: Families and/or significant others may be included in diabetes education to assist with adjustment to the diabetic regimen. Although options 2 and 3 may be accurate, they are not the most appropriate response. Option 4 devalues the client and disregards the issue of independence and promotes powerlessness.

Test-Taking Strategy: Use the process of elimination and therapeutic communication techniques. Eliminate option 4 first because it devalues the client. From the remaining options, note that option 1 is the umbrella (global) option. Review therapeutic communication techniques if you had difficulty with this question.

Level of Cognitive Ability: Application
Client Needs: Psychosocial Integrity
Integrated Process: Communication and Documentation
Content Area: Adult Health/Endocrine

References:

Ignatavicius, D., & Workman, M. (2002). *Medical surgical nursing: Critical thinking for collaborative care* (4th ed.). Philadelphia: Saunders, p. 1488.

Lewis, S., Heitkemper, M., & Dirksen, S. (2004). *Medical-surgical nursing: Assessment and management of clinical problems* (6th ed.). St. Louis: Mosby, p. 1288.

---

190. A 22-year-old female client has recently been diagnosed with polycystic kidney disease. The nurse has a series of discussions with the client, which are intended to help her adjust to the disorder. The nurse plans to include which item as part of one of these discussions?

1 Ongoing fluid restriction
2 Depression about massive edema
3 Risk of hypotensive episodes
4 Need for genetic counseling

Answer: 4

Rationale: Adult polycystic kidney disease is a hereditary disorder that is inherited as an autosomal dominant trait. Because of this, the client should have genetic counseling, as should the extended family. The client is likely to have hypertension, not hypotension. Massive edema is not part of the clinical picture for this disorder. Ongoing fluid restriction is unnecessary.

Test-Taking Strategy: Use the process of elimination. Because massive edema and the need for fluid restriction are not part of the clinical picture for the client with polycystic kidney disease, eliminate options 1 and 2. From the remaining options, recalling either that this disorder is hereditary in nature or that the client would exhibit hypertension, not hypotension, will direct you to option 4. Review psychosocial aspects related to polycystic kidney disease if you had difficulty with this question.

Level of Cognitive Ability: Application
Client Needs: Psychosocial Integrity
Integrated Process: Nursing Process/Planning
Content Area: Adult Health/Renal

Reference:
Black, J., & Hawks, J. (2005). *Medical-surgical nursing: Clinical management for positive outcomes* (7th ed.). Philadelphia: Saunders, p. 937.

191. A nurse is admitting a client to the hospital who is to undergo ureterolithotomy for urinary calculi removal. The nurse understands that it is unnecessary to assess which of the following in determining the client's readiness for surgery?

1 Understanding of the surgical procedure
2 Knowledge of postoperative activities
3 Feelings or anxieties about the surgical procedure
4 Need for a visit from a support group

Answer: 4

Rationale: Ureterolithotomy is removal of a calculus from the ureter using either a flank or abdominal incision. Because no urinary diversion is created during this procedure, the client has no need for a visit from a member of a support group. The client should have an understanding of the same items as for any surgery, which includes knowledge of the procedures, expected outcome, and postoperative routines and discomfort. The client should also be assessed for any concerns or anxieties before surgery.

Test-Taking Strategy: Use the process of elimination, noting the key word "unnecessary." Eliminate options 1, 2, and 3 because they are assessments that should be performed before any surgery. Also, recalling that a urinary diversion is not needed in this type of surgery will direct you to option 4. Review preoperative assessments if you had difficulty with this question.

Level of Cognitive Ability: Application
Client Needs: Psychosocial Integrity
Integrated Process: Nursing Process/Assessment
Content Area: Adult Health/Renal

Reference:
Black, J., & Hawks, J. (2005). *Medical-surgical nursing: Clinical management for positive outcomes* (7th ed.). Philadelphia: Saunders, pp. 889-890.

192. The spouse of a client who is dying says to the nurse, "I don't think I can come any-more and watch her die. It's chewing me up too much!" The nurse makes which therapeutic response to the spouse?

1 "I wish you'd focus on your wife's pain rather than yours. I know it's hard, but this isn't about what's happening to you, you know."

2 "I know it's hard for you, but she would know if you're not there and you'd feel guilty all the rest of your days."

3 "It's hard to watch someone you love die. You've been here with your wife every day. Are you taking any time for yourself?"

4 "I think you're making the right decision. Your wife knows you love her. You don't have to come. I'll take care of her."

Answer: 3

Rationale: The most therapeutic response is the one that is empathic and reflects the nurse's understanding of the client's (the husband) stress and emotional pain. In the correct option, the nurse suggests that the client take time for himself. Option 1 is an example of a nontherapeutic, judgmental attitude that places blame. Option 2 makes statements that the nurse cannot know are true (the client may, in fact, not know if the husband visits) and predicts guilt feelings, which is inappropriate. Option 4 fosters dependency and gives advice, which is nontherapeutic.

Test-Taking Strategy: Use therapeutic communication techniques to answer the question. Note that the client of the question is the husband. Option 3 is the only option that is therapeutic and addresses the husband's feelings. Review therapeutic communication techniques if you had difficulty with this question.

Level of Cognitive Ability: Application
Client Needs: Psychosocial Integrity
Integrated Process: Communication and Documentation
Content Area: Mental Health

References:

Stuart, G., & Laraia, M. (2005). *Principles and practice of psychiatric nursing* (8th ed.). St. Louis: Mosby, pp. 30-34.
Varcarolis, E.M. (2002). *Foundations of psychiatric mental health nursing* (4th ed.). Philadelphia: Saunders, pp. 837-838.

193. An older adult client at the Retirement Center spits her food out and throws it on the floor at a Thanksgiving dinner held in the community dining room. The client yells, "This turkey is dry and cold! I can't stand the food here!" The nurse makes which therapeutic response to the client?

1 "Let me get you another serving that is more to your liking. Would you like to come visit the chef and select your own serving?"

2 "I think you had better return to your apartment, where a new meal will be served to you there."

3 "Now look what you've done! You're ruining this meal for the whole community. Aren't you ashamed of yourself?"

4 "One of the things that the residents of this group agreed was that anyone who did not use appropriate behavior would be asked to leave the dining room. Please leave now."

Answer: 1

Rationale: Asking the client to accompany the nurse to the kitchen respects the client's need for control, removes the angry client from the dining room, and may offer the nurse an opportunity to assess what is happening to the client. Option 2 could provoke a regressive struggle between the nurse and client and cause more anger in the client. Option 3 is angry and aggressive and nontherapeutic. In option 4, the nurse is authoritative, and it would not be appropriate to ask the client to leave. This action might set up an aggressive struggle between the nurse and the client.

Test-Taking Strategy: Use therapeutic communication techniques and knowledge about care of an angry client. Option 1 is the only option that addresses the client's angry feelings. It also provides the nurse an opportunity to further assess the client. Review therapeutic communication techniques if you had difficulty with this question.

Level of Cognitive Ability: Application
Client Needs: Psychosocial Integrity
Integrated Process: Communication and Documentation
Content Area: Mental Health

References:

Stuart, G., & Laraia, M. (2005). *Principles and practice of psychiatric nursing* (8th ed.). St. Louis: Mosby, pp. 30-34.
Varcarolis, E.M. (2002). *Foundations of psychiatric mental health nursing* (4th ed.). Philadelphia: Saunders, p. 667.

194. A physician orders a follow-up home care visit for an older adult client with emphysema. When the home care nurse arrives, the client is smoking. Which statement by the nurse would be most therapeutic?

1 "Well, I can see you never got to the Stop Smoking clinic!"
2 "I notice that you are smoking. Did you explore the Stop Smoking Program at the Senior Citizens Center?"
3 "I wonder if you realize that you are slowly killing yourself? Why prolong the agony? You can just jump off the bridge!"
4 "I'm glad I caught you smoking! Now that your secret is out, let's decide what you are going to do."

Answer: 2

Rationale: Emphysema clients need to avoid smoking and all airborne irritants. The nurse who observes a maladaptive behavior in a client should not make judgmental comments and should explore an adaptive strategy with the client without being overly controlling. This will place the decision making in the client's hands and provide an avenue for the client to share what may be expressions of frustration about an inability to stop what is essentially a physiological addiction. Option 1 is an intrusive use of sarcastic humor that is degrading to the client. In Option 3, the nurse preaches and is judgmental. Option 4 is a disciplinary remark and places a barrier between the nurse and client within the therapeutic relationship.

Test-Taking Strategy: Use therapeutic communication techniques. Option 2 recognizes and addresses the client's behavior and explores an avenue to deal with the behavior. Review therapeutic communication techniques if you had difficulty with this question.

Level of Cognitive Ability: Application
Client Needs: Psychosocial Integrity
Integrated Process: Communication and Documentation
Content Area: Adult Health/Respiratory

References:
Black, J., & Hawks, J. (2005). *Medical-surgical nursing: Clinical management for positive outcomes* (7th ed.). Philadelphia: Saunders, p. 1818.
Potter, P., & Perry, A. (2005). *Fundamentals of nursing* (6th ed.). St. Louis: Mosby, p. 437.

195. A client is to have arterial blood gases drawn. While the nurse is performing the Allen test, the client says to the nurse, "What are you doing? No one else has done that!" The nurse makes which therapeutic response to the client?

1 "This is a routine precautionary step that simply makes certain your circulation is intact before obtaining a blood sample."
2 "Oh? You have questions about this? You should insist that they all do this procedure before drawing up your blood."
3 "I assure you that I am doing the correct procedure. I cannot account for what others do."
4 "This step is crucial to safe blood withdrawal. I would not let anyone take my blood until they did this."

Answer: 1

Rationale: The Allen test is performed to assess collateral circulation in the hand before drawing a radial artery blood specimen. The therapeutic response provides information to the client. Option 2 is aggressive and controlling as well as nontherapeutic in its disapproving stance. Option 3 is defensive and nontherapeutic in offering false reassurance. Option 4 identifies client advocacy but is overly controlling and aggressive and undermining of treatment.

Test-Taking Strategy: Use therapeutic communication techniques and the process of elimination. Option 1 addresses the issue of the question and provides information to the client. Review therapeutic communication techniques if you had difficulty with this question.

Level of Cognitive Ability: Application
Client Needs: Psychosocial Integrity
Integrated Process: Communication and Documentation
Content Area: Adult Health/Cardiovascular

References:
Black, J., & Hawks, J. (2005). *Medical-surgical nursing: Clinical management for positive outcomes* (7th ed.). Philadelphia: Saunders, p. 1764.
Potter, P., & Perry, A. (2005). *Fundamentals of nursing* (6th ed.). St. Louis: Mosby, p. 437.

196. A client is complaining of difficulty concentrating, having outbursts of anger, and feeling "keyed up" all the time. The nurse obtaining the client's history discovers that the symptoms started about 6 months ago. The client reveals that a best friend was killed in a drive-by shooting while they were sitting on the porch talking. The nurse suspects that the client is experiencing:
1 Obsessive-compulsive disorder (OCD)
2 Panic disorder
3 Post-traumatic stress disorder (PTSD)
4 Social phobia

Answer: 3
Rationale: PTSD is a response to an event that would be markedly distressing to almost anyone. Characteristic symptoms include sustained level of anxiety, difficulty sleeping, irritability, difficulty concentrating, or outbursts of anger. OCD refers to some repetitive thoughts or behaviors. Panic disorders and social phobia are characterized by a specific fear of an object or situation.

Test-Taking Strategy: Focus on the data in the question and use the process of elimination. Eliminate options 2 and 4 first because they are similar. From the remaining options, recalling that OCD relates to a repetitive thought or behavior will direct you to option 3. Review this disorder if you had difficulty with this question.

Level of Cognitive Ability: Analysis
Client Needs: Psychosocial Integrity
Integrated Process: Nursing Process/Analysis
Content Area: Mental Health

Reference:
Stuart, G., & Laraia, M. (2005). *Principles and practice of psychiatric nursing* (8th ed.). St. Louis: Mosby, p. 273.

197. A client who is reported by the staff to be very demanding says to the nurse, "I can't get any help with my care! I call and call but the nurses never answer my light. Last night one of them told me she had other patients besides me! I'm very sick, but the nurses don't care!" The nurse makes which therapeutic response to the client?
1 "I think you are being very impatient. The nurses work very hard and come as quickly as they can."
2 "I can hear your anger. That nurse had no right to speak to you that way. I will report her to the Director. It won't happen again."
3 "It's hard to be in bed and have to ask for help. You ring for a nurse who never seems to help?"
4 "You poor thing! I'm so sorry this happened to you. That nurse should be fired."

Answer: 3
Rationale: Empathy is a term that describes the nurse's capacity to enter into the life of another person and to perceive how the client is feeling and what meaning this has for the client. In option 3, the nurse displays empathy and shares perceptions. Sharing perceptions asks the client to validate the nurse's understanding of what the client is feeling and thinking. It opens the door for the client to share concerns, fears, and anxieties. In option 1, the nurse is assertive and certainly defends the nursing staff as well. In option 2, the nurse expresses the client's frustration by labeling the client's feelings as "angry" and disapproving of the nursing staff. This is splitting and is nontherapeutic. Option 4 is a social response and is demeaning to the client.

Test-Taking Strategy: Use therapeutic communication techniques and the process of elimination. Focus on the client's statement in the question. Note the relation between the client's statement and option 3. Also, in this option the nurse validates the client's feelings. Review therapeutic communication techniques if you had difficulty with this question.

Level of Cognitive Ability: Application
Client Needs: Psychosocial Integrity
Integrated Process: Communication and Documentation
Content Area: Mental Health

Reference:
Stuart, G., & Laraia, M. (2005). *Principles and practice of psychiatric nursing* (8th ed.). St. Louis: Mosby, pp. 30-34.

198. An English-speaking Hispanic male with a newly applied long leg cast has a right proximal fractured tibia. During rounds at night, the nurse finds the client restless, withdrawn, and quiet. Which initial nursing statement would be most appropriate?

1 "Are you uncomfortable?"

2 "Tell me what you are feeling."

3 "I'll get you pain medication right away."

4 "You'll feel better in the morning."

Answer: 2

Rationale: Option 2 is open-ended and makes no assumptions about the client's psychological or emotional state. Option 1 is incorrect because males in traditional standard Hispanic cultures practice "machismo" in which stoicism is valued, so this client may deny any pain when asked. Option 3 is incorrect because an assessment is necessary before administering medication for pain. False reassurance is never therapeutic, which makes option 4 incorrect.

Test-Taking Strategy: Use therapeutic communication techniques. Recalling that the client's feelings are the priority will direct you to option 2. Review therapeutic communication techniques if you had difficulty with this question.

Level of Cognitive Ability: Application
Client Needs: Psychosocial Integrity
Integrated Process: Communication and Documentation
Content Area: Adult Health/Musculoskeletal

Reference:
Potter, P., & Perry, A. (2005). *Fundamentals of nursing* (6th ed.). St. Louis: Mosby, p. 437.

---

199. A client was started on oral anticoagulant therapy while hospitalized. The client is now being discharged to home and is intermittently confused. The nurse determines that the client has the best support system for successful anticoagulant therapy monitoring if the client:

1 Has a good friend living next door who would take the client to the doctor

2 Has a home health aide coming to the house for 9 weeks

3 Was going to stay with a daughter in the daughter's home indefinitely

4 Was going to have blood work drawn in the home by a local laboratory

Answer: 3

Rationale: The client taking anticoagulant therapy should be informed about the medication, its purpose, and the necessity of taking the proper dose at the specified times. If the client is unwilling or unable to comply with the medication regimen, the continuance of the regime should be questioned. Clients may need support systems in place to enhance compliance with therapy. Option 1 facilitates medical care, option 2 facilitates reminding the client to take the medication, and option 4 facilitates blood work only. Option 3 provides a direct support system.

Test-Taking Strategy: Use the process of elimination. Note the issue: the best support system. Note that option 3 is the only option that indicates direct support for the client. Review the concepts surrounding support systems for the client if you had difficulty with this question.

Level of Cognitive Ability: Analysis
Client Needs: Psychosocial Integrity
Integrated Process: Nursing Process/Evaluation
Content Area: Adult Health/Cardiovascular

References:
Black, J., & Hawks, J. (2005). *Medical-surgical nursing: Clinical management for positive outcomes* (7th ed.). Philadelphia: Saunders, p. 489.
Ignatavicius, D., & Workman, M. (2002). *Medical surgical nursing: Critical thinking for collaborative care* (4th ed.). Philadelphia: Saunders, p. 717.

200. A client who has undergone successful femoral-popliteal bypass grafting to the leg says to the nurse, "I hope everything goes well after this, and I don't lose my leg. I'm so afraid that I'll have gone through this for nothing." The nurse makes which therapeutic response to the client?

1 "I can understand what you mean. I'd be nervous too, if I were in your shoes."

2 "Stress isn't helpful for you. You should probably just relax and try not to worry unless something actually happens."

3 "Complications are possible, but you have a good deal of control if you make the lifestyle adjustments we talked about."

4 "This surgery is so successful, that I wouldn't be concerned at all if I were you."

Answer: 3

Rationale: Clients frequently fear that they will ultimately lose a limb or become debilitated in some other way. Option 1 feeds into the client's anxiety and is not therapeutic. Option 4 gives false reassurance. Option 2 is meant to be reassuring, but offers no suggestions to empower the client. Option 3 acknowledges the client's concerns and empowers the client to improve health, which will ultimately reduce concern about the risk of complications.

Test-Taking Strategy: Use the process of elimination and therapeutic communication techniques. Option 3 is the only option that acknowledges the client's concerns and addresses the client's control over the situation. Review therapeutic communication techniques if you had difficulty with this question.

Level of Cognitive Ability: Application
Client Needs: Psychosocial Integrity
Integrated Process: Communication and Documentation
Content Area: Adult Health/Cardiovascular

Reference:
Potter, P., & Perry, A. (2005). *Fundamentals of nursing* (6th ed.). St. Louis: Mosby, p. 437.

---

201. A client in the coronary care unit is about to have a pericardiocentesis done for a rapidly accumulating pericardial effusion. The nurse best plans to alleviate the apprehension of the client by:

1 Staying beside the client and giving information and encouragement during the procedure

2 Talking to the client from the foot of the bed to be available to get added supplies

3 Telling the client that he or she (the nurse) will take care of another assigned client at this time, so as to be available once the procedure is complete

4 Telling the client to watch television during the procedure as a distraction

Answer: 1

Rationale: Clients who develop sudden complications are in situational crisis and need therapeutic intervention. Staying with the client and giving information and encouragement is part of building and maintaining trust in the nurse-client relationship. Options 3 and 4 distance the nurse from the client in a psychosocial as well as physical sense. The nurse should ask another caregiver to be available to get extra supplies if needed.

Test-Taking Strategy: Use the process of elimination and therapeutic communication techniques. Option 1 is the only option that provides direct contact and assistance to the client. Review therapeutic communication techniques if you had difficulty with this question.

Level of Cognitive Ability: Application
Client Needs: Psychosocial Integrity
Integrated Process: Caring
Content Area: Adult Health/Cardiovascular

Reference:
Black, J., & Hawks, J. (2005). *Medical-surgical nursing: Clinical management for positive outcomes* (7th ed.). Philadelphia: Saunders, p. 1622.

202. A nurse has formulated a nursing diagnosis of Disturbed Body Image for the male client taking spironolactone (Aldactone). The nurse based this diagnosis on assessment of which of the following side effects of the medication?
1 Edema
2 Hair loss
3 Alopecia
4 Decreased libido

Answer: 4

Rationale: The nurse should be alert to the fact that the client taking spironolactone may experience body image changes resulting from threatened sexual identity. These are related to decreased libido, gynecomastia in males, and hirsutism in females. Edema and hair loss are not specifically associated with the use of this medication.

Test-Taking Strategy: Use the process of elimination and knowledge regarding the side effects of spironolactone. Eliminate options 2 and 3 because they are similar. From the remaining options, focusing on the nursing diagnosis in the question will direct you to option 4. Review the side effects of this medication if you had difficulty with this question.

Level of Cognitive Ability: Analysis
Client Needs: Psychosocial Integrity
Integrated Process: Nursing Process/Analysis
Content Area: Pharmacology

Reference:
Hodgson, B., & Kizior, R. (2004). *Saunders nursing drug handbook 2004.* Philadelphia: Saunders, p. 932.

---

203. A nurse is caring for a client who is recovering from the signs and symptoms of autonomic dysreflexia (hyperreflexia). The nurse makes which therapeutic statement to the client?
1 "I'm sure you now understand the importance of preventing this from occurring."
2 "Now that this problem is taken care of, I'm sure you'll be fine."
3 "How could your home care nurse let this happen?"
4 "I have some time if you would like to talk about what happened to you."

Answer: 4

Rationale: Option 4 encourages the client to discuss feelings. Options 1 and 3 show disapproval and option 2 provides false reassurance. These are nontherapeutic techniques.

Test-Taking Strategy: Use the process of elimination and therapeutic communication techniques. Remembering to always address the client's concerns and feelings first will direct you to option 4. Review therapeutic communication techniques if you had difficulty with this question.

Level of Cognitive Ability: Application
Client Needs: Psychosocial Integrity
Integrated Process: Communication and Documentation
Content Area: Adult Health/Neurological

References:
Black, J., & Hawks, J. (2005). *Medical-surgical nursing: Clinical management for positive outcomes* (7th ed.). Philadelphia: Saunders, p. 2229.
Potter, P., & Perry, A. (2005). *Fundamentals of nursing* (6th ed.). St. Louis: Mosby, p. 437.

---

204. While assisting a spinal cord injury client with activities of daily living, the client states, "I can't do this; I wish I were dead." The nurse makes which therapeutic response to the client?
1 "Let's wash your back now."
2 "You wish you were dead?"
3 "I'm sure you are frustrated, but things will work out just fine for you."
4 "Why do you say that?"

Answer: 2

Rationale: Clarifying is a therapeutic technique involving restating what was said to obtain additional information. Option 1 changes the subject. In option 3, false reassurance is offered. By asking "why" (option 4), the nurse puts the client on the defensive. Options 1, 3, and 4 are nontherapeutic and block communication.

Test-Taking Strategy: Use the process of elimination and therapeutic communication techniques. Remember to focus on the client's feelings. Option 2 identifies clarifying and restating and is the only option that will encourage the client to verbalize feelings and concerns. Review therapeutic communication techniques if you had difficulty with this question.

Level of Cognitive Ability: Application
Client Needs: Psychosocial Integrity
Integrated Process: Communication and Documentation
Content Area: Adult Health/Neurological

References:
Black, J., & Hawks, J. (2005). *Medical-surgical nursing: Clinical management for positive outcomes* (7th ed.). Philadelphia: Saunders, p. 2234.
Potter, P., & Perry, A. (2005). *Fundamentals of nursing* (6th ed.). St. Louis: Mosby, p. 437.

205. Family members who are awaiting the outcome of a suicide attempt are tearful. Which statement by the nurse would be therapeutic to the family at this time?
   1 "Don't worry, you have nothing to feel guilty about."
   2 "Everything possible is being done."
   3 "Let me check to see how long it will be before you can see your loved one."
   4 "I can see you are worried."

Answer: 4
Rationale: Options 1, 2, and 3 are communication blocks. Option 1 labels the family's behavior without their validation. Option 2 uses clichés and false reassurance. Option 3 focuses on an important issue at an inappropriate time. Option 4 addresses the family's feelings and displays empathy.

Test-Taking Strategy: Use the process of elimination and therapeutic communication techniques. Option 4 identifies clarifying and is the only option that will encourage the family to verbalize feelings and concerns. Review therapeutic communication techniques if you had difficulty with this question.

Level of Cognitive Ability: Application
Client Needs: Psychosocial Integrity
Integrated Process: Caring
Content Area: Mental Health

References:
Fortinash, K., & Holoday-Worret, P. (2004). *Psychiatric mental health nursing* (3rd ed.). St. Louis: Mosby, pp. 561-562.
Stuart, G., & Laraia, M. (2005). *Principles and practice of psychiatric nursing* (8th ed.). St. Louis: Mosby, pp. 30-34.

206. A nurse is caring for an 11-year-old child who has been abused. The nurse includes which therapeutic action in the plan of care?

1 Encourage the child to fear the abuser
2 Provide a care environment that allows for the development of trust
3 Teach the child to make wise choices when confronted with an abusive situation
4 Have the child point out the abuser if he or she should visit while the child is hospitalized

Answer: 2

Rationale: The abused child usually requires long-term therapeutic support. The environment provided during the child's healing must include one in which trust and empathy are modeled and provided for the child. Option 1 reinforces fear, which should not be encouraged. Options 3 and 4 ask the child to behave with a maturity beyond that which would be expected for an 11-year-old. Option 2 is therapeutic because it provides the child with a nurturing and supportive environment in which to begin the healing process.

Test-Taking Strategy: Use the process of elimination and therapeutic techniques. Option 2 is the only option that provides support to the child. Review therapeutic interventions for a child who has been abused if you had difficulty with this question.

Level of Cognitive Ability: Application
Client Needs: Psychosocial Integrity
Integrated Process: Caring
Content Area: Child Health

Reference:
Wong, D., & Hockenberry, M. (2003). *Wong's nursing care of infants and children* (7th ed.). St. Louis: Mosby, p. 687.

207. A nurse assesses an older client for signs of potential abuse. Which of the following psychosocial factors obtained during the assessment place the client at risk for abuse?

1 The client is completely dependent upon family members for receiving food and medicine.
2 The client shows signs and symptoms of depression.
3 The client resides in a low-income neighborhood.
4 The client has a chronic illness.

Answer: 1

Rationale: Elder abuse is sometimes the result of frustrated adult children who find themselves caring for dependent parents. Increasing demands by parents for care and financial support can cause resentment and burden. Option 2 relates to depression rather than the risk for abuse. Option 4 relates to a physical factor, not a psychosocial factor. The issues of abuse are not bound to socioeconomic status.

Test-Taking Strategy: Use the process of elimination. Note the key words "psychosocial factors" and focus on the issue: at risk for abuse. Noting the key words "completely dependent" in option 1 will direct you to this option. Review the risk factors associated with elder abuse if you had difficulty with this question.

Level of Cognitive Ability: Analysis
Client Needs: Psychosocial Integrity
Integrated Process: Nursing Process/Assessment
Content Area: Mental Health

References:
Stuart, G., & Laraia, M. (2005). *Principles and practice of psychiatric nursing* (8th ed.). St. Louis: Mosby, pp. 810-811.
Varcarolis, E.M. (2002). *Foundations of psychiatric mental health nursing* (4th ed.). Philadelphia: Saunders, p. 711.

208. A nurse is caring for a dying client who says, "What would you say if I asked you to be the executor for my will?" Which nursing response would be therapeutic?
  1 "Why, I'd be honored to be the executor of your will."
  2 "Is there any money in it? I adore money, but I am honest."
  3 "Your confidence in me is an honor, but I would like to understand more about your thinking."
  4 "I'd say, great! No worries. I'll carry out your will just as you want me to."

Answer: 3
Rationale: In option 3, this nurse is seeking clarification and empathy. The client's question reflects the fact that the client has been thinking about the will and how best to obtain an executor. What is unknown is why the client is asking the nurse to be executor of the will and other specific and important information. In addition, the nurse would want to investigate the legal ramifications, which could arise if such a position was accepted. In option 1, the nurse responds with a social communication with no assessment of the consequences, which is lacking critical thinking and exploration of motivation or client needs. In option 2, the nurse uses histrionic language and crass ideation. In option 4, the nurse provides false reassurance, which is nontherapeutic.

Test-Taking Strategy: Use therapeutic communication techniques and the process of elimination. Option 3 is the only option that addresses the client's thoughts and feelings. Review therapeutic communication techniques if you had difficulty with this question.

Level of Cognitive Ability: Application
Client Needs: Psychosocial Integrity
Integrated Process: Communication and Documentation
Content Area: Fundamental Skills

References:
Brent, N. (2001). *Nurses and the law* (2nd ed.). Philadelphia: Saunders, p. 215.
Potter, P., & Perry, A. (2005). *Fundamentals of nursing* (6th ed.). St. Louis: Mosby, p. 437.

209. A client who is suffering from urticaria (hives) and pruritus says to the nurse, "What am I going to do? I'm getting married next week and I'll probably be covered in this rash and itching like crazy." The nurse makes which therapeutic response to the client?
  1 "You're very troubled that this will extend into your wedding?"
  2 "It's probably just due to prewedding jitters."
  3 "The antihistamine will help a great deal, just you wait and see."
  4 "I hope your husband-to-be has a sense of humor."

Answer: 1
Rationale: The therapeutic communication technique that the nurse uses in option 1 is reflection. In option 2, the nurse minimizes the client's anxiety and fears. In option 3, the nurse talks about antihistamines and asks the client to "wait and see." This is nontherapeutic because the nurse is making promises that may not be kept and because the response is close-ended and shuts off the client's expression of feelings. In option 4, the nurse uses humor inappropriately and with insensitivity.

Test-Taking Strategy: Use the process of elimination and therapeutic communication techniques. Options 2, 3, and 4 are nontherapeutic responses. Option 1 addresses the client's feelings. Use therapeutic communication techniques if you had difficulty with this question.

Level of Cognitive Ability: Application
Client Needs: Psychosocial Integrity
Integrated Process: Communication and Documentation
Content Area: Mental Health

Reference:
Stuart, G., & Laraia, M. (2005). *Principles and practice of psychiatric nursing* (8th ed.). St. Louis: Mosby, pp. 30-34.

210. A client with a spinal cord injury makes the following comments. Which comment warrants additional intervention by the nurse?
  1 "I'm so angry this happened to me."
  2 "I know I will have to make major adjustments in my life."
  3 "I would like my family members to be here for my teaching sessions."
  4 "I'm really looking forward to going home."

Answer: 1
Rationale: It is important to allow the client with a spinal cord injury to verbalize his or her feelings. If the client indicates a desire to discuss feelings, the nurse should respond therapeutically. Options 2 and 3 indicate that the client understands changes that will be occurring and that family involvement is best. No data in the question indicates that the client will not be going home, therefore this comment does not require further intervention.

Test-Taking Strategy: Use the process of elimination, noting the key words "warrants additional intervention." Noting the word "angry" in option 1 will direct you to this option. Review psychosocial issues related to the care of a client with a spinal cord injury if you had difficulty with this question.

Level of Cognitive Ability: Analysis
Client Needs: Psychosocial Integrity
Integrated Process: Nursing Process/Analysis
Content Area: Adult Health/Neurological

Reference:
Black, J., & Hawks, J. (2005). *Medical-surgical nursing: Clinical management for positive outcomes* (7th ed.). Philadelphia: Saunders, p. 2224.

211. A nurse is caring for a client with a grade II (mild) cerebral aneurysm rupture. The client becomes restless and anxious before visiting hours. The nurse determines that the client's behavior is likely related to:
  1 The severity of the aneurysm rupture
  2 Disabled family coping
  3 Disturbed body image
  4 Spiritual distress

Answer: 3
Rationale: A grade II cerebral aneurysm rupture is a mild bleed in which the client remains alert but has nuchal rigidity with possible neurological deficits, depending on the area of the bleed. Because these clients remain alert, they are acutely aware of the neurological deficits and frequently have some degree of body image disturbance. No data in the question indicates that the client's behavior is related to options 1, 2, or 4.

Test-Taking Strategy: Focus on the client's behavior and note the key words "before visiting hours." Using knowledge of the effects of this disorder and focusing on the client's behavior will direct you to option 3. Review the effects of a grade II cerebral aneurysm rupture if you had difficulty with this question.

Level of Cognitive Ability: Analysis
Client Needs: Psychosocial Integrity
Integrated Process: Nursing Process/Analysis
Content Area: Adult Health/Neurological

Reference:
Phipps, W., Monahan, F., Sands, J., Marek, J., & Neighbors, M. (2003). *Medical-surgical nursing: Health and illness perspectives* (7th ed.). St. Louis: Mosby, p. 1385.

212. In planning care for the client with thromboangiitis obliterans (Buerger's disease), the nurse incorporates measures to help the client cope with the lifestyle changes needed to control the disease process. The nurse can accomplish this by recommending a:

1 Smoking cessation program
2 Pain management clinic
3 Consult with a dietician
4 Referral to a medical social worker

Answer: 1

Rationale: Smoking is highly detrimental to the client with Buerger's disease, and clients are recommended to stop completely. Because smoking is a form of chemical dependency, referral to a smoking cessation program may be helpful for many clients. For many clients, symptoms are relieved or alleviated once smoking stops. Options 2, 3, and 4 are not directly related to the physiology associated with this condition.

Test-Taking Strategy: Use the process of elimination and focus on the client's diagnosis. Recalling that the treatment goals are the same as for peripheral vascular disease will direct you to option 1. Review the treatment goals for this disorder if you had difficulty with this question.

Level of Cognitive Ability: Application
Client Needs: Psychosocial Integrity
Integrated Process: Nursing Process/Implementation
Content Area: Adult Health/Cardiovascular

Reference:
Black, J., & Hawks, J. (2005). *Medical-surgical nursing: Clinical management for positive outcomes* (7th ed.). Philadelphia: Saunders, p. 1534.

---

213. A nurse is performing an assessment on a 14-year-old client. On assessment, the nurse notes bruises and bleeding in the genital area, cigarette burns on the chest, rope burns on the buttocks, and multiple old fractures. The child states, "I'm afraid to go home! My stepfather will be angry with me for telling on him!" The nurse makes which therapeutic response to the child?

1 "I am sorry that this has happened to you, but you will be safe here. Your physician has admitted you until further plans can be made."
2 "You can't go back there with that man. How do you think your mother will react?"
3 "You must know that your presence in the house will only tease your stepfather more."
4 "Let's keep this between you, me, and the physician until we can formulate further plans to assist you."

Answer: 1

Rationale: A child who has been physically and sexually abused should be admitted to the hospital. This will provide time for a more comprehensive evaluation while protecting the child from further abusiveness. The correct option also provides an empathic statement that supports the child to appropriately perceive self as the victim, while assuring the child of protection from abuse. In option 2, the nurse does not respond with a calm and reassuring communication style, nor does the nurse maintain a professional attitude. Option 3, which holds an innuendo, appears to accuse the victim of teasing the stepfather and is incorrect. It is also judgmental, controlling, and demeaning. The nurse's suggestion in option 4 is not only incorrect but is also passive in its stance.

Test-Taking Strategy: Use the process of elimination, therapeutic communication techniques, and knowledge of care of the child who has been physically abused. Recalling that the priority is safety to the victim will direct you to option 1. Review care of the child who has been abused if you had difficulty with this question.

Level of Cognitive Ability: Application
Client Needs: Psychosocial Integrity
Integrated Process: Caring
Content Area: Mental Health

Reference:
Stuart, G., & Laraia, M. (2005). *Principles and practice of psychiatric nursing* (8th ed.). St. Louis: Mosby, p. 808.

214. A nurse is caring for a 12-year-old female client who has been admitted to the hospital with a diagnosis of physical and sexual abuse by her father. That evening, the father angrily approaches the nurse and says, "I'm taking my daughter home. She's told me what you people are up to and we're out of here!" The nurse makes which therapeutic response to the child's father?

1 "Over my dead body you will! She's here and here she stays until the doctor says different. So get off my floor or I'll call hospital security and the police!"

2 "Listen to me. If you attempt to take your daughter from this unit, the police will only bring her back."

3 "Your daughter is ill and needs to be here. I know you want to help her to recover and that you will work to help everyone straighten out the circumstances that caused this. Go to the chapel and pray for your daughter and for your soul."

4 "You seem very upset. Let's talk at the nurse's station. I want to help you. I know you're very concerned and want to help your daughter. It will be best if you agree to let your daughter stay here for now."

Answer: 4

Rationale: When a suspected abused child is admitted to the hospital for further evaluation and protection, the physician will usually work with the parents so they will agree to the admission. If the parents refuse to agree to the admission, the hospital can request an immediate court order to retain the child for a specific length of time. In option 1, the nurse is angry and verbally abusive. It is clear that the nurse has decided that the father is guilty of child abuse. In addition, the nurse is aggressive and challenging and may antagonize the father and become a victim of violence as well. In option 2, the command to listen is somewhat demanding. Option 3 seems somewhat pompous and lecturing.

Test-Taking Strategy: Use the process of elimination and therapeutic communication techniques. Note that the client of the question is the child's father. Note that option 4 addresses the father's behavior yet protects the child. Review psychosocial issues related to child abuse if you had difficulty with this question.

Level of Cognitive Ability: Application
Client Needs: Psychosocial Integrity
Integrated Process: Communication and Documentation
Content Area: Mental Health

References:
Stuart, G., & Laraia, M. (2005). *Principles and practice of psychiatric nursing* (8th ed.). St. Louis: Mosby, p. 808.
Varcarolis, E.M. (2002). *Foundations of psychiatric mental health nursing* (4th ed.). Philadelphia: Saunders, pp. 694-695.

---

215. A client with peripheral arterial disease is being discharged to home. The client is occasionally forgetful about medication, exercise, and diet instructions; needs daily dressing changes to a small open area on the leg; has limited endurance for activities of daily living (ADLs); and lives alone in a one-story house. To best assist the client to adapt to self-care and disease management, the nurse initiates a request to the physician for which follow-up services to be provided in the home?

1 Nursing, home health aide, physical therapy

2 Nursing, home health aide, speech therapy

3 Home health aide, physical therapy, and occupational therapy

4 Nursing, physical therapy, and occupational therapy

Answer: 1

Rationale: Home health care agencies provide a variety of services to clients, depending on the individual need. The multidisciplinary team includes nurse, home health aides, social workers, and physical, occupational, and speech therapists. Nurses provide skilled nursing services including assessments. Home health aides can assist clients with ADLs, and physical therapists assist in rehabilitation and increasing musculoskeletal endurance. The occupational therapist would train clients to adapt to physical handicaps through new vocational skills and adaptive techniques for ADLs.

Test-Taking Strategy: Use the process of elimination and focus on the client's needs identified in the question. Recalling the role of each of these health care members and focusing on the client's needs will direct you to option 1. Review the roles of these health care members if you had difficulty with this question.

Level of Cognitive Ability: Application
Client Needs: Psychosocial Integrity
Integrated Process: Nursing Process/Implementation
Content Area: Fundamental Skills

Reference:
Potter, P., & Perry, A. (2005). *Fundamentals of nursing* (6th ed.). St. Louis: Mosby, p. 36.

216. A client with chronic arterial leg ulcers complains of pain and tells the nurse "I'm so discouraged. I have had this pain for over a year now. The pain never seems to go away. I can't do anything, and I feel as though I'll never get better." The nurse formulates which nursing diagnosis for this client?

1 Acute Pain, related to the effects of leg ischemia
2 Chronic Pain, related to the nonhealing arterial ulcerations
3 Fatigue, related to lack of sleep and frustration with illness
4 Ineffective Coping, related to chronic illness

Answer: 2

Rationale: The major focus of the client's complaint is the experience of pain. Pain that has a duration of greater than 6 months is defined as chronic pain, not acute pain. The North American Nursing Diagnosis Association (NANDA) defines Fatigue as "a sense of exhaustion and decreased capacity for physical and mental work." NANDA defines Ineffective Coping as "impairment of adaptive behaviors and abilities of a person in meeting life's demands and roles."

Test-Taking Strategy: Use the process of elimination. Focus on the client's statement, "I have had this pain for over a year now." This statement and noting the word "chronic" in the question and in option 2 will direct you to this option. Review the defining characteristics for this nursing diagnosis if you had difficulty with this question.

Level of Cognitive Ability: Analysis
Client Needs: Psychosocial Integrity
Integrated Process: Nursing Process/Analysis
Content Area: Adult Health/Cardiovascular

Reference:
Gulanick, M., Myers, J., Klopp, A., Gradishar, D., Galanes, S., & Puzas, M. (2003). *Nursing care plans: Nursing diagnosis and intervention* (5th ed.). St. Louis: Mosby, pp. 47; 56; 121; 126.

---

217. A client with valvular heart disease is being considered for mechanical valve replacement. Which item is essential to assess before the surgery is done?

1 The likelihood of the client experiencing body image problems
2 The ability to participate in a cardiac rehabilitation program
3 The physical demands of the client's lifestyle
4 The ability to comply with anticoagulant therapy for life

Answer: 4

Rationale: Mechanical valves carry the associated risk of thromboemboli, which requires long-term anticoagulation with warfarin (Coumadin). No data in the question indicates that physical demands in the client's lifestyle exist. Body image problems are important but not critical. Not all clients who undergo cardiac surgery need cardiac rehabilitation.

Test-Taking Strategy: Use the process of elimination, focusing on the key word "essential." Recalling that mechanical valves are thrombogenic will direct you to option 4. Review care of the client undergoing a mechanical valve replacement if you had difficulty with this question.

Level of Cognitive Ability: Application
Client Needs: Psychosocial Integrity
Integrated Process: Nursing Process/Assessment
Content Area: Adult Health/Cardiovascular

Reference:
Black, J., & Hawks, J. (2005). *Medical-surgical nursing: Clinical management for positive outcomes* (7th ed.). Philadelphia: Saunders, p. 1605.

218. A client who has a history of depression has been prescribed nadolol (Corgard) in the management of angina pectoris. Which item is most important when the nurse plans to counsel this client about the effects of this medication?
1 High incidence of hypoglycemia
2 Possible exacerbation of depression
3 Risk of tachycardia
4 Probability of fatigue

Answer: 2
Rationale: Clients with depression or a history of depression have experienced an exacerbation of depression after beginning therapy with beta-adrenergic blocking agents. These clients should be monitored carefully if these agents are prescribed. The medication would cause bradycardia, not tachycardia. Fatigue is a possible side effect but is not the most important item. Hypoglycemia is a sign that is masked with beta-blockers.

Test-Taking Strategy: Use the process of elimination. Noting the relationship between the client's history and option 2 will direct you to this option. Review this medication if you had difficulty with this question.

Level of Cognitive Ability: Application
Client Needs: Psychosocial Integrity
Integrated Process: Teaching/Learning
Content Area: Pharmacology

Reference:
Hodgson, B., & Kizior, R. (2004). *Saunders nursing drug handbook 2004.* Philadelphia: Saunders, p. 701.

219. The nurse is caring for a client with terminal cancer of the throat. The family approaches the nurse and tells the nurse that they have spoken to the physician regarding taking their loved one home. The nurse plans to coordinate discharge planning. Which of the following services would be most supportive to the client and family?
1 American Cancer Society
2 Lung Association
3 Hospice care
4 Local religious and social organizations

Answer: 3
Rationale: Hospice care provides an environment that emphasizes caring rather than curing. The emphasis is on palliative care. One of the major goals of hospice care is that the client is free of pain and other symptoms that do not allow clients to maintain a quality life. An interdisciplinary approach is utilized. Options 1, 2, and 4 would be helpful but are not the most supportive of the options provided.

Test-Taking Strategy: Note the key words, "most supportive." Knowledge regarding the goals and services provided by hospice care will assist in answering the question. Think about what each support service presented in the options will provide in meeting this client's needs. This will assist in directing you to option 3. Review the goals of these support systems and hospice care if you had difficulty with this question.

Level of Cognitive Ability: Analysis
Client Needs: Psychosocial Integrity
Integrated Process: Caring
Content Area: Adult Health/Oncology

Reference:
Black, J., & Hawks, J. (2005). *Medical-surgical nursing: Clinical management for positive outcomes* (7th ed.). Philadelphia: Saunders, p. 187.

220. A home care nurse is caring for a client with acute cancer pain. The most appropriate assessment of the client's pain would include which of the following?
1 The client's pain rating
2 The nurse's impression of the client's pain
3 Verbal and nonverbal clues from the client
4 Pain relief after appropriate nursing intervention

Answer: 1
Rationale: The client's perception of pain is the hallmark of pain assessment. Usually noted by the client rating on a scale of 1 to 10, the assessment is documented and followed with appropriate medical and nursing intervention. The nurse's impression and the verbal and nonverbal clues are subjective data. Pain relief following intervention is appropriate but relates to evaluation.

Test-Taking Strategy: Use the process of elimination. Eliminate option 4 first because it relates to evaluation. Next, eliminate options 2 and 3 because they relate to subjective data. Also, option 1 is client focused. Review the techniques of pain assessment if you had difficulty with this question.

Level of Cognitive Ability: Application
Client Needs: Psychosocial Integrity
Integrated Process: Caring
Content Area: Adult Health/Oncology

Reference:
Ignatavicius, D., & Workman, M. (2002). *Medical surgical nursing: Critical thinking for collaborative care* (4th ed.). Philadelphia: Saunders, p. 73.

---

221. A prenatal client has been told during a physician office visit that she is positive for human immunodeficiency virus (HIV). The client cried and was significantly distressed regarding this news. Which nursing diagnosis would this data best support?
1 Acute Pain
2 Noncompliance
3 High Risk for Infection
4 Anticipatory Grieving

Answer: 4
Rationale: A life-threatening diagnosis such as HIV will stimulate the anticipatory grief response. Anticipatory grief occurs when the client, family, and loved ones know that the client will die. The prenatal HIV client is forced to make important changes in her life, frequently resulting in grief related to lost future dreams and diminished self-esteem because of an inability to achieve life goals. Although options 1, 2, and 3 may be appropriate nursing diagnoses at some point, they do not address the information in the question

Test-Taking Strategy: Note the key words "best support." Use the process of elimination, focusing on the data in the question. A client who is distressed and crying is supporting data for the nursing diagnosis of Anticipatory Grieving. Review this nursing diagnosis if you had difficulty with this question.

Level of Cognitive Ability: Analysis
Client Needs: Psychosocial Integrity
Integrated Process: Caring
Content Area: Adult Health/Immune

Reference:
Lowdermilk, D., & Perry, A. (2004). *Maternity & women's health care* (8th ed.). St. Louis: Mosby, p. 205; 1145.

222. A nurse is assessing a client's suicide potential. The nurse asks the client which most important question?
1 "Why do you want to hurt yourself?"
2 "Can you describe how you are feeling right now?"
3 "Has anyone in your family committed suicide?"
4 "Do you have a plan to commit suicide?"

Answer: 4
Rationale: When assessing for suicide risk, the nurse must evaluate if the client has a suicide plan. Clients who have a definitive plan pose a greater risk for suicide. Options 2 and 3 may also be questions that the nurse would ask but are not the most important. The nurse avoids the use of the word "why" when communicating with a client. The use of this word may place the client on the defensive; additionally, the client may not even know the reason "why" he or she wants to hurt self.

Test-Taking Strategy: Use the process of elimination, noting the key words "most important." Recalling the importance of assessing for a suicide plan will direct you to option 4. If you are unfamiliar with assessment of suicide potential, review this content.

Level of Cognitive Ability: Application
Client Needs: Psychosocial Integrity
Integrated Process: Nursing Process/Assessment
Content Area: Mental Health

Reference:
Keltner, N., Schwecke, L., & Bostrom, C. (2003). *Psychiatric nursing* (4th ed.). St. Louis: Mosby, pp. 359; 361-362.

223. A nurse is caring for a client who is receiving electroconvulsive therapy (ECT) for a major depressive disorder. Which assessment finding would the nurse identify as an unexpected side effect of ECT requiring notifying the physician?
1 Memory loss
2 Disorientation
3 Confusion
4 Hypertension

Answer: 4
Rationale: The major side effects of ECT are confusion, disorientation, and memory loss. A change in blood pressure would not be an anticipated side effect and would be a cause for concern. If hypertension occurred following ECT, the physician should be notified.

Test-Taking Strategy: Use the process of elimination, focusing on the issue: an unexpected side effect. Recall the side effects of ECT and note that options 1, 2, and 3 are similar. Review the expected and unexpected side effects of ECT if you had difficulty with this question.

Level of Cognitive Ability: Analysis
Client Needs: Psychosocial Integrity
Integrated Process: Nursing Process/Assessment
Content Area: Mental Health

Reference:
Keltner, N., Schwecke, L., & Bostrom, C. (2003). *Psychiatric nursing* (4th ed.). St. Louis: Mosby, p. 529.

224. During the admission assessment of a client admitted to the hospital for esophageal varices, the client says, "I deserve this. I brought it on myself." The nurse makes which therapeutic response to the client?
1 "Would you like to talk to the chaplain?"
2 "Not all esophageal varices are caused by alcohol."
3 "Is there some reason you feel you deserve this?"
4 "That is something to think about when you leave the hospital."

Answer: 3

Rationale: Ruptured esophageal varices are often a complication of cirrhosis of the liver, and the most common type of cirrhosis is caused by chronic alcohol abuse. It is important to obtain an accurate history about alcohol intake from the client. If the client is ashamed or embarrassed, he or she may not respond accurately. Option 3 is open-ended and allows the client to discuss feelings about drinking. Option 1 blocks the nurse-client communication process. Options 2 and 4 are somewhat judgmental.

Test-Taking Strategy: Use the process of elimination and therapeutic communication techniques to direct you to option 3. Remember that the client's feelings should be addressed first. Review therapeutic communication techniques if you had difficulty with this question.

Level of Cognitive ability: Application
Client Needs: Psychosocial Integrity
Integrated Process: Communication and Documentation
Content Area: Adult Health/Gastrointestinal

References:
Ignatavicius, D., & Workman, M. (2002). *Medical surgical nursing: Critical thinking for collaborative care* (4th ed.). Philadelphia: Saunders, p. 1299.
Potter, P., & Perry, A. (2005). *Fundamentals of nursing* (6th ed.). St. Louis: Mosby, p. 437.

---

225. A nurse is performing a neurological assessment on a client with dementia and is assessing the function of the frontal lobes of the brain. Assessment of which of the following items by the nurse would yield the best information about this area of functioning?
1 Level of consciousness
2 Insight, judgment, and planning
3 Feelings or emotions
4 Eye movements

Answer: 2

Rationale: Insight, judgment, and planning are part of the function of the frontal lobe. Level of consciousness is controlled by the reticular activating system. Feelings and emotions are part of the role of the limbic system. Eye movements are under the control of cranial nerves III, IV, and VI.

Test-Taking Strategy: A specific understanding of the function of the frontal lobe of the brain will direct you to option 2. Review the function of this lobe if you had difficulty with this question.

Level of Cognitive Ability: Application
Client Needs: Psychosocial Integrity
Integrated Process: Nursing Process/Assessment
Content Area: Adult Health/Neurological

Reference:
Ignatavicius, D., & Workman, M. (2002). *Medical surgical nursing: Critical thinking for collaborative care* (4th ed.). Philadelphia: Saunders, p. 874.

CRITICAL THINKING: ALTERNATE FORMAT QUESTIONS

1. An emergency room nurse is caring for a female client who is in the acute phase of rape trauma syndrome. Select all nursing interventions that apply to the care of the client:

___ Leave the client alone so that she will feel more comfortable to cry and express sorrow

___ Encourage the client to talk about what she did to cause the rape

___ Obtain the client's written permission for examination and treatment

___ Inform the client that she needs to press charges if the offender is caught

___ Explain to the client that her emotional responses to the attack are normal and may continue for weeks after the rape

___ Assess the degree of injury sustained during the rape

Answer:
Obtain the client's written permission for examination and treatment
Explain to the client that her emotional responses to the attack are normal and may continue for weeks after the rape
Assess the degree of injury sustained during the rape

Rationale: Rape trauma syndrome refers to the acute or immediate phase of psychological disorganization and the long-term process of reorganization that occurs as a result of attempted or actual assault. During the acute phase, immediately after the assault, emergency assessment and treatment are provided and forensic evidence is collected. The nurse would always assess the degree of injury sustained during the rape and immediately treat any injury that is life-threatening. The client should not be left alone at this time and should be provided with calm and supportive interventions. Encouraging the client to talk about the cause of the rape is inappropriate. The nurse needs to encourage the client to talk about any mixed feelings that she may have and remind the client that she is in no way responsible for the rape. The nurse would obtain the client's written permission for examination and treatment. This is necessary because two types of specimens will be collected during the examination. One part of the specimen will be sent to the laboratory for evaluation, and another part will be sent to a forensic laboratory and will be considered evidence in the event that the offender is caught and the client presses charges. The decision to press charges is made by the client, and the nurse needs to support the client in the decision-making process. Sexual assault is the ultimate invasion of privacy and safety. The nurse needs to explain to the client that her emotional responses to the attack are normal and may continue for weeks after the rape. Time and counseling are needed before the victim feels safe, secure, and in control.

Test-Taking Strategy: Read each intervention carefully. Use the principles of a therapeutic nurse-client relationship and ethical and legal guidelines to select the correct interventions. Review these principles and guidelines and care of the rape victim if you had difficulty with this question.

Level of Cognitive Ability: Application
Client Needs: Psychosocial Integrity
Integrated Process: Caring
Content Area: Mental Health

Reference:
Gulanick, M., Myers, J., Klopp, A., Gradishar, D., Galanes, S., & Puzas, M. (2003). *Nursing care plans: Nursing diagnosis and intervention* (5th ed.). St. Louis: Mosby, pp. 1082-1087.

2. Diazepam (Valium) 7.5 mg intravenously has been prescribed for a client with acute alcohol withdrawal. The nurse draws how many mL into the syringe to administer the correct dose?

Answer: _____

Answer: 1.5

Rationale: Use the formula for calculating medication dosages.

Formula:

$$\frac{\text{Desired}}{\text{Available}} \times \text{Volume} = \text{mL per dose}$$

$$\frac{7.5 \text{ mg}}{5 \text{ mg}} \times 1 \text{ mL} = 1.5 \text{ mL}$$

Test-Taking Strategy: Identify the key components of the question and what the question is asking. In this case, the question asks for mL per dose. Set up the formula knowing that the desired dose is 7.5 mg, available is 5 mg per 1 mL. Review medication calculations if you had difficulty with this question.

Level of Cognitive Ability: Application
Client Needs: Psychosocial Integrity
Integrated Process: Nursing Process/Implementation
Content Area: Mental Health

Reference:
Kee, J. & Marshall, S. (2004). *Clinical calculations: With applications to general and specialty areas* (4th ed.). Philadelphia: Saunders, pp. 80-81; 180.

3. Haloperidol (Haldol) 3 mg intramuscularly has been prescribed for a client with delirium. The medication label reads 5 mg/mL. The nurse prepares how many mL to administer the correct dose?

Answer: _____

Answer: 0.6
Rationale: Use the formula for calculating medication dosages.

Formula:

$$\frac{\text{Desired}}{\text{Available}} \times \text{Volume} = \text{mL per dose}$$

$$\frac{3 \text{ mg}}{5 \text{ mg}} \times 1 \text{ mL} = 0.6 \text{ mL}$$

Test-Taking Strategy: Identify the key components of the question and what the question is asking. In this case, the question asks for mL per dose. Set up the formula knowing that the desired dose is 3 mg, available is 5 mg per 1 mL. Review medication calculations if you had difficulty with this question.

Level of Cognitive Ability: Application
Client Needs: Psychosocial Integrity
Integrated Process: Nursing Process/Implementation
Content Area: Mental Health

Reference:
Hodgson, B., & Kizior, R. (2004). *Saunders nursing drug handbook 2004.* Philadelphia: Saunders, pp. 489-490.

---

4. The nurse is caring for a client who is dying and formulates a nursing diagnosis of Fear and appropriate nursing interventions. List the nursing interventions in order of priority. (Number 1 is the first priority.)

___ Document verbal and nonverbal expressions of fear and other significant data

___ Assess the nature of the client's fears

___ Help the client express his fears

___ Help the client identify methods that he used to cope with fear in the past

Answer: 4123

Rationale: Fear can range from a paralyzing, overwhelming feeling to a mild concern. Therefore, the nurse would first assess the nature of the client's fears in order to know how best to help the client. Next, the nurse would help the client express his fears. The client's fear may not be limited to the fear of dying, and the nurse needs this information in order to help the client. Once the nurse is aware of the client's fears, the methods that the client used to cope with fear in the past are identified. From the interventions listed, the nurse would lastly document verbal and nonverbal expressions of fear and any other significant data.

Test-Taking Strategy: Use the steps of the nursing process to assist in determining the order of priority of the nursing interventions. This will assist in determining that assessing the nature of the client's fears is the first priority. Identify the last priority as documenting verbal and nonverbal expressions of fear and other significant data. The nurse would not be aware of this information until the nurse performed an assessment and provided care to the client. From the remaining two interventions, it would be necessary to help the client express his fears before methods used to cope with fear can be determined. Review care of the dying client who is experiencing fear if you had difficulty with this question.

Level of Cognitive Ability: Application
Client Needs: Psychosocial Integrity
Integrated Process: Nursing Process/Implementation
Content Area: Delegating/Prioritizing

Reference:
Gulanick, M., Myers, J., Klopp, A., Gradishar, D., Galanes, S., & Puzas, M. (2003). *Nursing care plans: Nursing diagnosis and intervention* (5th ed.). St. Louis: Mosby, pp. 1074-1076.

REFERENCES

Brent, N. (2001). *Nurses and the law* (2nd ed.). Philadelphia: Saunders.

Black, J., & Hawks, J. (2005). *Medical-surgical nursing: Clinical management for positive outcomes* (7th ed.). Philadelphia: Saunders.

Chernecky, C., & Berger, B. (2004). *Laboratory tests and diagnostic procedures* (4th ed.). Philadelphia: Saunders.

Fortinash, K., & Holoday-Worret, P. (2004). *Psychiatric mental health nursing* (3rd ed.). St. Louis: Mosby.

Gulanick, M., Myers, J., Klopp, A., Gradishar, D., Galanes, S., & Puzas, M. (2003). *Nursing care plans: Nursing diagnosis and intervention* (5th ed.). St. Louis: Mosby.

Harkreader, H., & Hogan, M.A. (2004). *Fundamentals of nursing: Caring and clinical judgment* (2nd ed.). Philadelphia: Saunders.

Hodgson, B., & Kizior, R. (2004). *Saunders nursing drug handbook 2004.* Philadelphia: Saunders.

Ignatavicius, D., & Workman, M. (2005). *Medical surgical nursing: Critical thinking for collaborative care* (5th ed.). Philadelphia: Saunders.

James, S., Ashwill, J., & Droske, S. (2002). *Nursing care of children: Principles & practice* (2nd ed.). Philadelphia:Saunders.

Keltner, N., Schwecke, L., & Bostrom, C. (2003). *Psychiatric nursing* (4th ed.). St. Louis: Mosby.

Lehne, R. (2004). *Pharmacology for nursing care* (5th ed.). Philadelphia: Saunders.

Lewis, S., Heitkemper, M., & Dirksen, S. (2004). *Medical-surgical nursing: Assessment and management of clinical problems* (6th ed.). St. Louis: Mosby.

Lowdermilk, D., & Perry, A. (2004). *Maternity & women's health care* (8th ed.). St. Louis: Mosby.

Matteson, P. (2001). *Women's health during the childbearing years: A community-based approach.* St. Louis: Mosby.

McKenry, L., & Salerno, E. (2003). *Mosby's pharmacology in nursing* (21st ed.). St. Louis: Mosby.

McKinney, E., James, S., Murray, S., & Ashwill, J. (2005). *Maternal-child nursing* (2nd ed.). St. Louis: Elsevier.

Murray, S., McKinney, E., & Gorrie, T. (2002). *Foundations of maternal-newborn nursing* (3rd ed.). Philadelphia: Saunders.

Phipps, W., Monahan, F., Sands, J., Marek, J., & Neighbors, M. (2003). *Medical-surgical nursing: Health and illness perspectives* (7th ed.). St. Louis: Mosby.

Potter, P., & Perry, A. (2005). *Fundamentals of nursing* (6th ed.). St. Louis: Mosby.

Stuart, G., & Laraia, M. (2005). *Principles and practice of psychiatric nursing* (8th ed.). St. Louis: Mosby.

Varcarolis, E.M. (2002). *Foundations of psychiatric mental health nursing* (4th ed.). Philadelphia: Saunders.

Wong, D., & Hockenberry, M. (2003). *Wong's nursing care of infants and children* (7th ed.). St. Louis: Mosby.

Integrated Processes

Integrated Processes and the NCLEX-RN® Test Plan

INTEGRATED PROCESSES

In the new test plan implemented in April 2004, the National Council of State Boards of Nursing (NCSBN) has identified a test plan framework based on Client Needs. This framework was selected based on the analysis of the findings in a practice analysis study of newly licensed registered nurses in the United States. This study identified the nursing activities performed by entry-level nurses across all settings for all clients. The NCSBN identifies four major categories of Client Needs. The Client Needs categories, which include Safe, Effective Care Environment; Health Promotion and Maintenance; Psychosocial Integrity; and Physiological Integrity, are described in Chapter 6.

The 2004 NCLEX-RN test plan also identifies four processes that are fundamental to the practice of nursing. These processes are integrated throughout the four major categories of Client Needs. The test plan for NCLEX-RN identifies these components as Integrated Processes. The Integrated Processes include Nursing Process; Caring; Communication and Documentation; and Teaching/Learning (Box 11-1).

NURSING PROCESS

The steps of the nursing process provide a systematic and organized method of problem solving and providing care to clients. These steps include assessment, analysis, planning, implementation, and evaluation (Box 11-2).

Assessment

Assessment is the first step of the nursing process. It involves a systematic method of collecting data about a client in order to identify actual and potential client health problems and establish a database. The database provides the foundation for the remaining steps of the nursing process; therefore, a thorough and adequate database is essential. Data collection begins with the first contact with the client. During all successive contacts, the nurse continues to collect information that is significant and relevant to the needs of the client.

During the assessment process, the nurse collects data about the client from a variety of sources. The client is the primary source of data. Family members and/or significant others are secondary sources of assessment data, and these sources may supplement or verify information provided by the client. Data may also be obtained from the client's record through the medical history, laboratory results, and diagnostic reports. Medical records from previous admissions may provide additional information about the client. The nurse may also obtain information through consultation with other health care team members who have had contact with the client.

A thorough database is obtained through a health history and physical assessment. The information collected by the nurse includes both subjective and objective data. Subjective data include the information that the client states. Objective data are the observable, measurable pieces of information about the client. Objective data include measurements, such as vital signs and laboratory findings, and information obtained from observing the client. Objective data also include clinical manifestations such as the signs and symptoms of an illness or disease.

The process of assessment additionally consists of confirming and verifying client data, communicating information obtained through the assessment process, and documenting assessment findings in a thorough and accurate manner.

On NCLEX-RN, remember that assessment is the first step in the nursing process. When answering these types of questions, focus on the data in the question and select the option that addresses an assessment action. Also, use skills of prioritizing and the ABCs—airway, breathing, and circulation—to answer the question (Box 11-3).

BOX 11-1

Integrated Processes

Nursing Process
Caring
Communication and Documentation
Teaching/Learning

BOX 11-2

Steps of the Nursing Process

Assessment
Analysis
Planning
Implementation
Evaluation

Analysis

Analysis is the second step of the nursing process. In this step, the nurse focuses on the data gathered during the assessment process and identifies actual or potential health care needs, problems, or both. During this process, the nurse summarizes and interprets the assessment data, organizes and validates the data, and determines the need for additional data. Client assessment data are compared with the normal expected findings and behaviors for the client's age, education, and cultural background. The nurse then draws conclusions regarding the client's unique needs and health care risks or problems.

Client health problems are categorized as potential problems requiring prevention or actual problems being managed or requiring interventions. The nurse reports the results of analysis to relevant members of

BOX 11-3

Nursing Process: Assessment

A child with hemophilia is brought into the emergency room after being hit on the neck with a baseball. The nurse immediately assesses the child for:
1. Spontaneous hematuria
2. Airway obstruction
3. Headache and slurred speech
4. Factor VIII deficiency

Answer: 2

Rationale: Trauma to the neck may cause bleeding into the tissues of the neck, which may compromise the airway. Although hematuria is a symptom of hemophilia, it is not associated with neck injury. Headache and slurred speech are associated with head trauma. Factor VIII deficiency is not a symptom of hemophilia but rather a common form of the disease. Use the ABCs—airway, breathing, and circulation—to answer this question. Airway assessment is always a first priority!

the health care team and documents the client's unique health care problems, needs, or both.

On NCLEX-RN, questions that address the process of analysis are difficult questions because they require an understanding of the principles of physiological responses and require an interpretation of the data based on assessment findings. Analysis questions require critical thinking and determining the rationale for therapeutic interventions that may be addressed in the case situation. Analysis questions may address the formulation of a nursing diagnosis and the communication and documentation of the results of the process of analysis (Box 11-4).

Planning

Planning is the third step of the nursing process. This step involves the functions of setting priorities, determining goals of care, planning actions, collaborating with other health team members, establishing evaluative criteria, and communicating the plan of care.

Setting priorities assists the nurse in organizing and planning care that solves the most urgent problems. Priorities may change as the client's level of wellness changes. Both actual and potential problems should be considered when establishing priorities. Actual problems are usually more important than potential problems. However, potential problems may at times take precedence over actual problems.

Once priorities are established, the client and nurse mutually decide on the expected goals. The selected goals serve as a guide in the selection of nursing interventions and in determining the criteria for evaluation. Before nursing actions are implemented, mechanisms

BOX 11-4

Nursing Process: Analysis

A client is admitted to the cardiac unit and placed on telemetry. A nurse reviews the client's laboratory values and notes that the client's potassium level is 6.3 mEq/L. In analyzing the cardiac rhythm, the nurse would expect to note which electrocardiogram (ECG) finding?
1. A sinus rhythm with a depressed ST segment
2. A sinus tachycardia with a prolonged QT interval
3. A sinus tachycardia with an extra U wave
4. A sinus rhythm with a tall, peaked T wave

Answer: 4

Rationale: A potassium level greater than 5.1 mEq/L indicates hyperkalemia, which can be detected on ECG by the presence of a tall, peaked T wave. A U wave and a depressed ST segment are present with hypokalemia. A prolonged QT interval indicates hypocalcemia. In this question, it is necessary to know that the client is experiencing hyperkalemia, as evidenced by the potassium level of 6.3 mEq/L. Once this has been determined, it is necessary to know the ECG changes (tall, peaked T wave) that occur with hyperkalemia.

to determine goal achievement and the effectiveness of nursing interventions are established. Unless criteria have been predetermined, it is difficult to know whether the goal has been achieved and the problem is resolved.

It is important for the nurse both to identify health or social resources available to the client and to collaborate with other health care team members when planning the delivery of care. The nurse needs to communicate the plan of care, review the plan of care with the client, and document the plan of care thoroughly and accurately.

When answering questions on NCLEX-RN, remember that this is a nursing examination, and the answer to the question most likely involves something that is included in the nursing care plan, rather than the medical plan. Also, remember that actual problems are usually more important than potential problems and that physiological needs are usually the priority (Box 11-5).

Implementation

Implementation is the fourth step of the nursing process. It includes initiating and completing nursing actions required to accomplish the defined goals. This step is the action phase that involves counseling, teaching, organizing and managing client care, providing care to achieve established goals, supervising and coordinating the delivery of client care, and communicating and documenting the nursing interventions and client responses.

During implementation, the nurse uses intellectual skills, interpersonal skills, and technical skills. Intellectual skills involve critical thinking, problem solving, and making judgments. Interpersonal skills involve the ability to communicate, listen, and convey compassion. Technical skills relate to the performance of treatments, performance of procedures, and the use of necessary equipment when providing care to the client.

The nurse independently implements actions that include activities that do not require a physician's order. The nurse also implements actions collaboratively based on the physician's orders. Sound nursing judgment and working with other health care members is incorporated into the process of implementation. The implementation step concludes when the nurse's actions are completed and these actions, including their effects and the client's response, are communicated and documented.

NCLEX-RN is an examination about nursing, so focus on the nursing action rather than on the medical action, unless the question is asking what prescribed medical action is anticipated (Box 11-6).

Evaluation

Evaluation is the fifth and final step of the nursing process. The process of evaluation identifies the degree to which the nursing diagnoses, plans for care, and interventions have been successful.

Although evaluation is the final step of the nursing process, it is an ongoing and integral component of each step. The process of data collection and assessment is reviewed to determine if sufficient information was obtained and whether the information obtained was specific and appropriate. The nursing diagnoses are evaluated for accuracy and completeness based on the client's specific needs. The plan and expected outcomes are examined to determine whether they are realistic, achievable, measurable, and effective. Interventions are

---

BOX 11-5
Nursing Process: Planning

A nurse is caring for a client with dementia who has a nursing diagnosis of Self-Care Deficit. The nurse plans for which most appropriate goal for this client?
1. Client will be oriented to place by the time of discharge
2. Client will correctly identify objects in his or her room by the time of discharge
3. Client will be free of hallucinations
4. Client will feed self with cueing within 24 hours

Answer: 4

Rationale: Option 4 identifies a goal that is directly related to the client's ability to care for self. Options 1, 2, and 3 are not related to the nursing diagnosis of Self-Care Deficit. Remember, based on Maslow's hierarchy of needs theory, physiological needs take precedence. Option 4 is the only option that addresses a physiological need.

BOX 11-6
Nursing Process: Implementation

A client with heart failure is receiving furosemide (Lasix) and digoxin (Lanoxin) daily. When the nurse enters the room to administer the morning doses, the client complains of anorexia, nausea, and yellow vision. The nurse should do which of the following first?
1. Administer the medications
2. Contact the physician
3. Check the morning serum potassium level
4. Check the morning serum digoxin level

Answer: 4

Rationale: The nurse should check for the result of the digoxin level that was drawn, because the symptoms are compatible with digitalis toxicity. Knowing that a low potassium level may contribute to digoxin toxicity, checking the serum potassium level may give useful additive information, but the digoxin level is checked first. The medications should be withheld until both levels are known. If the digoxin level is elevated and/or if the potassium level is not within normal range, then the physician is notified. If the morning digoxin level is within therapeutic range, then the client's complaints are unrelated to the digoxin. Additionally, noting the key word "first" will assist in determining that the nurse's action is to further investigate the cause of the client's complaints.

examined to determine their effectiveness in achieving the expected outcomes.

Because evaluation is an ongoing process, it is vital to all steps of the nursing process. It is the continuous process of comparing actual outcomes with expected outcomes of care, and provides the means for determining the need to modify the plan of care. Inherent in this step of the nursing process is the communication of evaluation findings and the process of documenting the client's response to treatment, care, and/or teaching. Evaluation-type questions on NCLEX-RN may be written to address a client's response to treatment measures or to determine a client's understanding of the prescribed treatment measures (Box 11-7).

CARING

Caring is the essence of nursing and is basic to any helping relationship. Caring is central to every encounter that a nurse may have with a client. Through caring, the nurse humanizes the client. Treating the client with respect and dignity is a true expression of caring. In the technological environment of health care, emphasizing the client's individuality counteracts any potential process of depersonalization. Caring is an Integrated Process of the test plan for NCLEX-RN. This means that this concept is nuclear to all Client Needs components of the test plan.

On NCLEX-RN, the concept of caring is primary. It is very easy to become involved with looking at a question from a technological viewpoint. The concept of caring needs to be addressed when reading a test question and when selecting an option. Always address the client's feelings and provide support. Remember: this examination is all about nursing, and Nursing is Caring! (Box 11-8).

COMMUNICATION AND DOCUMENTATION

The process of communication occurs as a nurse interacts either verbally or nonverbally with a client. Therapeutic communication techniques are key to an effective nurse-client relationship. Communication-type test questions are integrated throughout the NCLEX-RN test plan and may address a client situation in any health care setting.

When answering a question on NCLEX-RN, use of therapeutic communication techniques indicates a correct option, and use of nontherapeutic communication techniques indicates an incorrect option. Additionally, some communication-type questions may focus on psychosocial issues or issues related to client anxiety, fears, or concerns. In communication-type questions, always focus on the client's feelings *first*. If an option reflects the client's feelings, anxiety, or concerns, select that option.

Documentation is a critical component of a nurse's responsibility. The process of documentation serves many purposes and provides a comprehensive representation of the client's health status and the care given by all members of the health care team. There are many methods for documenting, but the responsibilities surrounding this practice remain the same.

When answering a question on NCLEX-RN related to documenting, consider the ethical and legal responsibilities related to documentation and the specific guidelines related to both narrative and computerized documentation systems (Box 11-9).

BOX 11-7

Nursing Process: Evaluation

A home care nurse visits a child with a diagnosis of celiac disease. Which finding would indicate that a gluten-free diet is being maintained and has been effective?
1. The child is free of diarrhea.
2. The child is free of bloody stools.
3. The child tolerates dietary wheat and rye.
4. A balanced fluid and electrolyte status as noted on the laboratory results.

Answer: 1

Rationale: This question addresses the child's response to prescribed dietary measures for celiac disease. Watery diarrhea is a frequent clinical manifestation of celiac disease. The absence of diarrhea indicates effective treatment. The grains of wheat and rye contain gluten and are not allowed. A balance in fluids and electrolytes does not necessarily demonstrate improved status of celiac disease. Remember: an evaluation-type question addresses a client's response to a treatment measure.

BOX 11-8

Caring

A female client and her infant have undergone testing for human immunodeficiency virus (HIV), and both clients were found to be positive. The news is devastating and the mother is crying. Using crisis intervention techniques, the nurse determines that which intervention will meet the client's needs at this time?
1. Calling an HIV counselor and making an appointment for them
2. Describing the progressive stages and treatments for HIV
3. Examining with the mother how she got HIV
4. Listening quietly while the mother talks and cries

Answer: 4

Rationale: This client has just received devastating news and needs to have someone present with her as she begins to cope with this issue. The nurse needs to sit and actively listen while the mother talks and cries. Calling an HIV counselor may be helpful, but it is not what the client needs at this time. The other options are not appropriate for this stage of coping with the news that both she and the baby are HIV positive. Remember to address the client's feelings and to support the client. The nurse should sit and listen and provide support because this is the most caring response.

BOX 11-9

Communication and Documentation

COMMUNICATION

A client says to the nurse, "I'm going to die and I wish my family would stop hoping for a cure! I get so angry when they carry on like this! After all, I'm the one who's dying." The nurse makes which therapeutic response to the client?
1. "You're feeling angry that your family continues to hope for you to be cured?"
2. "I think we should talk more about your anger with your family."
3. "Well, it sounds like you're being pretty pessimistic. After all, years ago before antibiotics were discovered, people died of pneumonia."
4. "Have you shared your feelings with your family?"

Answer: 1

Rationale: Reflection is the therapeutic communication technique that redirects the client's feelings back in order to validate what the client is saying. Option 1 uses the therapeutic technique of reflection. In option 2, the nurse attempts to use focusing, but the attempt to discuss central issues seems premature. In option 3, the nurse makes a judgment and is nontherapeutic in the one-to-one relationship. In option 4, the nurse is attempting to assess the client's ability to openly discuss feelings with family members. While this is an appropriate assessment of this client, the timing is somewhat premature and closes off facilitation of the client's feelings. Remember: the use of therapeutic communication techniques indicates a correct option.

DOCUMENTATION

A nurse hears a client calling out for help. The nurse hurries down the hallway to the client's room and finds the client lying on the floor. The nurse performs a thorough assessment and assists the client back to bed. The nurse notifies the physician of the incident and completes an incident report. Which of the following would the nurse document on the incident report?
1. The client was found lying on the floor.
2. The client climbed over the side rails.
3. The client fell out of bed.
4. The client became restless and tried to get out of bed.

Answer: 1

Rationale: The incident report should contain the client's name, age, and diagnosis. It should contain a factual description of the incident, any injuries experienced by those involved, and the outcome of the situation. Option 1 is the only option that describes the facts as observed by the nurse. Options 2, 3, and 4 are interpretations of the situation and are not factual data as observed by the nurse. Remember to focus on factual information when documenting and avoid including interpretations.

BOX 11-10

Teaching/Learning

A nurse provides instructions to a client about administering nitroglycerin ointment (Nitrobid). The nurse determines that the client is using the correct technique when applying the ointment if the client:
1. Applies additional ointment if chest pain occurs
2. Applies the ointment directly to the skin and then gently rubs the ointment into skin
3. Applies the ointment to any nonhairy area of the body
4. Washes the ointment off when bathing and reapplies after the bath

Answer: 3

Rationale: Nitroglycerin ointment is used on a scheduled basis and is not prescribed specifically for the occurrence of chest pain. The ointment is not rubbed into the skin. It is reapplied only as directed. The correct client action (option 3) indicates the acquisition of knowledge in regard to administering the prescribed medication.

The principles related to the teaching/learning process are used when the nurse functions in the role of a teacher. The nurse needs to remember that assessment of the client's readiness and motivation to learn is the initial step in the teaching/learning process.

When answering a question on NCLEX-RN related to the teaching/learning process, use the principles related to teaching/learning theory. If a test question addresses client education, remember that client motivation and readiness to learn is the *first* priority (Box 11-10).

REFERENCES

Harkreader, H., & Hogan, M.A. (2004). *Fundamentals of nursing: Caring and clinical judgment* (2nd ed.). Philadelphia: Saunders.

Hodgson, B., & Kizior, R. (2004). *Saunders nursing drug handbook 2004.* Philadelphia: Saunders.

Ignatavicius, D., & Workman, M. (2005). *Medical surgical nursing: Critical thinking for collaborative care* (5th ed.). Philadelphia: Saunders.

Keltner, N., Schwecke, L., & Bostrom, C. (2003). *Psychiatric nursing* (4th ed.). St. Louis: Mosby.

Lewis, S., Heitkemper, M., & Dirksen, S. (2004). *Medical-surgical nursing: Assessment and management of clinical problems* (6th ed.). St. Louis: Mosby.

National Council of State Boards of Nursing (eds.). (2003). *Test Plan for the National Council Licensure Examination for Registered Nurses.* (Effective Date: April 2004). Chicago: Author.

National Council of State Boards of Nursing (eds.). (2004). *Detailed Test Plan for the National Council Licensure Examination for Registered Nurses.* Chicago: Author.

National Council of State Boards of Nursing. Web Site: www.ncsbn.org

Phipps, W., Monahan, F., Sands, J., Marek, J., & Neighbors, M. (2003). *Medical-surgical nursing: Health and illness perspectives* (7th ed.). St. Louis: Mosby.

Potter, P., & Perry, A. (2005). *Fundamentals of nursing* (6th ed.). St. Louis: Mosby.

Stuart, G., & Laraia, M. (2005). *Principles and practice of psychiatric nursing* (8th ed.). St. Louis: Mosby.

TEACHING/LEARNING

Client and family education is a primary nursing responsibility. The NCSBN describes this process as facilitating the acquisition of knowledge, skills, and attitudes that lead to a change in behavior.

Integrated Processes

NURSING PROCESS
Nursing Process: Assessment

---

1. A nurse reviews the record of a client receiving external radiation therapy and notes documentation of a skin finding noted as moist desquamation. The nurse expects to note which of the following on assessment of the client?
   1 Reddened skin
   2 A rash
   3 Weeping of the skin
   4 Dermatitis

Answer: 3
Rationale: Moist desquamation occurs when the basal cells of the skin are destroyed. The dermal level is exposed, which results in the leakage of serum. Reddened skin, a rash, and dermatitis may occur with external radiation but is not described as a moist desquamation.

Test-Taking Strategy: Use the process of elimination. Options 1, 2, and 4 are eliminated because they are similar and describe a dry rather than a moist skin alteration. Also, note the relationship between the word "moist" in the question and the word "weeping" in the correct option. Review the signs associated with a moist desquamation if you had difficulty with this question.

Level of Cognitive Ability: Analysis
Client Needs: Physiological Integrity
Integrated Process: Nursing Process/Assessment
Content Area: Adult Health/Oncology

Reference:
Black, J., & Hawks, J. (2005). *Medical-surgical nursing: Clinical management for positive outcomes* (7th ed.). Philadelphia: Saunders, p. 386.

---

2. A nurse is performing an assessment on a pregnant client with a history of cardiac disease and is assessing for venous congestion. The nurse checks which body area, knowing that venous congestion is most commonly noted in this area?
   1 Vulva
   2 Fingers of the hands
   3 Around the eyes
   4 Around the abdomen

Answer: 1
Rationale: Assessment of the cardiovascular system includes observation for venous congestion that can develop into varicosities. Venous congestion is most commonly noted in the legs, vulva, or rectum. It would be difficult to assess for edema in the abdominal area of a client who is pregnant. Although edema may be noted in the fingers and around the eyes, edema in these areas would not be directly associated with venous congestion.

Test-Taking Strategy: Focus on the key words "venous congestion." From the options provided, the only body area that is associated with this problem is the vulva. Review physical assessment of the cardiovascular system in a pregnant client if you had difficulty with this question.

Level of Cognitive Ability: Application
Client Needs: Physiological Integrity
Integrated Process: Nursing Process/Assessment
Content Area: Maternity/Antepartum

Reference:
Murray, S., McKinney, E., & Gorrie, T. (2002). *Foundations of maternal-newborn nursing* (3rd ed.). Philadelphia: Saunders, p. 143.

---

3. A client who has been receiving long-term diuretic therapy is admitted to the hospital with a diagnosis of dehydration. The nurse would assess for which sign or symptom that correlates with this fluid imbalance?
  1 Increased blood pressure
  2 Decreased pulse
  3 Decreased central venous pressure (CVP)
  4 Bibasilar crackles

Answer: 3
Rationale: A client with dehydration has a low CVP. The normal CVP is between 4 to 11 mm H_2O. Other assessment findings with fluid volume deficit are increased pulse and respirations, weight loss, poor skin turgor, dry mucous membranes, decreased urine output, concentrated urine with increased specific gravity, increased hematocrit, and altered level of consciousness. The assessment signs in options 1, 2, and 4 occur with excess fluid volume.

Test-Taking Strategy: Use the process of elimination, focusing on the client's diagnosis. Remember that central venous pressure reflects the pressure under which blood is returned to the right atrium, and that pressure (volume) decreases with deficient fluid volume. Review the signs and symptoms of deficient fluid volume if you had difficulty with this question.

Level of Cognitive Ability: Analysis
Client Needs: Physiological Integrity
Integrated Process: Nursing Process/Assessment
Content Area: Fundamental Skills

Reference:
Black, J., & Hawks, J. (2005). *Medical-surgical nursing: Clinical management for positive outcomes* (7th ed.). Philadelphia: Saunders, pp. 208-209; 2494.

---

4. A nurse is preparing a plan of care for a child with Reye's syndrome. The nurse identifies nursing interventions and plans to monitor the child for:
  1 Signs of increased intracranial pressure (ICP)
  2 The presence of protein in the urine
  3 Signs of a bacterial infection
  4 Signs of hyperglycemia

Answer: 1
Rationale: Intracranial pressure, encephalopathy, and hepatic dysfunction are major symptoms of Reye's syndrome. Protein is not present in the urine. Reye's syndrome is related to a history of viral infections, and hypoglycemia is a symptom of this disease.

Test-Taking Strategy: Focus on the diagnosis. Recalling that increased ICP is a major symptom of Reyes's syndrome will direct you to option 1. Review the care of the child with Reye's syndrome if you had difficulty with this question.

Level of Cognitive Ability: Application
Client Needs: Physiological Integrity

Integrated Process: Nursing Process/Assessment
Content Area: Child Health

Reference:
Wong, D., & Hockenberry, M. (2003). *Wong's nursing care of infants and children* (7th ed.). St. Louis: Mosby, p. 1683.

---

5. A clinic nurse reads the chart of a client who was seen by the physician and notes that the physician has documented that the client has Lyme disease stage III. On assessment of the client, which clinical manifestation would the nurse expect to note?
 1 A generalized skin rash
 2 A cardiac dysrhythmia
 3 Enlarged and inflamed joints
 4 Palpitations

Answer: 3
Rationale: Stage III develops within a month to several months after initial infection. It is characterized by arthritic symptoms, such as arthralgia and enlarged or inflamed joints, which can persist for several years after the initial infection. Cardiac and neurological dysfunction occurs in stage II. A rash occurs in stage I.

Test-Taking Strategy: Use the process of elimination. Eliminate options 2 and 4 first because they are both cardiac related. From the remaining options, recalling that a rash occurs in stage I will direct you to option 3. Review the clinical manifestations associated with Lyme disease if you had difficulty with this question.

Level of Cognitive Ability: Analysis
Client Needs: Physiological Integrity
Integrated Process: Nursing Process/Assessment
Content Area: Adult Health/Integumentary

References:
Black, J., & Hawks, J. (2005). *Medical-surgical nursing: Clinical management for positive outcomes* (7th ed.). Philadelphia: Saunders, p. 2372.
Ignatavicius, D., & Workman, M. (2002). *Medical surgical nursing: Critical thinking for collaborative care* (4th ed.). Philadelphia: Saunders, p. 361.

---

6. A female client with narcolepsy has been prescribed dextroamphetamine (Dexedrine). The client complains to the nurse that she cannot sleep well anymore at night and does not want to take the medication any longer. The nurse then asks the client if the medication is taken at which appropriate time?
 1 At least 6 hours before bedtime
 2 Two hours before bedtime
 3 Before a bedtime snack
 4 Just before going to sleep

Answer: 1
Rationale: Dextroamphetamine is a central nervous system (CNS) stimulant that acts by releasing norepinephrine from nerve endings. The client should take the medication at least 6 hours before going to bed at night to prevent disturbances with sleep. Therefore, options 2, 3, and 4 are incorrect.

Test-Taking Strategy: Use the process of elimination. Recall that this medication causes CNS stimulation and interferes with sleep. Evaluate each of the options in terms of how far removed the scheduled dose is from the client's bedtime. This will direct you to option 1. Review this medication if you had difficulty with this question.

Level of Cognitive Ability: Application
Client Needs: Physiological Integrity
Integrated Process: Nursing Process/Assessment
Content Area: Pharmacology

Reference:
Hodgson, B., & Kizior, R. (2004). *Saunders nursing drug handbook 2004.* Philadelphia: Saunders, p. 297.

7. A nurse is assessing the level of consciousness in a child with a head injury and documents that the child is obtunded. Based on this documentation, which observation did the nurse note?

1 The child is unable to recognize place or person.
2 The child is unable to think clearly and rapidly.
3 The child requires considerable stimulation for arousal.
4 The child sleeps unless aroused and once aroused has limited interaction with the environment.

Answer: 4

Rationale: If the child is obtunded, the child sleeps unless aroused and once aroused has limited interaction with the environment. Option 1 describes disorientation. Option 2 describes confusion. Option 3 describes stupor.

Test-Taking Strategy: Note the key word "obtunded." Knowledge regarding the standard terms used to identify level of consciousness will direct you to option 4. Review this content if you are unfamiliar with assessment of level of consciousness.

Level of Cognitive Ability: Analysis
Client Needs: Physiological Integrity
Integrated Process: Nursing Process/Assessment
Content Area: Child Health

Reference:
Wong, D., & Hockenberry, M. (2003). *Wong's nursing care of infants and children* (7th ed.). St. Louis: Mosby, p. 1648.

---

8. A nurse is assessing a client with Addison's disease for signs of hyperkalemia. The nurse expects to note which of the following if hyperkalemia is present?

1 Polyuria
2 Dry mucous membranes
3 Cardiac dysrhythmias
4 Prolonged bleeding time

Answer: 3

Rationale: The inadequate production of aldosterone in Addison's disease causes inadequate excretion of potassium and results in hyperkalemia. The clinical manifestations of hyperkalemia are the result of altered nerve transmission. The most harmful consequence of hyperkalemia is its effect on cardiac function. Options 1, 2, and 4 are not manifestations associated with Addison's disease or hyperkalemia.

Test-Taking Strategy: Use the process of elimination and focus on the issue: hyperkalemia. Remember that hyperkalemia has a direct effect on cardiac function. This will direct you to option 3. Review the pathophysiology associated with Addison's disease and the effects of hyperkalemia if you had difficulty with this question.

Level of Cognitive Ability: Analysis
Client Needs: Physiological Integrity
Integrated Process: Nursing Process/Assessment
Content Area: Adult Health/Endocrine

Reference:
Black, J., & Hawks, J. (2005). *Medical-surgical nursing: Clinical management for positive outcomes* (7th ed.). Philadelphia: Saunders, p. 1220.

---

9. A client goes into respiratory distress, and an arterial blood gas (ABG) is drawn from the radial artery. The nurse performs the Allen test before the ABGs to determine the adequacy of the:

1 Femoral circulation
2 Brachial circulation
3 Carotid circulation
4 Ulnar circulation

Answer: 4

Rationale: Before radial puncture for obtaining an arterial specimen for ABGs, an Allen test is performed to determine adequate ulnar circulation. Failure to assess collateral circulation could result in severe ischemic injury to the hand, if damage to the radial artery occurs with arterial puncture. The Allen test does not determine adequacy of femoral, brachial, or carotid circulation.

Test-Taking Strategy: Use the process of elimination and note the key words "radial artery" in the question. Using knowledge of anatomy of the cardiovascular system, eliminate options 1, 2, and 3. Review the purpose and procedure of the Allen test if you had difficulty with this question.

Level of Cognitive Ability: Application
Client Needs: Physiological Integrity
Integrated Process: Nursing Process/Assessment
Content Area: Adult Health/Respiratory

Reference:
Black, J., & Hawks, J. (2005). *Medical-surgical nursing: Clinical management for positive outcomes* (7th ed.). Philadelphia: Saunders, pp. 1764-1765.

---

10. A pregnant client with diabetes mellitus arrives at the health care clinic for a follow-up visit. In this client, the nurse most importantly monitors:
1 Urine for glucose and ketones
2 Blood pressure, pulse, and respirations
3 Urine for specific gravity
4 For the presence of edema

Answer: 1
Rationale: The nurse assesses the pregnant client with diabetes mellitus for glucose and ketones in the urine at each prenatal visit because the physiological changes of pregnancy can drastically alter insulin requirements. Assessment of blood pressure, pulse, respirations, urine for specific gravity, and the presence of edema are more related to the client with pregnancy-induced hypertension.

Test-Taking Strategy: Use the process of elimination, focusing on the client's diagnosis. The only option that specifically addresses diabetes mellitus is option 1. Review prenatal care of the client with diabetes mellitus if you had difficulty with this question.

Level of Cognitive Ability: Application
Client Needs: Physiological Integrity
Integrated Process: Nursing Process/Assessment
Content Area: Maternity/Antepartum

Reference:
Lowdermilk, D., & Perry, A. (2004). *Maternity & women's health care* (8th ed.). St. Louis: Mosby, pp. 887; 892.

---

11. A home care nurse is visiting a client who is in a body cast. The nurse is performing an assessment of the psychosocial adjustment of the client to the cast. During the assessment, the nurse would most appropriately assess:
1 The type of transportation available for follow-up care
2 The ability to perform activities of daily living
3 The need for sensory stimulation
4 The amount of home care support available

Answer: 3
Rationale: A psychosocial assessment of the client who is immobilized would most appropriately include the need for sensory stimulation. This assessment should also include such factors as body image, past and present coping skills, and the coping methods used during the period of immobilization. Although transportation, home care support, and the ability to perform activities of daily living are components of an assessment, they are not specifically related to psychosocial adjustment, as is the need for sensory stimulation.

Test-Taking Strategy: Use the process of elimination and focus on the key words "psychosocial adjustment" and "most appropriately." Option 2 can be eliminated first because it relates to physiological integrity rather than psychosocial integrity. Next eliminate options 1 and 4 because they are most closely related to physical supports rather than psychosocial needs of the client. Review the components of a psychosocial assessment if you had difficulty with this question.

Level of Cognitive Ability: Analysis
Client Needs: Psychosocial Integrity
Integrated Process: Nursing Process/Assessment
Content Area: Adult Health/Musculoskeletal

Reference:
Black, J., & Hawks, J. (2005). *Medical-surgical nursing: Clinical management for positive outcomes* (7th ed.). Philadelphia: Saunders, p. 645.

---

12. A nurse is caring for a client with acquired immunodeficiency syndrome (AIDS). Which finding noted in the client indicates the presence of an opportunistic respiratory infection?
1 White plaques located on the oral mucosa
2 Fever, exertional dyspnea, and nonproductive cough
3 Loss of sight
4 Ulcerated perirectal lesions

Answer: 2
Rationale: Fever, exertional dyspnea, and a nonproductive cough are signs of pneumocystis pneumonia, a common, life-threatening opportunistic infection afflicting those with AIDS. Options 1, 3, and 4 are not associated with a respiratory infection. Option 1 describes the fungal infection oral candidiasis (*Candida albicans*), called thrush. Option 3 describes the viral infection, herpes zoster (shingles), when it has spread to involve the ophthalmic nerve. Option 4 describes herpes simplex, which can occur in homosexual men.

Test-Taking Strategy: Use the process of elimination and focus on the issue: respiratory infection. Option 2 is the only option that identifies symptoms related to the respiratory system. Review the signs of respiratory infection if you had difficulty with this question.

Level of Cognitive Ability: Analysis
Client Needs: Physiological Integrity
Integrated Process: Nursing Process/Assessment
Content Area: Adult Health/Immune

Reference:
Black, J., & Hawks, J. (2005). *Medical-surgical nursing: Clinical management for positive outcomes* (7th ed.). Philadelphia: Saunders, p. 2392.

---

13. An adult client seeks treatment in an ambulatory care clinic for complaints of a left earache, nausea, and a full feeling in the left ear. The client has an elevated temperature. The nurse first questions the client about:
1 A history of a recent brain abscess
2 A history of a recent upper respiratory infection (URI)
3 Whether acetaminophen (Tylenol) relieves the pain
4 Whether hearing is magnified in that ear

Answer: 2
Rationale: Otitis media in the adult is typically one-sided and presents as an acute process with earache, nausea and possible vomiting, fever, and fullness in the ear. The client may complain of diminished hearing in that ear. The nurse takes a client history first, assessing whether the client has had a recent URI. It is unnecessary to question the client about a brain abscess. The nurse may ask the client if anything relieves the pain, but ear infection pain is usually not relieved until antibiotic therapy is initiated.

Test-Taking Strategy: Use the process of elimination. Recalling the relationship between a URI and otitis media will direct you to option 2. Review otitis media if you had difficulty with this question.

Level of Cognitive Ability: Analysis
Client Needs: Physiological Integrity
Integrated Process: Nursing Process/Assessment
Content Area: Adult Health/Ear

Reference:
Black, J., & Hawks, J. (2005). *Medical-surgical nursing: Clinical management for positive outcomes* (7th ed.). Philadelphia: Saunders, p. 1984.

---

14. A home care nurse is making home visits to an older client with urinary incontinence who is very disturbed by the incontinent episodes. The nurse assesses the client's home situation to determine environmental barriers to normal voiding. The nurse determines that which item may be contributing to the client's problem?
  1 Presence of hand railings in the bathroom
  2 Having one bathroom on each floor of the home
  3 Nightlight present in the hall between the bedroom and bathroom
  4 Bathroom located on the second floor, bedroom on the first floor

Answer: 4
Rationale: Having a bathroom on the second floor and the bedroom on the first floor may pose a problem for an older client with incontinence. The need to negotiate the stairs and the distance may interfere with reaching the bathroom in a timely fashion. It is more helpful to the incontinent client to have a bathroom on the same floor as the bedroom or to have a commode rented for use. The presence of nightlights and hand railings are helpful to the client in reaching the bathroom quickly and safely.

Test-Taking Strategy: Focus on the issue: an environmental barrier to normal voiding. Note that options 1, 2, and 3 are similar in that they all are helpful and safe. Review measures that promote normal voiding if you had difficulty with this question.

Level of Cognitive Ability: Analysis
Client Needs: Health Promotion and Maintenance
Integrated Process: Nursing Process/Assessment
Content Area: Fundamental Skills

Reference:
Ebersole, P., & Hess, P. (2001). *Geriatric nursing & healthy aging.* St. Louis: Mosby, pp. 190-191.

---

15. A nurse is preparing to administer continuous intravenous (IV) fluid replacement through a peripheral IV site to a client with a diagnosis of dehydration. Which item is essential for the nurse to assess before initiating the IV fluid?
  1 Usual sleep patterns
  2 Ability to ambulate
  3 Body weight
  4 Intake and output

Answer: 3
Rationale: Body weight is an accurate indicator of fluid status. As a client is hydrated with IV fluids, the nurse monitors for increasing body weight. Accurate body weight is a better measurement of gains and losses than intake and output records. An IV should not greatly alter sleep patterns, and clients will still be able to ambulate with a peripheral IV site.

Test-Taking Strategy: Use the process of elimination. Note the relationship between the client's diagnosis and option 3. Remember that body weight is an accurate measurement of gains and losses. Review care of the dehydrated client if you had difficulty with this question.

Level of Cognitive Ability: Analysis
Client Needs: Physiological Integrity

Integrated Process: Nursing Process/Assessment
Content Area: Fundamental Skills

Reference:
Black, J., & Hawks, J. (2005). *Medical-surgical nursing: Clinical management for positive outcomes* (7th ed.). Philadelphia: Saunders, p. 209.

---

16. A client is scheduled for an arteriogram using a radiopaque dye. The nurse assesses which most critical item before the procedure?
1 Intake and output
2 Vital signs
3 Height and weight
4 Allergy to iodine or shellfish

Answer: 4
Rationale: This procedure requires a signed informed consent, because it involves injection of a radiopaque dye into the blood vessel. Although options 1, 2, and 3 are components of the preprocedure assessment, the risk of allergic reaction and possible anaphylaxis is most critical.

Test-Taking Strategy: Use the process of elimination, noting the key words "most critical." Recalling the risk of anaphylaxis related to the dye will direct you to option 4. Review preprocedure care for angiography if you had difficulty with this question.

Level of Cognitive Ability: Application
Client Needs: Physiological Integrity
Integrated Process: Nursing Process/Assessment
Content Area: Delegating/Prioritizing

Reference:
Chernecky, C., & Berger, B. (2004). *Laboratory tests and diagnostic procedures* (4th ed.). Philadelphia: Saunders, p. 201.

---

17. A nurse is performing a cardiovascular assessment on a client. Which item would the nurse assess to obtain the best information about the client's left-sided heart function?
1 Status of breath sounds
2 Presence of peripheral edema
3 Presence of jugular vein distention
4 Presence of hepatojugular reflux

Answer: 1
Rationale: The client with heart failure may present different symptoms depending on whether the right or the left side of the heart is failing. Peripheral edema, jugular vein distention, and hepatojugular reflux are all signs of right-sided heart function. Assessment of breath sounds provides information about left-sided heart function.

Test-Taking Strategy: Use the process of elimination and focus on the issue: the status of left-sided heart function. Remember "left" and "lungs." Options 2, 3, and 4 reflect right-sided heart failure. Review the signs of right- and left-sided heart failure if you had difficulty with this question.

Level of Cognitive Ability: Application
Client Needs: Physiological Integrity
Integrated Process: Nursing Process/Assessment
Content Area: Adult Health/Cardiovascular

Reference:
Ignatavicius, D., & Workman, M. (2002). *Medical surgical nursing: Critical thinking for collaborative care* (4th ed.). Philadelphia: Saunders, p. 701.

18. A nurse is obtaining a history on a client admitted to the hospital with a thrombotic cerebrovascular accident (CVA). The nurse assesses the client, knowing that before the CVA occurred, the client most likely experienced:
   1 Transient hemiplegia and loss of speech
   2 Throbbing headaches
   3 Unexplained episodes of loss of consciousness
   4 No symptoms at all

Answer: 1
Rationale: Cerebral thrombosis does not occur suddenly. In the few hours or days preceding a thrombotic CVA, the client may experience a transient loss of speech, hemiplegia, or paresthesias on one side of the body. Other signs and symptoms of thrombotic CVA vary, but may include dizziness, cognitive changes, or seizures. Headache is rare, and loss of consciousness is not likely to occur.

Test-Taking Strategy: Use the process of elimination. Option 4 is eliminated first because the client experiencing a CVA will likely experience symptoms. From the remaining options, focus on the type of stroke addressed in the question to direct you to option 1. Review the signs and symptoms of a thrombotic CVA if you had difficulty with this question.

Level of Cognitive Ability: Application
Client Needs: Physiological Integrity
Integrated Process: Nursing Process/Assessment
Content Area: Adult Health/Neurological

Reference:
Black, J., & Hawks, J. (2005). *Medical-surgical nursing: Clinical management for positive outcomes* (7th ed.). Philadelphia: Saunders, p. 2111.

19. A client in a long-term care facility has had a series of gastrointestinal (GI) diagnostic tests, including an upper GI series and endoscopies. Upon return to the long-term care facility, the priority nursing assessment should focus on:
   1 Level of consciousness
   2 Activity tolerance
   3 Hydration and nutrition status
   4 Comfort level

Answer: 3
Rationale: Many of the diagnostic studies to identify GI disorders require that the GI tract be cleaned (usually with laxatives and enemas) before testing. In addition, the client is most often NPO before and during the testing period. Because the studies may be done over a period exceeding 24 hours, the client may become dehydrated and/or malnourished. Although options 1, 2, and 4 may be a component of the assessment, option 3 is the priority.

Test-Taking Strategy: Note the key words "priority nursing assessment." Use Maslow's hierarchy of needs theory to direct you to option 3. Hydration and nutrition are a priority. Review care of the client following diagnostic GI tests if you had difficulty with this question.

Level of Cognitive Ability: Application
Client Needs: Physiological Integrity
Integrated Process: Nursing Process/Assessment
Content Area: Delegating/Prioritizing

References:
Chernecky, C., & Berger, B. (2004). *Laboratory tests and diagnostic procedures* (4th ed.). Philadelphia: Saunders, p. 1109.
Lewis, S., Heitkemper, M., & Dirksen, S. (2004). *Medical-surgical nursing: Assessment and management of clinical problems* (6th ed.). St. Louis: Mosby, p. 407.

20. A nurse plans to assess a client for the vegetative signs of depression. The nurse assesses for these signs by determining the client's:
1 Ability to think, concentrate, and make decisions
2 Appetite, weight, sleep patterns, and psychomotor activity
3 Level of self-esteem
4 Level of suicidal ideation

Answer: 2

Rationale: The vegetative signs of depression are changes in physiological functioning during depression. These include appetite, weight, sleep patterns, and psychomotor activity. Options 1, 3, and 4 represent psychological assessment categories.

Test-Taking Strategy: Focus on the issue: vegetative signs of depression. Recalling that the vegetative signs of depression refer to physiological changes will direct you to option 2. Review assessment of depression if you had difficulty with this question.

Level of Cognitive Ability: Analysis
Client Needs: Physiological Integrity
Integrated Process: Nursing Process/Assessment
Content Area: Mental Health

Reference:
Keltner, N., Schwecke, L., & Bostrom, C. (2003). *Psychiatric nursing* (4th ed.). St. Louis: Mosby, pp. 356; 358.

---

21. A nurse is caring for a client diagnosed with cirrhosis of the liver. The client is receiving spironolactone (Aldactone) 50 mg orally daily. Which of the following would indicate to the nurse that the client is experiencing a side effect related to the medication?
1 Excitability
2 Hyperkalemia
3 Constipation
4 Dry skin

Answer: 2

Rationale: Spironolactone (Aldactone) is a potassium-sparing diuretic. Side effects include hyperkalemia, dehydration, hyponatremia, and lethargy. Although the concern with most diuretics is hypokalemia, this medication is potassium-sparing, which means that the concern with the administration of this medication is hyperkalemia. Additional side effects include nausea, vomiting, cramping, diarrhea, headache, ataxia, drowsiness, confusion, and fever.

Test-Taking Strategy: Focus on the name of the medication. Recalling that this medication is potassium-sparing will direct you to option 2. Review those medications in the classification of potassium-sparing diuretics if you had difficulty with this question.

Level of Cognitive Ability: Analysis
Client Needs: Physiological Integrity
Integrated Process: Nursing Process/Assessment
Content Area: Pharmacology

Reference:
Hodgson, B., & Kizior, R. (2004). *Saunders nursing drug handbook 2004.* Philadelphia: Saunders, pp. 931; 933.

---

22. A nurse is preparing a woman in labor for an amniotomy. The nurse would assess which priority data before the procedure?
1 Maternal blood pressure
2 Maternal heart rate
3 Fetal heart rate
4 Fetal scalp sampling

Answer: 3

Rationale: Fetal well-being must be confirmed before and after amniotomy. Fetal heart rate should be checked by Doppler or by the application of the external fetal monitor. Although maternal vital signs may be assessed, fetal heart rate is the priority. A fetal scalp sampling cannot be done when the membranes are intact.

Test-Taking Strategy: Note the key word "priority." Eliminate option 4 first, knowing that a fetal scalp sampling cannot be done before an amniotomy. Eliminate options 1 and 2 next, noting that they are both similar and address maternal vital signs. Option 3 addresses fetal well-being. Review preprocedure care for amniotomy if you had difficulty with this question.

Level of Cognitive Ability: Application
Client Needs: Physiological Integrity
Integrated Process: Nursing Process/Assessment
Content Area: Maternity/Antepartum

Reference:
Lowdermilk, D., & Perry, A. (2004). *Maternity & women's health care* (8th ed.). St. Louis: Mosby, p. 1009.

---

23. A nurse is monitoring a client receiving an oxytocin (Pitocin) infusion for the induction of labor. The nurse would suspect water intoxication if which of the following were noted?
  1 Sleepiness
  2 Lethargy
  3 Tachycardia
  4 Fatigue

Answer: 3
Rationale: During an oxytocin infusion, the woman is monitored closely for water intoxication. Signs of water intoxication include tachycardia, cardiac dysrhythmias, shortness of breath, nausea, and vomiting.

Test-Taking Strategy: Focus on the issue of the question: water intoxication. Think about the physiological response that occurs when fluid overload exists to direct you to option 3. Also note the similarity in options 1, 2, and 4 and eliminate these options. Review the signs of water intoxication if you had difficulty with this question.

Level of Cognitive Ability: Analysis
Client Needs: Physiological Integrity
Integrated Process: Nursing Process/Assessment
Content Area: Maternity/Intrapartum

References:
Lowdermilk, D., & Perry, A. (2004). *Maternity & women's health care* (8th ed.). St. Louis: Mosby, p. 1010.
McKenry, L., & Salerno, E. (2003). *Mosby's pharmacology in nursing* (21st ed.). St. Louis: Mosby, p. 908.

---

24. A clinic nurse in a well baby clinic is collecting data regarding the motor development of a 15-month-old child. Which of the following is the highest level of development that the nurse would expect to observe in a 15-month-old child?
  1 The child builds a tower of two blocks
  2 The child opens a doorknob
  3 The child unzips a large zipper
  4 The child puts on simple clothes independently

Answer: 1
Rationale: At age 15 months, the nurse would expect that the child could build a tower of two blocks. A 24-month-old would be able to open a doorknob and unzip a large zipper. At age 30 months, the child would be able to put on simple clothes independently.

Test-Taking Strategy: Note the age of the child and the key words "highest level of development." Visualize each of the motor skills presented in the options to assist in selecting the correct option. Review these developmental milestones if you had difficulty with this question.

Level of Cognitive Ability: Analysis
Client Needs: Health Promotion and Maintenance
Integrated Process: Nursing Process/Assessment
Content Area: Child Health

Reference:
Wong, D., & Hockenberry, M. (2003). *Wong's nursing care of infants and children* (7th ed.). St. Louis: Mosby, pp. 593; 595.

---

25. A nurse is admitting a child with a diagnosis of irritable bowel syndrome to the hospital. Which data would the nurse expect to obtain on assessment of the child?
1 Reports of frothy diarrhea
2 Reports of profuse, watery diarrhea and vomiting
3 Reports of foul-smelling ribbon stools
4 Reports of diffuse abdominal pain unrelated to meals or activity

Answer: 4
Rationale: Irritable bowel syndrome causes diffuse abdominal pain unrelated to meals or activity. Alternating constipation and diarrhea with the presence of undigested food and mucus in the stools may also be noted. Option 1 is a clinical manifestation of lactose intolerance. Option 2 is a clinical manifestation of celiac disease. Option 3 is a clinical manifestation of Hirschsprung's disease.

Test-Taking Strategy: Focus on the child's diagnosis. Noting the name of the syndrome will direct you to option 4, because you would expect abdominal pain to occur in this disorder. Review the clinical manifestations associated with this disorder if you had difficulty with this question.

Level of Cognitive Ability: Analysis
Client Needs: Physiological Integrity
Integrated Process: Nursing Process/Assessment
Content Area: Child Health

Reference:
Wong, D., & Hockenberry, M. (2003). *Wong's nursing care of infants and children* (7th ed.). St. Louis: Mosby, p. 1432.

---

26. A nurse is caring for a child diagnosed with rubeola (measles). The nurse notes that the physician has documented the presence of Koplik spots. Based on this documentation, which of the following would the nurse expect to note on assessment of the child?
1 Petechiae spots that are reddish and pinpoint on the soft palate
2 Whitish vesicles located across the chest
3 Small, blue-white spots with a red base found on the buccal mucosa
4 Pinpoint petechiae noted on both legs

Answer: 3
Rationale: Koplik spots appear approximately 2 days before the appearance of the rash. These are small, blue-white spots with a red base found on the buccal mucosa. The spots last approximately 3 days, after which time they slough off. Options 1, 2, and 4 are incorrect.

Test-Taking Strategy: Use the process of elimination. Eliminate options 1 and 4 first because they are similar and address petechiae spots. From the remaining options, recalling that Koplik spots are located on the buccal mucosa will direct you to option 3. Review this content if you are unfamiliar with these characteristics.

Level of Cognitive Ability: Analysis
Client Needs: Physiological Integrity
Integrated Process: Nursing Process/Assessment
Content Area: Child Health

Reference:
Wong, D., & Hockenberry, M. (2003). *Wong's nursing care of infants and children* (7th ed.). St. Louis: Mosby, p. 657.

27. A child is hospitalized with a diagnosis of nephrotic syndrome. Which assessment finding would the nurse expect to note in the child?
  1 Weight loss
  2 Hypotension
  3 Abdominal pain
  4 Constipation

Answer: 3
Rationale: Clinical manifestations associated with nephrotic syndrome include edema, anorexia, fatigue, and abdominal pain from the presence of extra fluid in the peritoneal cavity. Diarrhea caused by edema of the bowel occurs and may cause decreased absorption of nutrients. Increased weight and a normal blood pressure are noted.

Test-Taking Strategy: Think about the physiology associated with nephrotic syndrome. Recalling that edema is a clinical manifestation will direct you to option 3. Review this content if you had difficulty with this question or are unfamiliar with the clinical manifestations associated with this disorder.

Level of Cognitive Ability: Analysis
Client Needs: Physiological Integrity
Integrated Process: Nursing Process/Assessment
Content Area: Child Health

Reference:
Wong, D., & Hockenberry, M. (2003). *Wong's nursing care of infants and children* (7th ed.). St. Louis: Mosby, p. 1275.

28. A child is admitted to the hospital with a suspected diagnosis of von Willebrand's disease. On assessment of the child, which symptom would most likely be noted?
  1 Bleeding from the mucous membranes
  2 Presence of hemarthrosis
  3 Hematuria
  4 Presence of hematomas

Answer: 1
Rationale: The primary clinical manifestations of von Willebrand's disease are bruising and mucous membrane bleeding from the nose, mouth, and gastrointestinal tract. Prolonged bleeding after trauma and surgery, including tooth extraction, may be the first evidence of abnormal hemostasis in those with mild disease. In females, menorrhagia and profuse postpartum bleeding may occur. Bleeding associated with von Willebrand's disease may be severe and lead to anemia and shock, but unlike the situation in hemophilia, deep bleeding into joints and muscles is rare. Options 2, 3, and 4 are characteristic of those signs found in hemophilia.

Test-Taking Strategy: Specific knowledge regarding the clinical manifestations associated with von Willebrand's disease is required to answer this question. Recalling that options 2, 3, and 4 are characteristic of hemophilia will assist in eliminating these options and direct you to option 1. Review this content if you are unfamiliar with this disorder.

Level of Cognitive Ability: Analysis
Client Needs: Physiological Integrity
Integrated Process: Nursing Process/Assessment
Content Area: Child Health

Reference:
Wong, D., & Hockenberry, M. (2003). *Wong's nursing care of infants and children* (7th ed.). St. Louis: Mosby, p. 1566.

29. A nurse is assigned to care for a child with a basilar skull fracture. The nurse reviews the child's record and notes that the physician has documented the presence of Battle sign. Which of the following would the nurse expect to note in the child?

1 Bruising behind the ear
2 Edematous periorbital area
3 Bruised periorbital area
4 Presence of epistaxis

Answer: 1

Rationale: The most serious type of skull fracture is a basilar skull fracture. Two classic findings associated with this type of skull fracture are Battle sign and raccoon eyes. Battle sign is the presence of bruising or ecchymosis behind the ear caused by leaking of blood into the mastoid sinuses. Raccoon eyes occur as a result of blood leaking into the frontal sinus and cause an edematous and bruised periorbital area.

Test-Taking Strategy: Use the process of elimination. Eliminate options 2 and 3 first because they are similar. From the remaining options, recalling the description of Battle sign will direct you to option 1. Review this content if you are unfamiliar with this sign and its description.

Level of Cognitive Ability: Analysis
Client Needs: Physiological Integrity
Integrated Process: Nursing Process/Assessment
Content Area: Child Health

Reference:
Wong, D., & Hockenberry, M. (2003). *Wong's nursing care of infants and children* (7th ed.). St. Louis: Mosby, p. 1667.

30. A mother brings a child to the health care clinic. The child has been complaining of severe headaches and has been vomiting. The child has a high fever, and the nurse notes the presence of nuchal rigidity in the child. The nurse suspects a possible diagnosis of bacterial meningitis. The nurse continues to assess the child for the presence of Kernig's sign. Which finding would indicate the presence of this sign?

1 Inability of the child to extend the legs fully when lying supine
2 Flexion of the hips when the neck is flexed from a lying position
3 Pain when the chin is pulled down to the chest
4 Calf pain when the foot is dorsiflexed

Answer: 1

Rationale: Kernig's sign is the inability of the child to extend the legs fully when lying supine. Brudzinski's sign is flexion of the hips when the neck is flexed from a supine position. Both of these signs are frequently present in bacterial meningitis. Nuchal rigidity is also present in bacterial meningitis and occurs when pain prevents the child from touching the chin to the chest. Homan's sign is elicited when pain occurs in the calf region when the foot is dorsiflexed. Homan's sign is present in thrombophlebitis.

Test-Taking Strategy: Use the process of elimination, focusing on the child's diagnosis. Option 4 is eliminated first because this is an assessment test for presence of thrombophlebitis, not meningitis. Next eliminate option 3 because this option identifies the presence of nuchal rigidity. From the remaining options, it is necessary to be able to distinguish between Kernig's sign and Brudzinski's sign. Review the assessment findings in meningitis if you had difficulty with this question.

Level of Cognitive Ability: Analysis
Client Needs: Physiological Integrity
Integrated Process: Nursing Process/Assessment
Content Area: Child Health

Reference:
Wong, D., & Hockenberry, M. (2003). *Wong's nursing care of infants and children* (7th ed.). St. Louis: Mosby, pp. 226; 228; 1678.

31. A home care nurse is assessing an older client's functional abilities and ability to perform activities of daily living (ADLs). The nurse focuses the assessment on:
1   Self-care needs, such as toileting, feeding, and ambulating
2   The normal everyday routine in the home
3   Ability to do light housework, heavy housework, and pay the bills
4   Ability to drive a car

Answer: 1
Rationale: Activities of daily living refer to the client's ability to bath, toilet, ambulate, dress, and feed oneself. These functional abilities are always assessed by the home care nurse. The normal routine in the home is not a component of functional assessment. The ability to do housework and drive a car relates to instrumental activities of daily living.

Test-Taking Strategy: Use the process of elimination, focusing on the issue: ability to perform ADLs. Recalling that ADLs refer to self-care needs will direct you to option 1. Review the concepts of ADLs if you had difficulty with this question.

Level of Cognitive Ability: Application
Client Needs: Health Promotion and Maintenance
Integrated Process: Nursing Process/Assessment
Content Area: Fundamental Skills

Reference:
Potter, P., & Perry, A. (2005). *Fundamentals of nursing* (6th ed.). St. Louis: Mosby, pp. 256; 347.

NURSING PROCESS: ANALYSIS

1. A nonstress test is performed on a client, and the results are documented in the chart. The results are documented as "two or more fetal heart rate (FHR) accelerations of 15 beats per minute, lasting 15 seconds in association with fetal movement." The nurse interprets these findings as:
1   A reactive nonstress test
2   A nonreactive nonstress test
3   Unclear for accurate interpretation
4   Unsatisfactory

Answer: 1
Rationale: A reactive nonstress test (normal/negative) indicates a healthy fetus. It is described as two or more FHR accelerations of at least 15 beats per minute, lasting at least 15 seconds from the beginning of the acceleration to the end in association with fetal movement, during a 20-minute period. A nonreactive nonstress test (abnormal) is described as no accelerations or accelerations of less than 15 beats per minute or lasting less than 15 seconds in duration throughout any fetal movement during the testing period. An unsatisfactory test cannot be interpreted because of the poor quality of the FHR.

Test-Taking Strategy: Use the process of elimination. Eliminate options 3 and 4 first because they are similar. From the remaining options, remembering that a reactive nonstress test is a normal or negative test will assist in directing you to option 1. Review the nonstress test if you had difficulty answering this question.

Level of Cognitive Ability: Analysis
Client Needs: Physiological Integrity
Integrated Process: Nursing Process/Analysis
Content Area: Maternity/Antepartum

Reference:
Lowdermilk, D., & Perry, A. (2004). *Maternity & women's health care* (8th ed.). St. Louis: Mosby, pp. 830; 831.

2. A nurse is developing a plan of care for a client in Buck's traction regarding measures to prevent complications. The nurse determines that the priority nursing diagnosis to be included in the plan is which of the following?
1 Deficient diversional activity related to bed rest
2 Bathing/hygiene self-care deficit related to the need for traction
3 Impaired physical mobility related to traction
4 Potential for infection at pin sites

Answer: 3
Rationale: The priority nursing diagnosis for the client in Buck's traction is impaired physical mobility. Options 1 and 2 may also be appropriate for the client in traction, but immobility presents the greatest risk for the development of complications. Buck's traction is a skin traction, and there are no pin sites.

Test-Taking Strategy: Use the process of elimination and eliminate option 4 first because there are no pin sites with Buck's traction. From the remaining options, focus on the key word "priority," recalling that the client experiences immobility when in traction. This will direct you to option 3. Review care of the client in Buck's traction if you had difficulty with this question.

Level of Cognitive Ability: Analysis
Client Needs: Physiological Integrity
Integrated Process: Nursing Process/Analysis
Content Area: Adult Health/Musculoskeletal

Reference:
Black, J., & Hawks, J. (2005). *Medical-surgical nursing: Clinical management for positive outcomes* (7th ed.). Philadelphia: Saunders, p. 637.

3. A pregnant client with mitral valve prolapse is receiving anticoagulant therapy during pregnancy. The nurse reviews the client's medical record, expecting to note that which medication is prescribed?
1 Oral intake of 15 mg of warfarin (Coumadin) daily
2 Intravenous infusion of heparin sodium 5000 units daily
3 Subcutaneous administration of heparin sodium 5000 units daily
4 Subcutaneous administration of terbutaline (Brethine) daily

Answer: 3
Rationale: Pregnant women with mitral valve prolapse are frequently given anticoagulant therapy during pregnancy because they are at greater risk for thromboembolic disease during the antenatal, intrapartal, and postpartum periods. Warfarin (Coumadin) is contraindicated during pregnancy because it passes the placental barrier, causing potential fetal malformations and hemorrhagic disorders. Heparin, which does not pass the placental barrier, is a safe anticoagulant therapy during pregnancy and would be administered by the subcutaneous route. Terbutaline is a medication that is indicated for preterm labor management.

Test-Taking Strategy: Use the process of elimination and knowledge regarding the medications that are safe during pregnancy to assist in answering the question. Eliminate options 1 and 4 first because warfarin is contraindicated and terbutaline is indicated for preterm labor management. From the remaining options, select option 3 because of the word "subcutaneous." Review the treatment measures for the pregnant client with mitral valve prolapse if you had difficulty with this question.

Level of Cognitive Ability: Analysis
Client Needs: Health Promotion and Maintenance
Integrated Process: Nursing Process/Analysis
Content Area: Maternity/Antepartum

Reference:
Murray, S., McKinney, E., & Gorrie, T. (2002). *Foundations of maternal-newborn nursing* (3rd ed.). Philadelphia: Saunders, p. 714.

4. A nurse continues to assess a client who is in the late first stage of labor for progress and fetal well-being. At the last vaginal exam, the client was fully effaced, 8 centimeters dilated, vertex presentation, and station -1. Which observation would indicate that the fetus was in fetal distress?

1 Vaginal exam continues to reveal some old meconium staining, and the fetal monitor demonstrates a U-shaped pattern of deceleration during contractions, recovering to a baseline of 140 beats per minute

2 Fresh thick meconium is passed with a small gush of liquid, and the fetal monitor shows late decelerations with a variable descending baseline

3 Fresh meconium is found on the examiner's gloved fingers after a vaginal exam, and the fetal monitor pattern remains essentially unchanged

4 The fetal heart rate slowly drops to 110 beats per minute during strong contractions, recovering to 138 beats per minute immediately afterward

Answer: 2

Rationale: Meconium staining alone is not a sign of fetal distress. Meconium passage is a normal physiological function, frequently noted with a fetus over 38 weeks' gestation. Old meconium staining may be the result of a prenatal trauma that is resolved. It is not unusual for the fetal heart rate to drop below the 140 to 160 beats per minute range in late labor during contractions, and in a healthy fetus the fetal heart rate will recover between contractions. Fresh meconium in combination with late decelerations and a variable descending baseline is an ominous signal of fetal distress caused by fetal hypoxia.

Test-Taking Strategy: Use the process of elimination, noting the issue: fetal distress. Eliminate options 1 and 4 first because they both indicate a recovering fetal heart rate. From the remaining options, eliminate option 3 because of the words "fetal monitor pattern remains essentially unchanged." Review signs of fetal distress if you had difficulty with this question.

Level of Cognitive Ability: Analysis
Client Needs: Physiological Integrity
Integrated Process: Nursing Process/Analysis
Content Area: Maternity/Intrapartum

References:
Lowdermilk, D., & Perry, A. (2004). *Maternity & women's health care* (8th ed.). St. Louis: Mosby, pp. 826-827.
Murray, S., McKinney, E., & Gorrie, T. (2002). *Foundations of maternal-newborn nursing* (3rd ed.). Philadelphia: Saunders, p. 353.

5. A nurse is caring for a child with complex partial seizures who is being treated with carbamazepine (Tegretol). The nurse reviews the laboratory report for the results of the drug plasma level and determines that the plasma level is in a therapeutic range if which of the following is noted?

1 1 mcg/mL
2 10 mcg/mL
3 18 mcg/mL
4 20 mcg/mL

Answer: 2

Rationale: When carbamazepine is administered, plasma levels of the medication need to be monitored periodically to check for the child's absorption of the medication. The amount of the medication prescribed is based on the results of this laboratory test. The therapeutic plasma level of carbamazepine is 3 to 14 mcg/mL. Option 1 indicates a low level, possibly requiring an increased medication dose. Options 3 and 4 identify elevated levels, indicating the need to decrease the medication dose.

Test-Taking Strategy: Use the process of elimination and knowledge of the therapeutic plasma level of carbamazepine to answer the question. Recalling that the therapeutic plasma level is 3 to 14 mcg/mL will direct you to option 2. Review the therapeutic plasma level of carbamazepine if you had difficulty with this question.

Level of Cognitive Ability: Analysis
Client Needs: Physiological Integrity
Integrated Process: Nursing Process/Analysis
Content Area: Pharmacology

References:
Hodgson, B., & Kizior, R. (2004). *Saunders nursing drug handbook 2004.* Philadelphia: Saunders, p. 148.
McKenry, L., & Salerno, E. (2003). *Mosby's pharmacology in nursing* (21st ed.). St. Louis: Mosby, p. 369.

6. A nurse performs an assessment on a client with a history of congestive heart failure. The client has been taking diuretics on a long-term basis. The nurse reviews the medication record, knowing that which medication, if prescribed for this client, would place the client at risk for hypokalemia?
1 Spironolactone (Aldactone)
2 Bumetanide (Bumex)
3 Triamterene (Dyrenium)
4 Amiloride HCL (Midamor)

Answer: 2
Rationale: Bumetanide (Bumex) is a loop diuretic. The client on this medication would be at risk for hypokalemia. Spironolactone (Aldactone), triamterene (Dyrenium), and amiloride HCL (Midamor) are potassium-sparing diuretics.

Test-Taking Strategy: Use the process of elimination and knowledge regarding the diuretics that are in the classification of potassium-sparing. Recalling that bumetanide is a loop diuretic will direct you to option 2. Review these medications if you had difficulty with this question.

Level of Cognitive Ability: Analysis
Client Needs: Physiological Integrity
Integrated Process: Nursing Process/Analysis
Content Area: Pharmacology

Reference:
Hodgson, B., & Kizior, R. (2004). *Saunders nursing drug handbook 2004.* Philadelphia: Saunders, p. 127.

---

7. A home care nurse is preparing to visit a client with a diagnosis of Ménière's disease. The nurse reviews the physician orders and expects to note that which of the following dietary measures is prescribed?
1 Low-fiber diet with decreased fluids
2 Low-sodium diet and fluid restriction
3 Low-carbohydrate diet and the elimination of red meats
4 Low-fat diet with restriction of citrus fruits

Answer: 2
Rationale: Dietary changes such as salt and fluid restrictions that reduce the amount of endolymphatic fluid is sometimes prescribed for clients with Ménière's disease. Options 1, 3, and 4 are not prescribed for this disorder.

Test-Taking Strategy: Use the process of elimination and focus on the client's diagnosis. Recalling that salt and fluid restrictions are sometimes necessary to reduce the amount of endolymphatic fluid will assist in directing you to option 2. Review the pathophysiology related to this condition and the treatment if you had difficulty with this question.

Level of Cognitive Ability: Analysis
Client Needs: Health Promotion and Maintenance
Integrated Process: Nursing Process/Analysis
Content Area: Adult Health/Ear

Reference:
Ignatavicius, D., & Workman, M. (2002). *Medical surgical nursing: Critical thinking for collaborative care* (4th ed.). Philadelphia: Saunders, p. 1068.

---

8. A nurse is caring for a client diagnosed with tuberculosis. The client is receiving rifampin (Rifadin) 600 mg orally daily. Which laboratory finding would indicate to the nurse that the client is experiencing an adverse reaction?
1 A white blood cell count of 6000/ul
2 An alkaline phosphatase of 25 units/dL
3 A sedimentation rate of 15 mm/hour
4 A total bilirubin of 0.5 mg/dL

Answer: 2
Rationale: Adverse reactions or toxic effects of rifampin include hepatotoxicity, hepatitis, blood dyscrasias, Stevens-Johnson syndrome, and antibiotic-related colitis. The nurse monitors for increased liver function, bilirubin, blood urea nitrogen, and uric acid levels because elevations indicate an adverse reaction. A normal white blood cell count is 4500 to 11,000/ul. The normal sedimentation rate is 0 to 30 mm/hour. The normal total bilirubin level is less than 1.5 mg/dL. The normal alkaline phosphatase is 4.5 to 13 King-Armstrong units/dL.

Test-Taking Strategy: Use the process of elimination. Recalling that the medication is metabolized in the liver will assist in eliminating options 1 and 3 because these laboratory studies are not directly related to assessing liver function. From the remaining options, knowledge of normal laboratory values will direct you to option 2. Review this content if you are unfamiliar with this medication or these laboratory values.

Level of Cognitive Ability: Analysis
Client Needs: Physiological Integrity
Integrated Process: Nursing Process/Analysis
Content Area: Pharmacology

References:
Hodgson, B., & Kizior, R. (2004). *Saunders nursing drug handbook 2004.* Philadelphia: Saunders, p. 886.
McKenry, L., & Salerno, E. (2003). *Mosby's pharmacology in nursing* (21st ed.). St. Louis: Mosby, p. 1059.

---

9. A home care nurse is assessing a client who is taking prazosin (Minipress). Which statement by the client would support the nursing diagnosis of noncompliance with medication therapy?
   1 "I don't understand why I have to keep taking the pills when my blood pressure is normal."
   2 "I can't see the numbers on the label to know how much salt is in food."
   3 "If I feel dizzy, I'll skip my dose for a few days."
   4 "If I have a cold, I shouldn't take any over-the-counter remedies without consulting my doctor."

Answer: 3
Rationale: Side effects of prazosin are dizziness and impotence. The client needs to be instructed to call the physician if these side effects occur. Holding (skipping) medication will cause an abrupt rise in blood pressure. Option 1 indicates a knowledge deficit. Option 2 indicates a self-care deficit. Option 4 indicates client understanding regarding the medication.

Test-Taking Strategy: Focus on the nursing diagnosis, noncompliance, to select the correct option. Noting the key words "I'll skip my dose" will direct you to option 3. Review the defining characteristics of noncompliance if you had difficulty with this question.

Level of Cognitive Ability: Analysis
Client Needs: Health Promotion and Maintenance
Integrated Process: Nursing Process/Analysis
Content Area: Pharmacology

Reference:
Hodgson, B., & Kizior, R. (2004). *Saunders nursing drug handbook 2004.* Philadelphia: Saunders, p. 828.

---

10. A client with a history of self-managed peptic ulcer disease has frequently used excessive amounts of oral antacids. The nurse interprets that this client is at risk for which acid-base disturbance?
    1 Metabolic acidosis
    2 Metabolic alkalosis
    3 Respiratory alkalosis
    4 Respiratory acidosis

Answer: 2
Rationale: Oral antacids commonly contain bicarbonate or other alkaline components. These bind onto the hydrochloric acid in the stomach to neutralize the acid. Excessive use of oral antacids containing bicarbonate can cause a metabolic alkalosis over time. Options 1, 3, and 4 are incorrect.

Test-Taking Strategy: Note that the question indicates that the problem is not respiratory in nature. With this in mind, eliminate options 3 and 4 first. Choose correctly from the remaining options, knowing that the word "antacid" must work "against" acids. Review the causes of metabolic alkalosis if you had difficulty with the question.

Level of Cognitive Ability: Analysis
Client Needs: Physiological Integrity
Integrated Process: Nursing Process/Analysis
Content Area: Fundamental Skills

Reference:
Ignatavicius, D., & Workman, M. (2002). *Medical surgical nursing: Critical thinking for collaborative care* (4th ed.). Philadelphia: Saunders, p. 230.

---

11. A nurse is assessing a 39-year-old Caucasian female client. The client has a blood pressure (BP) of 152/92 mmHg at rest, total cholesterol of 190 mg/dL, and a fasting blood glucose level of 110 mg/dL. The nurse would place priority on which risk factor for coronary heart disease (CHD) in this client?
1 Age
2 Hyperlipidemia
3 Hypertension
4 Glucose intolerance

Answer: 3
Rationale: Hypertension, cigarette smoking, and hyperlipidemia are major risk factors of CHD. Glucose intolerance, obesity, and response to stress are also contributing factors. Age greater than 40 is a nonmodifiable risk factor. A cholesterol level of 190 mg/dL and a blood glucose level of 110 mg/dL are within the normal range. The nurse places priority on major risk factors that need modification.

Test-Taking Strategy: Focus on the data in the question and note the key word "priority." Note that the only abnormal value is the BP. Review the risk factors associated with CHD if you had difficulty with this question.

Level of Cognitive Ability: Analysis
Client Needs: Health Promotion and Maintenance
Integrated Process: Nursing Process/Analysis
Content Area: Delegating/Prioritizing

Reference:
Ignatavicius, D., & Workman, M. (2002). *Medical surgical nursing: Critical thinking for collaborative care* (4th ed.). Philadelphia: Saunders, p. 792.

---

12. A nurse is caring for a client who has just returned to the nursing unit after an intravenous pyelogram (IVP). The nurse determines that which of the following is the most important priority in the post-procedure care of this client?
1 Encouraging increased intake of oral fluids
2 Ambulating the client in the hallway
3 Encouraging the client to try to void frequently
4 Maintaining the client on bed rest

Answer: 1
Rationale: Following IVP, the client should take in increased fluids to aid in clearance of the dye used for the procedure. It is unnecessary to void frequently after the procedure. The client is usually allowed activity as tolerated, without any specific activity guidelines.

Test-Taking Strategy: Use the process of elimination and note the key word "important." Option 3 has no useful purpose and is eliminated first. From the remaining options, recall that there are no activity guidelines after this procedure. Also, recall that fluids are necessary to promote clearance of the dye from the client's system. Review this procedure if you had difficulty with this question.

Level of Cognitive Ability: Analysis
Client Needs: Physiological Integrity
Integrated Process: Nursing Process/Analysis
Content Area: Adult Health/Renal

Reference:
Chernecky, C., & Berger, B. (2004). *Laboratory tests and diagnostic procedures* (4th ed.). Philadelphia: Saunders, p. 697.

13. A client had arterial blood gases drawn. The results are: pH 7.34, $PaCO_2$ of 37 mmHg, PaO_2 of 79, HCO_3 of 19 mEq/L. The nurse interprets that the client is experiencing:

1 Respiratory acidosis
2 Respiratory alkalosis
3 Metabolic acidosis
4 Metabolic alkalosis

Answer: 3

Rationale: Metabolic acidosis occurs when the pH falls below 7.35 and the bicarbonate level falls below 22 mEq/L. With respiratory acidosis, the pH drops below 7.35 and the carbon dioxide level rises above 45 mmHg. With respiratory alkalosis, the pH rises above 7.45 and the carbon dioxide level falls below 35 mmHg. With metabolic alkalosis, the pH rises above 7.45 and the bicarbonate level rises above 27 mEq/L.

Test-Taking Strategy: Use the process of elimination. Knowing that a pH of 7.34 is acidotic assists you to eliminate options 2 and 4 first. From the remaining options, knowing that a metabolic condition exists when the bicarbonate follows the same up or down pattern as the pH helps you choose option 3 over option 1. Review the analysis of arterial blood gas results if you had difficulty with this question.

Level of Cognitive Ability: Analysis
Client Needs: Physiological Integrity
Integrated Process: Nursing Process/Analysis
Content Area: Adult Health/Respiratory

References:

Pagana, K., & Pagana, T. (2003). *Mosby's diagnostic and laboratory test reference* (6th ed.). St. Louis: Mosby, pp. 116-117.
Chernecky, C., & Berger, B. (2004). *Laboratory tests and diagnostic procedures* (4th ed.). Philadelphia: Saunders, p. 245.

14. A client with advanced cirrhosis of the liver is not tolerating protein well, as evidenced by abnormal laboratory values. The nurse anticipates that which of the following medications will be prescribed for the client?

1 Lactulose (Chronulac)
2 Ethacrynic acid (Edecrin)
3 Folic acid (Folvite)
4 Thiamine (Vitamin B_1)

Answer: 1

Rationale: The client with cirrhosis has impaired ability to metabolize protein because of liver dysfunction. Administration of lactulose aids in the clearance of ammonia via the gastrointestinal (GI) tract. Ethacrynic acid is a diuretic. Folic acid and thiamine are vitamins, which may be used in clients with liver disease as supplemental therapy.

Test-Taking Strategy: To answer this question correctly, it is necessary to know that ammonia levels are elevated with advanced liver disease, and that lactulose is a standard form of medication therapy for this condition. Review this disorder and the purpose of this medication if you had difficulty with this question.

Level of Cognitive Ability: Analysis
Client Needs: Physiological Integrity
Integrated Process: Nursing Process/Analysis
Content Area: Pharmacology

Reference:

Hodgson, B., & Kizior, R. (2004). *Saunders nursing drug handbook 2004.* Philadelphia: Saunders, p. 578.

15. A nurse is caring for a child with renal disease and is analyzing the laboratory results. The nurse notes a sodium level of 148 mEq/L. Based on this finding, which clinical manifestation would the nurse expect to note in the child?
1 Diaphoresis
2 Cold, wet skin
3 Dry, sticky mucous membranes
4 Lethargy

Answer: 3
Rationale: Hypernatremia occurs when the sodium level is greater that 145 mEq/L. Clinical manifestations include intense thirst, oliguria, agitation and restlessness, flushed skin, peripheral and pulmonary edema, dry sticky mucous membranes, and nausea and vomiting. Options 1, 2, and 4 are not associated with the clinical manifestations of hypernatremia.

Test-Taking Strategy: First, determine that the sodium level is elevated and that the child is experiencing hypernatremia. Next, eliminate options 1 and 2 because they are similar. From the remaining options, recalling that agitation and restlessness are associated with hypernatremia will direct you to option 3. Review the normal sodium level and the clinical manifestations associated with an imbalance if you had difficulty with this question.

Level of Cognitive Ability: Analysis
Client Needs: Physiological Integrity
Integrated Process: Nursing Process/Analysis
Content Area: Child Health

Reference:
Wong, D., & Hockenberry, M. (2003). *Wong's nursing care of infants and children* (7th ed.). St. Louis: Mosby, pp. 1176; 1901.

16. A nurse is caring for an infant who is admitted to the hospital with a diagnosis of hemolytic disease. The nurse reviews the laboratory results, expecting to note which of the following in this infant?
1 Decreased red blood cell count
2 Decreased bilirubin count
3 Elevated blood glucose level
4 Decreased white blood cell count

Answer: 1
Rationale: The two primary pathophysiologic alterations associated with hemolytic disease are anemia and hyperbilirubinemia. The red blood cell count is decreased because the red blood cell production cannot keep pace with red blood cell destruction. Hyperbilirubinemia results from the red blood cell destruction accompanying this disorder as well as from the normally decreased ability of the neonate's liver to conjugate and excrete bilirubin efficiently from the body. Hypoglycemia is associated with hypertrophy of the pancreatic islet cells and increased levels of insulin. The white blood cell count is not related to this disorder.

Test-Taking Strategy: Focus on the infant's diagnosis. Noting the name "hemolytic" in the diagnosis will direct you to option 1. Review the clinical manifestations associated with hemolytic disease if you had difficulty with this question.

Level of Cognitive Ability: Analysis
Client Needs: Physiological Integrity
Integrated Process: Nursing Process/Analysis
Content Area: Child Health

References:
Wong, D., & Hockenberry, M. (2003). *Wong's nursing care of infants and children* (7th ed.). St. Louis: Mosby, p. 310.
James, S., Ashwill, J., & Droske, S. (2002). *Nursing care of children: Principles & practice* (2nd ed.). Philadelphia: Saunders, pp. 765-766.

17. A nurse is performing on assessment on a child who is to receive a measles, mumps, and rubella (MMR) vaccine. The nurse notes that the child is allergic to eggs. Which of the following would the nurse anticipate to be prescribed for this child?

1 Administration of diphenhydramine (Benadryl) and acetaminophen (Tylenol) before the administration of the MMR vaccine

2 Administration of a killed measles vaccine

3 Eliminating this vaccine from the immunization schedule

4 Administration of epinephrine (Adrenalin) before the administration of the MMR

Answer: 2

Rationale: Live measles vaccine is produced by chick embryo cell culture, so the possibility of an anaphylactic hypersensitivity in children with egg allergies should be considered. If there is a question of sensitivity, children should be tested before the administration of MMR vaccine. If a child tests positive for sensitivity, the killed measles vaccine may be given as an alternative.

Test-Taking Strategy: Use the process of elimination. Option 3 can be eliminated first because a vaccine would not be eliminated from the immunization schedule. Options 1 and 4 can be eliminated next, knowing that the use of medications before a vaccine is not normal procedure. Also, recalling that live measles vaccine is produced by chick embryo cell culture will direct you to option 2. Review the procedures related to the administration of vaccines if you had difficulty with this question.

Level of Cognitive Ability: Analysis
Client Needs: Health Promotion and Maintenance
Integrated Process: Nursing Process/Analysis
Content Area: Child Health

References:
James, S., Ashwill, J., & Droske, S. (2002). *Nursing care of children: Principles & practice* (2nd ed.). Philadelphia: Saunders, p. 88.
Lehne, R. (2004). *Pharmacology for nursing care* (5th ed.). Philadelphia: Saunders, pp. 714; 720.

18. Intravenous immune globulin (IVIG) therapy is prescribed for a child with immune thrombocytopenic purpura (ITP). The nurse determines that this medication is prescribed for the child to:

1 Provide immunity to the child against infection

2 Increase the number of circulating platelets

3 Decrease the production of antiplatelet antibodies

4 Prevent infection following exposure to communicable diseases

Answer: 2

Rationale: IVIG is usually effective in rapidly increasing the platelet count. It is thought to act by interfering with the attachment of antibody-coded platelets to receptors on the macrophage cells of the reticuloendothelial system. Corticosteroids may be prescribed to enhance vascular stability and decrease the production of antiplatelet antibodies. Options 1, 3, and 4 are unrelated to the administration of this medication.

Test-Taking Strategy: Note the relationship between the name of the diagnosis "thrombocytopenic purpura" and the word "platelets" in the correct option. This relationship may assist in directing you to the correct option. Review this content if you are unfamiliar with ITP and the purpose of IVIG.

Level of Cognitive Ability: Analysis
Client Needs: Physiological Integrity
Integrated Process: Nursing Process/Analysis
Content Area: Child Health

Reference:
Hodgson, B., & Kizior, R. (2004). *Saunders nursing drug handbook 2004.* Philadelphia: Saunders, p. 528.

19. A child was diagnosed with acute post-streptococcal glomerulonephritis and renal insufficiency. Which laboratory result will the nurse expect to note in the child?
  1 An elevated white blood cell (WBC) count
  2 Negative red blood cells in the urinalysis
  3 Negative protein in the urinalysis
  4 An elevated blood urea nitrogen (BUN) and creatinine

Answer: 4
Rationale: In post-streptococcal glomerulonephritis, a urinalysis will reveal hematuria with red cell casts. Proteinuria is also present. If renal insufficiency is severe, the BUN and creatinine levels will be elevated. The WBC is usually within normal limits, and mild anemia is common.

Test-Taking Strategy: Use the process of elimination, focusing on the child's diagnosis. Recalling that the BUN and creatinine are laboratory studies that relate to the renal system will direct you to option 4. Review the clinical manifestations associated with this disorder if you had difficulty with this question.

Level of Cognitive Ability: Analysis
Client Needs: Physiological Integrity
Integrated Process: Nursing Process/Analysis
Content Area: Child Health

Reference:
Wong, D., & Hockenberry, M. (2003). *Wong's nursing care of infants and children* (7th ed.). St. Louis: Mosby, p. 1274.

20. A nurse is assigned to care for a child with juvenile rheumatoid arthritis (JRA). The nurse reviews the plan of care, knowing that which of the following is a priority nursing diagnosis?
  1 Disturbed body image, related to activity intolerance
  2 Potential for self-care deficit, related to immobility
  3 High risk for injury, related to impaired physical mobility
  4 Acute pain, related to the inflammatory process

Answer: 4
Rationale: All of the nursing diagnoses are appropriate for the child with JRA; however, acute pain needs to be managed before other problems can be addressed.

Test-Taking Strategy: Note the key word "priority." Use Maslow's hierarchy of needs theory, remembering that physiological needs (option 4) receive highest priority. Option 3 addresses safety and security needs. Options 1 addresses self-esteem needs. Option 2 identifies a potential, not an actual problem. Review care of a child with JRA if you had difficulty with this question.

Level of Cognitive Ability: Analysis
Client Needs: Physiological Integrity
Integrated Process: Nursing Process/Analysis
Content Area: Delegating/Prioritizing

Reference:
Wong, D., & Hockenberry, M. (2003). *Wong's nursing care of infants and children* (7th ed.). St. Louis: Mosby, pp. 1823; 1826.

21. A child is admitted to the hospital with a suspected diagnosis of immune thrombocytopenic purpura (ITP), and diagnostic studies are performed. Which of the following diagnostic results are indicative of this disorder?

   1 Bone marrow examination indicating an increased number of immature white blood cells

   2 Bone marrow examination showing an increased number of megakaryocytes

   3 An elevated platelet count

   4 An elevated hemoglobin and hematocrit level

Answer: 2

Rationale: The laboratory manifestations of ITP include the presence of a low platelet count usually less than 50,000 cells per mm^3. Thrombocytopenia is the only laboratory abnormality expected with ITP. If there has been significant blood loss, there is evidence of anemia in the blood cell count. If a bone marrow examination is performed, the results with ITP show a normal or increased number of megakaryocytes, the precursors of platelets. Option 1 indicates the bone marrow result that would be found in leukemia.

Test-Taking Strategy: Focus on the diagnosis. Recalling that megakaryocytes are the precursors of platelets will assist in directing you to option 2. Review this content if you are unfamiliar with this disorder or the associated clinical manifestations.

Level of Cognitive Ability: Analysis
Client Needs: Physiological Integrity
Integrated Process: Nursing Process/Analysis
Content Area: Child Health

Reference:
Wong, D., & Hockenberry, M. (2003). *Wong's nursing care of infants and children* (7th ed.). St. Louis: Mosby, pp. 1566-1567.

22. An infant is brought to the health care clinic, and the mother tells the nurse that her infant has been vomiting after meals. The mother explains that the vomiting is now becoming more frequent and forceful and the infant seems to be constipated. On assessment, the nurse notes visible peristaltic waves moving from left to right across the abdomen. Based on this finding, the nurse would suspect which of the following?

   1 Colic

   2 Intussusception

   3 Pyloric stenosis

   4 Congenital megacolon

Answer: 3

Rationale: In pyloric stenosis, the vomitus contains sour, undigested food, but no bile, the child is constipated, and visible peristaltic waves move from left to right across the abdomen. A movable, palpable, firm olive-shaped mass in the right upper quadrant may be noted. Crying during the evening hours, appearing to be in pain, but eating well and gaining weight are clinical manifestations of colic. An infant who suddenly becomes pale, cries out, and draws the legs up to the chest is demonstrating physical signs of intussusception. Ribbon-like stool, bile-stained emesis, absence of peristalsis, and abdominal distension are symptoms of congenital megacolon (Hirschsprung's disease).

Test-Taking Strategy: Focus on the data provided in the question. Consider each condition presented in the options and think about the clinical manifestations of each. Recalling the manifestations associated with pyloric stenosis will direct you to option 3. Review the clinical manifestations of this disorder if you had difficulty with this question.

Level of Cognitive Ability: Analysis
Client Needs: Physiological Integrity
Integrated Process: Nursing Process/Analysis
Content Area: Child Health

Reference:
Wong, D., & Hockenberry, M. (2003). *Wong's nursing care of infants and children* (7th ed.). St. Louis: Mosby, p. 1446.

23. A nurse is reviewing the laboratory analysis of cerebrospinal fluid (CSF) obtained during a lumbar puncture from a child suspected of having bacterial meningitis. Which of the following results would most likely confirm this diagnosis?
  1 Cloudy CSF with low protein and low glucose
  2 Cloudy CSF with high protein and low glucose
  3 Clear CSF with low protein and low glucose
  4 Decreased pressure, cloudy CSF with high protein

Answer: 2
Rationale: A diagnosis of meningitis is made by testing CSF obtained by lumbar puncture. In the case of bacterial meningitis, findings usually include increased pressure, cloudy CSF, high protein, and low glucose. Options 1, 3, and 4 are incorrect.

Test-Taking Strategy: Use the process of elimination. Eliminate options 3 and 4 first because clear CSF and decreased pressure is not likely to be found with an infectious process such as meningitis. From the remaining options, recalling that high protein indicates a possible diagnosis of meningitis will direct you to option 2. Review this diagnostic test if you had difficulty with this question.

Level of Cognitive Ability: Analysis
Client Needs: Physiological Integrity
Integrated Process: Nursing Process/Analysis
Content Area: Child Health

Reference:
Wong, D., & Hockenberry, M. (2003). *Wong's nursing care of infants and children* (7th ed.). St. Louis: Mosby, p. 1681.

---

24. A child is admitted to the pediatric unit with a diagnosis of acute gastroenteritis. The nurse monitors the child for signs of hypovolemic shock as a result of fluid and electrolyte losses that have occurred in the child. Which finding would indicate the presence of compensated shock?
  1 Bradycardia
  2 Hypotension
  3 Profuse diarrhea
  4 Capillary refill time greater than 2 seconds

Answer: 4
Rationale: Shock may be classified as compensated or decompensated. In compensated shock, the child becomes tachycardic in an effort to increase the cardiac output. The blood pressure remains normal. Capillary refill time may be prolonged and greater than 2 seconds, and the child may become irritable because of increasing hypoxia. The most prevalent cause of hypovolemic shock is fluid and electrolyte losses associated with gastroenteritis. Diarrhea is not a sign of shock, but rather it is a cause of the fluid and electrolyte imbalance.

Test-Taking Strategy: Use the process of elimination, focusing on the key words "compensated shock." Recalling that hypotension is a late sign of shock in children will assist in eliminating option 2. Recalling that tachycardia rather than bradycardia occurs in shock will assist in eliminating option 1. From the remaining options, focusing on the issue, signs of shock, will direct you to option 4. Review the signs of compensated shock in a child if you had difficulty with this question.

Level of Cognitive Ability: Analysis
Client Needs: Physiological Integrity
Integrated Process: Nursing Process/Analysis
Content Area: Child Health

Reference:
Wong, D., & Hockenberry, M. (2003). *Wong's nursing care of infants and children* (7th ed.). St. Louis: Mosby, p. 1219.

25. A mother brings her child to the health care clinic for a routine examination. The mother tells the nurse that the teacher has reported that the child appears to be daydreaming and staring off into space. The teacher tells the mother that this occurs numerous times throughout the day, yet during the remainder of the day the child is alert and participates in classroom activity. The nurse documents the findings and suspects that which of the following are occurring with this child?

1 The child has attention deficit hyperactivity syndrome and is in need of medication.
2 The child probably has school phobia.
3 The child is experiencing absence seizures.
4 The child is showing signs of a behavioral problem.

Answer: 3

Rationale: Absence seizures are a type of generalized seizure. They consist of a sudden, brief (no longer than 30 seconds) arrest of the child's motor activities accompanied by a blank stare and loss of awareness. The child's posture is maintained at the end of the seizure. The child returns to activity that was in process as though nothing has happened. A child with attention deficit hyperactivity syndrome becomes easily distracted, is fidgety, and has difficulty following directions. School phobia includes physical symptoms that usually occur at home and may prevent the child from attending school. Behavior problems would be noted by more overt symptoms than described in this question.

Test-Taking Strategy: Use the process of elimination, focusing on the information provided in the question. Note the relationship of the information and option 3. Review this content if you are unfamiliar with the characteristics associated with absence seizures.

Level of Cognitive Ability: Analysis
Client Needs: Physiological Integrity
Integrated Process: Nursing Process/Analysis
Content Area: Child Health

Reference:
Wong, D., & Hockenberry, M. (2003). *Wong's nursing care of infants and children* (7th ed.). St. Louis: Mosby, p. 1688.

---

26. A mother and her 3-week-old infant arrive at the well baby clinic for a rescreening test for phenylketonuria (PKU). The nurse reviews the results of the serum phenylalanine levels and notes that the level is 1.0 mg/dL. The nurse interprets this level as:

1 Normal
2 Elevated, indicating PKU
3 Inconclusive
4 Requiring a repeat study

Answer: 1

Rationale: The normal PKU level is less the 2 mg/dL. With early postpartum discharge, screening is often performed at less than 2 days of age because of the concern that the infant will be lost to follow-up. Infants should be rescreened by 14 days of age if the initial screen was done at 24 to 48 hours of age.

Test-Taking Strategy: Use the process of elimination and knowledge regarding the normal phenylalanine level. Recalling that the normal level is less than 2 mg/dL will direct you to option 1. Review this content if you are unfamiliar with this screening test.

Level of Cognitive Ability: Analysis
Client Needs: Physiological Integrity
Integrated Process: Nursing Process/Analysis
Content Area: Maternity/Postpartum

Reference:
Wong, D., & Hockenberry, M. (2003). *Wong's nursing care of infants and children* (7th ed.). St. Louis: Mosby, p. 323.

27. A child is admitted to the hospital with a suspected diagnosis of bacterial endocarditis. The child has been experiencing fever, malaise, anorexia, and a headache, and diagnostic studies are performed on the child. Which of the following studies will primarily confirm the diagnosis?
1 An electrocardiogram (ECG)
2 A white blood cell count
3 A blood culture
4 A sedimentation rate

Answer: 3
Rationale: The diagnosis of bacterial endocarditis is primarily established on the basis of a positive blood culture of the organisms and visualization of vegetation on echocardiographic studies. Other laboratory tests that may help confirm the diagnosis are an elevated sedimentation rate and C-reactive protein level. An ECG is not usually helpful in the diagnosis of bacterial endocarditis.

Test-Taking Strategy: Note the key words "primarily confirm" in the stem of the question. Use the process of elimination, recalling that bacterial endocarditis is caused by an organism. The only test that will confirm the presence of an organism is the blood culture. Review this content if you are unfamiliar with the diagnostic studies associated with bacterial endocarditis.

Level of Cognitive Ability: Analysis
Client Needs: Physiological Integrity
Integrated Process: Nursing Process/Analysis
Content Area: Child Health

Reference:
Wong, D., & Hockenberry, M. (2003). *Wong's nursing care of infants and children* (7th ed.). St. Louis: Mosby, p. 1510.

28. A nurse is caring for a client with intracranial aneurysm. The nurse interprets that which of the following is related to dysfunction of cranial nerve III?
1 Mild drowsiness
2 Less frequent spontaneous speech
3 Slight slurring of speech
4 Ptosis of the left eyelid

Answer: 4
Rationale: Ptosis of the eyelid is caused by pressure on and dysfunction of cranial nerve III. Options 1, 2, and 3 identify early signs of a deteriorating level of consciousness.

Test Taking Strategy: Note the key words "cranial nerve III." Recalling the function of this nerve will direct you to option 4. Review the function of cranial nerve III if you had difficulty with this question.

Level of Cognitive Ability: Analysis
Client Needs: Physiological Integrity
Integrated Process: Nursing Process/Analysis
Content Area: Adult Health/Neurological

Reference:
Ignatavicius, D., & Workman, M. (2002). *Medical surgical nursing: Critical thinking for collaborative care* (4th ed.). Philadelphia: Saunders, p. 994.

29. A client with thrombotic cerebrovascular accident (CVA) experiences periods of emotional lability. The client alternately laughs and cries, and intermittently becomes irritable and demanding. The nurse interprets that this behavior indicates:

1 That the problem is likely to get worse before it gets better
2 That the client is experiencing the usual sequelae of a CVA
3 The client is not adapting well to the disability
4 The client is experiencing side effects of prescribed anticoagulants

Answer: 2

Rationale: Following CVA, the client often experiences periods of emotional lability, which is characterized by sudden bouts of laughing or crying, or by irritability, depression, confusion, or being demanding. This is a normal part of the clinical picture for the client with this health problem, although it may be difficult for health care personnel and family members to deal with. The other options are incorrect.

Test-Taking Strategy: Use the process of elimination. Eliminate options 1 and 4 first. Anticoagulants do not cause emotional lability, and there is no data in the question to support option 1. From the remaining options, recalling the emotional changes that accompany a CVA will direct you to option 2. Review the effects of a CVA if you had difficulty with this question.

Level of Cognitive Ability: Analysis
Client Needs: Psychosocial Integrity
Integrated Process: Nursing Process/Analysis
Content Area: Adult Health/Neurological

Reference:
Ignatavicius, D., & Workman, M. (2002). *Medical surgical nursing: Critical thinking for collaborative care* (4th ed.). Philadelphia: Saunders, p. 982.

30. A nurse is caring for a client with myasthenia gravis. The client is vomiting and complaining of abdominal cramps and diarrhea. The nurse also notes that the client is hypotensive and is experiencing facial muscle twitching. The nurse interprets that these symptoms are compatible with:

1 Systemic infection
2 A reaction to plasmapheresis
3 Cholinergic crisis
4 Myasthenic crisis

Answer: 3

Rationale: Signs and symptoms of cholinergic crisis include nausea, vomiting, abdominal cramping, diarrhea, blurred vision, pallor, facial muscle twitching, pupillary myosis, and hypotension. It is caused by overmedication with cholinergic (anticholinesterase) medications and is treated by withholding medications. Myasthenic crisis is an exacerbation of myasthenic symptoms caused by undermedication with anticholinesterase medications. There is no data in the question to support options 1, 2, and 4.

Test-Taking Strategy: Use the process of elimination. Note the client's diagnosis and think about the treatment for this disorder. Recalling the effects of cholinergic medications and focusing on the data in the question will direct you to option 3. Review the clinical manifestations associated with cholinergic crisis if you had difficulty with this question.

Level of Cognitive Ability: Analysis
Client Needs: Physiological Integrity
Integrated Process: Nursing Process/Analysis
Content Area: Adult Health/Neurological

Reference:
Ignatavicius, D., & Workman, M. (2002). *Medical surgical nursing: Critical thinking for collaborative care* (4th ed.). Philadelphia: Saunders, pp. 961-962.

Nursing Process: Planning

1. A nurse is caring for a client who is receiving total parental nutrition (TPN). The nurse plans for which nursing intervention to prevent infection in the client?
1 Using strict aseptic technique for intravenous site dressing changes
2 Monitoring serum blood urea nitrogen (BUN) levels
3 Weighing the client daily
4 Encouraging fluid intake

Answer: 1

Rationale: Strict aseptic technique is vital during dressing changes because the IV catheter can serve as a direct entry for microorganisms. Options 2, 3, and 4 are not measures that will prevent infection.

Test-Taking Strategy: Focus on the issue: to prevent infection. Note the relationship between "infection" in the question and "aseptic" in the correct option. Additionally, the only option that will prevent infection is option 1. Review care of a client receiving TPN if you had difficulty with this question.

Level of Cognitive Ability: Application
Client Needs: Safe, Effective Care Environment
Integrated Process: Nursing Process/Planning
Content Area: Fundamental Skills

Reference:
Ignatavicius, D., & Workman, M. (2002). *Medical surgical nursing: Critical thinking for collaborative care* (4th ed.). Philadelphia: Saunders, pp. 202; 1372.

2. A nurse develops a plan of care for a client with a spica cast that covers a lower extremity and documents that the client has a potential for impaired bowel elimination. When planning for bowel elimination needs, the nurse includes which of the following in the plan of care?
1 Use a fracture pan for bowel elimination
2 Use a regular bedpan to prevent spilling of contents in the bed
3 Use a bedside commode for all elimination needs
4 Administer an enema daily

Answer: 1

Rationale: A fracture pan is designed for use in clients with body or leg casts. A client with a spica cast (body cast) that covers a lower extremity cannot bend at the hips to sit up. Therefore, a regular bedpan and a commode would be inappropriate. Daily enemas are not a part of routine care.

Test-Taking Strategy: Focus on the words "covers a lower extremity." Use the process of elimination, noting the key word "fracture" in the correct option. Review care of the client with a spica cast if you had difficulty with this question.

Level of Cognitive Ability: Application
Client Needs: Physiological Integrity
Integrated Process: Nursing Process/Planning
Content Area: Fundamental Skills

Reference:
Potter, P., & Perry, A. (2005). *Fundamentals of nursing* (6th ed.). St. Louis: Mosby, p. 1395.

3. A nurse is caring for a postpartum client with thromboembolitic disease. When planning care to prevent the complication of pulmonary embolism, the nurse prepares specifically to:
1 Administer and monitor anticoagulant therapy as prescribed
2 Assess breath sounds frequently
3 Enforce bed rest
4 Monitor vital signs frequently

Answer: 1

Rationale: The purpose of anticoagulant therapy to treat thromboembolitic disease is to prevent the formation of a clot and prevent a clot from moving to another area, thus preventing pulmonary embolism. Although options 2, 3, and 4 may be implemented for a client with thromboembolitic disease, option 1 will specifically assist in preventing pulmonary embolism.

Test-Taking Strategy: Focus on the issue: preventing the complication of pulmonary embolism. Note the key word "specifically" in the stem of the question. Recall that anticoagulant therapy is prescribed to treat thromboembolitic disease. Also, noting the words "as prescribed" in option 1 will direct you to this option. Review interventions for the client with thromboembolitic disease that will prevent pulmonary embolism if you had difficulty with this question.

Level of Cognitive Ability: Application
Client Needs: Physiological Integrity
Integrated Process: Nursing Process/Planning
Content Area: Maternity/Postpartum

Reference:
Lowdermilk, D., & Perry, A. (2004). *Maternity & women's health care* (8th ed.). St. Louis: Mosby, pp. 1045-1046.

4. After reviewing a client's serum electrolytes, the physician states that the client would benefit most from an isotonic intravenous (IV) solution. The nurse plans care, anticipating that the order will indicate that which of the following solutions should be administered?
1 0.45% normal saline
2 5% dextrose in water
3 10% dextrose in water
4 5% dextrose in 0.9% normal saline

Answer: 2

Rationale: 5% dextrose in water is an isotonic solution. Another example of an isotonic solution is 0.9% normal saline. 0.45% normal saline is a hypotonic solution. 10% dextrose in water and 5% dextrose in 0.9% normal saline are hypertonic solutions.

Test-Taking Strategy: To answer this question accurately, you must be familiar with the tonicity of various IV solutions. Note the key word "isotonic" and recall that 5% dextrose in water and 0.9% normal saline are isotonic. Review the tonicity of IV fluids if you had difficulty with this question.

Level of Cognitive Ability: Analysis
Client Needs: Physiological Integrity
Integrated Process: Nursing Process/Planning
Content Area: Fundamental Skills

Reference:
Potter, P., & Perry, A. (2005). *Fundamentals of nursing* (6th ed.). St. Louis: Mosby, p. 1160.

5. A nurse is admitting a client to the hospital who recently had a bilateral adrenalectomy. Which intervention is essential for the nurse to include in the client's plan of care?
   1 Prevent social isolation
   2 Discuss changes in body image
   3 Consider occupational therapy
   4 Avoid stress-producing situations and procedures

Answer: 4
Rationale: Adrenalectomy can lead to adrenal insufficiency. Adrenal hormones are essential in maintaining homeostasis in response to stressors. Options 1, 2, and 3 are not essential interventions specific to this client's problem.

Test-Taking Strategy: Note the key word "essential" in the stem of the question. This indicates the need to prioritize. Remember that according to Maslow's hierarchy of needs theory, physiological needs come first. The stress reaction involves physiological processes. Review the postoperative effects following an adrenalectomy if you had difficulty with this question.

Level of Cognitive Ability: Application
Client Needs: Physiological Integrity
Integrated Process: Nursing Process/Planning
Content Area: Adult Health/Endocrine

Reference:
Black, J., & Hawks, J. (2005). *Medical-surgical nursing: Clinical management for positive outcomes* (7th ed.). Philadelphia: Saunders, p. 1227.

6. A perinatal client is admitted to the obstetric unit during an exacerbation of a heart condition. When planning for the nutritional requirements of the client, the nurse would consult with the dietitian to ensure which of the following?
   1 A low-calorie diet to ensure absence of weight gain
   2 A diet low in fluids and fiber to decrease blood volume
   3 A diet adequate in fluids and fiber to decrease constipation
   4 Unlimited sodium intake to increase circulating blood volume

Answer: 3
Rationale: Constipation can cause the client to use the Valsalva maneuver. This maneuver can cause blood to rush to the heart and overload the cardiac system. A low-calorie diet is not recommended during pregnancy. Diets low in fluid and fiber can cause a decrease in blood volume that can deprive the fetus of nutrients. Therefore, adequate fluid intake and high-fiber foods are important. Sodium should be restricted to some degree as prescribed by the physician because this will cause an overload to the circulating blood volume and contribute to cardiac complications.

Test Taking Strategy: Use the process of elimination. Think about the physiology of the cardiac system, the maternal and fetus needs, and the factors that increase the workload on the heart to answer the question. Review nursing measures for the pregnant client with cardiac disease if you had difficulty with this question.

Level of Cognitive Ability: Analysis
Client Needs: Physiological Integrity
Integrated Process: Nursing Process/Planning
Content Area: Maternity/Antepartum

Reference:
Murray, S., McKinney, E., & Gorrie, T. (2002). *Foundations of maternal-newborn nursing* (3rd ed.). Philadelphia: Saunders, p. 716.

7. A nurse is developing a plan of care for a client with a hip spica cast. In the planning, the nurse includes measures to limit complications of prolonged immobility. The nurse includes which essential item in the plan to prevent these complications?

1 Provide a daily fluid intake of 1000 mL
2 Monitor for signs of low serum calcium
3 Maintain the client in a supine position
4 Limit the intake of milk and milk products

Answer: 4

Rationale: The formation of renal and urinary calculi is a complication of immobility. Daily fluid intake should be 2000 mL or greater a day. The nurse should monitor for signs and symptoms of hypercalcemia, such as nausea, vomiting, polydipsia, polyuria, and lethargy. A supine position increases urinary stasis; therefore, this position should be limited or avoided. Limiting milk and milk products is the best measure to prevent the formation of calcium stones.

Test-Taking Strategy: Focus on the issue: a complication of prolonged immobility. Option 3 should be eliminated immediately because it refers to maintaining an immobile client in one position. Eliminate option 1 next, noting the amount of fluid in this option. From the remaining options, recalling the effect of the movement of calcium into the blood from the bones will direct you to option 4. Review the complications of immobility if you had difficulty with this question.

Level of Cognitive Ability: Application
Client Needs: Physiological Integrity
Integrated Process: Nursing Process/Planning
Content Area: Adult Health/Musculoskeletal

Reference:
Black, J., & Hawks, J. (2005). *Medical-surgical nursing: Clinical management for positive outcomes* (7th ed.). Philadelphia: Saunders, pp. 644-645.

---

8. A nurse determines that a Mantoux tuberculin skin test is positive. In order to most accurately diagnose tuberculosis (TB), the nurse plans to consult with the physician to follow-up the skin test with a:

1 Chest X-ray
2 Computed tomography scan of the chest
3 Sputum culture
4 Complete blood cell count

Answer: 3

Rationale: Although the findings on chest X-ray examination are important, it is not possible to make a diagnosis of TB solely on the basis of this examination, because other diseases can mimic the appearance of TB. The demonstration of tubercle bacilli bacteriologically is essential for establishing a diagnosis. Microscopic examination of sputum for acid-fast bacilli is usually the first bacteriologic evidence of the presence of tubercle bacilli. Options 2 and 4 will not diagnosis TB.

Test-Taking Strategy: Note the key words "most accurately diagnose tuberculosis." Recalling that the presence of tubercle bacilli indicates TB will direct you to option 3. Review the tests used in diagnosing tuberculosis if you had difficulty with this question.

Level of Cognitive Ability: Application
Client Needs: Physiological Integrity
Integrated Process: Nursing Process/Planning
Content Area: Adult Health/Respiratory

Reference:
Black, J., & Hawks, J. (2005). *Medical-surgical nursing: Clinical management for positive outcomes* (7th ed.). Philadelphia: Saunders, p. 1846.

9. A home care nurse is preparing a plan of care for a client with Ménière's disease who is experiencing severe vertigo. Which nursing intervention would the nurse include in the plan of care to assist the client in controlling the vertigo?
   1 Encourage the client to increase daily fluid intake
   2 Encourage the client to avoid sudden head movements
   3 Instruct the client to cut down on cigarette smoking
   4 Instruct the client to increase sodium in the diet

Answer: 2
Rationale: The nurse instructs the client to make slow head movements to prevent worsening of the vertigo. Dietary changes such as salt and fluid restrictions that reduce the amount of endolymphatic fluid are sometimes prescribed. Clients are advised to stop smoking because of its vasoconstrictive effects.

Test-Taking Strategy: Identify the issue of the question: severe vertigo. Note the relationship between the words "severe vertigo" and the correct option, which states to avoid sudden head movements. Recalling that salt and fluid restrictions are sometimes prescribed will also assist in eliminating options 1 and 4. Noting the words "cut down" in option 3 will assist in eliminating this option. Review measures that will reduce vertigo in the client with Ménière's disease if you had difficulty with this question.

Level of Cognitive Ability: Application
Client Needs: Health Promotion and Maintenance
Integrated Process: Nursing Process/Planning
Content Area: Adult Health/Ear

Reference:
Ignatavicius, D., & Workman, M. (2002). *Medical surgical nursing: Critical thinking for collaborative care* (4th ed.). Philadelphia: Saunders, p. 1068.

10. An 18-year-old woman is admitted to a mental health unit with the diagnosis of anorexia nervosa. The nurse plans care, knowing that health promotion should focus on:
    1 Helping the client identify and examine dysfunctional thoughts and beliefs
    2 Emphasizing social interaction with clients who are withdrawn
    3 Providing a supportive environment
    4 Examining intrapsychic conflicts and past issues

Answer: 1
Rationale: Health promotion focuses on helping clients identify and examine dysfunctional thoughts as well as identify and examine values and beliefs that maintain these thoughts. Providing a supportive environment is important but is not as primary as option 1 for this client. Emphasizing social interaction is not appropriate at this time. Examining intrapsychic conflicts and past issues is not directly related to the client's problem.

Test-Taking Strategy: Use the process of elimination, focusing on the issue of health promotion. Option 1 is the only option that is specifically client-centered. This option also focuses on assessment, the first step of the nursing process. Review care of the client with anorexia nervosa if you had difficulty with this question.

Level of Cognitive Ability: Application
Client Needs: Health Promotion and Maintenance
Integrated Process: Nursing Process/Planning
Content Area: Mental Health

Reference:
Keltner, N., Schwecke, L., & Bostrom, C. (2003). *Psychiatric nursing* (4th ed.). St. Louis: Mosby, pp. 504-505.

11. A nurse is preparing discharge plans for a hospitalized client who attempted suicide. The nurse includes which of the following in the plan?
1 Weekly follow-up appointments
2 Contracts and immediately available crisis resources
3 Encouraging family and friends to always be present
4 Providing phone numbers for the hospital and physician

Answer: 2
Rationale: Crisis times may occur between appointments. Contracts facilitate clients feeling a responsibility for keeping a promise. This gives the client control. Family and friends cannot always be present. Providing phone numbers will not ensure available and immediate crisis intervention.

Test-Taking Strategy: Focus on the issue: the availability of immediate resources for the client. Eliminate option 3 first because this is unrealistic. Options 1 and 4 will not necessarily provide immediate resources. Also, note the word "immediately" in the correct option. Review discharge plans for the client who attempted suicide if you had difficulty with this question.

Level of Cognitive Ability: Application
Client Needs: Psychosocial Integrity
Integrated Process: Nursing Process/Planning
Content Area: Mental Health

Reference:
Keltner, N., Schwecke, L., & Bostrom, C. (2003). *Psychiatric nursing* (4th ed.). St. Louis: Mosby, p. 357.

12. A nurse is developing a plan of care for a newborn infant diagnosed with bilateral club feet. The nurse includes instructions in the plan to tell the parents that:
1 Genetic testing is wise for future pregnancies, because other children born to this couple may also be affected
2 If casting is needed, it will begin at birth and continue for 12 weeks, and then the condition will be reevaluated
3 Surgery performed immediately after birth has been found to be most effective in achieving a complete recovery
4 The regimen of manipulation and casting is effective in all cases of bilateral club feet

Answer: 2
Rationale: Casting should begin at birth and continue for at least 12 weeks or until maximum correction is achieved. At this time, corrective shoes may provide support to maintain alignment, or surgery can be performed. Surgery is usually delayed until 4 to 12 months of age. Options 3 and 4 are inaccurate. Option 1 does not specifically address the issue of the question.

Test-Taking Strategy: Focus on the issue: parental instructions for the child with bilateral club feet. Eliminate option 1 because it does not specifically address the issue of the question and relates to the future. Eliminate option 3 because of the word "immediately." From the remaining options, note that option 2 provides accurate information and that option 4 contains the absolute word "all." Review the treatment plan for bilateral club feet if you had difficulty with this question.

Level of Cognitive Ability: Application
Client Needs: Health Promotion and Maintenance
Integrated Process: Nursing Process/Planning
Content Area: Child Health

Reference:
Wong, D., & Hockenberry, M. (2003). *Wong's nursing care of infants and children* (7th ed.). St. Louis: Mosby, pp. 452-453.

13. A nurse is planning to assist with obtaining a set of arterial blood gases on a client. The nurse plans to provide which of the following items to optimally maintain the integrity of the specimen?
  1 A syringe containing a preservative
  2 A syringe containing a preservative and a bag of ice
  3 A heparinized syringe and a preservative
  4 A heparinized syringe and a bag of ice

Answer: 4
Rationale: The arterial blood gas sample is obtained using a heparinized syringe. The sample of blood is placed on ice and sent to the laboratory immediately. A preservative is not used.

Test-Taking Strategy: Specific knowledge regarding this procedure is needed to answer this question. Review this content if you are unfamiliar with this procedure.

Level of Cognitive Ability: Application
Client Needs: Physiological Integrity
Integrated Process: Nursing Process/Planning
Content Area: Adult Health/Respiratory

Reference:
Chernecky, C., & Berger, B. (2004). *Laboratory tests and diagnostic procedures* (4th ed.). Philadelphia: Saunders, p. 248.

14. A client is experiencing diabetes insipidus secondary to cranial surgery. The nurse who is caring for the client plans to implement which of these anticipated therapies?
  1 Fluid restriction
  2 Intravenous (IV) replacement of fluid losses
  3 Increased sodium intake
  4 Administering diuretics

Answer: 2
Rationale: The client with diabetes insipidus excretes large amounts of extremely dilute urine. This usually occurs as a result of decreased synthesis or release of antidiuretic hormone (ADH) in conditions such as head injury, surgery near the hypothalamus, or increased intracranial pressure. Corrective measures include allowing ample oral fluid intake, administering IV fluid as needed to replace sensible and insensible losses, and administering vasopressin (Pitressin). Sodium is not administered because the serum sodium level is usually high, as is the serum osmolality. Option 4 is incorrect.

Test-Taking Strategy: Focus on the client's diagnosis, recalling that a large fluid loss is the problem in this client. This will assist in eliminating options 1 and 4. From the remaining options, recalling that the serum sodium level is already elevated in this disorder, or by knowing that fluid replacement is the most direct form of therapy for fluid loss, will direct you to option 2. Review the treatment for diabetes insipidus if you had difficulty with this question.

Level of Cognitive Ability: Analysis
Client Needs: Physiological Integrity
Integrated Process: Nursing Process/Planning
Content Area: Adult Health/Neurological

Reference:
Ignatavicius, D., & Workman, M. (2002). *Medical surgical nursing: Critical thinking for collaborative care* (4th ed.). Philadelphia: Saunders, pp. 996-997.

15. A nurse is planning care for a child with an infectious and communicable disease. The nurse determines that the primary goal is that the:
1 Child will experience only minor complications
2 Child will not spread the infection to others
3 Public health department will be notified
4 Child will experience mild discomfort

Answer: 2
Rationale: The primary goal is to prevent the spread of the disease to others. The child should experience no complications. Although the health department may need to be notified at some point, it is not the primary goal. It is also important to prevent discomfort as much as possible.

Test-Taking Strategy: Use the process of elimination. Note the key words "primary goal." Note the relationship between "infectious and communicable disease" in the question and "infection" in the correct option. Review goals of care for the child with an infectious and communicable disease if you had difficulty with this question.

Level of Cognitive Ability: Analysis
Client Needs: Health Promotion and Maintenance
Integrated Process: Nursing Process/Planning
Content Area: Child Health

Reference:
Wong, D., & Hockenberry, M. (2003). *Wong's nursing care of infants and children* (7th ed.). St. Louis: Mosby, pp. 650-651.

---

16. A nurse is preparing to care for an infant with pertussis. In planning care, the nurse addresses which critical problem?
1 Ineffective airway clearance
2 Excess fluid volume
3 Disturbed sleep pattern
4 Risk for infection

Answer: 1
Rationale: The most important problem relates to adequate air exchange. Because of the copious, thick secretions that occur with pertussis and the small airways of an infant, air exchange is critical. A deficient fluid volume is more likely to occur in this infant because of the thick secretions and vomiting. Sleep patterns may be disturbed because of the coughing, but it is not the critical issue. Infection is an important consideration, but airway is the priority.

Test-Taking Strategy: Use the process of elimination and the ABCs —airway, breathing, and circulation. Airway is always the most critical concern. This should direct you to option 1. Review care of the infant with pertussis if you had difficulty with this question.

Level of Cognitive Ability: Application
Client Needs: Physiological Integrity
Integrated Process: Nursing Process/Planning
Content Area: Child Health

Reference:
Wong, D., & Hockenberry, M. (2003). *Wong's nursing care of infants and children* (7th ed.). St. Louis: Mosby, pp. 656-657.

17. A nurse is planning care for an infant who has pyloric stenosis. In order to most effectively meet the infant's preoperative needs, the nurse includes which of the following in the plan of care?

1 Monitor the intravenous (IV) infusion, intake and output, and weight

2 Provide small frequent feedings of glucose, water, and electrolytes

3 Administer enemas until returns are clear

4 Provide the mother privacy to breast-feed every 2 hours

Answer: 1

Rationale: Preoperatively, important nursing responsibilities include monitoring the IV infusion, intake and output, weight, and obtaining urine specific gravity measurements. Additionally, weighing the infant's diapers provides information regarding output. Preoperatively, the infant is kept NPO unless the physician prescribes a thickened formula. Enemas until clear would further compromise the fluid volume status.

Test-Taking Strategy: Use the process of elimination, noting the key word "preoperative." Eliminate options 2 and 4 because the infant needs to be NPO in the preoperative period. Eliminate option 3 because enemas would further compromise the fluid balance status. Review preoperative care of the infant with pyloric stenosis if you had difficulty with this question.

Level of Cognitive Ability: Application
Client Needs: Physiological Integrity
Integrated Process: Nursing Process/Planning
Content Area: Child Health

References:

James, S., Ashwill, J., & Droske, S. (2002). *Nursing care of children: Principles & practice* (2nd ed.). Philadelphia: Saunders, p. 569.

Wong, D., & Hockenberry, M. (2003). *Wong's nursing care of infants and children* (7th ed.). St. Louis: Mosby, p. 1447.

18. A client who was a victim of a gunshot incident states, "I feel like I am losing my mind. I keep hearing the gunshots and seeing my friend lying on the ground." The nurse most appropriately plans strategies to formulate a therapeutic relationship that will include:

1 Asking the psychiatrist to order an antianxiety medication

2 Encouraging the client to talk about the incident and feelings related to it

3 Encouraging the client to think about how lucky he is to be alive

4 Teaching the client relaxation techniques

Answer: 2

Rationale: In developing a therapeutic relationship, it is important to acknowledge and validate the client's feelings. Although teaching the client relaxation techniques may be helpful at some point, it is not related to the issue of the question. Options 1 and 3 are nontherapeutic techniques and do not promote a therapeutic relationship.

Test-Taking Strategy: Use therapeutic communication techniques. Eliminate options 1 and 3 because they do not encourage further discussion about the client's feelings. Teaching the client how to relax may be helpful at some point, but not in the beginning of the therapeutic relationship. Remember to address the client's feelings. Review therapeutic communication techniques if you had difficulty with this question.

Level of Cognitive Ability: Application
Client Needs: Psychosocial Integrity
Integrated Process: Nursing Process/Planning
Content Area: Mental Health

Reference:

Keltner, N., Schwecke, L., & Bostrom, C. (2003). *Psychiatric nursing* (4th ed.). St. Louis: Mosby, p. 93.

19. A nurse is caring for a hospitalized child with a diagnosis of rheumatic fever who has developed carditis. The mother asks the nurse to explain the meaning of carditis. The nurse plans to respond, knowing that which of the following most appropriately describes this complication of rheumatic fever?

1 Tender painful joints, especially in the elbows, knees, ankles, and wrists
2 Inflammation of all parts of the heart, primarily the mitral valve
3 Involuntary movements affecting the legs, arms, and face
4 Red skin lesions that start as flat or slightly raised macules usually over the truck and spread peripherally

Answer: 2

Rationale: Carditis is the inflammation of all parts of the heart, primarily the mitral valve, and is a complication of rheumatic fever. Option 1 describes polyarthritis. Option 3 describes chorea. Option 4 describes erythema marginatum.

Test-Taking Strategy: Use the process of elimination. Note the relationship between the word "carditis" in the question and "heart" in the correct option. Review this content if you are unfamiliar with this complication that is associated with rheumatic fever.

Level of Cognitive Ability: Application
Client Needs: Physiological Integrity
Integrated Process: Nursing Process/Planning
Content Area: Child Health

Reference:
Wong, D., & Hockenberry, M. (2003). *Wong's nursing care of infants and children* (7th ed.). St. Louis: Mosby, p. 1511.

20. A nurse receives a telephone call from the emergency room and is told that a 7-month-old infant with febrile seizures will be admitted to the pediatric unit. In planning care for the admission of the infant, the nurse would anticipate the need for which of the following?

1 A padded tongue taped to the head of the bed
2 A code cart at the bedside
3 Restraints at the bedside
4 Suction equipment at the bedside

Answer: 4

Rationale: A padded tongue blade should never be used; in fact, nothing should be placed in the mouth during a seizure. During a seizure, the infant should be placed in a side-lying position, but should not be restrained. Suctioning may be required during a seizure to remove secretions that obstruct the airway. It is not necessary to place a code cart at the bedside, but a cart should be readily available on the nursing unit.

Test-Taking Strategy: Use the process of elimination and the ABCs—airway, breathing, and circulation—to answer the question. Option 4 is the only option that specifically relates to airway. Review nursing interventions for an infant with seizures if you had difficulty with this question.

Level of Cognitive Ability: Application
Client Needs: Physiological Integrity
Integrated Process: Nursing Process/Planning
Content Area: Child Health

Reference:
James, S., Ashwill, J., & Droske, S. (2002). *Nursing care of children: Principles & practice* (2nd ed.). Philadelphia: Saunders, p. 976.

21. A 10-month-old infant is hospitalized for respiratory syncytial virus (RSV). The nurse develops a plan of care for the infant. Based on the developmental stage of the infant, the nurse includes which of the following in the plan of care?
1 Wash hands, wear a mask when caring for the infant, and keep the infant as quiet as possible
2 Follow the home feeding schedule and only allow the infant to be held when the parents visit
3 Restrain the infant with a total body restraint to prevent any tubes from being dislodged
4 Provide a consistent routine, as well as touching, rocking, and cuddling throughout the hospitalization

Answer: 4

Rationale: A 10-month-old infant is in the Trust vs. Mistrust stage of psychosocial development (Erik Erikson) and in the sensorimotor period of cognitive development (Jean Piaget). RSV is not airborne (mask is not required) and is usually transmitted by the hands. Touching and holding the infant only when the parents visit will not provide adequate stimulation and interpersonal contact for the infant. Total body restraint is unnecessary and an incorrect action. Hospitalization may have an adverse effect. A consistent routine accompanied by touching, rocking, and cuddling will help the child develop trust and provide sensory stimulation.

Test-Taking Strategy: Note the age and diagnosis of the infant. Focusing on the key words "developmental stage of the infant" will direct you to option 4. Review the psychosocial needs of an infant if you had difficulty with this question.

Level of Cognitive Ability: Application
Client Needs: Physiological Integrity
Integrated Process: Nursing Process/Planning
Content Area: Child Health

Reference:
Wong, D., & Hockenberry, M. (2003). *Wong's nursing care of infants and children* (7th ed.). St. Louis: Mosby, pp. 501-502.

---

22. A pediatric nurse receives a telephone call from the admission office and is informed that a child with a diagnosis of Reye's syndrome is being admitted to the hospital. The nurse develops a plan of care for the child and includes which critical nursing action in the plan?
1 Provide a quiet environment with low dimmed lighting
2 Monitor for hearing loss
3 Monitor intake and output (I&O)
4 Reposition the child every 2 hours

Answer: 1

Rationale: Cerebral edema is a progressive part of the disease process in Reye's syndrome. A major component of care for a child with Reye's syndrome is to maintain effective cerebral perfusion and control intracranial pressure. Decreasing stimuli in the environment would decrease the stress on the cerebral tissue and neuron responses. Hearing loss does not occur in this disorder. Although monitoring I&O may be a component of the plan, it is not the critical nursing action. Changing the body position every 2 hours would not affect the cerebral edema and intracranial pressure directly. The child should be in a head-elevated position to decrease the progression of cerebral edema and promote drainage of cerebrospinal fluid.

Test-Taking Strategy: Note the key word "critical." Recalling that increased intracranial pressure is a concern will direct you to option 1. Review the plan of care for the child with Reye's syndrome if you had difficulty with this question.

Level of Cognitive Ability: Application
Client Needs: Physiological Integrity
Integrated Process: Nursing Process/Planning
Content Area: Child Health

Reference:
Wong, D., & Hockenberry, M. (2003). *Wong's nursing care of infants and children* (7th ed.). St. Louis: Mosby, pp. 1662; 1684.

23. A nursing student is preparing to conduct a clinical conference regarding cerebral palsy. Which characteristic related to this disorder will the student plan to include in the discussion?

1 Cerebral palsy is a chronic disability characterized by a difficulty in controlling muscles.
2 Cerebral palsy is an infectious disease of the central nervous system.
3 Cerebral palsy is an inflammation of the brain as a result of a viral illness.
4 Cerebral palsy is a congenital condition that results in moderate to severe retardation.

Answer: 1

Rationale: Cerebral palsy is a chronic disability characterized by a difficulty in controlling muscles because of an abnormality in the extrapyramidal or pyramidal motor system. Meningitis is an infectious process of the central nervous system. Encephalitis is an inflammation of the brain that occurs as a result of viral illness or central nervous system infections. Down syndrome is an example of a congenital condition that results in moderate to severe retardation.

Test-Taking Strategy: Use the process of elimination. Eliminate options 2 and 3 first, noting that they are similar and basically stating the same thing. From the remaining options, note the relationship between "palsy" in the question and "muscles" in the correct option. Review the characteristics associated with cerebral palsy if you had difficulty with this question.

Level of Cognitive Ability: Application
Client Needs: Physiological Integrity
Integrated Process: Nursing Process/Planning
Content Area: Child Health

References:
James, S., Ashwill, J., & Droske, S. (2002). *Nursing care of children: Principles & practice* (2nd ed.). Philadelphia: Saunders, p. 962.
Wong, D., & Hockenberry, M. (2003). *Wong's nursing care of infants and children* (7th ed.). St. Louis: Mosby, p. 1836.

24. A nursing student is asked to conduct a clinical conference regarding autism. The student plans to include in the discussion that the primary characteristic associated with autism is:

1 The consistent imitation of others actions
2 Normal social play
3 Lack of social interaction and awareness
4 Normal verbal but abnormal nonverbal communication

Answer: 3

Rationale: Autism is a severe developmental disorder that begins in infancy or toddlerhood. A primary characteristic is lack of social interaction and awareness. Social behaviors in autism include lack of or abnormal imitations of others' actions and the lack of or abnormal social play. Additional characteristics include lack of or impaired verbal communication and marked abnormal nonverbal communication.

Test-Taking Strategy: Use the process of elimination. Eliminate options 2 and 4 first because they address normal behaviors. From the remaining options, recalling that the autistic child lacks social interaction and awareness will direct you to option 3. Review the characteristics associated with autism if you had difficulty with this question.

Level of Cognitive Ability: Analysis
Client Needs: Psychosocial Integrity
Integrated Process: Nursing Process/Planning
Content Area: Child Health

Reference:
Wong, D., & Hockenberry, M. (2003). *Wong's nursing care of infants and children* (7th ed.). St. Louis: Mosby, pp. 1008-1009.

25. A charge nurse reviews the plan of care formulated by a new nursing graduate for a child returning from the operating room following a tonsillectomy. The charge nurse assists the new nursing graduate in changing the plan if which incorrect intervention is documented?

1 Offer clear, cool liquids when awake
2 Eliminate milk or milk products from the diet
3 Monitor for bleeding from the surgical site
4 Suction whenever necessary

Answer: 4

Rationale: Following tonsillectomy, suction equipment should be available, but suctioning is not performed unless there is an airway obstruction. Clear, cool liquids are encouraged. Milk and milk products are avoided initially because they coat the throat, causing the child to clear the throat, thus increasing the risk of bleeding. Option 3 is an important intervention following any type of surgery.

Test-Taking Strategy: Use the process of elimination, noting the key words "incorrect intervention." Eliminate option 3 first because this is an expected general nursing procedure. From the remaining options, thinking about the anatomical location of the surgery will direct you to option 4. Suctioning following tonsillectomy will disrupt the integrity of the surgical site and can cause bleeding. Review postoperative care following tonsillectomy if you had difficulty with this question.

Level of Cognitive Ability: Application
Client Needs: Physiological Integrity
Integrated Process: Nursing Process/Planning
Content Area: Leadership/Management

Reference:
Wong, D., & Hockenberry, M. (2003). *Wong's nursing care of infants and children* (7th ed.). St. Louis: Mosby, p. 1354.

---

26. A nurse is preparing a plan of care for a child being admitted to the hospital with a diagnosis of congestive heart failure (CHF). The nurse avoids including which of the following in the plan?

1 Limiting the time the child is allowed to bottle-feed
2 Elevating the head of the bed
3 Waking the child for feeding to ensure adequate nutrition
4 Providing oxygen during stressful periods

Answer: 3

Rationale: Measures that will decrease the workload on the heart include limiting the time the child is allowed to bottle-feed or breast-feed, elevating the head of the bed, allowing for uninterrupted rest periods, and providing oxygen during stressful periods.

Test-Taking Strategy: Note the key word "avoids" in the stem of the question. Review each option carefully, recalling that the goal for a child with CHF is to decrease the workload on the heart. Option 3 is the only option that will not ensure this goal. Review this content if you are unfamiliar with the measures associated with caring for the child with CHF.

Level of Cognitive Ability: Application
Client Needs: Physiological Integrity
Integrated Process: Nursing Process/Planning
Content Area: Child Health

Reference:
Wong, D., & Hockenberry, M. (2003). *Wong's nursing care of infants and children* (7th ed.). St. Louis: Mosby, p. 1485.

27. A nurse is preparing a plan of care for a child with leukemia who is scheduled to receive chemotherapy. Which intervention will the nurse include in the plan of care?
1 Monitor rectal temperatures every 4 hours
2 Monitor mouth and anus each shift for signs of breakdown
3 Provide meticulous mouth care several times daily using an alcohol-based mouthwash and a toothbrush
4 Encourage the child to consume fresh fruits and vegetables to maintain nutritional status

Answer: 2

Rationale: When the child is receiving chemotherapy, the nurse should avoid taking rectal temperatures. Oral temperatures are also avoided if mouth ulcers are present. Axillary temperatures should be taken to prevent alterations in skin integrity. Meticulous mouth care should be performed, but the nurse should avoid alcohol-based mouthwash and should use a soft-bristled toothbrush. The nurse should assess the mouth and anus each shift for ulcers, erythema, or breakdown. Bland, nonirritating foods and liquids should be provided to the child. Fresh fruits and vegetables need to be avoided because they can harbor organisms. Chemotherapy can cause neutropenia, and the child should be maintained on a low-bacteria diet if the white blood cell count is low.

Test-Taking Strategy: Use the process of elimination, reading each option carefully. Thinking about the side effects that can occur with chemotherapy will direct you to option 2. Review these important nursing measures if you had difficulty with this question.

Level of Cognitive Ability: Application
Client Needs: Physiological Integrity
Integrated Process: Nursing Process/Planning
Content Area: Child Health

Reference:
James, S., Ashwill, J., & Droske, S. (2002). *Nursing care of children: Principles & practice* (2nd ed.). Philadelphia: Saunders, p. 783.

---

28. A nurse is assisting in preparing to admit a client from the post-anesthesia care unit who has had microvascular decompression of the trigeminal nerve. The nurse asks the nursing assistant to make sure that which of the following equipment is at the bedside when the client arrives?
1 Flashlight and pulse oximeter
2 Cardiac monitor and suction equipment
3 Padded bedrails and suction equipment
4 Blood pressure cuff and cardiac monitor

Answer: 1

Rationale: The postoperative care of the client having microvascular decompression of the trigeminal nerve is the same as for the client undergoing craniotomy. This client requires hourly neurological assessment, as well as monitoring of cardiovascular and respiratory status. Cardiac monitoring and padded bedrails are not indicated unless there is a special need based on a client history of cardiac disease or seizures, respectively. Suctioning is done cautiously and only when necessary after craniotomy, to avoid increasing the intracranial pressure.

Test-Taking Strategy: Use the process of elimination, focusing on the data in the question. The client is not necessarily at risk for seizures postoperatively, so option 3 is eliminated first. Next eliminate options 2 and 4 because no data in the question indicates the client had a history of a cardiac problem. Also, knowing that the procedure is done by craniotomy enables you to recall that suctioning is done cautiously and only when necessary and that neurological assessment is needed and a flashlight would be required to perform a neurological assessment. Review care of the client following this procedure if you had difficulty with this question.

Level of Cognitive Ability: Application
Client Needs: Physiological Integrity

Integrated Process: Nursing Process/Planning
Content Area: Adult Health/Neurological

References:
Lewis, S., Heitkemper, M., & Dirksen, S. (2004). *Medical-surgical nursing: Assessment and management of clinical problems* (6th ed.). St. Louis: Mosby, p. 1603.
Phipps, W., Monahan, F., Sands, J., Marek, J., & Neighbors, M. (2003). *Medical-surgical nursing: Health and illness perspectives* (7th ed.). St. Louis: Mosby, p. 1347.

---

29. A nurse is receiving a client in transfer from the emergency room who has a diagnosis of Guillain-Barré syndrome. The client's chief complaint is an ascending paralysis that has reached the level of the waist. The nurse plans to have which item available for emergency use?
  1 Cardiac monitor and intubation tray
  2 Blood pressure cuff and flashlight
  3 Nebulizer and pulse oximeter
  4 Flashlight and incentive spirometer

Answer: 1
Rationale: The client with Guillain-Barré syndrome is at risk for respiratory failure because of ascending paralysis. An intubation tray should be available for emergency use. Another complication of this syndrome is cardiac dysrhythmias, which necessitates the need for cardiac monitoring. Although some of the items in options 2, 3, and 4 may be kept at the bedside (e.g., blood pressure cuff, flashlight, pulse oximeter), they are not necessarily needed for emergency use in this situation.

Test-Taking Strategy: Use the process of elimination. Note the key words "emergency use." This tells you that the correct answer will be an option that contains equipment that is not routinely used in providing care. With this in mind, eliminate options 2 and 4 first, because a flashlight is needed for routine neurological assessment. From the remaining options, recalling the complications of this syndrome will direct you to option 1. Review nursing care measures for the client with Guillain-Barré syndrome if you had difficulty with this question.

Level of Cognitive Ability: Application
Client Needs: Physiological Integrity
Integrated Process: Nursing Process/Planning
Content Area: Adult Health/Neurological

Reference:
Phipps, W., Monahan, F., Sands, J., Marek, J., & Neighbors, M. (2003). *Medical-surgical nursing: Health and illness perspectives* (7th ed.). St. Louis: Mosby, p. 1402.

---

30. A nurse in the newborn nursery receives a telephone call and is informed that a newborn infant whose mother is Rh negative will be admitted to the nursery. In planning care for the infant's arrival, the nurse takes which important action?
  1 Obtains the necessary equipment from the blood bank needed for an exchange transfusion
  2 Calls the maintenance department and asks for a phototherapy unit to be brought to the nursery
  3 Obtains the newborn infant's blood type and direct Coombs' results from the laboratory
  4 Obtains a vial of vitamin K from the pharmacy and prepares to administer an injection to prevent isoimmunization

Answer: 3
Rationale: To further plan for the newborn infant's care, the infant's blood type and direct Coombs' must be known. Umbilical cord blood is taken at the time of delivery to determine blood type, Rh factor, and antibody titer (direct Coombs' test) of the newborn infant. The nurse should obtain these results from the laboratory. Options 1 and 2 are inappropriate at this time, and additional data is needed to determine if these actions are needed. Option 4 is incorrect because vitamin K is given to prevent hemorrhagic disease of the newborn infant.

Test-Taking Strategy: Use the process of elimination and focus on the issue: that the mother is RH negative. Note the relationship between the issue of the question and option 3. Also, note that option 3 is the only option that addresses assessment. Review Rh incompatibilities if you had difficulty with this question.

Level of Cognitive Ability: Application
Client Needs: Physiological Integrity
Integrated Process: Nursing Process/Planning
Content Area: Maternity/Postpartum

Reference:
Murray, S., McKinney, E., & Gorrie, T. (2002). *Foundations of maternal-newborn nursing* (3rd ed.). Philadelphia: Saunders, p. 696.

---

31. A nurse is planning to instruct a client with chronic vertigo about safety measures to prevent exacerbation of symptoms or injury. The nurse plans to teach the client that it is important to:
1 Drive at times when the client does not feel dizzy
2 Go to the bedroom and lie down when vertigo is experienced
3 Remove throw rugs and clutter in the home
4 Turn the head slowly when spoken to

Answer: 3
Rationale: The client with chronic vertigo should avoid driving and using public transportation. The sudden movements involved in each could precipitate an attack. To further prevent vertigo attacks, the client should change positions slowly and should turn the entire body, not just the head, when spoken to. If vertigo does occur, the client should immediately sit down or grasp the nearest piece of furniture. The client should maintain the home in a state that is free of clutter and has throw rugs removed, because the effort of trying to regain balance after slipping could trigger the onset of vertigo.

Test-Taking Strategy: Use the process of elimination and focus on the issue: safety. Begin to answer this question by eliminating options 1 and 2 first, because they put the client at greatest risk of injury secondary to vertigo. Choose option 3 over option 4 because it is the safer intervention of the remaining options. Review safety measures for the client with vertigo if you had difficulty with this question.

Level of Cognitive Ability: Application
Client Needs: Health Promotion and Maintenance
Integrated Process: Nursing Process/Planning
Content Area: Adult Health/Ear

Reference:
Black, J., & Hawks, J. (2005). *Medical-surgical nursing: Clinical management for positive outcomes* (7th ed.). Philadelphia: Saunders, p. 1991.

---

32. A male client being discharged from the mental health unit who initially denied that he drank "2 six-packs of beer a day" is now willing to admit that he has a problem drinking. The client states he will "get some help" in order to live a healthier lifestyle. The nurse plans for a meeting with a representative of which of the following groups to meet with the client before discharge?
1 Al-Anon
2 Alcoholics Anonymous
3 Families Anonymous
4 Fresh Start

Answer: 2
Rationale: Alcoholics Anonymous is a major self-help organization for the treatment of alcoholism. Option 1 is a group for families of alcoholics. Option 3 is for parents of children who abuse substances. Option 4 is for nicotine addicts.

Test-Taking Strategy: Use the process of elimination. Note the relationship between "drinking" in the question and "Alcoholics" in the correct option. Review the purpose of specific support groups if you had difficulty with this question.

Level of Cognitive Ability: Application
Client Needs: Health Promotion and Maintenance
Integrated Process: Nursing Process/Planning
Content Area: Mental Health

Reference:
Keltner, N., Schwecke, L., & Bostrom, C. (2003). *Psychiatric nursing* (4th ed.). St. Louis: Mosby, pp. 485; 496.

---

33. A client with a cerebral vascular accident (CVA) is prepared for discharge from the hospital. The physician has prescribed range-of-motion (ROM) exercises for the client's right side. In planning for the client's care, the home care nurse:

1 Considers the use of active, passive, or active-assisted exercises in the home
2 Implements ROM exercises to the point of pain for the client
3 Encourages the client to be dependent on the home care nurse to complete the exercise program
4 Develops a schedule of ROM exercises every 2 hours while awake even if the client is fatigued

Answer: 1

Rationale: The home care nurse must consider all forms of ROM for the client. Even if the client has right hemiplegia, the client can assist in some of his or her own rehabilitative care. In addition, the goal in home care nursing is for the client to assume as much self-care and independence as possible. The nurse needs to teach so that the client becomes self-reliant. Options 2 and 4 are incorrect from a physiological standpoint.

Test-Taking Strategy: Use the process of elimination. Options 2 and 4 can be eliminated first because these actions can be harmful to the client. From the remaining options, recall that dependency is not in the best interest of a client's sense of health promotion, which eliminates option 3. Also, note that option 1 is the umbrella (global) option. Review basic knowledge related to ROM exercises if you had difficulty with this question.

Level of Cognitive Ability: Application
Client Needs: Health Promotion and Maintenance
Integrated Process: Nursing Process/Planning
Content Area: Adult Health/Neurological

Reference:
Ignatavicius, D., & Workman, M. (2002). *Medical surgical nursing: Critical thinking for collaborative care* (4th ed.). Philadelphia: Saunders, p. 127.

Nursing Process: Implementation

---

1. A client in late active first stage labor has just reported a gush of vaginal fluid. The nurse observes a fetal monitor pattern of variable decelerations during contractions followed by a brief acceleration. Then, there is a return to baseline until the next contraction, when the pattern is repeated. Based on this data, the nurse prepares to initially:

1 Take the client's vital signs
2 Perform a manual sterile vaginal exam
3 Perform a Leopold's maneuver
4 Test the vaginal fluid with a nitrazine strip

Answer: 2

Rationale: Variable deceleration with brief acceleration after a gush of amniotic fluid is a common clinical manifestation of cord compression caused by occult or frank prolapse of the umbilical cord. A manual vaginal exam can detect the presence of the cord in the vagina, confirming the problem. Based on the data in the question, options 1, 3, and 4 are not initial actions.

Test-Taking Strategy: Use the process of elimination and note the word "initially." Focusing on the data in the question and determining the significance of the data will direct you to option 2. Review the signs of cord compression if you had difficulty with this question.

Level of Cognitive Ability: Application
Client Needs: Physiological Integrity
Integrated Process: Nursing Process/Implementation
Content Area: Maternity/Intrapartum

Reference:
Lowdermilk, D., & Perry, A. (2004). *Maternity & women's health care* (8th ed.). St. Louis: Mosby, p. 1030.

---

2. A nurse is preparing to administer a feeding to a client receiving enteral nutrition through a nasogastric tube. The nurse takes which most important action before administering the feeding?
   1 Measuring intake and output
   2 Weighing the client
   3 Adding blue food coloring to the formula
   4 Determining tube placement

Answer: 4

Rationale: Initiating a tube feeding before determining tube placement can lead to serious complications such as aspiration. Options 1 and 2 are part of the total plan of care for a client on enteral feedings. Option 3 is instituted for a client who has been identified as a high risk for aspiration. Option 4 is the priority nursing action.

Test-Taking Strategy: Note the key words "most important." Use the ABCs—airway, breathing, and circulation—and the nursing process to answer the question. Option 4 relates to assessment and to the risk of aspiration. Review nursing interventions when initiating a tube feeding if you had difficulty with this question.

Level of Cognitive Ability: Application
Client Needs: Physiological Integrity
Integrated Process: Nursing Process/Implementation
Content Area: Fundamental Skills

Reference:
Lewis, S., Heitkemper, M., & Dirksen, S. (2004). *Medical-surgical nursing: Assessment and management of clinical problems* (6th ed.). St. Louis: Mosby, pp. 982; 984.

---

3. A nurse teaches a client with a rib fracture to cough and deep breathe. The client resists directions by the nurse because of the pain. The nurse most appropriately:
   1 Continues to give the client gentle encouragement to do so
   2 Requests that the physician perform a nerve block to deaden the pain
   3 Explains in detail the potential complications from lack of coughing and deep breathing
   4 Premedicates the client and assists the client to splint the area during these exercises

Answer: 4

Rationale: Shallow respirations that occur with rib fracture predispose the client to developing atelectasis and pneumonia. It is essential that the client perform coughing and deep breathing exercises to prevent these complications. The nurse accomplishes this most effectively by premedicating the client with pain medication and assisting the client with splinting during the exercises. Options 2 and 3 are inappropriate. Option 2 is an extreme measure, and the nurse would not explain in detail potential complications as identified in option 3. Because the client is resisting directions, "gentle encouragement" may not be adequate.

Test-Taking Strategy: Use the process of elimination, noting the key words "most appropriately." Options 2 and 3 are likely to be the most extreme or unrealistic options, respectively, and should be eliminated first. From the remaining options, premedication and assistance are more likely to be effective than continued gentle encouragement. Review care of the client with rib fracture if you had difficulty with this question.

Level of Cognitive Ability: Application
Client Needs: Physiological Integrity
Integrated Process: Nursing Process/Implementation
Content Area: Adult Health/Respiratory

Reference:
Lewis, S., Heitkemper, M., & Dirksen, S. (2004). *Medical-surgical nursing: Assessment and management of clinical problems* (6th ed.). St. Louis: Mosby, p. 621.

4. A nurse is caring for a 14-year-old child who is hospitalized and placed in Crutchfield traction. The child is having difficulty adjusting to the length of the hospital confinement. Which nursing action would be most appropriate to meet the child's needs?
1 Allow the child to have his or her hair dyed if the parent agrees
2 Allow the child to play loud music in the hospital room
3 Let the child wear his or her own clothing when friends visit
4 Allow the child to keep the shades closed and the room darkened at all times

Answer: 3

Rationale: An adolescent needs to identify with peers and has a strong need to belong to a group. The child should be allowed to wear his or her own clothes to feel a sense of belonging to the group. The adolescent likes to dress like the group and wear similar hairstyles. Because Crutchfield traction uses skeletal pins, hair dye is not appropriate. Loud music may disturb others in the hospital. The child's request for a darkened room is indicative of a possible problem with depression that may need further evaluation and intervention.

Test-Taking Strategy: Use the process of elimination and focus on the issues: Crutchfield traction and a 14-year-old child. Knowledge regarding Crutchfield traction and its limitations, and knowledge of growth and development concepts, will direct you to option 3. Review growth and development and care of the child in traction if you had difficulty with this question.

Level of Cognitive Ability: Application
Client Needs: Psychosocial integrity
Integrated Process: Nursing Process/Implementation
Content Area: Child Health

Reference:
Potter, P., & Perry, A. (2005). *Fundamentals of nursing* (6th ed.). St. Louis: Mosby, pp. 208-209.

5. A nurse receives a telephone call from the emergency room and is told that a client in leg traction will be admitted to the nursing unit. The nurse prepares for the arrival of the client and asks the nursing assistant to obtain which item that will be essential for helping the client move in bed while in the leg traction?
1 An electric bed
2 A bed trapeze
3 Extra pillows
4 A foot board

Answer: 2

Rationale: A trapeze is essential to allow the client to lift straight up while being moved so the amount of pull exerted on the limb in traction is not altered. Either an electric bed or manual bed can be used for traction, but this does not specifically assist the client to move in bed. A foot board and extra pillows do not facilitate moving.

Test-Taking Strategy: Note the key words "essential" and "move in bed." Attempt to visualize the items in the options, focusing on the issue: helping the client move in bed. Using the process of elimination will direct you to option 2. Review care of the client in traction if you had difficulty with this question.

Level of Cognitive Ability: Application
Client Needs: Physiological Integrity
Integrated Process: Nursing Process/Implementation
Content Area: Leadership/Management

Reference:
Potter, P., & Perry, A. (2005). *Fundamentals of nursing* (6th ed.). St. Louis: Mosby, pp. 1455-1456.

6. A pregnant client is receiving rehabilitative services for alcohol abuse. The nurse would provide supportive care by:

1 Encouraging the client to participate in care and identifying supportive strategies that are helpful

2 Avoiding discussion of the alcohol problem and recovery with the client

3 Minimizing communication with supportive family members

4 Encouraging the client to stop counseling once the infant is born

Answer: 1

Rationale: The nurse provides supportive care by encouraging the client to participate in care. The nurse should not avoid discussing the client's problem with the client, and communication with family members is important. Counseling needs to continue after the infant is born.

Test-Taking Strategy: Use the process of elimination, noting the key words "supportive care." Option 1 provides the client with an active role in care. Options 2, 3, and 4 create barriers for long-term success in dealing with the problem. Review measures that provide supportive nursing care for the pregnant client who abuses alcohol if you had difficulty with this question.

Level of Cognitive Ability: Application
Clients Needs: Health Promotion and Maintenance
Integrated Process: Nursing Process/Implementation
Content Area: Maternity/Antepartum

Reference:
Lowdermilk, D., & Perry, A. (2004). *Maternity & women's health care* (8th ed.). St. Louis: Mosby, p. 969.

---

7. A client in the second trimester of pregnancy is being assessed at the health care clinic. The nurse performing the assessment notes that the fetal heart rate is 100 beats per minute. Which nursing action would be most appropriate?

1 Document the findings

2 Inform the mother that the assessment is normal and everything is fine

3 Notify the physician

4 Instruct the mother to return to the clinic in 1 week for reevaluation of the fetal heart rate

Answer: 3

Rationale: The fetal heart rate should be between 120 to 160 beats per minute during pregnancy. A fetal heart rate of 100 beats per minute would require that the physician be notified and the client be further evaluated. Although the nurse would document the findings, the most appropriate nursing action is to notify the physician. Options 2 and 4 are inaccurate nursing actions.

Test-Taking Strategy: Use the process of elimination. Options 2 and 4 are similar, inaccurate, and can be eliminated first. From the remaining options, focus on the words "most appropriate." Knowing that the range for the fetal heart rate is between 120 and 160 beats per minute will direct you to option 3. Review the normal findings in the pregnant client if you had difficulty with this question.

Level of Cognitive Ability: Application
Client Needs: Physiological Integrity
Integrated Process: Nursing Process/Implementation
Content Area: Maternity/Antepartum

Reference:
Murray, S., McKinney, E., & Gorrie, T. (2002). *Foundations of maternal-newborn nursing* (3rd ed.). Philadelphia: Saunders, pp. 338; 978.

8. A client is admitted to the hospital with a diagnosis of a leaking cerebral aneurysm and is scheduled for surgery. The nurse implements which of the following during the preoperative period?
  1 Encourages the client to be up at least twice per day
  2 Allows the client to ambulate to the bathroom
  3 Obtains a bedside commode for the client's use
  4 Places the client on strict bed rest

Answer: 4
Rationale: The client's activity is kept to a minimum to prevent Valsalva maneuver. Clients often hold their breath and strain while pulling up to get out of bed. This exertion may cause a rise in blood pressure, which increases bleeding. Clients who have bleeding aneurysms in any vessel will have activity curtailed. Therefore, options 1, 2, and 3 are incorrect actions.

Test-Taking Strategy: Use the process of elimination, focusing on the client's diagnosis and the key words "preoperative period." Eliminate options 1, 2, and 3 because they are similar in that they all involve out-of-bed activity. Review aneurysm precautions if you had difficulty with this question.

Level of Cognitive Ability: Application
Client Needs: Physiological Integrity
Integrated Process: Nursing Process/Implementation
Content Area: Adult Health/Neurological

Reference:
Phipps, W., Monahan, F., Sands, J., Marek, J., & Neighbors, M. (2003). *Medical-surgical nursing: Health and illness perspectives* (7th ed.). St. Louis: Mosby, p. 1385.

9. A physician calls a nurse to obtain the daily laboratory results of a client receiving total parenteral nutrition (TPN). Which laboratory result would the nurse obtain from the client's record because it would provide the most valuable information regarding the client's status related to the TPN?
  1 Serum electrolyte levels
  2 Arterial blood gas (ABG) levels
  3 White blood cell count (WBC)
  4 Complete blood cell count (CBC)

Answer: 1
Rationale: TPN solutions contain amino acid and dextrose solutions, with electrolyte and trace elements added. The physician uses the electrolyte values to determine whether changes are needed in the composition of the TPN solutions that will be administered over the next 24 hours. This prevents the client from developing electrolyte imbalance. Options 2, 3, and 4 are not directly related to evaluating client status regarding TPN.

Test-Taking Strategy: Use the process of elimination. Eliminate options 3 and 4 first because a CBC includes a WBC count. From the remaining options, focusing on the issue and considering the composition of TPN solutions will direct you to option 1. Review the composition of TPN if you had difficulty with this question.

Level of Cognitive Ability: Application
Client Needs: Physiological Integrity
Integrated Process: Nursing Process/Implementation
Content Area: Fundamental Skills

Reference:
Black, J., & Hawks, J. (2005). *Medical-surgical nursing: Clinical management for positive outcomes* (7th ed.). Philadelphia: Saunders, p. 706.

10. A client who has episodes of bronchospasm and a history of tachydysrhythmias is admitted to the hospital. The nurse reviews the physician's orders and contacts the physician to verify which medication, if prescribed by the physician?
1   Metaproterenol (Alupent)
2   Albuterol (Proventil)
3   Epinephrine (Primatene Mist)
4   Salmeterol (Serevent)

Answer: 3
Rationale: A client with a history of tachydysrhythmias should not be given bronchodilators that contain catecholamines, such as epinephrine and isoproterenol hydrochloride (Isuprel). Other sympathomimetics that are noncatecholamines should be used instead. These include metaproterenol, albuterol, and salmeterol.

Test-Taking Strategy: Focus on the client's diagnosis, tachydysrhythmias, and use the process of elimination. Recalling that epinephrine is a catecholamine will direct you to option 3. Review the effects of epinephrine if you had difficulty with this question.

Level of Cognitive Ability: Analysis
Client Needs: Safe, Effective Care Environment
Integrated Process: Nursing Process/Implementation
Content Area: Pharmacology

Reference:
Hodgson, B., & Kizior, R. (2004). *Saunders nursing drug handbook 2004.* Philadelphia: Saunders, pp. 358-359.

11. A client has a compulsive bed-making ritual in which the client makes and remakes a bed numerous times. The client often misses breakfast and some of the morning activities because of the ritual. Which nursing action would be most helpful?
1   Verbalize tactful, mild disapproval of the behavior
2   Help the client to make the bed so that the task can be finished quicker
3   Discuss the ridiculousness of the behavior
4   Offer reflective feedback, such as "I see you have made your bed several times."

Answer: 4
Rationale: Verbalizing minimal disapproval would increase the client's anxiety and reinforce the need to perform the ritual. Helping with the ritual is nontherapeutic and also reinforces the behavior. The client is usually aware of the irrationality (ridiculousness) of the behavior. Reflective feedback acknowledges the client's behavior.

Test-Taking Strategy: Use the process of elimination. Recalling that the purpose of the ritual is to relieve anxiety would assist to eliminate options 1 and 3 because these actions would increase the client's anxiety. Eliminate option 2 because there is no therapeutic value in participating in the ritual. Review the appropriate interventions for the client with compulsive behavior if you had difficulty with this question.

Level of Cognitive Ability: Application
Client Needs: Psychosocial Integrity
Integrated Process: Nursing Process/Implementation
Content Area: Mental Health

Reference:
Varcarolis, E.M. (2002). *Foundations of psychiatric mental health nursing* (4th ed.). Philadelphia: Saunders, p. 313.

12. An older client who has undergone internal fixation after fracturing a left hip has developed a reddened left heel. The nurse obtains which of the following as a priority item to manage this problem?
  1 Bed cradle
  2 Sheepskin
  3 Trapeze
  4 Draw sheet

Answer: 2
Rationale: The reddened heel results from pressure of the foot against the mattress. The nurse obtains a sheepskin, heel protectors, or an alternating pressure mattress. The bed cradle will keep the linens off the client's lower extremities but not assist in managing a reddened heel. A draw sheet and trapeze are of general use for this client but are not specific in dealing with the reddened heel.

Test-Taking Strategy: Note the issue of the question: a reddened left heel. Eliminate option 1 first as an unnecessary and nonhelpful measure. Eliminate options 3 and 4 next, because although they are generally helpful in aiding the client's mobility, they are not related to the issue of the question. Option 2 addresses the problem stated in the question. Review measures that prevent skin breakdown in the immobile client if you had difficulty with this question.

Level of Cognitive Ability: Application
Client Needs: Physiological Integrity
Integrated Process: Nursing Process/Implementation
Content Area: Adult Health/Musculoskeletal

References:
Black, J., & Hawks, J. (2005). *Medical-surgical nursing: Clinical management for positive outcomes* (7th ed.). Philadelphia: Saunders, pp. 1406; 1410-1411.
Ignatavicius, D., & Workman, M. (2002). *Medical surgical nursing: Critical thinking for collaborative care* (4th ed.). Philadelphia: Saunders, p. 1583.

13. A nurse is caring for an infant following pyloromyotomy performed to treat hypertropic pyloric stenosis. The nurse places the infant in which position following surgery?
  1 Flat on the unoperative side
  2 Flat on the operative side
  3 Prone with the head of the bed elevated
  4 Supine with the head of the bed elevated

Answer: 3
Rationale: Following pyloromyotomy, the head of the bed is elevated and the infant is placed prone to reduce the risk of aspiration. Options 1, 2, and 4 are incorrect positions following this type of surgery.

Test-Taking Strategy: Consider the anatomical location of the surgical procedure and the risks associated with the procedure to answer the question. Visualize each of the positions identified in the options. Keeping in mind that aspiration is a major concern will direct you to option 3. Review nursing care measures following pyloromyotomy if you had difficulty with this question.

Level of Cognitive Ability: Application
Client Needs: Physiological Integrity
Integrated Process: Nursing Process/Implementation
Content Area: Child Health

Reference:
James, S., Ashwill, J., & Droske, S. (2002). *Nursing care of children: Principles & practice* (2nd ed.). Philadelphia: Saunders, p. 569.

14. A mother of a child with mumps calls the health care clinic to tell the nurse that the child has been lethargic and vomiting. The nurse most appropriately tells the mother:
1 To continue to monitor the child
2 That lethargy and vomiting are normal manifestations of mumps
3 To bring the child to the clinic to be seen by the physician
4 That as long as there is no fever, there is nothing to be concerned about

Answer: 3
Rationale: Mumps generally affect the salivary glands but can also affect multiple organs. The most common complication is septic meningitis, with the virus being identified in the cerebrospinal fluid. Common signs include nuchal rigidity, lethargy, and vomiting. The child should be seen by the physician.

Test-Taking Strategy: Focus on the signs and symptoms presented in the question. Recalling that meningitis is a complication of mumps will direct you to option 3. Review the complications of mumps and the associated clinical manifestations if you had difficulty with this question.

Level of Cognitive Ability: Application
Client Needs: Physiological Integrity
Integrated Process: Nursing Process/Implementation
Content Area: Child Health

Reference:
Wong, D., & Hockenberry, M. (2003). *Wong's nursing care of infants and children* (7th ed.). St. Louis: Mosby, pp. 541; 657.

15. A nurse is reviewing the physician's orders for a child admitted to the hospital with vaso-occlusive pain crisis from sickle cell anemia. Which of the following physician orders would the nurse question?
1 Intravenous fluids
2 Supplemental oxygen
3 Bed rest
4 Meperidine hydrochloride (Demerol) for pain

Answer: 4
Rationale: Meperidine hydrochloride is contraindicated for ongoing pain management because of the increased risk of seizures associated with the use of the medication. Management for severe pain generally includes the use of strong narcotic analgesics such as morphine sulfate or hydromorphone (Dilaudid). These medications are usually most effective when given as a continuous infusion or at regular intervals around the clock. Options 1, 2, and 3 are appropriate prescriptions for treating vaso-occlusive pain crisis.

Test-Taking Strategy: Use the process of elimination. Note the key words "orders would the nurse question." Recalling that oxygen, fluids, and bed rest are components of care will direct you to option 4. Also remember that meperidine hydrochloride is associated with an increased risk of seizures. Review care of a child with sickle cell anemia if you had difficulty with this question

Level of Cognitive Ability: Application
Client Needs: Safe, Effective Care Environment
Integrated Process: Nursing Process/Implementation
Content Area: Child Health

Reference:
Wong, D., & Hockenberry, M. (2003). *Wong's nursing care of infants and children* (7th ed.). St. Louis: Mosby, pp. 1550; 1552.

16. A nurse is caring for an infant with laryngomalacia (congenital laryngeal stridor). Which position would the nurse place the infant in to decrease the incidence of stridor?
  1 Supine
  2 Supine with the neck flexed
  3 Prone
  4 Prone with the neck hyperextended

Answer: 4
Rationale: The prone position with the neck hyperextended improves the child's breathing. Options 1, 2, and 3 are not appropriate positions.

Test-Taking Strategy: Use the process of elimination, noting the key words "decrease the incidence of stridor." Visualize each of the positions identified in the options to assist in directing you to option 4. Review this content if you had difficulty with this question.

Level of Cognitive Ability: Application
Client Needs: Physiological Integrity
Integrated Process: Nursing Process/Implementation
Content Area: Child Health

Reference:
James, S., Ashwill, J., & Droske, S. (2002). *Nursing care of children: Principles & practice* (2nd ed.). Philadelphia: Saunders, p. 638.

---

17. A nurse in the newborn nursery prepares to admit a newborn infant with spina bifida, meningomyelocele type. Which nursing action is most important in the care for this infant?
  1 Monitoring blood pressure
  2 Monitoring specific gravity of the urine
  3 Inspecting the anterior fontanel for bulging
  4 Monitoring temperature

Answer: 3
Rationale: Intracranial pressure is a complication associated with spina bifida. A sign of intracranial pressure in the newborn infant with spina bifida is a bulging anterior fontanel. The newborn infant is at risk for infection before the surgical procedure and closure of the gibbus, and monitoring the temperature is an important intervention; however, assessing the anterior fontanel for bulging is most important. A normal saline dressing is placed over the affected site to maintain moisture of the gibbus and its contents. This prevents tearing or breakdown of skin integrity at the site. Blood pressure is difficult to assess during the newborn period, and it is not the best indicator of infection or a potential complication. Urine concentration is not well developed in the newborn stage of development.

Test-Taking Strategy: Use the process of elimination, focusing on the key words "most important." Eliminate options 1 and 2 first because blood pressure and specific gravity are common assessments, but are not as reliable an indicator of changes in the newborn status as they would be for an older child. From the remaining options, focusing on the key words will direct you to option 3. Review care of the infant with spina bifida if you had difficulty with this question.

Level of Cognitive Ability: Application
Client Needs: Physiological Integrity
Integrated Process: Nursing Process/Implementation
Content Area: Maternity/Postpartum

Reference:
Wong, D., & Hockenberry, M. (2003). *Wong's nursing care of infants and children* (7th ed.). St. Louis: Mosby, pp. 425; 435; 437.

18. On assessment of a child, a nurse notes that the child's genitals are swollen. The nurse suspects that the child is being sexually abused. Which action by the nurse is of primary importance?

1 Document the child's physical findings

2 Report the case in which the abuse is suspected

3 Refer the family to appropriate support groups

4 Assist the family in identifying resources and support systems

Answer: 2

Rationale: The primary legal responsibility of the nurse when child abuse is suspected is to report the case. All 50 states require health care professionals to report all cases of suspected abuse. Although documentation of assessment findings, assisting the family, and referring the family to appropriate resources and support groups is important, the primary legal responsibility is to report the case.

Test-Taking Strategy: Use the process of elimination. In addition to the many implications associated with child abuse, recall that abuse is a crime. Keeping this in mind will direct you to option 2. Review the responsibilities of the nurse when child abuse is suspected if you had difficulty with this question.

Level of Cognitive Ability: Application
Client Needs: Psychosocial Integrity
Integrated Process: Nursing Process/Implementation
Content Area: Child Health

Reference:
Wong, D., & Hockenberry, M. (2003). *Wong's nursing care of infants and children* (7th ed.). St. Louis: Mosby, pp. 690; 692.

---

19. A nurse is planning care for an infant with a diagnosis of encephalocele located in the occipital area. Which item would the nurse use to assist in positioning the child to avoid pressure on the encephalocele?

1 Sheep skin

2 Foam half donut

3 Feather pillows

4 Sand bags

Answer: 2

Rationale: The infant is positioned to avoid pressure on the lesion. If the encephalocele is in the occipital area, a foam half donut may be useful in positioning to prevent this pressure. A sheepskin, feather pillow, or sandbag will not protect the encephalocele from pressure.

Test-Taking Strategy: Note the key word "occipital" and use the process of elimination. Note the similarities in options 1, 3, and 4 in that they would require the head to remain flat and therefore would not protect the lesion. Review nursing care associated with a child with an encephalocele if you have difficulty with this question.

Level of Cognitive Ability: Application
Client Needs: Physiological Integrity
Integrated Process: Nursing Process/Implementation
Content Area: Child Health

Reference:
Wong, D., & Hockenberry, M. (2003). *Wong's nursing care of infants and children* (7th ed.). St. Louis: Mosby, pp. 424; 434.

20. A nurse is caring for a child with a head injury. On review of the record, the nurse notes that the physician has documented decorticate posturing. On assessment of the child, the nurse notes extension of the upper extremities and internal rotation of the upper arm and wrist. The nurse also notes that the lower extremities are extended, with some internal rotation noted at the knees and feet. Based on these findings, which of the following is the appropriate nursing action?
1 Document the findings
2 Continue to monitor for posturing of the child
3 Attempt to flex the child's lower extremities
4 Notify the physician

Answer: 4
Rationale: Decorticate posturing refers to flexion of the upper extremities and extension of the lower extremities. Plantar flexion of the feet may also be observed. Decerebrate posturing involves extension of the upper extremities with internal rotation of the upper arm and wrist. The lower extremities will extend with some internal rotation noted at the knees and feet. The progression from decorticate to decerebrate posturing usually indicates deteriorating neurological function and warrants physician notification.

Test-Taking Strategy: Focus on the data in the question and use knowledge regarding the assessment findings associated with decerebrate and decorticate positioning. Recalling that progression from decorticate to decerebrate posturing usually indicates deteriorating neurological function will direct you to option 4. Review this content if you had difficulty with this question or are unfamiliar with these assessment findings.

Level of Cognitive Ability: Application
Client Needs: Physiological Integrity
Integrated Process: Nursing Process/Implementation
Content Area: Child Health

Reference:
Wong, D., & Hockenberry, M. (2003). *Wong's nursing care of infants and children* (7th ed.). St. Louis: Mosby, pp. 1651; 1669-1670.

---

21. A child with a diagnosis of hepatitis B is being cared for at home. The mother of the child calls the health care clinic and tells the nurse that the jaundice seems to be worsening. The nurse makes which response to the mother?
1 "The hepatitis may be spreading."
2 "You need to bring the child to the health care clinic to see the physician."
3 "The jaundice may appear to get worse before it resolves."
4 "It is necessary to isolate the child from the others."

Answer: 3
Rationale: The parents should be instructed that jaundice may appear to get worse before it resolves. The parents of a child with hepatitis should also be taught the danger signs that could indicate a worsening of the child's condition, specifically changes in neurological status, bleeding, and fluid retention. The statements in options 1, 2, and 4 are incorrect.

Test-Taking Strategy: Use knowledge regarding the physiology associated with hepatitis to answer this question. Remember that jaundice worsens before it resolves. This will direct you to the correct option. Review the instructions to the parents of a child with hepatitis if you had difficulty with this question.

Level of Cognitive Ability: Application
Client Needs: Physiological Integrity
Integrated Process: Nursing Process/Implementation
Content Area: Child Health

References:
James, S., Ashwill, J., & Droske, S. (2002). *Nursing care of children: Principles & practice* (2nd ed.). Philadelphia: Saunders, p. 580.
Wong, D., & Hockenberry, M. (2003). *Wong's nursing care of infants and children* (7th ed.). St. Louis: Mosby, pp. 1458-1459.

22. A nurse is preparing to suction a tracheotomy on an infant. The nurse prepares the equipment for the procedure and turns the suction to which setting?
1 60 mmHg
2 90 mmHg
3 110 mmHg
4 120 mmHg

Answer: 2
Rationale: The suctioning procedure for pediatric clients varies from that which is used in adults. Suctioning in infants and children requires the use of a smaller suction catheter and lower suction settings than in the adult. Suction settings for a neonate is 60 to 80 mmHg, for an infant is 80 to 100 mmHg, and for larger children is 100 to 120 mmHg.

Test-Taking Strategy: Use the process of elimination, noting the key word "infant." Recalling the procedure that is used in an adult will assist in directing you to option 2. Review this content if you are unfamiliar with this procedure.

Level of Cognitive Ability: Application
Client Needs: Physiological Integrity
Integrated Process: Nursing Process/Implementation
Content Area: Child Health

Reference:
Wong, D., & Hockenberry, M. (2003). *Wong's nursing care of infants and children* (7th ed.). St. Louis: Mosby, p. 1326.

23. A nurse is caring for a client who begins to experience seizure activity while in bed. The nurse implements which action to prevent aspiration?
1 Loosens restrictive clothing
2 Removes the pillow and raises the padded side rails
3 Raises the head of the bed
4 Positions the client on the side if possible, with the head flexed forward

Answer: 4
Rationale: Positioning the client on one side with the head flexed forward allows the tongue to fall forward and facilitates drainage of secretions, which could help prevent aspiration. The nurse would also remove restrictive clothing and the pillow, and raise the padded side rails, if present, but these actions would not decrease the risk of aspiration. Rather, they are general safety measures to use during seizure activity. The nurse would not raise the client's head of bed.

Test Taking Strategy: Note the key words "prevent aspiration." Eliminate option 2 first because it is unrelated to the issue of the question. Visualize the effect that each of the remaining options would have on airway and aspiration to direct you to option 4. Review care of the client with seizures to prevent aspiration if you had difficulty with this question.

Level of Cognitive Ability: Application
Client Needs: Physiological Integrity
Integrated Process: Nursing Process/Implementation
Content Area: Adult Health/Neurological

References:
Black, J., & Hawks, J. (2005). *Medical-surgical nursing: Clinical management for positive outcomes* (7th ed.). Philadelphia: Saunders, p. 2077.
Lewis, S., Heitkemper, M., & Dirksen, S. (2004). *Medical-surgical nursing: Assessment and management of clinical problems* (6th ed.). St. Louis: Mosby, p. 1561.

24. A client with a cerebrovascular accident (CVA) has episodes of coughing while swallowing liquids. The client has developed a temperature of 101°F, oxygen saturation of 91% (down from 98% previously), slight confusion, and noticeable dyspnea. The nurse would take which most appropriate action?
  1 Administer a bronchodilator ordered on a prn basis
  2 Administer an acetaminophen (Tylenol) suppository
  3 Encourage the client to cough and deep breathe
  4 Notify the physician

Answer: 4
Rationale: The client is exhibiting clinical signs and symptoms of aspiration, which include fever, dyspnea, decreased arterial oxygen levels, and confusion. Other symptoms that occur with this complication are difficulty in managing own saliva, or coughing or choking while eating. Because the client has developed a complication requiring medical intervention, the most appropriate action is to contact the physician.

Test-Taking Strategy: Focusing on the data in the question will indicate that aspiration has most likely occurred. Eliminate options 1, 2, and 3 because these actions will not assist in alleviating this life-threatening condition. Review the findings in the client who is aspirating and the appropriate nursing interventions if you had difficulty with this question.

Level of Cognitive Ability: Application
Client Needs: Physiological Integrity
Integrated Process: Nursing Process/Implementation
Content Area: Adult Health/Neurological

References:
Black, J., & Hawks, J. (2005). *Medical-surgical nursing: Clinical management for positive outcomes* (7th ed.). Philadelphia: Saunders, pp. 2124-2125.
Phipps, W., Monahan, F., Sands, J., Marek, J., & Neighbors, M. (2003). *Medical-surgical nursing: Health and illness perspectives* (7th ed.). St. Louis: Mosby, p. 1379.

25. A nurse is providing care to a client following a bone biopsy. Which action would the nurse take as part of aftercare for this procedure?
  1 Keep the area in a dependent position
  2 Monitor vital signs once per day
  3 Monitor the site for swelling, bleeding, or hematoma formation
  4 Administer intramuscular narcotic analgesics

Answer: 3
Rationale: Nursing care after bone biopsy includes monitoring the site for swelling, bleeding, or hematoma formation. The biopsy site is elevated for 24 hours to reduce edema. The vital signs are monitored every 4 hours for 24 hours. The client usually requires mild analgesics; more severe pain usually indicates that complications are arising.

Test-Taking Strategy: Begin to answer this question by recalling that after this procedure the client must have periodic assessments. With this in mind, eliminate option 2 because the time frame is too infrequent. Knowing that the procedure is done under local anesthesia helps you to eliminate option 4 next. From the remaining options, recall the principles related to circulation and positioning to direct you to option 3. Review care of a client following bone biopsy if you had difficulty with this question.

Level of Cognitive Ability: Application
Client Needs: Physiological Integrity
Integrated Process: Nursing Process/Implementation
Content Area: Adult Health/Musculoskeletal

Reference:
Black, J., & Hawks, J. (2005). *Medical-surgical nursing: Clinical management for positive outcomes* (7th ed.). Philadelphia: Saunders, p. 577.

26. A nurse is caring for a client who is going to have an arthrogram using a contrast medium. Which action by the nurse is the highest priority?
1 Determining the presence of client allergies
2 Telling the client that he will need to remain still during the procedure
3 Asking if the client has any last-minute questions
4 Telling the client to try to void before leaving the unit

Answer: 1
Rationale: Because of the risk of allergy to contrast medium, the nurse places highest priority on assessing whether the client has an allergy to iodine or shellfish. The nurse also reinforces information about the test and reminds the client about the need to remain still during the procedure. It is helpful to have the client void before the procedure for comfort.

Test-Taking Strategy: Use the process of elimination, noting the key words "contrast medium" and "highest priority." Recalling the risk associated with the administration of contrast medium will direct you to option 1. Review preprocedure care for an arthrogram if you had difficulty with this question.

Level of Cognitive Ability: Application
Client Needs: Physiological Integrity
Integrated Process: Nursing Process/Implementation
Content Area: Delegating/Prioritizing

Reference:
Chernecky, C., & Berger, B. (2004). *Laboratory tests and diagnostic procedures* (4th ed.). Philadelphia: Saunders, p. 202

---

27. A nurse responds to a call bell and finds a client lying on the floor after a fall. The nurse suspects that the client's arm may be broken. The nurse takes which immediate action?
1 Tells the client that there is no permanent damage
2 Immobilizes the arm
3 Takes a set of vital signs
4 Calls the radiology department

Answer: 2
Rationale: When a fracture is suspected, it is imperative that the area is splinted before the client is moved. Emergency help should be called for if the client is external to a hospital, and a physician is called if the client is hospitalized. The nurse should remain with the client and provide realistic reassurance. The client would not be told that there is no permanent damage. Vital signs would be taken, but this is not the immediate action. The physician (not the nurse) prescribes X-rays.

Test-Taking Strategy: Use the process of elimination, noting the key word "immediate." Eliminate option 4 because the physician will order radiology films. Option 1 is eliminated next because the nurse does not make statements to the client that could provide false reassurance. From the remaining options, noting that a fracture is suspected will direct you to option 2. Review care of the client with a suspected extremity fracture if you had difficulty with this question.

Level of Cognitive Ability: Application
Client Needs: Physiological Integrity
Integrated Process: Nursing Process/Implementation
Content Area: Adult Health/Musculoskeletal

Reference:
Black, J., & Hawks, J. (2005). *Medical-surgical nursing: Clinical management for positive outcomes* (7th ed.). Philadelphia: Saunders, p. 2501.

28. A nurse in the postpartum unit checks a client's temperature who delivered a healthy newborn infant 4 hours ago. The mother's temperature is 100.8°F. The nurse provides oral hydration to the mother and encourages fluids. Four hours later, the nurse rechecks the temperature and notes that it is still 100.8°F. Which nursing action is most appropriate?
1 Notify the physician
2 Continue hydration and recheck the temperature 4 hours later
3 Document the temperature
4 Increase the intravenous fluids

Answer: 1

Rationale: A temperature greater than 100.4°F in two consecutive readings is considered febrile, and the physician should be notified. Options 2, 3, and 4 are inappropriate actions at this time.

Test-Taking Strategy: Use the process of elimination. Option 4 can be eliminated first because this action requires a physician order. From the remaining options, noting that the temperature has remained unchanged following nursing intervention should provide you with the clue that further intervention is necessary and direct you to option 1. Review normal and abnormal findings in the postpartum period if you had difficulty with this question.

Level of Cognitive Ability: Application
Client Needs: Physiological Integrity
Integrated Process: Nursing Process/Implementation
Content Area: Maternity/Postpartum

Reference:
Murray, S., McKinney, E., & Gorrie, T. (2002). *Foundations of maternal-newborn nursing* (3rd ed.). Philadelphia: Saunders, pp. 440-441.

29. A nurse is checking the fundus in a postpartum woman and notes that the uterus is soft and spongy. Which nursing action is appropriate initially?
1 Massage the fundus gently until firm
2 Document fundal position and consistency and height
3 Encourage the mother to ambulate
4 Notify the physician

Answer: 1

Rationale: If the fundus is boggy (soft), it should be massaged gently until firm, observing for increased bleeding or clots. Option 3 is an inappropriate action at this time. The nurse should document fundal position, consistency and height, the need to perform fundal massage, and the client's response to the intervention. The physician will need to be notified if uterine massage is not helpful.

Test-Taking Strategy: Note the key words "appropriate initially." Note the relationship of the data in the question (soft and spongy) and the data in the correct option (massage the fundus gently until firm). Review nursing interventions related to this occurrence if you had difficulty with this question.

Level of Cognitive Ability: Application
Client Needs: Physiological Integrity
Integrated Process: Nursing Process/Implementation
Content Area: Maternity/Postpartum

Reference:
Lowdermilk, D., & Perry, A. (2004). *Maternity & women's health care* (8th ed.). St. Louis: Mosby, 619.

30. A primipara is being evaluated in the clinic during her second trimester of pregnancy. The nurse checks the fetal heart rate (FHR) and notes that it is 190 beats per minute. The appropriate nursing action would be to:
1 Document the finding
2 Consult with the physician
3 Tell the client that the FHR is normal
4 Recheck the FHR with the client in the standing position

Answer: 2
Rationale: The fetal heart rate should be 120 to 160 beats per minute throughout pregnancy. In this situation, the FHR is elevated from the normal range, and the nurse should consult with the physician. The FHR would be documented, but option 2 is the appropriate action. The nurse would not tell the client that the FHR is normal because this is not true information. Option 4 is an inappropriate action.

Test-Taking Strategy: Focus on the data in the question. Recalling that the normal FHR is 120 to 160 beats per minute will direct you to option 2. Review the normal FHR if you had difficulty with this question.

Level of Cognitive Ability: Application
Client Needs: Physiological Integrity
Integrated Process: Nursing Process/Implementation
Content Area: Maternity/Antepartum

Reference:
Murray, S., McKinney, E., & Gorrie, T. (2002). *Foundations of maternal-newborn nursing* (3rd ed.). Philadelphia: Saunders, p. 978.

---

31. A female client tells the clinic nurse that her skin is very dry and irritated. Which product would the nurse suggest that the client apply to the dry skin?
1 Glycerin emollient
2 Aspercreame
3 Myoflex
4 Acetic acid solution

Answer: 1
Rationale: Glycerin is an emollient that is used for dry, cracked, and irritated skin. Aspercreame and Myoflex are used to treat muscular aches. Acetic acid solution is used for irrigating, cleansing, and packing wounds infected by *Pseudomonas aeruginosa*.

Test-Taking Strategy: Use the process of elimination. Noting the key words "skin is very dry and irritated" will direct you to option 1. Review these products if you had difficulty with this question.

Level of Cognitive Ability: Application
Client Needs: Health Promotion and Maintenance
Integrated Process: Nursing Process/Implementation
Content Area: Pharmacology

Reference:
McKenry, L., & Salerno, E. (2003). *Mosby's pharmacology in nursing* (21st ed.). St. Louis: Mosby, p. 1124.

---

32. A client with a history of hypertension has been prescribed triamterene (Dyrenium). The nurse provides information to the client about the medication and tells the client to avoid consuming which of the following fruits?
1 Apples
2 Pears
3 Bananas
4 Cranberries

Answer: 3
Rationale: Triamterene is a potassium-sparing diuretic, and the client should avoid foods high in potassium. Fruits that are naturally higher in potassium include avocado, bananas, fresh oranges, mangoes, nectarines, papayas, and dried prunes.

Test-Taking Strategy: Recall that triamterene is a potassium-sparing diuretic. Then, identify the high-potassium food. Review this medication and those food items high in potassium if you had difficulty with this question.

Level of Cognitive Ability: Analysis
Client Needs: Health Promotion and Maintenance
Integrated Process: Nursing Process/Implementation
Content Area: Adult Health/Cardiovascular

References:
Hodgson, B., & Kizior, R. (2004). *Saunders nursing drug handbook 2004.* Philadelphia: Saunders, p. 1020.
McKenry, L., & Salerno, E. (2003). *Mosby's pharmacology in nursing* (21st ed.). St. Louis: Mosby, p. 679.

---

33. Breathing exercises and postural drainage is prescribed for a child with cystic fibrosis. A nurse implements these procedures by telling the child to:
1 Perform the postural drainage, then the breathing exercises
2 Perform the breathing exercises, then the postural drainage
3 Schedule the procedures so they are 4 hours apart
4 Perform postural drainage in the morning and breathing exercises in the evening

Answer: 1
Rationale: Breathing exercises are recommended for children with cystic fibrosis, even for those with minimal pulmonary involvement. The exercises are usually performed twice daily, and they are preceded with postural drainage. The postural drainage will mobilize secretions, and the breathing exercises will then assist with expectoration. Exercises to assist with posture and to mobilize the thorax are included, such as swinging the arms and bending and twisting the trunk. The ultimate aim of these exercises is to establish a good habitual breathing pattern.

Test-Taking Strategy: Use the process of elimination. Recalling that postural drainage and breathing exercises are most effective when performed together will assist in eliminating options 3 and 4. From the remaining options, consider the effectiveness that each procedure will have on the mobilization of secretions to direct you to option 1. Review these procedures if you had difficulty with this question.

Level of Cognitive Ability: Application
Client Needs: Health Promotion and Maintenance
Integrated Process: Nursing Process/Implementation
Content Area: Child Health

Reference:
Wong, D., & Hockenberry, M. (2003). *Wong's nursing care of infants and children* (7th ed.). St. Louis: Mosby, pp. 1407-1408.

Nursing Process: Evaluation

---

1. A nurse has been encouraging the intake of oral fluids in a woman in labor to improve hydration. Which of the following indicates a successful outcome of this action?
1 A urine specific gravity of 1.020
2 Continued leaking of amniotic fluid during labor
3 Blood pressure of 150/90 mmHg
4 Ketones in the urine

Answer: 1
Rationale: Urine specific gravity measures the concentration of the urine. During the first stage of labor, the renal system has a tendency to concentrate urine. Labor and birth require hydration and caloric intake to replenish energy expenditure and promote efficient uterine function. An elevated blood pressure and ketones in the urine are not expected outcomes related to labor and hydration. Once membranes are ruptured, it is expected that amniotic fluid may continue to leak.

Test-Taking Strategy: Use the process of elimination, focusing on the issue: a successful outcome related to oral intake. Recalling the relationship of oral intake to urine concentration will direct you to option 1. Review the importance of hydration in the woman in labor if you had difficulty with this question.

Level of Cognitive Ability: Analysis
Client Needs: Health Promotion and Maintenance
Integrated Process: Nursing Process/Evaluation
Content Area: Maternity/Intrapartum

Reference:
Lowdermilk, D., & Perry, A. (2004). *Maternity & women's health care* (8th ed.). St. Louis: Mosby, pp. 564; 571; 572.

---

2. A postpartum client has a nursing diagnosis of Risk for Infection. A goal has been developed that states: "The client will remain free of infection during her hospital stay." Which assessment data would support that the goal has been met?
  1 Presence of chills
  2 Abdominal tenderness
  3 Absence of fever
  4 Loss of appetite

Answer: 3
Rationale: Fever is the first indication of an infection. Chills, abdominal tenderness, and loss of appetite can indicate the presence of an infection. Therefore, the absence of a fever indicates that an infection is not present.

Test-Taking Strategy: Use the process of elimination, noting the key words "that the goal has been met." The question is asking for a means of evaluating the effectiveness of a goal that relates to infection. Options 1, 2, and 4 indicate possible signs of infection and that the goal has not been met. Review the signs of postpartum infection if you had difficulty with this question.

Level of Cognitive Ability: Analysis
Client Needs: Physiological Integrity
Integrated Process: Nursing Process/Evaluation
Content Area: Maternity/Postpartum

Reference:
Lowdermilk, D., & Perry, A. (2004). *Maternity & women's health care* (8th ed.). St. Louis: Mosby, p. 1048.

---

3. A nurse is monitoring the nutritional status of the client receiving enteral nutrition because of dysphagia that resulted from a head injury. The nurse monitors which of the following to best determine the effectiveness of the feedings for this client?
  1 Calorie count
  2 Daily intake and output
  3 Daily weight
  4 Serum protein level

Answer: 3
Rationale: The most accurate measurement of the effectiveness of nutritional management of the client is through monitoring of daily weight. This should be done at the same time (preferably early morning), in the same clothes, and using the same scale. Options 1, 2, and 4 assist in measuring nutrition and hydration status. However, the effectiveness of the diet is measured by maintenance of body weight.

Test-Taking Strategy: Note the key word "effectiveness." This tells you that the correct option is an outcome. With this in mind, eliminate options 1 and 2 first because these are tools the nurse uses to measure nutrition and fluid status. Eliminate option 4 next because it reflects only one component of the diet, namely protein. Review the methods of monitoring nutritional status if you had difficulty with this question.

Level of Cognitive Ability: Analysis
Client Needs: Physiological Integrity
Integrated Process: Nursing Process/Evaluation
Content Area: Fundamental Skills

References:

Black, J., & Hawks, J. (2005). *Medical-surgical nursing: Clinical management for positive outcomes* (7th ed.). Philadelphia: Saunders, pp. 672; 707; 2195.
Lewis, S., Heitkemper, M., & Dirksen, S. (2004). *Medical-surgical nursing: Assessment and management of clinical problems* (6th ed.). St. Louis: Mosby, p. 985.

---

4. An adult client with a critically high potassium level has received sodium polystyrene sulfonate (Kayexalate). The nurse evaluates that the medication was most effective if the client's repeat serum potassium level is:

1 6.2 mEq/L
2 5.8 mEq/L
3 5.4 mEq/L
4 4.9 mEq/L

Answer: 4

Rationale: The normal serum potassium level in the adult is 3.5 to 5.1 mEq/L. Option 4 is the only option reflecting a value that has dropped down into the normal range. Options 1, 2, and 3 identify elevated potassium levels.

Test-Taking Strategy: Use the process of elimination. Note the key words "critically high." You would expect that this medication is administered to lower the potassium level. Recalling the normal serum potassium level will direct you to option 4. Review the expected effects of this medication and the normal potassium level if you had difficulty with this question.

Level of Cognitive Ability: Analysis
Client Needs: Physiological Integrity
Integrated Process: Nursing Process/Evaluation
Content Area: Fundamental Skills

References:

Chernecky, C., & Berger, B. (2004). *Laboratory tests and diagnostic procedures* (4th ed.). Philadelphia: Saunders, p. 887.
Hodgson, B., & Kizior, R. (2004). *Saunders nursing drug handbook 2004.* Philadelphia: Saunders, p. 926.

---

5. A nurse assesses a client after abdominal surgery who has a nasogastric tube (NG) in place that is connected to suction. Which observation by the nurse indicates most reliably that the tube is functioning properly?

1 The suction gauge reads low intermittent suction.
2 The distal end of the NG tube is pinned to the client's gown.
3 The client indicates that pain is a 3 on a scale of 1 to 10.
4 The client denies nausea and has 250 mL of fluid in the suction collection container.

Answer: 4

Rationale: An NG tube connected to suction is used postoperatively to decompress and rest the bowel. The gastrointestinal tract lacks peristaltic activity because of manipulation during surgery. Although the nurse makes pertinent observations of the tube to ensure that it is secure and connected to suction properly, the client is assessed for the effect. The client should not experience symptoms of ileus (nausea and vomiting) if the tube is functioning properly. A pain indicator of 3 is an expected finding in a postoperative client.

Test-Taking Strategy: Focus on the issue that the tube is functioning properly. Recalling the purpose of the NG tube in a postoperative client will direct you to option 4. Review care of the client with an NG tube if you had difficulty with this question.

Level of Cognitive Ability: Analysis
Client Needs: Physiological Integrity
Integrated Process: Nursing Process/Evaluation
Content Area: Adult Health/Gastrointestinal

References:
Ignatavicius, D., & Workman, M. (2002). *Medical surgical nursing: Critical thinking for collaborative care* (4th ed.). Philadelphia: Saunders, pp. 290; 1228; 1230.
Potter, P., & Perry, A. (2005). *Fundamentals of nursing* (6th ed.). St. Louis: Mosby, p. 1408.

---

6. A nurse is caring for the client who has returned from the post-anesthesia care unit following prostatectomy. The client has a three-way Foley catheter with an infusion of continuous bladder irrigation (CBI). The nurse determines that the flow rate is adequate if the color of the urinary drainage is:
  1 Dark cherry colored
  2 Concentrated yellow with small clots
  3 Clear as water
  4 Pale yellow or slightly pink

Answer: 4
Rationale: The infusion of bladder irrigant is not at a preset rate, but rather it is increased or decreased to maintain urine that is a clear pale yellow color or that has just a slight pink tinge. The infusion rate should be increased if the drainage is cherry colored or if clots are seen. Correspondingly, the rate can be slowed down slightly if the returns are as clear as water.

Test-Taking Strategy: Use the process of elimination. Note the issue of the question: an adequate flow rate. With this in mind, eliminate option 2 because clots are not expected. Next, eliminate options 1 and 3 as reflecting inadequate and excessive irrigation flow, respectively. Review care of the client with CBI if you had difficulty with this question.

Level of Cognitive Ability: Analysis
Client Needs: Physiological Integrity
Integrated Process: Nursing Process/Evaluation
Content Area: Adult Health/Renal

Reference:
Ignatavicius, D., & Workman, M. (2002). *Medical surgical nursing: Critical thinking for collaborative care* (4th ed.). Philadelphia: Saunders, p. 1787.

---

7. A nurse who is caring for a client with Graves' disease notes a nursing diagnosis of "Imbalanced Nutrition: less than body requirements related to the effects of the hypercatabolic state" in the care plan. Which of the following indicates a successful outcome for this diagnosis?
  1 The client maintains his normal weight or gradually gains weight if it is below normal.
  2 The client demonstrates knowledge regarding the need to consume a diet high in fat and low in protein.
  3 The client verbalizes the need to avoid snacking between meals.
  4 The client discusses the relationship between mealtime and the blood glucose level.

Answer: 1
Rationale: Graves' disease causes a state of chronic nutritional and caloric deficiency caused by the metabolic effects of excessive T3 and T4. Clinical manifestations are weight loss and increased appetite. It is therefore a nutritional goal that the client will not lose additional weight and will gradually return to ideal body weight if necessary. To accomplish this, the client must be encouraged to eat frequent high-calorie, high-protein, and high-carbohydrate meals and snacks.

Test-Taking Strategy: Use the process of elimination, focusing on the key words "hypercatabolic state." Options 2 and 3 would not be beneficial for a client in a hypercatabolic state. Option 4 can be eliminated because discussing the fluctuation in the blood glucose level will not assist a client who is hypermetabolic. Review imbalanced nutrition and Graves' disease if you had difficulty with this question.

Level of Cognitive Ability: Analysis
Client Needs: Health Promotion and Maintenance
Integrated Process: Nursing Process/Evaluation
Content Area: Adult Health/Endocrine

Reference:
Black, J., & Hawks, J. (2005). *Medical-surgical nursing: Clinical management for positive outcomes* (7th ed.). Philadelphia: Saunders, p. 1196.

8. A nurse has developed a plan of care for a client who is in traction and documents a nursing diagnosis of Bathing/Hygiene Self-Care Deficit. The nurse evaluates the plan of care and determines that which observation indicates a successful outcome?

1 The client allows the nurse to complete the care on a daily basis.
2 The client allows the family to assist in the care.
3 The client refuses care .
4 The client assists in self-care as much as possible.

Answer: 4

Rationale: A successful outcome for the nursing diagnosis of Bathing/Hygiene Self-Care Deficit is for the client to do as much of the self-care as possible. The nurse should promote independence in the client and allow the client to perform as much self-care as is optimal considering the client's condition. The nurse would determine that the outcome is unsuccessful if the client refused care or allows others to do the care.

Test-Taking Strategy: Focus on the key words "successful outcome." Option 3 can be eliminated first because the client is refusing care. Note that options 1 and 2 are similar in that they indicate relying on others to perform care. Review successful outcomes related to the nursing diagnosis of Bathing/Hygiene Self-Care Deficit if you had difficulty with this question.

Level of Cognitive Ability: Analysis
Client Needs: Health Promotion and Maintenance
Integrated Process: Nursing Process/Evaluation
Content Area: Adult Health/Musculoskeletal

Reference:
Ignatavicius, D., & Workman, M. (2002). *Medical surgical nursing: Critical thinking for collaborative care* (4th ed.). Philadelphia: Saunders, p. 128.

9. A nurse instructs a parent regarding the appropriate actions to take when the toddler has a temper tantrum. Which statement by the parent indicates a successful outcome of the teaching?

1 "I will send my child to a room alone for 10 minutes after every tantrum."
2 "I will reward my child with candy at the end of each day without a tantrum."
3 "I will give frequent reminders that only bad children have tantrums."
4 "I will ignore the tantrums as long as there is no physical danger."

Answer: 4

Rationale: Ignoring a negative attention-seeking behavior is considered the best way to extinguish it, provided the child is safe from injury. Option 1 gives attention to the tantrum and also exceeds the recommended time of 1 minute per year of age for time-out. Providing candy for rewards is unhealthy and unlikely to be effective at the end of a day. Option 3 is untrue and negative.

Test-Taking Strategy: Use the process of elimination. Recalling that ignoring a tantrum is the best way to extinguish it will direct you to option 4. Review interventions for the child who has temper tantrums if you had difficulty with this question.

Level of Cognitive Ability: Analysis
Client Needs: Health Promotion and Maintenance
Integrated Process: Nursing Process/Evaluation
Content Area: Child Health

Reference:
Wong, D., & Hockenberry, M. (2003). *Wong's nursing care of infants and children* (7th ed.). St. Louis: Mosby, p. 607.

10. A nurse is caring for a client in seclusion. The nurse determines that the client is safe to come out of seclusion when the nurse hears the client say which of the following?
1 "I am no longer a threat to myself or others."
2 "I need to use the restroom right away."
3 "I'd like to go back to my room and be alone for a while."
4 "I can't breathe in here. The walls are closing in on me."

Answer: 1
Rationale: Option 1 indicates that the client may be safely removed from seclusion. The client in seclusion must be assessed at regular intervals (usually every 15 to 30 minutes) for physical needs, safety, and comfort. Option 2 indicates a physical need that could be met with a urinal, bedpan, or commode. It does not indicate that the client has calmed down enough to leave the seclusion room. Option 3 could be an attempt to manipulate the nurse. It gives no indication that the client will control him or herself when alone in the room. Option 4 could be handled by supportive communication or a prn medication, if indicated. It does not necessitate discontinuing seclusion.

Test-Taking Strategy: Focus on the issue of the question: removing a client from seclusion. Recalling the purpose and the use of seclusion will direct you to option 1. Review seclusion procedures if you had difficulty with this question.

Level of Cognitive Ability: Analysis
Client Needs: Psychosocial Integrity
Integrated Process: Nursing Process/Evaluation
Content Area: Mental Health

Reference:
Stuart, G., & Laraia, M. (2005). *Principles and practice of psychiatric nursing* (8th ed.). St. Louis: Mosby, p. 646.

11. A client has had a laryngectomy for throat cancer and has started oral intake. The nurse evaluates that the client has tolerated the first stage of dietary advancement if the client takes which of the following types of diet without aspiration or choking?
1 Bland
2 Clear liquids
3 Full liquids
4 Semi-solid foods

Answer: 4
Rationale: Oral intake after laryngectomy is started with semi-solid foods. Once the client can manage this type of food, liquids may be introduced. Thin liquids are not given until the risk of aspiration is negligible. A bland diet is not appropriate. The client may not be able to tolerate the texture of some of the solid foods that would be included in a bland diet.

Test-Taking Strategy: Use the process of elimination. Eliminate options 2 and 3 first, recalling that a client with swallowing difficulty will be unable to manage liquids. From the remaining options, recall that a bland diet provides no control over the consistency or texture of the food. Review dietary measures for a client following laryngectomy if you had difficulty with this question.

Level of Cognitive Ability: Analysis
Client Needs: Physiological Integrity
Integrated Process: Nursing Process/Evaluation
Content Area: Adult Health/Oncology

Reference:
Black, J., & Hawks, J. (2005). *Medical-surgical nursing: Clinical management for positive outcomes* (7th ed.). Philadelphia: Saunders, p. 1791.

12. An older male client who is a victim of elder abuse and his family have been seen in the counseling center weekly for the past month. Which statement, if made by the abusive family member, would indicate that he or she has learned more positive coping skills?

1 "I will be more careful to make sure that my father's needs are 100 percent met."

2 "I am so sorry and embarrassed that the abusive event occurred. It won't happen again."

3 "I feel better equipped to care for my father now that I know where to turn if I need assistance."

4 "Now that my father is moving into my home, I will have to stop drinking alcohol."

Answer: 3

Rationale: Elder abuse is sometimes the result of family members who are being expected to care for their aging parents. This care can cause the family to become overextended, frustrated, or financially depleted. Knowing where to turn in the community for assistance in caring for an aging family member can bring much-needed relief. Using these alternatives is a positive coping skill for many families. Options 1, 2, and 4 are statements of good faith or promises, which may or may not be kept in the future.

Test-Taking Strategy: Focus on the issue, a positive coping skill, and use the process of elimination. Option 3 is the only option that identifies a means of coping with the issues and outlines a definitive plan for how to handle the pressure associated with the father's care. Review the concepts related to elder abuse if you had difficulty with this question.

Level of Cognitive Ability: Analysis
Client Needs: Psychosocial Integrity
Integrated Process: Nursing Process/Evaluation
Content Area: Mental Health

Reference:
Varcarolis, E.M. (2002). *Foundations of psychiatric mental health nursing* (4th ed.). Philadelphia: Saunders, p. 710.

13. A nurse is caring for a term infant who is 24 hours old who had a confirmed episode of hypoglycemia at 1 hour of age. Which observation by the nurse would indicate the need for further evaluation?

1 Blood glucose level of 40 mg/dL before the last feeding

2 High-pitched cry, eating 10 to 15 mL of formula per feeding

3 Weight loss of 4 ounces and dry, peeling skin

4 Breast-feeding for 20 minutes or greater, strong sucking

Answer: 2

Rationale: At 24 hours of age, a term infant should be able to consume at least one ounce of formula per feeding. A high-pitched cry is indicative of neurological involvement. Blood glucose levels are acceptable at 40 mg/dL in the first few days of life. Weight loss over the first few days of life and dry, peeling skin are normal findings for term infants. Breast-feeding for 20 minutes with a strong suck is an excellent finding. Hypoglycemia causes central nervous system symptoms (high-pitched cry) and also is exhibited by lack of strength in eating enough for growth.

Test-Taking Strategy: Use the process of elimination, noting the key words "need for further evaluation." Eliminate options 1, 3, and 4 because these are normal findings. Also, the words "high-pitched cry" should direct you to option 2. Review normal newborn findings and the indications of hypoglycemia if you had difficulty with this question.

Level of Cognitive Ability: Analysis
Client Needs: Physiological Integrity
Integrated Process: Nursing Process/Evaluation
Content Area: Maternity/Postpartum

Reference:
Wong, D., & Hockenberry, M. (2003). *Wong's nursing care of infants and children* (7th ed.). St. Louis: Mosby, p. 317.

14. A home care nurse visits a child with a diagnosis of celiac disease. Which finding best indicates that a gluten-free diet is being maintained and has been effective?

1 The child is free of diarrhea.
2 The child is free of bloody stools.
3 The child tolerates dietary wheat and rye.
4 A balanced fluid and electrolyte status is noted on the laboratory results.

Answer: 1
Rationale: Watery diarrhea is a frequent clinical manifestation of celiac disease. The absence of diarrhea indicates effective treatment. Bloody stools is not associated with this disease. The grains of wheat and rye contain gluten and are not allowed. A balance in fluids and electrolytes does not necessarily demonstrate improved status of celiac disease.

Test-Taking Strategy: Focus on the issue: a lack of signs and symptoms related to celiac disease. Recalling that watery diarrhea is a manifestation of celiac disease will direct you to option 1. Review the manifestations of this disorder if you had difficulty with this question.

Level of Cognitive Ability: Analysis
Client Needs: Health Promotion and Maintenance
Integrated Process: Nursing Process/Evaluation
Content Area: Child Health

Reference:
Wong, D., & Hockenberry, M. (2003). *Wong's nursing care of infants and children* (7th ed.). St. Louis: Mosby, p. 1451.

15. A nurse is assisting in caring for a woman in labor who is receiving oxytocin (Pitocin) by intravenous (IV) infusion. The nurse monitors the client, knowing that which of the following indicates an adequate contraction pattern?

1 Three to five contractions in a 10-minute period, with resultant cervical dilatation
2 One contraction per minute, with resultant cervical dilatation
3 Four contractions every 5 minutes, with resultant cervical dilatation
4 One contraction every 10 minutes without resultant cervical dilatation

Answer: 1
Rationale: The preferred oxytocin dosage is the minimal amount necessary to maintain an adequate contraction pattern characterized by three to five contractions in a 10-minute period, with resultant cervical dilatation. If contractions are more frequent than every 2 minutes, contraction quality may be decreased.

Test-Taking Strategy: Use the process of elimination. Focusing on the issue, an adequate contraction pattern, will assist you in eliminating option 4. Next, eliminate options 2 and 3 because they are similar. Review the expected effects of this medication if you had difficulty with this question.

Level of Cognitive Ability: Analysis
Client Needs: Physiological Integrity
Integrated Process: Nursing Process/Evaluation
Content Area: Maternity/Intrapartum

Reference:
Lowdermilk, D., & Perry, A. (2004). *Maternity & women's health care* (8th ed.). St. Louis: Mosby, pp. 1011; 1013.

16. A home care nurse is assigned to visit a preschooler who has a diagnosis of scarlet fever and is on bed rest. What data obtained by the nurse would indicate that the child is coping with the illness and bed rest?
  1 The mother keeps providing new activities for the child to do.
  2 The child is coloring and drawing pictures in a notebook.
  3 The child insists that the mother stay in the room.
  4 The child sucks the thumb whenever the child does not get what is asked for.

Answer: 2
Rationale: According to Jean Piaget, for the preschooler, play is the best way for children to understand and adjust to life's experiences. They are able to use pencils and crayons. They can draw stick figures and other rudimentary things. A child with scarlet fever needs quiet play, and drawing will provide that. Options 1, 3, and 4 do not address positive coping mechanisms.

Test-Taking Strategy: Think about the developmental level of a preschooler. Note the issue: an analysis of data by the nurse to determine if the child is coping with the disease and bed rest. Option 2 is a positive coping mechanism for preschoolers. Options 1, 3, and 4 do not address positive coping mechanisms. Review the expected developmental level of a preschooler and the effects of bed rest on the child if you had difficulty with this question.

Level of Cognitive Ability: Analysis
Client Needs: Health Promotion and Maintenance
Integrated Process: Nursing Process/Evaluation
Content Area: Child Health

Reference:
Wong, D., & Hockenberry, M. (2003). *Wong's nursing care of infants and children* (7th ed.). St. Louis: Mosby, p. 631.

17. A client has just taken a dose of trimethobenzamide (Tigan). The nurse evaluates that the medication has been effective if the client states relief of:
  1 Heartburn
  2 Constipation
  3 Nausea and vomiting
  4 Abdominal pain

Answer: 3
Rationale: Trimethobenzamide (Tigan) is an antiemetic agent used in the treatment of nausea and vomiting. The medication is not used to treat heartburn, constipation, or abdominal pain.

Test-Taking Strategy: Use the process of elimination. Recalling that this medication is an antiemetic will direct you to option 3. Review the action of this medication if you had difficulty with this question.

Level of Cognitive Ability: Analysis
Client Needs: Physiological Integrity
Integrated Process: Nursing Process/Evaluation
Content Area: Pharmacology

Reference:
Hodgson, B., & Kizior, R. (2004). *Saunders nursing drug handbook 2004.* Philadelphia: Saunders, p. 1025.

18. A nurse is providing instructions to the mother of a child with a diagnosis of strabismus of the left eye, and the nurse reviews the procedure for patching the child. The nurse determines that the mother understands the procedure if the mother makes which statement?

1 "I will place the patch on the right eye."
2 "I will place the patch on both eyes."
3 "I will place the patch on the left eye."
4 "I will alternate the patch from the right to the left eye every hour."

Answer: 1

Rationale: Patching may be used in the treatment of strabismus to strengthen the weak eye. In this treatment, the good eye is patched. This encourages the child to use the weaker eye. It is most successful when done during the preschool years. The schedule for patching is individualized and prescribed by the ophthalmologist.

Test-Taking Strategy: Use the process of elimination. Remembering that this condition is a lazy eye will direct you to the correct option. It makes sense to patch the unaffected eye in order to strengthen the muscles in the affected eye. Review the procedure for patching if you had difficulty with this question.

Level of Cognitive Ability: Analysis
Client Needs: Physiological Integrity
Integrated Process: Nursing Process/Evaluation
Content Area: Child Health

Reference:
James, S., Ashwill, J., & Droske, S. (2002). *Nursing care of children: Principles & practice* (2nd ed.). Philadelphia: Saunders, p. 1045.

19. A nurse is assessing a client with pregnancy-induced hypertension (PIH) who was admitted to the hospital 48 hours ago. Which of the following data obtained would indicate that the condition has not yet resolved?

1 Blood pressure reading at prenatal baseline
2 Urinary output is increased
3 Client complaints of blurred vision
4 Presence of trace urinary protein

Answer: 3

Rationale: Client complaints of headache or blurred vision indicate a worsening of the condition and warrant immediate further evaluation. Options 1, 2, and 4 are all signs that the PIH is being resolved.

Test-Taking Strategy: Note the key words "has not yet resolved." These words indicate a false-response question and that you need to select the option that identifies a symptom of PIH. Options 1 and 2 can be eliminated first because they are normal findings. From the remaining options, note that option 4 contains the word "trace" and is the most normal finding of these two options. Review the clinical manifestations associated with PIH if you had difficulty with this question.

Level of Cognitive Ability: Analysis
Client Needs: Physiological Integrity
Integrated Process: Nursing Process/Evaluation
Content Area: Maternity/Antepartum

Reference:
Murray, S., McKinney, E., & Gorrie, T. (2002). *Foundations of maternal-newborn nursing* (3rd ed.). Philadelphia: Saunders, p. 681.

20. A client has begun medication therapy with betaxolol (Kerlone). The nurse determines that the client is experiencing the intended effects of therapy if which of the following is noted?
  1 Weight loss of 5 pounds
  2 Pulse rate increased from 58 to 74 beats per minute
  3 Blood pressure decreased from 142/94 mmHg to 128/82 mmHg
  4 Edema present at 3+

Answer: 3
Rationale: Betaxolol is a beta-adrenergic blocking agent used to lower blood pressure, relieve angina, or eliminate dysrhythmias. Side effects include bradycardia and symptoms of congestive heart failure, such as weight gain and increased edema.

Test-Taking Strategy: Note that the question asks for the "intended effect" of the medication. Remember that beta-adrenergic blocking agent medication names end with the suffix "lol." Recalling the action of the medication will direct you to option 3. Review the intended effects of this medication if you had difficulty with this question.

Level of Cognitive Ability: Analysis
Client Needs: Physiological Integrity
Integrated Process: Nursing Process/Evaluation
Content Area: Pharmacology

Reference:
Hodgson, B., & Kizior, R. (2004). *Saunders nursing drug handbook 2004.* Philadelphia: Saunders, p. 105.

21. A nurse has taught a client taking a xanthine bronchodilator about beverages to avoid. The nurse determines that the client understands the information if the client chooses which of the following beverages from the dietary menu?
  1 Chocolate milk
  2 Cranberry juice
  3 Coffee
  4 Cola

Answer: 2
Rationale: Cola, coffee, and chocolate contain xanthine and should be avoided by the client taking a xanthine bronchodilator. This could lead to an increased incidence of cardiovascular and central nervous system side effects that can occur with the use of these types of bronchodilators.

Test-Taking Strategy: Use the process of elimination. Note the similarity between options 1, 3, and 4 in that they all contain some form of stimulant. Review dietary measures for a client taking a xanthine bronchodilator if you had difficulty with this question.

Level of Cognitive Ability: Analysis
Client Needs: Health Promotion and Maintenance
Integrated Process: Nursing Process/Evaluation
Content Area: Pharmacology

Reference:
McKenry, L., & Salerno, E. (2003). *Mosby's pharmacology in nursing* (21st ed.). St. Louis: Mosby, p. 724.

22. A client is started on tolbutamide (Orinase) once daily. The nurse observes for which of the following intended effects of this medication?
  1 Decreased blood pressure
  2 Decreased blood glucose
  3 Weight loss
  4 Resolution of infection

Answer: 2
Rationale: Tolbutamide is an oral hypoglycemic agent that is taken in the morning. It is not used to decrease blood pressure, enhance weight loss, or treat infection.

Test-Taking Strategy: Note the key words "intended effects." Recalling that this medication is an oral hypoglycemic will direct you to option 2. Review the action of this medication if you had difficulty with this question.

Level of Cognitive Ability: Analysis
Client Needs: Physiological Integrity

Integrated Process: Nursing Process/Evaluation
Content Area: Pharmacology

Reference:
McKenry, L., & Salerno, E. (2003). *Mosby's pharmacology in nursing* (21st ed.). St. Louis: Mosby, pp. 880; 1218.

---

23. A client who regularly takes nonsteroidal antiinflammatory drugs (NSAIDs) has been taking misoprostol (Cytotec). The nurse would monitor the client to see if the client experienced relief of which of the following symptoms?
  1 Epigastric pain
  2 Diarrhea
  3 Bleeding
  4 Infection

Answer: 1
Rationale: The client who regularly takes NSAIDs is prone to gastric mucosal injury, which gives the client epigastric pain as a symptom. Misoprostol is administered to prevent this occurrence. Diarrhea can be a side effect of the medication, but is not an intended effect. Bleeding and infection are unrelated to the question.

Test-Taking Strategy: Note key words "NSAIDs" and "relief." This tells you that the medication is being given to treat or prevent the occurrence of a specific symptom. Recalling that NSAIDs can cause gastric mucosal injury will direct you to option 1. Review the action and indications for the use of misoprostol if you had difficulty with this question.

Level of Cognitive Ability: Analysis
Client Needs: Physiological Integrity
Integrated Process: Nursing Process/Evaluation
Content Area: Pharmacology

Reference:
McKenry, L., & Salerno, E. (2003). *Mosby's pharmacology in nursing* (21st ed.). St. Louis: Mosby, pp. 769-770.

---

24. A client has received a dose of a prn medication called loperamide (Imodium). The nurse evaluates the client after administration to see if the client has relief of:
  1 Constipation
  2 Diarrhea
  3 Tarry stools
  4 Abdominal pain

Answer: 2
Rationale: Loperamide is an antidiarrheal agent. It is commonly administered after loose stools. It is used in the management of acute diarrhea and also in chronic diarrhea, such as with inflammatory bowel disease. It can also be used to reduce the volume of drainage from an ileostomy.

Test-Taking Strategy: Use the process of elimination. Recalling that this medication is an antidiarrheal agent will direct you to option 2. Review the purpose of this medication if you had difficulty with this question.

Level of Cognitive Ability: Analysis
Client Needs: Physiological Integrity
Integrated Process: Nursing Process/Evaluation
Content Area: Pharmacology

Reference:
McKenry, L., & Salerno, E. (2003). *Mosby's pharmacology in nursing* (21st ed.). St. Louis: Mosby, p. 223.

25. A nurse has reinforced discharge instructions to a parent of a child following heart surgery. Which statement by the parent would indicate a need for further instructions?

 1 "I should call the physician if my child develops faster or harder breathing than normal."
 2 "My child can return to school for full days in 2 weeks following discharge."
 3 "I should have my child avoid crowds and people for 1 week after discharge."
 4 "I should allow my child to play inside but omit play outside at this time."

Answer: 2

Rationale: The child may return to school the third week after hospital discharge, but the child should go to school for half days for the first week. Play should be omitted for several weeks, allowing inside play as tolerated. The child should avoid crowds of people for 1 week after discharge, including crowds at day care centers and churches. If any difficulty with breathing occurs, the parent should notify the physician.

Test-Taking Strategy: Note the key words "indicate a need for further instructions." These words indicate a false-response question and that you need to select the incorrect parent statement. Recalling the principles related to the prevention of infection and the complications of surgery will direct you to option 2. Review home care instructions for the child following heart surgery if you had difficulty with this question.

Level of Cognitive Ability: Analysis
Client Needs: Health Promotion and Maintenance
Integrated Process: Nursing Process/Evaluation
Content Area: Child Health

Reference:
Wong, D., & Hockenberry, M. (2003). *Wong's nursing care of infants and children* (7th ed.). St. Louis: Mosby, p. 1509.

26. A client has been given a prescription for a course of azithromycin (Zithromax). The nurse determines that the medication is having the intended effect if which of the following is noted?

 1 Signs and symptoms of infection are relieved.
 2 Pain is relieved.
 3 Joint discomfort is reduced.
 4 Blood pressure is lowered.

Answer: 1

Rationale: Azithromycin is a macrolide antibiotic, which is used to treat infection. It is not ordered for the treatment of pain, joint discomfort, or blood pressure.

Test-Taking Strategy: Use the process of elimination. Eliminate options 2 and 3 first because they are similar. From the remaining options, recalling the action of this medication will direct you to option 1. Review the action and purpose of azithromycin if you had difficulty with this question.

Level of Cognitive Ability: Analysis
Client Needs: Physiological Integrity
Integrated Process: Nursing Process/Evaluation
Content Area: Pharmacology

References:
Lehne, R. (2004). *Pharmacology for nursing care* (5th ed.). Philadelphia: Saunders, p. 911.
McKenry, L., & Salerno, E. (2003). *Mosby's pharmacology in nursing* (21st ed.). St. Louis: Mosby, p. 995.

27. A nurse is assigned to care for a client with acquired immunodeficiency syndrome (AIDS) who is receiving amphotericin B (Fungizone) for a fungal respiratory infection. Which of the following would indicate an adverse reaction to the medication?
1 Hypocalcemia
2 Hypokalemia
3 Hypercalcemia
4 Hyperkalemia

Answer: 2
Rationale: Clients receiving amphotericin B may develop hypokalemia, which can be severe and lead to extreme muscle weakness and electrocardiogram (ECG) changes. Distal renal tubular acidosis commonly occurs, contributing to the development of hypokalemia. High potassium levels do not occur. The medication does not cause calcium levels to fluctuate.

Test-Taking Strategy: Note that the medication is an antifungal. Recalling that an adverse reaction to amphotericin B is hypokalemia is necessary to answer the question. Review this medication if you had difficulty with this question.

Level of Cognitive Ability: Analysis
Client Needs: Physiological Integrity
Integrated Process: Nursing Process/Evaluation
Content Area: Pharmacology

Reference:
McKenry, L., & Salerno, E. (2003). *Mosby's pharmacology in nursing* (21st ed.). St. Louis: Mosby, p. 1015.

28. A client is seen in the health care clinic, and a diagnosis of conjunctivitis is made. The nurse provides instructions to the client regarding care of the disorder while at home. Which statement by the client indicates a need for further instructions?
1 "I should apply warm compresses before instilling antibiotic drops if purulent discharge is present in my eye."
2 "I do not need to be concerned about spreading this infection to others in my family."
3 "I should perform a saline eye irrigation before instilling the antibiotic drops into my eye if purulent discharge is present."
4 "I can use an ophthalmic analgesic ointment at nighttime if I have eye discomfort."

Answer: 2
Rationale: Conjunctivitis is highly contagious. Antibiotic drops are usually administered four times a day. When purulent discharge is present, saline eye irrigations or eye applications of warm compresses may be necessary before instilling the medication. Ophthalmic analgesic ointment or drops may be instilled, especially at bedtime, because discomfort becomes more noticeable when the eyelids are closed.

Test-Taking Strategy: Use the process of elimination, noting the key words "need for further instructions." Knowing that this disorder is considered highly contagious will direct you to option 2. Review management of the client with this disorder if you have difficulty with this question.

Level of Cognitive Ability: Analysis
Client Needs: Health Promotion and Maintenance
Integrated Process: Nursing Process/Evaluation
Content Area: Adult Health/Eye

References:
Black, J., & Hawks, J. (2005). *Medical-surgical nursing: Clinical management for positive outcomes* (7th ed.). Philadelphia: Saunders, p. 1963.
Ignatavicius, D., & Workman, M. (2002). *Medical surgical nursing: Critical thinking for collaborative care* (4th ed.). Philadelphia: Saunders, p. 1029.

29. A nurse reviews the nursing care plan of a hospitalized child who is immobilized because of skeletal traction. The nurse notes a nursing diagnosis of Delayed Growth and Development related to immobilization and hospitalization. Which evaluative statement indicates a positive outcome for the child?

1 The fracture heals without complications.
2 The child displays age-appropriate developmental behaviors.
3 The caregivers verbalize safe and effective home care.
4 The child maintains normal joint and muscle integrity.

Answer: 2

Rationale: Regression and inappropriate developmental behaviors may be displayed in response to immobilization and hospitalization. With individualized care planning, a positive outcome of age-appropriate behavior can be achieved. Options 1, 3, and 4 are appropriate evaluative statements for an immobilized child but do not directly address the nursing diagnosis, Delayed Growth and Development.

Test-Taking Strategy: Focus on the issue: "Delayed Growth and Development." Recalling that Delayed Growth and Development is the state in which an individual is not performing age-appropriate tasks will direct you to option 2. All options are evaluative statements, but only option 2 addresses this nursing diagnosis. Review the defining characteristics and the appropriate outcomes for this nursing diagnosis if you had difficulty with this question.

Level of Cognitive Ability: Analysis
Client Needs: Health Promotion and Maintenance
Integrated Process: Nursing Process/Evaluation
Content Area: Child Health

Reference:
Wong, D., & Hockenberry, M. (2003). *Wong's nursing care of infants and children* (7th ed.). St. Louis: Mosby, pp. 1761-1762.

---

30. A nurse is evaluating the effects of care for the client with nephrotic syndrome. The nurse determines that the client showed the least amount of improvement if which of the following information was obtained serially over 2 days of care?

1 Initial weight 208 pounds, down to 203 pounds
2 Daily intake and output record of 2100 mL intake and 1900 mL output, and 2000 mL intake and 2900 mL output
3 Blood pressure 160/90 mmHg, down to 130/78 mmHg
4 Serum albumin 1.9 g/dL, up to 2.0 g/dL

Answer: 4

Rationale: The goal of therapy in nephrotic syndrome is to heal the leaking glomerular membrane. This would then control edema by stopping the loss of protein in the urine. Fluid balance and albumin levels are monitored to determine effectiveness of therapy. Option 1 represents a loss of fluid that slightly exceeds 2 liters and represents a significant improvement. Option 2 represents a total fluid loss of 700 mL over the 2 days, which is also helpful. Option 3 shows improvement because both systolic and diastolic blood pressures are lower. The least amount of improvement is in the serum albumin level, because the normal albumin level is 3.5 to 5.0 g/dL.

Test-Taking Strategy: Use the process of elimination, noting the key words "least amount of improvement." Option 1 illustrates the greatest improvement and is eliminated first. Option 2 is also a significant improvement and is eliminated next. From the remaining options, noting that the blood pressure has decreased significantly will direct you to option 4. Review care of the client with nephrotic syndrome if you had difficulty with this question.

Level of Cognitive Ability: Analysis
Client Needs: Physiological Integrity
Integrated Process: Nursing Process/Evaluation
Content Area: Adult Health/Renal

Reference:
Ignatavicius, D., & Workman, M. (2002). *Medical surgical nursing: Critical thinking for collaborative care* (4th ed.). Philadelphia: Saunders, p. 1654.

31. A client is being discharged to home after application of a plaster leg cast. The nurse determines that the client understands proper care of the cast if the client states to:
1 Avoid getting the cast wet
2 Use the fingertips to lift and move the leg
3 Cover the casted leg with warm blankets
4 Use a padded coat hanger end to scratch under the cast

Answer: 1
Rationale: A plaster cast must remain dry to keep its strength. The cast should be handled using the palms of the hands, not the fingertips, until fully dry. Air should circulate freely around the cast to help it dry. Additionally, the cast also gives off heat as it dries. The client should never scratch under the cast. A cool hair dryer may be used to relieve an itch.

Test-Taking Strategy: Use the process of elimination, noting the key word "plaster." Option 4 is dangerous to skin integrity and is eliminated first. Knowing that a wet cast can be dented with the fingertips causing pressure underneath helps eliminate option 2. Recalling that the cast needs to dry eliminates option 3. Remember that plaster casts, once they have dried after application, should not become wet. Review home care instructions for a client with a plaster cast if you had difficulty with this question.

Level of Cognitive Ability: Analysis
Client Needs: Health Promotion and Maintenance
Integrated Process: Nursing Process/Evaluation
Content Area: Adult Health/Musculoskeletal

Reference:
Black, J., & Hawks, J. (2005). *Medical-surgical nursing: Clinical management for positive outcomes* (7th ed.). Philadelphia: Saunders, p. 631.

32. A client is being discharged to home while recovering from acute renal failure (ARF). The client indicates an understanding of the therapeutic dietary regimen if the client states to eat foods that are lower in:
1 Vitamins
2 Potassium
3 Carbohydrates
4 Fats

Answer: 2
Rationale: Most of the excretion of potassium and the control of potassium balance are normal functions of the kidneys. In the client with renal failure, potassium intake must be restricted as much as possible (30 to 50 mEq/day). The primary mechanism of potassium removal during ARF is dialysis. Options 1, 3, and 4 are not normally restricted in the client with ARF unless a secondary health problem warrants the need to do so.

Test-Taking Strategy: Noting the diagnosis of the client will assist in answering the question. Recalling that potassium balance and excretion is controlled by the kidney will direct you to option 2. Review the therapeutic diet in the client with ARF if you had difficulty with this question.

Level of Cognitive Ability: Analysis
Client Needs: Health Promotion and Maintenance
Integrated Process: Nursing Process/Evaluation
Content Area: Adult Health/Renal

Reference:
Black, J., & Hawks, J. (2005). *Medical-surgical nursing: Clinical management for positive outcomes* (7th ed.). Philadelphia: Saunders, p. 946.

33. A client being discharged from the mental health unit has a history of anxiety and command hallucinations to harm self or others. The nurse teaches the client about interventions for hallucinations and anxiety. The nurse determines that the client understands these measures when the client says:

1 "If I take my medication, I won't be anxious."

2 "I can call my clinical specialist when I'm hallucinating so that I can talk about my feelings and plans and not hurt anyone."

3 "I can go to group and talk about my feelings."

4 "If I get enough sleep and eat well, I won't get anxious and hear things."

Answer: 2

Rationale: There may be an increased risk for impulsive and/or aggressive behavior if a client is receiving command hallucinations to harm self or others. The client should be asked if he or she has intentions to hurt self or others. Talking about auditory hallucinations can interfere with subvocal muscular activity associated with a hallucination. Options 1, 3, and 4 are general interventions but are not specific to anxiety and hallucinations.

Test-Taking Strategy: Use the process of elimination. Focus on the issue: anxiety and hallucinations. Options 1, 3, and 4 are all interventions that a client can do to aid wellness. Option 2 is specific to the issue and indicates self-responsible commitment and control over own behavior. Review interventions for anxiety and hallucinations if you had difficulty with this question.

Level of Cognitive Ability: Analysis
Client Needs: Psychosocial Integrity
Integrated Process: Nursing Process/Evaluation
Content Area: Mental Health

Reference:
Keltner, N., Schwecke, L., & Bostrom, C. (2003). *Psychiatric nursing* (4th ed.). St. Louis: Mosby, pp. 107; 109.

34. A perinatal client has been instructed on the prevention of genital tract infections. Which statement by the client indicates an understanding of these preventive measures?

1 "I should avoid the use of condoms."

2 "I can douche anytime I want."

3 "I can wear my tight-fitting jeans."

4 "I should wear underwear with a cotton panel liner."

Answer: 4

Rationale: Condoms should be used to minimize the spread of genital tract infections. Wearing tight clothes irritates the genital area and does not allow for air circulation. Douching is to be avoided. Wearing items with a cotton panel liner allows for air movement in and around the genital area.

Test-Taking Strategy: Use the process of elimination, noting the key words "indicates an understanding." Options 1, 2, and 3 are all incorrect statements regarding client self-care. Review prevention measures associated with genital tract infections if you had difficulty with this question.

Level of Cognitive Ability: Analysis
Client Needs: Health Promotion and Maintenance
Integrated Process: Nursing Process/Evaluation
Content Area: Maternity/Antepartum

Reference:
Lowdermilk, D., & Perry, A. (2004). *Maternity & women's health care* (8th ed.). St. Louis: Mosby, p. 209.

35. A nurse has given a client information about the use of nitroglycerin sublingual tablets. The client has an order for prn use if chest pain occurs. The nurse determines that the client understands how to self-administer the medication if the client stated to:

1 Avoid using the medication until chest pain actually begins and intensifies

2 Take acetylsalicylic acid (aspirin) to treat a headache that occurs with early use of nitroglycerin

3 Discard unused nitroglycerin tablets 6 to 9 months after the bottle is opened and obtain a new prescription

4 Keep nitroglycerin in a shirt pocket close to the body

Answer: 3

Rationale: Nitroglycerin may be self-administered sublingually 5 to 10 minutes before an activity that triggers chest pain. Tablets should be discarded 6 to 9 months after opening the bottle, and a new bottle of pills should be obtained from the pharmacy. Nitroglycerin is unstable and is affected by heat and cold, so it should not be kept close to the body (warmth) in a shirt pocket, but rather it should be kept in a jacket pocket or purse. Headache often occurs with early use and diminishes in time. Acetaminophen (Tylenol) may be used to treat headache.

Test-Taking Strategy: Use the process of elimination, noting the key words "understands how to self-administer the medication." Recalling that nitroglycerin loses its potency in 6 to 9 months will direct you to option 3. Review the client teaching points related to nitroglycerin if you had difficulty with this question.

Level of Cognitive Ability: Analysis
Client Needs: Health Promotion and Maintenance
Integrated Process: Nursing Process/Evaluation
Content Area: Pharmacology

References:
Lehne, R. (2004). *Pharmacology for nursing care* (5th ed.). Philadelphia: Saunders, p. 541.
McKenry, L., & Salerno, E. (2003). *Mosby's pharmacology in nursing* (21st ed.). St. Louis: Mosby, pp. 89-90; 609-610.

CARING

1. A woman comes into the emergency room in a severe state of anxiety following a car accident. The most important nursing intervention at this time would be to:

1 Remain with the client

2 Put the client in a quiet room

3 Teach the client deep breathing exercises

4 Encourage the client to talk about her feelings and concerns

Answer: 1

Rationale: If the client is left alone with severe anxiety, she or he may feel abandoned and become overwhelmed. Placing the client in a quiet room is also indicated, but the nurse must stay with the client. It is not possible to teach the client deep breathing or relaxation exercises until the anxiety decreases. Encouraging the client to discuss concerns and feelings would not take place until the anxiety has decreased.

Test-Taking Strategy: Note the key words "severe state of anxiety." Because the anxiety state is "severe," eliminate options 3 and 4. From the remaining options, consider the words "most important" in the stem of the question. This should direct you to option 1. Review care of the client with severe anxiety if you had difficulty with this question.

Level of Cognitive Ability: Application
Client Needs: Psychosocial Integrity
Integrated Process: Caring
Content Area: Mental Health

Reference:
Varcarolis, E.M. (2002). *Foundations of psychiatric mental health nursing* (4th ed.). Philadelphia: Saunders, p. 288.

2. A nurse has cared for a client who died a few minutes ago. The nurse reflects on the care given to the client. Which statement supports the nurse's belief that the client died with dignity?
   1 The family thanks the nurse and states that the client was not in pain and was peaceful at the end.
   2 The physician recognizes that all the orders were carried out and there were no questions.
   3 A new nurse states it is difficult to give that kind of care to a dying client.
   4 The nurse gave increasing doses of pain medication to keep the client well sedated.

Answer: 1

Rationale: The family response is an external perception and is extremely important. Families derive a great deal of comfort from knowing their loved one received the best care possible. Option 1 provides external validation that the client received comprehensive, quality care. Option 2 focuses on physician's orders rather than client care. Option 3 focuses on the feelings of a new nurse, who may be expressing his or her own anxiety. Option 4 reflects on only one aspect of caring for a dying client.

Test-Taking Strategy: Use the process of elimination and focus on the issue: that the client died with dignity. The only option that addresses this issue is option 1. Review the concepts related to death and dying if you had difficulty with this question.

Level of Cognitive Ability: Analysis
Client Needs: Psychosocial Integrity
Integrated Process: Caring
Content Area: Fundamental Skills

Reference:
Phipps, W., Monahan, F., Sands, J., Marek, J., & Neighbors, M. (2003). *Medical-surgical nursing: Health and illness perspectives* (7th ed.). St. Louis: Mosby, p. 101.

3. The family of a client with Parkinson's disease tells the nurse that the client is having difficulty adjusting to the disorder and that they do not know what to do to help. The nurse advises the family that which of the following would be therapeutic in assisting the client to cope with the disease?
   1 Encourage and praise client efforts to exercise and perform activities of daily living (ADLs)
   2 Cluster activities at the end of the day when the client is restless and bored
   3 Plan only a few activities for the client during the day
   4 Assist the client with ADLs as much as possible

Answer: 1

Rationale: The client with Parkinson's disease has a tendency to become withdrawn and depressed, which can be limited by encouraging the client to be an active participant in his or her own care. The family should also give the client encouragement and praise for perseverance in these efforts. The family should plan activities intermittently throughout the day to inhibit daytime sleeping and boredom.

Test-Taking Strategy: Use the process of elimination. Eliminate option 2 first because clustering activities at one time will tire the client. Eliminate option 3 next because of the use of the absolute word "only." From the remaining options, recalling that the client should be an active participant in his or her own care will direct you to option 1. Review therapeutic techniques for the client with Parkinson's disease to assist with adjustment to the disease if you had difficulty with this question.

Level of Cognitive Ability: Application
Client Needs: Psychosocial Integrity
Integrated Process: Caring
Content Area: Adult Health/Neurological

Reference:
Phipps, W., Monahan, F., Sands, J., Marek, J., & Neighbors, M. (2003). *Medical-surgical nursing: Health and illness perspectives* (7th ed.). St. Louis: Mosby, p. 1393.

4. A community health nurse is caring for a group of homeless people in a certain area of a city. In planning for the potential needs of this group, what is the most immediate concern?

1 Peer support through structured groups
2 Setting up a 24-hour crisis center and hotline
3 Meeting the basic needs to ensure that adequate food, shelter, and clothing are available
4 Finding affordable housing for the group

Answer: 3

Rationale: The question asks about the immediate concern. The ABCs of community health are always attending to people's basic needs of food, shelter, and clothing. Options 1, 2, and 4 are other activities that may be carried out at a later time.

Test-Taking Strategy: Use Maslow's hierarchy of needs theory to answer the question. Option 3 addresses basic physiological needs. Although options 1, 2, and 4 are also appropriate actions, option 3 is the immediate concern. Review the needs of the homeless population if you had difficulty with this question.

Level of Cognitive Ability: Analysis
Client Needs: Physiological Integrity
Integrated Process: Caring
Content Area: Delegating/Prioritizing

Reference:

Keltner, N., Schwecke, L., & Bostrom, C. (2003). *Psychiatric nursing* (4th ed.). St. Louis: Mosby, p. 84.

---

5. A stillborn was delivered a few hours ago. After the birth, the family has remained together, holding and touching the baby. Which statement by the nurse would further assist the family in their initial period of grief?

1 "I feel so bad. I don't understand why this happened either."
2 "You can hold the baby for another 15 minutes, but then I need to take the baby away."
3 "What did you name your baby?"
4 "You seem upset. Do you need a tranquilizer?"

Answer: 3

Rationale: Nurses should be able to explore measures that assist the family to create memories of an infant so that the existence of the child is confirmed and the parents can complete the grieving process. Option 3 identifies this measure and also demonstrates a caring and empathetic response. Option 1 is inappropriate and reflects a lack of knowledge on the nurse's part. Option 2 is uncaring. Option 4 devalues the parents' feelings and is inappropriate.

Test-Taking Strategy: Note the key words "further assist the family in their initial period of grief." Use the process of elimination and therapeutic communication techniques. Choose the option that demonstrates a caring and empathetic response by the nurse and meets the psychosocial needs of the client and family. Review therapeutic communication techniques and the grief process if you had difficulty with this question.

Level of Cognitive Ability: Application
Client Needs: Psychosocial Integrity
Integrated Process: Caring
Content Area: Maternity/Postpartum

References:

Murray, S., McKinney, E., & Gorrie, T. (2002). *Foundations of maternal-newborn nursing* (3rd ed.). Philadelphia: Saunders, p. 649.
Wong, D., & Hockenberry, M. (2003). *Wong's nursing care of infants and children* (7th ed.). St. Louis: Mosby, pp. 369-370.

6. While counseling a prenatal client about her dietary and alcohol drinking habits, the nurse observes that the client has difficulty concentrating and appears agitated. The nurse should proceed with the assessment using which guideline?
1 Discussion of possible consequences to drinking alcohol during pregnancy should be avoided
2 Women respond negatively to a hopeful message of the potential benefits of drinking cessation during pregnancy
3 A nonjudgmental approach may help gain maternal trust
4 Provoking maternal guilt may help a woman recognize her problem and seek support services

Answer: 3
Rationale: The potential effects of alcohol abuse during pregnancy for both the mother and fetus have been well documented. The nurse who expresses genuine concern with suspected abusers may motivate positive behavioral changes during the prenatal period. The maternal behaviors of lack of concentration and agitation are frequently seen in childbearing women abusing alcohol. Options 1, 2, and 4 are inappropriate guidelines for the nurse to follow in this situation, and they do not address a caring approach.

Test-Taking Strategy: Use therapeutic communication techniques and the process of elimination. Remember that it is important to display a caring and nonjudgmental attitude. This will direct you to option 3. Review therapeutic communication techniques if you had difficulty with this question.

Level of Cognitive Ability: Application
Clients Needs: Psychosocial Integrity
Integrated Process: Caring
Content Area: Maternity/Antepartum

Reference:
Lowdermilk, D., & Perry, A. (2004). *Maternity & women's health care* (8th ed.). St. Louis: Mosby, p. 126.

7. A client was injured in an automobile accident as a result of passing out from drinking alcohol and falling asleep at the wheel of the car. The client's only daughter, who was a passenger in the car, was killed instantly. In report, the nurse is told that the client is upset and withdrawn. When caring for the client, what is the nurse's appropriate initial action?
1 Let the client have some time alone to grieve over the loss
2 Tell the client that the injury and the daughter's death was a result of alcohol abuse and refer the client for counseling
3 Inform the physician of the client's depression and request medication to assist the client in coping with the loss
4 Reflect back to the client that he or she appears upset

Answer: 4
Rationale: The nurse needs to encourage the client to express feelings. Reflection statements tend to elicit deeper awareness of feelings. Additionally, option 4 validates the perception that the client is upset. A well-timed reflection can reveal an emotion that has escaped the client's notice. Option 2 is inappropriate and is a block to communication. Options 1 and 3 address interventions before assessing the situation.

Test-Taking Strategy: Note the key words "appropriate initial." Use therapeutic communication techniques and the process of elimination. Select the option that encourages the client to express feelings and talk more. Remember to always address the client's feelings. Review therapeutic communication techniques if you had difficulty with this question.

Level of Cognitive Ability: Application
Client Needs: Psychosocial Integrity
Integrated Process: Caring
Content Area: Mental Health

Reference:
Keltner, N., Schwecke, L., & Bostrom, C. (2003). *Psychiatric nursing* (4th ed.). St. Louis: Mosby, p. 96.

8. An emergency room nurse is assigned to care for an older client who has been identified as a victim of physical abuse. In planning care for this client, the nurse's priority is focused toward:

1 Referring the abusing family member for treatment
2 Adhering to the mandatory abuse reporting laws
3 Encouraging the client to file charges against the abuser
4 Removing the client from any immediate danger

Answer: 4

Rationale: Whenever the abused client remains in the abusive environment, priority must be placed on ascertaining whether the person is in any immediate danger. If so, emergency action must be taken to remove the person from the abusing situation. Options 1 and 2 may be appropriate interventions but are not the priority. Option 3 is not an appropriate intervention at this time and may produce increased fear and anxiety in the client.

Test-Taking Strategy: Use the process of elimination and eliminate option 3 first, knowing that this action may produce increased fear and anxiety in the client. Use Maslow's hierarchy of needs theory to select from the remaining options, remembering that if a physiological need is not present, then safety is the priority. This guide should direct you to option 4, the only option that directly addresses client safety. Review the principles related to caring for the abused client if you had difficulty with this question.

Level of Cognitive Ability: Application
Client Needs: Safe, Effective Care Environment
Integrated Process: Caring
Content Area: Mental Health

Reference:
Varcarolis, E.M. (2002). *Foundations of psychiatric mental health nursing* (4th ed.). Philadelphia: Saunders, p. 703.

9. A community health nurse is working with older residents involved in a recent flood. Many of the residents were emotionally despondent and refused to leave their homes for days. In planning for the rescue and relocation of these older residents, what is the first item the nurse needs to consider?

1 Attending to the emotional needs of the older residents
2 Attending to the nutritional status and basic needs of the older residents
3 Contacting the older residents' families
4 Arranging for ambulance transportation for the older residents

Answer: 2

Rationale: The question asks about the first thing that the nurse needs to consider. The ABCs of community health are always attending to people's basic needs of food, shelter, and clothing. Options 1, 3, and 4 are other activities that may or may not be needed at a later date.

Test-Taking Strategy: Use Maslow's hierarchy of needs theory to answer the question. Option 2 addresses basic physiological needs. Although options 1, 3, and 4 may be appropriate actions at a later time, option 2 is the immediate concern. Review care of clients experiencing crisis if you had difficulty with this question.

Level of Cognitive Ability: Application
Client Needs: Physiological Integrity
Integrated Process: Caring
Content Area: Delegating/Prioritizing

Reference:
Stuart, G., & Laraia, M. (2005). *Principles and practice of psychiatric nursing* (8th ed.). St. Louis: Mosby, pp. 234-235; 244.

10. A nurse is assisting in planning care for a suicidal client newly admitted to the mental health unit. In order to provide a caring, therapeutic environment, which of the following is included in the nursing care plan?

1 Placing the client in a private room to ensure privacy and confidentiality

2 Establishing a therapeutic relationship and conveying unconditional positive regard

3 Placing the client in charge of a meaningful unit activity, such as the morning chess tournament

4 Maintaining a distance of 10 inches at all times to ensure the client that control will be provided

Answer: 2

Rationale: The establishment of a therapeutic relationship with the suicidal client increases feelings of acceptance. While the suicidal behavior and thinking of the client is unacceptable, the use of unconditional positive regard acknowledges the client in a human-to-human context and increases the client's sense of self-worth. The client would not be placed in a private room because this is an unsafe action and may intensify the client's feelings of worthlessness. Placing the client in charge of the morning chess game is a premature intervention that can overwhelm and cause the client to fail. This can reinforce the client's feelings of worthlessness. Distances of 18 inches or less between two individuals constitutes intimate space. Invasion of this space may be misinterpreted by the client and increase the client's tension and feelings of helplessness.

Test-Taking Strategy: Use the process of elimination. Eliminate option 1 because isolation (private room) is not the safe and therapeutic intervention. Option 3 may produce feelings of worthlessness. Eliminate option 4 because a distance of 10 inches is restrictive. Option 2 is the only option that addresses a caring and therapeutic environment. Review care of the suicidal client if you had difficulty with this question.

Level of Cognitive Ability: Application
Client Needs: Psychosocial Integrity
Integrated Process: Caring
Content Area: Mental Health

References:
Keltner, N., Schwecke, L., & Bostrom, C. (2003). *Psychiatric nursing* (4th ed.). St. Louis: Mosby, p. 356.
Varcarolis, E.M. (2002). *Foundations of psychiatric mental health nursing* (4th ed.). Philadelphia: Saunders, p. 487.

11. A client has died, and when the nurse asks a family member about the funeral arrangements, the family member refuses to discuss the issue. The nurse's most appropriate action is to:

1 Provide information needed for decision making

2 Refer the family member to a mental health professional because the family member may be at risk of self-harm

3 Demonstrate acceptance of the family member's feelings

4 Remain with the family member without discussing funeral arrangements

Answer: 4

Rationale: The family member is exhibiting the first stage of grief, denial. Option 1 may be an appropriate intervention for the bargaining stage. Option 2 may be an appropriate intervention for the depression stage. Option 3 is an appropriate intervention for the acceptance or reorganization and restitution stage.

Test-Taking Strategy: Note the key words "most appropriate action." Focus on the issue: that the family member refuses to discuss the funeral arrangements. Eliminate options 1 and 2 because they do not address the issue of the question. From the remaining options, noting the key words "refuses to discuss the issue" will direct you to option 4. Acceptance of feelings is important, but in this situation, remaining with the family member is most appropriate. Review the grieving process if you had difficulty with this question.

Level of Cognitive Ability: Application
Client Needs: Psychosocial Integrity
Integrated Process: Caring
Content Area: Fundamental Skills

Reference:
Phipps, W., Monahan, F., Sands, J., Marek, J., & Neighbors, M. (2003). *Medical-surgical nursing: Health and illness perspectives* (7th ed.). St. Louis: Mosby, p. 112.

---

12. A 39-year-old man learned today that his 36-year-old wife has an incurable cancer and is expected to live not more than a few weeks. The nurse explores the client's feelings and identifies which of these responses by the husband as indicative of a normal and expected individual coping response?

1 He states that he will not allow his wife to come home to die.

2 He immediately arranges for their three teenaged children to live with relatives in another state.

3 He expresses his anger at God and the physicians for allowing this to happen.

4 He refuses to visit his wife in the hospital or to discuss her illness.

Answer: 3

Rationale: The expression of anger is known to be a normal response to impending loss, and the anger may be directed toward self, the dying person, God or other spiritual being, or the caregivers. Options 1 and 2 indicate possibly rash and unilateral decisions made by the husband, without taking into consideration anyone else's feelings. There is evidence of denial in option 4, because he refuses to visit or discuss his wife's illness. The only response that indicates a normal and expected individual coping response by the husband is option 3.

Test-Taking Strategy: Note the key words "a normal and expected individual coping response." Recalling the stages of grief associated with loss will direct you to option 3. Review effective coping mechanisms if you had difficulty with this question.

Level of Cognitive Ability: Analysis
Client Needs: Psychosocial Integrity
Integrated Process: Caring
Content Area: Fundamental Skills

Reference:
Black, J., & Hawks, J. (2005). *Medical-surgical nursing: Clinical management for positive outcomes* (7th ed.). Philadelphia: Saunders, p. 390.

---

13. A nurse is providing care to a Cuban American client who is terminally ill. Numerous family members are present most of the time, and many of the family members are very emotional. The appropriate nursing action is to:

1 Restrict the number of family members visiting at one time

2 Inform the family that emotional outbursts must be avoided

3 Request permission to move the client to a private room and allow the family members to visit

4 Contact the physician to speak to the family regarding their behaviors

Answer: 3

Rationale: In the Cuban American culture, loud crying and other physical manifestations of grief are considered socially acceptable. Of the options provided, option 3 is the only option that identifies a culturally sensitive and caring approach on the part of the nurse. Options 1, 2, and 4 are inappropriate nursing interventions.

Test-Taking Strategy: Focus on the client(s) of the question, which are the family members of a Cuban American client. Use the process of elimination, recalling the characteristics of this culture and the importance of cultural sensitivity. This will direct you to option 3. Review the characteristics of this culture if you had difficulty with this question.

Level of Cognitive Ability: Application
Client Needs: Psychosocial Integrity
Integrated Process: Caring
Content Area: Fundamental Skills

References:
Lewis, S., Heitkemper, M., & Dirksen, S. (2004). *Medical-surgical nursing: Assessment and management of clinical problems* (6th ed.). St. Louis: Mosby, pp. 20-21.
Riley, J. (2004). *Communication in nursing* (5th ed.). St. Louis: Mosby, pp. 54; 57-58.

14. A nurse is caring for an older client who has been recently admitted to a long-term care facility from home. The client has a diagnosis of end-stage renal cancer. The nurse recognizes that the client is coping with many losses. The best way to address the client's psychosocial needs is to:
1 Provide total care for the client
2 Medicate the client for pain every 4 hours as prescribed
3 Sit with the client to allow the client to verbalize feelings
4 Encourage the client to participate in daily social activities

Answer: 3

Rationale: Clients admitted into a long-term care facility from home are dealing with losses in control over their environment, independence, and privacy. Providing total care does not facilitate independence. Medicating for pain will keep the client comfortable, but this does not address psychosocial needs. Sitting with the client to allow the client to express feelings is the best way to address psychosocial needs. Participation in daily social activities will not meet the special psychosocial needs of this client.

Test-Taking Strategy: Focus on the key words: "psychosocial needs." Eliminate options 1 and 2 first because these options deal with physiological needs. From the remaining options, recall that the client's feelings should be addressed first. This will direct you to option 3. Review care of the client experiencing loss if you had difficulty with this question.

Level of Cognitive Ability: Application
Client Needs: Psychosocial Integrity
Integrated Process: Caring
Content Area: Fundamental Skills

Reference:
Potter, P., & Perry, A. (2005). *Fundamentals of nursing* (6th ed.). St. Louis: Mosby, pp. 573; 605.

---

15. A client with diabetes mellitus is told that amputation of the leg is necessary to sustain life. The client is very upset and states to the nurse: "This is all the doctor's fault! I have done everything that the doctor has asked me to do!" The nurse interprets the client's statement as:
1 An expected coping mechanism
2 A need to notify the hospital lawyer
3 An expression of guilt on the part of the client
4 An ineffective coping mechanism

Answer: 1

Rationale: The expression of anger is known to be a normal response to impending loss, and the anger may be directed toward self, God or other spiritual being, or the caregivers. The nurse needs to be aware of the effective and ineffective coping mechanisms that can occur in a client when loss is anticipated. Notifying the hospital lawyer is inappropriate. Guilt may or may not be a component of the client's feelings, and the data in the question does not provide an indication that guilt is present.

Test-Taking Strategy: Focus on the data provided in the question. Note that options 1 and 4 address coping mechanisms. This may provide you with the clue that one of these may be the correct option. Noting that the client is blaming the doctor and knowledge of the stages of grief associated with loss will direct you to option 1. Review these stages and expected client expressions if you had difficulty with this question.

Level of Cognitive Ability: Analysis
Client Needs: Psychosocial Integrity
Integrated Process: Caring
Content Area: Fundamental Skills

Reference:
Black, J., & Hawks, J. (2005). *Medical-surgical nursing: Clinical management for positive outcomes* (7th ed.). Philadelphia: Saunders, p. 1524.

16. A nurse has been caring for a terminally ill client whose death is imminent. The nurse has developed a close relationship with the family of the client. Which nursing intervention will the nurse avoid in dealing with the family during this difficult time?
1 Making decisions for the family during the difficult moments
2 Encouraging family discussion of feelings
3 Facilitating the use of spiritual practices identified by the family
4 Accepting the family's expressions of anger

Answer: 1

Rationale: Maintaining effective and open communication among family members affected by death and grief is of utmost importance. The nurse needs to maintain and enhance communication as well as preserve the family's sense of self-direction and control. Option 2 is likely to enhance communications. Option 3 is also an effective intervention, because spiritual practices give meaning to life and affect how people react to crisis. Option 4 is also an effective technique, and the family needs to know that someone will be there who is supportive and nonjudgmental. Option 1 removes autonomy and decision making from the family at a time when they are already experiencing feelings of loss of control. This is an ineffective intervention that can impair communication.

Test-Taking Strategy: Note the key word "avoid" in the stem of the question. This word indicates a false-response question and that you need to select the incorrect intervention. Using therapeutic communication techniques will direct you to option 1. Review therapeutic techniques for individuals in crisis if you had difficulty with this question.

Level of Cognitive Ability: Application
Client Needs: Psychosocial Integrity
Integrated Process: Caring
Content Area: Fundamental Skills

Reference:
Black, J., & Hawks, J. (2005). *Medical-surgical nursing: Clinical management for positive outcomes* (7th ed.). Philadelphia: Saunders, p. 500.

17. A client brought to the emergency room is dead on arrival (DOA). The family of the client tells the physician that the client had terminal cancer. The emergency room physician examines the client and asks the nurse to contact the medical examiner regarding an autopsy. The family of the client tells the nurse that they do not want an autopsy performed. The nurse makes which response to the family?
1 "It is required by federal law. Why don't we talk about it and why don't you tell me how you feel?"
2 "The decision is made by the medical examiner."
3 "I will contact the medical examiner regarding your request."
4 "An autopsy is mandatory for any client who is DOA."

Answer: 3

Rationale: An autopsy is required by state law in certain circumstances, including the sudden death of a client and a death that occurs under suspicious circumstances. It is not a requirement by federal law. It is not mandatory that every client who is DOA have an autopsy. If a family requests not to have an autopsy performed on a family member, then the nurse should contact the medical examiner about the request.

Test-Taking Strategy: Use knowledge regarding the laws and issues surrounding autopsy and therapeutic communication techniques to answer the question. Eliminate options 1 and 4 because these statements are not accurate. From the remaining options, option 3 is the most therapeutic and caring response to the family. Review the issues and laws surrounding autopsy if you had difficulty with this question.

Level of Cognitive Ability: Application
Client Needs: Safe, Effective Care Environment
Integrated Process: Caring
Content Area: Fundamental Skills

Reference:
Potter, P., & Perry, A. (2005). *Fundamentals of nursing* (6th ed.). St. Louis: Mosby, pp. 412; 589.

18. An older client with coronary heart disease is scheduled for hospital discharge and lives alone. The client states, "I don't know how I'll be able to remember all these instructions and take care of myself once I get home." The nurse plans to take which action to assist the client?

1 Ask an out-of-town relative to stay with the client for a day or so

2 Ask the physician to delay the discharge until the client is better able to manage self-care

3 Suggest that the social worker follow up with a telephone call after discharge to ensure that the client is progressing

4 Suggest that the physician be asked for a referral to a home health agency for nursing and home health aide support

Answer: 4

Rationale: With earlier hospital discharge, clients are returning home with greater acuity of problems than was previously true, and they may require support from a home health agency until they are independent in functioning. Option 3 does nothing to actively assist the client, and option 2 is not realistic in the current health care environment. Although option 1 is a viable option, it does not ensure the client continued care until the client is able to be independent in managing own care.

Test-Taking Strategy: Focus on the issue of the question and the client's concern. Use the process of elimination, noting that option 4 is the only action that will ensure that the client has the necessary assistance until independence is achieved. Review home care support services if you had difficulty with this question.

Level of Cognitive Ability: Application
Client Needs: Safe, Effective Care Environment
Integrated Process: Caring
Content Area: Fundamental Skills

Reference:
Potter, P., & Perry, A. (2005). *Fundamentals of nursing* (6th ed.). St. Louis: Mosby, pp. 35-36.

---

19. A nurse is interacting with the family of a client who is unconscious as a result of a head injury. Which approach should the nurse use to help the family cope with this situation?

1 Enforce adherence to visiting hours to ensure the client's rest

2 Encourage the family not to "give in" to their feelings of grief

3 Discourage the family from touching the client

4 Explain equipment and procedures on an ongoing basis

Answer: 4

Rationale: Families often need assistance to cope with the sudden severe illness of a loved one. The nurse should explain all equipment, treatments, and procedures, and supplement or reinforce information given by the physician. Family should be encouraged to touch and speak to the client and to become involved in the client's care in some way if they are comfortable with this. The nurse should allow the family to stay with the client whenever possible. The nurse also encourages the family to eat properly and to obtain enough sleep to maintain their strength.

Test-Taking Strategy: Use therapeutic communication techniques to answer this question. Each of the incorrect options puts distance between the family and the client. Review therapeutic techniques that assist the family to deal with a sudden illness if you had difficulty with this question.

Level of Cognitive Ability: Application
Client Needs: Psychosocial Integrity
Integrated Process: Caring
Content Area: Adult Health/Neurological

Reference:
Potter, P., & Perry, A. (2005). *Fundamentals of nursing* (6th ed.). St. Louis: Mosby, pp. 103; 437.

20. A nurse is performing an assessment on a client being admitted to the hospital. The client has right-sided weakness, aphasia, and urinary incontinence. One of the client's family members states, "If this is a stroke, it's the kiss of death." The nurse makes which response to the family member?
1 "Wait until the doctor gets here to think like that."
2 "A stroke is not the kiss of death."
3 "You feel as if your parent is dying?"
4 "These symptoms may be reversible."

Answer: 3
Rationale: Option 3 allows the family member to verbalize and begin to cope and adapt to what is happening. By restating, the nurse is able to clarify the family member's feelings and begin to offer information that will help ease some of the fears that he or she may face at the moment. Options 1 and 2 offer disapproval and put the family member's feeling on hold. Option 4 provides false hope at this point.

Test-Taking Strategy: Use therapeutic communication techniques. Option 3 is the only option that addresses the family member's feelings. Review therapeutic communication techniques if you had difficulty with this question.

Cognitive Level of Ability: Application
Client Needs: Psychosocial Integrity
Integrated Process: Caring
Content Area: Fundamental Skills

Reference:
Potter, P., & Perry, A. (2005). *Fundamentals of nursing* (6th ed.). St. Louis: Mosby, p. 437.

COMMUNICATION AND DOCUMENTATION

1. A nurse is trying to determine the client's adjustment to a new diagnosis of coronary heart disease before discharge from the hospital. Of the following questions, which one should the nurse ask to elicit the most useful response by the client in determining adjustment?
1 "Do you have anyone at home to help with housework and shopping?"
2 "How do you feel about the lifestyle changes you are planning to make?"
3 "Do you understand the use of your new medications?"
4 "Are you going to book your follow-up physician visit?"

Answer: 2
Rationale: All questions relate to aspects of post-hospital care, but only option 2 explores the client's feelings about the disease. Exploring feelings as the initial assessment will assist in determining the individualized plan of care for the client.

Test-Taking Strategy: Use therapeutic communication techniques. Open-ended questions are needed to explore the client's reactions or feelings to an identified situation. Close-ended responses generally elicit a "yes" or "no" response exclusively. All of the incorrect options are closed-ended responses. Review therapeutic communication techniques if you had difficulty with this question.

Level of Cognitive Ability: Application
Client Needs: Health Promotion and Maintenance
Integrated Process: Communication and Documentation
Content Area: Fundamental Skills

Reference:
Potter, P., & Perry, A. (2005). *Fundamentals of nursing* (6th ed.). St. Louis: Mosby, p. 437.

2. A female client with a long leg cast has been using crutches to ambulate for one week. She comes to the clinic with complaints of pain, fatigue, and frustration with crutch walking. She states, "I feel like I have a crippled leg." The nurse makes which response to the client?
   1 "I know how you feel. I had to use crutches before too."
   2 "Just remember, you'll be done with the crutches in another month."
   3 "Why don't you take a couple of days off work and rest."
   4 "Tell me what is bothersome for you."

Answer: 4
Rationale: Option 4 is the therapeutic communication technique of clarification and validation and indicates that the nurse is dealing with the client's problem from the client's perspective. Option 1 devalues the client's feelings and thus blocks communication. Option 2 provides false reassurances because the client may not be done with the crutches in another month. Additionally, it does not focus on the present problem. Option 3 gives advice and is a communication block.

Test-Taking Strategy: Use therapeutic communication techniques. Option 4 is the only response that encourages communication. Review therapeutic communication techniques if you had difficulty with this question.

Level of Cognitive Ability: Application
Client Needs: Psychosocial Integrity
Integrated Process: Communication and Documentation
Content Area: Adult Health/Musculoskeletal

Reference:
Potter, P., & Perry, A. (2005). *Fundamentals of nursing* (6th ed.). St. Louis: Mosby, p. 437.

3. An 18-year-old client is being discharged from the hospital after surgery and will need to ambulate with a cane for the next 6 months. The nurse asks the client which question that will provide data about the psychosocial status of the client regarding the use of the cane?
   1 "How do you feel about having to ambulate with a cane for the next six months?"
   2 "Do you have any questions about how to ambulate with the cane?"
   3 "Time will pass quickly, don't you think?"
   4 "You are not worried about what your friends will think, are you?"

Answer: 1
Rationale: How a client feels is an important part of the psychosocial assessment. Option 2 deals with a physical issue. Option 3 gives an opinion. Option 4 can be intimidating to the client. Additionally, options 2, 3, and 4 are closed-ended responses and are barriers to effective communication.

Test-Taking Strategy: Use therapeutic communication techniques. Avoid responses that include communication blocks. Eliminate options 2, 3, and 4 because they are closed-ended responses and are blocks to communication. Remember to address the client's feelings first. Review therapeutic communication techniques if you had difficulty with this question.

Level of Cognitive Ability: Application
Client Needs: Psychosocial Integrity
Integrated Process: Communication and Documentation
Content Area: Fundamental Skills

Reference:
Potter, P., & Perry, A. (2005). *Fundamentals of nursing* (6th ed.). St. Louis: Mosby, p. 437.

4. An 85-year-old client is hospitalized for a right fractured hip. During the postoperative period, the client's appetite is poor and the client refuses to get out of bed. The nurse makes which therapeutic and accurate statement to the client?

1 "It is important for you to get out of bed to be sure that calcium moves back into the bone."

2 "We need to increase your calcium intake because you are spending too much time in bed."

3 "We need to give you iodine so that it will help in hemoglobin synthesis."

4 "You need to remember to turn yourself in bed every 2 hours to keep from getting so stiff."

Answer: 1

Rationale: Early ambulation in the postoperative period is important because if a client does not increase activity, the bones will lose calcium. Increasing calcium intake in the immobile client would cause elevated amounts of calcium in the blood that could lead to kidney stones. Iron, not iodine, is recommended for hemoglobin synthesis because oxygen is necessary for wound healing. Clients who are not turned in bed will develop pressure ulcers. A client who is immobile and is 85 years old needs to be turned every 2 hours by the nursing staff. The client should not be expected to turn self.

Test-Taking Strategy: Use therapeutic communication techniques and knowledge regarding the effects of immobility. Option 4 is eliminated first because in this statement, the nurse is not accepting any responsibility for the client's care. Next, eliminate option 3 because it is an incorrect statement. From the remaining options, noting the key words "refuses to get out of bed" will direct you to option 1. Review the complications associated with immobility if you had difficulty with this question.

Level of Cognitive Ability: Application
Client Needs: Physiological Integrity
Integrated Process: Communication and Documentation
Content Area: Fundamental Skills

References:
Black, J., & Hawks, J. (2005). *Medical-surgical nursing: Clinical management for positive outcomes* (7th ed.). Philadelphia: Saunders, pp. 642; 645.
Lewis, S., Heitkemper, M., & Dirksen, S. (2004). *Medical-surgical nursing: Assessment and management of clinical problems* (6th ed.). St. Louis: Mosby, pp. 1254; 1677.

---

5. A client is diagnosed with thrombophlebitis of the left leg. The nurse documents in the nursing care plan that the client should be placed on bed rest with:

1 The left leg kept flat
2 Elevation of the left leg
3 The left leg in a dependent position
4 Bathroom privileges

Answer: 2

Rationale: Elevation of the affected leg facilitates blood flow by the force of gravity and also decreases venous pressure, which in turn relieves edema and pain. Bed rest is indicated to prevent emboli and to prevent pressure fluctuations in the venous system that occurs with walking. Thus, the nurse documents to elevate the left leg. Options 1 and 3 are inappropriate positions, and option 4 is an inappropriate activity; these options will not facilitate blood flow.

Test-Taking Strategy: Use the process of elimination. Focus on the client's diagnosis and think about the principles related to gravity flow and edema. This will direct you to option 2. Review nursing care for clients with a venous disorder if you had difficulty with this question.

Level of Cognitive Ability: Application
Client Needs: Physiological Integrity
Integrated Process: Communication and Documentation
Content Area: Fundamental Skills

Reference:
Black, J., & Hawks, J. (2005). *Medical-surgical nursing: Clinical management for positive outcomes* (7th ed.). Philadelphia: Saunders, pp. 1537; 1541.

6. A female client who is experiencing disordered thinking about food being poisoned is admitted to the mental health unit. The nurse uses which communication technique to encourage the client to eat dinner?
  1 Using open-ended questions and silence
  2 Offering opinions about the need to eat
  3 Verbalizing reasons that the client may not choose to eat
  4 Focusing on self-disclosure of own food preferences

Answer: 1
Rationale: Open-ended questions and silence are strategies used to encourage clients to discuss their problem in a descriptive manner. Options 2 and 3 are not helpful to the client because they do not encourage the client to express feelings. Option 4 is not a client-centered intervention.

Test-Taking Strategy: Use the process of elimination and therapeutic communication techniques. Eliminate options 2 and 3 first because they do not support client expression of feelings. Eliminate option 4 next because it is not a client-centered response. Review therapeutic communication techniques if you had difficulty with this question.

Level of Cognitive Ability: Application
Client Needs: Physiological Integrity
Integrated Process: Communication and Documentation
Content Area: Mental Health

Reference:
Varcarolis, E.M. (2002). *Foundations of psychiatric mental health nursing* (4th ed.). Philadelphia: Saunders, p. 253.

---

7. A nurse is engaged in preparing a client for electroconvulsive therapy (ECT). Following a thorough discussion with the client and family, the client signs the informed consent. Upon departure from the session, a family member states, "I don't know . . . I don't think that this ECT will be helpful if it makes people's memories worse." The nurse would then:
  1 Involve the family member in a dialogue to ascertain how the family member arrived at this conclusive statement
  2 Inquire with other family members and the client if they thought the same way about ECT making people worse
  3 Immediately reassure the client that the decision to receive ECT will help and that memory loss or confusion is minimal and temporary
  4 Reinforce with the family member that depression causes more memory impairment than ECT

Answer: 1
Rationale: In option 1, the nurse is exploring for data to assist in clarifying information about the procedure with the family. Option 2 may place family members on the defensive and promote conflict among family members. Option 3 would not acknowledge the family member's statement and concern. Option 4 addresses content clarification but not the assessment process and is not the most therapeutic action.

Test-Taking Strategy: Use therapeutic communication techniques and the nursing process. Remember that assessment is the first step in the nursing process. In option 1, the nurse gathers more data and addresses the family member's thoughts and feelings. Review therapeutic communication techniques if you had difficulty with this question.

Level of Cognitive Ability: Application
Client Needs: Psychosocial Integrity
Integrated Process: Communication and Documentation
Content Area: Mental Health

Reference:
Stuart, G., & Laraia, M. (2005). *Principles and practice of psychiatric nursing* (8th ed.). St. Louis: Mosby, pp. 30-34.

8. A client with type 2 diabetes mellitus was recently hospitalized for hyperglycemic hyperosmolar nonketotic syndrome (HHNS). Upon discharge from the hospital, the client expresses concerns about the recurrence of HHNS. The nurse makes which statement to the client?

1 "Don't worry. Your family will help you."
2 "I'm sure this won't happen again."
3 "You have concerns about the treatment for your condition?"
4 "I think you might need to go to the nursing home."

Answer: 3

Rationale: The nurse should provide time and listen to the client's concerns. In option 3, the nurse is attempting to clarify the client's feelings. Option 1 and 2 provide inappropriate false hope. Additionally, the nurse does not tell the client not to worry. Option 4 is not an appropriate nursing response, disregards the client's concerns, and gives advice.

Test-Taking Strategy: Use therapeutic communication techniques. Remembering to always address the client's feelings will direct you to option 3. Review these therapeutic techniques if you had difficulty with this question.

Level of Cognitive Ability: Application
Client Needs: Psychosocial Integrity
Integrated Process: Communication and Documentation
Content Area: Adult Health/Endocrine

Reference:
Potter, P., & Perry, A. (2005). *Fundamentals of nursing* (6th ed.). St. Louis: Mosby, p. 437.

---

9. The husband of a client who has a Sengstaken-Blakemore tube states to the nurse, "I thought having this tube down her nose the first time would convince my wife to quit drinking." The nurse makes which response to the client's husband?

1 "Alcoholism is a disease that affects the whole family."
2 "You sound frustrated in dealing with your wife's drinking problem."
3 "Have you discussed this subject at the Al-Anon meetings?"
4 "I think you are a good person to stay with your wife."

Answer: 2

Rationale: In option 2, the nurse uses the therapeutic communication techniques of clarifying and focusing in assisting the client (the husband) to express feelings concerning the wife's chronic illness. Stereotyping (option 1), changing the subject (option 3), and showing approval (option 4) are nontherapeutic techniques and block communication.

Test-Taking Strategy: Use therapeutic communication techniques. Remembering to always address the client's feelings will direct you to option 2. Review these therapeutic techniques if you had difficulty with this question.

Level of Cognitive Ability: Application
Client Needs: Psychosocial Integrity
Integrated Process: Communication and Documentation
Content Area: Adult Health/Gastrointestinal

Reference:
Potter, P., & Perry, A. (2005). *Fundamentals of nursing* (6th ed.). St. Louis: Mosby, p. 437.

---

10. A nurse has an order to institute aneurysm precautions for a client with a cerebral aneurysm. Which item should the nurse document on the plan of care for this client?

1 Encourage the client to take own daily bath
2 Allow the client to read and watch television
3 Limit out-of-bed activities to twice daily
4 Instruct the client not to strain with bowel movements

Answer: 4

Rationale: Aneurysm precautions include placing the client on bed rest in a quiet setting. Lights are kept dim to minimize environmental stimulation. Any activity that increases the blood pressure (BP) or impedes venous return from the brain is prohibited, such as pushing, pulling, sneezing, coughing, or straining. The nurse provides all physical care to minimize increases in the BP. For the same reason, visitors, radio, television, and reading materials are prohibited or limited. Stimulants such as caffeine and nicotine are prohibited. The nurse documents that the client is instructed to avoid straining with bowel movements.

Test-Taking Strategy: Recall that the components of aneurysm precautions are to limit the amount of stimulation (in any form) that the client receives and to prevent increased intracranial pressure (ICP). With this in mind, eliminate options 1 and 3 first. From the remaining options, recall that straining can increase ICP, so it is appropriate to tell the client not to do so. Review the components of aneurysm precautions if you had difficulty with this question.

Level of Cognitive Ability: Application
Client Needs: Physiological Integrity
Integrated Process: Communication and Documentation
Content Area: Adult Health/Neurological

Reference:
Phipps, W., Monahan, F., Sands, J., Marek, J., & Neighbors, M. (2003). *Medical-surgical nursing: Health and illness perspectives* (7th ed.). St. Louis: Mosby, p. 1385.

---

11. A client with myasthenia gravis is having difficulty with the motor aspects of speech. The client has difficulty forming words, and the voice has a nasal tone. The nurse would use which communication strategy when working with this client?
  1 Repeat what the client said to verify the message
  2 Encourage the client to speak quickly
  3 Nod continuously while the client is speaking
  4 Engage the client in lengthy discussions to strengthen the voice

Answer: 1
Rationale: The client has speech that is nasal in tone and dysarthritic because of cranial nerve involvement of the muscles governing speech. The nurse listens attentively and verbally verifies what the client has said. Other helpful techniques are to ask questions requiring a yes or no response, and to develop alternative communication methods (e.g., letter board, picture board, pen and paper, flash cards). Encouraging the client to speak quickly is inappropriate and counterproductive. Continuous nodding may be distracting and is unnecessary. Lengthy discussions will tire the client rather than strengthen the voice.

Test-Taking Strategy: Use the process of elimination and basic principles of communication techniques to answer this question. This will direct you to option 1. Review this disorder and effective communication strategies if you had difficulty with this question.

Level of Cognitive Ability: Application
Client Needs: Psychosocial Integrity
Integrated Process: Communication and Documentation
Content Area: Adult Health/Neurological

Reference:
Ignatavicius, D., & Workman, M. (2002). *Medical surgical nursing: Critical thinking for collaborative care* (4th ed.). Philadelphia: Saunders, p. 963.

12. A client with a peripheral intravenous (IV) site calls the nurse to the room and tells the nurse that the IV site is swollen. The nurse inspects the IV site and notes that it is also cool and pale and that the IV has stopped running. The nurse documents in the client's record that which of the following has probably occurred?
1 Infiltration
2 Phlebitis
3 Thrombosis
4 Infection

Answer: 1
Rationale: An infiltrated IV is one that has dislodged from the vein and is lying in subcutaneous tissue. The pallor, coolness, and swelling are the result of IV fluid being deposited in the subcutaneous tissue. When the pressure in the tissues exceeds the pressure in the tubing, the flow of the IV solution will stop. The corrective action will be to remove the catheter and have a new IV line started. The other three options are likely to be accompanied by warmth at the site, not coolness. The nurse would document that the client's IV has infiltrated.

Test-Taking Strategy: Use the process of elimination and knowledge regarding the signs of the complications associated with IV therapy. Focusing on the data in the question and noting the words "swollen, cool, and pale" will direct you to option 1. Review the signs of infiltration if you had difficulty with this question.

Level of Cognitive Ability: Application
Client Needs: Physiological Integrity
Integrated Process: Communication and Documentation
Content Area: Fundamental Skills

Reference:
Potter, P., & Perry, A. (2005). *Fundamentals of nursing* (6th ed.). St. Louis: Mosby, p. 1189.

13. A nurse is observing a nursing assistant talking to a client who is hearing impaired. The nurse would intervene if which of the following were performed by the nursing assistant during communication with the client?
1 The nursing assistant is facing the client when speaking.
2 The nursing assistant is speaking clearly to the client.
3 The nursing assistant is speaking directly into the impaired ear.
4 The nursing assistant is speaking in a normal tone.

Answer: 3
Rationale: When communicating with a hearing-impaired client, the nurse should speak in a normal tone to the client and should not shout. The nurse should talk directly to the client while facing the client and speak clearly. If the client does not seem to understand what is said, the nurse should express the statement differently. Moving closer to the client and toward the better ear may facilitate communication, but the nurse needs to avoid talking directly into the impaired ear.

Test-Taking Strategy: Note the key words "the nurse would intervene." These words indicate a false-response question and that you need to select the incorrect action by the nursing assistant. Knowledge regarding effective communication techniques for the hearing-impaired client will direct you to option 3. Review these therapeutic communication techniques if you had difficulty with this question.

Level of Cognitive Ability: Analysis
Client Needs: Safe, Effective Care Environment
Integrated Process: Communication and Documentation
Content Area: Leadership/Management

Reference:
Lewis, S., Heitkemper, M., & Dirksen, S. (2004). *Medical-surgical nursing: Assessment and management of clinical problems* (6th ed.). St. Louis: Mosby, p. 470.

14. A nurse is assigned to care for a client diagnosed with catatonic stupor. When the nurse enters the client's room, the client is found lying on the bed with the body pulled into a fetal position. The nurse should:
1 Leave the client alone and continue with providing care to other clients
2 Take the client into the dayroom to be with other clients
3 Sit beside the client in silence and occasionally ask open-ended questions
4 Ask the client direct questions to encourage talking

Answer: 3
Rationale: Clients who are withdrawn may be immobile and mute, and require consistent, repeated approaches. Intervention includes establishment of interpersonal contact. Communication with withdrawn clients requires much patience from the nurse. The nurse facilitates communication with the client by sitting in silence, asking open-ended questions, and pausing to provide opportunities for the client to respond. The client would not be left alone. Asking direct questions to the client is not therapeutic. It is not appropriate at this time to place the client in a public place, such as a dayroom.

Test Taking Strategy: Use the process of elimination. Eliminate option 1 because you would not leave the client alone. Eliminate option 2 because it is not appropriate to place the client in a public place. Eliminate option 4 because asking direct questions to this client is not therapeutic. Option 3 is the best action because it provides client supervision and communication with the client. Review care of the client with catatonic stupor if you had difficulty with this question.

Level of Cognitive Ability: Application
Client Needs: Psychosocial Integrity
Integrated Process: Communication and Documentation
Content Area: Mental Health

Reference:
Keltner, N., Schwecke, L., & Bostrom, C. (2003). *Psychiatric nursing* (4th ed.). St. Louis: Mosby, p. 344.

15. A nurse is developing a plan of care for an older client and includes strategies that will facilitate effective communication. The nurse would include which strategy to accomplish this goal?
1 Use an authoritarian approach
2 Use active listening
3 React enthusiastically during the conversation
4 React only to the facts during conversation

Answer: 2
Rationale: For effective communication, the nurse uses active listening and creates an environment in which the client feels comfortable expressing feelings. An authoritarian approach is directive and not permissive and will not create an environment for verbal exchange from the client. Reacting only to the facts are examples of inactive listening. Reacting enthusiastically is not the most effective strategy.

Test-Taking Strategy: Use the process of elimination and therapeutic communication techniques. This will direct you to option 2. Review this content if you had difficulty with this question or are unfamiliar with therapeutic communication techniques.

Level of Cognitive Ability: Application
Client Needs: Psychosocial Integrity
Integrated Process: Communication and Documentation
Content Area: Fundamental Skills

Reference:
Potter, P., & Perry, A. (2005). *Fundamentals of nursing* (6th ed.). St. Louis: Mosby, p. 439.

16. The nurse has made an error in documenting vital signs on a client and obtains the client's record to correct the error. The nurse corrects the error by:
1 Using whiteout
2 Erasing the error
3 Documenting a late entry
4 Drawing one line through the error, initialing and dating the line

Answer: 4
Rationale: If a nurse makes an error in documenting in the client's record, the nurse should follow agency policies to correct the error. This includes drawing one line through the error, initialing and dating the line, and then providing the correct information. Erasing data from the client's record and the use of whiteout is prohibited. A late entry is used to document additional information not remembered at the initial time of documentation.

Test-Taking Strategy: Use the process of elimination and principles related to documentation. Recalling that alterations to a client's record are avoided will eliminate options 1 and 2. From the remaining options, focusing on the issue of the question will direct you to option 4. Review the principles related to documentation if you had difficulty with this question.

Level of Cognitive Ability: Application
Client Needs: Safe, Effective Care Environment
Integrated Process: Communication and Documentation
Content Area: Fundamental Skills

Reference:
Potter, P., & Perry, A. (2005). *Fundamentals of nursing* (6th ed.). St. Louis: Mosby, p. 480.

17. A nurse hears a client calling out for help. The nurse hurries down the hallway to the client's room and finds a client lying on the floor. The nurse performs a thorough assessment and assists the client back to bed. The physician is notified of the incident and the nurse completes an incident report. The nurse documents which of the following on the incident report?
1 The client was found lying on the floor.
2 The client climbed over the side rails.
3 The client fell out of bed.
4 The client became restless and tried to get out of bed.

Answer: 1
Rationale: The incident report should contain the client's name, age, and diagnosis. It should contain a factual description of the incident, any injuries experienced by those involved, and the outcome of the situation. Option 1 is the only option that describes the facts as observed by the nurse. Options 2, 3, and 4 are interpretations of the situation and are not factual data as observed by the nurse.

Test-Taking Strategy: Use general documentation guidelines and principles to answer the question. Remember to focus on factual information when documenting and avoid including interpretations. This will direct you to option 1. Review documentation principles related to incident reports if you had difficulty with this question.

Level of Cognitive Ability: Application
Client Needs: Safe, Effective Care Environment
Integrated Process: Communication and Documentation
Content Area: Fundamental Skills

Reference:
Potter, P., & Perry, A. (2005). *Fundamentals of nursing* (6th ed.). St. Louis: Mosby, pp. 419; 497.

18. A client diagnosed with angina pectoris appears to be very anxious and states, "So, I had a heart attack, right?" The nurse makes which response to the client?

1 "No, and we will see to it that you do not have a heart attack."

2 "Yes, this is why you are here."

3 "No, but the doctor wants to monitor you and control or eliminate your pain."

4 "Yes, but there is minimal damage to your heart."

Answer: 3

Rationale: Angina pectoris occurs as a result of an inadequate blood supply to the myocardium. A myocardial infarction refers to a heart attack. Option 1 provides false reassurance. Neither the nurse nor the physician can guarantee that a heart attack will not occur.

Test-Taking Strategy: Use therapeutic communication techniques and knowledge regarding the definition of angina pectoris to eliminate options 2 and 4. From the remaining options, eliminate option 1 because it provides false reassurance. Review the pathophysiology associated with angina pectoris and therapeutic communication techniques if you had difficulty with this question.

Level of Cognitive Ability: Application
Client Needs: Psychosocial Integrity
Integrated Process: Communication and Documentation
Content Area: Adult Health/Cardiovascular

Reference:
Ignatavicius, D., & Workman, M. (2002). *Medical surgical nursing: Critical thinking for collaborative care* (4th ed.). Philadelphia: Saunders, p. 794.

---

19. A nurse is caring for a hospitalized client with a diagnosis of depression who is silent and not communicating. The nurse develops a plan of care and incorporates strategies for communicating with the client. Which statement would be most appropriate for the nurse to make when caring for the client?

1 "Can you tell me how you are feeling today?"

2 "Do you feel like talking today?"

3 "You are wearing your new shoes."

4 "Can you tell me how you slept last night?"

Answer: 3

Rationale: When a depressed client is mute or silent, the nurse should use the communication technique of making observations. A statement such as "you are wearing your new shoes" is an appropriate statement to make to the client. When the client is not ready to talk, direct questions (options 1, 2, and 4) can raise the client's anxiety level. Pointing to commonalties in the environment draws the client into and reinforces reality.

Test-Taking Strategy: Use therapeutic communication techniques. Eliminate options 1, 2, and 4 because they are similar. These options are direct questions requiring a response from the client. Review communication techniques for the depressed client if you had difficulty with this question.

Level of Cognitive Ability: Application
Client Needs: Psychosocial Integrity
Integrated Process: Communication and Documentation
Content Area: Mental Health

Reference:
Varcarolis, E.M. (2002). *Foundations of psychiatric mental health nursing* (4th ed.). Philadelphia: Saunders, pp. 463; 467.

20. A nurse is caring for a client with delirium who states, "Look at the spiders on the wall." The nurse makes which response to the client?

1 "I can see the spiders on the wall, but they are not going to hurt you."

2 "Would you like me to kill the spiders for you?"

3 "I know you are frightened, but I do not see spiders on the wall."

4 "You're having a hallucination; there are no spiders in this room at all."

Answer: 3

Rationale: When hallucinations are present, the nurse should reinforce reality with the client. In option 3, the nurse addresses the client's feelings and reinforces reality. Options 1 and 2 do not reinforce reality. Option 4 reinforces reality but does not address the client's feelings.

Test-Taking Strategy: Use therapeutic communication techniques. Eliminate options 1 and 2 because they reinforce the client's hallucination. Eliminate option 4 because, although it reinforces reality, it diminishes the importance of the client's feelings. Review therapeutic communication techniques for the client experiencing disturbed thought processes if you had difficulty with this question.

Level of Cognitive Ability: Application
Client Needs: Psychosocial Integrity
Integrated Process: Communication and Documentation
Content Area: Mental Health

Reference:
Stuart, G., & Laraia, M. (2005). *Principles and practice of psychiatric nursing* (8th ed.). St. Louis: Mosby, pp. 30-34.

TEACHING/LEARNING

1. A nurse has given instructions on site care to a hemodialysis client who had an implantation of an arteriovenous (AV) fistula in the right arm. The nurse determines that the client needs further instructions if the client states to:

1 Avoid carrying heavy objects on the right arm

2 Sleep on the right side

3 Report an increased temperature, redness, or drainage at the site

4 Perform range of motion exercises routinely on the right arm

Answer: 2

Rationale: Routine instructions to the client with an AV fistula, graft, or shunt includes reporting signs and symptoms of infection, performing routine range of motion to the affected extremity, avoiding sleeping with the body weight on the extremity with the access site, and avoiding carrying heavy objects or compressing the extremity that has the access site.

Test-Taking Strategy: Use the process of elimination, noting the key words "needs further instructions." These words indicate a false-response question and that you need to select the incorrect client statement. Recalling the importance of maintaining the patency of the AV fistula will direct you to option 2. Review home care instructions for a client with an AV fistula if you had difficulty with this question.

Level of Cognitive Ability: Analysis
Client Needs: Health Promotion and Maintenance
Integrated Process: Teaching/Learning
Content Area: Adult Health/Renal

Reference:
Ignatavicius, D., & Workman, M. (2002). *Medical surgical nursing: Critical thinking for collaborative care* (4th ed.). Philadelphia: Saunders, p. 1692.

2. A nurse provides instructions to a client about administering nitroglycerin ointment (Nitrobid). The nurse determines that the client is using correct technique when applying the ointment if the client:
1 Applies additional ointment if chest pain occurs
2 Applies the ointment directly to the skin, then gently rubs the ointment into the skin
3 Applies the ointment to any nonhairy area of the body
4 Washes the ointment off when bathing and reapplies after the bath

Answer: 3
Rationale: Nitroglycerin ointment is used on a scheduled basis and is not prescribed specifically for the occurrence of chest pain. The ointment is not rubbed into the skin. It is reapplied only as directed.

Test-Taking Strategy: Use the process of elimination and focus on the issue: using correct technique. Recalling medication principles related to the application of ointments will direct you to option 3. Review these client teaching points if you had difficulty with this question.

Level of Cognitive Ability: Analysis
Client Needs: Health Promotion and Maintenance
Integrated Process: Teaching/Learning
Content Area: Pharmacology

Reference:
McKenry, L., & Salerno, E. (2003). *Mosby's pharmacology in nursing* (21st ed.). St. Louis: Mosby, pp. 609-610.

3. A nurse is giving medication instructions to a client receiving furosemide (Lasix). The nurse determines that further teaching is necessary if the client makes which of the following statements?
1 "I need to avoid the use of salt substitutes because they contain potassium."
2 "I need to change positions slowly."
3 "I need to talk to my physician about the use of alcohol."
4 "I need to be careful not to get overheated in warm weather."

Answer: 1
Rationale: Furosemide is a potassium-losing diuretic, so there is no need to avoid high-potassium products, such as a salt substitute. Orthostatic hypotension is a risk, and the client must use caution with changing positions and with exposure to warm weather. The client needs to discuss the use of alcohol with the physician.

Test-Taking Strategy: Use the process of elimination, noting the key words "further teaching is necessary." These words indicate a false-response question and that you need to select the incorrect client statement. Recalling that furosemide is a potassium-losing diuretic and that diuretic therapy can induce orthostatic hypotension will direct you to option 1. Review this medication if you had difficulty with this question.

Level of Cognitive Ability: Analysis
Client Needs: Health Promotion and Maintenance
Integrated Process: Teaching/Learning
Content Area: Pharmacology

Reference:
McKenry, L., & Salerno, E. (2003). *Mosby's pharmacology in nursing* (21st ed.). St. Louis: Mosby, pp. 676-677.

4. A client has been prescribed a clonidine patch (Catapres TTS), and the nurse has instructed the client on the use of the patch. The nurse determines that further instruction is needed if the nurse noted that the client:
1 Verbalized to leave the patch in place during bathing or showering
2 Verbalized to change the patch every 7 days
3 Trimmed the patch because one edge was loose
4 Selected a hairless site on the torso for application

Answer: 3
Rationale: The clonidine patch should be applied to a hairless site on the torso or upper arm. It is changed every 7 days and is left in place when bathing or showering. The patch should not be trimmed because it will alter the medication dose. If it becomes slightly loose, it should be covered with an adhesive overlay from the medication package. If it becomes very loose or falls off, it should be replaced. The patch is discarded by folding it in half with the adhesive sides together.

Test-Taking Strategy: Use the process of elimination, noting the key words "further instruction is needed." These words indicate a false-response question and that you need to select the incorrect client statement. Noting the words "trimmed the patch" will direct you to this option because this client action would alter the medication dose. Review this medication if you had difficulty with this question.

Level of Cognitive Ability: Analysis
Client Needs: Physiological Integrity
Integrated Process: Teaching/Learning
Content Area: Pharmacology

Reference:
McKenry, L., & Salerno, E. (2003). *Mosby's pharmacology in nursing* (21st ed.). St. Louis: Mosby, pp. 576-579.

5. Cholestyramine (Questran) is prescribed, and the nurse provides instructions to the client about the medication. The nurse determines that further instructions are needed if the client makes which statement?
1 "I need to mix the medicine with juice or applesauce."
2 "I should call my doctor immediately if it causes constipation."
3 "I should increase my fluid intake while taking this medication."
4 "I should take this medication with meals."

Answer: 2
Rationale: This medication should not be taken dry and can be mixed in water, juice, carbonated beverage, applesauce, or soup. Common side effects include constipation, nausea, indigestion, and flatulence. Increasing fluids will minimize the constipating effects of the medication. Questran must be administered with food to be effective.

Test-Taking Strategy: Use the process of elimination, noting the key words "further instructions are needed." These words indicate a false-response question and that you need to select the incorrect client statement. Select option 2 because of the word "immediately" and because normally measures can be taken to prevent constipation rather than immediately calling the physician. Review this medication if you are unfamiliar with it.

Level of Cognitive Ability: Analysis
Client Needs: Health Promotion and Maintenance
Integrated Process: Teaching/Learning
Content Area: Pharmacology

Reference:
McKenry, L., & Salerno, E. (2003). *Mosby's pharmacology in nursing* (21st ed.). St. Louis: Mosby, pp. 654-656.

6. A nurse is preparing written medication instructions for a client receiving colestipol hydrochloride (Colestid). The nurse includes instructions about the need for the client to take which of the following to counteract unintended medication effects?
  1 Vitamin D
  2 Fat-soluble vitamins
  3 B-complex vitamins
  4 Vitamin C

Answer: 2
Rationale: Colestipol, a bile-sequestering agent, is used to lower blood cholesterol levels. However, the bile salts (rich in cholesterol) interfere with the absorption of the fat-soluble vitamins A, D, E, and K, as well as folic acid. With ongoing therapy, the client is at risk of deficiency of these vitamins and is counseled to take supplements of these vitamins.

Test-Taking Strategy: Use the process of elimination. Recalling that bile-sequestering agents interfere with the absorption of fat-soluble vitamins will assist in eliminating options 3 and 4. From the remaining options, select option 2 because it is the umbrella (global) option. Review client teaching points regarding this medication if you had difficulty with this question.

Level of Cognitive Ability: Application
Client Needs: Physiological Integrity
Integrated Process: Teaching/Learning
Content Area: Pharmacology

Reference:
McKenry, L., & Salerno, E. (2003). *Mosby's pharmacology in nursing* (21st ed.). St. Louis: Mosby, 653.

7. A client with tuberculosis (TB) is preparing for discharge from the hospital, and the nurse provides instructions to the client about home care. Which client statement indicates that further instructions are necessary?
  1 "If I miss a dose of medication because of nausea, I just skip that dose and resume my regular schedule."
  2 "I need to eat foods that are high in iron, protein, and vitamin C."
  3 "I need to place used tissues in a plastic bag when I am home."
  4 "It is not necessary to maintain respiratory isolation when I am home."

Answer: 1
Rationale: Because of the resistant strains of tuberculosis, the nurse must emphasize that noncompliance regarding medication could lead to an infection that is difficult to treat and may cause total drug resistance. Clients may prevent nausea related to the medications by taking the daily dose at bedtime. Antinausea medications may also prevent this symptom. Medication doses should not be skipped. Options 2, 3, and 4 are correct statements.

Test-Taking Strategy: Note the key words "further instructions are necessary." These words indicate a false-response question and that you need to select the incorrect client statement. General principles related to medication administration will direct you to option 1. Review medication therapy and its importance in TB if you had difficulty with this question.

Level of Cognitive Ability: Analysis
Client Needs: Health Promotion and Maintenance
Integrated Process: Teaching/Learning
Content Area: Adult Health/Respiratory

References:
Ignatavicius, D., & Workman, M. (2002). *Medical surgical nursing: Critical thinking for collaborative care* (4th ed.). Philadelphia: Saunders, p. 588.
McKenry, L., & Salerno, E. (2003). *Mosby's pharmacology in nursing* (21st ed.). St. Louis, Mosby, p 1050.

8. A nurse is planning to teach a client who is newly diagnosed with tuberculosis (TB) on how to prevent the spread of TB. Which instruction would be least effective in preventing the spread of TB?

1 Teach the client to cover the mouth when coughing
2 Teach the client to sterilize dishes at home
3 Teach the client to properly dispose of facial tissues
4 Teach the client that close contacts should be tested for TB

Answer: 2

Rationale: Options 1, 3, and 4 would assist in breaking the chain of infection. Option 2 would not only be impractical, but no evidence suggests that sterilizing dishes would break the chain of infection with pulmonary TB.

Test-Taking Strategy: Note the key words "least effective." These words indicate a false-response question and that you need to select the action that is not helpful in preventing the spread of TB. Recalling the methods of transmission of TB will direct you to option 2. Review home care principles related to TB if you had difficulty with this question.

Level of Cognitive Ability: Application
Client Needs: Safe, Effective Care Environment
Integrated Process: Teaching/Learning
Content Area: Adult Health/Respiratory

Reference:
Ignatavicius, D., & Workman, M. (2002). *Medical surgical nursing: Critical thinking for collaborative care* (4th ed.). Philadelphia: Saunders, p. 587.

---

9. A client is being discharged to home with a heparin lock (intermittent IV catheter) to receive a week of antibiotic IV therapy at home following abdominal surgery. The nurse determines that the client needs further home care instructions about the heparin lock if the client makes which statement?

1 "I'll examine the IV site frequently."
2 "If the IV site becomes wet or moist, it can air dry."
3 "Pain, redness, and swelling need to be reported to the physician."
4 "If the lock or catheter accidentally comes out, I'll apply pressure to the site."

Answer: 2

Rationale: The client needs to be instructed on site assessment as well as complications (such as signs of infection) that need to be reported to the physician. Clients should also know how to treat complications, such as a dislodged catheter or bleeding at the IV site. Clients often are expected to change dressings and need to be aware that if the dressing is wet or soiled, it needs to be changed immediately in order to prevent infection.

Test-Taking Strategy: Note the key words "needs further home care instructions." These words indicate a false-response question and that you need to select the incorrect client statement. Using the process of elimination and principles related to asepsis will direct you to option 2. Review these principles if you had difficulty with this question.

Level of Cognitive Ability: Analysis
Client Needs: Safe, Effective Care Environment
Integrated Process: Teaching/Learning
Content Area: Fundamental Skills

Reference:
Potter, P., & Perry, A. (2005). *Fundamentals of nursing* (6th ed.). St. Louis: Mosby, p. 1194.

10. A home care nurse provides instructions to a client with jaundice who is experiencing pruritus. The nurse determines that the client needs additional instructions if the client stated to:

1 Wear loose cotton clothing
2 Use tepid water for bathing
3 Maintain a warm house temperature
4 Take the prescribed antihistamines to relieve the itch

Answer: 3

Rationale: Pruritus is caused by the accumulation of bile salts in the skin and results from obstructed biliary excretion. Antihistamines may relieve the itching, as will tepid water or emollient baths. The client should avoid the use of alkaline soap and wear loose, soft cotton clothing. The client is instructed to keep the house temperature cool.

Test-Taking Strategy: Use the process of elimination, noting the key words "needs additional instructions." These words indicate a false-response question and that you need to select the incorrect client statement. Recalling that heat causes vasodilation will assist in directing you to option 3. Review the measures that assist in alleviating pruritus if you had difficulty with this question.

Level of Cognitive Ability: Analysis
Client Needs: Health Promotion and Maintenance
Integrated Process: Teaching/Learning
Content Area: Adult Health/Gastrointestinal

Reference:
Ignatavicius, D., & Workman, M. (2002). *Medical surgical nursing: Critical thinking for collaborative care* (4th ed.). Philadelphia: Saunders, p. 1515.

---

11. A nurse provides home care instructions to a client hospitalized for a transurethral resection of the prostate (TURP). Which statement by the client indicates the need for further instructions?

1 "I need to avoid strenuous activity for 4 to 6 weeks."
2 "I need to maintain a daily intake of 6 to 8 glasses of water daily."
3 "I can lift and push objects up to 30 pounds in weight."
4 "I need to include prune juice in my diet."

Answer: 3

Rationale: The client needs to be advised to avoid strenuous activity for 4 to 6 weeks and to avoid lifting items weighing greater than 20 pounds. The client needs to consume a daily intake of at least 6 to 8 glasses of nonalcoholic fluids to minimize clot formation. Straining during defecation is avoided to prevent bleeding. Prune juice is a satisfactory bowel stimulant.

Test-Taking Strategy: Note the key words "need for further instructions." These words indicate a false-response question and that you need to select the incorrect client statement. Options 1 and 2 can be eliminated first because they are general postoperative teaching points. Considering the anatomical location of the surgical procedure, it is reasonable to think that constipation needs to be avoided; therefore, eliminate option 4. Also note that lifting items weighing 30 pounds is excessive. Review TURP discharge teaching points if you had difficulty with this question.

Level of Cognitive Ability: Analysis
Client Needs: Health Promotion and Maintenance
Integrated Process: Teaching/Learning
Content Area: Adult Health/Renal

Reference:
Ignatavicius, D., & Workman, M. (2002). *Medical surgical nursing: Critical thinking for collaborative care* (4th ed.). Philadelphia: Saunders, p. 1789.

12. A nurse is providing home care instructions to a client who will be receiving intravenous (IV) therapy at home. The nurse teaches the client that the most important action to prevent an infection at the IV site is to:

1 Assess the IV site carefully every day for redness and edema

2 Redress the IV site daily, cleansing it with alcohol

3 Carefully wash hands with antibacterial soap before working with the IV site or equipment

4 Change IV tubing and fluid containers daily

Answer: 3

Rationale: While assessment of the IV site is important, it will not actively prevent an infection. IV sites do not need to be redressed daily unless the dressing becomes soiled, wet, or loose. While IV containers should be changed daily, tubing only needs to be changed every 48 to 72 hours based on the Centers for Disease Control guidelines. It is extremely important for the client to understand the absolute necessity of handwashing before working with IV fluids and equipment.

Test-Taking Strategy: Note the key words "most important" and focus on the issue: preventing infection. Remember that the top priority in infection prevention always includes proper handwashing technique. Review standard precautions and their role in preventing infection if you had difficulty with this question.

Level of Cognitive Ability: Application
Client Needs: Safe, Effective Care Environment
Integrated Process: Teaching/Learning
Content Area: Fundamental Skills

Reference:
Potter, P., & Perry, A. (2005). *Fundamentals of nursing* (6th ed.). St. Louis: Mosby, p. 1194.

---

13. A 64-year-old client is being treated for an atrial dysrhythmia with quinidine gluconate (Duraquin), and the nurse provides instructions to the client about the medication. Which statement by the client indicates that the client understands the instructions?

1 "If I miss a dose, I take two doses of the medication at the next scheduled time."

2 "If I miss a dose, I should call my doctor."

3 "If I miss a dose, I should take the dose in the evening if I remember."

4 "If I miss a dose, I should take the next prescribed dose as usual."

Answer: 4

Rationale: The client should be instructed not to take an extra dose. The client should be instructed to take the medication if remembered within 2 hours of the missed dose, or to omit the dose and then resume the normal schedule. Quinidine gluconate needs to be taken exactly as prescribed. There is no need to call the doctor.

Test-Taking Strategy: Use the process of elimination and general principles related to medication administration. Eliminate option 1 because this action is inaccurate and could cause toxic effects. There is no need to call the doctor unless toxic effects occur, therefore eliminate option 2. From the remaining options, recalling that a missed dose can be taken within 2 hours if remembered will direct you to option 4. Review the basic principles associated with medication administration if you had difficulty with this question.

Level of Cognitive Ability: Analysis
Client Needs: Health Promotion and Maintenance
Integrated Process: Teaching/Learning
Content Area: Pharmacology

Reference:
Lehne, R. (2004). *Pharmacology for nursing care* (5th ed.). Philadelphia: Saunders, p. 504.

14. A client asks the nurse for a recommendation about how to prevent fires and burn injury. The nurse tells the client that the one single intervention that has been shown to decrease the risk of dying in a residential fire is:

1 The installation of a sprinkler system
2 Fire extinguishers placed in key areas such as the kitchen, near the furnace, and near the hot water heater
3 The use of operable smoke detectors
4 Installation of fire-resistant drywall panels throughout the house

Answer: 3

Rationale: Early detection of smoke and, subsequently, immediate evacuation from the house have been shown to significantly impact mortality. The installation of a sprinkler system is very expensive and not usually used in residential situations. Fire extinguishers are a good idea to have in the kitchen for small fires, but they are unrealistic and dangerous to use to attempt to extinguish large fires. Although fire-resistant products may help slow down a blaze, even fire-resistant products can eventually catch on fire.

Test-Taking Strategy: Use the process of elimination. Look for the health prevention measure that is simple to implement and will alert individuals of the need to evacuate a residence. This will direct you to option 3. Review fire safety if you had difficulty with this question.

Level of Cognitive Ability: Application
Client Needs: Safe, Effective Care Environment
Integrated Process: Teaching/Learning
Content Area: Fundamental Skills

Reference:
Potter, P., & Perry, A. (2005). *Fundamentals of nursing* (6th ed.). St. Louis: Mosby, pp. 991-992.

15. A client has had same-day surgery to insert a ventilating tube in the tympanic membrane. The nurse determines that the client understands the discharge instructions if the client states to:

1 Use a shower cap if taking a shower
2 Swim only with the head above water
3 Wash the hair quickly in 2 minutes or less
4 Avoid taking any medication for pain

Answer: 1

Rationale: Following insertion of tubes in the tympanic membrane, it is important to avoid getting water in the ears. For this reason, swimming, showering, or washing the hair is avoided after surgery until the time frame designated for each is identified by the surgeon. A shower cap or ear plug may be used when showering, if allowed by the physician. The client should take medication as advised for postoperative discomfort.

Test-Taking Strategy: Use the process of elimination, noting the key words "understands the discharge instructions." Eliminate option 2 because of the absolute word "only" and option 3 because of the word "quickly." From the remaining options, focusing on the anatomical location of the surgery will direct you to option 1. Review client instructions following this type of surgery if you had difficulty with this question.

Level of Cognitive Ability: Analysis
Client Needs: Health Promotion and Maintenance
Integrated Process: Teaching/Learning
Content Area: Adult Health/Ear

Reference:
Ignatavicius, D., & Workman, M. (2002). *Medical surgical nursing: Critical thinking for collaborative care* (4th ed.). Philadelphia: Saunders, p. 1066.

16. A nurse has completed diet teaching for a client on a low-sodium diet for the treatment of hypertension. The nurse determines that further teaching is necessary if the client makes which statement?
1   "This diet will help lower my blood pressure."
2   "The reason I need to lower my salt intake is to reduce fluid retention."
3   "This diet is not a replacement for my antihypertensive medications."
4   "Frozen foods are lowest in sodium."

Answer: 4
Rationale: A low-sodium diet is used as an adjunct to antihypertensive medications for the treatment of hypertension. Sodium retains fluid, which leads to hypertension secondary to increased fluid volume. Frozen foods use salt as a preservative and should not be encouraged as part of a low-sodium diet. Fresh foods are best.

Test-Taking Strategy: Note the key words "further teaching is necessary." These words indicate a false-response question and that you need to select the incorrect client statement. Use the process of elimination and eliminate options 1, 2, and 3 because these are accurate statements related to hypertension. Review the treatment of hypertension and foods high in sodium if you had difficulty with this question.

Level of Cognitive Ability: Analysis
Client Needs: Health Promotion and Maintenance
Integrated Process: Teaching/Learning
Content Area: Adult Health/Cardiovascular

Reference:
Williams, S. (2001). *Basic nutrition & diet therapy* (11th ed.). St. Louis: Mosby, p. 185.

---

17. A nurse is preparing a plan regarding home care instructions for the parents of a child with generalized tonic-clonic seizures who is being treated with oral phenytoin (Dilantin). The nurse includes instructions in the plan regarding:
1   Monitoring the child's intake and output daily
2   Checking the child's blood pressure before the administration of the medication
3   Providing oral hygiene, especially care of the gums
4   Administering the medication one hour before food intake

Answer: 3
Rationale: Phenytoin causes gum bleeding and hyperplasia and, therefore, a soft toothbrush and gum massage should be instituted to diminish this complication and prevent trauma. Intake and output and blood pressure are not affected by this medication. Directions for administration of this medication include administering it with food to minimize gastrointestinal upset.

Test-Taking Strategy: Use the process of elimination. Correlate phenytoin with gum bleeding and hyperplasia. Also, note the word "oral" in the question and in the correct option. Review the side effects and the method of administration of this medication if you had difficulty with this question.

Level of Cognitive Ability: Application
Client Needs: Health Promotion and Maintenance
Integrated Process: Teaching/Learning
Content Area: Pharmacology

Reference:
McKenry, L., & Salerno, E. (2003). *Mosby's pharmacology in nursing* (21st ed.). St. Louis: Mosby, p. 358.

18. A nurse performs an initial assessment on a pregnant client and determines that the client is at risk for toxoplasmosis. The nurse would teach the client which of the following to prevent exposure to this disease?

1 Wash hands only before meals
2 Eat raw meats
3 Avoid exposure to litter boxes used by cats
4 Use topical corticosteroid treatments prophylactically

Answer: 3

Rationale: Infected house cats transmit toxoplasmosis through the feces. Handling litter boxes can transmit the disease to the pregnant client. Meats that are undercooked can harbor microorganisms that can cause infection. Hands should be washed frequently throughout the day. The use of topical corticosteroids will not prevent exposure to the disease.

Test-Taking Strategy: Use the process of elimination. Eliminate option 1 because of the absolute word "only." Option 2 represents an extreme statement and can also be eliminated. From the remaining options, focusing on the key words "prevent exposure" in the question will direct you to option 3. Review the causes of toxoplasmosis if you had difficulty with this question.

Level of Cognitive Ability: Application
Client Needs: Health Promotion and Maintenance
Integrated Process: Teaching/Learning
Content Area: Maternity/Antepartum

Reference:
Murray, S., McKinney, E., & Gorrie, T. (2002). *Foundations of maternal-newborn nursing* (3rd ed.). Philadelphia: Saunders, p. 729.

---

19. A home care nurse is instructing the mother of a child with cystic fibrosis (CF) about the appropriate dietary measures. The nurse tells the mother that the child needs to consume a:

1 Low-calorie, low-fat diet
2 High-calorie, high-protein diet
3 Low-calorie, low-protein diet
4 High-calorie, restricted fat

Answer: 2

Rationale: Children with CF are managed with a high-calorie, high-protein diet. Pancreatic enzyme replacement therapy and fat-soluble vitamin supplements are administered. Fat restriction is not necessary.

Test-Taking Strategy: Use the process of elimination. Eliminate options 1 and 4 first because they both indicate restricting fat in the diet. From the remaining options, thinking about the pathophysiology related to CF will direct you to option 2. Review these measures if you are unfamiliar with the diet plan for the child with CF.

Level of Cognitive Ability: Application
Client Needs: Physiological Integrity
Integrated Process: Teaching/Learning
Content Area: Child Health

Reference:
Wong, D., & Hockenberry, M. (2003). *Wong's nursing care of infants and children* (7th ed.). St. Louis: Mosby, p. 1410.

20. A nurse in the ambulatory care unit is reviewing the surgical instructions with a client who will be admitted for knee replacement surgery. The nurse informs the client that crutches will be needed for ambulation after surgery and that the client will be instructed in the use of the crutches:

1 At the time of discharge following surgery
2 Before surgery
3 On the second postoperative day
4 On the first postoperative day

Answer: 2
Rationale: It is best to assess crutch-walking ability and instruct the client in the use of the crutches before surgery, because this task can be difficult to learn when the client is in pain and not used to the imbalance that may occur following surgery. Options 1, 3, and 4 are not the appropriate times to teach a client about crutch walking.

Test-Taking Strategy: Use the process of elimination. Note the similarity between options 1, 3, and 4 in that they all address the postoperative period. Review preoperative teaching principles if you had difficulty with this question.

Level of Cognitive Ability: Application
Client Needs: Health Promotion and Maintenance
Integrated Process: Teaching/Learning
Content Area: Adult Health/Musculoskeletal

References:
Black, J., & Hawks, J. (2005). *Medical-surgical nursing: Clinical management for positive outcomes* (7th ed.). Philadelphia: Saunders, p. 596.
Ignatavicius, D., & Workman, M. (2002). *Medical surgical nursing: Critical thinking for collaborative care* (4th ed.). Philadelphia: Saunders, p. 237.

21. A client with a short leg plaster cast complains of an intense itching under the cast. The nurse provides instructions to the client regarding relief measures for the itching. Which statement by the client indicates an understanding of the measures to relieve the itching?

1 "I can use the blunt part of a ruler to scratch the area."
2 "I need to obtain assistance when placing an object into the cast for the itching."
3 "I can use a hair dryer on the low setting and allow the air to blow into the cast."
4 "I can trickle small amounts of water down inside the cast."

Answer: 3
Rationale: Itching is a common complaint of clients with casts. Objects should not be put inside a cast because of the risk of scratching the skin and providing a point of entry for bacteria. A plaster cast can break down when wet. Therefore, the best way to relieve itching is with a forceful injection of air inside the cast.

Test-Taking Strategy: Use the process of elimination and eliminate options 1 and 2 first because they both involve the use of an object being placed inside the cast. Recalling that water can soften a plaster cast and cause maceration of the skin will direct you to option 3 from the remaining options. Review client teaching regarding cast care if you had difficulty with this question.

Level of Cognitive Ability: Analysis
Client Needs: Health Promotion and Maintenance
Integrated Process: Teaching/Learning
Content Area: Adult Health/Musculoskeletal

Reference:
Phipps, W., Monahan, F., Sands, J., Marek, J., & Neighbors, M. (2003). *Medical-surgical nursing: Health and illness perspectives* (7th ed.). St. Louis: Mosby, p. 1481.

22. Antabuse (Disulfiram) has been prescribed for a client, and the nurse provides instructions to the client about the medication. Which statement by the client indicates the need for further instructions?
  1 "As long as I don't drink alcohol, I'll be fine."
  2 "I must be careful taking cold medicines."
  3 "I'll have to check my aftershave lotion."
  4 "I'll have to be more careful with the ingredients I use for cooking."

Answer: 1
Rationale: Clients who are taking antabuse (Disulfiram) must be taught that substances containing alcohol can trigger an adverse reaction. Sources of hidden alcohol include foods (soups, sauces, vinegars), medicine (cold medicine), mouthwashes, and skin preparations (alcohol rubs, aftershave lotions).

Test-Taking Strategy: Note the key words "need for further instructions." These words indicate a false-response question and that you need to select the incorrect client statement. Remember that antabuse is used for clients who have alcoholism and that any form of alcohol needs to be avoided with this medication. Review this content if you are unfamiliar with this medication and the health teaching that is indicated when this medication is prescribed.

Level of Cognitive Ability: Analysis
Client Needs: Health Promotion and Maintenance
Integrated Process: Teaching/Learning
Content Area: Pharmacology

Reference:
McKenry, L., & Salerno, E. (2003). *Mosby's pharmacology in nursing* (21st ed.). St. Louis: Mosby, pp. 170; 175.

23. A nurse has provided instructions to a client receiving external radiation therapy. Which statement by the client indicates a need for further instructions regarding self-care related to the radiation therapy?
  1 "I need to avoid exposure to sunlight."
  2 "I need to wash my skin with a mild soap and pat it dry."
  3 "I need to apply pressure on the irritated area to prevent bleeding."
  4 "I need to eat a high-protein diet."

Answer: 3
Rationale: The client should avoid pressure on the irritated area and should wear loose-fitting clothing. Specific physician instructions would be necessary to obtain if an alteration in skin integrity occurred as a result of the radiation therapy. Options 1, 2, and 4 are accurate measures regarding radiation therapy.

Test-Taking Strategy: Note the key words "need for further instructions." These words indicate a false-response question and that you need to select the incorrect client statement. The word "pressure" in option 3 is an indication that this is an inappropriate measure. Review client teaching points related to skin care and radiation therapy if you had difficulty with this question.

Level of Cognitive Ability: Application
Client Needs: Health Promotion and Maintenance
Integrated Process: Teaching/Learning
Content Area: Adult Health/Oncology

Reference:
Phipps, W., Monahan, F., Sands, J., Marek, J., & Neighbors, M. (2003). *Medical-surgical nursing: Health and illness perspectives* (7th ed.). St. Louis: Mosby, pp. 336-337.

24. A nurse has provided instructions to a client regarding the Testicular Self-Examination (TSE). Which statement by the client indicates that the client needs further instructions regarding TSE?

1 "I feel the spermatic cord in back and going up."
2 "I know to report any small lumps."
3 "I examine myself after I take a warm shower."
4 "I examine myself every two months."

Answer: 4

Rationale: TSE should be performed every month. Small lumps or abnormalities should be reported. The spermatic cord finding is normal. After a warm bath or shower, the scrotum is relaxed, making it easier to perform TSE.

Test-Taking Strategy: Use the process of elimination. Remembering that Breast Self-Examination needs to be performed monthly may assist in recalling that TSE is also performed monthly. Review the procedure for TSE if you had difficulty with this question.

Level of Cognitive Ability: Analysis
Client Needs: Health Promotion and Maintenance
Integrated Process: Teaching/Learning
Content Area: Adult Health/Oncology

Reference:
Black, J., & Hawks, J. (2005). *Medical-surgical nursing: Clinical management for positive outcomes* (7th ed.). Philadelphia: Saunders, p. 1005.

---

25. A client with acquired immunodeficiency syndrome (AIDS) has a nursing diagnosis of Fatigue. The nurse teaches the client which strategy to conserve energy after discharge from the hospital?

1 Stand in the shower instead of taking a bath
2 Bathe before eating breakfast
3 Sit for as many activities as possible
4 Group all tasks to be performed early in the morning

Answer: 3

Rationale: The client is taught to conserve energy by sitting for as many activities as possible, including dressing, shaving, preparing food, ironing, and so on. The client should also sit in a shower chair instead of standing while bathing. The client needs to prioritize activities such as eating breakfast before bathing, and should intersperse each major activity with a period of rest.

Test-Taking Strategy: Focus on the issue: conserve energy. Think about the amount of exertion required by the client in performing each of the activities in the options. Options 1 and 4 are obviously taxing for the client and are eliminated first. From the remaining options, recall that bathing may take away energy that could be used for eating and is not helpful. Review measures that conserve energy if you had difficulty with this question.

Level of Cognitive Ability: Application
Client Needs: Health Promotion and Maintenance
Integrated Process: Teaching/Learning
Content Area: Adult Health/Immune

Reference:
Ignatavicius, D., & Workman, M. (2002). *Medical surgical nursing: Critical thinking for collaborative care* (4th ed.). Philadelphia: Saunders, p. 382.

26. A nurse has provided self-care activity instructions to a client after insertion of an automatic internal cardioverter-defibrillator (AICD). The nurse determines that further instruction is needed if the client makes which statement?

1 "I should try to avoid doing strenuous things that would make my heart rate go up to or above the rate cutoff on the AICD."

2 "I should keep away from electromagnetic sources such as transformers, large electrical generators, metal detectors, and leaning over running motors."

3 "I can perform activities such as swimming, driving, or operating heavy equipment as I need too."

4 "I need to avoid doing anything where there would be rough contact with the AICD insertion site."

Answer: 3

Rationale: Post-discharge instructions typically include avoiding tight clothing or belts over AICD insertion sites, rough contact with the AICD insertion site, electromagnetic fields such as with electrical transformers, radio/TV/radar transmitters, metal detectors, and running motors of cars or boats. Clients must also alert physicians or dentists of the device, because certain procedures such as diathermy, electrocautery, and magnetic resonance imaging may need to be avoided to prevent device malfunction. Clients should follow the specific advice of a physician regarding activities that are potentially hazardous to self or others, such as swimming, driving, or operating heavy equipment.

Test-Taking Strategy: Use the process of elimination, noting the key words "further instruction is needed." These words indicate a false-response question and that you need to select the incorrect client statement. Options 2 and 4 can be eliminated first, because they are similar to standard post-pacemaker insertion instructions. From the remaining options, noting the words "heavy equipment" in option 3 will direct you to this option. Review client teaching points for AICD if you had difficulty with this question.

Level of Cognitive Ability: Analysis
Client Needs: Health Promotion and Maintenance
Integrated Process: Teaching/Learning
Content Area: Adult Health/Cardiovascular

References:
Lewis, S., Heitkemper, M., & Dirksen, S. (2004). *Medical-surgical nursing: Assessment and management of clinical problems* (6th ed.). St. Louis: Mosby, p. 876.
Ignatavicius, D., & Workman, M. (2002). *Medical surgical nursing: Critical thinking for collaborative care* (4th ed.). Philadelphia: Saunders, pp. 695-696.

27. A 10-year-old child who is very active socially and is often away from the parents has been diagnosed with type 1 diabetes mellitus. The nurse prepares to educate the family about the disorder and plans to teach:

1 The child's school teacher to monitor insulin requirements and administer the child's insulin

2 The child to monitor insulin requirements and administer own insulin

3 The parents to always be available to monitor the child's insulin requirements

4 All the friends and family involved with the child's activities to monitor the child's insulin requirements

Answer: 2

Rationale: Most children nine years old or older can understand the principles of monitoring their own insulin requirements. They are usually responsible enough to determine the appropriate intervention needed to maintain their health. The school teacher will not take responsibility for health care interventions. Parents, friends, and family can not always be available.

Test-Taking Strategy: Noting the age of the child will indicate that the child is able to take control and responsibility regarding the health care situation. Eliminate option 4 first because of the absolute word "all." From the remaining options, note that options 1 and 3 rely on other individuals to care for the child. Review growth and development of a 10-year-old if you had difficulty with this question.

Level of Cognitive Ability: Application
Client Needs: Health Promotion and Maintenance
Integrated Process: Teaching/Learning
Content Area: Child Health

Reference:
Wong, D., & Hockenberry, M. (2003). *Wong's nursing care of infants and children* (7th ed.). St. Louis: Mosby, pp. 1750; 1753.

---

28. A nurse instructs a client with candidiasis (thrush) of the oral cavity about how to care for the disorder. The nurse determines that the client needs additional instructions if the client stated to:
1 Rinse the mouth four times daily with a commercial mouthwash
2 Eliminate spicy foods from the diet
3 Eliminate citrus juices and hot liquids from the diet
4 Eat foods that are liquid or pureed

Answer: 1
Rationale: Clients with thrush cannot tolerate commercial mouthwashes because the high alcohol concentration in these products can cause pain and discomfort to the lesions. A solution of warm water or mouthwash formulas without alcohol are better tolerated and may promote healing. A change in diet to liquid or pureed food often eases the discomfort of eating. The client should avoid spicy foods, citrus juice, and hot liquids.

Test-Taking Strategy: Use the process of elimination and note the key words "needs additional instructions." These words indicate a false-response question and that you need to select the incorrect client statement. Also, noting the words "commercial mouthwash" in option 1 will direct you to this option. Review the client teaching points related to candidiasis (thrush) if you had difficulty with this question.

Level of Cognitive Ability: Application
Client Needs: Health Promotion and Maintenance
Integrated Process: Teaching/Learning
Content Area: Adult Health/Immune

Reference:
Ignatavicius, D., & Workman, M. (2002). *Medical surgical nursing: Critical thinking for collaborative care* (4th ed.). Philadelphia: Saunders, pp. 1180-1181.

CRITICAL THINKING: ALTERNATE FORMAT QUESTIONS

---

1. The physician's order reads: tobramycin sulfate (Nebcin), 7.5 mg intramuscularly twice daily. The medication label reads: 10 mg/mL. The nurse prepares how many milliliters to administer one dose?

Answer: _____

Answer: 0.75

Rationale: Use the formula for calculating a medication dose.

Formula:

$$\frac{\text{Desired}}{\text{Available}} \times \text{Volume} = \text{mL per dose}$$

$$\frac{7.5 \text{ mg}}{10 \text{ mg}} \times 1.0 \text{ mL} = 0.75 \text{ mL}$$

Test-Taking Strategy: Identify the key components of the question and what the question is asking. In this case, the question asks for the mL per dose. Use the formula to determine the correct dosage and use a calculator to verity your answer. Review the formula for calculating a medication dose if you had difficulty with this question.

Level of Cognitive Ability: Application
Client Needs: Physiological Integrity
Integrated Process: Nursing Process/Implementation
Content Area: Fundamental Skills

Reference:
Kee, J., & Marshall, S. (2004). *Clinical calculations: With applications to general and specialty areas* (4th ed.). Philadelphia: Saunders, p. 80.

---

2. A nurse is asked to assist another health care member in providing care for a client. On entering the client's room, the nurse notes that the client is placed in this position. The nurse interprets that the client is most likely being treated for:

  1 A head injury
  2 Respiratory insufficiency
  3 Shock
  4 Increased intracranial pressure

Answer: 3

Rationale: A client in shock is placed in a modified Trendelenburg position that includes elevating the legs, leaving the trunk flat, and elevating the head and shoulders slightly. This position promotes increased venous return from the lower extremities without compressing the abdominal organs against the diaphragm. Options 1, 2, and 4 identify conditions in which the client's head of the bed would be elevated.

Test-Taking Strategy: Focus on the position identified in the question. Eliminate options 1 and 4 first because they are similar and both relate to a neurological condition. From the remaining options, eliminate option 2 recalling that the head of the bed is elevated in respiratory conditions. Review care of the client with shock if you had difficulty with this question.

Level of Cognitive Ability: Analysis
Client Needs: Physiological Integrity
Integrated Process: Nursing Process/Analysis
Content Area: Adult Health/Cardiovascular

Reference:
Black, J., & Hawks, J. (2005). *Medical-surgical nursing: Clinical management for positive outcomes* (7th ed.). Philadelphia: Saunders, p. 2461.

---

3. A clinic nurse is performing a complete physical assessment on a client. During respiratory assessment, the nurse is using which physical assessment technique? (See illustration to determine the answer.)

  1 Auscultation
  2 Palpation
  3 Percussion
  4 Inspection

Answer: 3

Answer: To perform percussion, the nurse places the middle finger of the nondominant hand against the body's surface. The tip of the middle finger of the dominant hand strikes the top of the middle finger of the nondominant hand. Auscultation is listening to sounds produced by the body. Palpation is performed through the sense of touch. Inspection is the process of observation.

Test-Taking Strategy: Use the process of elimination. Recalling the definition of each technique in the options will direct you to option 3. Remember that inspection is observing, palpation uses the sense of touch, and inspection is observation. Review physical assessment techniques if you had difficulty with this question.

Level of Cognitive Ability: Application
Client Needs: Health Promotion and Maintenance
Integrated Process: Nursing Process/Assessment
Content Area: Adult Health/Respiratory

Reference:
Potter, P., & Perry, A. (2005). *Fundamentals of nursing* (6th ed.). St. Louis: Mosby, p. 677.

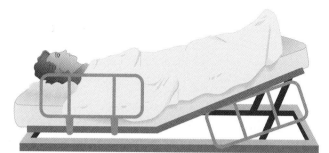

From: Black & Hawks (2005) *Medical surgical nursing* (7th ed). Philadelphia : WB (Saunders).

4. A client arrives in the postanesthesia care unit following colectomy. After receiving a verbal report from the anesthesia care provider, the nurse performs an initial assessment. List in order of priority the initial assessment actions. (Number 1 is the first assessment action.)

_____ Assesses level of consciousness

_____ Checks for airway patency

_____ Counts the heart rate and determines the rhythm

_____ Counts the respiratory rate and determines the quality of respirations

Answer: 4132

Rationale: Postoperative assessment should begin with an evaluation of the ABCs—airway, breathing, and circulation—status of the client. Airway patency is always assessed first to ensure adequate oxygenation to body organs and tissues. Next, the rate and quality of the client's respirations are determined, and breath sounds are auscultated throughout all lung fields to ensure adequate respiratory status. The client's heart rate and rhythm are determined and the client's blood pressure is checked following respiratory assessment. A neurological assessment is then performed along with other assessments such as assessment of the urinary status, dressings, drains, and tubes, and pain assessment as needed.

Test-Taking Strategy: Note the words "order of priority." Use the ABCs (i.e., airway, breathing, and circulation). This will assist in determining the correct order of action. Review initial care of the postoperative client if you had difficulty with this question.

Level of Cognitive Ability: Application
Client Needs: Physiological Integrity
Integrated Process: Nursing Process/Assessment
Content Area: Fundamental Skills

Reference:
Lewis, S., Heitkemper, M., & Dirksen, S. (2004). *Medical-surgical nursing: Assessment and management of clinical problems* (6th ed.). St. Louis: Mosby, pp. 393-394.

5. A nurse is providing home care instructions to the spouse of a client who is confused and will be cared for at home. Select all instructions that the nurse provides to the spouse:

___ Display a calendar and a clock around the client's room

___ Encourage frequent visits from family and friends

___ Limit the number of choices given to the client

___ Turn the lights off at dusk

___ Maintain a predictable routine

___ Use simple, clear communication

Answer:

Display a calendar and a clock around the house

Limit the number of choices given to the client

Maintain a predictable routine

Use simple, clear communication

Rationale: The caregiver of a confused client is taught measures and techniques that will keep the client oriented and calm. Sensory overload or tasks and activities that are overwhelming for the client will cause disorientation and additional confusion. Therefore, any measures or activities that will increase sensory overload are avoided. Some helpful techniques include displaying a calendar and a clock around the house and in the client's room; maintaining a predictable routine; limiting the number of visitors who come to see the client; limiting the number of choices given to the client; using simple, clear communication; and turning the lights on at dusk to avoid the sundown syndrome of increased confusion and combative behavior.

Test-Taking Strategy: Focus on the issue: measures that will keep the client oriented and calm. Think about each listed intervention, and remember that measures or activities that will increase sensory overload or are overwhelming for the client are avoided. This principle will assist in selecting the correct measures. Review care of the confused client if you had difficulty with this question.

Level of Cognitive Ability: Application
Client Needs: Psychosocial Integrity
Integrated Process: Teaching/Learning
Content Area: Mental Health

Reference:

Harkreader, H., & Hogan, M.A. (2004) *Fundamentals of nursing: Caring and clinical judgment.* (2nd ed.). Philadelphia: Saunders. p. 1028.

REFERENCES

Black, J., & Hawks, J. (2005). *Medical-surgical nursing: Clinical management for positive outcomes* (7th ed.). Philadelphia: Saunders.

Chernecky, C., & Berger, B. (2004). *Laboratory tests and diagnostic procedures* (4th ed.). Philadelphia: Saunders.

Ebersole, P., & Hess, P. (2001). *Geriatric nursing & healthy aging.* St. Louis: Mosby.

Harkreader, H., & Hogan, M.A. (2004) *Fundamentals of nursing: Caring and clinical judgment.* (2nd ed.). Philadelphia: Saunders.

Hodgson, B., & Kizior, R. (2004). *Saunders nursing drug handbook 2004.* Philadelphia: Saunders.

Ignatavicius, D., & Workman, M. (2005). *Medical surgical nursing: Critical thinking for collaborative care* (5th ed.). Philadelphia: Saunders.

James, S., Ashwill, J., & Droske, S. (2002). *Nursing care of children: Principles & practice* (2nd ed.). Philadelphia: Saunders.

Kee, J., & Marshall, S. (2004). *Clinical calculations: With applications to general and specialty areas* (5th ed.). Philadelphia: Saunders.

Keltner, N., Schwecke, L., & Bostrom, C. (2003). *Psychiatric nursing* (4th ed.). St. Louis: Mosby.

Lehne, R. (2004). *Pharmacology for nursing care* (5th ed.). Philadelphia: Saunders.

Lewis, S., Heitkemper, M., & Dirksen, S. (2004). *Medical-surgical nursing: Assessment and management of clinical problems* (6th ed.). St. Louis: Mosby.

Lowdermilk, D., & Perry, A. (2004). *Maternity & women's health care* (8th ed.). St. Louis: Mosby.

McKenry, L., & Salerno, E. (2003). *Mosby's pharmacology in nursing* (21st ed.). St. Louis: Mosby.

McKinney, E., James, S., Murray, S., & Ashwill, J. (2005). *Maternal-child nursing* (2nd ed.). St. Louis: Elsevier.

Murray, S., McKinney, E., & Gorrie, T. (2002). *Foundations of maternal-newborn nursing* (3rd ed.). Philadelphia: Saunders.

Pagana, K., & Pagana, T. (2003). *Mosby's diagnostic and laboratory test reference* (6th ed.). St. Louis: Mosby.

Phipps, W., Monahan, F., Sands, J., Marek, J., & Neighbors, M. (2003). *Medical-surgical nursing: Health and illness perspectives* (7th ed.). St. Louis: Mosby.

Potter, P., & Perry, A. (2005). *Fundamentals of nursing* (6th ed.). St. Louis: Mosby.

Riley, J. (2004). *Communication in nursing* (5th ed.). St. Louis: Mosby.

Stuart, G., & Laraia, M. (2005). *Principles and practice of psychiatric nursing* (8th ed.). St. Louis: Mosby.

Varcarolis, E.M. (2002). *Foundations of psychiatric mental health nursing* (4th ed.). Philadelphia: Saunders.

Williams, S. (2001). *Basic nutrition & diet therapy* (11th ed.). St Louis: Mosby.

Wong, D., & Hockenberry, M. (2003). *Wong's nursing care of infants and children* (7th ed.). St. Louis: Mosby.

Comprehensive Test

1. A nurse is performing an assessment on a 6-month-old infant suspected of having hydrocephalus. Which finding is associated with this diagnosis?
1 The presence of protein in the urine
2 An elevated apical heart rate
3 A drop in blood pressure from baseline
4 A bulging anterior fontanel

Answer: 4
Rationale: A bulging anterior fontanel indicates an increase in cerebrospinal fluid collection in the cerebral ventricle, which occurs in hydrocephalus. Proteinuria, an elevated apical pulse, and a drop in blood pressure are not specifically related to increasing cerebrospinal fluid in the brain tissue.

Test-Taking Strategy: Use the principles associated with excessive fluid buildup in the cranial cavity to answer this question. Remember that fluid accumulation in the cranial cavity will exert pressure on the soft brain tissue. This will cause the anterior fontanel to expand. Additionally, correlate the word "hydrocephalus" in the question with "anterior fontanel" in option 4. Review the findings associated with hydrocephalus if you had difficulty with this question.

Level of Cognitive Ability: Analysis
Client Needs: Physiological Integrity
Integrated Process: Nursing Process/Assessment
Content Area: Child Health

Reference:
Wong, D., & Hockenberry, M. (2003). *Wong's nursing care of infants and children* (7th ed.). St. Louis: Mosby, p. 437.

2. A 10-day postpartum breastfeeding client telephones the postpartum unit complaining of a reddened, painful breast and elevated temperature. Based on assessment of the client's complaints, the nurse tells the client to:
1 "Stop breastfeeding because you probably have an infection."
2 "Notify your physician because you may need medication."
3 "Continue breastfeeding because this is a normal response in breastfeeding mothers."
4 "Breastfeed only with the unaffected breast."

Answer: 2
Rationale: Based on the signs and symptoms presented by the client (particularly the elevated temperature), the physician needs to be notified because an antibiotic that is tolerated by the infant as well as the mother may be prescribed. The mother should continue to nurse on both breasts, but should start the infant on the unaffected breast while the affected breast lets down.

Test-Taking Strategy: Focus on the data in the question and note that the client has an elevated temperature. Option 3 can be eliminated first because the client's complaints are not normal. Eliminate option 1 because it does not encourage the continuation of breastfeeding or notification of the physician. Option 4 also does not encourage continuation of normal breastfeeding and could possibly lead to engorgement, creating more discomfort and pain for the mother. Review postpartum complications if you had difficulty with this question.

Level of Cognitive Ability: Application
Client Needs: Physiological Integrity
Integrated Process: Nursing Process/Implementation
Content Area: Maternity/Postpartum

Reference:
Lowdermilk, D., & Perry, A. (2004). *Maternity & women's health care* (8th ed.). St. Louis: Mosby, p. 779.

3. The nurse notes that the physician has written an order for prednisone (Deltasone) for a client. The nurse contacts the physician about revision of the client's medication plan if which medication is noted on the client's medication record?
1 Oxycodone (Oxycontin)
2 Propoxyphene (Darvon)
3 Acetaminophen (Tylenol)
4 Acetylsalicylic acid (aspirin)

Answer: 4
Rationale: Prednisone is irritating to the gastrointestinal (GI) tract, which could be worsened by the use of other products that have the same side effect. Therefore, products such as aspirin and nonsteroidal antiinflammatory drugs are not used during corticosteroid therapy.

Test-Taking Strategy: Use the process of elimination and think about the side effects of prednisone. Recalling that aspirin is irritating to the GI tract will assist in answering the question. Review the side effects of prednisone if you had difficulty with this question.

Level of Cognitive Ability: Application
Client Needs: Safe, Effective Care Environment
Integrated Process: Nursing Process/Implementation
Content Area: Pharmacology

Reference:
Lehne, R. (2004). *Pharmacology for nursing care* (5th ed.). Philadelphia: Saunders, pp. 766-767.

---

4. A nurse is asked to go to a local high school to talk to students about sexually transmitted diseases (STDs). The nurse plans to tell the students that:
1 Birth control pills are the only way to prevent STDs
2 A diaphragm provides a barrier to prevent STDs
3 The use of condoms does not provide any protection at all
4 The use of condoms and avoiding casual sex with multiple partners prevent STDs

Answer: 4
Rationale: The use of condoms and avoiding casual sex with multiple partners should be the focus of discussion because these measures prevent STDs. The use of condoms does provide some protection against STDs. Birth control pills and the use of a diaphragm help prevent pregnancy but do not provide protection from STDs.

Test-Taking Strategy: Focus on the issue, which relates to STDs, not pregnancy. This focus will eliminate options 1, 2, and 3. Review the methods of protection against STDs if you had difficulty with this question.

Level of Cognitive Ability: Application
Client Needs: Safe, Effective Care Environment
Integrated Process: Teaching/Learning
Content Area: Fundamental Skills

Reference:
Black, J., & Hawks, J. (2005). *Medical-surgical nursing: Clinical management for positive outcomes* (7th ed.). Philadelphia: Saunders, pp. 1127-1128.

---

5. A home care nurse is caring for a client who has just been discharged from the hospital after implantation of a permanent pacemaker. A priority nursing action to maintain a safe environment for the client would be to assess the client's home for the presence of:
1 Hair dryers
2 Electric toothbrushes
3 Electrical items that have strong electric currents or magnetic fields
4 Electric blankets

Answer: 3
Rationale: A pacemaker is shielded from interference from most electrical devices. Radios, TVs, electric blankets, toasters, microwave ovens, heating pads, and hair dryers are considered to be safe. Devices to be forewarned about include those with a strong electric current or magnetic field, such as antitheft devices in stores, metal detectors used in airports, and radiation therapy (if applicable and which might require relocation of the pacemaker).

Test-Taking Strategy: Use the process of elimination. Note that option 3 uses the word "strong" and is the umbrella (global) option addressing items with strong electric currents or magnetic fields. Review home care measures for the client with a pacemaker if you had difficulty with this question.

Level of Cognitive Ability: Application
Client Needs: Safe, Effective Care Environment
Integrated Process: Nursing Process/Assessment
Content Area: Adult Health/Cardiovascular

Reference:
Phipps, W., Monahan, F., Sands, J., Marek, J., & Neighbors, M. (2003). *Medical-surgical nursing: Health and illness perspectives* (7th ed.). St. Louis: Mosby, p. 700.

---

6. A client with low back pain asks the nurse which type of exercise will best strengthen the lower back muscles. The nurse tells the client to participate in which beneficial exercise?

1 Tennis
2 Diving
3 Canoeing
4 Swimming

Answer: 4
Rationale: Walking and swimming are very beneficial in strengthening back muscles for the client with low back pain. The other options involve twisting and pulling of the back muscles, which is not helpful to the client experiencing back pain.

Test-Taking Strategy: Recalling that low back pain is aggravated by any activity that twists or turns the spine, evaluate each of the options according to this guideline. This will enable you to eliminate options 1, 2, and 3. Review home care measures for the client with low back pain if you had difficulty with this question.

Level of Cognitive Ability: Application
Client Needs: Health Promotion and Maintenance
Integrated Process: Teaching/Learning
Content Area: Adult Health/Neurological

Reference:
Phipps, W., Monahan, F., Sands, J., Marek, J., & Neighbors, M. (2003). *Medical-surgical nursing: Health and illness perspectives* (7th ed.). St. Louis: Mosby, p. 1577.

---

7. A nurse is caring for a child with a diagnosis of Kawasaki disease, and the mother of the child asks the nurse about the disorder. The nurse bases the response to the mother on which description of this disorder?

1 It is an acquired cell-mediated immunodeficiency disorder.
2 It is an inflammatory autoimmune disease that affects the connective tissue of the heart, joints, and subcutaneous tissues.
3 It is a chronic multisystem autoimmune disease characterized by the inflammation of connective tissue.
4 It is also called mucocutaneous lymph node syndrome and is a febrile generalized vasculitis of unknown etiology.

Answer: 4
Rationale: Kawasaki disease, also called mucocutaneous lymph node syndrome, is a febrile generalized vasculitis of unknown etiology. Option 1 describes human immunodeficiency virus (HIV) infection. Option 2 describes rheumatic fever. Option 3 describes systemic lupus erythematosus.

Test-Taking Strategy: Knowledge regarding the description of Kawasaki disease is required to answer this question. Review this content if you are unfamiliar with this disorder.

Level of Cognitive Ability: Application
Client Needs: Physiological Integrity
Integrated Process: Nursing Process/Implementation
Content Area: Child Health

Reference:
Wong, D., & Hockenberry, M. (2003). *Wong's nursing care of infants and children* (7th ed.). St. Louis: Mosby, p. 1514.

8. A nurse is preparing to teach the parents of a child with anemia about the dietary sources of iron that are easy for the body to absorb. Which food item would the nurse include in the teaching plan?
1 Apricots
2 Poultry
3 Fruits
4 Vegetables

Answer: 2

Rationale: Dietary sources of iron that are easy for the body to absorb include meat, poultry, and fish. Vegetables, fruits, cereals, and breads are also dietary sources of iron, but they are harder for the body to absorb.

Test-Taking Strategy: Focus on the issue: food sources that are high in iron and easy to absorb. Options 1 and 3 are similar and should be eliminated first. From the remaining options, focusing on the key words "easy for the body to absorb" assists in eliminating option 4. Review food items high in iron if you had difficulty with this question.

Level of Cognitive Ability: Application
Client Needs: Health Promotion and Maintenance
Integrated Process: Teaching/Learning
Content Area: Child Health

Reference:
Wong, D., & Hockenberry, M. (2003). *Wong's nursing care of infants and children* (7th ed.). St. Louis: Mosby, pp. 562; 564.

9. A nurse is caring for a child with a patent ductus arteriosus. The nurse reviews the child's assessment data, knowing that which of the following is characteristic of this disorder?
1 It involves an opening between the two atria.
2 It involves an opening between the two ventricles.
3 It produces abnormalities in the atrial septum.
4 It involves an artery that connects the aorta and the pulmonary artery during fetal life.

Answer: 4

Rationale: Patent ductus arteriosus is described as an artery that connects the aorta and the pulmonary artery during fetal life. It generally closes spontaneously within a few hours to several days after birth. It allows abnormal blood flow from the high-pressure aorta to the low-pressure pulmonary artery, resulting in a left-to-right shunt. Options 1, 2, and 3 are not characteristics of this cardiac defect.

Test-Taking Strategy: Knowledge regarding the characteristics associated with patent ductus arteriosus is required to answer this question. Review this content if you are unfamiliar with this cardiac defect.

Level of Cognitive Ability: Analysis
Client Needs: Physiological Integrity
Integrated Process: Nursing Process/Analysis
Content Area: Child Health

Reference:
Wong, D., & Hockenberry, M. (2003). *Wong's nursing care of infants and children* (7th ed.). St. Louis: Mosby, pp. 1490; 1494.

10. A nurse is caring for a client who has returned to the physician's office for follow-up after a parathyroidectomy with autotransplantation of some parathyroid tissue into the forearm. The client has been taking oral calcium and vitamin D supplements since discharge 2 weeks ago. Which statement by the client indicates an understanding of the medical management following this type of surgical procedure?

1 "Well, I guess the transplant isn't working because my calcium levels are still low."

2 "The thought of taking these pills for the rest of my life makes me shudder!"

3 "I can't wait for the transplant to start working. I'm tired of taking all these pills!"

4 "Do you think I'll always have to take these pills?"

Answer: 3

Rationale: The purpose of autotransplantation of some parathyroid tissue is to regain function of the parathyroid gland. Autotransplantation of parathyroid tissue takes some time to mature. Oral calcium and vitamin D supplements must be taken to prevent hypoparathyroidism until the transplant matures and becomes an active endocrine gland.

Test-Taking Strategy: Use the process of elimination. Options 2 and 4 can be eliminated first because they are similar and both seem to negate the purpose of transplants, that being gaining function of the organ. From the remaining options, eliminate option 1 because the question does not address low calcium levels. Review the purpose of parathyroid transplant surgery if you had difficulty with this question.

Level of Cognitive Ability: Analysis
Client Needs: Health Promotion and Maintenance
Integrated Process: Teaching/Learning
Content Area: Adult Health/Endocrine

Reference:
Black, J., & Hawks, J. (2005). *Medical-surgical nursing: Clinical management for positive outcomes* (7th ed.). Philadelphia: Saunders, p. 1213.

11. Desmopressin acetate (DDAVP) is prescribed via intranasal route for a child with von Willebrand's disease, and the nurse instructs the parents regarding the administration of this medication. Which statement by the parents indicates a need for further instructions?

1 "We need to restrict our child's fluid intake."

2 "We need to refrigerate the DDAVP."

3 "Nausea and abdominal cramps can occur as a side effect of the medication."

4 "Headache and drowsiness may be a sign of water intoxication that can occur with the medication."

Answer: 1

Rationale: The parents should be instructed to monitor intake and output and to avoid overhydration, but fluids should not be restricted. The medication should be refrigerated, but freezing should be avoided. Side effects of the medication include facial flushing, nasal congestion, increased blood pressure, nausea, abdominal cramps, decreased urination, and vulval pain. Signs and symptoms of water intoxication include headache, drowsiness and confusion, weight gain, seizures, and coma.

Test-Taking Strategy: Note the key words "need for further instructions." These words indicate a false-response question and that you need to select the incorrect client statement. Noting the word "restrict" in option 1 will direct you to this option. Review the action, use, and side effects of this medication if you had difficulty with this question.

Level of Cognitive Ability: Analysis
Client Needs: Health Promotion and Maintenance
Integrated Process: Teaching/Learning
Content Area: Child Health

References:
Hodgson, B., & Kizior, R. (2004). *Saunders nursing drug handbook 2004.* Philadelphia: Saunders, p. 288.
McKenry, L., & Salerno, E. (2003). *Mosby's pharmacology in nursing* (21st ed.). St. Louis: Mosby, p. 834.

12. A child is brought to the emergency room after being bitten in the arm by a neighborhood dog. The nurse performs a focused assessment, cleanses the wound as prescribed, and continues to perform a thorough assessment on the child. Which of the following is the priority question for the nurse to ask the mother of the child?
1 "Did the dog have rabies?"
2 "Are the child's immunizations up-to-date?"
3 "How old is the dog?"
4 "Did the dog have all of its recommended shots?"

Answer: 2
Rationale: When a bite occurs, the injury site of the bite should be cleansed carefully and the child should be given tetanus prophylaxis if immunizations are not up-to-date. Option 2 is the priority consideration. Options 1, 3, and 4 identify information that may have to be obtained, but are not the priority questions. Additionally, the mother may not have the answers to these questions.

Test-Taking Strategy: Use the process of elimination and note the key word "priority." Option 2 is the only option that focuses on the needs of the child. Review this content if you are unfamiliar with the assessment and care of a child who receives a dog bite.

Level of Cognitive Ability: Application
Client Needs: Health Promotion and Maintenance
Integrated Process: Nursing Process/Assessment
Content Area: Child Health

Reference:
James, S., Ashwill, J., & Droske, S. (2002). *Nursing care of children: Principles & practice* (2nd ed.). Philadelphia: Saunders, p. 295.

---

13. A nurse is providing instructions to the mother of a child who had a myringotomy with insertion of tympanostomy tubes. The nurse tells the mother that if the tubes fall out:
1 It is important to replace them immediately so that the surgical opening does not close
2 To bring the child to the emergency room immediately
3 It is not an emergency, but it is best to call the health care clinic
4 Clean the tubes with half-strength hydrogen peroxide for 30 minutes and then replace them into the child's ears

Answer: 3
Rationale: The mother should be assured that if the tympanostomy tubes fall out, it is not an emergency, but it is best if the physician or health care clinic is notified. The size and appearance of the tympanostomy tubes should be described to the mother following surgery so that she will be familiar with their appearance. Options 1, 2, and 4 are incorrect.

Test-Taking Strategy: Use the process of elimination. Option 2 is eliminated first because it will cause concern in the mother. Next eliminate options 1 and 4 because they are similar and relate to replacing the tubes. Review home care instructions following this procedure if you had difficulty with this question.

Level of Cognitive Ability: Application
Client Needs: Physiological Integrity
Integrated Process: Teaching/Learning
Content Area: Child Health

Reference:
Wong, D., & Hockenberry, M. (2003). *Wong's nursing care of infants and children* (7th ed.). St. Louis: Mosby, p. 1360.

14. The mother of a child calls the health care clinic and tells a nurse that the child has developed a bloody nose. The nurse instructs the mother to do which of the following?
1 Maintain the child in a sitting position with the head tilted backward
2 Pinch the nostrils for 5 minutes and then recheck for bleeding
3 Lay the child down with a pillow tucked under the neck and stay with the child to keep the child calm
4 Have the child sit with the head tilted forward and hold pressure on the soft part of the nose for a period of 10 minutes

Answer: 4

Rationale: The child should be positioned erect, sitting with head tilted forward to avoid blood dripping posteriorly to the pharynx. The soft part of the nose should be tightly pinched against the center wall for 10 minutes, and the mother should be instructed that this pinch should be timed by a clock, not estimated. The mother should be told not to release pressure for 10 minutes. The child is encouraged to remain calm and quiet and to breathe through the mouth.

Test-Taking Strategy: Use the process of elimination, focusing on the issue: controlling a bloody nose. Visualize the positions presented in the options to direct you to option 4. Review the interventions used when epistaxis occurs if you had difficulty with question.

Level of Cognitive Ability: Application
Client Needs: Physiological Integrity
Integrated Process: Nursing Process/Implementation
Content Area: Child Health

Reference:
Wong, D., & Hockenberry, M. (2003). *Wong's nursing care of infants and children* (7th ed.). St. Louis: Mosby, p. 1567.

---

15. A nurse is assessing a child admitted to the hospital with a diagnosis of rheumatic fever. The nurse asks the child's mother which significant question during the assessment?
1 "Has your child had difficulty urinating?"
2 "Has any family member had a sore throat within the past few weeks?"
3 "Has any family member had a gastrointestinal disorder in the past few weeks?"
4 "Has your child been exposed to anyone with chickenpox?"

Answer: 2

Rationale: Rheumatic fever characteristically presents 2 to 6 weeks following an untreated or partially treated group A beta hemolytic streptococcal infection of the respiratory tract. Initially, the nurse determines whether any family member has had a sore throat or unexplained fever within the past few weeks. Options 1, 3, and 4 are unrelated to the assessment findings of rheumatic fever.

Test-Taking Strategy: Note the key word "significant." Recalling that rheumatic fever characteristically presents 2 to 6 weeks following a streptococcal infection of the respiratory tract will direct you to the correct option. Review this content if you are unfamiliar with the etiology and the pathophysiology associated with this disorder.

Level of Cognitive Ability: Application
Client Needs: Physiological Integrity
Integrated Process: Nursing Process/Assessment
Content Area: Child Health

Reference:
Wong, D., & Hockenberry, M. (2003). *Wong's nursing care of infants and children* (7th ed.). St. Louis: Mosby, p. 1512.

16. The parents of a child with mumps express concern that their child will develop orchitis as a result of having mumps and ask the nurse about the signs of this complication. The nurse tells the parents that which of the following is a sign of this complication?

1 Swollen glands
2 Facial swelling
3 Fever
4 Difficulty urinating

Answer: 3

Rationale: Unilateral orchitis occurs more frequently than bilateral orchitis. About one week after the appearance of parotitis, there is an abrupt onset of testicular pain, tenderness, fever, chills, headache, and vomiting. The affected testicle becomes red, swollen, and tender. Atrophy, resulting in sterility, occurs only in a small number of cases. Difficulty urinating is not a sign of this complication. Swollen glands and facial swelling normally occurs in mumps.

Test-Taking Strategy: Use the process of elimination. Eliminate options 1 and 2 first because they are similar. From the remaining options, focus on the word "orchitis." Recalling that "itis" indicates inflammation will direct you to option 3. Review the characteristics of orchitis if you had difficulty with this question.

Level of Cognitive Ability: Application
Client Needs: Health Promotion and Maintenance
Integrated Process: Teaching/Learning
Content Area: Child Health

References:
James, S., Ashwill, J., & Droske, S. (2002). *Nursing care of children: Principles & practice* (2nd ed.). Philadelphia: Saunders, pp. 455-456.
Wong, D., & Hockenberry, M. (2003). *Wong's nursing care of infants and children* (7th ed.). St. Louis: Mosby, p. 657.

17. A maternity nurse is teaching a pregnant woman about the physiological effects and hormone changes that occurs in pregnancy, and a woman asks the nurse about the purpose of estrogen. The nurse bases the response on which of the following?

1 It maintains the uterine lining for implantation.
2 It stimulates metabolism of glucose and converts the glucose to fat.
3 It prevents the involution of the corpus luteum and maintains the production of progesterone until the placenta is formed.
4 It stimulates uterine development to provide an environment for the fetus and stimulates the breasts to prepare for lactation.

Answer: 4

Rationale: Estrogen stimulates uterine development to provide an environment for the fetus and stimulates the breasts to prepare for lactation. Progesterone maintains the uterine lining for implantation and relaxes all smooth muscle. Human placental lactogen stimulates the metabolism of glucose and converts the glucose to fat. Human chorionic gonadotropin prevents involution of the corpus luteum and maintains the production of progesterone until the placenta is formed.

Test-Taking Strategy: Knowledge regarding the functions of various hormones related to pregnancy is required to answer this question. Review this content if you had difficulty with this question or are unfamiliar with these hormones.

Level of Cognitive Ability: Application
Client Needs: Physiological Integrity
Integrated Process: Teaching/Learning
Content Area: Maternity/Antepartum

Reference:
Murray, S., McKinney, E., & Gorrie, T. (2002). *Foundations of maternal-newborn nursing* (3rd ed.). Philadelphia: Saunders, p. 130.

18. A nurse has explained the reason that the physician has chosen laser surgery to treat a client's cervical cancer. Which statement by the client indicates an understanding of the explanation?
1 "I have too much cancer to be removed with surgery."
2 "I want to be asleep during my procedure."
3 "The doctor is able to see all the edges of my cancer clearly."
4 "I am young and the laser prevents cancer tissue from regrowing."

Answer: 3
Rationale: Laser therapy is performed in an outpatient setting and is used when all boundaries of the lesion are visible. Option 1 is not the reason for performing laser surgery. Laser surgery is painless, and the client would not receive general anesthesia. Laser therapy does not prevent regrowth.

Test-Taking Strategy: Use the process of elimination and focus on the issue: laser surgery. Thinking about the procedure involved in laser surgery will direct you to option 3. Review this type of treatment for cervical cancer if you had difficulty with this question.

Level of Cognitive Ability: Analysis
Client Needs: Physiological Integrity
Integrated Process: Teaching/Learning
Content Area: Adult Health/Oncology

Reference:
Black, J., & Hawks, J. (2005). *Medical-surgical nursing: Clinical management for positive outcomes* (7th ed.). Philadelphia: Saunders, pp. 1075-1076.

---

19. A 9-year-old child is newly diagnosed with type 1 diabetes mellitus. The nurse is planning for home care with the child and his family and determines that an age-appropriate activity for this child for health maintenance is:
1 Independently self-administering insulin
2 Making independent decisions regarding sliding-scale coverage of insulin
3 Having an adult assist in self-administration of insulin and glucose monitoring
4 Administering insulin drawn up by an adult

Answer: 1
Rationale: School-aged children have the cognitive and motor skills to independently administer insulin with adult supervision. Developmentally, they do not yet have the maturity to make situational decisions without adult validation. Options 3 and 4 suppress the maximum level of independence appropriate to the level of this child.

Test-Taking Strategy: Use the process of elimination. Focusing on the age of the child will assist in eliminating options 3 and 4. From the remaining options, recalling that in this age group decision making is a cognitive skill that develops later than motor skills will direct you to option 1. Review growth and development of the 9-year-old if you had difficulty with this question.

Level of Cognitive Ability: Analysis
Client Needs: Health Promotion and Maintenance
Integrated Process: Nursing Process/Planning
Content Area: Child Health

References:
James, S., Ashwill, J., & Droske, S. (2002). *Nursing care of children: Principles & practice* (2nd ed.). Philadelphia: Saunders, pp. 928-929.
Wong, D., & Hockenberry, M. (2003). *Wong's nursing care of infants and children* (7th ed.). St. Louis: Mosby, pp. 1750-1751.

20. A nurse is reviewing a plan of care formulated by a nursing student who is working in the health care clinic and is preparing to instruct a pregnant woman to perform Kegel exercises. The nurse asks the student to explain the purpose of the Kegel exercises. Which response by the student indicates an understanding of the purpose of these types of exercises?
1 "The exercises will help strengthen the pelvic floor in preparation for delivery."
2 "The exercises will help prevent urinary tract infections."
3 "The exercises will help reduce backache."
4 "The exercises will help prevent ankle edema."

Answer: 1
Rationale: Kegel exercises will assist to strengthen the pelvic floor (pubococcygeal muscle). Pelvic tilt exercises will help reduce backaches. Instructing a client to drink 8 ounces of fluids six times a day will help prevent urinary tract infections. Leg elevation will assist in preventing ankle edema.

Test-Taking Strategy: Focus on the issue of the question: Kegel exercises. Remember that Kegel exercises will help strengthen the pelvic floor muscles. Review the purpose of Kegel exercises if you had difficulty with this question.

Level of Cognitive Ability: Analysis
Client Needs: Health Promotion and Maintenance
Integrated Process: Teaching/Learning
Content Area: Maternity/Antepartum

Reference:
Lowdermilk, D., & Perry, A. (2004). *Maternity & women's health care* (8th ed.). St. Louis: Mosby, p. 124.

---

21. The physician's order reads: piperacillin sodium (Pipracil), 650 mg intravenously every 6 hours. The medication label reads: 2 g and reconstitute with 5 mL of bacteriostatic water. The nurse draws up how many mL to administer one dose? (Round answer to the tenth position.)

Answer: _____

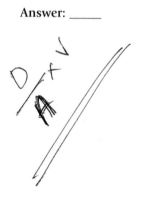

Answer: 1.6
Rationale: Convert 2 g to mg and then use the formula for calculating medication doses. In the metric system, to convert larger to smaller, multiply by 1000 or move the decimal three places to the right. Therefore, 2 g = 2000 mg.

Formula:

$$\frac{Desired}{Available} \times Volume = mL\ per\ dose$$

$$\frac{650\,mg}{2000\,mg} \times 5\,mL = 1.625\,mL = 1.6\,mL$$

Test-Taking Strategy: Identify the key components of the question and what the question is asking. In this case, the question asks for the milliliters per dose. Convert grams to milligrams first. Next, use the formula to determine the correct dose, knowing that 2000 mg = 5.0 mL. Finally, round the answer to the nearest tenth.

Level of Cognitive Ability: Application
Client Needs: Physiological Integrity
Integrated Process: Nursing Process/Implementation
Content Area: Fundamental Skills

Reference:
Kee, J., & Marshall, S. (2004). *Clinical calculations: With applications to general and specialty areas* (5th ed.). Philadelphia: Saunders, p. 80.

22. A child with sickle cell disease is admitted to the hospital for treatment of vaso-occlusive pain crisis. A nursing student is assigned to care for the child, and the nurse reviews the plan of care with the student. Which intervention, if included in the plan of care, indicates a need for further research by the student?

1 IV fluids for rehydration
2 Meperidine hydrochloride (Demerol) for pain management
3 Oxygen administration
4 Increased fluid intake

Answer: 2

Rationale: Management of the severe pain that occurs with vaso-occlusive crisis includes the use of strong narcotic analgesics, such as morphine sulfate and hydromorphone hydrochloride (Dilaudid). Meperidine hydrochloride is contraindicated because of its side effects and increased risk of seizures. Oxygen is administered to increase tissue perfusion. Fluids are necessary to promote hydration.

Test-Taking Strategy: Note the key words "need for further research." These words indicate a false-response question and that you need to select the incorrect intervention. Eliminate options 1 and 4 first, knowing that hydration is necessary, and because these options are similar. From the remaining options, use the ABCs—airway, breathing, and circulation—to eliminate option 3. Review care of the client with sickle cell disease if you had difficulty with this question.

Level of Cognitive Ability: Analysis
Client Needs: Physiological Integrity
Integrated Process: Teaching/Learning
Content Area: Child Health

Reference:
Wong, D., & Hockenberry, M. (2003). *Wong's nursing care of infants and children* (7th ed.). St. Louis: Mosby, p. 1553.

23. A newborn infant receives the first dose of hepatitis B vaccine within 12 hours of birth. The nurse instructs the mother regarding the immunization schedule for this vaccine and tells the mother that the second vaccine is administered at:

1 1 to 2 months of age and then 4 months after the initial dose
2 6 months of age and then 8 months after the initial dose
3 8 months of age and then 1 year after the initial dose
4 3 years of age and then during the adolescent years

Answer: 1

Rationale: The vaccination schedule for an infant whose mother tests negative for hepatitis B consists of a series of three immunizations given at 0 months (birth), 1 to 2 months of age, and then 4 months after the initial dose. An infant whose mother tests positive receives hepatitis B immune globulin along with the first dose of the hepatitis vaccine within 12 hours of birth.

Test-Taking Strategy: Knowledge regarding the immunization schedule for hepatitis B vaccine is required to answer this question. Review this schedule if you are unfamiliar with it.

Level of Cognitive Ability: Application
Client Needs: Health Promotion and Maintenance
Integrated Process: Teaching/Learning
Content Area: Child Health

Reference:
Lowdermilk, D., & Perry, A. (2004). *Maternity & women's health care* (8th ed.). St. Louis: Mosby, p. 1065.

24. A nurse assesses the client with a diagnosis of thyroid storm. Which classic signs and symptoms associated with thyroid storm would indicate the need for immediate nursing intervention?
1 Polyuria, nausea, and severe headaches
2 Fever, tachycardia, and systolic hypertension
3 Profuse diaphoresis, flushing, and constipation
4 Hypotension, translucent skin, and obesity

Answer: 2

Rationale: The excessive amounts of thyroid hormone cause a rapid increase in the metabolic rate, thereby causing the classic signs and symptoms of thyroid storm such as fever, tachycardia, and hypertension. When these signs present themselves, the nurse must take quick action to prevent deterioration of the client's health because death can ensue. Priority interventions include maintaining a patent airway and stabilizing the hemodynamic status. Options 1, 3, and 4 do not indicate the need for immediate nursing intervention.

Test-Taking Strategy: Note the words "the need for immediate nursing intervention" and use the process of elimination. Tachycardia, hypertension, and a fever indicate hemodynamic instability and take precedence over the signs and symptoms identified in options 1, 3, and 4. Additionally, option 2 is the only option that identifies all the signs and symptoms of thyroid storm. Review thyroid storm if you had difficulty with this question.

Level of Cognitive Ability: Analysis
Client Needs: Physiological Integrity
Integrated Process: Nursing Process/Assessment
Content Area: Adult Health/Endocrine

Reference:
Black, J., & Hawks, J. (2005). *Medical-surgical nursing: Clinical management for positive outcomes* (7th ed.). Philadelphia: Saunders, p. 1202.

---

25. A client is hospitalized for ingesting an overdose of acetaminophen (Tylenol). The nurse prepares to administer which specific antidote for this medication overdose?
1 Protamine sulfate
2 Naloxone hydrochloride (Narcan)
3 Acetylcysteine (Mucomyst)
4 Vitamin K (AquaMephyton)

Answer: 3

Rationale: Acetylcysteine restores sulfhydryl groups that are depleted by acetaminophen metabolism. Vitamin K is the antidote for warfarin sodium (Coumadin). Naloxone hydrochloride reverses respiratory depression. Protamine sulfate is the antidote for heparin.

Test-Taking Strategy: Use the process of elimination. Recalling the specific antidotes for both heparin and warfarin sodium will assist in eliminating options 1 and 4. Next, recalling that naloxone hydrochloride reverses respiratory depression will assist in eliminating option 2. Review these antidotes if you had difficulty with this question.

Level of Cognitive Ability: Analysis
Client Needs: Physiological Integrity
Integrated Process: Nursing Process/Planning
Content Area: Pharmacology

Reference:
Hodgson, B., & Kizior, R. (2004). *Saunders nursing drug handbook 2004.* Philadelphia: Saunders, p. 8.

26. A nurse is caring for a client at risk for suicide. Which client behavior is most indicative that the client may be contemplating suicide?
   1 The client tells the nurse that he plans to use his shoelaces to strangle himself.
   2 The client cries for long periods of time.
   3 The client spends long periods of time alone.
   4 The client reports sleep disturbances.

Answer: 1
Rationale: If a client displays a suicidal ideation and is able to share a plan, the client should be taken very seriously and suicide precautions should be implemented. Option 1 clearly states such a plan. Options 2, 3 and 4 are indicative of depression but are not as definitive as option 1 in regard to suicide.

Test-Taking Strategy: Note the key words "most indicative" and focus on the issue: suicide. Recalling that a cardinal sign of suicidal ideation is the formulation of a specific suicidal plan will direct you to option 1. Review assessment of the client at risk for suicide if you had difficulty with this question.

Level of Cognitive Ability: Analysis
Client Needs: Physiological Integrity
Integrated Process: Nursing Process/Analysis
Content Area: Mental Health

Reference:
Keltner, N., Schwecke, L., & Bostrom, C. (2003). *Psychiatric nursing* (4th ed.). St. Louis: Mosby, pp. 359-361.

---

27. A nurse is reviewing the record of a client who was admitted to the hospital for diagnostic studies following a fainting spell. The nurse notes that the client is receiving olanzapine (Zyprexia). Which disorder or condition would the nurse suspect in the client?
   1 History of schizophrenia
   2 History of diabetes mellitus
   3 History of diabetes insipidus
   4 History of coronary artery disease

Answer: 1
Rationale: Zyprexia is an antipsychotic medication used in the management of manifestations associated with psychotic disorders. It is the first-line treatment for schizophrenia targeting both the positive and the negative symptoms. Options 2, 3, and 4 are not indicated uses for this medication.

Test-Taking Strategy: Focus on the name of the medication. Recalling that this medication is an antipsychotic will direct you to option 1. Review this content if you are unfamiliar with the action and use of this medication.

Level of Cognitive Ability: Analysis
Client Needs: Physiological Integrity
Integrated Process: Nursing Process/Analysis
Content Area: Pharmacology

Reference:
Lehne, R. (2004). *Pharmacology for nursing care.* (5th ed). Philadelphia: Saunders, pp. 292-293.

---

28. A client is admitted to the hospital for a thyroidectomy. While preparing the client for surgery, the nurse assesses the client for psychosocial problems that may cause preoperative anxiety, knowing that a realistic source of anxiety is fear of:
   1 Developing gynecomastia and hirsutism postoperatively
   2 Sexual dysfunction and infertility
   3 Imposed dietary restrictions post discharge
   4 Changes in body image secondary to the location of the incision

Answer: 4
Rationale: Because the incision is in the neck area, the client may be fearful of having a large scar postoperatively. Having all or part of the thyroid gland removed will not cause the client to experience gynecomastia or hirsutism. Sexual dysfunction and infertility could possibly occur if the entire thyroid gland was removed and if the client was not placed on thyroid replacement medications. The client will not have specific dietary restrictions postdischarge.

Test-Taking Strategy: Use the process of elimination, focusing on the surgical procedure. Recalling the location of the thyroid gland will direct you to option 4. Review the psychosocial concerns of the client following thyroidectomy if you had difficulty with this question.

Level of Cognitive Ability: Analysis
Client Needs: Psychosocial Integrity
Integrated Process: Nursing Process/Assessment
Content Area: Adult Health/Endocrine

Reference:
Lewis, S., Heitkemper, M., & Dirksen, S. (2004). *Medical-surgical nursing: Assessment and management of clinical problems* (6th ed.). St. Louis: Mosby, p. 1317.

---

29. A physician prescribes intralipids (fat emulsion) intravenously for a client. Before initiating the solution, the nurse should assess which of the following?
1 Blood pressure
2 Hypersensitivity to eggs
3 Fingerstick blood glucose level
4 History of seizures

Answer: 2
Rationale: Before administering any medication, the nurse must assess for allergy or hypersensitivity to substances used in producing the medication. Fat emulsions such as intralipids contain an emulsifying agent obtained from egg yolks. Clients sensitive to eggs are at risk for developing hypersensitivity reactions. Options 1, 3, and 4 are unrelated to administering fat emulsion.

Test-Taking Strategy: Knowledge regarding the administration of fat emulsion is required to answer this question. Review the content related to the administration of this solution if you had difficulty with this question.

Level of Cognitive Ability: Application
Client Needs: Physiological Integrity
Integrated Process: Nursing Process/Assessment
Content Area: Fundamental Skills

Reference:
Gahart, B., & Nazareno, A. (2005). *Intravenous medications* (21st ed.). St. Louis: Mosby, p. 524.

---

30. A client is admitted to the hospital with a myocardial infarction and is not experiencing chest pain at this time. The nurse reviews the ECG rhythm strip and notes that the P-R interval is 0.16 seconds. The nurse determines that this rhythm indicates:
1 First-degree AV block
2 An abnormal finding
3 An impending reinfarction
4 A normal finding

Answer: 4
Rationale: The P-R interval represents the time it takes for the cardiac impulse to spread from the atria to the ventricles. The P-R interval range is 0.12 to 0.2 seconds. Therefore, the finding is normal.

Test-Taking Strategy: Use the process of elimination and knowledge regarding ECG readings. Eliminate options 1, 2, and 3 because they are similar and all indicate an abnormal finding. Review basic ECG findings if you had difficulty with this question.

Level of Cognitive Ability: Analysis
Client Needs: Physiological Integrity
Integrated Process: Nursing Process/Analysis
Content Area: Adult Health/Cardiovascular

Reference:
Black, J., & Hawks, J. (2005). *Medical-surgical nursing: Clinical management for positive outcomes* (7th ed.). Philadelphia: Saunders, p. 1584.

31. A nurse administers 30 units of NPH insulin at 7:00 AM to a client with a blood glucose level of 200 mg/dL. The nurse monitors the client for a hypoglycemic reaction, knowing that NPH insulin peaks in approximately how many hours following administration?

 1 2 hours
 2 3 to 4 hours
 3 6 to 14 hours
 4 16 to 24 hours

Answer: 3
Rationale: NPH is an intermediate-acting insulin with an onset of action in 60 to 120 minutes, a peak time in 6 to 14 hours, and a duration time of 16 to 24 hours.

Test-Taking Strategy: Knowledge of the onset, peak, and duration of NPH insulin is required. Recalling that NPH is an intermediate-acting insulin will direct you to option 3. Review the various types of insulin if you had difficulty with this question.

Level of Cognitive Ability: Application
Client Needs: Physiological Integrity
Integrated Process: Nursing Process/Assessment
Content Area: Pharmacology

Reference:
Lehne, R. (2004). *Pharmacology for nursing care* (5th ed.). Philadelphia: Saunders, p. 602.

---

32. A client with a psychotic disorder is being treated with haloperidol (Haldol). The nurse monitors the client for which of the following that indicates the presence of an adverse effect of this medication?

 1 Hypotension
 2 Nausea
 3 Excessive salivation
 4 Blurred vision

Answer: 3
Rationale: Adverse effects of this medication include extrapyramidal symptoms such as marked drowsiness and lethargy, excessive salivation, a fixed stare, akathisia, acute dystonias, and tardive dyskinesia. Hypotension, nausea, and blurred vision are occasional side effects.

Test-Taking Strategy: Focus on the issue: an adverse effect. Use the process of elimination and select option 3 because of the word "excessive" in this option. Review the adverse effects of this medication if you had difficulty with this question.

Level of Cognitive Ability: Application
Client Needs: Physiological Integrity
Integrated Process: Nursing Process/Assessment
Content Area: Pharmacology

Reference:
Hodgson, B., & Kizior, R. (2004). *Saunders nursing drug handbook 2004.* Philadelphia: Saunders, p. 491.

---

33. A home care nurse visits an older client who has acute gouty arthritis. Indomethacin (Indocin) has been prescribed for the client, and the nurse teaches the client about the medication. Which statement by the client indicates that further teaching is necessary?

 1 " I can take a pill whenever I need to for pain."
 2 "I need to call the doctor if I notice a rash."
 3 "I'll rest if I am having pain."
 4 "I'll watch for any swollen feet or fingers or any stomach distress."

Answer: 1
Rationale: Indomethacin (Indocin) may be prescribed to treat gouty arthritis. It may alleviate pain but is administered on a scheduled time frame, not a prn schedule. When pain occurs, the client will usually limit movement and rest. A rash should be reported because it could indicate hypersensitivity to the medication. The client should be instructed to monitor for swelling and gastric distress, which can be caused by the medication.

Test-Taking Strategy: Note the key words "further teaching is necessary." These words indicate a false-response question and that you need to select the incorrect client statement. Recalling the action and purpose of indomethacin will direct you to option 1. Review this medication if you had difficulty with this question.

Level of Cognitive Ability: Analysis
Client Needs: Health Promotion and Maintenance
Integrated Process: Teaching/Learning
Content Area: Pharmacology

Reference:
McKenry, L., & Salerno, E. (2003). *Mosby's pharmacology in nursing* (21st ed.). St. Louis: Mosby, p. 295.

---

34. A nurse is providing information to a community group about violence in the family. Which statement by a group member would indicate a need to provide additional information?

1 "Abusers usually have poor self-esteem."
2 "Abusers use fear and intimidation."
3 "Abusers are often jealous or self-centered."
4 "Abuse occurs more in low-income families."

Answer: 4
Rationale: Personal characteristics of abusers include low self-esteem, immaturity, dependence, insecurity, and jealousy. Abusers will often use fear and intimidation to the point where their victims will do anything just to avoid further abuse. The statement that abuse occurs more in low-income families is inaccurate.

Test-Taking Strategy: Note the key words "need to provide additional information." These words indicate a false-response question and that you need to select the incorrect statement. Use knowledge regarding the characteristics related to family violence to direct you to option 4. Review the characteristics of an abuser and family violence if you had difficulty with this question.

Level of Cognitive Ability: Analysis
Client Needs: Psychosocial Integrity
Integrated Process: Teaching/Learning
Content Area: Mental Health

Reference:
Keltner, N., Schwecke, L., & Bostrom, C. (2003). *Psychiatric nursing* (4th ed.). St. Louis: Mosby, p. 568.

---

35. A nurse is caring for a client with possible cholelithiasis who is being prepared for an intravenous (IV) cholangiogram, and the nurse tells the client about the procedure. Which client statement indicates that the client understands the purpose of this procedure?

1 "They are going to look at my gallbladder and ducts."
2 "This procedure will drain my gallbladder."
3 "My gallbladder will be irrigated."
4 "They will put medication in my gallbladder."

Answer: 1
Rationale: An IV cholangiogram is for diagnostic purposes. It outlines both the gallbladder and the ducts, so gallstones that have moved into the ductal system can be detected. X-rays are used to visualize the biliary duct system after IV injection of a radiopaque dye.

Test-Taking Strategy: Use the process of elimination and recall the pathophysiology of cholelithiasis and the purpose of the cholangiogram. Note that options 2, 3, and 4 are similar because they involve some form of treatment. Option 1 involves assessment of the gallbladder. Review the purpose of this procedure if you had difficulty with this question.

Level of Cognitive Ability: Analysis
Client Needs: Physiological Integrity
Integrated Process: Teaching/Learning
Content Area: Adult Health/Gastrointestinal

Reference:
Chernecky, C., & Berger, B. (2004). *Laboratory tests and diagnostic procedures* (4th ed.). Philadelphia: Saunders, p. 695.

36. A registered nurse asks a nursing student about suicide and suicide intentions. The registered nurse determines that the student understands the concepts associated with this topic if the student makes which statement?

1 "Suicide runs in the family, so there is nothing that health care personnel can do about it."

2 "Suicidal attempts are just attention-seeking behaviors."

3 "Many individuals who commit suicide have talked about their suicidal intentions to others."

4 "Only psychotic individuals commit suicide."

Answer: 3

Rationale: Most people who do commit suicide have given definite clues or warnings about their intentions. Suicide is not an inherited condition. A suicide attempt is not an attention-seeking behavior, and each act should be taken very seriously. The individual who is suicidal is not necessarily psychotic. Options 1, 2, and 4 are considered myths regarding suicide.

Test-Taking Strategy: Use the process of elimination. Eliminate option 1 because of the statement "there is nothing that health care personnel can do about it." Eliminate option 2 because of the statement "just attention-seeking behaviors." Eliminate option 4 because of the word "only." Review concepts related to suicide if you had difficulty with this question.

Level of Cognitive Ability: Analysis
Client Needs: Psychosocial Integrity
Integrated Process: Teaching/Learning
Content Area: Mental Health

Reference:
Keltner, N., Schwecke, L., & Bostrom, C. (2003). *Psychiatric nursing* (4th ed.). St. Louis: Mosby, p. 359.

37. A hospitalized 19-year-old famous pianist wanders in and out of other client rooms taking their possessions while singing to herself, and then giggling for no apparent reason. The nurse, recognizing the severe regression of the client and the difficulty with limit setting, implements which action?

1 Putting arms around the client saying, "You're okay. You just need a hug."

2 Taking the client to seclusion until she cooperates with unit rules

3 Saying, "I can see you are very anxious today. Let's go and play the piano."

4 Taking the client to the lounge and saying, "Sit here and behave yourself."

Answer: 3

Rationale: The use of a defense mechanism allows a person to avoid the painful experience of anxiety or to transform it into a more tolerable symptom, such as regression. Regression allows the threatened client to move backward developmentally to a stage in which more security is felt. The recognition of regression is a signal that the client feels anxious. Option 3 will help the client feel less anxious. Options 2 and 4 are restrictive and degrading. Option 1 does not address the client's anxiety.

Test-Taking Strategy: Use the process of elimination. Recall that because anxiety consumes energy, it should be redirected into a healthier task. Also, note the relation of the word "pianist" in the question and the words "Let's go and play the piano" in the correct option. Review defense mechanisms if you had difficulty with this question.

Level of Cognitive Ability: Application
Client Needs: Psychosocial Integrity
Integrated Process: Nursing Process/Implementation
Content Area: Mental Health

Reference:
Keltner, N., Schwecke, L., & Bostrom, C. (2003). *Psychiatric nursing* (4th ed.). St. Louis: Mosby, pp. 24-25.

38. A nurse is caring for a human immunodeficiency virus (HIV)-positive pregnant client. To help prevent the transmission of HIV from the woman to her fetus during the intrapartum period, the nurse plans to initiate measures to avoid:
1 Cesarean birth
2 External fetal monitoring
3 Epidural anesthesia
4 Direct (internal) fetal heart rate monitoring

Answer: 4

Rationale: Health care professionals must use caution during the intrapartal period to reduce the risk of the transmission of HIV to the fetus. Any procedure that exposes blood or body fluids from the mother to the fetus should be avoided. Direct (internal) fetal monitoring is a procedure that may expose the fetus to maternal blood or body fluids and therefore should be avoided. Options 1, 2, and 3 are not invasive measures that place the fetus at risk in the intrapartum period.

Test-Taking Strategy: Note the key word "avoid." This word indicates a false-response question and that you need to select the incorrect intervention. All of the options address invasive procedures that may take place during the intrapartum period, but only option 4 is invasive with regard to the fetus. Recalling that transmission of HIV occurs primarily by the exchange of body fluids will direct you to option 4. Review this content area if you had difficulty with this question.

Level of Cognitive Ability: Application
Client Needs: Safe, Effective Care Environment
Integrated Process: Nursing Process/Implementation
Content Area: Maternity/Intrapartum

Reference:
Lowdermilk, D., & Perry, A. (2004). *Maternity & women's health care* (8th ed.). St. Louis: Mosby, pp. 205; 813; 1066.

39. During electroconvulsive therapy (ECT), the client receives oxygen by mask via positive pressure ventilation. The nurse assisting with this procedure knows that positive pressure ventilation is necessary because:
1 Grand mal seizure activity depresses respirations
2 Muscle relaxants given to prevent injury during seizure activity depress respirations
3 Anesthesia is administered during the procedure
4 Decreased oxygen to the brain increases confusion and disorientation

Answer: 2

Rationale: A short-acting skeletal muscle relaxant such as succinylcholine (Anectine) is administered during this procedure to prevent injuries during the seizure. The client receives positive pressure ventilation until the muscle relaxant is metabolized, usually within 2 to 3 minutes. Options 1, 3, and 4 do not address the issue of the question and the specific reason for positive pressure ventilation.

Test-Taking Strategy: Use the process of elimination and focus on the issue. Recalling that a muscle relaxant is administered will direct you to option 2. Review this content if you are unfamiliar with the procedure for ECT.

Level of Cognitive Ability: Analysis
Client Needs: Physiological Integrity
Integrated Process: Nursing Process/Analysis
Content Area: Mental Health

Reference:
Keltner, N., Schwecke, L., & Bostrom, C. (2003). *Psychiatric nursing* (4th ed.). St. Louis: Mosby, pp. 525-526.

40. A client is in a coma of unknown cause, and the physician has written several orders for the client including the need for intubation. Which procedure would the nurse withhold until the client was properly intubated?
1 Gastric feeding
2 Fingerstick for blood glucose level
3 Urethral catheterization
4 Venipuncture for complete blood cell (CBC) count

Answer: 1
Rationale: Intubation should always precede gastric feeding to prevent pulmonary aspiration. All other options identify procedures that can be initiated before intubation of the client.

Test-Taking Strategy: Use the process of elimination and the ABCs—airway, breathing, and circulation. Recalling that the comatose client is at risk for aspiration will direct you to option 1. Review care of the comatose client if you had difficulty with this question.

Level of Cognitive Ability: Application
Client Needs: Physiological Integrity
Integrated Process: Nursing Process/Implementation
Content Area: Adult Health/Neurological

References:
Black, J., & Hawks, J. (2005). *Medical-surgical nursing: Clinical management for positive outcomes* (7th ed.). Philadelphia: Saunders, pp. 2058; 2060.
Phipps, W., Monahan, F., Sands, J., Marek, J., & Neighbors, M. (2003). *Medical-surgical nursing: Health and illness perspectives* (7th ed.). St. Louis: Mosby, p. 517.

41. A manic client is placed in a seclusion room after an outburst of violent behavior that included a physical assault on another client. As the client is secluded, the nurse should:
1 Remain silent because verbal interaction would be too stimulating
2 Tell the client that he will be allowed to rejoin the others when he can behave
3 Ask the client if he understands why the seclusion is necessary
4 Inform the client that he is being secluded to help regain control of self

Answer: 4
Rationale: The client is removed to a nonstimulating environment as a result of behavior. Options 1, 2, and 3 are nontherapeutic. In addition, option 2 implies punishment. It is best to directly inform the client of the purpose of the seclusion.

Test-Taking Strategy: Use the process of elimination. Look for the option that presents reality most clearly to the client. Option 4 is the only option that provides a clear and direct purpose of the seclusion. Review care of the client requiring seclusion if you had difficulty with this question.

Level of Cognitive Ability: Application
Client Needs: Psychosocial Integrity
Integrated Process: Nursing Process/Implementation
Content Area: Mental Health

Reference:
Keltner, N., Schwecke, L., & Bostrom, C. (2003). *Psychiatric nursing* (4th ed.). St. Louis: Mosby, p. 141.

42. A client with a ruptured cerebral aneurysm who also has a history of essential hypertension exhibits a sudden elevation in blood pressure. The nurse immediately contacts the physician and immediate treatment is prescribed for the client. Which medication would the nurse expect to prescribed?
1 Epinephrine (Adrenaline)
2 Dobutamine (Dobutrex)
3 Sodium nitroprusside (Nipride)
4 Dopamine (Intropin)

Answer: 3
Rationale: Sodium nitroprusside decreases the blood pressure by vasodilation, thus reducing pressure in the aneurysm. The other medications increase blood pressure, which may disrupt an existing cerebral clot and precipitate bleeding.

Test-Taking Strategy: Focus on the issue: a sudden elevation in blood pressure. Remember that nitroglycerin compounds are vasodilators and that they decrease the blood pressure. Review the actions of these medications if you had difficulty with this question.

Level of Cognitive Ability: Analysis
Client Needs: Physiological Integrity
Integrated Process: Nursing Process/Analysis
Content Area: Adult Health/Neurological

References:
Black, J., & Hawks, J. (2005). *Medical-surgical nursing: Clinical management for positive outcomes* (7th ed.). Philadelphia: Saunders, p. 1659.
Hodgson, B., & Kizior, R. (2004). *Saunders nursing drug handbook 2004.* Philadelphia: Saunders, p. 736.

---

43. A nurse is providing instructions to a client regarding quinapril hydrochloride (Accupril). The nurse tells the client:
   1 To take the medication with food only
   2 To rise slowly from a lying to a sitting position
   3 To discontinue the medication if nausea occurs
   4 That a therapeutic effect will be noted immediately

Answer: 2
Rationale: Accupril is an angiotensin-converting enzyme (ACE) inhibitor. It is used in the treatment of hypertension. The client should be instructed to rise slowly from a lying to sitting position and to permit the legs to dangle from the bed momentarily before standing to reduce the hypotensive effect. The medication does not need to be taken with meals. It may be given without regard to food. If nausea occurs, the client should be instructed to take a noncola carbonated beverage and salted crackers or dry toast. A full therapeutic effect may be noted in 1 to 2 weeks.

Test-Taking Strategy: Use the process of elimination. Eliminate option 1 because of the absolute word "only." From the remaining options, focus on the medication classification. Recalling that medication names that end with "pril" indicate that the medication is an ACE inhibitor and that ACE inhibitors are used in the treatment of hypertension will direct you to option 2. Review the action of this medication and the associated client teaching points if you had difficulty with this question.

Level of Cognitive Ability: Application
Client Needs: Health Promotion and Maintenance
Integrated Process: Teaching/Learning
Content Area: Pharmacology

Reference:
Hodgson, B., & Kizior, R. (2004). *Saunders nursing drug handbook 2004.* Philadelphia: Saunders, p. 863.

---

44. A nurse is providing emergency treatment for a client in ventricular tachycardia and is preparing to defibrillate the client. Which nursing action provides for the safest environment during a defibrillation attempt?
   1 Placing the charged paddles one at a time on the client's chest
   2 Ensuring that no lubricant is on the paddles
   3 Holding the client's upper torso stable while the defibrillation is performed
   4 Performing a visual and verbal check that all assisting personnel are clear of the client and the client's bed

Answer: 4
Rationale: Safety during defibrillation is essential for preventing injury to the client and to the personnel assisting with the procedure. The person performing the defibrillation ensures that all personnel are standing clear of the bed by a verbal and visual check of "all clear." For the shock to be effective, some type of conductive medium (e.g., lubricant, gel) must be placed between the paddles and the skin. Both paddles are placed on the client's chest.

Test-Taking Strategy: Use the process of elimination, focusing on the issue: safest environment. Option 4 involves a verbal and visual check of "all clear" providing for the safety of all involved. Review the procedure for defibrillation if you had difficulty with this question.

Level of Cognitive Ability: Application
Client Needs: Safe, Effective Care Environment
Integrated Process: Nursing Process/Implementation
Content Area: Adult Health/Cardiovascular

Reference:
Black, J., & Hawks, J. (2005). *Medical-surgical nursing: Clinical management for positive outcomes* (7th ed.). Philadelphia: Saunders, pp. 1685; 1689.

---

45. A client is admitted to the emergency department with complaints of severe, radiating chest pain. The client is extremely restless, frightened, and dyspneic. Immediate admission orders include oxygen by nasal cannula at 4 liters per minute, troponin, creatinine phosphokinase (CPK), and isoenzymes blood levels, a chest X-ray, and a 12-lead ECG. Which action would the nurse take first?

1 Obtain the 12-lead ECG
2 Draw the blood specimens
3 Call radiology to order the chest X-ray
4 Apply the oxygen to the client

Answer: 4
Rationale: The first action would be to apply the oxygen because the client can be experiencing myocardial ischemia. The ECG can provide evidence of cardiac damage and the location of myocardial ischemia. However, oxygen is the priority to prevent further cardiac damage. Drawing the blood specimens would be done after oxygen administration and just before or after the ECG, depending on the situation. Although the chest X-ray can show cardiac enlargement, having the chest X-ray would not influence immediate treatment.

Test-Taking Strategy: Note the key word "first." Remember that the immediate goal of therapy is to prevent myocardial ischemia. The only option that will achieve that goal is option 4. Also, use the ABCs—airway, breathing, and circulation—to direct you to option 4. Review care of the client with a myocardial infarction if you had difficulty with this question.

Level of Cognitive Ability: Application
Client Needs: Physiological Integrity
Integrated Process: Nursing Process/Implementation
Content Area: Adult Health/Cardiovascular

Reference:
Black, J., & Hawks, J. (2005). *Medical-surgical nursing: Clinical management for positive outcomes* (7th ed.). Philadelphia: Saunders, p. 1721.

---

46. Chemical cardioversion is prescribed for the client with atrial fibrillation. The nurse who is assisting in preparing the client would expect that which medication specific for chemical cardioversion will be needed?

1 Verapamil (Calan)
2 Nifedipine (Procardia)
3 Quinidine (Quinidex)
4 Bretylium (Bretylol)

Answer: 3
Rationale: Quinidine is an antidysrhythmic. Verapamil is generally used to control heart rate. Nifedipine is a vasodilator. Bretylium is generally used for control of ventricular dysrhythmia.

Test-Taking Strategy: Note the key words "chemical cardioversion." Recalling the action of these medications and that quinidine is an antidysrhythmic will direct you to option 3. Review this content if you are unfamiliar with these medications or with pre-procedure care.

Level of Cognitive Ability: Analysis
Client Needs: Physiological Integrity
Integrated Process: Nursing Process/Analysis
Content Area: Adult Health/Cardiovascular

References:

Black, J., & Hawks, J. (2005). *Medical-surgical nursing: Clinical management for positive outcomes* (7th ed.). Philadelphia: Saunders, p. 1679.

Hodgson, B., & Kizior, R. (2004). *Saunders nursing drug handbook 2004.* Philadelphia: Saunders, p. 864.

---

47. A registered nurse is observing a nursing student auscultate the breath sounds of a client. The registered nurse intervenes if the nursing student performs which incorrect action?
1 Asks the client to sit straight up
2 Has the client breathe slowly and deeply through the mouth
3 Places the stethoscope directly on the client's skin
4 Uses the bell of the stethoscope

Answer: 4
Rationale: The bell of the stethoscope is not used to auscultate breath sounds. The client ideally should sit up and breathe slowly and deeply through the mouth. The diaphragm of the stethoscope, which is warmed before use, is placed directly on the client's skin, not over a gown or clothing.

Test-Taking Strategy: Note the key words "intervenes" and "incorrect." These words indicate a false-response question and that you need to select the incorrect action by the nursing student. Visualizing each action and the procedure for auscultating breath sounds will direct you to option 4. Review auscultation as a basic physical assessment technique if you had difficulty with this question.

Level of Cognitive Ability: Application
Client Needs: Health Promotion and Maintenance
Integrated Process: Nursing Process/Assessment
Content Area: Leadership/Management

Reference:

Potter, P. , & Perry, A. (2005). *Fundamentals of nursing* (6th ed.). St. Louis: Mosby, p. 720.

---

48. A home care nurse is caring for an obese adult client who is at home after receiving treatment for a sprained right ankle. The client is using a cane to ambulate but has not exercised for more than 1 week and has missed the last two rehabilitation appointments. The client says, "I'm getting therapy for my ankle and I do my exercises three times a day." The nurse makes which therapeutic response to the client?
1 "Sounds good to me. Have you made all of your appointments?"
2 "You say you are following your exercise plan, yet you've missed the last two appointments with the physical therapist?"
3 "Show me how you do your exercises. I want to determine if you're doing them correctly."
4 "You must keep your appointments. I already know that you've missed two appointments with the therapist."

Answer: 2
Rationale: In option 2, the nurse employs the therapeutic communication technique of sharing perceptions. Sharing perceptions involves asking the client to verify the nurse's understanding of what the client is feeling, thinking, or doing. In this situation, the client is employing avoidance. By sharing perceptions, the nurse is assisting the client to begin problem solving. In option 1, the nurse is nontherapeutic in giving approval and is mirroring the client's avoidance and passivity by not dealing directly with the problem of missed appointments. In option 3, the nurse is therapeutic in the attempt to engage the client in exercises, but this nursing action does not occur in a helpful manner. In this option, the nurse is "telling" the client to perform the exercises, which could lead to resistance and eventually, a regressive struggle. In option 4, the nurse is empathic but does so by giving advice and using inappropriate timing.

Test-Taking Strategy: Use therapeutic communication techniques and the process of elimination. Option 2 is the only option that is addressing what the client is feeling, thinking, or doing. Review therapeutic communication techniques if you had difficulty with this question.

Level of Cognitive Ability: Application
Client Needs: Psychosocial Integrity

Integrated Process: Communication and Documentation
Content Area: Fundamental Skills

Reference:
Keltner, N., Schwecke, L., & Bostrom, C. (2003). *Psychiatric nursing* (4th ed.). St. Louis: Mosby, pp. 94-95.

---

49. A client with unstable ventricular tachycardia (VT) loses consciousness and becomes pulseless after an initial treatment with a dose of lidocaine (Xylocaine) intravenously. The nurse caring for the client would immediately obtain which of the following needed items?
1 A second dose of lidocaine
2 A pacemaker
3 An electrocardiogram (ECG) machine
4 A defibrillator

Answer: 4
Rationale: For the client with VT who becomes pulseless, the physician or qualified advanced cardiac life support (ACLS) personnel immediately defibrillates the client. In the absence of this equipment, cardiopulmonary resuscitation (CPR) is initiated immediately. Options 1, 2, and 3 are not items that are needed immediately in this situation.

Test-Taking Strategy: Use the process of elimination, noting the key word "immediately" and that the client is in VT. Options 1 and 3 should be eliminated first, because option 1 was unsuccessful and option 3 is of no use. From the remaining options, focusing on the issue will direct you to option 4. Review the immediate measures for VT if you had difficulty with this question.

Level of Cognitive Ability: Application
Client Needs: Physiological Integrity
Integrated Process: Nursing Process/Implementation
Content Area: Adult Health/Cardiovascular

Reference:
Phipps, W., Monahan, F., Sands, J., Marek, J., & Neighbors, M. (2003). *Medical-surgical nursing: Health and illness perspectives* (7th ed.). St. Louis: Mosby, p. 689.

---

50. A nurse has done preoperative teaching with a client scheduled for percutaneous insertion of an inferior vena cava (IVC) filter. The nurse determines that the client needs further clarification if the client stated that the procedure:
1 Is rarely associated with complications
2 Eliminates the need for anticoagulant therapy
3 Is done under general anesthesia
4 May cause congestion when clots get trapped at the filter

Answer: 3
Rationale: Complications after insertion of an IVC filter are rare. When they do occur, they include air embolism, improper placement, and filter migration. The percutaneous approach uses local anesthesia. There is usually no need for anticoagulant therapy after surgery. Venous congestion can occur from accumulation of thrombi on the filter, but the process usually occurs gradually.

Test-Taking Strategy: Note the key words "needs further clarification." These words indicate a false-response question and that you need to select the incorrect client statement. Noting the words "percutaneous insertion" in the question should direct you to option 3. General anesthesia is not used in this procedure. Review this procedure if you had difficulty with this question.

Level of Cognitive Ability: Analysis
Client Needs: Physiological Integrity
Integrated Process: Teaching/Learning
Content Area: Adult Health/Cardiovascular

Reference:
Phipps, W., Monahan, F., Sands, J., Marek, J., & Neighbors, M. (2003). *Medical-surgical nursing: Health and illness perspectives* (7th ed.). St. Louis: Mosby, p. 603.

51. A client with a head injury and a feeding tube continuously tries to remove the tube. The nurse contacts the physician who prescribes the use of restraints. After checking the agency's policy and procedure regarding the use of restraints, the nurse uses which method in restraining the client?
1 Mitten restraints
2 Wrist restraints
3 Waist restraint
4 Vest restraint

Answer: 1

Rationale: Mitten restraints are useful for this client because the client cannot pull against them, creating resistance that could lead to increased intracranial pressure (ICP). Wrist restraints cause resistance. Vest and waist restraints prevent the client from getting up or falling out of bed but do nothing to limit hand movement.

Test-Taking Strategy: Use the process of elimination and focus on the issue: a restraint that safely limits hand movement for this client. Eliminate options 3 and 4 because they do not address this issue. From the remaining options, thinking about the concern of ICP in a client with a head injury will direct you to option 1. Review care of the client with a head injury if you had difficulty with this question.

Level of Cognitive Ability: Application
Client Needs: Physiological Integrity
Integrated Process: Nursing Process/Implementation
Content Area: Adult Health/Neurological

References:
Ignatavicius, D., & Workman, M. (2002). *Medical surgical nursing: Critical thinking for collaborative care* (4th ed.). Philadelphia: Saunders, p. 997.
Potter, P. , & Perry, A. (2005). *Fundamentals of nursing* (6th ed.). St. Louis: Mosby, p. 986.

52. A nurse has oriented a new employee to basic procedures for continuous ECG monitoring. The nurse would intervene if the new employee did which of the following while initiating cardiac monitoring on a client?
1 Cleansed the skin with betadine (povidone iodine) before applying the electrodes
2 Clipped small areas of hair under the area planned for electrode placement
3 Stated the need to change the electrodes and inspect the skin every 24 hours
4 Stated the need to use hypoallergenic electrodes for clients who are sensitive

Answer: 1

Rationale: The skin is cleansed with soap and water (not betadine), denatured with alcohol, and allowed to air dry before electrodes are applied. The other three options are correct.

Test-Taking Strategy: Note the key word "intervene." This word indicates a false-response question and that you need to select the incorrect action. Eliminate options 3 and 4 because they are correct. From the remaining options, remember that betadine is used to cleanse the skin usually before some type of invasive procedure that breaks the skin barrier. ECG monitoring does not break the skin. Review the procedure for initiating cardiac monitoring if you had difficulty with this question.

Level of Cognitive Ability: Application
Client Needs: Safe, Effective Care Environment
Integrated Process: Teaching/Learning
Content Area: Leadership/Management

Reference:
Black, J., & Hawks, J. (2005). *Medical-surgical nursing: Clinical management for positive outcomes* (7th ed.). Philadelphia: Saunders, p. 1583.

53. A client has been defibrillated three times using an automatic external defibrillator (AED). The nurse observes that the attempts to convert the ventricular fibrillation (VF) were unsuccessful. Based on an evaluation of the situation, the nurse determines that which action would be best?

1 Performing CPR for 1 minute, then defibrillating up to three more times at 360 joules
2 Performing CPR for 5 minutes, then defibrillating three more times at 400 joules
3 Preparing for the administration of sodium bicarbonate intravenously
4 Terminating the resuscitation effort

Answer: 1

Rationale: After three unsuccessful defibrillation attempts, CPR should be done for 1 minute, followed by three more shocks, each delivered at 360 joules. There is no information in the question to indicate that life support should be terminated. Sodium bicarbonate may be prescribed but is not the best action. Giving CPR for 5 minutes may not help oxygenation to the brain and myocardium and is not the best action. It would be best to administer CPR for 1 minute and then resume attempts to convert the rhythm to a viable one.

Test-Taking Strategy: Use the process of elimination and knowledge regarding the treatment for VF. There is no information in the question to indicate that life support should be terminated, so option 4 is eliminated first. From the remaining options, focusing on the key word "best" and recalling the treatment for VF will direct you to option 1. Review the treatment for VF if you had difficulty with this question.

Level of Cognitive Ability: Analysis
Client Needs: Physiological Integrity
Integrated Process: Nursing Process/Analysis
Content Area: Adult Health/Cardiovascular

Reference:
Phipps, W., Monahan, F., Sands, J., Marek, J., & Neighbors, M. (2003). *Medical-surgical nursing: Health and illness perspectives* (7th ed.). St. Louis: Mosby, p. 689.

54. A nurse is inserting an oropharyngeal airway into an assigned client. The nurse plans to use which correct insertion procedure?

1 Leave any dentures in place
2 Flex the client's neck
3 Insert the airway with the tip pointed upward
4 Suction the client's mouth once per shift

Answer: 3

Rationale: Before insertion of an oropharyngeal airway, any dentures or partial plates should be removed from the client's mouth. An airway should be selected that is an appropriate size. The client should be positioned supine, with the neck hyperextended if possible. The airway is inserted with the tip pointed upward and is then rotated downward once the flange has reached the client's teeth. Following insertion, the client's mouth is suctioned every hour or as necessary. The airway is removed for inspection of the mouth every 2 to 4 hours.

Test-Taking Strategy: Note the key words "correct insertion procedure." Eliminate option 4 because this is not part of the insertion procedure. Next eliminate option 2, because the neck is hyperextended (unless contraindicated) to open the airway. From the remaining options, recall that dentures should be removed because they are a potential source of airway obstruction. Review this procedure if you had difficulty with this question.

Level of Cognitive Ability: Application
Client Needs: Physiological Integrity
Integrated Process: Nursing Process/Planning
Content Area: Adult Health/Respiratory

Reference:
Phipps, W., Monahan, F., Sands, J., Marek, J., & Neighbors, M. (2003). *Medical-surgical nursing: Health and illness perspectives* (7th ed.). St. Louis: Mosby, p. 510.

55. A home care nurse is caring for an older female adult client at home. The nurse is told that the client was found wandering the highway in her nightgown last night. Her daughter, who lives with her, says to the nurse, "This wandering started last week, but this is the first time she got out of the house. She always seems to do it around 10:00 PM. What can I do?" Based on an evaluation of the situation, the nurse makes which response to the client's daughter?

1 "This is probably sundowners syndrome, a common occurrence in older adults."

2 "Since this is the first time your mother has gotten away from you, what has worked to prevent this before this time?"

3 "I think you need to consider a nursing home immediately. Put your mother's name in, and when an empty bed comes up, let the doctor admit her. You can't handle this alone, and she could get killed!"

4 "Try approaching your mother before it happens so she doesn't wander. This could be seen as neglect, and you could be prosecuted."

Answer: 2

Rationale: The nurse should first assess the situation and collect data regarding this change in behavior. The best response is the one that focuses on the daughter's problem solving so that the nurse can then suggest strategies to try. Option 1 does not help at this time, and other factors may be causing confusion. Option 3 is histrionic, and no data indicates that this action is necessary. Option 4 is inappropriate and may cause resentment if the nurse assumes that the caregiver did not think critically.

Test-Taking Strategy: Use the steps of the nursing process. Option 2 is the only option that addresses assessment. Review therapeutic communication techniques and interventions for caregivers if you had difficulty with this question.

Level of Cognitive Ability: Application
Client Needs: Psychosocial Integrity
Integrated Process: Communication and Documentation
Content Area: Fundamental Skills

Reference:
Keltner, N., Schwecke, L., & Bostrom, C. (2003). *Psychiatric nursing* (4th ed.). St. Louis: Mosby, p. 94; 612.

---

56. A nurse is assigned to visit an older adult client at home. During the visit, the client says to the nurse, "I wonder if you could do a little grocery shopping for me? I usually go, but I'm feeling so punk that I don't think I can manage." Which statement by the nurse would be a therapeutic response?

1 "I'm sorry, but I'm not allowed to do that; it's against agency policy."

2 "Do you have any family or support systems you can call on when you're feeling punk?"

3 "Nurses don't have the time to do these things with their heavy caseloads. Please call a grocery store with home delivery."

4 "Not having someone to help on those punk days is a problem. Let's discuss how we can solve it."

Answer: 4

Rationale: The nurse has the commitment of helping the client. It is important that the nurse collect data first and then find an immediate solution and a solution for the long-term problem. In option 1, the nurse hides behind policy and rules, and this is a passive approach. In option 2, the nurse asks a closed-ended question. Option 3 is inappropriate and indicates that the nurse thinks more of status than of helping the client. Option 4 reflects the client's situation and begins to work with the client in a mutual way, which preserves the client's locus of control.

Test-Taking Strategy: Use the process of elimination and therapeutic communication techniques. Option 4 is the only option that addresses the client's problem and provides the means to problem solve. Review therapeutic communication techniques if you had difficulty with this question.

Level of Cognitive Ability: Application
Client Needs: Psychosocial Integrity
Integrated Process: Communication and Documentation
Content Area: Fundamental Skills

Reference:
Keltner, N., Schwecke, L., & Bostrom, C. (2003). *Psychiatric nursing* (4th ed.). St. Louis: Mosby, p. 94.

57. A nurse is caring for a client who is being treated with an intravenous (IV) bolus of lidocaine hydrochloride (Xylocaine). The nurse understands the actions and the effects of the medication and plans to monitor which of the following?
1 Respiratory status and blood pressure
2 Urinary pH
3 Radial pulse
4 Temperature

Answer: 1
Rationale: The nurse is responsible for monitoring the client's respiratory status and blood pressure while the client is being treated with an IV bolus of lidocaine hydrochloride. The urinary pH and temperature are not related to this medication. It is best to monitor the apical pulse in this client.

Test-Taking Strategy: Use the ABCs—airway, breathing, and circulation—to answer the question. This should direct you to option 1. Review nursing responsibilities when a client receives lidocaine hydrochloride if you had difficulty with this question.

Level of Cognitive Ability: Application
Client Needs: Physiological Integrity
Integrated Process: Nursing Process/Implementation
Content Area: Pharmacology

Reference:
Hodgson, B., & Kizior, R. (2004). *Saunders nursing drug handbook 2004.* Philadelphia: Saunders, p. 601.

58. When planning the discharge of a client with chronic anxiety, the nurse evaluates achievement of the discharge maintenance goals. Which goal would most appropriately have been included in the plan of care requiring evaluation?
1 The client maintains contact with a crisis counselor.
2 The client identifies anxiety-producing situations.
3 The client ignores feelings of anxiety.
4 The client eliminates all anxiety from daily situations.

Answer: 2
Rationale: Recognizing situations that produce anxiety allows the client to prepare to cope with anxiety or avoid specific stimulus. Counselors will not be available for all anxiety-producing situations, and this option does not encourage the development of internal strengths. Ignoring feelings will not resolve anxiety. It is impossible to eliminate all anxiety from life.

Test-Taking Strategy: Use the process of elimination. Eliminate option 1 because it promotes dependence on a counselor. Eliminate options 3 and 4 because of the words "ignores" and "all" in these options. Option 2 is the only realistic option. Review care of the client with chronic anxiety if you had difficulty with this question.

Level of Cognitive Ability: Analysis
Client Needs: Psychosocial Integrity
Integrated Process: Nursing Process/Evaluation
Content Area: Mental Health

Reference:
Stuart, G., & Laraia, M. (2005). *Principles and practice of psychiatric nursing* (8th ed.). St. Louis: Mosby, p. 274.

59. A client has an order for seizure precautions, and a nursing student develops a plan of care for the client. The registered nurse reviews the plan of care with the student and identifies which incorrect intervention?

1 Monitor the client closely while the client is showering
2 Push the lock-out button on the electric bed to keep the bed in the lowest position
3 Keep all the lights on in the room at night
4 Assist the client to ambulate in the hallway

Answer: 3

Rationale: A quiet, restful environment is provided as part of seizure precautions. This includes undisturbed times for sleep, while using a nightlight for safety. The client should be accompanied during activities such as bathing and walking, so that assistance is readily available and injury is minimized if a seizure begins. The bed is maintained in low position for safety.

Test-Taking Strategy: Note the key words "incorrect intervention." These words indicate a false-response question and that you need to select the incorrect intervention. Focus on the issue: seizure precautions. Noting the word "all" in option 3 and thinking about the importance of a quiet, restful environment will direct you to this option. Review care of the client on seizure precautions if you had difficulty with this question.

Level of Cognitive Ability: Application
Client Needs: Safe, Effective Care Environment
Integrated Process: Nursing Process/Implementation
Content Area: Leadership/Management

References:
Ignatavicius, D., & Workman, M. (2002). *Medical surgical nursing: Critical thinking for collaborative care* (4th ed.). Philadelphia: Saunders, pp. 901-903.
Phipps, W., Monahan, F., Sands, J., Marek, J., & Neighbors, M. (2003). *Medical-surgical nursing: Health and illness perspectives* (7th ed.). St. Louis: Mosby, p. 1341.

60. A nurse is caring for a child who sustained a head injury from a fall. The nurse avoids which of the following in the care of this child?

1 Keeping the child in a sitting-up position
2 Forcing fluids
3 Keeping the child awake as much as possible
4 Performing neurological assessments

Answer: 2

Rationale: A child with a head injury is at risk for increased intracranial pressure (ICP). Sitting up will decrease fluid retention in cerebral tissue and promote drainage. Keeping the child awake will assist in accurate evaluation of any cerebral edema that is present and will detect early coma. Neurological assessments need to be performed to monitor for increased ICP. Forcing fluids may cause fluid overload and increased ICP. Additionally, the nurse would not "force" the client to do something.

Test-Taking Strategy: Note the key word "avoids." Use the process of elimination and knowledge regarding increased ICP. Eliminate options 1, 3, and 4 because they are correct in terms of monitoring for and preventing increased ICP. Additionally, noting the word "forcing" in option 2 will direct you to this option. Review measures to prevent increased ICP if you had difficulty with this question.

Level of Cognitive Ability: Application
Client Needs: Physiological Integrity
Integrated Process: Nursing Process/Implementation
Content Area: Child Health

Reference:
Wong, D., & Hockenberry, M. (2003). *Wong's nursing care of infants and children* (7th ed.). St. Louis: Mosby, pp. 1669; 1672.

61. A nurse has conducted a stress-management seminar for clients in an ambulatory care setting. Which statements by an attendee would indicate that further instruction is needed?

1 "Biofeedback might be nice, but I don't like the idea of having to use equipment."
2 "I can use guided imagery anywhere and anytime."
3 "The progressive muscle relaxation technique should ease my tension headaches."
4 "Using confrontation with coworkers should solve my problems at work quickly."

Answer: 4
Rationale: Biofeedback, progressive muscle relaxation, meditation, and guided imagery are techniques that the nurse can teach the client to reduce the physical impact of stress on the body and promote a feeling of self-control for the client. Biofeedback entails electronic equipment, whereas the others require no adjuncts, such as tapes, once the technique is learned. Confrontation is a communication technique, not a stress-management technique. It may also exacerbate stress, at least in the short term, rather than alleviate it.

Test-Taking Strategy: Note the key words "further instruction is needed." These words indicate a false-response question and that you need to select the incorrect statement. Recalling the methods of stress management techniques guides you to option 4, which is a communication technique rather than a stress-management technique. Review stress-management techniques if you had difficulty with this question.

Level of Cognitive Ability: Analysis
Client Needs: Psychosocial Integrity
Integrated Process: Teaching/Learning
Content Area: Mental Health

References:
Stuart, G., & Laraia, M. (2005). *Principles and practice of psychiatric nursing* (8th ed.). St. Louis: Mosby, pp. 292-293.
Varcarolis, E.M. (2002). *Foundations of psychiatric mental health nursing.* (4th ed.). Philadelphia: Saunders, pp. 270-274.

62. A nurse is caring for a client with a peptic ulcer. In assessing the client for gastrointestinal perforation (GI), the nurse monitors for:

1 Increase in bowel sounds
2 Sudden, severe abdominal pain
3 Positive guaiac stool tests
4 Slow, strong pulses

Answer: 2
Rationale: Sudden, severe abdominal pain is the most indicative sign of perforation. When perforation of an ulcer occurs, the nurse may be unable to hear bowel sounds at all. When perforation occurs, the pulse will more likely be weak and rapid. Positive guaiac stool results indicate the presence of bleeding but are not necessarily indicative of perforation.

Test-Taking Strategy: Use the process of elimination, focusing on the issue: the signs of perforation. Correlate perforation with sudden, severe abdominal pain. Remember that the nurse may be unable to hear bowel sounds and that the pulse will most likely be weak and rapid. Positive guaiac stool results are not specific to perforation. Review the signs of perforation if you had difficulty with this question.

Level of Cognitive Ability: Application
Client Needs: Physiological Integrity
Integrated Process: Nursing Process/Assessment
Content Area: Adult Health/Gastrointestinal

Reference:
Lewis, S., Heitkemper, M., & Dirksen, S. (2004). *Medical-surgical nursing: Assessment and management of clinical problems* (6th ed.). St. Louis: Mosby, p. 1031.

63. Human albumin (Albuminar) administered intravenously (IV) is prescribed for a client with second- and third-degree burns of the anterior chest and both legs. The nurse reviews the client's medical record to identify the presence of any existing conditions, which would be a contraindication in the use of human albumin. The nurse contacts the physician before administering the human albumin if which of the following is noted in the client's record?
1 Lymphocytic leukemia
2 Multiple myeloma
3 Diabetes mellitus
4 Renal insufficiency

Answer: 4
Rationale: Human albumin (Albuminar) is classified as a blood derivative and is contraindicated in severe anemia, cardiac failure, history of allergic reaction, renal insufficiency, and when no albumin deficiency is present. It is used with caution in clients with low cardiac reserve, pulmonary disease, or hepatic or renal failure.

Test-Taking Strategy: Use the process of elimination and focus on the issue: a contraindication. Eliminate options 1 and 2 first because they are similar in that they are oncological disorders. From the remaining options, recalling that albumin restores intravascular volume will assist in directing you to option 4. Review this blood derivative if you had difficulty with this question.

Level of Cognitive Ability: Application
Client Needs: Safe, Effective Care Environment
Integrated Process: Nursing Process/Implementation
Content Area: Pharmacology

References:
Hodgson, B., & Kizior, R. (2004). *Saunders nursing drug handbook 2004.* Philadelphia: Saunders, p. 15.
McKenry, L., & Salerno, E. (2003). *Mosby's pharmacology in nursing* (21st ed.). St. Louis: Mosby, pp. 533-534.

---

64. A male newborn is in the neonatal intensive care unit for respiratory distress syndrome (RDS) and surfactant replacement therapy has been given. The nurse evaluates the infant 1 hour after the surfactant therapy and determines that the infant's condition has improved somewhat. Which of the following, if observed by the nurse, indicates improvement?
1 Decreased need for supplemental oxygen
2 Increased work of breathing
3 Unequal breath sounds
4 Increased level of carbon dioxide (CO2) in the blood gas analysis

Answer: 1
Rationale: A decreased need for supplemental oxygen indicates an improvement in the infant's ability to use oxygen. The increased work of breathing indicates air hunger and the need for further support. Unequal breath sounds may indicate atelectasis or blocked airways. Increased levels of CO_2 would indicate increasing respiratory acidosis and not improvement of oxygenation.

Test-Taking Strategy: Use the process of elimination, focusing on the key word "improvement." Noting the word "increased" in options 2 and 4 will assist in eliminating these options. From the remaining options, recall that "unequal" does not indicate improvement. Review the expected effects of surfactant therapy if you had difficulty with this question.

Level of Cognitive Ability: Analysis
Client Needs: Physiological Integrity
Integrated Process: Nursing Process/Evaluation
Content Area: Child Health

Reference:
Lowdermilk, D., & Perry, A. (2004). *Maternity & women's health care* (8th ed.). St. Louis: Mosby, p. 684.

65. A nurse is evaluating the effectiveness of antimicrobial therapy for a client with infective endocarditis. The nurse determines that which finding documented in the client's health record is the least reliable indicator of effectiveness?
1 Clear breath sounds
2 Systolic heart murmur
3 Temperature of 98.8°F
4 Negative blood cultures

Answer: 2

Rationale: A systolic heart murmur, once present, will not resolve spontaneously and is therefore the least reliable indicator. Negative blood cultures and normothermia indicate resolution of infection. Clear breath sounds are a normal finding, and in this instance could mean resolution of heart failure, if that was accompanying the endocarditis.

Test-Taking Strategy: Note the key words "least reliable indicator." The question is worded to look for the finding that will not respond to antimicrobial therapy and that is an abnormal finding. The only option that meets these criteria is option 2, which does not resolve once it has developed. Review care of the client with infective endocarditis if you had difficulty with this question.

Level of Cognitive Ability: Analysis
Client Needs: Physiological Integrity
Integrated Process: Nursing Process/Evaluation
Content Area: Adult Health/Cardiovascular

Reference:

Phipps, W., Monahan, F., Sands, J., Marek, J., & Neighbors, M. (2003). *Medical-surgical nursing: Health and illness perspectives* (7th ed.). St. Louis: Mosby, pp. 708-709.

66. A nurse is caring for a client with continuous electrocardiogram (ECG) monitoring. The nurse notes that the ECG complexes are very small and hard to evaluate. The nurse checks which setting on the ECG monitor console?
1 Power button
2 Low rate alarm
3 Amplitude or "gain"
4 High rate alarm

Answer: 3

Rationale: The power button turns the machine on and off. The high and low alarm settings indicate the heart rate limits beyond which an alarm will sound. The amplitude, commonly called "gain," regulates the size of the complex and can be adjusted up and down to some degree.

Test-Taking Strategy: Focus on the issue: that the complexes are small and hard to evaluate. Eliminate options 2 and 4 first because they are similar. From the remaining options, noting the relation of the issue to the word "amplitude" (meaning size or strength) in option 3 will direct you to this option. Review the procedure for the use of an ECG monitor if you had difficulty with this question.

Level of Cognitive Ability: Application
Client Needs: Physiological Integrity
Integrated Process: Nursing Process/Implementation
Content Area: Adult Health/Cardiovascular

References:

Black, J., & Hawks, J. (2005). *Medical-surgical nursing: Clinical management for positive outcomes* (7th ed.). Philadelphia: Saunders, p. 1586.
Phipps, W., Monahan, F., Sands, J., Marek, J., & Neighbors, M. (2003). *Medical-surgical nursing: Health and illness perspectives* (7th ed.). St. Louis: Mosby, p. 636.

67. A nurse is monitoring a client who has received antidysrhythmic therapy for the treatment of premature ventricular contractions (PVCs). The nurse would determine this therapy as being less than optimal if the client's PVCs continued to:
1 Be fewer than six per minute
2 Be unifocal in appearance
3 Fall after the end of the T wave
4 Occurred in pairs

Answer: 4
Rationale: PVCs are considered dangerous when they are frequent (more than six per minute), occur in pairs or couplets, are multifocal (multiform), or fall on the T wave.

Test-Taking Strategy: Note the key words "less than optimal." These words indicate a false-response question and that you need to select the option that identifies ineffective treatment. Knowledge regarding the occurrence of PVCs and the situations in which they may be dangerous to the client will direct you to option 4. Review this basic information if you had difficulty with this question.

Level of Cognitive Ability: Analysis
Client Needs: Physiological Integrity
Integrated Process: Nursing Process/Evaluation
Content Area: Adult Health/Cardiovascular

Reference:
Black, J., & Hawks, J. (2005). *Medical-surgical nursing: Clinical management for positive outcomes* (7th ed.). Philadelphia: Saunders, p. 1682.

---

68. A nurse is reviewing the client's arterial blood gas (ABG) results. Which finding would indicate that the client had respiratory acidosis?
1 pH 7.5, Pco2 30
2 pH 7.3, Pco2 50
3 pH 7.3, Pco2 19
4 pH 7.5, Pco2 30

Answer: 2
Rationale: In respiratory acidosis, the pH is decreased and an opposite effect is seen in the Pco_2 (pH decreased, Pco_2 elevated). Option 1 indicates respiratory alkalosis; option 3 indicates possible metabolic acidosis; and option 4 indicates possible metabolic alkalosis.

Test-Taking Strategy: Use the process of elimination. Recalling that the pH is decreased in acidosis will assist in eliminating options 1 and 4. Next, remember in respiratory acidosis the Pco_2 has an opposite effect from the pH. This will direct you to option 2. Review these basic interpretations if you had difficulty with this question.

Level of Cognitive Ability: Analysis
Client Needs: Physiological Integrity
Integrated Process: Nursing Process/Analysis
Content Area: Adult Health/Respiratory

Reference:
Black, J., & Hawks, J. (2005). *Medical-surgical nursing: Clinical management for positive outcomes* (7th ed.). Philadelphia: Saunders, p. 254.

---

69. A nurse is assigned to care for a client with a chest tube attached to closed chest drainage. The nurse determines that the client's lung has completely expanded if:
1 The oxygen saturation is greater than 92%
2 Fluctuations in the water seal chamber ceased
3 Pleuritic chest pain has resolved
4 Suction in the chest drainage system is no longer needed

Answer: 2
Rationale: When the lung has completely expanded, there is no longer air or fluid in the pleural space to be drained into the water seal chamber. Thus, an indication that a chest tube is ready for removal is when fluctuations in the water seal chamber cease and drainage of fluid into the collection bottle/chamber ceases. Adequate oxygen saturation does not imply that the lung has fully reexpanded. Although air is known to be an irritant to pleural tissue, cessation of pleuritic pain does not indicate that the lung is expanded. The chest tube acts as an irritant and therefore contributes to pain. Use or nonuse of suction in the chest drainage system is not necessarily governed by the degree of lung

expansion. Suction is indicated when gravity is not sufficient to drain air and pleural fluid or if the client has a poor respiratory effort and cough. Suction increases the speed at which air and fluid is removed from the pleural space.

Test-Taking Strategy: Note the key words "completely expanded." Eliminate options 1 and 3 because they are not directly related to a chest tube drainage system. From the remaining options, recalling the functioning of chest tubes will direct you to option 2. Review chest tube drainage systems if you had difficulty with this question.

Level of Cognitive Ability: Analysis
Client Needs: Physiological Integrity
Integrated Process: Nursing Process/Evaluation
Content Area: Adult Health/Respiratory

Reference:
Black, J., & Hawks, J. (2005). *Medical-surgical nursing: Clinical management for positive outcomes* (7th ed.). Philadelphia: Saunders, p. 1866.

---

70. A nurse is caring for a child with leukemia and notes that the platelet count is 20,000/mm³. Based on this finding, the nurse deletes which of the following from the plan of care?
1 Monitor stools for blood
2 Clean oral cavity with soft swabs
3 Administer acetaminophen (Tylenol) suppositories for fever
4 Provide appropriate play activities

Answer: 3
Rationale: A platelet count of 20,000/mm³ places the child at risk for bleeding. Options 1, 2, and 4 are accurate interventions. The use of suppositories is avoided because of the risk of rectal bleeding.

Test-Taking Strategy: Note the key word "deletes." This word indicates a false-response question and that you need to select the intervention that is contraindicated. Noting the issue of the question, bleeding, and recalling the interventions related to bleeding precautions will direct you to option 3. Review interventions for the child at risk for bleeding if you had difficulty with this question.

Level of Cognitive Ability: Application
Client Needs: Physiological Integrity
Integrated Process: Nursing Process/Planning
Content Area: Child Health

References:
James, S., Ashwill, J., & Droske, S. (2002). *Nursing care of children: Principles & practice* (2nd ed.). Philadelphia: Saunders, pp. 783;785.
Wong, D., & Hockenberry, M. (2003). *Wong's nursing care of infants and children* (7th ed.). St. Louis: Mosby, p. 1612.

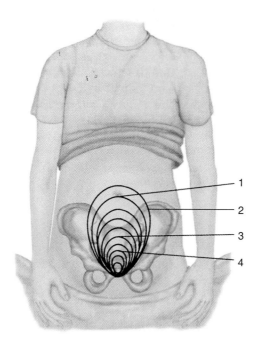

71. It has been 12 hours since the client's delivery of a newborn. The nurse assesses the mother for the process of involution and documents that it is progressing normally when palpation of the client's fundus is noted at which level?

Answer: 1

Rationale: The term "involution" is used to describe the rapid reduction in size and the return of the uterus to a normal condition similar to its pregnant state. Immediately following the delivery of the placenta, the uterus contracts to the size of a large grapefruit. The fundus is situated in the midline between the symphysis pubis and the umbilicus. Within 6 to 12 hours after birth, the fundus of the uterus rises to the level of the umbilicus. The top of the fundus remains at the level of the umbilicus for about a day and then descends into the pelvis approximately one fingerbreadth on each succeeding day.

Test-Taking Strategy: Note the key words "it has been 12 hours." Attempt to visualize the process of assessment of involution and the expected finding at this time to answer the question. Remember that within 6 to 12 hours after birth, the fundus of the uterus rises to the level of the umbilicus, remaining at this level for about a day, and then descends into the pelvis approximately one fingerbreadth on each succeeding day. Review this process if you had difficulty with this question.

Level of Cognitive Ability: Application
Client Needs: Health Promotion and Maintenance
Integrated Process: Nursing Process/Assessment
Content Area: Maternity/Postpartum

Reference:
Murray, S., McKinney, E., & Gorrie, T. (2002). *Foundations of maternal-newborn nursing* (3rd ed.). Philadelphia: Saunders, pp. 425-426.

72. A nurse evaluates the arterial blood gas (ABG) results of a client who is receiving supplemental oxygen. Which finding would indicate that the oxygen level was adequate?
1 A Po2 of 80 mmHg
2 A Po2 of 60 mmHg
3 A Po2 of 50 mmHg
4 A Po2 of 45 mmHg

Answer: 1

Rationale: The normal Po_2 level is 80 to 100 mmHg. Options 2, 3, and 4 are low values and do not indicate adequate oxygen levels.

Test-Taking Strategy: Focus on the issue: oxygen level was adequate. Use the process of elimination and select the option that identifies the highest oxygen level. This will direct you to option 1. Review interpretation of the results of ABGs if you had difficulty with this question.

Level of Cognitive Ability: Analysis
Client Needs: Physiological Integrity
Integrated Process: Nursing Process/Evaluation
Content Area: Adult Health/Respiratory

Reference:
Black, J., & Hawks, J. (2005). *Medical-surgical nursing: Clinical management for positive outcomes* (7th ed.). Philadelphia: Saunders, pp. 252; 1764.

73. A nurse assesses a client admitted to the hospital with rib fractures in order to identify the risk for potential complications. The nurse notes that the client has a history of emphysema. Following the assessment, the nurse ensures that which priority intervention is documented in the plan of care?
1 Have the client cough and breathe deeply 20 minutes after pain medication is given
2 Administer low-flow oxygen at 2 liters per minute as prescribed
3 Assist the client to a position of comfort
4 Administer small, frequent meals with plenty of fluids

Answer: 2

Rationale: Giving the client with emphysema a high flow of oxygen would halt the hypoxic drive and cause apnea. Although options 1, 3, and 4 may be appropriate nursing interventions, option 2 specifically addresses the issue of the question.

Test-Taking Strategy: Note the key word "priority." Focus on the data in the question and note that the client has emphysema. Recalling the care of a client with emphysema and use of the ABCs—airway, breathing, and circulation—will direct you to option 2. Review the complications that can occur in the client with emphysema if you had difficulty with this question.

Level of Cognitive Ability: Application
Client Needs: Physiological Integrity
Integrated Process: Communication and Documentation
Content Area: Delegating/Prioritizing

Reference:
Lewis, S., Heitkemper, M., & Dirksen, S. (2004). *Medical-surgical nursing: Assessment and management of clinical problems* (6th ed.). St. Louis: Mosby, p. 549.

74. A nurse is developing a plan of care for a client with acquired immunodeficiency syndrome (AIDS). The nurse documents which appropriate goal in the plan of care?
1 The client does not experience respiratory distress.
2 The client has no increased platelet aggregation.
3 The client has no evidence of dissecting aortic aneurysm.
4 The client has a urinary output of 50 mL per hour.

Answer: 1
Rationale: A common, life-threatening opportunistic infection that attacks clients with AIDS is pneumocystis carinii pneumonia. Its symptoms include fever, exertional dyspnea, and nonproductive cough. The absence of respiratory distress is one of the goals that the nurse sets as a priority. Options 2, 3, and 4 are not specifically related to the issue of the question.

Test-Taking Strategy: Note the issue of the question. Option 1 is the only option that is directly related to the client's diagnosis. In addition, use the ABCs—airway, breathing, and circulation—to answer the question. Review care of the client with AIDS if you had difficulty with this question.

Level of Cognitive Ability: Application
Client Needs: Physiological Integrity
Integrated Process: Communication and Documentation
Content Area: Adult Health/Respiratory

Reference:
Phipps, W., Monahan, F., Sands, J., Marek, J., & Neighbors, M. (2003). *Medical-surgical nursing: Health and illness perspectives* (7th ed.). St. Louis: Mosby, p. 1667.

---

75. A client with active tuberculosis is to be admitted to a medical-surgical unit. When planning a bed assignment, the nurse:
1 Plans to transfer the client to the intensive care unit
2 Assigns the client to a double room because intravenous antibiotics will be administered
3 Assigns the client to a double room and places a "strict handwashing" sign outside the door
4 Places the client in a private, well-ventilated room

Answer: 4
Rationale: According to category-specific (respiratory) isolation precautions, a client with TB requires a private room. The room needs to be well-ventilated and should have at least six exchanges of fresh air per hour and should be ventilated to the outside if possible. Therefore, option 4 is the only correct option.

Test-Taking Strategy: Note that the question states "active tuberculosis." Eliminate options 2 and 3 because they are similar in that they involve assignment to a double room. From the remaining options, recalling the need for respiratory isolation precautions will direct you to option 4. Review care of the client with active tuberculosis if you had difficulty with this question.

Level of Cognitive Ability: Application
Client Needs: Safe, Effective Care Environment
Integrated Process: Nursing Process/Planning
Content Area: Leadership/Management

Reference:
Phipps, W., Monahan, F., Sands, J., Marek, J., & Neighbors, M. (2003). *Medical-surgical nursing: Health and illness perspectives* (7th ed.). St. Louis: Mosby, p. 539.

76. A client has a diagnosis of an irregular heart rate. What question by the client would indicate that client teaching should begin?

1 "How is an ECG interpreted?"
2 "What is it like to have a pacemaker?"
3 "Can you tell me what a diagnosis of irregular heart rate means?"
4 "What is wrong with my roommate's heart?"

Answer: 3

Rationale: Learning depends on two things: physical and emotional readiness to learn. Without one or the other, teaching can occur, but learning may not take place. There is usually a time at which the client will indicate an interest in learning. Option 3 addresses the client's readiness because the client is directly asking about the disorder. At this point, the client's readiness and motivation to learn is present.

Test-Taking Strategy: Use the process of elimination. Note that option 3 directly addresses the client's diagnosis. Also note the similarity of "irregular heart rate" in the question and in the correct option. Review teaching-learning principles if you had difficulty with this question.

Level of Cognitive Ability: Analysis
Client Needs: Psychosocial Integrity
Integrated Process: Teaching/Learning
Content Area: Fundamental Skills

Reference:
Lewis, S., Heitkemper, M., & Dirksen, S. (2004). *Medical-surgical nursing: Assessment and management of clinical problems* (6th ed.). St. Louis: Mosby, pp. 44-45.

---

77. A physician orders intralipids, an intravenous fat emulsion, for a client who will be receiving total parenteral nutrition (TPN) for several months. The nurse explains to the client that the fat emulsion is administered:

1 To increase the amount of fluid given by the intravenous route
2 On a daily basis and must be administered at bedtime
3 To decrease the incidence of phlebitis in the vein where the TPN is administered
4 To provide essential fatty acids and additional calories

Answer: 4

Rationale: Intralipids is a brand of intravenous fat emulsion. Clients receiving TPN parenterally for a prolonged period are at risk for developing essential fatty acid deficiency. Fat emulsions are given to meet client nonprotein caloric needs that cannot be met by glucose administration alone. Fat emulsions are not administered to increase the amount of fluids administered, and they do not decrease the incidence of phlebitis. They may be prescribed daily but do not need to be administered at bedtime.

Test-Taking Strategy: Focus on the issue: intravenous fat emulsion. Eliminate option 2 because of the absolute word "must." From the remaining options, note the relationship between "fat emulsion" in the question and "fatty acids" in the correct option. Review the purpose of administering fat emulsion during TPN therapy if you had difficulty with this question.

Level of Cognitive Ability: Application
Client Needs: Physiological Integrity
Integrated Process: Teaching/Learning
Content Area: Fundamental Skills

References:
Gahart, B., & Nazareno, A. (2005). *Intravenous medications* (21st ed.). St. Louis: Mosby, p. 524.
McKenry, L., & Salerno, E. (2003). *Mosby's pharmacology in nursing* (21st ed.). St. Louis: Mosby, p. 1193.

78. A client with valvular heart disease is at risk for developing congestive heart failure. The nurse assesses which of the following most closely when monitoring for congestive heart failure?
1   Heart rate
2   Blood pressure
3   Breath sounds
4   Activity tolerance

Answer: 3
Rationale: Breath sounds are the best way to assess for the onset of congestive heart failure. The presence of crackles or rales or an increase in crackles is an indicator of fluid in the lungs caused by congestive heart failure. Options 1, 2, and 4 are components of the assessment but are less reliable indicators of congestive heart failure.

Test-Taking Strategy: Use the process of elimination, thinking about the pathophysiology that occurs with congestive heart failure. Use of the ABCs—airway, breathing, and circulation—will direct you to option 3. Review assessment of congestive heart failure if you had difficulty with this question.

Level of Cognitive Ability: Analysis
Client Needs: Physiological Integrity
Integrated Process: Nursing Process/Assessment
Content Area: Delegating/Prioritizing

Reference:
Black, J., & Hawks, J. (2005). *Medical-surgical nursing: Clinical management for positive outcomes* (7th ed.). Philadelphia: Saunders, p. 1655.

79. A nurse is caring for a client receiving fludrocortisone acetate (Florinef) for the treatment of Addison's disease. The nurse monitors the client for improvement, knowing that the anticipated therapeutic effect of this medication is to:
1   Stimulate the immune response
2   Promote electrolyte balance
3   Stimulate thyroid production
4   Stimulate thytrotropin production

Answer: 2
Rationale: Florinef is a long-acting oral medication with mineralocorticoid and moderate glucocorticoid activity that is used for long-term management of Addison's disease. Mineralocorticoids act on the renal distal tubules to enhance the reabsorption of sodium and chloride ions and the excretion of potassium and hydrogen ions. The client can rapidly develop hypotension and fluid and electrolyte imbalance if the medication is discontinued abruptly. The medication does not affect the immune response or thyroid or thyrotropin production.

Test-Taking Strategy: Remember that Addison's disease produces deficiencies of glucocorticoids, mineralocorticoids, and androgens. Eliminate options 3 and 4 first because they are similar. From the remaining options, recalling that Addison's disease is not related to the immune system will direct you to option 2. Review the action of this medication if you had difficulty with this question.

Level of Cognitive Ability: Analysis
Client Needs: Physiological Integrity
Integrated Process: Nursing Process/Evaluation
Content Area: Adult Health/Endocrine

Reference:
Hodgson, B., & Kizior, R. (2004). *Saunders nursing drug handbook 2004.* Philadelphia: Saunders, p. 419.

80. A nurse is assessing the leg pain of a client who has just undergone right femoral-popliteal artery bypass grafting. Which question would be most useful in determining whether the client is experiencing graft occlusion?
   1 "Can you rate the pain on a scale of 1 to 10?"
   2 "Can you describe what the pain feels like?"
   3 "Can you compare this pain to the pain you felt before surgery?"
   4 "Did you get any relief from the last dose of pain medication?"

Answer: 3
Rationale: The most frequent indication that a graft is occluding is the return of pain that is similar to that experienced preoperatively. Standard pain assessment techniques also include the items described in options 1, 2, and 4, but these will not help differentiate current pain from preoperative pain.

Test-Taking Strategy: Focus on the issue: the assessment question that will help differentiate expected postoperative pain from pain that indicates graft occlusion. Eliminate options 1, 2, and 4 because they are similar and are standard pain assessment questions. Review care of the client following this type of surgery if you had difficulty with this question.

Level of Cognitive Ability: Application
Client Needs: Physiological Integrity
Integrated Process: Nursing Process/Assessment
Content Area: Adult Health/Cardiovascular

Reference:
Black, J., & Hawks, J. (2005). *Medical-surgical nursing: Clinical management for positive outcomes* (7th ed.). Philadelphia: Saunders, pp. 1518-1519.

81. A client has implemented dietary and other lifestyle changes to manage hypertension. The nurse determines that the client has been most successful if the client has a follow-up blood pressure reading of:
   1 156/89 mmHg
   2 128/84 mmHg
   3 164/90 mmHg
   4 140/94 mmHg

Answer: 2
Rationale: Normal blood pressure readings are less than 120/80 mmHg. A blood pressure reading between 120/80 mmHg to 139/89 mmHg is considered to be a prehypertensive state. From the readings provided in the options, option 2 identifies the most successful outcome, although the reading indicates a prehypertensive state.

Test-Taking Strategy: Note the key words "most successful." Option 2 identifies a reading that is closest to normal even though it identifies a prehypertensive state. Review the definitions of prehypertension and hypertension if you had difficulty with this question.

Level of Cognitive Ability: Analysis
Client Needs: Physiological Integrity
Integrated Process: Nursing Process/Evaluation
Content Area: Adult Health/Cardiovascular

Reference:
Black, J., & Hawks, J. (2005). *Medical-surgical nursing: Clinical management for positive outcomes* (7th ed.). Philadelphia: Saunders, p. 1497.

82. A client is scheduled to have insertion of an inferior vena cava (IVC) filter. The nurse would place highest priority on determining whether the surgeon wants which of the following medications held in the preoperative period?
1 Famotidine (Pepcid)
2 Multivitamin with minerals
3 Warfarin (Coumadin)
4 Furosemide (Lasix)

Answer: 3

Rationale: The nurse is careful to question the surgeon about whether warfarin should be administered in the preoperative period before insertion of an IVC filter. This medication is often withheld for a period of time preoperatively to minimize the risk of hemorrhage during surgery. The other medications may also be withheld if specifically ordered, but usually they are discontinued as part of an NPO (nothing by mouth) after midnight order.

Test-Taking Strategy: Note the key words "highest priority." Recalling that warfarin is an anticoagulant and that when a client is taking an anticoagulant a risk for bleeding exists will direct you to option 3. Review anticoagulant medication therapy and preoperative nursing care if you had difficulty with this question.

Level of Cognitive Ability: Analysis
Client Needs: Safe, Effective Care Environment
Integrated Process: Nursing Process/Analysis
Content Area: Adult Health/Cardiovascular

Reference:
Black, J., & Hawks, J. (2005). *Medical-surgical nursing: Clinical management for positive outcomes* (7th ed.). Philadelphia: Saunders, pp. 1832-1833.

83. A client's medical record states a history of intermittent claudication. In collecting data about this symptom, the nurse would ask the client about which symptom?
1 Chest pain that is sudden and occurs with exertion
2 Chest pain that is dull and feels like heartburn
3 Leg pain that is achy and gets worse as the day progresses
4 Leg pain that is sharp and occurs with exercise

Answer: 4

Rationale: Intermittent claudication is a symptom characterized by a sudden onset of leg pain that occurs with exercise and is relieved by rest. It is the classic symptom of peripheral arterial insufficiency. Venous insufficiency is characterized by an achy type of leg pain that intensifies as the day progresses. Chest pain can occur for a variety of reasons, including angina pectoris (option 1) or indigestion (option 2).

Test-Taking Strategy: Use the process of elimination. Focusing on the key word "intermittent" in the question will direct you to option 4. Review this content area if you had difficulty with this question or if you are unfamiliar with the term intermittent claudication.

Level of Cognitive Ability: Application
Client Needs: Physiological Integrity
Integrated Process: Nursing Process/Assessment
Content Area: Adult Health/Cardiovascular

Reference:
Black, J., & Hawks, J. (2005). *Medical-surgical nursing: Clinical management for positive outcomes* (7th ed.). Philadelphia: Saunders, p. 1476.

84. A client has just been diagnosed with right leg deep vein thrombosis (DVT). The nurse immediately implements which intervention?
1 Elevation of the right leg
2 Ice packs to the right leg
3 Vigorous range of motion to the right leg
4 Hourly calf measurements

Answer: 1

Rationale: Treatment for DVT may require bed rest, leg elevation, and application of warm moist heat to the affected leg. The client may have calf measurements ordered once per shift or once per day, but they would not be obtained hourly. Option 2 is incorrect because heat may be prescribed, not cold. Option 3 is dangerous to the client, because vigorous activity after clot formation can cause pulmonary embolus.

Test-Taking Strategy: Focus on the client's diagnosis and use knowledge of the treatment for DVT as well as concepts related to gravity and the applications of heat and cold to answer the question. Review the interventions for this disorder if you had difficulty with this question.

Level of Cognitive Ability: Application
Client Needs: Physiological Integrity
Integrated Process: Nursing Process/Implementation
Content Area: Adult Health/Cardiovascular

Reference:
Black, J., & Hawks, J. (2005). *Medical-surgical nursing: Clinical management for positive outcomes* (7th ed.). Philadelphia: Saunders, pp. 1540-1541.

85. A client is scheduled to have a serum digoxin (Lanoxin) level obtained. The nurse would arrange to have the blood sample drawn:
1 Just before a dose is given
2 Just after a dose has been given
3 One-half hour after a dose is given
4 One hour after a dose is given

Answer: 1

Rationale: The purpose of a serum digoxin (Lanoxin) level is to record the serum concentration of the medication to ensure that it is in the therapeutic range. Serum digoxin levels are most often drawn before a dose, although they may be drawn 4 to 10 hours after a dose was administered. Drawing the medication before a dose ensures that the level is not falsely elevated.

Test-Taking Strategy: Eliminate options 2, 3, and 4 because they are similar. Each of these options requires the blood sample to be drawn within a relatively short period after the client has been given the medication. Review this laboratory test if you had difficulty with this question.

Level of Cognitive Ability: Application
Client Needs: Physiological Integrity
Integrated Process: Nursing Process/Planning
Content Area: Adult Health/Cardiovascular

References:
Black, J., & Hawks, J. (2005). *Medical-surgical nursing: Clinical management for positive outcomes* (7th ed.). Philadelphia: Saunders, p. 1685.
Chernecky, C., & Berger, B. (2004). *Laboratory tests and diagnostic procedures* (4th ed.). Philadelphia: Saunders, pp. 478-479.

86. A home care nurse is collecting data regarding the environmental safety for the client receiving home oxygen therapy. The nurse determines that the client needs instructions regarding safe use of oxygen if which observation is made?
1 Gas stove is lit in a room 30 feet from where the oxygen is used.
2 Oxygen concentrator is placed against a wall.
3 Oxygen tank is secured in holder.
4 A "no smoking" sign is in the window near the door of the client's home.

Answer: 2
Rationale: There should be no open flames or smoking within 10 feet of the oxygen source. The tank should remain secured in its holder, and the concentrator should be away from walls or other close quarters (to allow adequate air circulation around the unit). The oxygen source should also be removed from sources of heat or sunlight. A "no smoking" sign should be in visible view, such as in the window near the door of the client's home.

Test-Taking Strategy: Note the key words "the client needs instructions." These words indicate a false-response question and that you need to select the incorrect client action. Recalling the principles of safe oxygen use will direct you to option 2. Review these safety principles if you had difficulty with this question.

Level of Cognitive Ability: Analysis
Client Needs: Safe, Effective Care Environment
Integrated Process: Nursing Process/Evaluation
Content Area: Fundamental Skills

Reference:
Potter, P. , & Perry, A. (2005). *Fundamentals of nursing* (6th ed.). St. Louis: Mosby, p. 1122.

---

87. A nurse has finished suctioning the tracheostomy of a client. The nurse determines the effectiveness of the procedure by monitoring which item?
1 Respiratory rate
2 Oxygen saturation level
3 Breath sounds
4 Capillary refill

Answer: 3
Rationale: After suctioning a client either with or without an artificial airway, the breath sounds are auscultated to determine the extent to which the airways have been cleared of respiratory secretions. The other assessment items are not as precise as breath sounds for this purpose.

Test-Taking Strategy: Use the process of elimination, focusing on the issue: evaluating the effectiveness of suctioning. Recalling that the purpose of suctioning is to clear the airways of secretions will direct you to option 3. Review the procedure for suctioning if you had difficulty with this question.

Level of Cognitive Ability: Analysis
Client Needs: Physiological Integrity
Integrated Process: Nursing Process/Evaluation
Content Area: Adult Health/Respiratory

Reference:
Potter, P. , & Perry, A. (2005). *Fundamentals of nursing* (6th ed.). St. Louis: Mosby, pp. 1101; 1108-1109.

88. A nurse has given a client directions for proper use of aluminum hydroxide tablets (Alu-Caps). The client indicates an understanding of the medication if which statement is made?

1 "I should take the tablet at the same time as an antacid."
2 "I should take each dose with a laxative to prevent constipation."
3 "I should chew the tablet thoroughly and then drink four ounces of water."
4 "I should swallow the tablet whole with a full glass of water."

Answer: 3

Rationale: Aluminum hydroxide tablets should be chewed thoroughly before swallowing. This prevents them from entering the small intestine undissolved. They should not be swallowed whole. Antacids should be taken at least 2 hours apart from other medications to prevent interactive effects. Constipation is a side effect of the use of aluminum products, but the client should not take a laxative with each dose. This promotes laxative abuse. The client should first try other means to prevent constipation.

Test-Taking Strategy: Use the process of elimination. Eliminate option 2 first because it does not promote healthy bowel function. Next, eliminate option 1 using general knowledge of antacid interactive effects. From the remaining options, use principles of digestion and medication use to direct you to option 3. Review client teaching points related to the use of this medication if you had difficulty with this question.

Level of Cognitive Ability: Analysis
Client Needs: Physiological Integrity
Integrated Process: Teaching/Learning
Content Area: Pharmacology

Reference:
Lehne, R. (2004). *Pharmacology for nursing care.* (5th ed). Philadelphia: Saunders, p. 832.

89. A nurse is checking a client's disposable closed chest drainage system at the beginning of the shift and notes continuous bubbling in the water seal chamber. The nurse interprets that:

1 There is an air leak somewhere in the system
2 A pneumothorax is resolving
3 The system is intact
4 The suction to the system is shut off

Answer: 1

Rationale: Continuous bubbling in the water seal chamber through both inspiration and expiration indicates that air is leaking into the system. A resolving pneumothorax would show intermittent bubbling with respiration in the water seal chamber. Shutting the suction off to the system stops bubbling in the suction control chamber, but does not affect the water seal chamber.

Test-Taking Strategy: Use the process of elimination and focus on the issue: continuous bubbling in the water seal chamber. The words "continuous bubbling" should provide you with the clue that an air leak is present. Review the concepts associated with a chest tube drainage system if you had difficulty with this question.

Level of Cognitive Ability: Analysis
Client Needs: Physiological Integrity
Integrated Process: Nursing Process/Evaluation
Content Area: Adult Health/Respiratory

Reference:
Black, J., & Hawks, J. (2005). *Medical-surgical nursing: Clinical management for positive outcomes* (7th ed.). Philadelphia: Saunders, p. 1863.

90. A client is suspected of having pulmonary tuberculosis. The nurse assesses the client for which signs and symptoms of tuberculosis?
1 Weight gain, insomnia, and night sweats
2 Low-grade fever, fatigue, and productive cough
3 High fever and chest pain
4 Increased appetite, dyspnea, and chills

Answer: 2
Rationale: The client with pulmonary tuberculosis generally has a productive or nonproductive cough, anorexia and weight loss, fatigue, low-grade fever, chills and night sweats, dyspnea, hemoptysis, and chest pain. Breath sounds may reveal crackles.

Test-Taking Strategy: Use the process of elimination. Remember that when an option has more than one part, all of the parts of that option must be correct if the entire option is to be correct. Eliminate options 1 and 4 first because the client will not have an increased appetite or weight gain. From the remaining options, it is necessary to know that the fever will be low grade. Review findings related to tuberculosis if you had difficulty with this question.

Level of Cognitive Ability: Application
Client Needs: Physiological Integrity
Integrated Process: Nursing Process/Assessment
Content Area: Adult Health/Respiratory

Reference:
Black, J., & Hawks, J. (2005). *Medical-surgical nursing: Clinical management for positive outcomes* (7th ed.). Philadelphia: Saunders, pp. 1845-1846.

91. Auranofin (Ridaura) is prescribed for a client with rheumatoid arthritis, and the nurse monitors the client for signs of an adverse effect related to the medication. Which of the following indicates an adverse effect?
1 Nausea
2 Diarrhea
3 Anorexia
4 Proteinuria

Answer: 4
Rationale: Auranofin (Ridaura) is a gold preparation that is used as an antirheumatic. Gold toxicity is an adverse effect and is evidenced by decreased hemoglobin, leukopenia, reduced granulocyte counts, proteinuria, hematuria, stomatitis, glomerulonephritis, nephrotic syndrome, or cholestatic jaundice. Anorexia, nausea, and diarrhea are frequent side effects of the medication.

Test-Taking Strategy: Focus on the issue: an adverse effect. Eliminate options 1, 2, and 3 because they are similar and indicate gastrointestinal effects. Review toxicity related to gold compounds if you had difficulty with this question.

Level of Cognitive Ability: Analysis
Client Needs: Physiological Integrity
Integrated Process: Nursing Process/Analysis
Content Area: Pharmacology

Reference:
Hodgson, B., & Kizior, R. (2004). *Saunders nursing drug handbook 2004.* Philadelphia: Saunders, p. 84.

92. A nurse is preparing to implement emergency care measures for the client who has just experienced pulmonary embolism. The nurse implements which of the following physician orders first?
1 Administer morphine sulfate
2 Apply oxygen
3 Start an intravenous line
4 Obtain an electrocardiogram (ECG)

Answer: 2
Rationale: The client needs immediate oxygen because of hypoxemia, which is most often accompanied by respiratory distress and cyanosis. The client should have an IV line for the administration of emergency medications such as morphine sulfate. An ECG is useful in determining the presence of possible right ventricular hypertrophy. All of the interventions listed are appropriate, but the client needs the oxygen first.

Test-Taking Strategy: Note the key word "first." Use the process of elimination and the ABCs—airway, breathing, and circulation. This will direct you to option 2. Review care of the client with pulmonary embolism if you had difficulty with this question.

Level of Cognitive Ability: Application
Client Needs: Physiological Integrity
Integrated Process: Nursing Process/Implementation
Content Area: Delegating/Prioritizing

Reference:
Phipps, W., Monahan, F., Sands, J., Marek, J., & Neighbors, M. (2003). *Medical-surgical nursing: Health and illness perspectives* (7th ed.). St. Louis: Mosby, p. 604.

93. A client is scheduled for bronchoscopy, and the registered nurse reviews the plan of care written by a nursing student. The registered nurse discusses revision of the plan with the nursing student if which incorrect intervention was documented?
1 Obtaining a signed informed consent
2 Letting the client eat or drink
3 Removing contact lenses
4 Removing any dentures

Answer: 2
Rationale: The client is not allowed to eat or drink for usually 6 hours before the procedure. The client must sign an informed consent, because the procedure is invasive. If the client has any contact lenses, dentures, or other prostheses, they are removed before sedation is administered to the client.

Test-Taking Strategy: Note the key words "incorrect intervention." These words indicate a false-response question and that you need to select the incorrect intervention. Recalling that for many invasive procedures the client must be on nothing by mouth status (NPO) will direct you to option 2. Review care of the client undergoing bronchoscopy if you had difficulty with this question.

Level of Cognitive Ability: Application
Client Needs: Physiological Integrity
Integrated Process: Nursing Process/Implementation
Content Area: Leadership/Management

Reference:
Chernecky, C., & Berger, B. (2004). *Laboratory tests and diagnostic procedures* (4th ed.). Philadelphia: Saunders, p, 297

94. A client who has no history of immuno-suppressive disease and is at low risk for tuberculosis has a Mantoux test. The results indicate an area of induration that is 8 mm in size. The nurse interprets that the client:
1 Has active tuberculosis
2 Has a history of tuberculosis
3 Has been exposed to tuberculosis
4 Has a negative response

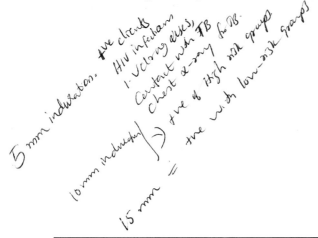

Answer: 4
Rationale: Induration of 15 mm or more is considered positive for clients in low-risk groups. More than 5 mm of induration is considered a positive result for clients with known or suspected human immunodeficiency virus infection, intravenous drug users, people in close contact with a known case of tuberculosis, and the client with a chest X-ray suggestive of previous tuberculosis. More than 10 mm of induration is considered positive in all other high-risk groups.

Test-Taking Strategy: Use the process of elimination and note the key words "at low risk." Noting that the area of induration measures 8 mm will direct you to option 4. Review the normal parameters for this test if you had difficulty with this question.

Level of Cognitive Ability: Analysis
Client Needs: Physiological Integrity
Integrated Process: Nursing Process/Analysis
Content Area: Adult Health/Respiratory

Reference:
Black, J., & Hawks, J. (2005). *Medical-surgical nursing: Clinical management for positive outcomes* (7th ed.). Philadelphia: Saunders, p. 1846.

---

95. A client has an order to have a set of arterial blood gases (ABGs) drawn, and the intended site is the radial artery. The nurse ensures that which of the following is positive before the ABGs are drawn?
1 Homan's sign
2 Brudzinski's sign
3 Babinski reflex
4 Allen test

Answer: 4
Rationale: The Allen test is performed before drawing ABGs. Each of the radial and ulnar arteries is occluded in turn and then released. Observation is made in the distal circulation. If the results are positive, then the client has adequate circulation, and that site may be used. Homan's sign tests for deep vein thrombosis with dorsiflexion of the foot. Brudzinski's sign tests for nuchal rigidity by bending the head down toward the chest. The Babinski reflex is checked by stroking upward on the sole of the foot.

Test-Taking Strategy: Note the key words "radial artery." Recalling the purpose of each test listed in the options will direct you to option 4. Review these tests if you had difficulty with this question.

Level of Cognitive Ability: Analysis
Client Needs: Physiological Integrity
Integrated Process: Nursing Process/Analysis
Content Area: Adult Health/Respiratory

Reference:
Chernecky, C., & Berger, B. (2004). *Laboratory tests and diagnostic procedures* (4th ed.). Philadelphia: Saunders, p. 248.

96. A client has been taking benzonatate (Tessalon) as ordered. The nurse tells the client that this medication should do which of the following?
1 Take away nausea and vomiting
2 Calm the persistent cough
3 Decrease anxiety level
4 Increase comfort level

Answer: 2
Rationale: Benzonatate is a locally acting antitussive. Its effectiveness is measured by the degree to which it decreases the intensity and frequency of cough, without eliminating the cough reflex. Options 1, 3, and 4 are not intended effects of this medication.

Test-Taking Strategy: Use the process of elimination and focus on the medication classification. Recalling that benzonatate is a locally acting antitussive will direct you to option 2. Review this content if you had difficulty with this question or if you are unfamiliar with this medication.

Level of Cognitive Ability: Application
Client Needs: Physiological Integrity
Integrated Process: Teaching/Learning
Content Area: Pharmacology

Reference:
Hodgson, B., & Kizior, R. (2004). *Saunders nursing drug handbook 2004.* Philadelphia: Saunders, p. 99.

97. A nurse is assessing a client with a suspected rib fracture. The nurse observes for which typical symptoms?
1 Pain on expiration, deep rapid respirations
2 Pain on expiration, shallow guarded respirations
3 Pain on inspiration, deep rapid respirations
4 Pain on inspiration, shallow guarded respirations

Answer: 4
Rationale: The client with fractured ribs typically has pain over the fracture site with inspiration and to palpation. Respirations are shallow, and guarding of the area is often noted. Bruising may or may not be present.

Test-Taking Strategy: Focus on the client's diagnosis. Think about the movement of the chest wall on inspiration and expiration. Remember that pain will occur on inspiration and respirations will be shallow. Review the signs related to a rib fracture if you had difficulty with this question.

Level of Cognitive Ability: Application
Client Needs: Physiological Integrity
Integrated Process: Nursing Process/Assessment
Content Area: Adult Health/Respiratory

Reference:
Phipps, W., Monahan, F., Sands, J., Marek, J., & Neighbors, M. (2003). *Medical-surgical nursing: Health and illness perspectives* (7th ed.). St. Louis: Mosby, p. 605.

98. A client with a flail chest caused by four fractured rib segments is experiencing severe pain when trying to breathe. The nurse observes the client for which characteristics of a flail chest?
1 Slight tachypnea with shallow breaths
2 Pallor and paradoxical chest movement
3 Severe dyspnea and paradoxical chest movement
4 Cyanosis and slow respirations

Answer: 3
Rationale: The client with flail chest is in obvious respiratory distress. The client has severe dyspnea and cyanosis accompanied by paradoxical chest movement. Respirations are shallow, rapid, and grunting in nature.

Test-Taking Strategy: Use the process of elimination. Remember that for an option to be correct, all of the parts of that option must also be correct. With this in mind, eliminate options 1 and 2 because of the words "slight" and "pallor." Choose between the remaining options, knowing that this client would be tachypneic, rather than having slow respirations. Review the clinical manifestations associated with flail chest if you had difficulty with this question.

Level of Cognitive Ability: Analysis
Client Needs: Physiological Integrity
Integrated Process: Nursing Process/Assessment
Content Area: Adult Health/Respiratory

Reference:

Phipps, W., Monahan, F., Sands, J., Marek, J., & Neighbors, M. (2003). *Medical-surgical nursing: Health and illness perspectives* (7th ed.). St. Louis: Mosby, p. 606.

---

99. A nurse is assigned to care for a client with pneumonia. The nurse reviews the nursing care plan and notes documentation of a nursing diagnosis of Activity Intolerance. The nurse implements which of the following in the client's care?
  1 Provides stimulation in the environment to maintain client alertness
  2 Encourages deep, rapid breathing during activity
  3 Schedules activities before giving respiratory medications or treatments
  4 Observes vital signs and oxygen saturation periodically during activity

Answer: 4
Rationale: The nurse monitors vital signs, including oxygen saturation, before, during, and after activity to gauge client response. Activities should be planned after giving the client respiratory medications or treatments to increase activity tolerance. The client should use pursed-lip and diaphragmatic breathing to lower oxygen consumption during activity. Finally, the environment should be conducive to rest, because the client is easily fatigued.

Test-Taking Strategy: Focus on the issue, Activity Intolerance, and note the client's diagnosis. Use the ABCs—airway, breathing, and circulation—to direct you to option 4. Review the interventions for a client with pneumonia and Activity Intolerance if you had difficulty with this question.

Level of Cognitive Ability: Application
Client Needs: Physiological Integrity
Integrated Process: Nursing Process/Implementation
Content Area: Adult Health/Respiratory

Reference:

Black, J., & Hawks, J. (2005). *Medical-surgical nursing: Clinical management for positive outcomes* (7th ed.). Philadelphia: Saunders, p. 1843.

---

100. A nurse is assisting in admitting a newborn infant to the nursery and notes that the physician has documented that the newborn has gastroschisis. The nurse plans care, knowing that in this condition the viscera are:
  1 Inside the abdominal cavity and under the dermis
  2 Inside the abdominal cavity and under the skin
  3 Outside the abdominal cavity but inside a translucent sac covered with peritoneum and amniotic membrane
  4 Outside the abdominal cavity and not covered with a sac

Answer: 4
Rationale: Gastroschisis is an abdominal wall defect in which the viscera are outside the abdominal cavity and not covered with a sac. Embryonal weakness in the abdominal wall causes herniation of the gut on one side of the umbilical cord during early development. Option 3 describes an omphalocele. Options 1 and 2 describe an umbilical hernia.

Test-Taking Strategy: Use the process of elimination. Eliminate options 1 and 2 first because they are similar. From the remaining options, recalling the definition of gastroschisis will direct you to option 4. Review this disorder if you are unfamiliar with it.

Level of Cognitive Ability: Application
Client Needs: Physiological Integrity
Integrated Process: Nursing Process/Planning
Content Area: Maternity/Postpartum

Reference:

Wong, D., & Hockenberry, M. (2003). *Wong's nursing care of infants and children* (7th ed.). St. Louis: Mosby, p. 473.

101. A home care nurse is providing instructions to a client who is taking zolpidem (Ambien) for insomnia. To produce a maximal effect of the medication, the nurse tells the client to take the medication:

1 With a full glass of water on an empty stomach
2 Following the evening meal
3 At bedtime with a snack
4 With milk or an antacid

Answer: 1

Rationale: The client should be instructed to take the medication at bedtime and to swallow the medication whole with a full glass of water. For faster onset of sleep, the client should be instructed not to administer the medication with milk or food, or immediately after a meal. Antacids should be avoided with the administration of the medication because of interactive effects.

Test-Taking Strategy: Use the process of elimination and note the key words "maximal effect" in the question. For maximal effectiveness of medications, medications should be taken on an empty stomach with water only. Also note that options 2, 3, and 4 are similar and indicate taking the medication with food or another substance. Review the principles related to the administration of zolpidem if you had difficulty with this question.

Level of Cognitive Ability: Application
Client Needs: Physiological Integrity
Integrated Process: Teaching/Learning
Content Area: Pharmacology

References:
Hodgson, B., & Kizior, R. (2004). *Saunders nursing drug handbook 2004.* Philadelphia: Saunders, p. 1078.
Lehne, R. (2004). *Pharmacology for nursing care* (5th ed.). Philadelphia: Saunders, p. 337.

102. A registered nurse is discussing treatment for a client who is hospitalized with acute systemic lupus erythematosus (SLE) with a nursing student assigned to care for the client. The registered nurse determines that the nursing student needs to research information about the disease if the student states that which of the following is a clinical manifestation of SLE?

1 Fever
2 Muscular aches and pains
3 Butterfly rash on the face
4 Bradycardia

Answer: 4

Rationale: Manifestations of acute SLE may include fever, musculoskeletal aches and pains, butterfly rash on the face, pleural effusion, basilar pneumonia, generalized lymphadenopathy, pericarditis, tachycardia, hepatosplenomegaly, nephritis, delirium, convulsions, psychosis, and coma.

Test-Taking Strategy: Note the key words "needs to research information." These words indicate a false-response question and that you need to select the incorrect clinical manifestation. Think about the pathophysiology associated with this disorder to direct you to option 4. Review its clinical manifestations if you are unfamiliar with this disorder.

Level of Cognitive Ability: Analysis
Client Needs: Physiological Integrity
Integrated Process: Teaching/Learning
Content Area: Leadership/Management

Reference:
Black, J., & Hawks, J. (2005). *Medical-surgical nursing: Clinical management for positive outcomes* (7th ed.). Philadelphia: Saunders, p. 2354.

103. A client is seen in the health care clinic and anemia has been diagnosed. On further assessment, the nurse notes that the client appears pale and complains of fatigue, weakness, dizziness, headache, loss of appetite, and palpitations. Based on the client's symptoms, the nurse would expect that the hemoglobin results would indicate which of the following?
1 Hemoglobin of 14 g/dL
2 Hemoglobin of 12 g/dL
3 Hemoglobin of 10 g/dL
4 Hemoglobin of 7 g/dL

Answer: 4
Rationale: Severely anemic persons (those with a hemoglobin below 8 g/dL) appear pale and always feel exhausted. They may have palpitations, sensitivity to cold, loss of appetite, profound weakness, dizziness, and headaches.

Test-Taking Strategy: Note that the client had numerous symptoms associated with anemia. Recalling the normal hemoglobin level will direct you to option 4. Review the normal hemoglobin level and the signs of anemia if you had difficulty with this question.

Level of Cognitive Ability: Analysis
Client Needs: Physiological Integrity
Integrated Process: Nursing Process/Analysis
Content Area: Fundamental Skills

References:
Black, J., & Hawks, J. (2005). *Medical-surgical nursing: Clinical management for positive outcomes* (7th ed.). Philadelphia: Saunders, p. 2273.
Chernecky, C., & Berger, B. (2004). *Laboratory tests and diagnostic procedures* (4th ed.). Philadelphia: Saunders, p. 637.

104. A nurse in the newborn nursery is performing vital signs on the newborn infant. Which finding would indicate a normal respiratory rate?
1 28 breaths per minute
2 50 breaths per minute
3 70 breaths per minute
4 80 breaths per minute

Answer: 2
Rationale: The normal respiratory rate for a newborn infant is 30 to 60 breaths per minute. Therefore, options 1, 3, and 4 are incorrect.

Test-Taking Strategy: Knowledge of the normal respiratory rate for a newborn infant is required to answer this question. Review this content if you are unfamiliar with the normal ranges for newborn vital signs.

Level of Cognitive Ability: Analysis
Client Needs: Physiological Integrity
Integrated Process: Nursing Process/Assessment
Content Area: Maternity/Postpartum

Reference:
Lowdermilk, D., & Perry, A. (2004). *Maternity & women's health care* (8th ed.). St. Louis: Mosby, p. 713.

105. A nurse is assessing a client with a diagnosis of polycythemia vera. Which clinical manifestation would the nurse expect to note in this client?
1 Pallor
2 Hypertension
3 Pale mucous membranes
4 A low hematocrit level

Answer: 2
Rationale: Manifestations of polycythemia vera include a ruddy complexion, dusky red mucosa, hypertension, dizziness, headache, and a sense of fullness in the head. Signs of congestive heart failure may also be present. The hematocrit level is usually greater than 54% in men and 49% in women.

Test-Taking Strategy: Focus on the client's diagnosis. Recalling that polycythemia vera is a myeloproliferative disease that causes increased blood viscosity and blood volume will direct you to option 2. Review this content if you are unfamiliar with the clinical manifestations associated with this disorder.

Level of Cognitive Ability: Analysis
Client Needs: Physiological Integrity
Integrated Process: Nursing Process/Assessment
Content Area: Adult Health/Cardiovascular

References:

Black, J., & Hawks, J. (2005). *Medical-surgical nursing: Clinical management for positive outcomes* (7th ed.). Philadelphia: Saunders, pp. 2299-2230.
Phipps, W., Monahan, F., Sands, J., Marek, J., & Neighbors, M. (2003). *Medical-surgical nursing: Health and illness perspectives* (7th ed.). St. Louis: Mosby, p. 828.

---

106. When reviewing the laboratory results of a client with leukemia who is receiving chemotherapy, the registered nurse notes that the neutrophil count is less than 500/mm^3. The registered nurse reviews the laboratory result with a nursing student caring for the client and asks the student to identify the appropriate precautions that need to be instituted. Which intervention identified by the student indicates a need for teaching?

1 Padding the side rails and removing all hazardous and sharp objects from the environment
2 Restricting visitors with colds or respiratory infections
3 Removing all live plants, flowers, and stuffed animals in the client's room
4 Placing the client on a low-bacteria diet that excludes raw foods and vegetables

Answer: 1

Rationale: When the neutrophil count is less than 500/mm^3, visitors should be screened for the presence of infection, and any visitors or staff with colds or respiratory infections should not be allowed in the client's room. All live plants, flowers, and stuffed animals are removed from the client's room. The client is placed on a low-bacteria diet that excludes raw fruits and vegetables. Padding the side rails and removing all hazardous and sharp objects from the environment would be instituted if the client is at risk for bleeding. This client is at risk for infection.

Test-Taking Strategy: Note the key words "indicates a need for teaching." These words indicate a false-response question and that you need to select the incorrect intervention. Recalling that a low neutrophil count places the client at risk for infection will direct you to option 1. Review this content if you are unfamiliar with the normal neutrophil count and the nursing interventions necessary when the count is low.

Level of Cognitive Ability: Analysis
Client Needs: Physiological Integrity
Integrated Process: Teaching/Learning
Content Area: Leadership/Management

Reference:

Black, J., & Hawks, J. (2005). *Medical-surgical nursing: Clinical management for positive outcomes* (7th ed.). Philadelphia: Saunders, pp. 382; 2408.

---

107. A nurse is delivering care to a client who was diagnosed with toxic shock syndrome (TSS). The nurse monitors the client for which complication of this syndrome?

1 Pulmonary embolism
2 Disseminated intravascular coagulopathy (DIC)
3 Vitamin K deficiency
4 Factor VIII deficiency

Answer: 2

Rationale: Toxic shock syndrome is caused by infection and is often associated with tampon use. DIC is a complication of TSS. The nurse monitors the client for signs of this complication, and notifies the physician promptly if signs and symptoms are noted. Options 1, 3, and 4 are not complications of TSS.

Test-Taking Strategy: Familiarity with TSS and knowledge that DIC is a complication is needed to answer this question. Review the complications of TTS if you had difficulty with this question.

Level of Cognitive Ability: Analysis
Client Needs: Physiological Integrity
Integrated Process: Nursing Process/Assessment
Content Area: Adult Health/Cardiovascular

Reference:
Ignatavicius, D., & Workman, M. (2002). *Medical surgical nursing: Critical thinking for collaborative care* (4th ed.). Philadelphia: Saunders, p. 1761.

---

108. A nurse is caring for a client with an acute head injury. The nurse carefully assesses which neurological sign as the most sensitive indicator of neurological status?
1 Vital signs
2 Level of consciousness
3 Sensory function
4 Motor function

Answer: 2

Rationale: The level of consciousness is the most sensitive indicator of neurological status. An alteration in the level of consciousness occurs before any other changes in neurologic signs or vital signs. Vital sign changes occur late.

Test-Taking Strategy: Noting the issue, neurological status, and the key words "most sensitive indicator" will direct you to option 2. Remember that the level of consciousness is the most sensitive indicator of neurological status. Review neurological assessment if you had difficulty with this question.

Level of Cognitive Ability: Application
Client Needs: Physiological Integrity
Integrated Process: Nursing Process/Assessment
Content Area: Adult Health/Neurological

Reference:
Black, J., & Hawks, J. (2005). *Medical-surgical nursing: Clinical management for positive outcomes* (7th ed.). Philadelphia: Saunders, p. 2034.

---

109. A client is admitted to the hospital with Cushing's syndrome. The nurse reviews the results of the client's laboratory studies for which manifestation of this disorder?
1 Hypokalemia
2 Hyperglycemia
3 Low white blood cell (WBC) count
4 Decreased plasma cortisol levels

Answer: 2

Rationale: The client with adrenocorticosteroid excess experiences hyperkalemia, hyperglycemia, elevated WBC count, and elevated plasma cortisol and adrenocorticotropic hormone (ACTH) levels. These abnormalities are caused by the effects of excess glucocorticoids and mineralocorticoids on the body.

Test-Taking Strategy: Recalling that an adrenocorticosteroid excess occurs in Cushing's syndrome will direct you to option 2. Also note that options 1, 3, and 4 identify low or decreased levels. Review the manifestations associated with Cushing's syndrome if you had difficulty with this question.

Level of Cognitive Ability: Analysis
Client Needs: Physiological Integrity
Integrated Process: Nursing Process/Assessment
Content Area: Adult Health/Endocrine

References:
Black, J., & Hawks, J. (2005). *Medical-surgical nursing: Clinical management for positive outcomes* (7th ed.). Philadelphia: Saunders, p. 1164.
Ignatavicius, D., & Workman, M. (2002). *Medical surgical nursing: Critical thinking for collaborative care* (4th ed.). Philadelphia: Saunders, p. 1417.

110. A nurse is going to suction an adult client with a tracheostomy who has copious amounts of secretions. The nurse does which of the following to accomplish this procedure safely and effectively?
  1 Occludes the Y-port of the catheter while advancing it into the tracheostomy
  2 Applies continuous suction in the airway for up to 20 seconds
  3 Hyperoxygenates the client after the procedure only
  4 Sets the wall suction pressure range between 80 to 120 mmHg

Answer: 4
Rationale: The safe wall suction range for an adult is 80 to 120 mmHg (120 to 150 mmHg with the tubing occluded), making option 4 the action that is consistent with safe and effective practice. The nurse should hyperoxygenate the client both before and after suctioning. The nurse should advance the catheter into the tracheostomy without occluding the Y-port to minimize mucosal trauma and aspiration of the client's oxygen. The nurse should use intermittent suction in the airway (not constant) for up to 10 to 15 seconds.

Test-Taking Strategy: Use the process of elimination. Eliminate option 3 because of the absolute word "only." From the remaining options, visualize the procedure to direct you to option 4. Review the procedure for suctioning if you had difficulty with this question.

Level of Cognitive Ability: Application
Client Needs: Physiological Integrity
Integrated Process: Nursing Process/Implementation
Content Area: Adult Health/Respiratory

References:
Lewis, S., Heitkemper, M., & Dirksen, S. (2004). *Medical-surgical nursing: Assessment and management of clinical problems* (6th ed.). St. Louis: Mosby, p. 579.
Potter, P., & Perry, A. (2005). *Fundamentals of nursing* (6th ed.). St. Louis: Mosby, p. 1102.

111. A nurse is caring for a hospitalized client who has been taking clozapine (Clozaril) for the treatment of a schizophrenic disorder, and the nurse reviews the laboratory studies that have been prescribed for the client. Which laboratory study will the nurse specifically review to monitor for an adverse effect associated with the use of this medication?
  1 White blood cell count
  2 Platelet count
  3 Cholesterol level
  4 Blood urea nitrogen

Answer: 1
Rationale: Hematological reactions can occur in the client taking clozapine and include agranulocytosis and mild leukopenia. The white blood cell count should be assessed before initiating treatment and should be monitored closely during the use of this medication. The client should also be monitored for signs indicating agranulocytosis, which may include sore throat, malaise, and fever. Options 2, 3, and 4 are unrelated to the use of this medication.

Test-Taking Strategy: Recalling that clozapine causes agranulocytosis will direct you to option 1. If you are unfamiliar with the adverse effects of this medication and the laboratory studies that need to be monitored, review this information.

Level of Cognitive Ability: Analysis
Client Needs: Physiological Integrity
Integrated Process: Nursing Process/Assessment
Content Area: Pharmacology

Reference:
Hodgson, B., & Kizior, R. (2004). *Saunders nursing drug handbook 2004.* Philadelphia: Saunders, p. 237.

112. A nurse is monitoring the function of a client's chest tube. The chest tube is attached to a Pleur-Evac drainage system. The nurse notes that the fluid in the water seal chamber is below the 2 cm mark. The nurse determines that:
1 Suction should be added to the system
2 There is a leak in the system
3 This is caused by client pneumothorax
4 Water should be added to the chamber

Answer: 4

Rationale: The water seal chamber should be filled to the 2 cm mark to provide an adequate water seal between the external environment and the client's pleural cavity. The water seal prevents air from reentering the pleural cavity. Because evaporation of water can occur, the nurse should remedy this problem by adding water until the level is again at the 2 cm mark. The other interpretations are incorrect.

Test-Taking Strategy: Focus on the issue: that the water seal chamber is below the 2cm mark. Recalling that the chamber needs to be filled to the 2 cm mark will direct you to option 4. Review the principles associated with care of chest tubes if you had difficulty with this question.

Level of Cognitive Ability: Analysis
Client Needs: Physiological Integrity
Integrated Process: Nursing Process/Analysis
Content Area: Adult Health/Respiratory

References:
Black, J., & Hawks, J. (2005). *Medical-surgical nursing: Clinical management for positive outcomes* (7th ed.). Philadelphia: Saunders, pp. 1862-1863.
Lewis, S., Heitkemper, M., & Dirksen, S. (2004). *Medical-surgical nursing: Assessment and management of clinical problems* (6th ed.). St. Louis: Mosby, pp. 623-624.

113. A client has decided to use a transcutaneous electrical nerve stimulation (TENS) as prescribed by the physician for the relief of chronic pain, and the nurse has provided instructions to the client regarding the TENS unit. Which statement by the client would indicate a need for further instructions regarding this pain relief measure?
1 "I am not sure that I am going to like those electrodes attached to my skin."
2 "I am not real happy that I have to stay in the hospital for this treatment."
3 "This unit will eliminate the need for taking so many pain medications."
4 "I understand that this will help relieve the pain."

Answer: 2

Rationale: The TENS unit is a portable unit, and the client controls the system for relieving pain and reducing the need for analgesics. It is attached to the skin of the body by electrodes. It is not necessary that the client remain in the hospital for this treatment.

Test-Taking Strategy: Note the words "need for further instructions." These words indicate a false-response question and that you need to select the incorrect client statement. Options 3 and 4 can be eliminated first because they are similar. From the remaining options, select option 2, because it would not be a very cost-effective pain management technique if the client required hospitalization. Review the principles related to the TENS unit if you had difficulty with this question.

Level of Cognitive Ability: Analysis
Client Needs: Physiological Integrity
Integrated Process: Teaching/Learning
Content Area: Pharmacology

Reference:
Phipps, W., Monahan, F., Sands, J., Marek, J., & Neighbors, M. (2003). *Medical-surgical nursing: Health and illness perspectives* (7th ed.). St. Louis: Mosby, p. 224.

114. A client with chronic renal failure has a protein restriction in the diet. The nurse would include in a teaching plan to avoid which of the following sources of incomplete protein in the diet?
1 Nuts
2 Eggs
3 Milk
4 Fish

Answer: 1
Rationale: The client whose diet has a protein restriction should be careful to ensure that the proteins eaten are complete proteins with the highest biologic value. Foods such as meat, fish, milk, and eggs are complete proteins, which are optimal for the client with chronic renal failure.

Test-Taking Strategy: Focus on the issue: protein composition of various foods. Eliminate options 2 and 3 first because they are similar and are dairy products. From the remaining options, note the key words "avoid" and "incomplete protein" to direct you to option 1. Review foods that are complete and incomplete proteins if you had difficulty with this question.

Level of Cognitive Ability: Application
Client Needs: Health Promotion and Maintenance
Integrated Process: Teaching/Learning
Content Area: Adult Health/Renal

References:
Lewis, S., Heitkemper, M., & Dirksen, S. (2004). *Medical-surgical nursing: Assessment and management of clinical problems* (6th ed.). St. Louis: Mosby, p. 1223.
Peckenpaugh, N. (2003). *Nutrition essentials and diet therapy* (9th ed.). Philadelphia: Saunders, p. 295.

115. A newborn infant is diagnosed with imperforate anus. The nurse plans care, knowing that which of the following most appropriately describes a characteristic of this disorder?
1 Incomplete development of the anus
2 Invagination of a section of the intestine into the distal bowel
3 The infrequent and difficult passage of dry stools
4 The presence of fecal incontinence

Answer: 1
Rationale: Imperforate anus (anal atresia, anal agenesis) is the incomplete development or absence of the anus in its normal position in the perineum. Option 2 describes intussusception. Option 3 describes constipation. Option 4 describes encopresis. Constipation can affect any child at any time, although it peaks at age 2 to 3 years. Encopresis generally affects preschool and school-aged children.

Test-Taking Strategy: Use the process of elimination. Noting the relationship between the disorder "imperforate anus" and "incomplete development of the anus" in option 1 should direct you to this option. Review this disorder if you had difficulty with this question.

Level of Cognitive Ability: Application
Client Needs: Physiological Integrity
Integrated Process: Nursing Process/Planning
Content Area: Maternity/Postpartum

Reference:
Wong, D., & Hockenberry, M. (2003). *Wong's nursing care of infants and children* (7th ed.). St. Louis: Mosby, p. 466; 469.

116. A nurse is providing bottle-feeding instructions to the mother of a newborn infant. The nurse provides instructions regarding the amount of formula to be given, knowing that the stomach capacity for a newborn infant is approximately:

1 5 to 10 mL
2 10 to 20 mL
3 30 to 90 mL
4 75 to 100 mL

Answer: 2

Rationale: The stomach capacity of a newborn infant is approximately 10 to 20 mL. It is 30 to 90 mL for a 1-week-old infant, and 75 to 100 mL for a 2- to 3-week-old infant.

Test-Taking Strategy: Use the process of elimination. Note the key words "newborn infant." This should assist in eliminating options 3 and 4. From the remaining options, visualize the amounts in options 1 and 2. Noting that 5 mL is a very small amount should assist in directing you to option 2. Review these pediatric differences if you had difficulty with this question.

Level of Cognitive Ability: Application
Client Needs: Health Promotion and Maintenance
Integrated Process: Teaching/Learning
Content Area: Maternity/Postpartum

References:
Lowdermilk, D., & Perry, A. (2004). *Maternity & women's health care* (8th ed.). St. Louis: Mosby, p. 689.
Murray, S., McKinney, E., & Gorrie, T. (2002). *Foundations of maternal-newborn nursing* (3rd ed.). Philadelphia: Saunders, p. 493.

---

117. A mother who is breastfeeding her newborn infant is experiencing nipple soreness, and the nurse provides instructions regarding measures to relieve the soreness. Which statement by the mother indicates an understanding of the instructions?

1 "I need to avoid rotating breastfeeding positions so that the nipple will toughen."
2 "I need to stop nursing during the period of nipple soreness to allow the nipples to heal."
3 "I need to nurse less frequently and substitute a bottle feeding until the nipples become less sore."
4 "I need to position my infant with her ear, shoulder, and hip in straight alignment and place her stomach against me."

Answer: 4

Rationale: Comfort measures for nipple soreness include positioning the infant with the ear, shoulder, and hip in straight alignment and with the infant's stomach against the mother's. Additional measures include rotating breastfeeding positions; breaking suction with the little finger; nursing frequently; beginning feeding on the less sore nipple; not allowing the infant to chew on the nipple or to sleep holding the nipple in the mouth; and applying tea bags soaked in warm water to the nipple. Options 1, 2, and 3 are incorrect.

Test-Taking Strategy: Use the process of elimination, focusing on the key words "indicates an understanding." Visualize each of the options in terms of how they may or may not lessen the nipple soreness to direct you to option 4. Review these measures if you had difficulty answering the question.

Level of Cognitive Ability: Analysis
Client Needs: Health Promotion and Maintenance
Integrated Process: Teaching/Learning
Content Area: Maternity/Postpartum

Reference:
Lowdermilk, D., & Perry, A. (2004). *Maternity & women's health care* (8th ed.). St. Louis: Mosby, p. 778.

118. A client with acute myocardial infarction receives therapy with alteplase recombinant, or tissue plasminogen activator (t-PA), and the nurse monitors the client for complications of this treatment. Which finding would indicate a possible complication?

1 Epistaxis
2 Vomiting
3 ECG changes
4 Absent pedal pulses

Answer: 1
Rationale: Bleeding is a major side effect of t-PA therapy. The bleeding can be superficial or internal and can be spontaneous. Options 2, 3, and 4 are not side or adverse effects of t-PA therapy.

Test-Taking Strategy: Use the process of elimination. Recalling that this medication is a thrombolytic and that epistaxis is a bloody nose will direct you to option 1. Review the side and adverse effects of t-PA if you had difficulty with this question.

Level of Cognitive Ability: Analysis
Client Needs: Physiological Integrity
Integrated Process: Nursing Process/Analysis
Content Area: Pharmacology

Reference:
Hodgson, B., & Kizior, R. (2004). *Saunders nursing drug handbook 2004.* Philadelphia: Saunders, p. 33.

---

119. A nurse is performing an assessment on a mother who just delivered a healthy newborn infant. The nurse checks the uterine fundus, expecting to note that the fundus is positioned:

1 At the level of the umbilicus
2 Above the level of the umbilicus
3 One fingerbreadth above the symphysis pubis
4 To the right of the abdomen

Answer: 1
Rationale: Immediately after delivery, the uterine fundus should be at the level of the umbilicus or one to three fingerbreadths below it and in the midline of the abdomen. If the fundus is above the umbilicus, this may indicate that blood clots in the uterus need to be expelled by fundal massage. A fundus that is not located in the midline may indicate a full bladder.

Test-Taking Strategy: Use the process of elimination, noting the key words "just delivered." Use knowledge regarding normal anatomy and visualize each description in the options to direct you to option 1. Review normal post-delivery findings if you had difficulty with this question.

Level of Cognitive Ability: Analysis
Client Needs: Physiological Integrity
Integrated Process: Nursing Process/Assessment
Content Area: Maternity/Postpartum

Reference:
Lowdermilk, D., & Perry, A. (2004). *Maternity & women's health care* (8th ed.). St. Louis: Mosby, p. 619.

---

120. A nurse obtains the vital signs on a mother who delivered a healthy newborn infant 2 hours ago and notes that the mother's temperature is 102°F. The most appropriate nursing action would be to:

1 Document the finding and recheck the temperature in 4 hours
2 Notify the physician
3 Administer acetaminophen (Tylenol) and recheck the temperature in 4 hours
4 Remove the blanket from the client's bed

Answer: 2
Rationale: Vital signs return to normal within the first hour postpartum if no complications arise. If the temperature is greater than 2°F above normal, this may indicate infection, and the physician should be notified. Options 1, 3, and 4 are inaccurate nursing interventions for a temperature of 102°F 2 hours following delivery.

Test-Taking Strategy: Note that the mother delivered 2 hours ago. Use the process of elimination and think about the normal postpartum findings. It is most appropriate in this situation to report the findings because a temperature of 102° F can indicate infection. Review normal vital signs following delivery and the appropriate nursing interventions if the vital signs are not within the normal range.

Level of Cognitive Ability: Application
Client Needs: Physiological Integrity
Integrated Process: Nursing Process/Implementation
Content Area: Maternity/Postpartum

References:
Lowdermilk, D., & Perry, A. (2004). *Maternity & women's health care* (8th ed.). St. Louis: Mosby, p. 1046.
Murray, S., McKinney, E., & Gorrie, T. (2002). *Foundations of maternal-newborn nursing* (3rd ed.). Philadelphia: Saunders, pp. 440-441.

---

121. A nurse in the postpartum unit is caring for a mother following vaginal delivery of a healthy newborn infant. The client received epidural anesthesia for the delivery. One-half hour after admission to the postpartum unit, the nurse checks the client and suspects the presence of a vaginal hematoma. Which finding would be the best indicator of the presence of this type of hematoma?
1 Client complaints of a tearing sensation
2 Client complaints of intense vaginal pressure
3 Changes in vital signs
4 Signs of vaginal bruising

Answer: 3
Rationale: Changes in vital signs indicate hypovolemia in the anesthetized postpartum woman with a vaginal hematoma. Because the client received anesthesia, she would not feel pain or pressure. Vaginal bruising may be present, but this may be a result of the delivery process and additionally is not the best indicator of the presence of a hematoma.

Test-Taking Strategy: Focus on the data presented in the question. Noting that the client received an epidural anesthetic will assist in eliminating options 1 and 2. From the remaining options, recalling the pathophysiology associated with the development of a hematoma and use of the ABCs—airway, breathing, and circulation—will direct you to option 3. Review the signs of a vaginal hematoma if you had difficulty with this question.

Level of Cognitive Ability: Analysis
Client Needs: Physiological Integrity
Integrated Process: Nursing Process/Assessment
Content Area: Maternity/Postpartum

Reference:
Lowdermilk, D., & Perry, A. (2004). *Maternity & women's health care* (8th ed.). St. Louis: Mosby, pp. 1039; 1042.

---

122. A client with acute renal failure has an elevated blood urea nitrogen (BUN). The client is experiencing difficulty remembering information due to uremia. The nurse avoids which of the following when communicating with this client?
1 Include the family in discussions related to care
2 Give thorough, lengthy explanations of procedures
3 Give simple, clear directions
4 Explain treatments using understandable language

Answer: 2
Rationale: The client with acute renal failure may have difficulty remembering information and instructions because of anxiety and the increased level of the BUN. The nurse should avoid giving lengthy explanations about procedures because this information may not be remembered by the client and could increase client anxiety. Communications should be clear, simple, and understandable. The family should be included whenever possible.

Test-Taking Strategy: Use the process of elimination and note the key word "avoids." Use knowledge of the basic principles of effective communication to eliminate each of the incorrect options. Review basic communication techniques if you had difficulty with this question.

Level of Cognitive Ability: Application
Client Needs: Psychosocial Integrity
Integrated Process: Communication and Documentation
Content Area: Adult Health/Renal

Reference:
Black, J., & Hawks, J. (2005). *Medical-surgical nursing: Clinical management for positive outcomes* (7th ed.). Philadelphia: Saunders, pp. 941; 948.

---

123. A nurse in the newborn nursery receives a telephone call from the delivery room and is told that a post-term small for gestational age (SGA) newborn will be admitted to the nursery. The nurse develops a plan of care for the newborn and documents that the priority nursing action is to monitor:
1 Urinary output
2 Total bilirubin levels
3 Blood glucose levels
4 Hemoglobin and hematocrit

Answer: 3
Rationale: The most common metabolic complication in the SGA newborn is hypoglycemia, which can produce central nervous system abnormalities and mental retardation if not corrected immediately. Urinary output, although important, is not the highest priority action because the post-term SGA newborn is typically dehydrated from placental dysfunction. Hemoglobin and hematocrit levels are monitored because the post-term SGA newborn exhibits polycythemia, although this also does not require immediate attention. The polycythemia contributes to increased bilirubin levels, usually beginning on the second day after delivery.

Test-Taking Strategy: Note the key words "priority nursing action." Recalling that the most common metabolic complication in the SGA newborn is hypoglycemia will direct you to option 3. Review the SGA newborn content if you had difficulty with this question.

Level of Cognitive Ability: Application
Client Needs: Physiological Integrity
Integrated Process: Nursing Process/Planning
Content Area: Maternity/Postpartum

References:
Lowdermilk, D., & Perry, A. (2004). *Maternity & women's health care* (8th ed.). St. Louis: Mosby, pp. 1141-1142.
Murray, S., McKinney, E., & Gorrie, T. (2002). *Foundations of maternal-newborn nursing* (3rd ed.). Philadelphia: Saunders, p. 835.

---

124. A nurse in the postpartum unit reviews a client's record and notes that a new mother was administered methylergonovine (Methergine) intramuscularly following delivery. The nurse determines that this medication was administered to:
1 Decrease uterine contractions
2 Maintain a normal blood pressure
3 Prevent postpartum hemorrhage
4 Reduce the amount of lochia drainage

Answer: 3
Rationale: Methylergonovine, an oxytocic, is an agent used to prevent or control postpartum hemorrhage by contracting the uterus. The first dose is usually administered intramuscularly, and then if it needs to be continued, it is given by mouth. It increases the strength and frequency of contractions and may elevate blood pressure. There is no relationship between the action of this medication and lochial drainage.

Test-Taking Strategy: Use the process of elimination, focus on the medication name, and note the client is postpartum. Recalling that this medication is an oxytocic agent will direct you to option 3. Review its action and use if you are unfamiliar with this medication.

Level of Cognitive Ability: Analysis
Client's Needs: Physiological Integrity

Integrated Process: Nursing Process/Analysis
Content Area: Pharmacology

Reference:
Hodgson, B., & Kizior, R. (2004). *Saunders nursing drug handbook 2004.* Philadelphia: Saunders, p. 654.

---

125. A nurse in the newborn nursery receives a telephone call and is informed that a newborn infant with Apgar scores of 1 and 4 will be brought to the nursery. The nurse quickly prepares for the arrival of the newborn and determines that the priority intervention is to:

1 Connect the resuscitation bag to the oxygen
2 Turn on the apnea and cardiorespiratory monitor
3 Prepare for the insertion of an intravenous line with 5% dextrose in water
4 Set up the radiant warmer control temperature at 36.5°C (97.6°F)

Answer: 1

Rationale: The priority action for a newborn infant with low Apgar scores is airway, which would involve preparing respiratory resuscitation equipment. Options 2, 3, and 4 are also important, although they are of lower priority. Setting up an IV with 5% dextrose in water would provide circulatory support. The radiant warmer will provide an external heat source, which is necessary to prevent further respiratory distress. The newborn infant's cardiopulmonary status would be monitored by a cardiorespiratory monitoring device.

Test-Taking Strategy: Note the key words "priority intervention." This question asks you to prioritize care planning based on information about a newborn infant's condition. Use the ABCs—airway, breathing, circulation to direct you to option 1. Although options 2, 3, and 4 are a component of the plan of care, option 1 is the priority. Review care of the newborn infant with a low Apgar score if you had difficulty with this question.

Level of Cognitive Ability: Application
Client Needs: Physiological Integrity
Integrated Process: Nursing Process/Implementation
Content Area: Delegating/Prioritizing

Reference:
Murray, S., McKinney, E., & Gorrie, T. (2002). *Foundations of maternal-newborn nursing* (3rd ed.). Philadelphia: Saunders, p. 324.

---

126. A nurse is caring for a client in labor who has butorphanol tartrate (Stadol) prescribed for the relief of labor pain. During the administration of the medication, the nurse would ensure that which priority item was readily available?

1 An intravenous form of an antiemetic
2 Naloxone (Narcan)
3 An intravenous (IV) solution of normal saline
4 Meperidine hydrochloride (Demerol)

Answer: 2

Rationale: Butorphanol tartrate is an opioid analgesic that provides systemic pain relief during labor. The nurse would ensure that naloxone and resuscitation equipment are readily available to treat respiratory depression, should it occur. Although an antiemetic may be prescribed for vomiting, antiemetics may enhance the respiratory depressant effects of the butorphanol tartrate. Although an IV access is desirable, the administration of normal saline is unrelated to the administration of this medication. Meperidine hydrochloride is also an opioid analgesic that may be used for pain relief, but it also causes respiratory depression.

Test-Taking Strategy: Use the process of elimination, focusing on the key words "readily available" in the question. Recalling that butorphanol tartrate causes respiratory depression will direct you to option 2. Review this medication and its use during labor if you had difficulty with this question.

Level of Cognitive Ability: Application
Client Needs: Physiological Integrity
Integrated Process: Nursing Process/Planning
Content Area: Maternity/Intrapartum

Reference:
Murray, S., McKinney, E., & Gorrie, T. (2002). *Foundations of maternal-newborn nursing* (3rd ed.). Philadelphia: Saunders, pp. 374-376.

---

127. Methylergonovine (Methergine) is prescribed for a woman who has just delivered a healthy newborn infant. The priority assessment before administering the medication is to check the client's:

1 Lochia
2 Blood pressure
3 Deep tendon reflexes
4 Uterine tone

Answer: 2
Rationale: Methergine, an oxytocic, is an agent used to prevent or control postpartum hemorrhage by contracting the uterus. The immediate dose is administered intramuscularly, and then if still needed, it is administered orally. It causes constant uterine contractions and may elevate the blood pressure. A priority assessment before administration of methylergonovine is blood pressure. Methylergonovine is to be administered cautiously in the presence of hypertension, and the physician should be notified if hypertension is present. Options 1 and 4 are general components of care in the postpartum period. Option 3 is most specifically related to the administration of magnesium sulfate.

Test-Taking Strategy: Use the process of elimination. Options 1 and 4 can be eliminated first because lochia and uterine tone are similar and are general assessments related to the postpartum period. Next, note the key word "priority" and use the ABCs—airway, breathing, circulation—to direct you to option 2. Blood pressure is a method of assessing circulation. Additionally, option 3 can be eliminated because it most specifically relates to the administration of magnesium sulfate. Review the nursing responsibilities related to the administration of methylergonovine if you had difficulty with this question.

Level of Cognitive Ability: Application
Client's Needs: Physiological Integrity
Integrated Process: Nursing Process/Assessment
Content Area: Maternity/Postpartum

Reference:
Lowdermilk, D., & Perry, A. (2004). *Maternity & women's health care* (8th ed.). St. Louis: Mosby, p. 1040.

---

128. A nurse reinforces instructions to a client who is taking allopurinol (Zyloprim) for the treatment of gout. Which statement by the client indicates an understanding of the medication?

1 "I can use an antihistamine lotion if I get a rash that is itchy."
2 "I need to drink at least eight glasses of fluid every day."
3 "I need to take the medication two hours after I eat."
4 "I should put ice on my lips if they swell."

Answer: 2
Rationale: Clients taking allopurinol are encouraged to drink 3000 mL of fluid a day. Allopurinol is to be given with or immediately following meals or milk. If the client develops a rash, irritation of the eyes, or swelling of the lips or mouth, he or she should contact the physician because this may indicate hypersensitivity.

Test-Taking Strategy: Use the process of elimination, noting the key words "indicates an understanding." Options 1 and 4 can be eliminated first because they indicate a hypersensitivity, which is not a normal expected response. From the remaining options, recalling that the medication should be taken with food or milk will direct you to option 2. Review client instructions related to allopurinol if you had difficulty with this question.

Level of Cognitive Ability: Analysis
Client Needs: Health Promotion and Maintenance
Integrated Process: Teaching/Learning
Content Area: Pharmacology

Reference:
Hodgson, B., & Kizior, R. (2004). *Saunders nursing drug handbook 2004.* Philadelphia: Saunders, p. 25.

---

129. A rubella vaccine is administered to a client who delivered a healthy newborn infant 2 days ago. The nurse provides instructions to the client regarding the potential risks associated with this vaccination. Which statement by the client indicates an understanding of the medication?

1 "I need to stay out of the sunlight for 3 days."
2 "The injection site may itch, but I can scratch it if I need to."
3 "I need to prevent becoming pregnant for 2 to 3 months after the vaccination."
4 "I need to avoid sexual intercourse for 2 to 3 months after the vaccination."

Answer: 3
Rationale: Rubella vaccine is a live attenuated virus that evokes an antibody response and provides immunity for approximately 15 years. Because rubella is a live vaccine, it will act as the virus and is potentially teratogenic in the organogenesis phase of fetal development. The client needs to be informed about the potential effects this vaccine may have and the need to avoid becoming pregnant for a period of 2 to 3 months afterward. Abstinence from sexual intercourse is not necessary, unless another form of effective contraception is not being used. The vaccine may cause local or systemic reactions, but all are mild and short-lived. Sunlight has no effect on the person who is vaccinated.

Test-Taking Strategy: Use the process of elimination, recalling the effect of live vaccines on pregnancy and fetal development. Remembering that viruses can cross the placental barrier will direct you to option 3. Review the potential risks associated with the administration of this vaccine if you had difficulty with this question.

Level of Cognitive Ability: Analysis
Client Needs: Physiological Integrity
Integrated Process: Teaching/Learning
Content Area: Maternity/Postpartum

References:
Lowdermilk, D., & Perry, A. (2004). *Maternity & women's health care* (8th ed.). St. Louis: Mosby, p. 636.
McKenry, L., & Salerno, E. (2003). *Mosby's pharmacology in nursing* (21st ed.). St. Louis: Mosby, p. 1090.

---

130. A school nurse is planning to give a class on testicular self-examination (TSE) at a local high school. The nurse plans to include which instruction on a written handout to be given to the students?

1 Roll the testicle between the thumb and forefinger
2 Perform the self-examination every other month
3 Perform the self-examination after a cold shower
4 Expect the self-examination to be slightly painful

Answer: 1
Rationale: Testicular self-examination is a self-screening examination for testicular cancer, which predominantly affects men in their late teens and twenties. The self-examination is performed once a month, as is breast-self examination. As an aid to remember to do it, the examination should be done on the same day each month. The scrotum is held in one hand and the testicle is rolled between the thumb and forefinger of the other hand. The self-examination should not be painful. It is easiest to do either during or after a warm shower (or bath) when the scrotum is relaxed.

Test-Taking Strategy: Focus on the issue, self-examination, and read each option carefully. Knowledge of physical examination techniques will direct you to option 1. Review this content if you are unfamiliar with the procedure for TSE.

Level of Cognitive Ability: Application
Client Needs: Health Promotion and Maintenance
Integrated Process: Teaching/Learning
Content Area: Adult Health/Oncology

Reference:
Black, J., & Hawks, J. (2005). *Medical-surgical nursing: Clinical management for positive outcomes* (7th ed.). Philadelphia: Saunders, p. 1005.

---

131. A 32-year-old female client has a history of fibrocystic disorder of the breasts. The nurse determines that the client understands the nature of the disorder if the client states that symptoms are more likely to occur:
1 Before menses
2 After menses
3 In the spring months
4 In the winter months

Answer: 1
Rationale: The client with fibrocystic breast disorder experiences worsening of symptoms (breast lumps, painful breasts, and possible nipple discharge) before the onset of menses. This is associated with cyclical hormone changes. Clients should understand that this is part of the clinical picture of this disorder. Options 2, 3, and 4 are incorrect.

Test-Taking Strategy: Note the key words "more likely." This implies that there is a predictable variation in symptoms. Focus on the disorder and use knowledge of the effects of the various hormonal changes that occur in the body to direct you to option 1. Review the cyclical hormonal changes that occur in the female and the characteristics of fibrocystic disorder of the breasts if you had difficulty with this question.

Level of Cognitive Ability: Analysis
Client Needs: Physiological Integrity
Integrated Process: Teaching/Learning
Content Area: Adult Health/Oncology

References:
Black, J., & Hawks, J. (2005). *Medical-surgical nursing: Clinical management for positive outcomes* (7th ed.). Philadelphia: Saunders, p. 1120.
Ignatavicius, D., & Workman, M. (2002). *Medical surgical nursing: Critical thinking for collaborative care* (4th ed.). Philadelphia: Saunders, p. 1735.
Lewis, S., Heitkemper, M., & Dirksen, S. (2004). *Medical-surgical nursing: Assessment and management of clinical problems* (6th ed.). St. Louis: Mosby, p. 1364.

---

132. A client has received a dose of dimenhydrinate (Dramamine). The nurse determines that the medication is effective if the client obtains relief of:
1 Nausea and vomiting
2 Ringing in the ears
3 Headache
4 Chills

Answer: 1
Rationale: Dimenhydrinate is used to treat and prevent the symptoms of dizziness, vertigo, and nausea and vomiting that accompany motion sickness. The other options are incorrect.

Test-Taking Strategy: Focus on the issue: medication effectiveness. Recalling that this medication is used to treat motion sickness will direct you to option 1. Review its action and uses if this medication is unfamiliar to you.

Level of Cognitive Ability: Analysis
Client Needs: Physiological Integrity
Integrated Process: Nursing Process/Evaluation
Content Area: Pharmacology

References:
Lehne, R. (2004). *Pharmacology for nursing care.* (5th ed). Philadelphia: Saunders, p. 842.
McKenry, L., & Salerno, E. (2003). *Mosby's pharmacology in nursing* (21st ed.). St. Louis: Mosby, p. 759.

---

133. A client is preparing for discharge 10 days after a radical vulvectomy. The nurse determines that the client has the best understanding of the measures to prevent complications if the client plans to do which of the following after discharge?
   1 Sit in a chair all day
   2 Drive a car
   3 Housework
   4 Walking

Answer: 4
Rationale: The client should resume activity slowly, and walking is a beneficial activity. The client should know to rest when fatigue occurs. Activities to be avoided include driving, heavy housework, wearing tight clothing, crossing the legs, and prolonged standing or sitting. Sexual activity is usually prohibited for 4 to 6 weeks after surgery.

Test-Taking Strategy: Note the key words "to prevent complications." With this in mind, evaluate each of the options in terms of the stress or harm it could cause to the perineal area. This will direct you to option 4. Review teaching points for the client following radical vulvectomy if you had difficulty with this question.

Level of Cognitive Ability: Analysis
Client Needs: Physiological Integrity
Integrated Process: Teaching/Learning
Content Area: Adult Health/Oncology

Reference:
Black, J., & Hawks, J. (2005). *Medical-surgical nursing: Clinical management for positive outcomes* (7th ed.). Philadelphia: Saunders, pp. 1086-1087.

---

134. A nurse is caring for the client with silicosis who has massive pulmonary fibrosis. The nurse monitors the client for emotional reactions related to the chronic respiratory disease. Which emotional reaction if expressed by the client would indicate a need for immediate intervention?
   1 Anxiety
   2 Ineffective coping
   3 Depression
   4 Suicidal ideation

Answer: 4
Rationale: Common emotional reactions to a disease such as massive pulmonary fibrosis may be the same as for chronic airflow limitation and include anxiety, ineffective coping, and depression. Suicidal ideation is not a normal emotional reaction with this condition. If it is expressed, it warrants immediate intervention.

Test-Taking Strategy: Use the process of elimination. Noting the key words "need for immediate intervention" will direct you to option 4. Review the common emotional reactions that occur in chronic diseases and nursing interventions if suicidal ideation is expressed by the client if you had difficulty with this question.

Level of Cognitive Ability: Analysis
Client Needs: Psychosocial Integrity
Integrated Process: Nursing Process/Analysis
Content Area: Adult Health/Respiratory

Reference:
Ignatavicius, D., & Workman, M. (2002). *Medical surgical nursing: Critical thinking for collaborative care* (4th ed.). Philadelphia: Saunders, p. 134.

135. At the beginning of the work shift, a nurse is checking a client who has returned from the post-anesthesia care unit following transurethral resection of the prostate (TURP). The client has a bladder irrigation running via a three-way Foley catheter. The nurse would notify the physician if which color of the urine were noted in the urinary drainage bag?
1 Pale pink
2 Dark pink
3 Bright red
4 Tea-colored

Answer: 3
Rationale: Bright red bleeding should be reported, because it could indicate complications related to active bleeding. If the bladder irrigation is infusing at a sufficient rate, the urinary drainage will be pale pink. A dark pink color (sometimes referred to as punch-colored) indicates that the speed of the irrigation should be increased. Tea-colored urine is not seen after TURP, but may be noted in the client with renal failure or other renal disorders.

Test-Taking Strategy: Use the process of elimination, recalling that hemorrhage is a complication following any surgical procedure. Remember also that the purpose of a bladder irrigation is to flush out blood and clots that could otherwise accumulate in the bladder following surgery. With this in mind, select option 3 because bright red drainage would indicate a potential complication such as bleeding. Review care of the client following TURP if you had difficulty with this question.

Level of Cognitive Ability: Analysis
Client Needs: Physiological Integrity
Integrated Process: Nursing Process/Analysis
Content Area: Adult Health/Renal

Reference:
Phipps, W., Monahan, F., Sands, J., Marek, J., & Neighbors, M. (2003). *Medical-surgical nursing: Health and illness perspectives* (7th ed.). St. Louis: Mosby, p. 1835.

136. Phenelzine sulfate (Nardil) is being administered to a client with depression. The client suddenly complains of a severe occipital headache radiating frontally, neck stiffness and soreness, and is vomiting. On further assessment, the client exhibits signs of hypertensive crisis. Which medication would the nurse prepare anticipating that it will be prescribed as the antidote for hypertensive crisis?
1 Phentolamine (Regitine)
2 Vitamin K
3 Protamine sulfate
4 Calcium gluconate

Answer: 1
Rationale: The manifestations of hypertensive crisis include hypertension, occipital headache radiating frontally, neck stiffness and soreness, nausea, vomiting, sweating, fever and chills, clammy skin, dilated pupils, and palpitations. Tachycardia and bradycardia and constricting chest pain may also be present. The antidote for hypertensive crisis is phentolamine (Regitine) and a dosage by intravenous injection is administered. Protamine sulfate is the antidote for heparin, and vitamin K is the antidote for warfarin (Coumadin) overdose. Calcium gluconate is used for magnesium overdose.

Test-Taking Strategy: Knowledge regarding the antidotes for various medications and disorders is required to answer this question. Review this content if you are unfamiliar with the antidotes associated with the use of certain medications and conditions.

Level of Cognitive Ability: Analysis
Client Needs: Physiological Integrity
Integrated Process: Nursing Process/Planning
Content Area: Pharmacology

Reference:
Hodgson, B., & Kizior, R. (2004). *Saunders nursing drug handbook 2004.* Philadelphia: Saunders, p. 801.

137. A nurse is caring for a 25-year-old single client who will undergo bilateral orchidectomy for testicular cancer. The nurse would make it a priority to explore which potential psychological concern with this client?
  1 Postoperative pain
  2 Postoperative swelling
  3 Length of recuperative period
  4 Loss of reproductive ability

Answer: 4
Rationale: Although the client will need factual information about the postoperative period and recuperation, the nurse would place priority on addressing loss of reproductive ability as a psychological concern. The radical effects of this surgery in the reproductive area make it likely that the client may have some difficulty in adjustment to this consequence of surgery.

Test-Taking Strategy: Use the process of elimination, focusing on the client's diagnosis and surgical procedure. Eliminate options 1, 2, and 3 because they are general concerns of any surgical procedure. Option 4 is specific to an orchidectomy. Review the psychosocial issues related to an orchidectomy if you had difficulty with this question.

Level of Cognitive Ability: Application
Client Needs: Psychosocial Integrity
Integrated Process: Caring
Content Area: Adult Health/Oncology

Reference:
Phipps, W., Monahan, F., Sands, J., Marek, J., & Neighbors, M. (2003). *Medical-surgical nursing: Health and illness perspectives* (7th ed.). St. Louis: Mosby, p. 1829.

138. A nurse is assisting in participating in a prostate screening clinic for men. The nurse questions each client about which sign of prostatism?
  1 Excessive force in urinary stream
  2 Hesitancy when initiating urinary stream
  3 Ability to stop voiding quickly
  4 Absence of post-void dribbling

Answer: 2
Rationale: Signs of prostatism that may be reported to the nurse are reduced force and size of urinary stream, intermittent stream, hesitancy in beginning the flow of urine, inability to stop urinating quickly, a sensation of incomplete bladder emptying after voiding, and an increase in episodes of nocturia. These symptoms are the result of pressure of the enlarging prostate on the client's urethra.

Test-Taking Strategy: Use the process of elimination. Eliminate options 1, 3, and 4 because they are similar and indicate no difficulty with proper emptying of the bladder. Review the signs of prostatism if you had difficulty with this question.

Level of Cognitive Ability: Application
Client Needs: Health Promotion and Maintenance
Integrated Process: Nursing Process/Assessment
Content Area: Adult Health/Renal

Reference:
Black, J., & Hawks, J. (2005). *Medical-surgical nursing: Clinical management for positive outcomes* (7th ed.). Philadelphia: Saunders, p. 1016.

139. A male client being seen in the ambulatory care clinic has a history of being treated for syphilis infection. The nurse interprets that the client has been reinfected if which characteristic is noted in a penile lesion?
1 Multiple vesicles, with some that have ruptured
2 Papular areas and erythema
3 Cauliflower-like appearance
4 Induration and absence of pain

Answer: 4
Rationale: The characteristic lesion of syphilis is painless and indurated. The lesion is referred to as a chancre. Genital herpes is accompanied by the presence of one or more vesicles that then rupture and heal. Scabies is characterized by erythematous, papular eruptions. Genital warts are characterized by cauliflower-like growths, or growths that are soft and fleshy.

Test-Taking Strategy: To answer this question accurately, it is necessary to be familiar with the characteristics of skin lesions of the various sexually transmitted diseases. Review the appearance of lesions associated with syphilis if you had difficulty with this question.

Level of Cognitive Ability: Analysis
Client Needs: Physiological Integrity
Integrated Process: Nursing Process/Assessment
Content Area: Adult Health/Integumentary

References:
Black, J., & Hawks, J. (2005). *Medical-surgical nursing: Clinical management for positive outcomes* (7th ed.). Philadelphia: Saunders, p. 1133.
Phipps, W., Monahan, F., Sands, J., Marek, J., & Neighbors, M. (2003). *Medical-surgical nursing: Health and illness perspectives* (7th ed.). St. Louis: Mosby, p. 1864.

140. An adult client has been admitted to the hospital with a 3-day history of uncontrolled vomiting and diarrhea. The nurse assesses for which of the following in this client?
1 Tenting of the skin
2 Bradycardia
3 Hypertension
4 Excitability

Answer: 1
Rationale: The client described in the question will most likely be dehydrated. The nurse assesses this client for weight loss, lethargy or headache, sunken eyes, poor skin turgor (such as tenting), flat neck and peripheral veins, tachycardia, and low blood pressure.

Test-Taking Strategy: Use the process of elimination, focusing on the data in the question. Recalling that a client who has a 3-day episode of uncontrolled vomiting and diarrhea is at risk for dehydration will direct you to option 1. Review the signs of dehydration if you had difficulty with this question.

Level of Cognitive Ability: Analysis
Client Needs: Physiological Integrity
Integrated Process: Nursing Process/Assessment
Content Area: Adult Health/Gastrointestinal

Reference:
Black, J., & Hawks, J. (2005). *Medical-surgical nursing: Clinical management for positive outcomes* (7th ed.). Philadelphia: Saunders, p. 208.

141. An adult client with renal insufficiency has been placed on a fluid restriction of 1200 mL per day. The nurse discusses the fluid restriction with the dietician and then plans to allow the client to have how many mL of fluid from 7:00 AM to 3:00 PM?

1 1000
2 800
3 600
4 400

Answer: 3

Rationale: When a client is on a fluid restriction, the nurse informs the dietary department and discusses the allotment of fluid per shift with the dietician. When calculating how to distribute a fluid restriction, the nurse usually allows half of the daily allotment (600 mL) during the day shift, when the client eats two meals and takes most medications. Another two-fifths (480 mL) is allotted to the evening shift, with the balance (120 mL) allowed during the nighttime.

Test-Taking Strategy: To answer this question accurately, you must be familiar with fluid restriction and the general principles related to fluid distribution over a 24-hour period. Review these principles and calculation of fluid distribution in the client with renal insufficiency if you had difficulty with this question.

Level of Cognitive Ability: Application
Client Needs: Physiological Integrity
Integrated Process: Nursing Process/Planning
Content Area: Adult Health/Renal

Reference:
Ignatavicius, D., & Workman, M. (2002). *Medical surgical nursing: critical thinking for collaborative care* (4th ed.). Philadelphia: Saunders, pp. 148-150.

142. A client with chronic renal failure has learned about managing diet and fluid restriction between dialysis treatments. The nurse determines that the client is compliant with the therapeutic regime if the client gains no more than how much weight between hemodialysis treatments?

1 0.5 to 1 kg
2 1 to 1.5 kg
3 2 to 4 kg
4 5 to 6 kg

Answer: 2

Rationale: A limit of 1 to 1.5 kg of weight gain between dialysis treatments helps prevent hypotension that tends to occur during dialysis with the removal of larger fluid loads. The nurse determines that the client is compliant with fluid restriction if this weight gain is not exceeded.

Test-Taking Strategy: It may be helpful in answering this question to recall that 1 liter of fluid weighs approximately 1 kg. Recalling that there are approximately 6 liters of blood circulating in the body will assist in eliminating options 3 and 4 as being amounts that are too large. Correspondingly, option 1 is eliminated because the amount is too small, representing only 500 to 1000 mL of fluid. Review teaching points for the client with chronic renal failure if you had difficulty with this question.

Level of Cognitive Ability: Analysis
Client Needs: Health Promotion and Maintenance
Integrated Process: Nursing Process/Evaluation
Content Area: Adult Health/Renal

References:
Black, J., & Hawks, J. (2005). *Medical-surgical nursing: Clinical management for positive outcomes* (7th ed.). Philadelphia: Saunders, pp. 926; 964.
Ignatavicius, D., & Workman, M. (2002). *Medical surgical nursing: Critical thinking for collaborative care* (4th ed.). Philadelphia: Saunders, p. 1684.

143. A client was admitted to the surgical unit following right total knee replacement performed 2 hours earlier. Which observation by the nurse indicates the need to contact the surgeon?
1. Ability to flex and extend the right foot
2. Pain relieved by a narcotic analgesic
3. Pale pink and warm right foot
4. Hemovac wound suction drainage of 175 mL per hour

Answer: 4
Rationale: Following total knee replacement, the neurovascular status of the affected leg is assessed, and findings should be within normal limits. The client should have intact capillary refill and adequate color, temperature, sensation, and motion to the limb. Incisional pain should be relieved by narcotic analgesic administration. The knee incision may have a wound suction drain in place, which is expected to drain up to 200 mL in the first 8 hours after surgery. Drainage of 175 mL per hour is excessive and should be reported.

Test-Taking Strategy: Note the key words "need to contact the surgeon." Options 1 and 3 represent normal neurovascular status and are eliminated first. Knowing that surgery causes the client pain, which is then relieved by analgesics, will assist in eliminating option 2. This leaves option 4 as the correct option given the wording of this question. Review expected findings following a total knee replacement if you had difficulty with this question.

Level of Cognitive Ability: Analysis
Client Needs: Physiological Integrity
Integrated Process: Nursing Process/Assessment
Content Area: Adult Health/Musculoskeletal

References:
Black, J., & Hawks, J. (2005). *Medical-surgical nursing: Clinical management for positive outcomes* (7th ed.). Philadelphia: Saunders, pp. 595-596.
Phipps, W., Monahan, F., Sands, J., Marek, J., & Neighbors, M. (2003). *Medical-surgical nursing: Health and illness perspectives* (7th ed.). St. Louis: Mosby, pp. 423; 452.

144. A client is being discharged from the hospital following removal of chest tubes that were inserted following thoracic surgery. The nurse provides home care instructions to the client and determines the need for further instructions if the client states:
1. "I need to remove the chest tube site dressing as soon as I get home."
2. "I need to report any difficulty with breathing to the physician."
3. "I need to avoid heavy lifting for the first 4 to 6 weeks."
4. "I need to take my temperature to detect a possible infection."

Answer: 1
Rationale: Upon removal of a chest tube, a dressing is placed over the chest tube site. This is maintained in place until the physician says it may be removed. The client is taught to monitor and report any respiratory difficulty or increased temperature. The client should avoid heavy lifting for the first 4 to 6 weeks after discharge to facilitate continued wound healing.

Test-Taking Strategy: Use the process of elimination, noting the key words "need for further instructions." These words indicate a false-response question and that you need to select the incorrect client statement. Recalling that signs of infection and respiratory difficulty should be monitored and reported helps eliminate options 2 and 4 first. From the remaining options, recalling that either heavy lifting should be avoided postoperatively or that removal of the chest tube site dressing disturbs the occlusive seal to the site will direct you to option 1. Review teaching points following removal of a chest tube if you had difficulty with this question.

Level of Cognitive Ability: Analysis
Client Needs: Health Promotion and Maintenance
Integrated Process: Teaching/Learning
Content Area: Adult Health/Respiratory

References:
Lewis, S., Heitkemper, M., & Dirksen, S. (2004). *Medical-surgical nursing: Assessment and management of clinical problems* (6th ed.). St. Louis: Mosby, p. 625.
Phipps, W., Monahan, F., Sands, J., Marek, J., & Neighbors, M. (2003). *Medical-surgical nursing: Health and illness perspectives* (7th ed.). St. Louis: Mosby, p. 557.

145. A nurse is administering epoetin alfa (Epogen) to a client with chronic renal failure (CRF). The nurse monitors the client for which adverse effect of this therapy?
1 Anemia
2 Hypertension
3 Iron intoxication
4 Bleeding tendencies

Answer: 2
Rationale: The client taking epoetin alfa is at risk of hypertension and seizure activity as the most serious adverse effects of therapy. This medication is used to treat anemia. The medication does not cause iron intoxication. Bleeding tendencies is not an adverse effect of this medication.

Test-Taking Strategy: Knowledge regarding the adverse effects of this medication is needed to answer this question. Review this medication if you had difficulty with this question.

Level of Cognitive Ability: Analysis
Client Needs: Physiological Integrity
Integrated Process: Nursing Process/Assessment
Content Area: Adult Health/Renal

References:
Hodgson, B., & Kizior, R. (2004). *Saunders nursing drug handbook 2004.* Philadelphia: Saunders, p. 364.
McKenry, L., & Salerno, E. (2003). *Mosby's pharmacology in nursing* (21st ed.). St. Louis: Mosby, p. 695.

146. A client is taking lansoprazole (Prevacid) for the chronic management of Zollinger-Ellison syndrome. The nurse determines that the client best understands this disorder and the medication regime if the client states to take which of the following products for pain?
1 Naprosyn (Aleve)
2 Acetylsalicylic acid (aspirin)
3 Acetaminophen (Tylenol)
4 Ibuprofen (Motrin)

Answer: 3
Rationale: Zollinger-Ellison syndrome is a hypersecretory condition of the stomach. The client should avoid taking medications that are irritating to the stomach lining. Irritants would include aspirin and nonsteroidal antiinflammatory medications (naprosyn and ibuprofen). The client should take acetaminophen for pain relief.

Test-Taking Strategy: Use the process of elimination. Eliminate options 1 and 4 first because they are both nonsteroidal antiinflammatory medications. From the remaining options, select acetaminophen over aspirin because it is least irritating to the stomach. Review these medications if you had difficulty with this question.

Level of Cognitive Ability: Analysis
Client Needs: Physiological Integrity
Integrated Process: Nursing Process/Evaluation
Content Area: Pharmacology

Reference:
Lehne, R. (2004). *Pharmacology for nursing care.* (5th ed). Philadelphia: Saunders, p. 823; 831.

147. The client scheduled for a transurethral prostatectomy (TURP) has listened to the surgeon's explanation of the surgery. The client later asks the nurse to explain again how the prostate is going to be removed. The nurse tells the client that the prostate will be removed through:
1 The urethra using a cutting wire
2 An incision made in the perineal area
3 An upper abdominal incision
4 A lower abdominal incision

Answer: 1
Rationale: A TURP is done through the urethra. An instrument called a resectoscope is used to cut the tissue using high-frequency current. An incision between the scrotum and anus is made when a perineal prostatectomy is performed. A lower abdominal incision is used for suprapubic or retropubic prostatectomy. An upper abdominal incision is not used.

Test-Taking Strategy: Use the process of elimination. Note the relationship between the name of the procedure "transurethral" in the question and the word "urethra" in the correct option. Review this procedure if you had difficulty with this question.

Level of Cognitive Ability: Application
Client Needs: Physiological Integrity
Integrated Process: Teaching/Learning
Content Area: Adult Health/Renal

Reference:
Phipps, W., Monahan, F., Sands, J., Marek, J., & Neighbors, M. (2003). *Medical-surgical nursing: Health and illness perspectives* (7th ed.). St. Louis: Mosby, pp. 1832-1833.

---

148. A client scheduled for a bone marrow aspiration asks the nurse about possible sites that could be used to perform the procedure. The nurse tells the client that, in addition to the iliac crest, the test may be done in which of the following areas?
1 Femur
2 Sternum
3 Scapula
4 Ribs

Answer: 2
Rationale: The most common sites for bone marrow aspiration in the adult are the iliac crest and the sternum. These areas are rich in bone marrow and are easily accessible for testing. The femur, scapula, and ribs are not sites for bone marrow aspiration.

Test-Taking Strategy: Focus on the issue: a bone marrow aspiration. Recalling the anatomy and physiology related to the bones and bone marrow will direct you to option 2. Review the procedure for a bone marrow aspiration if you had difficulty with this question.

Level of Cognitive Ability: Application
Client Needs: Physiological Integrity
Integrated Process: Nursing Process/Implementation
Content Area: Fundamental Skills

Reference:
Chernecky, C., & Berger, B. (2004). *Laboratory tests and diagnostic procedures* (4th ed.). Philadelphia: Saunders, p. 279.

---

149. A client is taking amiloride (Midamor) 10 mg orally daily for the treatment of hypertension. The nurse gives the client which instruction regarding its use?
1 Take the medication in the morning with breakfast
2 Take the medication 2 hours after lunch on an empty stomach
3 Eat foods with extra sodium while taking this medication
4 Withhold the medication if the blood pressure is high

Answer: 1
Rationale: Amiloride is a potassium-sparing diuretic used to treat edema or hypertension. A daily dose should be taken in the morning to avoid nocturia. The dose should be taken with food to increase bioavailability. Sodium should be restricted if used as an antihypertensive. Increased blood pressure is not a reason to hold the medication, and it may be an indication for its use.

Test-Taking Strategy: Use the process of elimination. Noting the client's diagnosis and recalling that this medication is a potassium-sparing diuretic will direct you to option 1. Review client teaching points related to this medication if you had difficulty with this question.

Level of Cognitive Ability: Application
Client Needs: Health Promotion and Maintenance
Integrated Process: Teaching/Learning
Content Area: Pharmacology

Reference:
Lehne, R. (2004). *Pharmacology for nursing care.* (5th ed). Philadelphia: Saunders, pp. 408-409.

---

150. A nurse is preparing a poster for a booth at a health fair to promote primary prevention of cervical cancer. The nurse includes which recommendation on the poster?
1 Perform monthly breast-self examination (BSE)
2 Use oral contraceptives as a preferred method of birth control
3 Use a commercial douche on a daily basis
4 Seek treatment promptly for infections of the cervix

Answer: 4
Rationale: Early treatment of cervical infection can help prevent chronic cervicitis, which can lead to dysplasia of the cervix. Cervical dysplasia is an early cell change that is considered to be premalignant. Oral contraceptives and douches do not decrease the risk for this type of cancer. BSE is useful for early detection of breast cancer, but is unrelated to cervical cancer.

Test-Taking Strategy: Note the key words "primary prevention" and "cervical cancer." Eliminate option 1 because it is unrelated to cervical cancer. From the remaining options, recalling the risk factors associated with this type of cancer will direct you to option 4. Review the risk factors associated with cervical cancer if you had difficulty with this question.

Level of Cognitive Ability: Application
Client Needs: Health Promotion and Maintenance
Integrated Process: Teaching/Learning
Content Area: Adult Health/Oncology

Reference:
Black, J., & Hawks, J. (2005). *Medical-surgical nursing: Clinical management for positive outcomes* (7th ed.). Philadelphia: Saunders, pp. 354; 1072.

---

151. One unit of packed red blood cells has been prescribed for a client postoperatively because the client's hemoglobin level is low. The physician prescribes diphenhydramine (Benadryl) to be administered before the administration of the transfusion. The nurse determines that this medication has been prescribed to:
1 Prevent an urticaria reaction
2 Prevent a fever
3 Assist in the absorption of the blood product
4 Promote movement of the red blood cells into the bone marrow

Answer: 1
Rationale: An urticaria reaction is characterized by a rash accompanied by pruritis. This type of transfusion reaction can be prevented by pretreating the client with an antihistamine, such as diphenhydramine. Options 2, 3, and 4 are incorrect. Acetaminophen (Tylenol), however, may be prescribed before the administration of blood to assist in preventing an elevated temperature.

Test-Taking Strategy: Use the process of elimination, focusing on the issue: the purpose of the diphenhydramine. Eliminate options 3 and 4 first because blood does not absorb or move into the bone marrow. From the remaining options, recalling the classification of diphenhydramine will direct you to option 1. Review the purpose of diphenhydramine if you had difficulty with this question.

Level of Cognitive Ability: Analysis
Client Needs: Physiological Integrity
Integrated Process: Nursing Process/Analysis
Content Area: Fundamental Skills

Reference:
Hodgson, B., & Kizior, R. (2004). *Saunders nursing drug handbook 2004.* Philadelphia: Saunders, p. 317.

152. A client is admitted to the hospital with a diagnosis of infiltrating ductal carcinoma of the breast. The nurse assesses the client for which expected manifestation?
  1 Bilateral palpable masses
  2 A fixed, irregularly shaped mass
  3 A round-shaped mass that is moveable
  4 Pain in the breast and edema

Answer: 2
Rationale: Infiltrating ductal carcinoma of the breast usually presents as a fixed, irregularly shaped mass. The mass is usually single and unilateral, and is painless, nontender, and hard to the touch.

Test-Taking Strategy: Using principles of anatomy and knowledge regarding the characteristics of a cancerous lesion will assist in eliminating options 1 and 3 first. Choose option 2 over option 4, recalling that pain is generally a late sign of a disorder and that involvement of the ducts makes it more likely that the mass does not move (fixed). Review the characteristics of breast cancer if you had difficulty with this question.

Level of Cognitive Ability: Application
Client Needs: Physiological Integrity
Integrated Process: Nursing Process/Assessment
Content Area: Adult Health/Oncology

Reference:
Black, J., & Hawks, J. (2005). *Medical-surgical nursing: Clinical management for positive outcomes* (7th ed.). Philadelphia: Saunders, p. 1099.

153. A mother of a 9-year-old child newly diagnosed with diabetes mellitus is very concerned about the child going to school and participating in social events. The nurse develops a plan of care and formulates which goal?
  1 The child's normal growth and development will be maintained.
  2 The child and family will discuss all aspects of the illness and its treatments.
  3 The child will use effective coping mechanisms to manage anxiety.
  4 The child and family will integrate diabetes care into patterns of daily living.

Answer: 4
Rationale: In order to effectively manage social events in the child's life, the family and the child need to integrate the care and management of diabetes into their daily living. The other options are goals for the family, but they do not deal with social issues.

Test-Taking Strategy: Use the process of elimination and focus on the issue: social events. Noting the relationship of this issue and the words "into patterns of daily living" will direct you to option 4. Review goals of care for a child with diabetes mellitus if you had difficulty with this question.

Level of Cognitive Ability: Application
Client Needs: Psychosocial Integrity
Integrated Process: Nursing Process/Planning
Content Area: Child Health

Reference:
Wong, D., & Hockenberry, M. (2003). *Wong's nursing care of infants and children* (7th ed.). St. Louis: Mosby, pp. 1743-1744.

154. A client has been taking metoclopramide (Reglan) on a long-term basis. A home care nurse calls the physician immediately if which side effect is noted in this client?

1 Excitability
2 Uncontrolled rhythmic movements of the face or limbs
3 Anxiety or irritability
4 Dry mouth not minimized by the use of sugar free hard candy

Answer: 2
Rationale: If the client experiences tardive dyskinesia (rhythmic movements of the face or limbs), the nurse should withhold the medication and call the physician. These side effects may be irreversible. Excitability is not a side effect of this medication. Anxiety, irritability, and dry mouth are milder side effects that are not harmful to the client.

Test-Taking Strategy: Note the key words "calls the physician immediately." Select the option that identifies the most serious effect. This will direct you to option 2. Review the side effects of this medication and the signs of tardive dyskinesia if you had difficulty with this question.

Level of Cognitive Ability: Application
Client Needs: Physiological Integrity
Integrated Process: Nursing Process/Implementation
Content Area: Pharmacology

Reference:
McKenry, L., & Salerno, E. (2003). *Mosby's pharmacology in nursing* (21st ed.). St. Louis: Mosby, p. 762.

155. A client has had a left mastectomy with axillary lymph node dissection. The nurse determines that the client understands postoperative restrictions and arm care if the client states to:

1 Use a straight razor to shave under the arms
2 Allow blood pressures to be taken only on the left arm
3 Carry a handbag and heavy objects on the left arm
4 Use gloves when working in the garden

Answer: 4
Rationale: The client is at risk for edema and infection as a result of lymph node dissection. The client should avoid activities that increase edema, such as carrying heavy objects or having blood pressures taken on the affected arm. The client should also use a variety of techniques to avoid trauma to the affected arm. Examples include using an electric razor to shave under the arm, gloves when working in the garden, and potholders when cooking to prevent burns.

Test-Taking Strategy: Note the surgical procedure and focus on the issue: postoperative restrictions and arm care. Keeping this issue in mind, read each option, noting the potential risk related to edema or trauma. This will direct you to option 4. Review teaching points for the client following mastectomy if you had difficulty with this question.

Level of Cognitive Ability: Analysis
Client Needs: Health Promotion and Maintenance
Integrated Process: Teaching/Learning
Content Area: Adult Health/Oncology

Reference:
Black, J., & Hawks, J. (2005). *Medical-surgical nursing: Clinical management for positive outcomes* (7th ed.). Philadelphia: Saunders, p. 1108.

156. A nurse is teaching a client about the modifiable risk factors that can reduce the risk for colorectal cancer. The nurse places highest priority on discussing which risk factor with this client?
   1 Personal history of ulcerative colitis or gastrointestinal (GI) polyps
   2 Distant relative with colorectal cancer
   3 Age over 30 years
   4 High-fat, low-fiber diet

Answer: 4
Rationale: Common risk factors for colorectal cancer that cannot be changed include age over 40, first-degree relative with colorectal cancer, and history of bowel problems such as ulcerative colitis or familial polyposis. Clients should be aware of modifiable risk factors as part of general health maintenance and primary disease prevention. Modifiable risk factors are those that can be reduced, and include a high-fat and low-fiber diet.

Test-Taking Strategy: Focus on the issue: modifiable risk factors related to colorectal cancer. Note the key words "reduce the risk" and "highest priority." Recalling that modifiable risk factors are those that can be changed will direct you to option 4. Review modifiable and nonmodifiable risk factors related to colorectal cancer if you had difficulty with this question.

Level of Cognitive Ability: Application
Client Needs: Health Promotion and Maintenance
Integrated Process: Teaching/Learning
Content Area: Adult Health/Gastrointestinal

Reference:
Phipps, W., Monahan, F., Sands, J., Marek, J., & Neighbors, M. (2003). *Medical-surgical nursing: Health and illness perspectives* (7th ed.). St. Louis: Mosby, p. 1100.

157. A client with gastroesophageal reflux disease (GERD) complains of chest discomfort that feels like heartburn, especially following each meal. After teaching the client to take antacids as prescribed, the nurse suggests that the client lie in which position during sleep?
   1 With the head of the bed elevated 6 to 8 inches
   2 Flat
   3 Supine with the head of the bed flat
   4 On the stomach with the head of the bed flat

Answer: 1
Rationale: The discomfort of reflux is aggravated by positions that allow the reflux of gastrointestinal contents. The client is instructed to remain upright for 1 to 2 hours after a meal and to sleep with the head of the bed elevated 6 to 8 inches. Lying flat will increase the episodes of reflux, resulting in chest discomfort.

Test-Taking Strategy: Use the process of elimination and think about the physiology associated with this disorder. Eliminate options 2, 3, and 4 because they are similar and all indicate flat positions. Review measures that will reduce discomfort in the client with GERD if you had difficulty with this question.

Level of Cognitive Ability: Application
Client Needs: Physiological Integrity
Integrated Process: Teaching/Learning
Content Area: Adult Health/Gastrointestinal

References:
Lewis, S., Heitkemper, M., & Dirksen, S. (2004). *Medical-surgical nursing: Assessment and management of clinical problems* (6th ed.). St. Louis: Mosby, p. 1015.
Phipps, W., Monahan, F., Sands, J., Marek, J., & Neighbors, M. (2003). *Medical-surgical nursing: Health and illness perspectives* (7th ed.). St. Louis: Mosby, p. 1010.

158. A nurse is providing instructions to a female client regarding the procedure for collecting a midstream urine sample for culture and sensitivity. Which statement by the client indicates an understanding of the procedure?
  1 "I need to douche before collecting the specimen."
  2 "I need to cleanse the perineum from front to back."
  3 "I need to collect the urine in the cup as soon as I begin to urinate."
  4 "I can collect the specimen tonight and drop it off at the clinic in the morning."

Answer: 2

Rationale: As part of correct procedure, the client should cleanse the perineum from front to back with the antiseptic swabs that are packaged with the specimen kit. The client should begin the flow of urine and collect the sample after starting the flow of urine. The specimen should be sent to the laboratory as soon as possible and not allowed to stand. Improper specimen handling can yield inaccurate test results. It is not normal procedure to douche before collecting the specimen.

Test-Taking Strategy: Use the process of elimination. Noting the name of the type of sample, "midstream," will assist in eliminating option 3. Recalling that the specimen should be brought to the laboratory after collection will assist in eliminating option 4. From the remaining options, use basic principles related to hygiene to assist in directing you to option 2. Review this procedure if you had difficulty with this question.

Level of Cognitive Ability: Analysis
Client Needs: Physiological Integrity
Integrated Process: Teaching/Learning
Content Area: Fundamental Skills

Reference:
Chernecky, C., & Berger, B. (2004). *Laboratory tests and diagnostic procedures* (4th ed.). Philadelphia: Saunders, p. 1124.

159. A nurse is preparing to care for a client who has undergone esophagogastroduodenoscopy (EGD). The nurse would do which of the following first after checking the client's vital signs?
  1 Monitor for sharp epigastric pain
  2 Monitor for complaints of heartburn
  3 Check for the return of the gag reflex
  4 Give warm gargles for sore throat

Answer: 3

Rationale: The nurse places highest priority on assessing for the return of the gag reflex, which is part of maintaining the client's airway. The nurse would monitor the client for sharp pain (may indicate a potential complication) and heartburn. The client would also receive warm gargles, but this cannot be done until the gag reflex has returned.

Test-Taking Strategy: Note the key word "first." Use the ABCs—airway, breathing, and circulation—to direct you to option 3. Review postprocedure care following an EGD if you had difficulty with question.

Level of Cognitive Ability: Application
Client Needs: Physiological Integrity
Integrated Process: Nursing Process/Implementation
Content Area: Adult Health/Gastrointestinal

References:
Chernecky, C., & Berger, B. (2004). *Laboratory tests and diagnostic procedures* (4th ed.). Philadelphia: Saunders, p. 510.
Lewis, S., Heitkemper, M., & Dirksen, S. (2004). *Medical-surgical nursing: Assessment and management of clinical problems* (6th ed.). St. Louis: Mosby, p. 963.

160. Methylphenidate (Ritalin) is prescribed for a child with a diagnosis of attention deficit hyperactivity disorder (ADHD). The nurse provides instructions to the mother regarding the administration of the medication and tells the mother to administer the medication:

1 Before dinner and at bedtime
2 Before breakfast and before the noontime meal
3 In the morning after breakfast and at bedtime
4 At the noontime and evening meals

Answer: 2

Rationale: Methylphenidate is a central nervous stimulant and should be taken before breakfast and before the noontime meal. It should not be taken in the afternoon or evening because the stimulating effect causes insomnia. Options 1, 3, and 4 are incorrect.

Test-Taking Strategy: Use the process of elimination. Noting the name of the medication and the disorder and recalling that this medication is a central nervous system stimulant will direct you to option 2. Review the client teaching points related to the administration of this medication if you had difficulty with this question.

Level of Cognitive Ability: Application
Client Needs: Health Promotion and Maintenance
Integrated Process: Teaching/Learning
Content Area: Pharmacology

Reference:

Hodgson, B., & Kizior, R. (2004). *Saunders nursing drug handbook 2004.* Philadelphia: Saunders, p. 656.

161. A client has been scheduled for a barium swallow (esophagography) the next day. The nurse determines that the client understands preprocedure instructions if the client states to do which of the following before the test?

1 Take all oral medications as scheduled
2 Monitor own bowel movement pattern for constipation
3 Remove metal objects and jewelry, especially from the neck and chest area
4 Eat a regular breakfast on the day of the test

Answer: 3

Rationale: A barium swallow, or esophagography, is an X-ray that uses a substance called barium for contrast to highlight abnormalities in the gastrointestinal (GI) tract. The client is told to remove metal objects such as medals and jewelry before the test, so they won't interfere with X-ray visualization of the field. The client should fast for 8 to 12 hours before the test, depending on physician instructions. Some oral medications are withheld before the test, and the client should follow the physician's instructions regarding medication administration. It is important after the procedure to monitor for constipation, which can occur as a result of the presence of barium in the GI tract.

Test-Taking Strategy: Note the key words "barium swallow" and "before the test." This tells you that the correct option is an item that the client needs to comply with before the test is done. Eliminate option 2 first, because it is a part of aftercare. Knowing that the procedure is a type of X-ray that involves barium and that the client needs to remain NPO will assist in eliminating options 1 and 4. Review preprocedure care for a barium swallow if you had difficulty with this question.

Level of Cognitive Ability: Analysis
Client Needs: Physiological Integrity
Integrated Process: Teaching/Learning
Content Area: Adult Health/Gastrointestinal

References:

Chernecky, C., & Berger, B. (2004). *Laboratory tests and diagnostic procedures* (4th ed.). Philadelphia: Saunders, pp. 219-220; 359-360.
Lewis, S., Heitkemper, M., & Dirksen, S. (2004). *Medical-surgical nursing: Assessment and management of clinical problems* (6th ed.). St. Louis: Mosby, p. 961.

162. A physician orders a chemotherapy medication dose that the nurse believes is too high. The nurse calls the physician, but the physician has left the office for the weekend. The nurse appropriately:
1 Checks with the pharmacist, who agrees the dose is too high, and then reduces the dose accordingly
2 Withholds giving the medication until the physician's partner makes rounds the following day
3 Reschedules the client's chemotherapy until the following week
4 Calls the answering service, and confers with the on-call physician

Answer: 4
Rationale: If the nurse believes a physician's order to be in error, the nurse is responsible for clarifying the order before carrying out the order. Checking with the pharmacist can assist the nurse in determining whether the dose ordered is incorrect, but the nurse or pharmacist cannot alter the dose without an order from the physician. Withholding the medication until the following day is incorrect. Chemotherapy agents must often be administered in the proper combinations or sequence in order to be effective. Rescheduling the client's chemotherapy is also incorrect. Chemotherapy must be administered on a specific schedule for maximum effect with minimum adverse effects. Additionally, the nurse cannot withhold or reschedule chemotherapy without a physician's order.

Test-Taking Strategy: Use the process of elimination and knowledge of the legal responsibilities of the nurse in regard to a physician's orders and medication administration. Remember that a nurse cannot alter, withhold, or reschedule a medication dose. Review these legal responsibilities if you had difficulty with this question.

Level of Cognitive Ability: Application
Client Needs: Safe, Effective Care Environment
Integrated Process: Nursing Process/Implementation
Content Area: Leadership/Management

Reference:
Potter, P. , & Perry, A. (2005). *Fundamentals of nursing* (6th ed.). St. Louis: Mosby, pp. 419; 842.

163. A nurse working in a long-term care setting has recently attended a workshop on creating a restraint-free environment for the residents. Several coworkers have been employed in this facility for many years and firmly believe that their current methods are satisfactory. The nurse can be effective in facilitating change by:
1 Informing the nursing supervisor that current restraint policies must be changed and requesting that all staff be required to comply
2 Writing a new restraint policy over the weekend and distributing it to coworkers for immediate implementation on Monday morning
3 Asking coworkers' to help gather data comparing the facility's restraint procedures and outcomes with those of others using revised procedures
4 Pointing out to coworkers the various mistakes that they are presently making in adhering to outdated restraint procedures

Answer: 3
Rationale: To be an effective leader, the nurse must work collaboratively with others to solve common problems. The nurse who works collaboratively with others to facilitate change has a much greater chance of success than one who unilaterally demands or implements change. By enlisting the assistance of others, there is a greater chance that they will support proposed changes in procedures. A punitive atmosphere is not effective in promoting change because it discourages people from taking risks. To focus on errors (perceived or real) serves only to alienate others and is not effective in promoting change.

Test-Taking Strategy: Use the process of elimination, remembering that to facilitate change, collaboration between the nurse and coworkers is important. Additionally, options 1, 2, and 4 focus on unilateral actions by the nurse. Review the change process if you had difficulty with this question.

Level of Cognitive Ability: Application
Client Needs: Safe, Effective Care Environment
Integrated Process: Nursing Process/Implementation
Content Area: Leadership/Management

Reference:
Potter, P., & Perry, A. (2005). *Fundamentals of nursing* (6th ed.). St. Louis: Mosby, p. 385.

164. A client being discharged from the hospital with a diagnosis of gastric ulcer has an order for sucralfate (Carafate) 1 gram by mouth four times daily. The nurse determines that the client understands proper use of the medication if the client states to take it:

1 Every 6 hours around the clock
2 One hour after meals and at bedtime
3 With meals and at bedtime
4 One hour before meals and at bedtime

Answer: 4

Rationale: Sucralfate (Carafate) is an antiulcer medication. The medication should be scheduled for administration 1 hour before meals and at bedtime. This timing will allow the medication to form a protective coating over the ulcer before it becomes irritated by food intake, gastric acid production, and mechanical movement. The other options are incorrect.

Test-Taking Strategy: Use the process of elimination. Recalling the action of this medication, to form a protective coating, will direct you to option 4. Review client teaching points regarding this medication if you had difficulty with this question.

Level of Cognitive Ability: Analysis
Client Needs: Physiological Integrity
Integrated Process: Teaching/Learning
Content Area: Pharmacology

Reference:
Hodgson, B., & Kizior, R. (2004). *Saunders nursing drug handbook 2004.* Philadelphia: Saunders, p. 940.

165. A nurse is assisting a physician with abdominal paracentesis. The nurse assists the client into what position for this procedure?

1 Supine
2 Prone
3 Upright
4 Low Fowler's on the right side

Answer: 3

Rationale: For abdominal paracentesis, the nurse should position the client in an upright position on the edge of the bed with the feet resting on a stool and the back well supported. This position allows the intestine to float posteriorly and helps prevent laceration during catheter insertion. Options 1, 2, and 4 are incorrect positions.

Test-Taking Strategy: Focus on the name and the purpose of the procedure. Eliminate options 1 and 2 because they are similar. From the remaining options, visualize this procedure and its associated complications to answer the question. Review the procedure for abdominal paracentesis if you had difficulty with this question.

Level of Cognitive Ability: Application
Client Needs: Physiological Integrity
Integrated Process: Nursing Process/Implementation
Content Area: Adult Health/Gastrointestinal

Reference:
Black, J., & Hawks, J. (2005). *Medical-surgical nursing: Clinical management for positive outcomes* (7th ed.). Philadelphia: Saunders, p. 1188.

166. A client was admitted to the hospital with a diagnosis of frequent symptomatic premature ventricular contractions (PVCs). After sitting up in a chair for a few minutes, the client complains of feeling lightheaded. On auscultation of the heartbeat, the nurse would most likely expect to note:

1 A regular apical pulse
2 An irregular apical pulse
3 A very rapid regular apical pulse
4 A very slow regular apical pulse

Answer: 2

Rationale: The most accurate means of assessing pulse rhythm is by auscultation of the apical pulse. When a client has PVCs, the rate is irregular and if the radial pulse is taken, a true picture of what is occurring is not obtained. A very fast regular apical pulse indicates tachycardia. A very slow regular apical pulse indicates bradycardia.

Test-Taking Strategy: Use the process of elimination, focusing on the issue: PVCs. Eliminate options 1, 3, and 4 because they are similar and indicate a regular pulse. Review the manifestations associated with PVCs if you had difficulty with this question.

Level of Cognitive Ability: Analysis
Client Needs: Physiological Integrity
Integrated Process: Nursing Process/Assessment
Content Area: Adult Health/Cardiovascular

References:

Black, J., & Hawks, J. (2005). *Medical-surgical nursing: Clinical management for positive outcomes* (7th ed.). Philadelphia: Saunders, p. 1682.
Potter, P., & Perry, A. (2005). *Fundamentals of nursing* (6th ed.). St. Louis: Mosby, pp. 642; 725.

167. A client with a history of duodenal ulcer is taking calcium carbonate chewable tablets. The nurse monitors the client for relief of which symptom?

1 Flatus
2 Rectal pain
3 Muscle twitching
4 Heartburn

Answer: 4

Rationale: Calcium carbonate is used as an antacid for the relief of heartburn and indigestion. It can also be used as a calcium supplement or to bind phosphorus in the gastrointestinal (GI) tract in clients with renal failure. Options 1, 2, and 3 are unrelated to this medication.

Test-Taking Strategy: Use the process of elimination. Focusing on the client's diagnosis will direct you to option 4. Review the action of this medication if you had difficulty with this question.

Level of Cognitive Ability: Analysis
Client Needs: Health Promotion and Maintenance
Integrated Process: Nursing Process/Evaluation
Content Area: Pharmacology

Reference:

Hodgson, B., & Kizior, R. (2004). *Saunders nursing drug handbook 2004.* Philadelphia: Saunders, p. 139.

168. A child with Hirschsprung's disease is scheduled for surgery, and a temporary colostomy is performed on the child. Postoperatively, the nurse reinforces instructions to the parents about colostomy care at home. Which statement by the parents indicates their understanding of the instructions?
1 "We will report signs of skin breakdown."
2 "We will apply a heat lamp to any moist red tissue around the stoma."
3 "We will give antidiarrheal medications."
4 "We will give saline water enemas if my child doesn't pass stool."

Answer: 1
Rationale: The parents are instructed to report signs of skin breakdown or stomal complications, such as ribbon-like stools, or failure to pass flatus or stools to the physician or the nurse. Moist, red granulation tissue may grow around an ostomy site and does not require special treatment. Options 3 and 4 are incorrect actions and are contraindicated.

Test-Taking Strategy: Use the process of elimination, noting the key words "indicates their understanding of the instructions." Focusing on the issue, colostomy care, and careful reading of each option will direct you to option 1. Review parent teaching and colostomy care if you had difficulty with this question.

Level of Cognitive Ability: Analysis
Client Needs: Health Promotion and Health Maintenance
Integrated Process: Teaching/Learning
Content Area: Child Health

Reference:
Wong, D., & Hockenberry, M. (2003). *Wong's nursing care of infants and children* (7th ed.). St. Louis: Mosby, pp. 1166-1167.

---

169. A client with Bell's palsy is distressed about the change in facial appearance. The nurse tells the client about which characteristic of Bell's palsy to help the client cope with the disorder?
1 The symptoms will completely go away once the tumor is removed.
2 It usually resolves when treated with vasodilator medications.
3 It is similar to stroke, but all symptoms will go away eventually.
4 It is not caused by stroke, and many clients recover in 3 to 5 weeks.

Answer: 4
Rationale: Clients with Bell's palsy should be reassured that they have not experienced a stroke and that symptoms often disappear spontaneously in 3 to 5 weeks. The client is given supportive treatment for symptoms. It is not usually caused by a tumor, and the treatment does not involve administering vasodilators.

Test-Taking Strategy: Focus on the issue: helping the client cope with the disorder. Recalling that Bell's palsy is not a cerebral vascular accident and is not caused by a tumor or vasoconstriction will eliminate options 1, 2, and 3. Review the characteristics associated with Bell's palsy if you had difficulty with this question.

Level of Cognitive Ability: Application
Client Needs: Psychosocial Integrity
Integrated Process: Caring
Content Area: Adult Health/Neurological

Reference:
Black, J., & Hawks, J. (2005). *Medical-surgical nursing: Clinical management for positive outcomes* (7th ed.). Philadelphia: Saunders, p. 2154.

---

170. A client has been given a prescription for propantheline (Pro-Banthine) as adjunctive treatment for peptic ulcer disease. The nurse tells the client to take this medication:
1 With antacids
2 30 minutes before meals
3 With meals
4 Just after meals

Answer: 2
Rationale: Propantheline is an antimuscarinic anticholinergic medication that decreases gastrointestinal secretions. It should be administered 30 minutes before meals. The other options are incorrect.

Test-Taking Strategy: Use the process of elimination. Option 1 can be eliminated first because most medications cannot be administered with antacids because of interactive effects. Eliminate options 3 and 4 next because they are similar and indicate administering the medication with food. Review this medication if you had difficulty with this question.

Level of Cognitive Ability: Application
Client Needs: Health Promotion and Maintenance
Integrated Process: Teaching/Learning
Content Area: Pharmacology

Reference:
Lehne, R. (2004). *Pharmacology for nursing care.* (5th ed). Philadelphia: Saunders, p. 119.

---

171. A nurse is assigned to care for a client who is receiving total parenteral nutrition (TPN). The nurse performs a fingerstick glucose, and the result indicates a glucose level of 400 mg/dL. Based on this finding, the nurse takes which action?
 1 Stops the TPN
 2 Decreases the flow rate of the TPN
 3 Increases the flow rate of the TPN
 4 Notifies the physician

Answer: 4
Rationale: Hyperglycemia is a complication associated with the administration of TPN. Because the glucose result is elevated, the nurse would immediately notify the physician for further instructions. Options 1, 2, and 3 are not implemented without a physician's order.

Test-Taking Strategy: Use the process of elimination. Eliminate options 1, 2, and 3 because they are not within the scope of nursing practice. Additionally, recalling the normal glucose level will direct you to option 4. Review this content if you are unfamiliar with the care of the client receiving TPN.

Level of Cognitive Ability: Application
Client Needs: Physiological Integrity
Integrated Process: Nursing Process/Implementation
Content Area: Fundamental Skills

References:
Black, J., & Hawks, J. (2005). *Medical-surgical nursing: Clinical management for positive outcomes* (7th ed.). Philadelphia: Saunders, p. 708.
Ignatavicius, D., & Workman, M. (2002). *Medical surgical nursing: Critical thinking for collaborative care* (4th ed.). Philadelphia: Saunders, p. 1372.

---

172. Carbamazepine (Tegretol) is prescribed for a client in the management of generalized tonic-clonic seizures. The nurse provides instructions to the client regarding the side effects associated with the use of the medication and tells the client to inform the physician if which of the following occurs?
 1 Drowsiness
 2 Dizziness
 3 Nausea
 4 Sore throat

Answer: 4
Rationale: Drowsiness, dizziness, nausea, and vomiting are frequent side effects associated with the medication. Adverse reactions include blood dyscrasias. If the client develops a fever, sore throat, mouth ulcerations, unusual bleeding or bruising, or joint pain, this may be indicative of a blood dyscrasia, and the physician should be notified.

Test-Taking Strategy: Note the key words "tells the client to inform the physician." Recalling that blood dyscrasias can occur with the use of carbamazepine will direct you to option 4. Also, noting the key words, "inform the physician," will direct you to option 4 because a sore throat is a sign of infection. Review this content if you are unfamiliar with the adverse effects of carbamazepine.

Level of Cognitive Ability: Application
Client Needs: Health Promotion and Maintenance
Integrated Process: Teaching/Learning
Content Area: Pharmacology

Reference:
Hodgson, B., & Kizior, R. (2004). *Saunders nursing drug handbook 2004.* Philadelphia: Saunders, p. 149.

173. A medication nurse is supervising a newly hired nurse who is administering pyridostigmine (Mestinon) orally to a client with myasthenia gravis. Which observation by the medication nurse indicates safe practice by the newly hired nurse before administering this medication?
1 Asking the client to lie down on her right side
2 Instructing the client to void before taking the medication
3 Asking the client to take sips of water
4 Asking the client to look up at the ceiling for 30 seconds

Answer: 3
Rationale: Myasthenia gravis can affect the client's ability to swallow. The primary assessment is to determine the client's ability to swallow. Options 1 and 4 are not appropriate. In this situation, there is no reason for the client to lie down to swallow medication or to look up at the ceiling. Additionally, lying down could place the client at risk for aspiration. There is no specific reason for the client to void before taking medication.

Test-Taking Strategy: Note the diagnosis of the client and that the question addresses an oral medication. Recalling that myasthenia gravis can affect the client's ability to swallow will direct you to option 3. Review nursing care of the client with myasthenia gravis if you had difficulty with this question.

Level of Cognitive Ability: Analysis
Client Needs: Safe, Effective Care Environment
Integrated Process: Nursing Process/Evaluation
Content Area: Leadership/Management

References:
Black, J., & Hawks, J. (2005). *Medical-surgical nursing: Clinical management for positive outcomes* (7th ed.). Philadelphia: Saunders, p. 2184.
Lewis, S., Heitkemper, M., & Dirksen, S. (2004). *Medical-surgical nursing: assessment and management of clinical problems* (6th ed.). St. Louis: Mosby, p. 1574.

174. A home care nurse visits a client with chronic obstructive pulmonary disease (COPD) who is on home oxygen at 2 liters per minute. The client's respiratory rate is 22 breaths per minute, and the client is complaining of increased dyspnea. The nurse would initially:
1 Determine the need to increase the oxygen
2 Collect additional information regarding the client's respiratory status
3 Call emergency services to come to the home
4 Reassure the client that there is no need to worry

Answer: 2
Rationale: Completing the assessment and collecting additional information regarding the client's respiratory status is the initial nursing action. Reassuring the client is appropriate, but it is inappropriate to tell the client not to worry. Calling emergency services is a premature action. The oxygen is not increased without the approval of the physician, especially because clients with COPD can retain carbon dioxide.

Test-Taking Strategy: Use the steps of the nursing process. Remember that assessment is the first step. Also, use the ABCs (i.e., airway, breathing, and circulation) to direct you to option 2. Review care of the client with COPD if you had difficulty with this question.

Level of Cognitive Ability: Application
Client Needs: Physiological Integrity
Integrated Process: Nursing Process/Implementation
Content Area: Adult Health/Respiratory

Reference:
Phipps, W., Monahan, F., Sands, J., Marek, J., & Neighbors, M. (2003). *Medical-surgical nursing: Health and illness perspectives* (7th ed.). St. Louis: Mosby, p. 579.

175. A new breastfeeding mother is seen in the clinic with complaints of breast discomfort. The nurse determines that the mother is experiencing breast engorgement and provides the mother with instructions regarding care for the condition. Which statement by the mother indicates an understanding of the measures that will provide comfort for the engorgement?

1 "I will breastfeed using only one breast."

2 "I will apply cold compresses to my breasts."

3 "I will massage my breasts before feeding to stimulate letdown."

4 "I will avoid the use of a bra while my breasts are engorged."

Answer: 3

Rationale: Comfort measures for breast engorgement include massaging the breasts before feeding to stimulate letdown; wearing a supportive well-fitting bra at all times; taking a warm shower or applying warm compresses just before feeding; and alternating the breasts during feeding. Options 1, 2, and 4 are incorrect measures.

Test-Taking Strategy: Use the process of elimination, noting the key words "indicates an understanding." Visualize each of the descriptions in the options to assist in directing you to option 3. Review the measures to alleviate breast engorgement if you had difficulty with this question.

Level of Cognitive Ability: Analysis
Client Needs: Health Promotion and Maintenance
Integrated Process: Nursing Process/Evaluation
Content Area: Maternity/Postpartum

Reference:
Lowdermilk, D., & Perry, A. (2004). *Maternity & women's health care* (8th ed.). St. Louis: Mosby, p. 777.

176. A client's vital signs have noticeably deteriorated over the past 4 hours following surgery. The nurse does not recognize the significance of these changes in vital signs and takes no action. The client later requires emergency surgery. The nurse could be liable for a lack of action according to the definition of which of the following?

1 Tort

2 Misdemeanor

3 Common law

4 Statutory law

Answer: 1

Rationale: A tort is a wrongful act intentionally or unintentionally committed against a person or his or her property. The nurse's inaction in the situation described is consistent with the definition of a tort offense. Option 2 is an offense under criminal law. Option 3 describes case law that has evolved over time via precedents. Option 4 describes laws that are enacted by state, federal, or local governments.

Test-Taking Strategy: Focus on the data in the question. Use knowledge regarding the definitions of the items identified in the options to answer this question. Review the definitions related to these items if you had difficulty with this question.

Level of Cognitive Ability: Analysis
Client Needs: Physiological Integrity
Integrated Process: Nursing Process/Analysis
Content Area: Fundamental Skills

Reference:
Potter, P. , & Perry, A. (2005). *Fundamentals of nursing* (6th ed.). St. Louis: Mosby, pp. 413-414.

177. A post-mastectomy client has been found to have an estrogen-receptor positive tumor. The nurse interprets after reading this information in the pathology report that the client will most likely have which common follow-up treatment prescribed?
1 Administration of estrogen
2 Administration of progesterone
3 Administration of tamoxifen (Nolvadex)
4 Removal of the ovaries

Answer: 3
Rationale: A common treatment for women with estrogen-receptor positive breast tumors is follow-up treatment with tamoxifen. This medication is classified as an antineoplastic agent and competes with estrogen for binding sites in the breast and other tissues. The medication may be administered for years following surgery. Options 1, 2, and 4 are incorrect.

Test-Taking Strategy: Note the key words "estrogen-receptor positive" and "common treatment." These key words will assist in eliminating option 1. From the remaining options, it is necessary to know the action of the tamoxifen. Review the action and use of this medication if you had difficulty with this question.

Level of Cognitive Ability: Analysis
Client Needs: Physiological Integrity
Integrated Process: Nursing Process/Analysis
Content Area: Adult Health/Oncology

Reference:
Black, J., & Hawks, J. (2005). *Medical-surgical nursing: Clinical management for positive outcomes* (7th ed.). Philadelphia: Saunders, pp. 1096-1097.

178. A nurse reviews the client's health care record and notes that the client is taking donepezil hydrochloride (Aricept). Which disorder does the nurse suspect this client may have based on the use of this medication?
1 Seizure disorder
2 Obsessive compulsive disorder
3 Dementia
4 History of schizophrenia

Answer: 3
Rationale: Donepezil hydrochloride (Aricept) is a cholinergic agent that is used in the treatment of mild to moderate dementia of the Alzheimer's type. It enhances cholinergic functions by increasing the concentration of acetylcholine. It slows the progression of Alzheimer's disease. Options 1, 2, and 4 are incorrect.

Test-Taking Strategy: Specific knowledge regarding the use of donepezil hydrochloride is required to answer this question. Review its action and use if you are unfamiliar with this medication.

Level of Cognitive Ability: Analysis
Client Needs: Physiological Integrity
Integrated Process: Nursing Process/Analysis
Content Area: Pharmacology

Reference:
Hodgson, B., & Kizior, R. (2004). *Saunders nursing drug handbook 2004.* Philadelphia: Saunders, p. 333.

179. A registered nurse (RN) is supervising a licensed practical nurse (LPN) providing care to a client with end-stage heart failure. The client is withdrawn, reluctant to talk, and shows little interest in participating in hygienic care or activities. Which statement by the LPN to the client indicates that the LPN needs instructions in the use of therapeutic communication skills?

1 "You are very quiet today."
2 "Why don't you feel like getting up?"
3 "What are your feelings right now?"
4 "Tell me more about your difficulty with sleeping at night."

Answer: 2

Rationale: When a "why" question is made to the client, an explanation for feelings and behaviors is requested, and the client may not know the reason. Requesting an explanation is a nontherapeutic communication technique. In option 1, the LPN is using the therapeutic communication technique of acknowledging the client's behavior. In option 3, the LPN is encouraging identification of emotions or feelings. In option 4, the LPN is using the therapeutic communication technique of exploring, which is asking the client to describe something in more detail or to discuss it more fully.

Test-Taking Strategy: Note the key words "needs instructions in the use of therapeutic communication skills." These words indicate a false-response question and that you need to select the incorrect statement by the LPN. Use the process of elimination, seeking the option that is a block to communication. The word "why" in option 2 should guide you to this option. Review therapeutic communication techniques if you had difficulty with this question.

Level of Cognitive Ability: Analysis
Client Needs: Psychosocial Integrity
Integrated Process: Teaching/Learning
Content Area: Leadership/Management

Reference:
Potter, P. , & Perry, A. (2005). *Fundamentals of nursing* (6th ed.). St. Louis: Mosby, p. 437.

180. A nurse is administering a dose of ondansetron hydrochloride (Zofran) to a client for nausea and vomiting. The nurse tells the client to report which frequent side effect of this medication?

1 A warm feeling
2 Dizziness
3 Blurred vision
4 Urinary frequency

Answer: 2

Rationale: Ondansetron hydrochloride (Zofran) is a selective receptor antagonist used as an antinausea and antiemetic. Frequent side effects include anxiety, drowsiness, dizziness, headache, fatigue, constipation, diarrhea, urinary retention, and hypoxia. Occasional side effects include abdominal pain, diminished saliva secretion, fever, feeling of cold, paresthesia, and weakness. Rare side effects include hypersensitivity reaction and blurred vision.

Test-Taking Strategy: Focus on the issue: a frequent side effect. Noting that the medication is used to treat nausea and vomiting and that this medication is a selective receptor antagonist will direct you to option 2. Review this content if you had difficulty with this question and are unfamiliar with the side effects associated with the use of this medication.

Level of Cognitive Ability: Application
Client Needs: Physiological Integrity
Integrated Process: Nursing Process/Implementation
Content Area: Pharmacology

Reference:
Hodgson, B., & Kizior, R. (2004). *Saunders nursing drug handbook 2004.* Philadelphia: Saunders, p. 756.

181. A nurse is reviewing a urinalysis report for a client with acute renal failure and notes that the results are highly positive for proteinuria. The nurse interprets that this client has which type of renal failure?
  1 Postrenal failure
  2 Prerenal failure
  3 Intrinsic renal failure
  4 Atypical renal failure

Answer: 3
Rationale: With intrinsic renal failure, there is a fixed specific gravity and the urine tests positive for proteinuria. In postrenal failure, there is a fixed specific gravity and little or no proteinuria. In prerenal failure, the specific gravity is high, and there is very little or no proteinuria. There is no such classification as atypical renal failure.

Test-Taking Strategy: Specific knowledge regarding the types of renal failure is required to answer this question. Review the manifestations associated with the classifications of renal failure if you had difficulty with this question.

Level of Cognitive Ability: Analysis
Client Needs: Physiological Integrity
Integrated Process: Nursing Process/Analysis
Content Area: Adult Health/Renal

Reference:
Ignatavicius, D., & Workman, M. (2002). *Medical surgical nursing: Critical thinking for collaborative care* (4th ed.). Philadelphia: Saunders, p. 1668.

---

182. A client has undergone a vaginal hysterectomy. The nurse writes on the client's nursing care plan that which of the following is to be avoided?
  1 Elevating the knees with the knee gatch on the bed
  2 Using pneumatic compression boots
  3 Removing antiembolism stockings twice daily
  4 Assisting with range of motion leg exercises

Answer: 1
Rationale: The client is at risk for deep vein thrombosis or thrombophlebitis after this surgery, as for any other major surgery. For this reason, the nurse implements measures that will prevent this complication. Range of motion exercises, antiembolism stockings, and pneumatic compression boots are all helpful. The nurse should avoid elevating the knees using the knee gatch in the bed, which inhibits venous return, and places the client more at risk for deep vein thrombosis or thrombophlebitis.

Test-Taking Strategy: Note the key word "avoided." This word indicates a false-response question and that you need to select the incorrect nursing action. Use basic nursing knowledge of postoperative care to direct you to option 1. Review care of the client following hysterectomy if you had difficulty with this question.

Level of Cognitive Ability: Application
Client Needs: Physiological Integrity
Integrated Process: Nursing Process/Planning
Content Area: Adult Health/Oncology

Reference:
Phipps, W., Monahan, F., Sands, J., Marek, J., & Neighbors, M. (2003). *Medical-surgical nursing: Health and illness perspectives* (7th ed.). St. Louis: Mosby, p. 1775.

183. Sertraline (Zoloft) is prescribed for a client in the treatment of depression. Before administering the medication, the nurse reviews the client's record and consults with the physician if which of the following were noted?
1 Use of phenelzine sulfate (Nardil)
2 A history of myocardial infarction
3 A history of irritable bowel syndrome
4 A history of diabetes mellitus

Answer: 1
Rationale: Sertraline (Zoloft) is a serotonin reuptake inhibitor. Serious potentially fatal reactions may occur if sertraline is administered concurrently with a monoamine oxidase inhibitor (MAOI). Phenelzine sulfate is an MAOI. MAOIs should be stopped at least 14 days before sertraline therapy. Sertraline should also be stopped at least 14 days before MAOI therapy. Options 2, 3, and 4 are not concerns with the administration of this medication.

Test-Taking Strategy: Knowledge regarding the interactions and contraindications associated with the use of sertraline is required to answer this question. Review this content if you are unfamiliar with the medication interactions and contraindications.

Level of Cognitive Ability: Application
Client Needs: Safe, Effective Care Environment
Integrated Process: Nursing Process/Implementation
Content Area: Pharmacology

Reference:
Hodgson, B., & Kizior, R. (2004). *Saunders nursing drug handbook 2004.* Philadelphia: Saunders, p. 912.

---

184. A 30-week gestation woman is admitted to the maternity unit in preterm labor. Betamethasone (Celestone) is prescribed to be administered to the mother, and the mother asks the nurse about the purpose of the medication. The nurse tells the mother that this medication will:
1 Stop the premature uterine contractions
2 Delay delivery for at least 48 hours
3 Promote fetal lung maturity
4 Prevent premature closure of the ductus arteriosus

Answer: 3
Rationale: Betamethasone (Celestone), a corticosteroid, is administered to increase the surfactant level and increase fetal lung maturity, reducing the incidence of respiratory distress syndrome in the newborn infant. Surfactant production does not become stable until after 32 weeks' gestation. If adequate amounts of surfactant are not present in the lungs, respiratory distress and death are possible consequences. Delivery needs to be delayed for at least 48 hours after the administration of betamethasone in order to allow time for the lungs to mature. Options 1, 2, and 4 are incorrect.

Test-Taking Strategy: Use the process of elimination. Eliminate options 1 and 2 first because they are similar and both relate to stopping labor. Recalling that respiratory distress syndrome caused by immature lungs is a major concern of prematurity will direct you to option 3 from the remaining options. Review the purpose of this medication if you had difficulty with this question.

Level of Cognitive Ability: Application
Client's Needs: Physiological Integrity
Integrated Process: Nursing Process/Implementation
Content Area: Maternity/Intrapartum

Reference:
Lowdermilk, D., & Perry, A. (2004). *Maternity & women's health care* (8th ed.). St. Louis: Mosby, p. 995.

185. A clinic nurse provides home care instructions to an adult client diagnosed with influenza. Select all instructions that the nurse provides to the client:
___ Remain at home until feeling better
___ Practice frequent handwashing
___ Return in 1 week for an influenza vaccine
___ Completely isolate self in a room from other family members and use a separate bathroom until feeling better
___ Cover the nose and mouth when sneezing and coughing
___ Take acetaminophen (Tylenol) for myalgia

Answer:
Remain at home until feeling better
Practice frequent handwashing
Cover the nose and mouth when sneezing and coughing
Take acetaminophen (Tylenol) for myalgia

Rationale: Influenza (commonly know as the flu) refers to an acute viral infection of the respiratory tract. It is a communicable disease spread by droplet infection, and measures are instituted to prevent its spread. The client is instructed to remain at home, practice frequent handwashing, and cover the nose and mouth when sneezing and coughing. Supportive measures to relieve fever and myalgia such as the use of acetaminophen are also encouraged. It is unrealistic to completely isolate oneself in a room from other family members, and there is no useful reason to use a separate bathroom because the infection is spread through droplets. Influenza immunization is administered before the start of the "flu" season, not after developing the infection.

Test-Taking Strategy: Focus on the client's diagnosis: influenza. Recalling that this infection is spread by droplets will assist in selecting the correct instructions. Also remember that the influenza immunization is administered before the start of the "flu" season, not after developing the infection. Review home care measures for treating influenza if you had difficulty with this question.

Level of Cognitive Ability: Analysis
Client Needs: Health Promotion and Maintenance
Integrated Process: Teaching/Learning
Content Area: Adult Health/Respiratory

Reference:
Black, J., & Hawks, J. (2005). *Medical-surgical nursing: Clinical management for positive outcomes* (7th ed.). Philadelphia: Saunders, p. 1839.

---

186. A client who has a positive sputum culture for mycobacterium tuberculosis is receiving streptomycin (Streptomycin) as part of the treatment. The nurse determines that the client is experiencing toxic effects of the medication if which laboratory result(s) is abnormal?
1 Hemoglobin and hematocrit
2 Blood urea nitrogen (BUN) and creatinine
3 Hepatic enzymes
4 Vision testing

Answer: 2
Rationale: BUN and creatinine are measured during therapy with streptomycin because the medication is nephrotoxic. The client taking isoniazid (INH) for tuberculosis is at risk for hepatotoxicity. Vision testing is done during treatment with ethambutol (Myambutol). Hemoglobin and hematocrit are not specifically related to tuberculosis.

Test-Taking Strategy: To answer this question accurately, you must be familiar with the various medications that are used to treat tuberculosis and their associated adverse or toxic effects. Review the adverse effects of streptomycin if you had difficulty with this question.

Level of Cognitive Ability: Analysis
Client Needs: Physiological Integrity
Integrated Process: Nursing Process/Analysis
Content Area: Adult Health/Respiratory

Reference:
Hodgson, B., & Kizior, R. (2004). *Saunders nursing drug handbook 2004.* Philadelphia: Saunders, p. 939.

---

187. A nurse is planning care for a client with a chest tube attached to a Pleur-Evac drainage system. The nurse avoids which action as part of routine chest tube care?
1 Keeps the collection chamber below the client's waist
2 Clamps the chest tube when the client gets out of bed
3 Adds water to the suction chamber as it evaporates
4 Tapes the connection between the chest tube and the drainage system

Answer: 2
Rationale: To avoid causing tension pneumothorax, the nurse avoids clamping the chest tube for any reason unless specifically ordered. In most instances, clamping of the chest tube is contraindicated by agency policy. The nurse keeps the drainage collection system below the level of the client's waist to prevent fluid or air from reentering the pleural space. Water is added to the suction control chamber as needed to maintain the full suction level ordered. Connections between the chest tube and system are taped to prevent accidental disconnection.

Test-Taking Strategy: Note the key word "avoids." This word indicates a false-response question and that you need to select the incorrect nursing action. Recalling that clamping chest tubes is contraindicated unless specifically ordered will direct you to option 2. Review care of the client with a chest tube if you had difficulty with this question.

Level of Cognitive Ability: Application
Client Needs: Physiological Integrity
Integrated Process: Nursing Process/Implementation
Content Area: Adult Health/Respiratory

References:
Lewis, S., Heitkemper, M., & Dirksen, S. (2004). *Medical-surgical nursing: Assessment and management of clinical problems* (6th ed.). St. Louis: Mosby, p. 624.
Phipps, W., Monahan, F., Sands, J., Marek, J., & Neighbors, M. (2003). *Medical-surgical nursing: Health and illness perspectives* (7th ed.). St. Louis: Mosby, p. 556.

---

188. Ibuprofen (Motrin) 400 mg orally four times daily has been prescribed for an older client with a diagnosis of rheumatoid arthritis. The client asks the nurse about the amount of medication prescribed. The nurse responds based on the understanding that this prescribed dosage is:
1 The normal adult dose
2 Lower than the normal adult dose
3 Higher than the normal adult dose
4 An unusual dosage for this diagnosis

Answer: 1
Rationale: For acute or chronic rheumatoid arthritis or osteoarthritis, the normal oral adult dose for an older client is 200 to 800 mg three to four times a day. Therefore, options 2, 3, and 4 are incorrect.

Test-Taking Strategy: Knowledge of the normal dosage for ibuprofen is required to answer this question. Review the normal dosage for this medication if you had difficulty with this question.

Level of Cognitive Ability: Analysis
Client Needs: Physiological Integrity
Integrated Process: Nursing Process/Implementation
Content Area: Pharmacology

Reference:
Hodgson, B., & Kizior, R. (2004). *Saunders nursing drug handbook 2004.* Philadelphia: Saunders, p. 517.

189. A nurse is monitoring a client with multiple sclerosis who is receiving baclofen (Lioresal). Which assessment finding would indicate a therapeutic response from the medication?

1 Increased muscle tone and strength
2 Decreased nausea
3 Decreased muscle spasms
4 Increased range of motion of all extremities

Answer: 3

Rationale: Baclofen is a skeletal muscle relaxant and acts at the spinal cord level to decrease the frequency and amplitude of muscle spasms in clients with spinal cord injuries or diseases, or multiple sclerosis. Options 1, 2, and 4 are unrelated to the effects of this medication.

Test-Taking Strategy: Focus on the client's diagnosis and the issue: a therapeutic response. Recalling that this medication is a skeletal muscle relaxant will direct you to option 3. Review the action of this medication if you had difficulty with this question.

Level of Cognitive Ability: Analysis
Client Needs: Physiological Integrity
Integrated Process: Nursing Process/Evaluation
Content Area: Pharmacology

Reference:
Hodgson, B., & Kizior, R. (2004). *Saunders nursing drug handbook 2004.* Philadelphia: Saunders, p. 92.

---

190. Lorazepam (Ativan) is prescribed for a client to manage anxiety. Which of the following, if noted on the client's record, would indicate the need to consult with the physician before administering the medication?

1 History of glaucoma
2 History of diabetes mellitus
3 History of hypothyroidism
4 History of coronary artery disease

Answer: 1

Rationale: Lorazepam is contraindicated if hypersensitivity or cross-sensitivity with other benzodiazepines exist. It is also contraindicated in clients who are comatose, with preexisting central nervous system (CNS) depression, with uncontrolled severe pain, and those with narrow-angle glaucoma. It is also not prescribed for clients who are pregnant or breastfeeding.

Test-Taking Strategy: Knowledge regarding the contraindications associated with the use of lorazepam is required to answer this question. Review this content if you are unfamiliar with these contraindications.

Level of Cognitive Ability: Analysis
Client Needs: Safe, Effective Care Environment
Integrated Process: Nursing Process/Implementation
Content Area: Pharmacology

Reference:
Hodgson, B., & Kizior, R. (2004). *Saunders nursing drug handbook 2004.* Philadelphia: Saunders, p. 617.

191. A hospitalized client with type 1 diabetes mellitus suddenly complains of hunger, shakiness, and sweating, and the nurse suspects that the client is experiencing a hypoglycemic reaction. List in order of priority the actions that the nurse takes. (Number 1 is the first action.)

___ Gives the client 4 ounces of orange juice to drink

___ Obtains a blood glucose reading with a glucose meter

___ Documents the client's complaints and other significant information related to the reaction

___ Determines the cause of the reaction

Answer: 2143

Rationale: The client's symptoms indicate mild hypoglycemia. If the hospitalized client complains of symptoms of hypoglycemia, a blood glucose test with a blood glucose meter should be performed. (In the nonhospitalized client, it is safer to assume and treat hypoglycemia if a blood glucose meter is unavailable.) The nurse then treats the reaction by administering a carbohydrate such as 4 ounces orange juice, 6 ounces regular soda, 6 to 8 ounces 2% milk, or a similar item containing 10 to 15 g of carbohydrate if the reaction is mild. Once the condition is corrected, the nurse would assess the client to determine the cause. The nurse should then document the client's complaints, the blood glucose level, treatment and response, the potential cause of the reaction, and other significant information related to the reaction.

Test-Taking Strategy: Noting that the client is hospitalized will assist in determining that a blood glucose reading should be obtained followed by immediate treatment. From the remaining actions provided, the nurse would next assess the cause of the reaction because this data would need to be part of the information documented. Review care of a client experiencing a hypoglycemic reaction if you had difficulty with this question.

Level of Cognitive Ability: Application
Client Needs: Physiological Integrity
Integrated Process: Nursing Process/Implementation
Content Area: Delegating/Prioritizing

References:
Black, J., & Hawks, J. (2005). *Medical-surgical nursing: Clinical management for positive outcomes* (7th ed.). Philadelphia: Saunders, p. 1275.
Lewis, S., Heitkemper, M., & Dirksen, S. (2004). *Medical-surgical nursing: Assessment and management of clinical problems* (6th ed.). St. Louis: Mosby, p. 1295.

192. A nurse caring for a client immediately following transurethral resection of the prostate (TURP) notices that the client has suddenly become confused and disoriented. The nurse determines that this may be a result of which potential complication of this surgical procedure?
1 Hypernatremia
2 Hyponatremia
3 Hyperchloremia
4 Hypochloremia

Answer: 2

Rationale: The client who suddenly becomes disoriented and confused following TURP could be experiencing early signs of hyponatremia. This may occur because the flushing solution used during the operative procedure is hypotonic. If enough solution is absorbed through the prostate veins during surgery, the client experiences increased circulating volume and dilutional hyponatremia. The nurse needs to report these symptoms.

Test-Taking Strategy: Note the key words "potential complication." Specific knowledge about the complications of this procedure will direct you to option 2. Also noting that options 1 and 2 are opposite findings may indicate that one of these options is the correct one. Review the complications related to TURP if you had difficulty with this question.

Level of Cognitive Ability: Analysis
Client Needs: Physiological Integrity
Integrated Process: Nursing Process/Analysis
Content Area: Adult Health/Renal

Reference:
Phipps, W., Monahan, F., Sands, J., Marek, J., & Neighbors, M. (2003). *Medical-surgical nursing: Health and illness perspectives* (7th ed.). St. Louis: Mosby, p. 1838.

---

193. A nurse is assessing a client hospitalized with a diagnosis of schizophrenia. Risperidone (Risperdal) is prescribed for the client for the treatment of this disorder. Which laboratory study would the nurse anticipate to be prescribed before the initiation of this medication therapy?
1 Complete blood count
2 Liver function studies
3 Blood clotting tests
4 Platelet count

Answer: 2

Rationale: Risperidone (Risperdal) is an antipsychotic medication that suppresses behavioral response in psychosis. Baseline assessment includes renal and liver function tests, and these studies should be done before the initiation of treatment. This medication is used with caution in clients with renal or hepatic impairment, clients with underlying cardiovascular disorders, and in older or debilitative clients. Options 1, 3, and 4 are unrelated to the administration of this medication.

Test-Taking Strategy: Use the process of elimination. Recalling that baseline liver and renal function studies should be done before therapy and that this medication is used cautiously in clients with renal or hepatic impairment will direct you to option 2. Review this content if you are unfamiliar with the contraindications associated with the use of this medication.

Level of Cognitive Ability: Analysis
Client Needs: Physiological Integrity
Integrated Process: Nursing Process/Analysis
Content Area: Pharmacology

Reference:
Hodgson, B., & Kizior, R. (2004). *Saunders nursing drug handbook 2004.* Philadelphia: Saunders, p. 891.

---

194. A nurse has been working with an obese man and is evaluating a weight-reduction plan designed for the client. Which statement by the client indicates the need for additional teaching?
1 "I wish my mother could have seen me lose the 60 pounds in the last 9 months."
2 "It is so difficult to find food exchanges that taste good and fill me up."
3 "My wife was kidding me the other night about my being a whole new husband."
4 "This diet doesn't let me go out for lunch with my friends at work anymore."

Answer: 4

Rationale: Both options 1 and 3 are responses indicating a positive perception of self, that another person has recognized these changes, and that the client wishes to have been able to share these changes with his mother. In the absence of other data, option 2 is a normal response to the changes in eating habits. Option 4 indicates that the client may be having difficulty in making appropriate dietary choices when going out for lunch or that he may perceive his coworkers are uncomfortable with his need to eat differently. A sense of not fitting in can leave the obese individual isolated and therefore make it more difficult for him to maintain his diet at work.

Test-Taking Strategy: Use the process of elimination, noting the key words "need for additional teaching." These words indicate a false-response question and that you need to select the option that indicates client difficulty with the diet regimen and the need for teaching. Read each option carefully and determine whether it is a positive indicator or a negative one. This will assist in eliminating options 1 and 3 first. Option 2 is a common response by persons who have had to make dietary changes. Option 4 clearly states that the client perceives a definite barrier in pursuing his accustomed lifestyle. Review dietary principles related to weight reduction if you had difficulty with this question.

Level of Cognitive Ability: Analysis
Client Needs: Health Promotion and Maintenance
Integrated Process: Nursing Process/Evaluation
Content Area: Fundamental Skills

References:
Lewis, S., Heitkemper, M., & Dirksen, S. (2004). *Medical-surgical nursing: Assessment and management of clinical problems* (6th ed.). St. Louis: Mosby, p. 994.
Potter, P., & Perry, A. (2005). *Fundamentals of nursing* (6th ed.). St. Louis: Mosby, pp. 437; 1279.

195. A client is complaining of skin irritation from the edges of a cast that was applied the previous day, and the nurse notes that the skin edges are pink and irritated. The nurse plans to do which of the following as a corrective action?
1 Use a hair dryer set on a cool high setting to soothe the irritation
2 Petal the edges of the cast with tape
3 Massage the skin at the rim of the cast
4 Shake a small amount of powder under the cast rim

Answer: 2
Rationale: The nurse should petal the edges of the cast with tape to minimize skin irritation. A hair dryer is used on a cool low setting if a nonplaster cast becomes wet or if the client's skin itches under a cast. Massaging the skin will not help the problem. Powder should not be shaken under the cast, because it could clump, become moist, and cause skin breakdown.

Test-Taking Strategy: Focus on the issue and note the cause of the client's skin irritation. Because the question tells you that the cast edges are the cause, you can eliminate options 1, 3, and 4. Review the principles of cast care if you had difficulty with this question.

Level of Cognitive Ability: Application
Client Needs: Physiological Integrity
Integrated Process: Nursing Process/Planning
Content Area: Adult Health/Musculoskeletal

Reference:
Phipps, W., Monahan, F., Sands, J., Marek, J., & Neighbors, M. (2003). *Medical-surgical nursing: Health and illness perspectives* (7th ed.). St. Louis: Mosby, p. 1481.

196. A nurse who has just begun the work shift is preparing to do tracheostomy care on a client. The nurse would obtain which tracheostomy care items from the supply area?
1 Tracheostomy care kit, sterile saline and water, and a suction kit
2 Bottle of sterile saline and a tracheostomy care kit
3 Bottles of sterile saline and water, and a tracheostomy dressing
4 Suction kit and tracheostomy dressing

Answer: 1
Rationale: Equipment needed to perform tracheostomy care includes a tracheostomy care kit, sterile water and saline solutions for cleansing and rinsing, and a suction kit for client suctioning. As part of tracheostomy care, the client's airway should be suctioned before cleansing the tracheostomy. New sterile solutions are obtained once per 24 hours, which is often done at the beginning of the work day. A tracheostomy care kit contains the needed supplies for cleaning the tracheostomy and for changing the dressing and tapes.

Test-Taking Strategy: Use the process of elimination. Remember when an option contains more than one part, all parts of the option must be complete and correct. Recalling that the key items needed are the tracheostomy kit and suction kit will direct you to option 1. Review the procedure for tracheostomy care if you had difficulty with this question.

Level of Cognitive Ability: Application
Client Needs: Physiological Integrity
Integrated Process: Nursing Process/Implementation
Content Area: Adult Health/Respiratory

References:
Lewis, S., Heitkemper, M., & Dirksen, S. (2004). *Medical-surgical nursing: Assessment and management of clinical problems* (6th ed.). St. Louis: Mosby, p. 579.
Potter, P., & Perry, A. (2005). *Fundamentals of nursing* (6th ed.). St. Louis: Mosby, pp. 1113-1114.

---

197. A nurse is observing a nursing assistant care for an older client who had a hip pinned following a fracture 4 days ago. To prevent client injury, the nurse intervenes in the care if the nursing assistant:
1 Places the call bell within reach
2 Answers the call bell promptly
3 Leaves the side rails down
4 Assures that the nightlight is working

Answer: 3
Rationale: Safe nursing actions intended to prevent injury to the client include keeping the side rails up, bed in low position, and providing a call bell that is within the client's reach. Responding promptly to the client's use of the call bell minimizes the chance that the client will try to get up alone, which could result in a fall. Nightlights are built into the lighting systems of most facilities, and these bulbs should be routinely checked to see that they are functional.

Test-Taking Strategy: Use the process of elimination, noting the key word "intervenes." This word indicates a false-response question and that you need to select the incorrect action by the nursing assistant. Because options 1 and 2 are standard safety measures, they are eliminated first. Use of a nightlight would help prevent falls, which is also helpful, and can be eliminated next. Review basic safety measures if you had difficulty with this question.

Level of Cognitive Ability: Application
Client Needs: Safe, Effective Care Environment
Integrated Process: Nursing Process/Implementation
Content Area: Leadership/Management

References:
Lewis, S., Heitkemper, M., & Dirksen, S. (2004). *Medical-surgical nursing: Assessment and management of clinical problems* (6th ed.). St. Louis: Mosby, pp. 384-385.
Potter, P., & Perry, A. (2005). *Fundamentals of nursing* (6th ed.). St. Louis: Mosby, p. 990.

---

198. A client with chronic renal failure has received dietary counseling about potassium restriction in the diet. The nurse determines that the client has learned the information correctly if the client states to do which of the following for preparation of vegetables?
1 Eat only fresh vegetables
2 Buy frozen vegetables whenever possible
3 Use salt substitute on them liberally
4 Boil them and discard the water

Answer: 4
Rationale: The potassium content of vegetables can be reduced by boiling them and discarding the cooking water. Options 1 and 2 are incorrect. Clients with renal failure should avoid the use of salt substitutes altogether, because they tend to be high in potassium content.

Test-Taking Strategy: Use the process of elimination, recalling which foods are high in potassium and how to reduce their potassium content. Options 2 and 3 can be eliminated first using basic principles of nutrition. Eliminate option 1 next, noting the word "only" in this option. Review client teaching points related to potassium restrictions if you had difficulty with this question.

Level of Cognitive Ability: Analysis
Client Needs: Health Promotion and Maintenance
Integrated Process: Teaching/Learning
Content Area: Adult Health/Renal

Reference:
Peckenpaugh, N. (2003). *Nutrition essentials and diet therapy* (9th ed.). Philadelphia: Saunders, p. 295.

199. A client with chronic renal failure has started receiving epoetin alfa (Epogen). The nurse reminds the client about the importance of taking which prescribed medication to enhance the effects of this therapy?
1 Calcium carbonate (Tums)
2 Aluminum hydroxide gel (Amphogel)
3 Iron supplement
4 Aluminum carbonate (Basaljel)

Answer: 3
Rationale: In order to form healthy red blood cells, which is the purpose of epoetin alfa, the body needs adequate stores of iron, folic acid, and vitamin B_{12}. The client should take these supplements regularly to enhance the hematocrit-raising benefit of this medication. The other options are incorrect.

Test-Taking Strategy: Use the process of elimination. Recall that this medication is used to stimulate red blood cell formation and that adequate body stores of vitamins and iron are needed to achieve this effect. Also, note that options 1, 2, and 4 are similar in that they are antacids. Review client teaching points regarding this medication if you had difficulty with this question.

Level of Cognitive Ability: Application
Client Needs: Physiological Integrity
Integrated Process: Teaching/Learning
Content Area: Adult Health/Renal

Reference:
McKenry, L., & Salerno, E. (2003). *Mosby's pharmacology in nursing* (21st ed.). St. Louis: Mosby, p. 695.

200. A client has just been diagnosed with acute renal failure. The laboratory calls the nurse to report a serum potassium level of 6.1 mEq/L on the client. The nurse takes which immediate action?
1 Calls the physician
2 Checks the sodium level
3 Encourages an extra 500 mL of fluid intake
4 Teaches the client about foods low in potassium

Answer: 1
Rationale: The client with hyperkalemia is at risk of developing cardiac dysrhythmias and resultant cardiac arrest. Because of this, the physician must be notified at once so that the client may receive definitive treatment. Fluid intake would not be increased because it would contribute to fluid overload and wouldn't effectively lower the serum potassium level. Dietary teaching may be necessary at some point, but this action is not the priority. The nurse might also check the result of a serum sodium level, but this is not a priority action of the nurse.

Test-Taking Strategy: Use the process of elimination, noting the key word "immediate." Recalling the normal potassium level and noting that the level identified in the question is elevated will direct you to option 1. Review the normal potassium level if you had difficulty with this question.

Level of Cognitive Ability: Application
Client Needs: Physiological Integrity
Integrated Process: Nursing Process/Implementation
Content Area: Adult Health/Renal

Reference:
Chernecky, C., & Berger, B. (2004). *Laboratory tests and diagnostic procedures* (4th ed.). Philadelphia: Saunders, p. 887.

201. A nurse in the postpartum unit is developing a nursing care plan for a client following cesarean delivery. The nurse documents which intervention in the plan of care that will assist in preventing thrombophlebitis?

1 Frequent ambulation
2 Applying warm moist packs to the legs
3 Remaining on bed rest with the legs elevated
4 Wearing support stockings

Answer: 1

Rationale: Stasis is believed to be a major predisposing factor in the development of thrombophlebitis. Because cesarean delivery is a risk factor for the development of thrombophlebitis, the mother should ambulate early and frequently to promote circulation and prevent stasis. Bed rest is discouraged. Warm moist packs will not prevent thrombophlebitis. Support stockings may be a helpful measure in treating thrombophlebitis.

Test-Taking Strategy: Focus on the issue of the question: to prevent thrombophlebitis. Also, use basic principles related to nursing care and the prevention of complications following any type of abdominal surgery to direct you to option 1. Remember that thrombophlebitis results from the stasis of blood. Review content related to the prevention of thrombophlebitis in the postoperative period if you had difficulty with this question.

Level of Cognitive Ability: Application
Client Needs: Physiological Integrity
Integrated Process: Nursing Process/Planning
Content Area: Maternity/Postpartum

Reference:
Lowdermilk, D., & Perry, A. (2004). *Maternity & women's health care* (8th ed.). St. Louis: Mosby, p. 1024.

---

202. A client with glomerulonephritis is at risk of developing acute renal failure. The nurse monitors the client for which sign of this complication?

1 Decreased cardiac output
2 Decreased central venous pressure
3 Hypertension
4 Bradycardia

Answer: 3

Rationale: Acute renal failure caused by glomerulonephritis is classified as intrinsic or intrarenal failure. This form of acute renal failure is commonly manifested by hypertension, tachycardia, oliguria, lethargy, edema, and other signs of fluid overload. Acute renal failure from prerenal causes is characterized by decreased blood pressure or a recent history of the same, tachycardia, and decreased cardiac output and central venous pressure. Bradycardia is not part of the clinical picture for renal failure.

Test-Taking Strategy: Use the process of elimination, focusing on the client's diagnosis. Eliminate option 4 first because bradycardia will not occur. Remember that renal failure is accompanied by fluid overload. This will help you eliminate option 2 next. From the remaining options, recall that hypertension accompanies acute renal failure resulting from intrarenal causes, whereas decreased cardiac output accompanies acute renal failure resulting from prerenal causes. Review the manifestations associated with acute renal failure if you had difficulty with this question.

Level of Cognitive Ability: Analysis
Client Needs: Physiological Integrity
Integrated Process: Nursing Process/Assessment
Content Area: Adult Health/Renal

Reference:
Ignatavicius, D., & Workman, M. (2002). *Medical surgical nursing: Critical thinking for collaborative care* (4th ed.). Philadelphia: Saunders, p. 1651.

203. A client has been prescribed metoprolol (Lopressor) for hypertension. The nurse monitors client compliance carefully because of which common side effect of the medication?
1 Increased appetite
2 Impotence
3 Difficulty swallowing
4 Mood swings

Answer: 2
Rationale: A common side effect of beta-adrenergic blocking agents, such as metoprolol, is impotence. Other common side effects include fatigue and weakness. Central nervous system side effects occur rarely and include mental status changes, nervousness, depression, and insomnia. Increased appetite, difficulty swallowing, and mood swings are not reported side effects.

Test-Taking Strategy: Focus on the medication name and recall that medication names that end with the letters "lol" are beta-adrenergic blocking agents. Next, focus on the issue, monitoring compliance, and the key words "common side effect." Remember that a common side effect of beta-adrenergic blocking agents is impotence. This will direct you to option 2. Review the expected side effects of this group of medications if you had difficulty with this question.

Level of Cognitive Ability: Analysis
Client Needs: Physiological Integrity
Integrated Process: Nursing Process/Assessment
Content Area: Pharmacology

Reference:
Hodgson, B., & Kizior, R. (2004). *Saunders nursing drug handbook 2004.* Philadelphia: Saunders, p. 665.

204. A nurse is caring for a client with cancer of the lung who is receiving chemotherapy. The nurse reviews the laboratory results and notes that the platelet count is 18,000/mm^3. Based on this laboratory result, which of the following would the nurse implement?
1 Neutropenic precautions
2 Bleeding precautions
3 Contact precautions
4 Respiratory precautions

Answer: 2
Rationale: When the platelet count is less than 20,000/mm^3, the client is at risk for bleeding, and the nurse would institute bleeding precautions. Neutropenic precautions would be instituted for a client with a low neutrophil count. Contact precautions is initiated in a client who has drainage from wounds that may be infectious. Respiratory precautions are instituted for a client with a respiratory infection that is transmitted by the airborne route.

Test-Taking Strategy: Use the process of elimination. Recalling that when the platelet count is low, the client is at risk for bleeding will direct you to option 2. Review the normal platelet count and the nursing interventions necessary when the platelet count is low if you had difficulty with this question.

Level of Cognitive Ability: Application
Client Needs: Physiological Integrity
Integrated Process: Nursing Process/Implementation
Content Area: Adult Health/Oncology

Reference:
Phipps, W., Monahan, F., Sands, J., Marek, J., & Neighbors, M. (2003). *Medical-surgical nursing: Health and illness perspectives* (7th ed.). St. Louis: Mosby, p. 831.

205. A client with a leaking intracranial aneurysm has been placed on aneurysm precautions. A visiting family member wants to take the client to the unit lounge for "just a few minutes." The nurse would use which of the following concepts when explaining why the client must remain in the room?

1 Clients with aneurysms need isolation to cope with photosensitivity.
2 Reduced environmental stimuli is needed to prevent aneurysm rupture.
3 A quiet environment promotes more rapid healing of the aneurysm.
4 The client has disturbed thought processes and needs reduced stimulation.

Answer: 2

Rationale: Subarachnoid precautions (or aneurysm precautions) are intended to minimize environmental stimuli, which could increase intracranial pressure and trigger bleeding or rupture of the aneurysm. The client does not need isolation to "cope" with photosensitivity (although photosensitivity may be a problem). The aneurysm will not heal more rapidly with reduced stimuli, and no data indicates that the client has disturbed thought processes.

Test-Taking Strategy: Focus on the issue: the purpose of aneurysm precautions. Recalling that the concern in this client is rupture will direct you to option 2. Review this content if you are unfamiliar with aneurysm precautions and their purpose.

Level of Cognitive Ability: Application
Client Needs: Psychosocial Integrity
Integrated Process: Nursing Process/Implementation
Content Area: Adult Health/Neurological

Reference:
Phipps, W., Monahan, F., Sands, J., Marek, J., & Neighbors, M. (2003). *Medical-surgical nursing: Health and illness perspectives* (7th ed.). St. Louis: Mosby, p. 1385.

206. A postoperative client is anemic from blood loss during a recent surgery. The nurse interprets that which symptom exhibited by the client is most likely associated with the anemia?

1 Bradycardia
2 Fatigue
3 Increased respiratory rate
4 Muscle cramps

Answer: 2

Rationale: The client with anemia is likely to complain of fatigue, caused by decreased ability of the body to carry oxygen to tissues to meet metabolic demands. The client is likely to have tachycardia, not bradycardia because of efforts by the body to compensate for the effects of anemia. Increased respiratory rate is not an associated finding, although some clients may have shortness of breath. Muscle cramps are an unrelated finding.

Test-Taking Strategy: Use the process of elimination, focusing on the issue: the symptoms associated with anemia. Recalling that anemia causes a reduction in the oxygen-carrying capacity to the tissues will direct you to option 2. Review the manifestations associated with anemia if you had difficulty with this question.

Level of Cognitive Ability: Analysis
Client Needs: Physiological Integrity
Integrated Process: Nursing Process/Analysis
Content Area: Fundamental Skills

References:
Black, J., & Hawks, J. (2005). *Medical-surgical nursing: Clinical management for positive outcomes* (7th ed.). Philadelphia: Saunders, pp. 2273; 2280; 2282.
Phipps, W., Monahan, F., Sands, J., Marek, J., & Neighbors, M. (2003). *Medical-surgical nursing: Health and illness perspectives* (7th ed.). St. Louis: Mosby, p. 816.

207. A nurse employed in a rehabilitation center is planning the client assignments for the day. Which client would the nurse assign to the nursing assistant?
1 A client who had a below-the-knee amputation
2 A client on a 24-hour urine collection who is also on strict bed rest
3 A client scheduled for transfer to the hospital for coronary artery bypass surgery
4 A client scheduled for transfer to the hospital for an invasive diagnostic procedure

Answer: 2
Rationale: The nurse must assign tasks based on the guidelines of Nursing Practice Acts and the job description of the employing agency. A client who had a below-the-knee amputation, a client scheduled to be transferred to the hospital for coronary artery bypass surgery, and a client scheduled for an invasive diagnostic procedure will require both physiological and psychosocial needs. The nursing assistant has been trained to care for a client on bed rest and on urine collections. The nurse would provide instructions to the nursing assistant regarding the tasks, but the tasks required for this client are within the role description of a nursing assistant.

Test-Taking Strategy: Note that the question asks for the assignment to be delegated to the nursing assistant. When asked questions related to delegation, think about the role description of the employee and the client needs. This will direct you to option 2. Review the responsibilities related to delegation and the job description of the nursing assistant if you had difficulty with this question.

Level of Cognitive Ability: Application
Client Needs: Safe, Effective Care Environment
Integrated Process: Nursing Process/Planning
Content Area: Delegating/Prioritizing

Reference:
Potter, P., & Perry, A. (2005). *Fundamentals of nursing* (6th ed.). St. Louis: Mosby, pp. 378-380.

---

208. A nurse is in the room with a client when a seizure begins. The client's entire body becomes rigid, and the muscles in all four extremities alternate between relaxation and contraction. Following the seizure, the nurse documents that the client has experienced a(n):
1 Absence seizure
2 Tonic-clonic seizure
3 Partial seizure
4 Complex partial seizure

Answer: 2
Rationale: Tonic-clonic seizures are characterized by body rigidity (tonic phase) followed by rhythmic jerky contraction and relaxation of all body muscles, especially those of the extremities (clonic phase). There are two types of complex partial seizures: complex partial seizures with automatisms and partial seizures evolving into generalized seizures. Complex partial seizures with automatisms include purposeless repetitive activities such as lip smacking, chewing, or patting the body. Partial seizures evolving into a generalized seizure begin locally and then spread through the body. Absence seizures are characterized by a sudden lapse of consciousness for approximately 2 to 10 seconds and a blank facial expression.

Test-Taking Strategy: Use the process of elimination. Eliminate options 3 and 4 first because they are similar. From the remaining options, focus on the characteristics of the seizure in the question and recall that no convulsion occurs in an absence seizure. This will direct you to option 2. Review the characteristics of the various types of seizures if you had difficulty with this question.

Level of Cognitive Ability: Analysis
Client Needs: Physiological Integrity
Integrated Process: Communication and Documentation
Content Area: Adult Health/Neurological

References:
Black, J., & Hawks, J. (2005). *Medical-surgical nursing: Clinical management for positive outcomes* (7th ed.). Philadelphia: Saunders, pp. 2075-2076.
Phipps, W., Monahan, F., Sands, J., Marek, J., & Neighbors, M. (2003). *Medical-surgical nursing: Health and illness perspectives* (7th ed.). St. Louis: Mosby, p. 1339.

209. A nurse is reviewing the nursing care plan for a client with a right cerebrovascular accident (CVA) who has left-sided deficits. The nurse notes a nursing diagnosis of Unilateral Neglect. The nurse would tell a family member who is assisting the client that it would be least helpful to do which of the following?
1 Approach the client from the right side
2 Teach the client to scan the environment
3 Move the commode and chair to the left side
4 Place bedside articles on the left side

Answer: 1
Rationale: Unilateral neglect is an unawareness of the paralyzed side of the body, which increases the client's risk for injury. The nurse's role is to refocus the client's attention to the affected side. Personal care items, belongings, a bedside chair, and a commode are all placed on the affected side. The client is taught to scan the environment to become aware of that half of the body and is approached on that side by family and caregivers as well.

Test-Taking Strategy: Use the process of elimination, noting the key words "left-sided deficits" and "unilateral neglect." Eliminate options 3 and 4 first because they are similar. From the remaining options, note the key words "least helpful." These words indicate a false-response question and that you need to select the incorrect intervention. This will direct you to option 1. Review care of the client with unilateral neglect if you had difficulty with this question.

Level of Cognitive Ability: Application
Client Needs: Safe, Effective Care Environment
Integrated Process: Nursing Process/Implementation
Content Area: Adult Health/Neurological

Reference:
Black, J., & Hawks, J. (2005). *Medical-surgical nursing: Clinical management for positive outcomes* (7th ed.). Philadelphia: Saunders, pp. 2115; 2131.

210. A nurse is evaluating the status of a client with myasthenia gravis. The nurse interprets that the client's medication regime may not be optimal if the client continues to experience fatigue that occurs:
1 Before meals and at the end of the day
2 Early in the morning and late in the day
3 Following exertion and at the end of the day
4 Early in the morning and before lunch

Answer: 3
Rationale: The client with myasthenia gravis has weakness after periods of exertion and near the end of the day. Medication therapy should assist in alleviating the weakness. The medication regime may not be optimal if the client continues to experience fatigue. The nurse also works with the client to space out activities to conserve energy and regain muscle strength by resting between activities. The client is also instructed to take medication as prescribed.

Test-Taking Strategy: Note the key words "may not be optimal if the client continues to experience fatigue." Also remember that when an option has two parts, both parts of the option must be correct in order for the option to be the correct answer. Remember that clients with any form of chronic condition characterized by fatigue experience the greatest amount of fatigue after exertion and at the end of the day. With this global concept in mind, eliminate options 1, 2, and 4. Review care of the client with myasthenia gravis if you had difficulty with this question.

Level of Cognitive Ability: Analysis
Client Needs: Physiological Integrity
Integrated Process: Nursing Process/Evaluation
Content Area: Adult Health/Neurological

Reference:
Phipps, W., Monahan, F., Sands, J., Marek, J., & Neighbors, M. (2003). *Medical-surgical nursing: Health and illness perspectives* (7th ed.). St. Louis: Mosby, p. 1399.

---

211. A nurse has just been told by a physician that an order has been written to administer an iron injection to an adult client. The nurse plans to administer the medication in which of the following locations?
1 In the gluteal muscle using Z-track technique
2 In the deltoid muscle using an air lock
3 In the subcutaneous tissue of the abdomen
4 In the anterolateral thigh using a 5/8-inch needle

Answer: 1
Rationale: The correct technique for administering parenteral iron is deep in the gluteal muscle using Z-track technique. This method minimizes the possibility that the injection will stain the skin a dark color. The medication is not given by the subcutaneous route (options 3 and 4), nor is it given in the arms, abdomen, or thighs (options 2, 3, 4). An air lock should not be used.

Test-Taking Strategy: Use principles of medication administration by the parenteral route and focus on the issue: an iron injection. Eliminate options 3 and 4 because they both indicate administering the medication by the subcutaneous route. From the remaining options, recalling that iron stains the skin will direct you to option 1. Review the procedure for the administration of iron if you had difficulty with this question.

Level of Cognitive Ability: Application
Client Needs: Physiological Integrity
Integrated Process: Nursing Process/Planning
Content Area: Fundamental Skills

Reference:
Hodgson, B., & Kizior, R. (2004). *Saunders nursing drug handbook 2004.* Philadelphia: Saunders, p. 557.

---

212. A client who has never had gastric surgery is diagnosed with pernicious anemia. The nurse reviews the client's health history for disorders involving which organ responsible for vitamin B_{12} absorption?
1 Stomach
2 Duodenum
3 Ileum
4 Colon

Answer: 3
Rationale: Pernicious anemia can occur in a client who has not had gastric surgery, such as when the client has a disease that involves the ileum, where vitamin B_{12} is absorbed. The nurse checks the client's history for small bowel disorders to detect this risk factor.

Test-Taking Strategy: Focus on the issue: vitamin B_{12} absorption. Recalling that vitamin B_{12} is absorbed in the small intestine will direct you to option 3. Review the physiology associated with the gastrointestinal tract if you had difficulty with this question.

Level of Cognitive Ability: Application
Client Needs: Physiological Integrity
Integrated Process: Nursing Process/Assessment
Content Area: Fundamental Skills

Reference:
Black, J., & Hawks, J. (2005). *Medical-surgical nursing: Clinical management for positive outcomes* (7th ed.). Philadelphia: Saunders, pp. 2289-2290.

213. A client had a positive Papanicolaou smear and underwent cryosurgery with laser therapy. The nurse would provide the client with which piece of information before letting the client go home?
1 There should be no odor or vaginal discharge.
2 Vaginal discharge should be clear and watery.
3 Sitz baths are soothing to the irritated tissues.
4 Pain can be relieved with narcotic analgesics.

Answer: 2
Rationale: Cryosurgery is a procedure that involves freezing cervical tissues. Vaginal discharge should be clear and watery following the procedure. The client will then begin to slough off dead cell debris, which may be odorous. This resolves within approximately 8 weeks. Tub and sitz baths are avoided while the area is healing, which takes about 10 weeks. There is mild pain following the procedure, and narcotic analgesics would not be required.

Test-Taking Strategy: Specific knowledge about the purpose and effects of this procedure is needed to answer the question. Review this surgical procedure and the client teaching points if you had difficulty with this question.

Level of Cognitive Ability: Application
Client Needs: Physiological Integrity
Integrated Process: Teaching/Learning
Content Area: Adult Health/Oncology

Reference:
Black, J., & Hawks, J. (2005). *Medical-surgical nursing: Clinical management for positive outcomes* (7th ed.). Philadelphia: Saunders, p. 1076.

---

214. A nurse is planning to do preoperative teaching with a client scheduled for a transurethral resection of the prostate (TURP). The nurse plans to include in the discussion that the most frequent cause of postoperative pain will be:
1 The lower abdominal incision
2 Bleeding within the bladder
3 Bladder spasms
4 Tension on the Foley catheter

Answer: 3
Rationale: Bladder spasms can occur after this surgery because of postoperative bladder distention or irritation from the balloon on the indwelling urinary catheter. The nurse administers antispasmodic medications, such as belladonna and opium, to treat this type of pain. There is no incision with a TURP (option 1). Options 2 and 4 are not frequent causes of pain. Some surgeons purposefully apply tension to the catheter for a few hours postoperatively to control bleeding.

Test-Taking Strategy: Use the process of elimination, focusing on the surgical procedure. Eliminate option 1, knowing that there is no incision with this procedure. Eliminate options 2 and 4 because they are unrelated to the cause of pain. Review the causes of pain following this type of surgery if you had difficulty with this question.

Level of Cognitive Ability: Application
Client Needs: Physiological Integrity
Integrated Process: Nursing Process/Planning
Content Area: Adult Health/Renal

Reference:
Phipps, W., Monahan, F., Sands, J., Marek, J., & Neighbors, M. (2003). *Medical-surgical nursing: Health and illness perspectives* (7th ed.). St. Louis: Mosby, p. 1835.

215. A client with gastroesophageal reflux disease (GERD) has just received a breakfast tray. The nurse setting up the tray for the client notices that which of the following foods is the only one that will increase the lower esophageal sphincter (LES) pressure and thus lessen the client's symptoms?
1 Fresh scrambled eggs
2 Nonfat milk
3 Whole wheat toast with butter
4 Coffee

Answer: 2
Rationale: Foods that increase the LES pressure will decrease reflux and lessen the symptoms of GERD. The food substance that will increase the LES pressure is nonfat milk. The other substances listed decrease the LES pressure, thus increasing reflux symptoms. Aggravating substances include chocolate, coffee, fatty foods, and alcohol and should be avoided in the diet of a client with GERD.

Test-Taking Strategy: Use the process of elimination and recall the effect of various food substances on LES pressure and GERD. Also, noting the word "nonfat" in option 2 will assist in directing you to this option. Review this content if you are unfamiliar with the LES pressure and the foods that will increase this pressure.

Level of Cognitive Ability: Analysis
Client Needs: Physiological Integrity
Integrated Process: Nursing Process/Analysis
Content Area: Adult Health/Gastrointestinal

Reference:
Phipps, W., Monahan, F., Sands, J., Marek, J., & Neighbors, M. (2003). *Medical-surgical nursing: Health and illness perspectives* (7th ed.). St. Louis: Mosby, p. 1010.

216. A nurse is reviewing the serum laboratory test results for a client with sickle cell anemia. The nurse anticipates finding that which of the following values is elevated?
1 Hemoglobin F
2 Hemoglobin S
3 Hemoglobin C
4 Hemoglobin A1

Answer: 2
Rationale: Sickle cell anemia is a severe anemia that predominantly affects African Americans. It is characterized by the presence of only hemoglobin S. The client must have two abnormal genes yielding hemoglobin S to have sickle cell anemia. A client could have sickle cell trait by carrying one hemoglobin A gene and one hemoglobin S gene. Options 1, 3, and 4 are unrelated to sickle cell anemia.

Test-Taking Strategy: To answer this question accurately, you must know the pathophysiology of sickle cell anemia and how it is reflected in common laboratory studies. If needed, review the pathophysiology of sickle cell anemia.

Level of Cognitive Ability: Analysis
Client Needs: Physiological Integrity
Integrated Process: Nursing Process/Assessment
Content Area: Fundamental Skills

Reference:
Phipps, W., Monahan, F., Sands, J., Marek, J., & Neighbors, M. (2003). *Medical-surgical nursing: Health and illness perspectives* (7th ed.). St. Louis: Mosby, p. 820.

217. A client wishes to donate blood for a family member for an upcoming surgery and asks the nurse, "How will I know if our blood types will match?" In formulating a response, the nurse incorporates that which test will be used to test compatibility?
1 Eosinophil count
2 Monocyte count
3 Direct Coombs'
4 Indirect Coombs'

Answer: 4
Rationale: The indirect Coombs' test detects circulating antibodies against red blood cells (RBCs) and is the "screening" component of the order to "type and screen" a client's blood. This test is used in addition to the ABO typing, which is normally done to determine blood type. The direct Coombs' test is used to detect idiopathic hemolytic anemia by detecting the presence of autoantibodies against the client's RBCs. Eosinophil and monocyte counts are part of a complete blood count, a routine hematologic screening test.

Test-Taking Strategy: Use the process of elimination. Eliminate options 1 and 2 because they are part of routine laboratory work. From the remaining options, it is necessary to know the difference between the two tests. Review the purpose of the direct and indirect Coombs' test if you had difficulty with this question.

Level of Cognitive Ability: Analysis
Client Needs: Physiological Integrity
Integrated Process: Nursing Process/Implementation
Content Area: Fundamental Skills

Reference:
Chernecky, C., & Berger, B. (2004). *Laboratory tests and diagnostic procedures* (4th ed.). Philadelphia: Saunders, p. 412.

---

218. A client is being discharged to home after undergoing a transurethral prostatectomy (TURP). The nurse teaches the client to expect which variation in normal urine color for several days following the procedure?
1 Clear yellow
2 Cloudy amber
3 Pink-tinged
4 Dark red

Answer: 3
Rationale: The client should expect that the urine will be pink-tinged for several days following this procedure. Dark red urine may be present initially, especially with inadequate bladder irrigation, and if it occurs, it must be corrected. Options 1 and 2 are incorrect because urine of these colors is not generally expected for several days following surgery.

Test-Taking Strategy: Note the issue: a client being discharged to home after a TURP. Eliminate options 1 and 2 first because they are similar. From the remaining options, focus on the issue to direct you to option 3. Review assessment of the urine for the client who has had this type of surgery if you had difficulty with this question.

Level of Cognitive Ability: Application
Client Needs: Health Promotion and Maintenance
Integrated Process: Teaching/Learning
Content Area: Adult Health/Renal

Reference:
Phipps, W., Monahan, F., Sands, J., Marek, J., & Neighbors, M. (2003). *Medical-surgical nursing: Health and illness perspectives* (7th ed.). St. Louis: Mosby, p. 1835.

---

219. A client is admitted to the hospital with sickle cell crisis. The nurse monitors this client for which most frequent symptom of the disorder?
1 Bradycardia
2 Pain
3 Diarrhea
4 Blurred vision

Answer: 2
Rationale: Sickle cell crisis often causes pain in the bones and joints, accompanied by joint swelling. Pain is a classic symptom and may require large doses of narcotic analgesics when it is severe. The symptoms listed in the other options are not associated with sickle cell crisis.

Test-Taking Strategy: Note the client's diagnosis. Recalling that the primary treatment of sickle cell crisis focuses on the administration of fluids and on pain management will direct you to option 2. Review the manifestations associated with sickle cell crisis if you had difficulty with this question.

Level of Cognitive Ability: Application
Client Needs: Physiological Integrity

Integrated Process: Nursing Process/Assessment
Content Area: Fundamental Skills

Reference:
Black, J., & Hawks, J. (2005). *Medical-surgical nursing: Clinical management for positive outcomes* (7th ed.). Philadelphia: Saunders, pp. 2295-2298.

---

220. Quinidine gluconate (Duraquin) is prescribed for a client. The nurse reviews the client's medical record, knowing that which of the following is a contraindication in the use of this medication?
1 Complete atrioventricular (AV) block
2 Muscle weakness
3 Asthma
4 Infection

Answer: 1
Rationale: Quinidine gluconate is an antidysrhythmic medication used as prophylactic therapy to maintain normal sinus rhythm after conversion of atrial fibrillation and/or atrial flutter. It is contraindicated in complete AV block, intraventricular conduction defects, abnormal impulses and rhythms caused by escape mechanisms, and in myasthenia gravis. It is used with caution in clients with preexisting asthma, muscle weakness, infection with fever, and hepatic or renal insufficiency.

Test-Taking Strategy: Note the key word "contraindication." Recalling that this medication is an antidysrhythmic medication and has a direct cardiac effect will direct you to option 1. Review this content if you are unfamiliar with this medication and its contraindications.

Level of Cognitive Ability: Analysis
Client Needs: Physiological Integrity
Integrated Process: Nursing Process/Analysis
Content Area: Pharmacology

Reference:
Hodgson, B., & Kizior, R. (2004). *Saunders nursing drug handbook 2004.* Philadelphia: Saunders, p. 865.

---

221. A client with a ruptured intracranial aneurysm has surgery delayed and is still maintained on bed rest with subarachnoid precautions in place. The nurse should question an order for which of the following medications if prescribed for this client?
1 Aminocaproic acid (Amicar)
2 Heparin sodium (Heparin)
3 Nimodipine (Nimotop)
4 Docusate sodium (Colace)

Answer: 2
Rationale: The nurse should question an order for heparin sodium, which is an anticoagulant. This medication could place the client at risk for rebleeding. Aminocaproic acid is an antifibrinolytic agent that prevents clot breakdown or dissolution. It may be prescribed after ruptured intracranial aneurysm and subarachnoid hemorrhage if surgery is delayed or contraindicated. Nimodipine is a calcium-channel blocking agent that is useful in the management of vasospasm associated with cerebral hemorrhage. Docusate sodium is a stool softener, which helps prevent straining. Straining would raise intracranial pressure.

Test-Taking Strategy: Use the process of elimination. Noting the key word "ruptured" in the question suggests that hemorrhage is occurring. It makes sense, knowing the action of heparin sodium, that this medication would be contraindicated. Review care of the client with a ruptured intracranial aneurysm if you had difficulty with this question.

Level of Cognitive Ability: Application
Client Needs: Safe, Effective Care Environment
Integrated Process: Nursing Process/Implementation
Content Area: Adult Health/Neurological

References:

Black, J., & Hawks, J. (2005). *Medical-surgical nursing: Clinical management for positive outcomes* (7th ed.). Philadelphia: Saunders, p. 2095.

Phipps, W., Monahan, F., Sands, J., Marek, J., & Neighbors, M. (2003). *Medical-surgical nursing: health and illness perspectives* (7th ed.). St. Louis: Mosby, p. 1385.

---

222. A client who has a history of chronic ulcerative colitis is diagnosed with anemia. The nurse interprets that which factor is most likely responsible for the anemia?
  1 Decreased intake of dietary iron
  2 Intestinal malabsorption
  3 Blood loss
  4 Intestinal hookworm

Answer: 3

Rationale: The client with ulcerative colitis is most likely anemic as a result of chronic blood loss in small amounts that occurs with exacerbations of the disease. These clients often have bloody stools and are at increased risk for anemia. There is no information in the question to support options 1 or 4. In ulcerative colitis, the large intestine is involved, not the small intestine where vitamin B_{12} and folic acid are absorbed (option 2).

Test-Taking Strategy: Note the issue: the cause of the anemia. Focusing on the client's diagnosis and recalling the pathophysiology that occurs in this disorder will direct you to option 3. Review the manifestations in ulcerative colitis if you had difficulty with this question.

Level of Cognitive Ability: Analysis
Client Needs: Physiological Integrity
Integrated Process: Nursing Process/Analysis
Content Area: Adult Health/Gastrointestinal

Reference:

Black, J., & Hawks, J. (2005). *Medical-surgical nursing: Clinical management for positive outcomes* (7th ed.). Philadelphia: Saunders, p. 815.

---

223. A physician has prescribed nimodipine (Nimotop) for a client with subarachnoid hemorrhage. The nurse administering the first dose tells the client that this medication is a:
  1 Calcium-channel blocker used to decrease the blood pressure
  2 Calcium-channel blocker used to decrease cerebral blood vessel spasm
  3 Beta-adrenergic blocker used to decrease blood pressure
  4 Vasodilator that has an affinity for cerebral blood vessels

Answer: 2

Rationale: Nimodipine is a calcium-channel blocking agent that has an affinity for cerebral blood vessels. It is used to prevent or control vasospasm in cerebral blood vessels, thereby reducing the chance for rebleeding of the aneurysm. Options 1, 3, and 4 are incorrect.

Test-Taking Strategy: Use the process of elimination. Recalling that nimodipine is a calcium-channel blocking agent (ends with the suffix "-pine") helps you eliminate options 3 and 4. Recalling that calcium-channel blockers decrease vasospasm helps you select option 2 from the remaining options. Review the action of this medication if you had difficulty with this question.

Level of Cognitive Ability: Application
Client Needs: Physiological Integrity
Integrated Process: Nursing Process/Implementation
Content Area: Adult Health/Neurological

Reference:

Hodgson, B., & Kizior, R. (2004). *Saunders nursing drug handbook 2004.* Philadelphia: Saunders, p. 730.

224. A nurse is monitoring a client who is receiving a blood transfusion. The client begins to complain of a sweaty and warm feeling and a backache. The nurse notes that the client's skin is flushed and suspects that the client is having a transfusion reaction. The nurse immediately stops the blood transfusion and then:

1 Discontinues the intravenous (IV) line
2 Changes the continuous IV to an intermittent needle device
3 Hangs an IV bag of 5% dextrose in water
4 Hang an IV bag of normal saline

Answer: 4

Rationale: If a transfusion reaction is suspected, the transfusion is stopped and then normal saline is infused pending further physician orders. This maintains a patent IV access line and aids in maintaining the client's intravascular volume. The IV line would not be discontinued because there would be no IV access route. Normal saline is the solution of choice over solutions containing dextrose because saline does not cause clumping of red blood cells.

Test-Taking Strategy: Use the process of elimination and knowledge regarding blood transfusions to answer the question. Recalling that normal saline is the solution that is compatible with blood will direct you to option 4. Review interventions if a blood transfusion occurs if you had difficulty with this question.

Level of Cognitive Ability: Application
Client Needs: Physiological Integrity
Integrated Process: Nursing Process/Implementation
Content Area: Fundamental Skills

Reference:
Lewis, S., Heitkemper, M., & Dirksen, S. (2004). *Medical-surgical nursing: Assessment and management of clinical problems* (6th ed.). St. Louis: Mosby, p. 747.

---

225. A client has been taking lisinopril (Prinivil) for 3 months. The client complains to the nurse of a persistent dry cough that began about 1 month ago. The nurse interprets that this is most likely:

1 Caused by a concurrent upper respiratory infection
2 Caused by neutropenia as a result of therapy
3 An expected, though bothersome, side effect of therapy
4 An indication that the client will show signs of heart failure

Answer: 3

Rationale: A frequent side effect of therapy with any of the angiotensin-converting enzyme (ACE) inhibitors, such as lisinopril, is the appearance of a persistent, dry cough. The cough generally does not improve while the client is taking the medication. Clients are advised to notify the physician if the cough becomes very troublesome to them. The other options are incorrect.

Test-Taking Strategy: Use the process of elimination. Eliminate options 1 and 2 first because they are similar and focus on infection. From the remaining options, it is necessary to know the frequent side effects of this medication to direct you to option 3. Review the side effects of ACE inhibitor therapy if you had difficulty with this question.

Level of Cognitive Ability: Analysis
Client Needs: Physiological Integrity
Integrated Process: Nursing Process/Analysis
Content Area: Pharmacology

Reference:
McKenry, L., & Salerno, E. (2003). *Mosby's pharmacology in nursing* (21st ed.). St. Louis: Mosby, p. 586.

226. A client has been given a prescription to begin using nitroglycerin transdermal patches in the management of angina pectoris. The nurse instructs the client about this medication administration system and tells the client to:
1 Apply a new system every 7 days
2 Apply the system in the morning and leave it in place for 12 to 16 hours as directed
3 Place the system in the area of a skin fold to promote better adherence
4 Wait 1 day to apply a new system if it becomes dislodged

Answer: 2
Rationale: Nitroglycerin is a coronary vasodilator used in the management of coronary artery disease. The client is generally advised to apply a new system each morning and leave it in place for 12 to 16 hours as per physician directions. This prevents the client from developing tolerance (as happens with 24-hour use). The client should avoid placing the system in skin folds or excoriated areas. The client can apply a new system if it becomes dislodged because the dose is released continuously in small amounts through the skin.

Test-Taking Strategy: Specific information related to this type of medication administration system is needed to answer this question. Recalling that tolerance can occur with this medication will direct you to option 2. Review the procedures related to transdermal medication systems if you had difficulty with this question.

Level of Cognitive Ability: Application
Client Needs: Physiological Integrity
Integrated Process: Teaching/Learning
Content Area: Pharmacology

References:
Hodgson, B., & Kizior, R. (2004). *Saunders nursing drug handbook 2004.* Philadelphia: Saunders, p. 735.
McKenry, L., & Salerno, E. (2003). *Mosby's pharmacology in nursing* (21st ed.). St. Louis: Mosby, p. 611.

---

227. A nurse is visiting a client who has been started on therapy with clotrimazole (Lotrimin). The nurse tells the client that this medication will alleviate:
1 Sneezing
2 Rash
3 Fever
4 Pain

Answer: 2
Rationale: Clotrimazole is a topical antifungal used in the treatment of cutaneous fungal infections. The nurse teaches the client that it is used for this purpose. It is not used for sneezing, fever, or pain.

Test-Taking Strategy: Focus on the name of the medication. Recalling that this medication is an antifungal will direct you to option 2. Review the purpose of this antiinfective if you had difficulty with this question.

Level of Cognitive Ability: Application
Client Needs: Physiological Integrity
Integrated Process: Teaching/Learning
Content Area: Pharmacology

Reference:
Hodgson, B., & Kizior, R. (2004). *Saunders nursing drug handbook 2004.* Philadelphia: Saunders, p. 235.

228. A nurse is providing care to the client who has received medication therapy with tissue plasminogen activator (t-PA, Activase). As part of standard nursing care for this client, the nurse plans to have which item available for use?

1 Pulse oximeter
2 Suction equipment
3 Flashlight
4 Occult blood test strips

Answer: 4

Rationale: Tissue plasminogen activator is a thrombolytic medication that is used to dissolve thrombi or emboli caused by thrombus. A frequent and potentially adverse effect of therapy is bleeding. The nurse monitors for signs of bleeding in clients receiving this therapy. Equipment needed by the nurse would include occult blood test strips to monitor for occult blood in the urine, stool, or nasogastric drainage. Pulse oximeter and suction equipment would be needed if the client had evidence of respiratory problems. A flashlight may be used for pupil assessment as part of the neurological exam in the client who is neurologically impaired.

Test-Taking Strategy: Focus on the name of the medication. Recalling that this medication is a thrombolytic and that bleeding is an adverse effect of this therapy will direct you to option 4. Review this medication and its adverse effects if you had difficulty with this question.

Level of Cognitive Ability: Application
Client Needs: Physiological Integrity
Integrated Process: Nursing Process/Planning
Content Area: Pharmacology

Reference:
Hodgson, B., & Kizior, R. (2004). *Saunders nursing drug handbook 2004.* Philadelphia: Saunders, p. 33.

229. A client newly diagnosed with angina pectoris has taken two sublingual nitroglycerin tablets for chest pain. The chest pain is relieved, but the client complains of a headache. The nurse interprets that this symptom most likely represents:

1 An allergic reaction to the nitroglycerin
2 An expected side effect of the medication
3 An early sign of medication tolerance
4 A warning that the medication should not be used again

Answer: 2

Rationale: Headache is a frequent side effect of nitroglycerin, because of the vasodilating action of the medication. It usually diminishes in frequency as the client becomes accustomed to the medication and is effectively treated with acetaminophen (Tylenol). The other options are incorrect.

Test-Taking Strategy: Use the process of elimination. Eliminate options 1 and 4 because they are similar and imply that the medication can no longer be used by the client. From the remaining options, recalling that the medication vasodilates will direct you to option 2. Review the effect of this medication if you had difficulty with question.

Level of Cognitive Ability: Analysis
Client Needs: Physiological Integrity
Integrated Process: Nursing Process/Analysis
Content Area: Pharmacology

Reference:
Hodgson, B., & Kizior, R. (2004). *Saunders nursing drug handbook 2004.* Philadelphia: Saunders, p. 735.

230. A nurse is caring for a client with atrial fibrillation. The physician has prescribed verapamil (Calan) 5 mg intravenously (IV). The nurse ensures that which most essential item is present when the administering this medication?
1 Pulse oximeter
2 Oxygen
3 Noninvasive blood pressure monitor
4 Cardiac monitor

Answer: 4
Rationale: Verapamil is a calcium-channel blocking agent that may be used to treat rapid-rate supraventricular tachydysrhythmias, such as atrial flutter or atrial fibrillation. The client must be placed on a cardiac monitor to evaluate the effectiveness of the medication. A noninvasive blood pressure monitor is also helpful but is not as essential as the cardiac monitor. Pulse oximeter and oxygen are related to respiratory care, and although they should be available, they are not directly related to the use of this medication.

Test-Taking Strategy: Note the key words "most essential." Eliminate options 1 and 2 first because there is no information about respiratory difficulty in the case situation. From the remaining options, noting the client's diagnosis will direct you to option 4. Review nursing interventions related to the administration of this medication if you had difficulty with this question.

Level of Cognitive Ability: Application
Client Needs: Physiological Integrity
Integrated Process: Nursing Process/Planning
Content Area: Pharmacology

Reference:
Hodgson, B., & Kizior, R. (2004). *Saunders nursing drug handbook 2004.* Philadelphia: Saunders, p. 1047.

---

231. A client is taking albuterol (Ventolin) by inhalation but cannot cough up secretions. The nurse teaches the client to do which of the following to best help clear the bronchial secretions?
1 Administer an extra dose before bedtime
2 Take in increased amounts of fluids every day
3 Get more exercise each day
4 Use a dehumidifier in the home

Answer: 2
Rationale: The client should take in increased fluids (2000 to 3000 mL/day unless contraindicated) to make secretions less viscous. This may help the client to expectorate secretions. This is standard advice given to clients receiving any of the adrenergic bronchodilators, such as albuterol, unless the client has another health problem that could be worsened by increased fluid intake. A dehumidifier will dry secretions. The client would not be advised to take additional medication. Additional exercise will not effectively clear bronchial secretions.

Test-Taking Strategy: Focus on the issue: clearing bronchial secretions. Use general guidelines related to administering medication to eliminate option 1. Next eliminate option 4, recalling that a dehumidifier will dry secretions. From the remaining options, recalling basic respiratory principles will direct you to option 2. Review client teaching points related to this medication if you had difficulty with this question.

Level of Cognitive Ability: Application
Client Needs: Health Promotion and Maintenance
Integrated Process: Teaching/Learning
Content Area: Pharmacology

Reference:
McKenry, L., & Salerno, E. (2003). *Mosby's pharmacology in nursing* (21st ed.). St. Louis: Mosby, p. 716.

232. A nurse reviews the serum laboratory results for a client taking chlorothiazide (Diuril). The nurse specifically monitors for which of the following most frequent medication side effects on a regular basis?
1 Hyperphosphatemia
2 Hypocalcemia
3 Hypernatremia
4 Hypokalemia

Answer: 4
Rationale: The client taking a potassium-wasting diuretic such as chlorothiazide (Diuril) needs to be monitored for decreased potassium levels. Other fluid and electrolyte imbalances that occur with the use of this medication include hyponatremia, hypercalcemia, hypomagnesemia, and hypophosphatemia.

Test-Taking Strategy: Focus on the name of the medication and recall that this medication is a potassium-wasting diuretic. Remember that hypokalemia is a concern when a client is taking a potassium-wasting diuretic. Review the side effects of this medication if you had difficulty with this medication.

Level of Cognitive Ability: Application
Client Needs: Physiological Integrity
Integrated Process: Nursing Process/Assessment
Content Area: Pharmacology

Reference:
McKenry, L., & Salerno, E. (2003). *Mosby's pharmacology in nursing* (21st ed.). St. Louis: Mosby, 673.

---

233. A nurse has administered a dose of diazepam (Valium) to the client. The nurse would take which most important action before leaving the client's room?
1 Draw the shades closed
2 Put up the side rails on the bed
3 Give the client a bedpan
4 Turn the volume on the television set down

Answer: 2
Rationale: Diazepam is a sedative/hypnotic with anticonvulsant and skeletal muscle relaxant properties. The nurse should institute safety measures before leaving the client's room to ensure that the client does not injure self. The most frequent side effects of this medication are dizziness, drowsiness, and lethargy. For this reason, the nurse puts the side rails up on the bed before leaving the room to prevent falls. Options 1, 3, and 4 may be helpful measures that provide a comfortable, restful environment. However, option 2 provides for the client's safety needs.

Test-Taking Strategy: Note the key words "most important" and "before leaving the client's room." Recalling that diazepam is a sedative/hypnotic and that safety is an issue will direct you to option 2. Review care of the client receiving this medication if you had difficulty with this question.

Level of Cognitive Ability: Application
Client Needs: Safe, Effective Care Environment
Integrated Process: Nursing Process/Implementation
Content Area: Pharmacology

Reference:
Hodgson, B., & Kizior, R. (2004). *Saunders nursing drug handbook 2004*. Philadelphia: Saunders, pp. 298; 1092.

234. A nurse provides home care instructions to a client who is taking lithium carbonate (Eskalith). Which statement by the client indicates a need for further instructions?
1 "My blood levels must be monitored very closely."
2 "I need to withhold the medication if I have excessive diarrhea, vomiting, or diaphoresis."
3 "I need to take the lithium with meals."
4 "I need to decrease my salt and fluid intake while taking the lithium."

Answer: 4
Rationale: Because therapeutic and toxic dosage ranges are so close, lithium blood levels must be monitored very closely, more frequently at first, then once every several months after that. The client should be instructed to withhold the medication if excessive diarrhea, vomiting, or diaphoresis occurs, and to inform the physician if any of these problems occur. Lithium is irritating to the gastric mucosa; therefore, lithium should be taken with meals. A normal diet and normal salt and fluid intake (1500 to 3000 mL per day) should be maintained because lithium decreases sodium reabsorption by the renal tubules, which could cause sodium depletion. A low-sodium intake causes a relative increase in lithium retention and could lead to toxicity.

Test-Taking Strategy: Note the key words "need for further instructions." These words indicate a false-response question and that you need to select the incorrect client statement. Remember that, generally, it is important that clients be taught to maintain an adequate fluid intake. This principle will direct you to option 4. Review the client teaching points related to the administration of this medication if you had difficulty with this question.

Level of Cognitive Ability: Analysis
Client Needs: Health Promotion and Maintenance
Integrated Process: Teaching/Learning
Content Area: Pharmacology

Reference:
Hodgson, B., & Kizior, R. (2004). *Saunders nursing drug handbook 2004.* Philadelphia: Saunders, p. 608.

235. A client is brought to the emergency room following a severe burn caused by a fire at home. The burns are extensive, covering greater than 25% of the total body surface area (TBSA). The nurse reviews the laboratory results drawn on the client and would most likely expect to note which of the following?
1 White blood cell (WBC) count 6,000/ul
2 Hematocrit 65%
3 Albumin 4.0g/dL
4 Sodium 140 mEq/L

Answer: 2
Rationale: Extensive burns covering greater than 25% of the TBSA result in generalized body edema in both burned and nonburned tissues and a decrease in circulating intravascular blood volume. Hematocrit levels elevate in the first 24 hours post-injury as a result of hemoconcentration from the loss of intravascular fluid. The normal WBC count is 5,000 to 10,000/ul. The normal sodium level is 135 to145 mEq/L. The normal albumin is 3.4 to 5 g/dL. The normal hematocrit is 40% to 54% in the male and 38% to 47% in the female.

Test-Taking Strategy: Use the process of elimination and knowledge regarding physiological alterations and fluid and electrolyte balance during the first 24 hours post-injury of a burn client. Note that the only abnormal laboratory value is option 2, the hematocrit. Review normal laboratory values and the immediate post-injury period of burns if you had difficulty with this question.

Level of Cognitive Ability: Analysis
Client Needs: Physiological Integrity
Integrated Process: Nursing Process/Analysis
Content Area: Adult Health/Integumentary

Reference:
Lewis, S., Heitkemper, M., & Dirksen, S. (2004). *Medical-surgical nursing: Assessment and management of clinical problems* (6th ed.). St. Louis: Mosby, pp 531; 560.

---

236. A nurse is caring for a client with Parkinson's disease who is taking ben-ztropine mesylate (Cogentin) daily. The nurse assesses the client for side effects of this medication and specifically monitors:

1 Pupil response
2 Skin temperature
3 Intake and output
4 Prothrombin time

Answer: 3

Rationale: Urinary retention is a side effect of benztropine mesylate. The nurse needs to observe for dysuria, distended abdomen, voiding in small amounts, and overflow incontinence. Options 1, 2, and 4 are not side effects of this medication.

Test-Taking Strategy: Focus on the name of the medication. It is necessary to know that urinary retention is a concern with this medication. Review this medication and its side effects if you had difficulty with this question.

Level of Cognitive Ability: Application
Client Needs: Physiological Integrity
Integrated Process: Nursing Process/Assessment
Content Area: Pharmacology

Reference:
Hodgson, B., & Kizior, R. (2004). *Saunders nursing drug handbook 2004.* Philadelphia: Saunders, p. 100.

---

237. A client has received electroconvulsive therapy (ECT). In the post-treatment area and upon the client's awakening, the nurse will perform which intervention first?

1 Orient the client and monitor the client's vital signs
2 Offer the client frequent reassurance and repeat orientation statements
3 Assist the client from the stretcher to a wheelchair
4 Check for a gag reflex and then encourage the client to eat breakfast and resume activity

Answer: 1

Rationale: The nurse would first monitor vital signs, orient the client, and review with the client that he or she just received an ECT treatment. The post-treatment area should include accessibility to the anesthesia staff, oxygen, suction, pulse oximeter, vital sign monitoring, and emergency equipment. The nursing interventions outlined in options 2, 3, and 4 will follow accordingly.

Test-Taking Strategy: Use the process of elimination and note the key word "first." Use the ABCs—airway, breathing, and circulation—remembering that vital signs are a method of assessing the ABCs. Review care of the client following ECT if you had difficulty with this question.

Level of Cognitive Ability: Application
Client Needs: Physiological Integrity
Integrated Process: Nursing Process/Implementation
Content Area: Delegating/Prioritizing

Reference:
Keltner, N., Schwecke, L., & Bostrom, C. (2003). *Psychiatric nursing* (4th ed.). St. Louis: Mosby, p. 526.

238. A client with acquired immunodeficiency syndrome (AIDS) who has cytomegalovirus (CMV) retinitis is receiving ganciclovir (Cytovene). The nurse plans to do which of the following while the client is taking this medication?
1 Provide the client with a soft toothbrush and an electric razor
2 Apply pressure to venipuncture sites for at least 2 minutes
3 Monitor blood glucose levels for elevation
4 Administer the medication on an empty stomach only

Answer: 1
Rationale: Ganciclovir causes neutropenia and thrombocytopenia as the most frequent side effects. For this reason, the nurse monitors the client for signs and symptoms of bleeding and implements the same precautions that are used for a client receiving anticoagulant therapy. These include providing a soft toothbrush and electric razor to minimize the risk of trauma that could result in bleeding. Venipuncture sites should be held for approximately 10 minutes. The medication does not have to be taken on an empty stomach. The medication may cause hypoglycemia, but not hyperglycemia.

Test-Taking Strategy: Use the process of elimination. Eliminate option 4 first because of the absolute word "only." Next eliminate option 2 because of the words "2 minutes." From the remaining options, recalling that ganciclovir causes thrombocytopenia will direct you to option 1. Review the side effects of this medication if you had difficulty with this question.

Level of Cognitive Ability: Application
Client Needs: Safe, Effective Care Environment
Integrated Process: Nursing Process/Planning
Content Area: Pharmacology

Reference:
Hodgson, B., & Kizior, R. (2004). *Saunders nursing drug handbook 2004.* Philadelphia: Saunders, pp. 457; 459.

239. A client is to be discharged from the hospital on quinidine gluconate (Quinaglute) to control ventricular ectopy, and the nurse provides medication instructions to the client. Which statement by the client would indicate the need for further instructions?
1 "I need to take this medication regularly, even if my heart feels strong."
2 "The best time to schedule this medication is with my meals."
3 "If I get diarrhea, nausea, or vomiting, I need to stop the medication immediately and then call my doctor."
4 "I should avoid alcohol, caffeine, and cigarettes while on this medication."

Answer: 3
Rationale: Diarrhea, nausea, vomiting, loss of appetite, and dizziness are all common side effects of quinidine. If these should occur, the physician or nurse should be notified, but the medication should never be stopped by the client. A rapid decrease in the medication level of an antidysrhythmic could precipitate dysrhythmia. Options 1, 2, and 4 are accurate client statements.

Test-Taking Strategy: Note the key words "need for further instructions." These words indicate a false-response question and that you need to select the incorrect client statement. Noting that quinidine is used to control ectopy and recalling that the client should not stop taking a medication without first consulting the physician will direct you to option 3. Review client teaching points related to this medication if you had difficulty with this question.

Level of Cognitive Ability: Analysis
Client Needs: Physiological Integrity
Integrated Process: Teaching/Learning
Content Area: Pharmacology

Reference:
Hodgson, B., & Kizior, R. (2004). *Saunders nursing drug handbook 2004.* Philadelphia: Saunders, p. 865.

240. A client having a mild panic attack has the following arterial blood gas (ABG) results: pH 7.49, P_{CO_2} 31 mmHg, P_{AO_2} 97 mmHg, HCO_3^- 22 mEq/L. The nurse reviews the results and determines that the client has which acid-base disturbance?

1 Respiratory acidosis
2 Respiratory alkalosis
3 Metabolic acidosis
4 Metabolic alkalosis

Answer: 2

Rationale: Acidosis is defined as a pH of less than 7.35, whereas alkalosis is defined as a pH of greater than 7.45. Respiratory alkalosis is present when the P_{CO_2} is less than 35, whereas respiratory acidosis is present when the P_{CO_2} is greater than 45. Metabolic acidosis is present when the HCO_3^- is less than 22 mEq/L, whereas metabolic alkalosis is present when the HCO_3^- is greater than 27 mEq/L. This client's ABGs are consistent with respiratory alkalosis.

Test-Taking Strategy: Note the key words "panic attack." This may help you anticipate that the client is having an increased respiratory rate, which makes the client prone to respiratory alkalosis. Otherwise, use the steps for interpreting blood gas results to answer the question. Review these steps if you had difficulty with this question.

Level of Cognitive Ability: Analysis
Client Needs: Physiological Integrity
Integrated Process: Nursing Process/Analysis
Content Area: Adult Health/Respiratory

Reference:
Phipps, W., Monahan, F., Sands, J., Marek, J., & Neighbors, M. (2003). *Medical-surgical nursing: Health and illness perspectives* (7th ed.). St. Louis: Mosby, p. 272.

241. Vasopressin (Pitressin) is prescribed for a client with diabetes insipidus, and the client asks the nurse about the purpose of the medication. The nurse responds, knowing that the action of the medication is to:

1 Inhibit contraction of smooth muscle
2 Produce vasodilation
3 Decrease urinary output
4 Decrease peristalsis

Answer: 3

Rationale: Vasopressin is a vasopressor and an antidiuretic. It directly stimulates contraction of smooth muscle, causes vasoconstriction, stimulates peristalsis, and increases reabsorption of water by the renal tubules, resulting in decreased urinary flow rate.

Test-Taking Strategy: Use the process of elimination. Eliminate options 1 and 4 first because they are similar. From the remaining options, recalling the pathophysiology associated with diabetes insipidus will direct you to option 3. Review the actions of this medication if you had difficulty with this question.

Level of Cognitive Ability: Application
Client Needs: Physiological Integrity
Integrated Process: Teaching/Learning
Content Area: Pharmacology

Reference:
Hodgson, B., & Kizior, R. (2004). *Saunders nursing drug handbook 2004.* Philadelphia: Saunders, p. 1043.

242. A client is seen in the health care clinic. The client has diabetes mellitus that has been well controlled with glyburide (Diabeta), but recently, the client's fasting blood glucose has been reported to be 180 to 200 mg/dL. Which of the following medications, if noted in the client's record, may be contributing to the elevated blood glucose level?
1 Cimetidine (Tagamet)
2 Ranitidine (Zantac)
3 Ciprofloxacin hydrochloride (Cipro)
4 Prednisone (Deltasone)

Answer: 4
Rationale: Corticosteroids, thiazide diuretics, and lithium may decrease the effect of glyburide, causing hyperglycemia. Options 1, 2, and 3 may increase the effect of glyburide, leading to hypoglycemia.

Test-Taking Strategy: Knowledge regarding the medications that have an adverse effect if taken concurrently with glyburide is required to answer this question. Review this content if you are unfamiliar with these medications.

Level of Cognitive Ability: Analysis
Client Needs: Physiological integrity
Integrated Process: Nursing Process/Analysis
Content Area: Pharmacology

Reference:
Hodgson, B., & Kizior, R. (2004). *Saunders nursing drug handbook 2004.* Philadelphia: Saunders, pp. 831-832.

243. A nurse is caring for a client in the postpartum unit who suddenly exhibits signs of a pulmonary embolism. The nurse immediately prepares to:
1 Administer oxygen by face mask at 8 to 10 liters per minute
2 Administer pain medication
3 Administer antianxiety medication
4 Monitor the vital signs

Answer: 1
Rationale: Because pulmonary circulation is compromised in the presence of an embolus, cardiorespiratory support is initiated by oxygen administration. Although option 4 may be a component of care for the client with pulmonary embolism, the immediate action is to prepare to administer oxygen. Options 2 and 3 are not immediate interventions.

Test-Taking Strategy: Note the key word "immediately." Use the ABCs—airway, breathing, and circulation. In this case, the airway and breathing may be adequate, but circulation of oxygenated blood can best be supported with oxygen administration. Review immediate care measures for a client with pulmonary embolism if you had difficulty with this question.

Level of Cognitive Ability: Application
Client Needs: Physiological Integrity
Integrated Process: Nursing Process/Implementation
Content Area: Maternity/Postpartum

Reference:
Murray, S., McKinney, E., & Gorrie, T. (2002). *Foundations of maternal-newborn nursing* (3rd ed.). Philadelphia: Saunders, p. 787.

244. Buspirone hydrochloride (BuSpar) is prescribed for a client with an anxiety disorder. The nurse instructs the client regarding the medication and tells the client that:
1 The medication can produce a sedating effect
2 Tolerance can occur with the medication
3 The medication is addicting
4 Dizziness and nervousness may occur

Answer: 4
Rationale: Buspirone hydrochloride is used in the management of anxiety disorders. The advantages of this medication is that it is not sedating, tolerance does not develop, and it is not addicting. The medication has a more favorable side effect profile than do the benzodiazepines. Dizziness, nausea, headaches, nervousness, lightheadedness, and excitement, which generally are not major problems, are side effects of the medication.

Test-Taking Strategy: Knowledge regarding the side effects and the advantages of buspirone hydrochloride is required to answer this question. Review its characteristics if you are unfamiliar with this medication and its use.

Level of Cognitive Ability: Application
Client Needs: Physiological Integrity
Integrated Process: Teaching/Learning
Content Area: Pharmacology

Reference:
Hodgson, B., & Kizior, R. (2004). *Saunders nursing drug handbook 2004.* Philadelphia: Saunders, pp. 130-131.

---

245. Neuroleptic malignant syndrome is suspected in a client who is taking chlorpromazine (Thorazine). Which medication would the nurse prepare in anticipation of being prescribed to treat this adverse reaction related to the use of chlorpromazine?
1 Phytonadione (Vitamin K)
2 Bromocriptine (Parlodel)
3 Enalapril maleate (Vasotec)
4 Protamine sulfate

Answer: 2
Rationale: Bromocriptine is an antiparkinson prolactin inhibitor used in the treatment of neuroleptic malignant syndrome. Vitamin K is the antidote for warfarin (Coumadin) overdose. Protamine sulfate is the antidote for heparin overdose. Enalapril maleate is an angiotensin-converting enzyme (ACE inhibitor) and an antihypertensive that is used in the treatment of hypertension.

Test-Taking Strategy: Use the process of elimination. Recalling that option 1 is the antidote for warfarin overdose and option 4 is the antidote for heparin will assist in eliminating these options. From the remaining options, focus on the medication classifications and eliminate option 3 because it is an antihypertensive. Review neuroleptic malignant syndrome if you had difficulty with this question.

Level of Cognitive Ability: Analysis
Client Needs: Physiological Integrity
Integrated Process: Nursing Process/Planning
Content Area: Pharmacology

Reference:
Lehne, R. (2004). *Pharmacology for nursing care.* (5th ed). Philadelphia: Saunders, pp. 180; 183; 297; 691.

---

246. A client with a fractured leg has learned how to use crutches to assist in ambulation. The nurse determines that the client misunderstood the information if the client states to:
1 Keep spare crutch tips available
2 Keep crutch tips dry so they don't slip
3 Keep the set of crutches found in the basement of the home as a spare pair
4 Inspect the crutch tips for wear from time to time

Answer: 3
Rationale: The client should use only crutches measured for the client. Crutches belonging to another person should not be used unless they have been adjusted to fit the client. Crutch tips should remain dry. Water could cause slipping by decreasing the surface friction of the rubber tip on the floor. If crutch tips get wet, the client should dry them with a cloth or paper towel. The tips should be inspected for wear, and spare tips and crutches fitted to the client should be available if needed.

Test-Taking Strategy: Note the key words "misunderstood the information." These words indicate a false-response question and that you need to select the incorrect client statement. Option 2 relates to safety and is eliminated first. Eliminate options 1 and 4 next because they are similar. Review client teaching points related to the use of crutches if you had difficulty with this question.

Level of Cognitive Ability: Analysis
Client Needs: Health Promotion and Maintenance
Integrated Process: Teaching/Learning
Content Area: Adult Health/Musculoskeletal

Reference:
Black, J., & Hawks, J. (2005). *Medical-surgical nursing: Clinical management for positive outcomes* (7th ed.). Philadelphia: Saunders, p. 2501.

---

247. Disulfiram (Antabuse) is prescribed for a client who is seen in the psychiatric health care clinic. The nurse is collecting data from the client and is providing instructions regarding the use of this medication. Which data is important for the nurse to obtain before beginning the administration of this medication?
  1 When the last alcoholic drink was consumed
  2 If the client has a history of diabetes insipidus
  3 If the client has a history of hyperthyroidism
  4 When the last full meal was consumed

Answer: 1
Rationale: Disulfiram is used as an adjunct treatment for selected clients with chronic alcoholism who want to remain in a state of enforced sobriety. Clients must abstain from alcohol intake for at least 12 hours before the initial dose of the medication is administered. Therefore, it is important for the nurse to determine when the last alcoholic drink was consumed. The medication is used with caution in clients with diabetes mellitus, hypothyroidism, epilepsy, cerebral damage, nephritis, and hepatic disease. It is also contraindicated in severe heart disease, psychosis, or hypersensitivity related to the medication.

Test-Taking Strategy: Use the process of elimination. Recalling that this medication is used as an adjunct treatment for chronic alcoholism will direct you to option 1. Review this medication if you are unfamiliar with it.

Level of Cognitive Ability: Analysis
Client Needs: Physiological integrity
Integrated Process: Nursing Process/Assessment
Content Area: Pharmacology

Reference:
McKenry, L., & Salerno, E. (2003). *Mosby's pharmacology in nursing* (21st ed.). St. Louis: Mosby, p. 172.

---

248. A client with nephrotic syndrome states to the nurse: "Why should I even bother trying to control my diet and the edema? It doesn't really matter what I do, if I can never get rid of this kidney problem anyway!" Based on the client's statement, the nurse addresses which potential client problem?
  1 Powerlessness
  2 Ineffective coping
  3 Anxiety
  4 Disturbed body image

Answer: 1
Rationale: Powerlessness is a problem when the client believes that personal actions will not affect an outcome in any significant way. Ineffective coping indicates that the client has impaired adaptive abilities or behaviors in meeting the demands or roles expected from the individual. Anxiety occurs when the client has a feeling of unease with a vague or undefined source. Disturbed body image occurs when the way the client perceives body image is altered.

Test-Taking Strategy: Use the process of elimination, focusing on the data in the question. Note the words "It doesn't really matter what I do . . ." This implies that the client has a sense of no control of the situation. This will direct you to option 1. Review the defining characteristics of powerlessness if you had difficulty with this question.

Level of Cognitive Ability: Analysis
Client Needs: Psychosocial Integrity

Integrated Process: Nursing Process/Analysis
Content Area: Adult Health/Renal

References:
Gulanick, M., Myers, J., Klopp, A., Gradishar, D., Galanes, S., & Puzas, M. (2003). *Nursing care plans: Nursing diagnosis and intervention* (5th ed.). St. Louis: Mosby, pp. 14; 19; 47; 129.
Phipps, W., Monahan, F., Sands, J., Marek, J., & Neighbors, M. (2003). *Medical-surgical nursing: Health and illness perspectives* (7th ed.). St. Louis: Mosby, p. 81.

---

249. Fluoxetine hydrochloride (Prozac) daily is prescribed for a client, and the nurse provides instructions to the client regarding the administration of the medication. Which statement by the client indicates an understanding regarding the administration of the medication?
1 "I should take the medication at bedtime with a snack."
2 "I should take the medication with food only."
3 "I should take the medication at noontime with an antacid."
4 "It is best to take the medication in the morning."

Answer: 4
Rationale: A daily dose of fluoxetine hydrochloride should be taken in the morning. If the medication is prescribed more than once daily, then the client is instructed to take the last dose of the day before 4:00 PM to avoid insomnia.

Test-Taking Strategy: Use the process of elimination. Eliminate option 2 because of the absolute word "only." Next eliminate option 3, recalling that generally medications should not be administered with an antacid. From the remaining options, recalling that the medication can cause insomnia will direct you to option 4. Review this content if you are unfamiliar with the use of this medication and the client teaching points.

Level of Cognitive Ability: Analysis
Client Needs: Health Promotion and Maintenance
Integrated Process: Teaching/Learning
Content Area: Pharmacology

Reference:
Hodgson, B., & Kizior, R. (2004). *Saunders nursing drug handbook 2004.* Philadelphia: Saunders, p. 427.

---

250. A nursing student is assigned to care for a client with a diagnosis of schizophrenia who is receiving haloperidol (Haldol). The registered nurse asks the student to describe the action of the medication. The student responds correctly by stating that this medication:
1 Blocks the uptake of norepinephrine and serotonin
2 Blocks the binding of dopamine to the post-synaptic dopamine receptors in the brain
3 Is a serotonin reuptake blocker
4 Inhibits the breakdown of released acetylcholine

Answer: 2
Rationale: Haloperidol acts by blocking the binding of dopamine to the post-synaptic dopamine receptors in the brain. Imipramine hydrochloride (Tofranil) blocks the reuptake of norepinephrine and serotonin. Donepezil hydrochloride (Aricept) inhibits the breakdown of released acetylcholine. Fluoxetine hydrochloride (Prozac) is a potent serotonin reuptake blocker.

Test-Taking Strategy: Knowledge regarding the action of haloperidol is required to answer this question. Review its action and use if you are unfamiliar with this medication.

Level of Cognitive Ability: Analysis
Client Needs: Physiological Integrity
Integrated Process: Teaching/Learning
Content Area: Pharmacology

Reference:
Hodgson, B., & Kizior, R. (2004). *Saunders nursing drug handbook 2004.* Philadelphia: Saunders, p. 489.

251. A nurse is teaching a client how to mix Regular insulin and NPH insulin in the same syringe. The nurse tells the client to:
1 Take all of the air out of the insulin bottle before mixing
2 Draw up the NPH insulin into the syringe first
3 Keep both bottles in the refrigerator at all times
4 Rotate the NPH insulin bottle in the hands before mixing

Answer: 4
Rationale: The NPH insulin bottle needs to be rotated for at least one minute between both hands. This resuspends the insulin. The nurse should not shake the bottles. Shaking causes foaming and bubbles to form, which may trap particles of insulin and alter the dosage. Insulin may be maintained at room temperature. Additional bottles of insulin for future use should be stored in the refrigerator. Regular insulin is drawn up before NPH insulin. Air does not need to be removed from the insulin bottle.

Test-Taking Strategy: Use the process of elimination. Visualizing the procedure for preparing the insulin will direct you to option 4. Review this procedure if you had difficulty with this question.

Level of Cognitive Ability: Application
Client Needs: Health Promotion and Maintenance
Integrated Process: Teaching/Learning
Content Area: Pharmacology

Reference:
Lehne, R. (2004). *Pharmacology for nursing care.* (5th ed). Philadelphia: Saunders, pp. 603; 616.

---

252. A client has undergone mastectomy. The nurse determines that the client is having the most difficulty adjusting to the loss of the breast if which behavior is observed?
1 Refusing to look at the dressing
2 Asking for pain medication when needed
3 Performing arm exercises
4 Reading the postoperative care booklet

Answer: 1
Rationale: The client demonstrates the most difficult adjustment to the loss if she refuses to look at the dressing. This indicates that the client is not ready or willing to begin to acknowledge and cope with the surgery. Asking for pain medication is an action-oriented option that is helpful, although there is no direct connection to adjustment to the loss of the breast. Reading the postoperative care booklet indicates an interest in self-care and is a positive sign indicating beginning adjustment. Performing arm exercises is also an action-oriented behavior on the part of the client and is considered a positive sign of adjustment.

Test-Taking Strategy: Note the key words "most difficulty adjusting" and focus on the issue. Note that options 2, 3, and 4 are similar and indicate a positive client action. Review psychosocial responses related to loss if you had difficulty with this question.

Level of Cognitive Ability: Analysis
Client Needs: Psychosocial Integrity
Integrated Process: Nursing Process/Evaluation
Content Area: Adult Health/Oncology

References:
Black, J., & Hawks, J. (2005). *Medical-surgical nursing: Clinical management for positive outcomes* (7th ed.). Philadelphia: Saunders, pp. 1106-1108.
Lewis, S., Heitkemper, M., & Dirksen, S. (2004). *Medical-surgical nursing: Assessment and management of clinical problems* (6th ed.). St. Louis: Mosby, pp. 1374-1375.

253. A client has been taking lansoprazole (Prevacid) for 4 weeks. The nurse monitors the client for relief of which of the following symptoms?
1 Constipation
2 Diarrhea
3 Flatulence
4 Heartburn

Answer: 4

Rationale: Lansoprazole is a gastric pump inhibitor and is classified as an antiulcer agent. The intended effect of the medication is relief of pain from gastric irritation, often referred to as heartburn by clients. The medication does not improve the other symptoms listed.

Test-Taking Strategy: Focus on the name of the medication. Recalling that medication names that end with the letters "zole" are gastric pump inhibitors will direct you to option 4. Review its actions and use if you are unfamiliar with this medication.

Level of Cognitive Ability: Analysis
Client Needs: Health Promotion and Maintenance
Integrated Process: Nursing Process/Evaluation
Content Area: Pharmacology

Reference:
Hodgson, B., & Kizior, R. (2004). *Saunders nursing drug handbook 2004.* *Philadelphia*: Saunders, p. 583.

254. A nurse is preparing a client who had a total knee replacement with a metal prosthesis for discharge to home and provides the client with discharge instructions. Which statement by the client indicates a need for further instructions?
1 "I need to report bleeding gums or tarry stools to the physician."
2 "I need to tell any future caregivers about the metal prosthesis."
3 "I need to report fever, redness, or increased pain to the physician."
4 "I can expect that changes in the shape of the knee will occur."

Answer: 4

Rationale: After total knee replacement, the client should be taught to report any changes in the shape of the knee. This is not an expected event during recuperation from surgery. Fever, redness, or increased pain may indicate infection. With a metal prosthesis, the client must be on anticoagulant therapy and should report adverse effects of this therapy, such as evidence of bleeding from a variety of sources. The client must also notify caregivers of the metal implant, because the client will need antibiotic prophylaxis for invasive procedures, and because the client will be ineligible for magnetic resonance imaging as a diagnostic procedure.

Test-Taking Strategy: Note the key words "metal prosthesis" and "need for further instructions." These words indicate a false-response question and that you need to select the incorrect client statement. Recalling that the client will be on prophylactic anticoagulant therapy will assist in eliminating option 1. Eliminate options 2 and 3 next because these are standard postoperative guidelines. Review client teaching points following total knee replacement if you had difficulty with this question.

Level of Cognitive Ability: Analysis
Client Needs: Health Promotion and Maintenance
Integrated Process: Teaching/Learning
Content Area: Adult Health/Musculoskeletal

References:
Black, J., & Hawks, J. (2005). *Medical-surgical nursing: Clinical management for positive outcomes* (7th ed.). Philadelphia: Saunders, pp. 595-596.
Ignatavicius, D., & Workman, M. (2002). *Medical surgical nursing: Critical thinking for collaborative care* (4th ed.). Philadelphia: Saunders, p. 341.
Phipps, W., Monahan, F., Sands, J., Marek, J., & Neighbors, M. (2003). *Medical-surgical nursing: Health and illness perspectives* (7th ed.). St. Louis: Mosby, p. 1537.

255. A nurse in the preoperative holding unit administers a dose of scopolamine to a client. The nurse monitors the client for which common side effect of the medication?
1 Dry mouth
2 Pupillary constriction
3 Excessive urination
4 Diaphoresis

Answer: 1
Rationale: Scopolamine is an anticholinergic medication that causes the frequent side effects of dry mouth, urinary retention, decreased sweating, and dilation of the pupils. Each of the incorrect options is the opposite of a side effect of this medication.

Test-Taking Strategy: Focus on the name of the medication. Recalling that this medication is an anticholinergic will direct you to option 1. Review the side effects of anticholinergics if you had difficulty with this question.

Level of Cognitive Ability: Application
Client Needs: Physiological Integrity
Integrated Process: Nursing Process/Assessment
Content Area: Pharmacology

Reference:
Lehne, R. (2004). *Pharmacology for nursing care.* (5th ed). Philadelphia: Saunders, pp. 118-119.

256. A nurse is providing medication instructions to a client who is taking imipramine (Tofranil) daily. Which statement by the client indicates a need for further instructions?
1 "If I miss a dose, I need to take it as soon as possible unless it is almost time for the next dose."
2 "I need to take the medication in the morning before breakfast."
3 "The effects of the medication may not be noticed for at least two weeks."
4 "I need to avoid alcohol while taking the medication."

Answer: 2
Rationale: The client should be instructed to take the medication (a single dose) at bedtime and not in the morning because it causes fatigue and drowsiness. The client is instructed to take the medication exactly as directed, and if a dose is missed to take it as soon as possible unless it is almost time for the next dose. The client is told that medication effects may not be noticed for at least 2 weeks, and to avoid alcohol or other central nervous system depressants during therapy.

Test-Taking Strategy: Note the key words "need for further instructions." These words indicate a false-response question and that you need to select the incorrect client statement. General principles related to medication administration will eliminate options 1 and 4. From the remaining options, recalling that this medication is an antidepressant will eliminate option 3. Review these client teaching points if you are unfamiliar with this medication.

Level of Cognitive Ability: Analysis
Client Needs: Health Promotion and Maintenance
Integrated Process: Teaching/Learning
Content Area: Pharmacology

References:
Lehne, R. (2004). *Pharmacology for nursing care* (5th ed.). Philadelphia: Saunders, p. 362.
Skidmore-Roth, L. (2005). *Mosby's drug guide for nurses* (6th ed.). St. Louis: Mosby, p. 440.

257. A nurse is preparing to assess a client who was admitted to the hospital with a diagnosis of trigeminal neuralgia (Tic Douloureux). On review of the client's record, the nurse would expect to note that the client experiences:
1 Chronic, intermittent pain in the seventh cranial nerve
2 Abrupt onset of pain in the fifth cranial nerve
3 Bilateral pain in the sixth cranial nerve
4 Unilateral pain in the sixth cranial nerve

Answer: 2
Rationale: Trigeminal neuralgia is a chronic syndrome characterized by an abrupt onset of pain. It involves one or more divisions of the trigeminal nerve or cranial nerve V. Options 1, 3, and 4 are incorrect.

Test-Taking Strategy: Focus on the client's diagnosis. Recalling that trigeminal neuralgia affects the fifth cranial nerve will assist in eliminating options 1, 3, and 4. Review the pathophysiology associated with trigeminal neuralgia if you had difficulty with this question.

Level of Cognitive Ability: Analysis
Client Needs: Physiological Integrity
Integrated Process: Nursing Process/Assessment
Content Area: Adult Health /Neurological

References:
Black, J., & Hawks, J. (2005). *Medical-surgical nursing: Clinical management for positive outcomes* (7th ed.). Philadelphia: Saunders, pp. 2153-2154.
Lewis, S., Heitkemper, M., & Dirksen, S. (2004). *Medical-surgical nursing: Assessment and management of clinical problems* (6th ed.). St. Louis: Mosby, p. 1601.

258. A client is taking docusate (Colace). The nurse tells the client to monitor for which of the following to ensure that the medication has the intended effect?
1 Decrease in fatty stools
2 Regular bowel movements
3 Abdominal pain
4 Decreased heartburn

Answer: 2
Rationale: Docusate is a stool softener that promotes absorption of water into the stool, producing a softer consistency of stool. The intended effect is relief or prevention of constipation. The medication does not relieve abdominal pain, relieve heartburn, or decrease the amount of fat in the stools.

Test-Taking Strategy: Focus on the name of the medication. Recalling that this medication is a stool softener will direct you to option 2. Review the action of this medication if you had difficulty with this question.

Level of Cognitive Ability: Application
Client Needs: Health Promotion and Maintenance
Integrated Process: Teaching/Learning
Content Area: Pharmacology

Reference:
Hodgson, B., & Kizior, R. (2004). *Saunders nursing drug handbook 2004.* Philadelphia: Saunders, p. 329.

259. A client's laboratory test results reveal a decreased serum transferrin and total iron-binding capacity (TIBC). The nurse interprets that this laboratory finding is compatible with anemia because of which of the following problems?
1 Malnutrition
2 Infection
3 Sickle cell disease
4 Iron deficiency

Answer: 1
Rationale: Malnutrition can cause reductions in both the serum transferrin and the TIBC. Infection is an unrelated option. Sickle cell anemia is diagnosed by determining that the client has hemoglobin S. Iron-deficiency anemia is usually characterized by decreased iron-binding capacity but increased transferrin levels. Additionally, in clinical practice, the hemoglobin level is routinely used to detect iron-deficiency anemia.

Test-Taking Strategy: Focus on the laboratory tests identified in the question. Use this data and knowledge regarding the findings in malnutrition to direct you to option 1. Review the findings in malnutrition if you had difficulty with this question.

Level of Cognitive Ability: Analysis
Client Needs: Physiological Integrity
Integrated Process: Nursing Process/Analysis
Content Area: Fundamental Skills

Reference:
Ignatavicius, D., & Workman, M. (2002). *Medical surgical nursing: Critical thinking for collaborative care* (4th ed.). Philadelphia: Saunders, p. 1367.

---

260. A nurse notes that the client has an order to have a Schilling test performed. The nurse reads the client's progress notes, looking for a tentative diagnosis of which of the following types of anemias?
1 Pernicious
2 Megaloblastic
3 Iron-deficiency
4 Aplastic

Answer: 1
Rationale: The Schilling test is used to determine the cause of vitamin B_{12} deficiency, which leads to pernicious anemia. This test involves the use of a small oral dose of radioactive B_{12} and a large nonradioactive intramuscular dose. A 24-hour urine specimen is then collected to measure the amount of radioactivity in the urine. This test is not helpful in diagnosing megaloblastic, iron-deficiency, or aplastic anemia.

Test-Taking Strategy: Specific knowledge regarding the Schilling test and its purpose is needed to answer this question. Review this test and the diagnostic tests associated with pernicious anemia if you had difficulty with this question.

Level of Cognitive Ability: Analysis
Client Needs: Physiological Integrity
Integrated Process: Nursing Process/Analysis
Content Area: Fundamental Skills

Reference:
Chernecky, C., & Berger, B. (2004). *Laboratory tests and diagnostic procedures* (4th ed.). Philadelphia: Saunders, pp. 982-983.

---

261. A physician has written an order for a client with diabetic gastroparesis to receive metoclopramide (Reglan) four times a day. The nurse schedules this medication to be given at which of the following times?
1 One hour after each meal and at bedtime
2 Every 6 hours spaced evenly around the clock
3 30 minutes before meals and at bedtime
4 With each meal and at bedtime

Answer: 3
Rationale: Metoclopramide stimulates the motility of the upper gastrointestinal tract and is used to treat gastroparesis (nausea, vomiting, and persistent fullness after meals). The client should be taught to take this medication 30 minutes before meals and at bedtime. The before-meals administration allows the medication time to begin working before the client consumes food requiring digestion. The other options are incorrect.

Test-Taking Strategy: Focus on the client's diagnosis. Noting that the medication is used to treat gastroparesis will direct you to option 3. Remember that it must be taken before meals to enhance digestion. Review the procedure for the administration of this medication if you had difficulty with this question.

Level of Cognitive Ability: Application
Client Needs: Physiological Integrity
Integrated Process: Nursing Process/Implementation
Content Area: Pharmacology

Reference:
Hodgson, B., & Kizior, R. (2004). *Saunders nursing drug handbook 2004*. Philadelphia: Saunders, p. 660.

---

262. A nurse is caring for a client who has just had a mastectomy. The nurse assists the client in doing which of the following exercises during the first 24 hours following surgery?
1 Elbow flexion and extension
2 Shoulder abduction and external rotation
3 Pendulum arm swings
4 Hand wall climbing

Answer: 1
Rationale: During the first 24 hours following surgery, the client is assisted to move the fingers and hands, and to flex and extend the elbow. The client may also use the arm for self-care provided that she does not raise the arm above shoulder level or abduct the shoulder. The exercises identified in options 2, 3, and 4 are done once surgical drains are removed and wound healing is well established.

Test-Taking Strategy: Note the key words "during the first 24 hours" and use the process of elimination. Remember that options that are similar are not likely to be correct. In this situation, each of the incorrect options involves movement of the shoulder joint. Review appropriate exercises for the client following mastectomy if you had difficulty with this question.

Level of Cognitive Ability: Application
Client Needs: Physiological Integrity
Integrated Process: Nursing Process/Implementation
Content Area: Adult Health/Oncology

Reference:
Black, J., & Hawks, J. (2005). *Medical-surgical nursing: Clinical management for positive outcomes* (7th ed.). Philadelphia: Saunders, p. 1109.

---

263. A nurse teaches a client about an upcoming endoscopic retrograde cholangiopancreatography (ERCP) procedure. The nurse determines that the client requires additional information if the client states that:
1 A signed informed consent is necessary
2 It is important to lie still during the procedure
3 Medication will be given orally for sedation
4 An anesthetic throat spray will be used

Answer: 3
Rationale: The client needs to lie still for ERCP, which takes about an hour to perform. The client also has to sign an informed consent form. Intravenous sedation (not oral) is given to relax the client, and an anesthetic throat spray is used to help keep the client from gagging as the endoscope is passed.

Test-Taking Strategy: Note the key word "requires additional information" in the stem of the question. Recalling that this procedure is endoscopic and noting the word "orally" in option 3 will direct you to this option. Review preprocedure care for an ERCP if you had difficulty with this question.

Level of Cognitive Ability: Application
Client Needs: Physiological Integrity
Integrated Process: Teaching/Learning
Content Area: Adult Health/Gastrointestinal

Reference:
Chernecky, C., & Berger, B. (2004). *Laboratory tests and diagnostic procedures* (4th ed.). Philadelphia: Saunders, p. 501.

264. A client has an order to take magnesium citrate to prevent constipation following upper and lower gastrointestinal (GI) barium studies. The nurse tells the client that this medication is best taken:
1 Chilled with a full glass of water
2 At room temperature
3 With a tepid glass of water
4 With fruit juice only

Answer: 1

Rationale: Magnesium citrate is available as an oral solution. It is commonly used as a laxative following certain studies of the GI tract. It should be served chilled and taken with a full glass of water. It should not be allowed to stand for prolonged periods. Allowing the medication to stand would reduce the carbonation and make the solution even less palatable. Options 2, 3, and 4 are incorrect.

Test-Taking Strategy: Use the process of elimination. Eliminate option 4 first because of the absolute word "only." Next eliminate options 2 and 3 because they identify similar temperatures. Review the procedure for administering this medication if you had difficulty with this question.

Level of Cognitive Ability: Application
Client Needs: Physiological Integrity
Integrated Process: Nursing Process/Implementation
Content Area: Pharmacology

References:
Hodgson, B., & Kizior, R. (2004). *Saunders nursing drug handbook 2004.* Philadelphia: Saunders, p. 623.
Lehne, R. (2004). *Pharmacology for nursing care* (5th ed). Philadelphia: Saunders, p. 838.
McKenry, L., & Salerno, E. (2003). *Mosby's pharmacology in nursing* (21st ed.). St. Louis: Mosby, p. 218.

265. An emergency room nurse is caring for a client with carbon monoxide poisoning from a suicide attempt. The nurse ensures that which most-needed service is put in place for the client?
1 Pulmonary rehabilitation
2 Occupational therapy
3 Psychiatric consult
4 Neurological consult

Answer: 3

Rationale: The client with carbon monoxide poisoning as a result of a suicide attempt should have a psychiatric consult. The necessity of a neurological consult would depend on the sequelae to the nervous system from the carbon monoxide poisoning. Occupational therapy and pulmonary rehabilitation are not indicated.

Test-Taking Strategy: Note the key words "suicide attempt" and "most needed" in the question. Eliminate occupational therapy first because there is no indication of the need for that service. The client will need respiratory therapy but not pulmonary rehabilitation, so option 1 is eliminated next. A neurological consult could be beneficial, but only if the client suffers long-term central nervous system damage from the suicide attempt. This client is most in need of a psychiatric consult at this time. Review care of the client who attempted suicide if you had difficulty with this question.

Level of Cognitive Ability: Application
Client Needs: Psychosocial Integrity
Integrated Process: Nursing Process/Implementation
Content Area: Mental Health

Reference:
Keltner, N., Schwecke, L., & Bostrom, C. (2003). *Psychiatric nursing* (4th ed.). St. Louis: Mosby, p 361.

266. A client has begun medication therapy with pancrelipase (Pancrease). The nurse teaches the client that this medication should:
1 Relieve heartburn
2 Help regulate blood glucose
3 Decrease the amount of fat in the stools
4 Eliminate abdominal pain

Answer: 3
Rationale: Pancrelipase is a pancreatic enzyme used in clients with pancreatitis as a digestive aid. The medication should reduce the amount of fatty stools (steatorrhea). Another intended effect could be improved nutritional status. It is not used to treat abdominal pain or heartburn. It does not regulate blood glucose; this is a function of insulin, a hormone produced in the beta cells of the pancreas.

Test-Taking Strategy: Focus on the name of the medication, which gives an indication of the possible uses of this medication. Also use knowledge of the physiology of the pancreas and recall that the suffix "-ase" in the medication name indicates an enzyme. This will assist in directing you to option 3. Review the action of this medication if you had difficulty with this question.

Level of Cognitive Ability: Application
Client Needs: Physiological Integrity
Integrated Process: Teaching/Learning
Content Area: Pharmacology

Reference:
McKenry, L., & Salerno, E. (2003). *Mosby's pharmacology in nursing* (21st ed.). St. Louis: Mosby, p. 758.

267. A nurse is performing tracheostomy care and has replaced the tracheostomy tube holder (tracheostomy ties). The nurse ensures that the holder is not too tight by checking to see if:
1 The client nods that he or she feels comfortable
2 The tracheostomy does not move more than 1/2 inch when the client is coughing
3 Four fingers can be slid comfortably under the holder
4 Two fingers can be slid comfortably under the holder

Answer: 4
Rationale: There should be enough room for two fingers to slide comfortably under the tracheostomy holder. This ensures that the holder is tight enough to prevent tracheostomy dislocation, while preventing excessive constriction around the neck. The other options are incorrect.

Test-Taking Strategy: Use the process of elimination, focusing on the issue: that the tracheostomy holder is not too tight. Visualize each of the descriptions in the options to direct you to option 4. Review the essentials of this fundamental nursing procedure if you had difficulty with this question.

Level of Cognitive Ability: Analysis
Client Needs: Physiological Integrity
Integrated Process: Nursing Process/Evaluation
Content Area: Adult Health/Respiratory

Reference:
Ignatavicius, D., & Workman, M. (2002). *Medical surgical nursing: Critical thinking for collaborative care* (4th ed.). Philadelphia: Saunders, p. 503.

268. A nurse has assisted the physician in placing a central (subclavian) catheter. Following the procedure, the nurse takes which priority action?
  1 Obtains a temperature reading to monitor for infection
  2 Monitors the blood pressure (BP) to check for fluid volume overload
  3 Labels the dressing with the date and time of catheter insertion
  4 Ensures that a chest X-ray is done

Answer: 4

Rationale: A major risk associated with central catheter placement is the possibility of a pneumothorax developing from an accidental puncture of the lung. Obtaining a chest X-ray and checking the results is the best method to determine if this complication has occurred and to verify catheter tip placement before initiating intravenous (IV) therapy. While a client may develop an infection at the central catheter site, a temperature elevation would not likely occur immediately after placement. While BP assessment is always important in checking a client's status after an invasive procedure, fluid volume overload is not a concern until IV fluids are started. Labeling the dressing site is important, but it is not a priority action in this situation.

Test-Taking Strategy: Use the process of elimination. Noting the key words "following the procedure" will assist in eliminating options 1 and 2. Next, noting the words "priority action" will direct you to option 4 from the remaining options. Review post-procedure care following central catheter insertion if you had difficulty with this question.

Level of Cognitive Ability: Application
Clinical Needs: Physiological Integrity
Integrated Process: Nursing Process/Implementation
Content Area: Delegating/Prioritizing

References:
Ignatavicius, D., & Workman, M. (2002). *Medical surgical nursing: Critical thinking for collaborative care* (4th ed.). Philadelphia: Saunders, p. 209.
Perry, A., & Potter, P. (2004). *Clinical nursing skills and techniques* (5th ed.). St. Louis: Mosby, p. 691.

269. A client is complaining of gas pains following surgery and requests medication. The nurse reviews the medication order sheet to see if which medication is ordered for the relief of gas pains?
  1 Acetaminophen (Tylenol)
  2 Simethicone (Mylicon)
  3 Magnesium hydroxide (MOM)
  4 Droperidol (Inapsine)

Answer: 2

Rationale: Simethicone is an antiflatulent used in the relief of pain caused by excessive gas in the gastrointestinal (GI) tract. Acetaminophen is a non-narcotic analgesic. Magnesium hydroxide is an antacid and laxative. Droperidol is used to treat postoperative nausea and vomiting.

Test-Taking Strategy: Focus on the key words "gas pains." Recalling the classifications of each of the medications listed in the options will direct you to option 2. Review the action and purpose of each of the medications listed if you had difficulty with this question.

Level of Cognitive Ability: Analysis
Client Needs: Physiological Integrity
Integrated Process: Nursing Process/Analysis
Content Area: Pharmacology

Reference:
McKenry, L., & Salerno, E. (2003). *Mosby's pharmacology in nursing* (21st ed.). St. Louis: Mosby, p. 215.

270. A home care nurse notes that an older client is taking cimetidine (Tagamet). On assessment of the client, the nurse checks for which side effect of this medication?
1 Constipation
2 Blurred vision
3 Confusion
4 Fatigue

Answer: 3

Rationale: Cimetidine is a gastric acid secretion inhibitor. Older clients are especially susceptible to the central nervous system side effects of cimetidine. The most frequent of these is confusion. Less common central nervous system side effects include headache, dizziness, drowsiness, agitation, and hallucinations. Options 1, 2, and 4 are not associated with the use of this medication.

Test-Taking Strategy: Focus on the medication. Recalling that cimetidine causes central nervous system side effects will direct you to option 3. Review the side effects of this medication if you had difficulty with this question.

Level of Cognitive Ability: Analysis
Client Needs: Health Promotion and Maintenance
Integrated Process: Nursing Process/Assessment
Content Area: Pharmacology

Reference:
McKenry, L., & Salerno, E. (2003). *Mosby's pharmacology in nursing* (21st ed.). St. Louis: Mosby, p. 773.

271. A client is admitted to the hospital after sustaining a fall from a roof. The client has multiple lacerations and a right leg fracture, which has been treated with a plaster cast. The nurse positions the client's leg in which manner to promote optimal circulation?
1 Elevated on pillows continuously for 24 to 48 hours
2 Elevated for 3 hours, and then flat for 1 hour
3 Flat or a level position
4 Flat for 3 hours and elevated for 1 hour

Answer: 1

Rationale: A casted extremity is elevated continuously for the first 24 to 48 hours to minimize swelling and to promote venous drainage. The other options are not part of standard positioning of the newly casted extremity.

Test-Taking Strategy: Focus on the issue: to promote optimal circulation. Recalling that edema occurs after a fracture and can be increased by casting and using the principles of gravity will direct you to option 1. Review appropriate positioning following casting of an extremity if you had difficulty with this question.

Level of Cognitive Ability: Application
Client Needs: Physiological Integrity
Integrated Process: Nursing Process/Implementation
Content Area: Adult Health/Musculoskeletal

Reference:
Phipps, W., Monahan, F., Sands, J., Marek, J., & Neighbors, M. (2003). *Medical-surkgical nursing: Health and illness perspectives* (7th ed.). St. Louis: Mosby, p. 1481.

272. A physical assessment is performed on a suicidal client on admission to the inpatient unit. The nurse understands that this is an important part of the admission process because it provides the nurse with information regarding:
1 The presence of abnormalities
2 Evidence of physical self-harm
3 Existing medical problems
4 Baseline data

Answer: 2

Rationale: The physical assessment of a suicidal client should be thorough and should focus on the evidence of self-harm or the client's formulation of a plan for the suicide attempt. Although all of the options are correct, option 2 is most appropriate in the context of the suicidal client. Clients with a history of self-harm are greater suicide risks.

Test-Taking Strategy: Use the process of elimination and focus on the client's diagnosis. Remember that assessing for physical evidence of harm is an important component of the assessment process of a suicidal client. Review the characteristics of the client at risk for suicide if you had difficulty with this question.

Level of Cognitive Ability: Analysis
Client Needs: Physiological Integrity
Integrated Process: Nursing Process/Assessment
Content Area: Mental Health

Reference:
Stuart, G., & Laraia, M. (2005). *Principles and practice of psychiatric nursing* (8th ed.). St. Louis: Mosby, p. 367.

---

273. A client being mechanically ventilated after experiencing a fat embolus is visibly anxious. The nurse takes which appropriate action?
1 Encourages the client to sleep until arterial blood gas results improve
2 Asks a family member to stay with the client at all times
3 Asks the physician to obtain an order for an antianxiety medication
4 Remains with the client and provides reassurance

Answer: 4
Rationale: The nurse always speaks to the client calmly and provides reassurance to the anxious client. Family members are also stressed. Therefore, it is not beneficial to ask the family to take on the burden of remaining with the client at all times. Encouraging the client to sleep will not assist in relieving the client's anxiety. Antianxiety medications are used only if necessary and if other interventions fail to relieve the client's anxiety.

Test-Taking Strategy: Note the key words "appropriate action." Use the process of elimination, remembering that it is most important to address the client's feelings. Review care of the client who is anxious if you had difficulty with this question.

Level of Cognitive Ability: Application
Client Needs: Psychosocial Integrity
Integrated Process: Caring
Content Area: Adult Health/Respiratory

Reference:
Phipps, W., Monahan, F., Sands, J., Marek, J., & Neighbors, M. (2003). *Medical-surgical nursing: Health and illness perspectives* (7th ed.). St. Louis: Mosby, p. 233.

---

274. A nurse is caring for a client who is receiving colchicine. The nurse plans to monitor for a decrease in which of the following to determine the effectiveness of this medication?
1 Headaches
2 Blood glucose level
3 Serum triglyceride level
4 Joint inflammation

Answer: 4
Rationale: Colchicine is classified as an antigout agent. It interferes with the ability of the white blood cells to initiate and maintain an inflammatory response to monosodium urate crystals. The client should report a decrease in pain and inflammation in affected joints, as well as a decrease in the number of gout attacks. The other options are not related to the use of this medication.

Test-Taking Strategy: Focus on the name of the medication. Recalling that this medication is used in the treatment of gout will direct you to option 4. Review the action of this medication if you had difficulty with this question.

Level of Cognitive Ability: Analysis
Client Needs: Physiological Integrity
Integrated Process: Nursing Process/Evaluation
Content Area: Pharmacology

Reference:
Hodgson, B., & Kizior, R. (2004). *Saunders nursing drug handbook 2004.* Philadelphia: Saunders, p. 241.

275. A client has an order to begin short-term therapy with enoxaparin (Lovenox). The nurse explains to the client that this medication is being ordered to:

1 Dissolve urinary calculi
2 Reduce the risk of deep vein thrombosis
3 Relieve migraine headaches
4 Stop progression of multiple sclerosis

Answer: 2

Rationale: Enoxaparin is an anticoagulant that is administered to prevent deep vein thrombosis and thromboembolism in selected clients at risk. It is not used to treat urinary calculi, migraine headaches, or multiple sclerosis.

Test-Taking Strategy: Focus on the name of the medication. Recalling that this medication is an anticoagulant will direct you to option 2. Review the action of this medication if you had difficulty with this question.

Level of Cognitive Ability: Application
Client Needs: Physiological Integrity
Integrated Process: Teaching/Learning
Content Area: Pharmacology

Reference:
Hodgson, B., & Kizior, R. (2004). *Saunders nursing drug handbook 2004.* Philadelphia: Saunders, p. 354.

276. A client takes aluminum hydroxide (Amphojel) as needed for heartburn. The nurse teaches the client that the most common side effect of this medication is:

1 Constipation
2 Excitability
3 Muscle pain
4 Dizziness

Answer: 1

Rationale: Because of the antacid's aluminum base, aluminum hydroxide causes constipation as a side effect. The other side effect is hypophosphatemia, which is noted by monitoring serum laboratory studies. The other options are not side effects of this medictation.

Test-Taking Strategy: Focus on the medication name and recall that this medication is an antacid. Recalling that aluminum-based antacids cause constipation will direct you to option 1. Review the side effects associated with this medication if you had difficulty with this question.

Level of Cognitive Ability: Application
Client Needs: Health Promotion and Maintenance
Integrated Process: Teaching/Learning
Content Area: Pharmacology

Reference:
Hodgson, B., & Kizior, R. (2004). *Saunders nursing drug handbook 2004.* Philadelphia: Saunders, p. 35.

277. A nurse is caring for a young adult client diagnosed with sarcoidiosis. The client is angry and tells the nurse that there is no point in learning disease management, because there is no possibility of ever being cured. Based on the client's statement, the nurse determines that the client is experiencing which potential problem?

1 Disturbed thought processes
2 Impaired health maintenance
3 Anxiety
4 Powerlessness

Answer: 4

Rationale: The client with powerlessness expresses feelings of having no control over a situation or outcome. Impaired health maintenance involves the inability to seek out help that is needed to maintain health. Anxiety is a vague sense of unease. Disturbed thought processes involves disruption in cognitive abilities or thought.

Test-Taking Strategy: Focus on the data in the question. Use the process of elimination, noting the key words "no point in learning disease management." This will direct you to option 4. Review the defining characteristics of powerlessness if you had difficulty with this question.

Level of Cognitive Ability: Analysis
Client Needs: Psychosocial Integrity
Integrated Process: Nursing Process/Analysis
Content Area: Adult Health/Respiratory

Reference:
Phipps, W., Monahan, F., Sands, J., Marek, J., & Neighbors, M. (2003). *Medical-surgical nursing: Health and illness perspectives* (7th ed.). St. Louis: Mosby, p. 81.

---

278. A nurse is providing instructions to the spouse of a client who is taking tacrine (Cognex) for the management of moderate dementia associated with Alzheimer's disease. The nurse tells the spouse:
1 If flu-like symptoms occur, it is necessary to notify the physician immediately
2 If a dose is missed, double up on the next dose
3 If a change in the color of the stools occurs, notify the physician
4 Do not administer the medication with food

Answer: 3
Rationale: Tacrine (Cognex) may be administered between meals on an empty stomach, and if gastrointestinal upset occurs, it may be administered with meals. Flu-like symptoms without fever is a frequent side effect that may occur with the use of the medication. The client or spouse should never be instructed to double the dose of any medication if it was missed, and the client and caregiver are instructed to notify the physician if nausea, vomiting, diarrhea, rash, jaundice, or changes in the color of the stool occur. This may be indicative of the potential occurrence of hepatitis.

Test-Taking Strategy: Use the process of elimination. Eliminate option 1 because of the word "immediately." Flu-like symptoms should not be a concern requiring immediate physician notification. Next eliminate option 2 because of the words "double up on the next dose." From the remaining options, recalling that an adverse effect associated with the use of the medication is hepatitis will direct you to option 3. Review this medication if you are unfamiliar with its use and potential adverse effects.

Level of Cognitive Ability: Application
Client Needs: Health Promotion and Maintenance
Integrated Process: Teaching/Learning
Content Area: Pharmacology

References:
Lehne, R. (2004). *Pharmacology for nursing care.* (5th ed). Philadelphia: Saunders, p. 189.
McKenry, L., & Salerno, E. (2003). *Mosby's pharmacology in nursing* (21st ed.). St. Louis: Mosby, pp. 724; 1510.

---

279. An older client has been using cascara sagrada on a long-term basis to treat constipation. The nurse determines that which laboratory result is a result of the side effects of this medication?
1 Sodium 135 mEq/L
2 Sodium 145 mEq/L
3 Potassium 3.1 mEq/L
4 Potassium 5.0 mEq/L

Answer: 3
Rationale: Hypokalemia can result from long-term use of casanthrol (cascara sagrada), which is a laxative. The medication stimulates peristalsis and alters fluid and electrolyte transport, thus helping fluid to accumulate in the colon. The normal range for potassium is 3.5 to 5.1 mEq/L. The normal range for sodium is 135 to 145 mEq/L. Options 1, 2, and 4 are normal values.

Test-Taking Strategy: Use the process of elimination and knowledge regarding the normal laboratory values for sodium and potassium. The only abnormal value is option 3. Review the effects of this medication if you had difficulty with this question.

Level of Cognitive Ability: Analysis
Client Needs: Physiological Integrity
Integrated Process: Nursing Process/Analysis
Content Area: Pharmacology

Reference:
Hodgson, B., & Kizior, R. (2004). *Saunders nursing drug handbook 2004.* Philadelphia: Saunders, p. 158.

---

280. A client has been started on cyclobenza-prine (Flexeril) for the management of muscle spasms. The nurse teaches the client to observe for which most frequent central nervous system side effects of this medication?
1 Drowsiness
2 Fatigue
3 Irritability
4 Excitability

Answer: 1
Rationale: The most frequent side effects of cyclobenzaprine are drowsiness, dizziness, and dry mouth. This medication is a centrally acting skeletal muscle relaxant used in the management of muscle spasms that accompany a variety of conditions. Fatigue, nervousness, and confusion are rare side effects of the medication.

Test-Taking Strategy: Note the key words "most frequent." Eliminate options 3 and 4 first because they are similar. Recalling that this medication is a centrally acting skeletal muscle relaxant will direct you to option 1 from the remaining options. Review this medication if you had difficulty with this question.

Level of Cognitive Ability: Application
Client Needs: Physiological Integrity
Integrated Process: Teaching/Learning
Content Area: Pharmacology

Reference:
Hodgson, B., & Kizior, R. (2004). *Saunders nursing drug handbook 2004.* Philadelphia: Saunders, p. 255.

---

281. A nurse is caring for a client following shoulder arthroplasty for rheumatoid arthritis and is checking the client for brachial plexus compromise. To assess the status of the median nerve, which of the following would the nurse perform?
1 Have the client move the thumb toward the palm and back to the neutral position
2 Have the client grasp the nurse's hand while noting the client's strength of the first and second fingers
3 Have the client spread all of the fingers wide and resist pressure
4 Monitor for flexion of the biceps by having the client raise the forearm

Answer: 2
Rationale: To assess the median nerve status, the client should be instructed to grasp the nurse's hand. The nurse should note the strength of the client's first and second fingers. A weak grip may indicate compromise of the median nerve. Asking the client to move the thumb toward the palm and back to neutral position is assessing the radial nerve status. Asking the client to spread all fingers wide and resisting pressure is assessing the ulnar nerve status. Monitoring for flexion of the biceps by raising the forearm is assessing for cutaneous nerve status.

Test-Taking Strategy: Focus on the issue: assessment of the median nerve. Recalling the location and function of the median nerve will direct you to option 2. Review this assessment technique if you are unfamiliar with this procedure.

Level of Cognitive Ability: Application
Client Needs: Health Promotion and Maintenance
Integrated Process: Nursing Process/Assessment
Content Area: Adult Health/Musculoskeletal

Reference:
Black, J., & Hawks, J. (2005). *Medical-surgical nursing: Clinical management for positive outcomes* (7th ed.). Philadelphia: Saunders, pp. 2010; 2351.

---

282. A nurse is preparing to administer heparin sodium (Liquaemin) 5000 units subcutaneously. Which of the following indicates the accurate procedure for administering the medication?
  1 Injecting the medication 1 inch from the umbilicus
  2 Massaging the injection site following administration
  3 Injecting the medication via an infusion device
  4 Changing the needle on the syringe after withdrawing the medication from the vial

Answer: 4
Rationale: Heparin administered by the subcutaneous route does not require an infusion device. The injection site is above the iliac crest or in the abdominal fat layer. It is injected at least 2 inches from the umbilicus. After administration, the needle is withdrawn, pressure is applied to the injection site, and the site is not massaged. Injection sites are rotated. After withdrawal of heparin from the vial, the needle is changed before injection to prevent leakage of the heparin along the needle tract, which can cause bruising and bleeding.

Test-Taking Strategy: Use the process of elimination, focusing on the issue: accurate procedure. Visualize the procedure as you read each option. Recalling the action and effects of heparin will direct you to option 4. Review this procedure if you had difficulty with this question.

Level of Cognitive Ability: Application
Client Needs: Physiological Integrity
Integrated Process: Nursing Process/Implementation
Content Area: Pharmacology

Reference:
Hodgson, B., & Kizior, R. (2004). *Saunders nursing drug handbook 2004.* Philadelphia: Saunders, p. 492.

---

283. A client is admitted to the hospital with a tentative diagnosis of pernicious anemia. The nurse assesses the client for which sign associated with this disorder?
  1 Constipation
  2 Dusky, mucous membranes
  3 Red tongue that is smooth and sore
  4 Shortness of breath

Answer: 3
Rationale: Classic signs of pernicious anemia include weakness, mild diarrhea, and a smooth, sore red tongue. The client may also have nervous system symptoms, such as paresthesias, difficulty with balance, and occasional confusion. The mucous membranes do not become dusky, and the client does not exhibit shortness of breath.

Test-Taking Strategy: To answer this question accurately, you must be familiar with the signs and symptoms that characterize pernicious anemia. Review the assessment data related to this disorder if you had difficulty with the question.

Level of Cognitive Ability: Application
Client Needs: Physiological Integrity
Integrated Process: Nursing Process/Assessment
Content Area: Fundamental Skills

Reference:
Phipps, W., Monahan, F., Sands, J., Marek, J., & Neighbors, M. (2003). *Medical-surgical nursing: Health and illness perspectives* (7th ed.). St. Louis: Mosby, p. 826.

284. Benztropine mesylate (Cogentin) is prescribed for a client with a diagnosis of Parkinson's disease. The clinic nurse is reinforcing instructions to the client regarding the medication and tells the client to:

1 Avoid driving if drowsiness or dizziness occurs
2 Expect difficulty swallowing while taking this medication
3 Spend one hour a day during rest periods sitting in the sun to enhance the effectiveness of the medication
4 Expect episodes of vomiting and constipation while taking this medication

Answer: 1

Rationale: The client taking benztropine mesylate should be instructed to avoid driving or operating hazardous equipment if drowsy or dizzy. The client's tolerance to heat may be reduced because of the diminished ability to sweat, and the client should be instructed to plan rest periods in cool places during the day. The client should be instructed to stop taking the medication if difficulty swallowing or speaking or vomiting occurs. The client should also inform the physician if central nervous system effects occur. The client is instructed to monitor urinary output and to watch for signs of constipation.

Test-Taking Strategy: Use the process of elimination. General principles related to safety and medications will direct you to option 1. Review client teaching points related to this medication if you had difficulty with this question.

Level of Cognitive Ability: Application
Client Needs: Health Promotion and Maintenance
Integrated Process: Teaching/Learning
Content Area: Pharmacology

Reference:
Hodgson, B., & Kizior, R. (2004). *Saunders nursing drug handbook 2004.* Philadelphia: Saunders, p. 101.

---

285. A nurse is preparing to do preoperative teaching with a client scheduled for radical neck dissection. The nurse initially focuses on:

1 Postoperative communication techniques
2 Client's coping behaviors
3 Client's support systems
4 Information given to the client by the surgeon

Answer: 4

Rationale: The first step in client education is establishing what the client already knows. This allows the nurse to not only correct any misinformation but also to determine the starting point for teaching and to implement the education at the client's level. Although options 1, 2, and 3 may be a component of the plan, the first step in client education is establishing what the client already knows.

Test-Taking Strategy: Note the key word "initially." It is likely that all of the options listed may be included in the teaching plan, but you need to determine what the nurse would initially focus on. Remember, in the teaching/learning process, client motivation and readiness to learn along with what the client already knows are initial assessment items. Review the teaching/learning process if you had difficulty with this question.

Level of Cognitive Ability: Application
Client Needs: Psychosocial Integrity
Integrated Process: Teaching/Learning
Content Area: Fundamental Skills

Reference:
Potter, P., & Perry, A. (2005). *Fundamentals of nursing* (6th ed.). St. Louis: Mosby, pp. 451-454.

286. A client with refractory myasthenia gravis is told by the physician that plasmapheresis therapy is indicated. After the physician leaves the room, the client asks the nurse to repeat the physician's reason for ordering this treatment. The nurse tells the client that this therapy will most likely improve which of the client's symptoms?

1 Urinary incontinence
2 Pins and needles sensation in the legs
3 Double vision
4 Difficulty breathing

Answer: 4

Rationale: Plasmapheresis is a process that separates the plasma from the blood elements, so that plasma proteins that contain antibodies can be removed. It is used as an adjunct therapy in myasthenia gravis and may give temporary relief to clients with actual or impending respiratory failure. Usually three to five treatments are required. This therapy is not indicated for the reasons listed in options 1, 2, and 3.

Test-Taking Strategy: Note the key word "refractory." This tells you that the client with myasthenia gravis has severe disease, which is not adequately controlled with medication and other measures. Recalling the purpose of plasmapheresis and knowledge of the complications of this disease will direct you to option 4. Review the purpose of this procedure if you had difficulty with this question.

Level of Cognitive Ability: Application
Client Needs: Physiological Integrity
Integrated Process: Nursing Process/Implementation
Content Area: Adult Health/Neurological

Reference:
Black, J., & Hawks, J. (2005). *Medical-surgical nursing: Clinical management for positive outcomes* (7th ed.). Philadelphia: Saunders, p. 2184.

---

287. A client is admitted to the hospital in myasthenic crisis. The nurse questions the family about the occurrence of which precipitating factor for this event?

1 Not taking prescribed medication
2 Taking excess prescribed medication
3 Getting more sleep than usual
4 A decrease in food intake recently

Answer: 1

Rationale: Myasthenic crisis is often caused by undermedication and responds to the administration of cholinergic medications such as neostigmine (Prostigmin) and pyridostigmine (Mestinon). Cholinergic crisis (the opposite problem) is caused by excess medication and responds to withholding of medications. Change in diet and increased sleep are not precipitating factors. However, overexertion and overeating could possibly trigger myasthenic crisis.

Test-Taking Strategy: Focus on the issue: myasthenic crisis. Recalling that myasthenia gravis is treated with medication will direct you to option 1. Review the causes of myasthenia gravis if you had difficulty with this question.

Level of Cognitive Ability: Analysis
Client Needs: Physiological Integrity
Integrated Process: Nursing Process/Assessment
Content Area: Adult Health/Neurological

Reference:
Black, J., & Hawks, J. (2005). *Medical-surgical nursing: Clinical management for positive outcomes* (7th ed.). Philadelphia: Saunders, p. 2183.

288. A client with trigeminal neuralgia asks the nurse what can be done to minimize the episodes of pain. The nurse's response is based on an understanding that the symptoms can be triggered by:
1 Infection or stress
2 Excessive watering of the eyes or nasal stuffiness
3 Sensations of pressure or extreme temperature
4 Hypoglycemia and fatigue

Answer: 3
Rationale: The paroxysms of pain that accompany this neuralgia are triggered by stimulation of the terminal branches of the trigeminal nerve. Symptoms can be triggered by pressure from washing the face, brushing the teeth, shaving, eating, and drinking. Symptoms can also be triggered by thermal stimuli such as a draft of cold air. The items listed in the other options do not trigger the spasm.

Test-Taking Strategy: Recall the pathophysiology of this disorder and that precipitating factors such as pressure or thermal stimuli trigger the spasm. This will direct you to option 3. Review this cranial nerve disorder if you had difficulty with this question.

Level of Cognitive Ability: Analysis
Client Needs: Physiological Integrity
Integrated Process: Nursing Process/Analysis
Content Area: Adult Health/Neurological

Reference:
Black, J., & Hawks, J. (2005). *Medical-surgical nursing: Clinical management for positive outcomes* (7th ed.). Philadelphia: Saunders, pp. 2153-2154.

289. A client has been diagnosed with Bell's palsy. The nurse assesses the client to see if which signs and symptoms are visible?
1 Speech difficulties and one-sided facial droop
2 Twitching of one side of the face and ruddy cheeks
3 Eye paralysis and ptosis of the eyelid
4 Fixed pupil and an elevated eyelid on one side

Answer: 1
Rationale: Bell's palsy is a one-sided facial paralysis resulting from compression of the facial nerve (CN VII). There is facial droop from paralysis of the facial muscles, increased lacrimation, painful sensations in the eye, face, or behind the ear, and speech or chewing difficulties. The other items listed are not associated with this disorder.

Test-Taking Strategy: Use the process of elimination. Remember that palsy is a type of paralysis. This will assist in eliminating option 2. Recalling that Bell's palsy results from dysfunction of the facial nerve (CN VII), not the nerves that govern eye movements (CN III, IV, VI), will eliminate options 3 and 4. Review the characteristics associated with Bell's palsy if you had difficulty with this question.

Level of Cognitive Ability: Analysis
Client Needs: Physiological Integrity
Integrated Process: Nursing Process/Assessment
Content Area: Adult Health/Neurological

Reference:
Black, J., & Hawks, J. (2005). *Medical-surgical nursing: Clinical management for positive outcomes* (7th ed.). Philadelphia: Saunders, p. 2154.

290. A female client arrives at the emergency room and states she was just raped. In preparing a plan of care, the priority intervention in addition to medical attention should include:

1　Providing instructions for medical follow-up

2　Obtaining counseling for the victim

3　Providing anticipatory guidance for police investigations, medical questions, and court proceedings

4　Exploring safety concerns by obtaining permission to notify significant others who can provide shelter

Answer: 4

Rationale: After the provision of medical treatment, the nurse's next priority would be obtaining support and planning for safety. Options 2 and 3 seek to meet the emotional needs related to the rape and emotional readiness for the process of discovery and legal action. Option 1 is concerned with ensuring that the victim understands the importance of and commits to the need for medical follow-up. From the options provided, this is not a priority intervention.

Test-Taking Strategy: Use Maslow's hierarchy of needs theory and note the key words "priority intervention." Remember that physiological needs are the priority, followed by safety needs. Because medical attention is addressed in the question, select option 4 because it addresses the safety needs. Review care of the rape victim if you had difficulty with this question.

Level of Cognitive Ability: Analysis
Client Needs: Safe, Effective Care Environment
Integrated Process: Nursing Process/Planning
Content Area: Mental Health

Reference:
Keltner, N., Schwecke, L., & Bostrom, C. (2003). *Psychiatric nursing* (4th ed.). St. Louis: Mosby, p. 559.

---

291. A home care nurse makes a home visit to a client. The client tells the nurse that the physician instructions state to take ibuprofen (Advil) 0.4 g for mild pain. The medication bottle states ibuprofen (Advil) 200 mg tablets. How many tablet(s) will the nurse instruct the client to take?

Answer: _____

Answer: 2

Rationale: Convert 0.4 g to mg. In the metric system, to convert larger to smaller, multiply by 1000 or move the decimal three places to the right. Then, follow the medication calculation formula.

0.4 g = 400 mg

$$\frac{400 \text{ mg}}{200 \text{ mg}} \times 1 \text{ tablet} = 2 \text{ tablets}$$

Test-Taking Strategy: Use the formula for the calculation of a medication dose. Remember to convert grams to milligrams. Make sure that the calculated dose makes sense, and recheck your answer using a calculator. Review conversions and calculations if you had difficulty with this question.

Level of Cognitive Ability: Application
Client Needs: Physiological Integrity
Integrated Process: Teaching/Learning
Content Area: Fundamental Skills

Reference:
Kee, J., & Marshall, S. (2004). *Clinical calculations: With applications to general and specialty areas* (4th ed.). Philadelphia: Saunders, p. 80.

292. A nurse is admitting a client to the hospital who has a diagnosis of Guillain-Barré syndrome. After ensuring that the client's vital signs are stable and that the client is comfortable in bed, the nurse asks a family member if the client has recently had:
1 A respiratory or gastrointestinal (GI) infection
2 Meningitis
3 A back injury or spinal cord trauma
4 Seizures or head trauma

Answer: 1

Rationale: Guillain-Barré syndrome is a clinical syndrome of unknown origin that involves cranial and peripheral nerves. Many clients report a history of respiratory or GI infection in the 1 to 4 weeks before the onset of neurological deficits. Occasionally, it has been triggered by vaccination or surgery. The other options are not associated with an incidence of this syndrome.

Test-Taking Strategy: Use the process of elimination. Eliminate options 2, 3, and 4 because they are similar and relate to neurological problems. Review the etiology associated with Guillain-Barré syndrome if you had difficulty with this question.

Level of Cognitive Ability: Analysis
Client Needs: Physiological Integrity
Integrated Process: Nursing Process/Assessment
Content Area: Adult Health/Neurological

References:

Black, J., & Hawks, J. (2005). *Medical-surgical nursing: Clinical management for positive outcomes* (7th ed.). Philadelphia: Saunders, p. 2182.
Phipps, W., Monahan, F., Sands, J., Marek, J., & Neighbors, M. (2003). *Medical-surgical nursing: Health and illness perspectives* (7th ed.). St. Louis: Mosby, p. 1401.

293. A client is using diphenhydramine (Benadryl) 1% as a topical agent for allergic dermatosis. The nurse evaluates that the medication is having the intended effect if the client reported relief of what complaint?
1 Headache
2 Skin redness
3 Pain
4 Urticaria

Answer: 4

Rationale: Diphenhydramine is an antihistamine medication that has many uses. When used as a topical agent on the skin, it reduces the symptoms of allergic reaction, such as itching or urticaria. It does not act to relieve headache, skin redness, or pain.

Test-Taking Strategy: Note the key words "intended effect." Recalling that diphenhydramine is an antihistamine medication will assist in directing you to option 4. Review the action of this medication if you had difficulty with this question.

Level of Cognitive Ability: Analysis
Client Needs: Health Promotion and Maintenance
Integrated Process: Nursing Process/Evaluation
Content Area: Pharmacology

Reference:

Hodgson, B., & Kizior, R. (2004). *Saunders nursing drug handbook 2004.* Philadelphia: Saunders, p. 317.

294. A client is treated in the ambulatory clinic for a sprained ankle. Before releasing the client home, the nurse instructs the client to do which of the following during the next 24 hours?
1 Apply ice to the site intermittently
2 Cover the foot with heavy blankets
3 Sit with the foot flat on the floor
4 Walk on the foot for 20 minutes every hour

Answer: 1

Rationale: Soft tissue injuries such as sprains are treated by RICE (Rest, Ice, Compression, Elevation) for the first 24 hours after the injury. Ice is applied intermittently for 20 to 30 minutes at a time. Heat (such as with heavy blankets) is not used in the first 24 hours because it could increase venous congestion, which would increase edema and pain. The client should rest the foot and not walk around on it. The foot should be elevated and not placed in a dependent position.

Test-Taking Strategy: Use the process of elimination. Recalling that sprains should not be aggravated eliminates options 3 and 4. From the remaining options, recall that ice is applied to an injury in the first 24 hours rather than heat. Also, remember that heavy blankets would be uncomfortable on an injured foot. Review measures related to treatment of a sprained ankle if you had difficulty with this question.

Level of Cognitive Ability: Application
Client Needs: Health Promotion and Maintenance
Integrated Process: Teaching/Learning
Content Area: Adult Health/Musculoskeletal

Reference:
Black, J., & Hawks, J. (2005). *Medical-surgical nursing: Clinical management for positive outcomes* (7th ed.). Philadelphia: Saunders, pp. 652; 2501.

---

295. A client who is being evaluated for tuberculosis has never had a chest X-ray. The nurse instructs the client about which item before the procedure?
  1 It is necessary to breathe slowly and deeply while the film is taken.
  2 The client must void in the bathroom before the procedure.
  3 The X-ray will cause only a small amount of pain.
  4 A metal neck chain must be removed while the film is taken.

Answer: 4
Rationale: An X-ray is a photographic image of a part of the body on a special film, which is used to diagnose a wide variety of conditions. The X-ray itself is painless; any discomfort would arise from repositioning a painful part for filming. The nurse may want to premedicate a client who is at risk for pain. Any radiopaque objects such as jewelry or other metal must be removed because they interfere with the photographic image. The client is asked to breathe in deeply and then hold the breath while the chest X-ray is taken. The client is not required to void before the procedure, but may do so to enhance comfort during the procedure.

Test-Taking Strategy: Use the process of elimination and focus on the issue: a chest X-ray. Note the relationship between the anatomical location of this diagnostic test and the words "metal neck chain" in option 4. Review client teaching points related to a chest X-ray if you had difficulty with this question.

Level of Cognitive Ability: Application
Client Needs: Physiological Integrity
Integrated Process: Nursing Process/Implementation
Content Area: Adult Health/Respiratory

Reference:
Pagana, K., & Pagana, T. (2003). *Mosby's diagnostic and laboratory test reference* (6th ed.). St. Louis: Mosby, p. 239.

---

296. A client is being treated in the emergency room for a fractured tibia. The skin is not broken, but the nurse can see on the X-ray viewer that the bone is completely fractured across the shaft and has small splintered pieces around it. The nurse interprets that this client's fracture is a:
  1 Compound fracture
  2 Simple fracture
  3 Greenstick fracture
  4 Comminuted fracture

Answer: 4
Rationale: A comminuted fracture is a complete fracture across the shaft of a bone, with splintering of the bone into fragments. A compound fracture, also called an open fracture, is one in which the skin or mucous membrane has been broken, and the wound extends to the depth of the fractured bone. A simple fracture is a fracture of the bone across its entire shaft with some possible displacement but without breaking the skin. A greenstick fracture is an incomplete fracture, which occurs through part of the cross section of a bone. One side of the bone is fractured, and the other side is bent.

Test-Taking Strategy: Use the process of elimination, focusing on the key words "small splintered pieces." Remember that a *comminuted* fracture is broken into *minute* (small) pieces. Review the characteristics of the types of fractures if you had difficulty with this question.

Level of Cognitive Ability: Analysis
Client Needs: Physiological Integrity
Integrated Process: Nursing Process/Analysis
Content Area: Adult Health/Musculoskeletal

Reference:
Phipps, W., Monahan, F., Sands, J., Marek, J., & Neighbors, M. (2003). *Medical-surgical nursing: Health and illness perspectives* (7th ed.). St. Louis: Mosby, pp. 1468-1469.

---

297. A nurse in the emergency room is providing care to a client with a leg fracture. The nurse ensures that which essential item is done first before the fracture is reduced in the casting room?
1 Obtaining an anesthesia consent
2 Obtaining an informed consent for treatment
3 Notifying the operating room staff
4 Administering a narcotic analgesic

Answer: 2
Rationale: Before a fracture is reduced, an informed consent for treatment is needed. The nurse would give the client explanations according to the client's needs and ability to understand. An analgesic would be administered as prescribed, because the procedure is painful, but the informed consent form needs to be obtained before administering the medication. Administration of anesthesia would only be done in the operating room for open reduction of fractures. Closed reductions may be done in the emergency room without anesthesia.

Test Taking Strategy: Note the key words "essential" and "first" in the stem of the question. Note that the question specifically states that the procedure is going to be done in the cast room. This will assist in eliminating options 1 and 3. Recalling that an informed consent form must be obtained before administering sedating medication will direct you to option 2 from the remaining options. Review the procedure related to a closed reduction if you had difficulty with this question.

Level of Cognitive Ability: Analysis
Client Needs: Physiological Integrity
Integrated Process: Nursing Process/Analysis
Content Area: Adult Health/Musculoskeletal

References:
Ignatavicius, D., & Workman, M. (2002). *Medical surgical nursing: Critical thinking for collaborative care* (4th ed.). Philadelphia: Saunders, pp. 247-248.
Phipps, W., Monahan, F., Sands, J., Marek, J., & Neighbors, M. (2003). *Medical-surgical nursing: Health and illness perspectives* (7th ed.). St. Louis: Mosby, p. 1471.

---

298. A nurse is monitoring a client with a fracture to the left arm. Which sign observed by the nurse is consistent with impaired venous return in the area?
1 Weakened distal pulse
2 Continued pain despite medication
3 Pallor or blotchy cyanosis
4 Increasing edema

Answer: 4
Rationale: Impaired venous return is characterized by increasing edema. In the client with a fracture, this is most often prevented by elevating the limb. The other options identify signs of arterial damage, which can occur if the artery is contused, thrombosed, lacerated, or becomes spastic.

Test-Taking Strategy: Note the key words "impaired venous return." Use principles of blood flow to answer the question. Each of the incorrect options identifies difficulty with circulation to the extremity and is an arterial sign. The correct option identifies a sign that is consistent with impaired venous return. Review the signs noted in impaired venous return if you had difficulty with this question.

Level of Cognitive Ability: Analysis
Client Needs: Physiological Integrity
Integrated Process: Nursing Process/Analysis
Content Area: Adult Health/Musculoskeletal

Reference:
Black, J., & Hawks, J. (2005). *Medical-surgical nursing: Clinical management for positive outcomes* (7th ed.). Philadelphia: Saunders, pp. 1535-1536.

---

299. The nurse receives in transfer from the post-anesthesia care unit a client who has had skeletal traction applied in the operating room. The nurse takes immediate action to correct which problem noted with the traction setup?
1 Weights are resting against the foot of the bed
2 Knots are secured tightly
3 Ropes are centered in the wheel grooves of the pulleys
4 Ropes are free of frays or shredding

Answer: 1
Rationale: The traction setup is checked to ensure that the ropes are in the grooves of the pulleys, ropes are not frayed, knots are tied securely, and weights are hanging freely from the ropes. Problems with any of these can interfere with maintenance of proper traction. If any problems are noted, they should be fixed immediately.

Test-Taking Strategy: Use the process of elimination, noting the key words "takes immediate action to correct." Recalling that weights exert the pulling force needed in a traction setup will direct you to option 1. Review the principles of setting up traction if you had difficulty with this question.

Level of Cognitive Ability: Application
Client Needs: Physiological Integrity
Integrated Process: Nursing Process/Implementation
Content Area: Adult Health/Musculoskeletal

Reference:
Phipps, W., Monahan, F., Sands, J., Marek, J., & Neighbors, M. (2003). *Medical-surgical nursing: Health and illness perspectives* (7th ed.). St. Louis: Mosby, p. 1480.

---

300. A nurse is monitoring for the presence of pitting edema in the prenatal client. The nurse presses the fingertips of the middle and index fingers against the shin and holds pressure for 2 to 3 seconds. The nurse notes that the indentation is approximately 1 inch deep. The nurse documents that the client has which level of pitting edema?
1 1+
2 2+
3 3+
4 4+

Answer: 4
Rationale: When evaluating the presence of pitting edema, the nurse presses the fingertips of the index and middle fingers against the shin and holds pressure for 2 to 3 seconds. An indentation of approximately 1 inch deep would be indicative of 4+ edema. A slight indentation would indicate 1+ edema. An indentation of approximately 1/4 inch deep indicates 2+ edema. An indentation of approximately 1/2 inch deep indicates 3+ edema.

Test-Taking Strategy: Focus on the words "indentation is approximately 1 inch." Knowledge regarding this technique and the interpretation of the findings will assist in directing you to option 4. Review this content if you are unfamiliar with this technique.

Level of Cognitive Ability: Application
Client Needs: Health Promotion and Maintenance
Integrated Process: Nursing Process/Assessment
Content Area: Maternity/Antepartum

Reference:
Lowdermilk, D., & Perry, A. (2004). *Maternity & women's health care* (8th ed.). St. Louis: Mosby, p. 845.

REFERENCES

Black, J., & Hawks, J. (2005). *Medical-surgical nursing: Clinical management for positive outcomes* (7th ed.). Philadelphia: Saunders.

Chernecky, C., & Berger, B. (2004). *Laboratory tests and diagnostic procedures* (4th ed.). Philadelphia: Saunders.

Gahart, B., & Nazareno, A. (2004). *Intravenous medications* (20th ed.). St. Louis: Mosby.

Gulanick, M., Myers, J., Klopp, A., Gradishar, D., Galanes, S., & Puzas, M. (2003). *Nursing care plans: Nursing diagnosis and intervention* (5th ed.). St. Louis: Mosby.

Hodgson, B., & Kizior, R. (2004). *Saunders nursing drug handbook 2004.* Philadelphia: Saunders.

Ignatavicius, D., & Workman, M. (2005). *Medical surgical nursing: Critical thinking for collaborative care* (5th ed.). Philadelphia: Saunders.

James, S., Ashwill, J., & Droske, S. (2002). *Nursing care of children: Principles & practice* (2nd ed.). Philadelphia: Saunders.

Kee, J., & Marshall, S. (2004). *Clinical calculations: With applications to general and specialty areas* (5th ed.). Philadelphia: Saunders.

Keltner, N., Schwecke, L., & Bostrom, C. (2003). *Psychiatric nursing* (4th ed.). St. Louis: Mosby.

Lehne, R. (2004). *Pharmacology for nursing care* (5th ed.). Philadelphia: Saunders.

Lewis, S., Heitkemper, M., & Dirksen, S. (2004). *Medical-surgical nursing: Assessment and management of clinical problems* (6th ed.). St. Louis: Mosby.

Lowdermilk, D., & Perry, A. (2004). *Maternity & women's health care* (8th ed.). St. Louis: Mosby.

McKenry, L., & Salerno, E. (2003). *Mosby's pharmacology in nursing* (21st ed.). St. Louis: Mosby.

McKinney, E., James, S., Murray, S., & Ashwill, J. (2005). *Maternal-child nursing* (2nd ed.). St. Louis: Elsevier.

Murray, S., McKinney, E., & Gorrie, T. (2002). *Foundations of maternal-newborn nursing* (3rd ed.). Philadelphia: Saunders.

Pagana, K., & Pagana, T. (2003). *Mosby's diagnostic and laboratory test reference* (6th ed.). St. Louis: Mosby.

Peckenpaugh, N. (2003). *Nutrition essentials and diet therapy* (9th ed.). Philadelphia: Saunders.

Perry, A., & Potter, P. (2004). *Clinical nursing skills and techniques* (5th ed.). St. Louis: Mosby.

Phipps, W., Monahan, F., Sands, J., Marek, J., & Neighbors, M. (2003). *Medical-surgical nursing: Health and illness perspectives* (7th ed.). St. Louis: Mosby.

Potter, P., & Perry, A. (2005). *Fundamentals of nursing* (6th ed.). St. Louis: Mosby.

Skidmore-Roth, L. (2005). *Mosby's drug guide for nurses* (6th ed.). St. Louis: Mosby.

Stuart, G., & Laraia, M. (2005). *Principles and practice of psychiatric nursing* (8th ed.). St. Louis: Mosby.

Varcarolis, E.M. (2002). *Foundations of psychiatric mental health nursing* (4th ed.). Philadelphia: Saunders.

Wong, D., & Hockenberry, M. (2003). *Wong's nursing care of infants and children* (7th ed.). St. Louis: Mosby.

Thomas scrambled to his feet and grabbed her wrist to help her upward.

She slapped his hand away, and reached her feet with a grace that made Thomas feel awkward.

Even without the hat that had always cast a shade over her face aboard the ship, the layers of dirt and the filthy hair cropped short still made it difficult to recognize her. Yet it truly was Katherine.

She glared hatred at him and spat on the ground beside him.

The puppy skidded to a halt between them. Thomas barely noticed.

"You . . . what the . . . how?"

He did not finish his stammered sentence.

Katherine looked over his shoulder and her eyes widened.

There was a slight rustle and the sound of rushing air. Then a terrible, black pain overwhelmed him.

When he woke, it only took several seconds to realize he was in a crude jail. Alone.

Thomas groaned. He touched the back of his head—a foolish move, for he already knew how badly it ached, and his gentle probing of a large lump brought renewed stabs of pain.

That it was a jail he had no doubt.

Early evening light filtered through a tiny hole hewn in the stone.

The dimming light showed a straw-littered floor, stone walls so confining that he could touch all four easily from the center of the cell, and a battered wooden door.

Thomas stood and groaned again.

He felt an incredible thirst and he staggered to the door. He thumped it weakly.

What evil has befallen me now?

As he waited for a response, he puzzled over this turn of events. *Who has thrown me here? Why? Did that devil's child, Katherine, have others to help her?*

There was no answer, so Thomas thumped the door again. The impact of the heel of his hand against wood worsened the throbbing of his head.

My cloak. My gold. The old man's book. My sword and sheath. Gone.

It finally dawned on Thomas that he had been stripped down to his undergarments.

In anger, he pounded the door again.

"Release me," he croaked through a parched throat. "Return my belongings."

Faint footsteps outside the door reached him as the echoes of his words faded in the twilight of his cell.

Then, a slight scraping of wood against wood, as someone outside slid back the cover of a small partition high in the door.

"Your majesty," a cackling voice called in sarcastic English heavily accented with thick Portuguese. "Come closer."

Thomas did.

"Do you stand before the door?" that voice queried. "Beneath the window?"

Thomas looked directly above him at the hole in the door which permitted the voice to float clearly through.

"Yes," Thomas answered.

"Good. Here's something to shut your mouth for the night."

Without warning, a cascade of filthy water arched through the opening. Thoroughly drenched, Thomas could only sputter.

"And I've got buckets more if *that* doesn't instruct you on manners. Now let me sleep."

The partition slammed shut, and the footsteps retreated.

Thomas moved back to the side of the cell and gathered straw around him. Already he was beginning to shiver.

Shortly after the first star appeared in the small, square patch of sky that Thomas could see from his huddled position, across his feet ran the first rat of many in a long, sleepless night.

"Your majesty has a visitor." That heavy Portuguese accent interrupted Thomas' dreams.

Thomas opened gritty eyes to look upward at the face of a wrinkled gnome. A toothless grin leered down at him.

"Why should you enjoy sleep?" the voice continued.

Thomas began to focus, and the ancient gnome became a tiny old man with blackened gums that smacked and slobbered each word. "If I'm to be wakened this early, so must you."

The gnomelike man pointed back over his shoulder at the open doorway. "Why a common thief like you would receive such a visitor is beyond any mortal's understanding."

Thomas ignored the man. And ignored the constant throbbing of his head, the itching of straw and flea bites, and the thirst that squeezed his throat.

He was transfixed by his visitor.

Katherine.

Not the Katherine he had seen in any form before. Not the Katherine as a noble friend, disguised as a freak in the wrapping of bandages. Not as the Katherine whose long, blond hair had flowed in the moonlight during her visits as a midnight messenger. Not the Katherine who had betrayed him first to the Druids, then the outlaws. Not the Katherine covered with grime as a cook's assistant.

Thomas gaped at the transformation. Gone was the filth. Gone were the rags.

Instead, a long cape of fine silk reached almost to her feet. Holding the cloak in place was an oval clasp, showing a sword engraved into fine metal. Her neck and wrists glittered with exquisite jewelry. Her hair, still short, had been trimmed and altered to highlight the delicate curves of her cheekbones.

A slight smile played across Katherine's face, as if she knew his thoughts.

She would put a queen to shame.

Thomas fought against the surge of warmth the struck him at that mysterious and aloof smile.

She is one of them, he warned himself, *one of the Druids who have taken Magnus.*

He opened his mouth to speak, and she shook her head slightly to caution him against it.

"This most certainly is my runaway servant," she said sternly. "I shall see he is whipped thoroughly."

Servant?

The gnomelike man nodded with understanding. "Feed them and clothe them, and still they show no gratitude."

Servant?

"I have spoken to the authorities," Katherine continued. "The boy that this—" Katherine sniffed scorn and pointed at Thomas "—scoundrel attacked has not reappeared to seek compensation. Given that, and the fortune in gold that changed from my hands to the magistrate's, I have been granted permission for his return."

The gnomelike man somehow shook his head in sympathy. "Is he worth this?"

"A promise to his mother, a faithful servant," Katherine answered. "She was dear to our family, and we vowed never to let her son stray."

"Aaah," the jailer said.

He kicked Thomas. "Be sure we don't see your face again."

Thomas pushed himself to his feet. His back felt like a board from leaning against the cold stone; his legs ached from shivering, and his head still throbbed. Now he was to be treated as her servant?

Yet, what were his alternatives? He shuffled forward meekly. *Wait,* he promised himself, *until she and I are away from listening ears.*

Not until the jailer retrieved Thomas' clothing did he realize how immodest it was to be standing there in his undergarments. He seethed with frustration as he dressed under her smirking gaze, stumbling awkwardly as he balanced on one leg and then the other.

Then Thomas followed her through the narrow corridor into the bright sunlight outside, not daring to wonder what poor souls wasted away behind the other silent, wooden prison doors.

They stood at the north end of the harbor, and the noise and the confusion of the chaos of men busy among ships reached them clearly.

"You were arrested yesterday," Katherine began, "as you lay there gasping like a stunned fish."

Thomas rubbed the back of his head. "What foul luck. Certainly a harbor like this has only a handful of men who guard and patrol for the townspeople."

"The guard was pleased to be such a hero," Katherine said. "Rarely do such bold crimes occur in broad daylight. He also seemed pleased at the accuracy of his blow."

She paused. "It cost fully a quarter of your gold to pay your ransom."

"*My* gold?" Thomas sputtered.

"Of course," Katherine said calmly. "I lifted your pouch as I helped them drag you away."

"My gold?"

"Had I not, the jailer certainly would have. After all, did he not keep your sword and sheath?"

Thomas ground his teeth in anger.

"Fear not," Katherine said sweetly. "As the cook's assistant, I spirited away your puppy. It remains safely waiting for you at the inn."

"And my remaining gold?" Thomas spat each word.

Her voice remained sweet. "Much of it purchased this fine clothing I needed to pose as a noblewoman retrieving an errant servant. Besides, it would serve neither of us for me to remain as a mere shiphand on our next voyage."

"*Much* of it? *Next* voyage?" He caught the implications. "*Our* next voyage?"

"Yes."

"Hardly," Thomas vowed. "I have my own path to follow."

"Not unless you jump ship," Katherine said smugly. "I need only say the word and you will be thrown in jail again. Until we leave Lisbon, you are mine; and under my orders, you will board the ship of my choice."

"You have much to explain." Thomas dared not trust himself to say more. His fists were clenched in fury.

"Perhaps. But as my penniless servant, you are in no position to dictate any terms."

She favored him with another radiant smile.

"And my first command is that you bathe. You smell wretched."

"You should find the servants' quarters somewhere below," Katherine said as they stepped onto the gangway.

Thomas gritted his teeth. Katherine had been shrewd enough to dispense an amount of gold that guaranteed eternal loyalty from the port authorities.

Twice, in fact, he had rebelled during this long day since his release from prison. Was it not bad enough she had refused to return his remaining gold? Was it not bad enough she had taken such enjoyment at his discomfort, before and after his time in the public bath? Twice he had stormed from her, uncaring that he was penniless in a strange town. And twice he had been overtaken by a pair of guards who offered him the alternative of jail or a return to his mistress, that wonderful noblewoman.

So now he stood on the gangway that led to the galley *Santa Magdalen,* an Italian merchant galley. This ship, unlike the *Dragon's Eye's* single mast with square sail, had two masts with lateens, triangular sails which, in the calmer seas of the mid-Atlantic and Mediterranean, enabled the ship to sail into winds with a minimum of tacking back and forth.

Thomas scowled at Katherine. But discreetly. He could see lurking behind her on the dock the two guards, and remembered they had not been gentle in the manner in which they had persuaded him to return to her.

She smiled back. Sweetly, of course.

He wanted to stitch her lips together, anything to rid her of that assured smile. He wanted to shake her by the shoulders and loosen the words from her mouth, words to explain how she had followed him, and how she had known his destination, to find passage on a galley which sailed to Israel, the Holy Land. Far worse, he wanted to be able to stare into those taunting green eyes for every heartbeat for the rest of his life. That confusion only served to deepen his foul mood.

She is one of them, he forced himself to remember, each time their eyes met. *I should not feel this insane warmth.*

So he growled surly agreement at her directions to the servants' area and began to march to the cramped and foul section of the ship which would be his home for several weeks.

"Thomas," she called, before he took three steps. He turned around and scowled again.

She pointed to the expensive leather bags at her feet which held her considerable array of travel possessions, all purchased with his gold. One of the bags held the smuggled puppy. Neither wanted trouble with this crew.

"Must you forget the simplest of duties?" Katherine

asked. "Surely you don't expect *me* to carry these bags to my quarters."

It took nearly an hour to leave the harbor. The galley was awkward at slow speeds, and the captain dared not raise the sails until they reached the open sea.

The crew used oars instead. Thomas was half surprised that Katherine had not volunteered his services as an oarsman.

In the hum of the activity of departure, Thomas moved unnoticed to the prow of the ship where Katherine stood, and enjoyed the breeze above the water.

Spray cascaded against the wooden bow as the galley rose and fell with the waves. That sound made it easy for him to approach her back without being heard.

"Have I not been tortured enough?" he asked.

She half turned and stepped back, not startled at his sudden presence. "I've hardly begun," she said. "But this is a long voyage, and I remember well your treatment of me as I hung by a rope."

"Do not hold those foolish dreams of revenge," Thomas said. "We are away from those wretched Lisbon watchdogs. I shall be my own man now."

She smiled. "If you glance over your shoulder, you will see unfriendly eyes watching closely your every move."

Thomas groaned. "Not so."

"Indeed," Katherine informed him. "Your gold has proven to work wonders with the ship's captain as well. He has promised to have you whipped, should you exhibit the same behavior which jailed you in Lisbon."

"My gold cannot last for eternity," Thomas protested. "Silks, perfumes, rich food, passage, and now protection! I had planned to live for a year on that gold."

"Wool," Katherine said.

"Wool?" Thomas stared at her as if she had lost her sanity.

"Silks, perfumes, rich food, passage, protection. And wool."

"Wool?" The despair of comprehension began to fill his voice.

"Wool," she repeated patiently. "This merchant ship

holds twenty tons of wool which I purchased with your gold. Even after the price of passage, I should profit handsomely with its sale when we arrive in the Holy Land."

"Impossible," Thomas said, through lips thinned with frustration.

"Oh, no," Katherine assured him. "Wool is much needed in far ports."

"I . . . meant . . . impossible . . . that . . . I . . . had . . . enough . . . gold . . . for . . . twenty . . . tons . . . of . . . wool." Thomas could hardly speak now, so difficult was it to remain in control.

Katherine dismissed that with a cheerful wave. "Have I neglected to inform you that I borrowed heavily from the supply of gold you have hidden in England?"

His mouth dropped.

"Remember?" she prompted. "Near the cave which contains your secret books?"

A strangled gasp left his throat. Thomas clutched his chest.

"It was child's play to follow you to Scarborough after your contest with the outlaw Robert Hood. All I needed to do was return to that cave and wait for your arrival."

She lifted an eyebrow and pretended surprise. "You expected that I would remain with the outlaws to share the ransom collected for Isabelle?"

Thomas closed his eyes briefly, as if fighting a spasm of pain.

"Thomas, Thomas," she chided. "Surely you don't believe it was your doing to win the contest with the outlaw?"

His eyes now widened.

"Robert Hood had been instructed to lose. I wanted you set free."

She moved closer to him and mockingly placed a consoling hand on his arm. "Take comfort, however. He admitted later the outcome was not certain, even had he wanted to defeat you."

Thomas slapped her hand away.

"Woman," he said fiercely, "you have pushed me too far."

He grew cold with rage as he continued. "My fight for Magnus was a deathbed promise to the nurse who raised and loved me more than my parents might ever had done. Every pain suffered to fulfill that pledge is a pain I would gladly have suffered ten times over."

He stepped closer but did not raise his voice.

"Yet even after victory, the strange secrets behind Magnus haunted me. And each new secret glimpsed has had your face. I fight enemies I cannot see, and I fight enemies I wish I could not see. Too many good men have sacrificed themselves for this fight."

He advanced while she backed to the railing.

"Yet the reason for this fight—a reason I am certain *you* know—has been kept from me. And even the reason it has been kept from me has been kept from me."

He paused for breath. "Your face and those secrets follow me here to the ends of the earth. And now I am your prisoner on a tiny ship in vast waters. You have stolen my gold. You have humiliated me."

He raised his forefinger and held it beneath her chin. "And now you mock me in tone and words. I will take no more."

Thomas stepped back and said in a whisper. "From this moment on, wherever you stand on this boat, I will choose the point farthest away from you. Threaten me, punish me, have me thrown overboard. I do not care. For I wash my hands of you."

He stared at her for a long moment, then let scorn fill his face before turning away.

She called to his back immediately.

"Forgive me," Katherine said. The mocking banter in her voice had disappeared. "Love leads one to do strange things."

He turned.

"Que je ne peux pas *ne pas* t'aimer," Katherine said.

Thomas was still stunned by her first words. So it took his befuddled brain a moment to translate. *"I cannot not love you," she just said. Why French?*

"And I have loved you fiercely since I was a child," she

was now saying. Although he understood those words clearly, it took Thomas another moment to realize her last sentence had been spoken in flawless German.

Loved me since she was a child?

"I see by the light in your eyes," Katherine said, now in English, "that you understand well my words. And that is part of why I cannot *not* love you."

"Truth and answers," Thomas replied, using Latin. "Only a fool would throw away love offered by you, but first I need truth and answers."

She smiled at his switch in language and answered him in Latin.

"Can you not now see we have received the same education? Have we not been driven mercilessly by our teachers to be literate and fluent in all the civilized languages, when few in this world can even read in their own tongue?"

She moved to Thomas again, and placed again her hand on his forearm. This touch, however, was tender, not mocking. "And have we not been trained to fight the same fight against the same enemies?"

She looked beyond Thomas and discreetly removed her hand from his arm. "The ship's captain approaches. Tonight, let us talk."

The five hours until moonlight seemed as long as the entire voyage from England to Lisbon.

Thomas had stood on the stern platform, staring at the coastline directly eastward that became little more than a faint haze with distance.

I dare not trust her. Her vow of love is merely a trick. For if she were not one of them, how else could I have been captured in my camp the morning after her arrival with the old man?

Yet, the old man spoke of Merlins, raised from birth to fight the evil spawned by generations of a secret society of Druids. I almost believed him, until my capture through their betrayal proved they were Druids posing as Merlins.

And yet, I must consider the alternative. If Katherine is a Merlin and can truly explain the apparent betrayal, she is my only hope to recapture Magnus, my only source to the secrets which have plagued me. If she is a Druid, I will play the game to find what she really wants. So I must pretend to believe her, and refuse to let my heart be fooled as it so desperately wants to be.

Thomas remained on the stern platform all those hours until she appeared.

Her hair was now silver in the moonlight, her face a haunting mixture of shadows.

I cannot read her eyes. How dare I trust her words?

"You know by now that a secret war rages," she began without greeting. "Between Druids, who have chosen darkness and secrecy as the way to power, and Merlins, who battle back in equal secrecy."

Thomas nodded.

"You and I were born to Merlin parents," Katherine said. "But not even birth destines a child to be a Merlin. Some, in fact, live and grow old unaware of their parents' mission."

Thomas held up a hand to interrupt.

"Certainly I know of the Druids," he said. "Their circle of evil is ancient. The Roman Emperor Julius Caesar observed them more than twelve hundred years ago, when they still reigned openly in Britain."

Katherine nodded. "Of course. You know that from your books in the cave. But of Merlins—"

"Of Merlins I know nothing more than their name, as mentioned by the old man and another I knew in Magnus. It is more than passing strange that they—we—bear the same name as King Arthur's wise man and trusted counselor."

"More than passing strange," Katherine agreed. "King Arthur and his knights ruled some hundreds of years after the Roman conquerers had taken Britain and forced the Druids into hiding openly."

"Hiding openly?"

"Openly. The safest way to hide. Blacksmiths, tanners, farmers, noblemen, knights, priests—during the day. But at night . . ." Katherine's voice trailed. "At night they would meet to continue their quest for power."

She shivered, although the air was warm. "Frightening, is it not? Any man or woman you might meet in England—a false sorcerer at night. And many strove for positions of power in society, the better to influence the direction of their secret plans."

Thomas spat disgust but said nothing. He knew too well the treachery of Druids.

"Merlin?" he prompted her.

"Yes. Merlin. Eight hundred years ago. The brightest and best of the Druids."

Thomas stood transfixed. The creaking of the ship passing through water, the clouds slipping past the moon, he was aware of none of it.

"Merlin a Druid?" he asked.

"It explains much, does it not? His powers have become legendary; some call him an enchanter. Equipped with the knowledge of a Druid—knowledge that is considerable and often seems magic to poor, ignorant peasants—he accomplished much through deception. And what better place for a Druid than at the right hand of Britain's finest king?"

Thomas shook his head, trying to understand. "Yet he battled—"

"Yet Merlin battled the same Druids who raised him to such power. Merlin founded generations of the Druids' greatest enemies, each person equipped with the knowledge of a Druid. In short, he turned their own powerful sword upon themselves."

"Why?" Thomas asked softly. He let his mind drift back those eight hundred years to the court of King Arthur—Sir Galahad, Sir Lancelot, and the other Knights of the Round Table. And Merlin, the man who established that Round Table, at the right hand of Britain's most powerful man. "Merlin had everything a man might desire. Why risk losing all by rejecting the same Druids who had given him that power?"

"It is legend among us," Katherine said, equally softly. "The Druids had waited generations for one of them to have the power in open society that Merlin did. With Merlin, there was finally one to set into motion the plan that would let them conquer the entire kingdom, a plan so evil that its success would establish the Druids forever. Merlin was the one man able to ensure success, until he became the one man to stop them. The legend is that a simple priest showed Merlin the power of faith in God by—"

"A bold plan to establish the Druids?" Thomas interrupted. "It failed with Merlin. Is it the plan they follow now that Magnus has been conquered?"

"Yes," Katherine said quietly. "Merlin stopped them once. And since then, we have fought them, generation by generation, at every turn. We have held them at bay, until they finally discovered where we had hidden ourselves."

"What is at the end of this evil plan?" Thomas asked.

Hesitation. Then Katherine said, "I . . . I do not know. The old man always promised to tell me . . . but never had that chance."

Does she lie? Or are her faltering words because of grief for the old man?

Thomas paced back and forth several times, then asked. "The Merlins also hide openly?"

"Yes."

"And seek positions of power to counteract the influence of Druids?"

"Yes." Katherine smiled. "Sometimes we reach fame through these efforts. And we reach far. Generations ago, Charles the Great, king of the Franks, sent for educated people from all over Christendom. He wanted his people to learn again, from books."

Katherine paused, trying to recall the story. "The Druids had arranged to send one of their people. What better way to spread evil in other countries? We intercepted the orders and replaced that Druid with a man named Alcuin. He rose quickly within the royal court of the Franks and did untold good, spreading knowledge and even introducing a new style of writing."

She waved her hand. "There are others, of course, through the ages. We have all been taught the stories of our history."

Thomas frowned. "How many of us are there?"

Katherine sighed. "Before Magnus fell twenty years ago,

hundreds. More than enough to keep the Druids from reaching their goal."

"And now?"

"I . . . I . . . do not know. I have only the stories they taught me."

She became quiet, the memory of the old man too hard to bear.

Thomas sensed her sadness and tried to occupy her with other thoughts. "Hundreds? How could hundreds be taught in secrecy? That would take hundreds of teachers!"

"Not so," Katherine replied, her voice not entirely free of sorrow. "Merlin devised a new method. He appointed his successor before he died. And each successor appointed another, so that Merlin's command was passed directly from generation to generation. Each leader was the finest among us. Each one selected teachers, who every generation shared knowledge with entire groups who sat together. One teacher had as many as thirty listeners."

Thomas whistled appreciation. "'Tis wondrous strange. Yet seems so simple. Now it strikes me odd this method is not followed elsewhere."

Katherine nodded. "Merlin called it 'school.' "

Thomas stumbled over the strange word. "*School.*"

Katherine nodded again. "Our legends tell us he so named it because of the schools of fish reminded him of the way we gather to listen, but this I must believe is a story invented for only the youngest Merlins."

Thomas barely heard her last words.

Much now made sense.

Magnus. Isolated in the moors north of England, far from the intrigues and attention of reigning monarchs.

Magnus. With only moderate wealth, not a prize worth seeking.

Magnus. Insignificant, nearly invisible.

Magnus. Hidden as it is, with the largest fortress in the north, a construction which must have cost a king's ransom, far more than the land itself could earn, even with the profit of centuries of income.

Magnus. Hidden as it is, with the largest fortress in the

north, yet with seemingly nothing to protect.

Magnus. Riddled with secret passageways.

Thomas understood. He stopped pacing abruptly and voiced his certainty to Katherine.

"Merlin established Magnus. Obscure and well protected, it has been the training ground for every generation to follow."

"Yes," she said. "Merlin chose Magnus and had the fortress built. He retired to the island in that remote land. From there, he taught the others and sent them throughout the country to combat the Druids in hidden warfare. And Magnus served us well for hundreds of years. Even after the Druids finally discovered its location and purpose, it took generations for them to conquer it. I was not there when that happened, of course, but the old man told me that their surprise attack and ruthless slaughter twenty years ago all but destroyed the Merlins. Only a few survived."

She stopped, and in the dim light, Thomas could see she was trying to search his face.

"And, Thomas," she finally whispered, "you were appointed shortly after your birth, chosen as Merlin's successor of this generation to reconquer Magnus for us."

Chapter Forty-Five

Thomas stood and squarely faced her, with feet braced and arms crossed. It was the only way he could stop the trembling which threatened to overwhelm him.

I want so badly to believe her.

"You weave a fanciful tale," he said scornfully. "Yet if it were true, why was I not told of this?"

"But you were, in a way," Katherine said softly. "Was it an accident you were hidden in that obscure abbey? Was it an accident that Sarah, your childhood nurse, gladly exiled herself there to raise and train you as thoroughly as if you had been raised in Magnus as son of the reigning earl?"

That startled Thomas into dropping his bluff of indifference.

"You jest! My father was a mason, a builder of churches. He and my mother died of the plague, but left behind money to pay for my education among the clergy."

"No, Thomas. Sarah had been commanded to keep the truth from you. Your father, the ruler of Magnus, was the appointed leader of *his* generation of Merlins. It was too important that no one ever discover your real identity, and it was feared that as a child, you might blurt it aloud in front of the wrong ears."

Thomas shook his head. "Sarah encouraged me to dream of reigning over Magnus, but she always told me it was *her* parents I should avenge."

Katherine disagreed, sadly. "Too many of the Merlins fell with Magnus. The old man often told me you were our only hope, that should the Druids discover the only son of the last leader of the Merlins was still alive, they would leave no stone in England unturned in their search to have you murdered."

Thomas took several moments to consider this staggering news. "My father reigned over Magnus? My father was the successor to Merlin? It was my father's death at Druid hands that I was raised to avenge?"

"Yes."

Thomas raised his hands helplessly. "I should have been told this. I stumbled in the darkness." His voice became accusing. "Alone."

Katherine put a finger to her own lips to silence his protests. "How old were you when Sarah died?"

"Nine."

"Too young to be trusted yet with that precious knowledge. And there was no one who could replace her at the abbey to instruct you more. The old man often told me that we could only trust her training had been a magnificent seed, that you would learn more from the books left with you, and that you would always remember Magnus."

Thomas shook his head again, more firmly. "Yet I ruled Magnus for three seasons. Neither you, nor the old man, nor Gervaise revealed this to me then."

Katherine moved to the edge of the ship and stared away. Thomas was forced to follow to be able to listen to her words before they were swallowed by the breeze.

"We could not," she said, still staring at the moon. "For you had been alone at the abbey for five years. We could not know if the Druids had found you and claimed you as one of their own."

"I conquered Magnus! I took it from them!"

Katherine sighed. "Yes. I argued that often with the old man. He told me that we played a terrible game of chess against unseen masters. He told me they might have artfully arranged a simple deception, that the more it seemed you were against them, the more likely we might be to tell you the final truth, and in so doing lose this centuries-old battle in the quickest of heartbeats."

Thomas pondered her words and spoke slowly. "What is the final truth?"

The constant splash of water against the side of the galley was his only reply.

"The final truth," he demanded.

"Not even I was told."

She lies. I can sense that, even with her face turned away from me. Yet I must pretend to believe.

So Thomas said, "There is a undeniable logic in that. How could you ever finally believe that I was not a Druid, posing as one of you? So I was watched. By Gervaise, who posed as a simple old caretaker. And by you, in your disguise beneath the bandages."

"I am relieved you understand."

There is a simple flaw with this entire story. And it breaks my heart. Yet, I cannot leave it lie.

So Thomas spun her to face him and squeezed both her wrists without mercy.

"But explain," he said fiercely, "why you finally tell me this now. And explain it well, for otherwise I believe nothing, and I shall cast you overboard."

"No, Thomas," she begged. "You must let go!"

His response was to pull her closer to the edge of the ship.

She must believe this terrible bluff.

Thomas had no chance to continue it.

"Speak now—" he started.

Her eyes widened and she called out, "No!"

But her cry was not directed at Thomas.

He heard a scuffling of feet and began to turn his head. *Late, much too late.* A familiar blackness crashed down upon him.

Thomas dreamed that gigantic court jesters juggled him like a tiny ball, laughing and yelling as they tossed him back and forth.

He woke with a muffled shout just as the most hideous jester dropped him, and discovered indeed he had been tossed back and forth, but in the confines of the brig in the belly of the ship.

Thomas propped out a hand to keep from pitching back

to the other side, and waited for his eyes to adjust to the dimness. The extent of his new prison—walls of rough wood and iron bars for a door—made the cell in Lisbon seem like a castle.

His head felt it might split.

Uncanny, he thought with a twisted grin, *how they managed to hit me in the exact spot of my previous lump. Do bumps grow atop bumps?*

He was able to contemplate this imprisonment for several hours before he had a visitor.

"No," he groaned at the scent of perfume. "Curse me with your arrival no longer."

"Hush," Katherine said. "I risk too much even now. A real noblewoman saved from the attack of a rebellious servant would never grace him with a visit."

Thomas shook his head slightly, but at the reverberations of pain, held it very still. "You had us watched as we spoke," he accused. "And they believed I would harm you."

"Would you have?" Katherine asked.

"Then, no." He touched the back of his head. "Now, yes."

She smiled. "I have little time. Yet I wish to answer your question."

Thomas studied her face throught the iron bars.

"In Scarborough," Katherine began, "you made an error. You sought advice from an old hag who sold fish, advice on how to reach the Holy Land."

Thomas shrugged, then winced. "Unfamiliar with the ways of the sea, I needed that advice. And I dared not ask any ship captain. I did not want him to know my destination. So I asked her, thinking she would never remember a passing stranger."

"A passing stranger with a tail sticking out of his cloak as he walked away?"

"The puppy."

"Yes," Katherine said. "Now safely hidden in my quarters. Thus I discovered your destination. There was only one ship in the harbor leaving for Lisbon. It was not difficult to sign on as a cook's assistant."

"Why—"

"Hush. Time flees too quickly."

She took a breath. "I had intended merely to follow you on both ships. Until you lured me into the trap and had the misfortune to be arrested." She stopped, puzzled. "How was it you guessed you had been followed aboard the ship?"

"The manner in which three hardened sailors fell at the wave of my sword. It was the same mysterious manner in which my soldiers fell at Magnus."

Katherine giggled. "The surprise on your face as they fell!" Then she sobered. "A Druid trick. Short thick hollow straws. A puff of breath directs a tiny pellet coated with a sleeping potion. I was in the shadows nearby, watching, because I had heard the crewmen speak and knew you were in danger."

A Druid trick. Either she tells the truth and is a Merlin who knows much about the enemy. Or she is the enemy. How do I decide?

Thomas nodded to conceal his doubt. There was yet the major flaw in her words. So he spoke the question aloud. "Why reveal what you did last night? Why now, if not ever before?"

"I will tell you now. And there is no need to threaten to throw me overboard," Katherine replied. "When you were arrested, desperate measures were needed. I had to help you out, and could only do so by playing the role I did. As a noblewoman. And by then, I had also decided you were not a Druid. Not if you were truly going to the Holy Land by yourself."

She hesitates. What does she hide?

Katherine must have caught the doubt in his eyes. "Hawkwood is gone. If you are a Merlin, I need your help as badly as you need mine. It was a risk worth taking. If you are a Druid . . . I knew I was safe, protected by your gold as a noblewoman in Lisbon, and on this ship."

Perhaps. But there must be more. It is obvious in her manner.

Thomas nodded pretended satisfaction.

He thrust his hands through the gap between the iron bars and spoke softly.

"Love," he said. "Since childhood?"

She took his hands in hers. Although he had meant it as an appearance of trust, the touch of her hands in his filled him with warmth.

Do not trust her, nor your heart. Yet remember the first time you met her, and how there was an instinctive reaching of your heart for hers, as if it was remembering a love deeply buried.

And he could not ignore the happiness that swelled his throat.

"Love. Since childhood and before you arrived at Magnus," she repeated. "I pray in the Holy Land that much more will be revealed to both of us."

A noise from behind startled her into dropping both her hands.

"Thomas," she said quickly, "if it is possible to return safely, I will. Otherwise . . ."

She picked up the ends of her long cape and disappeared in the opposite direction of an approaching crewman.

Thomas did not see her until the galley reached the harbor of St. Jean d'Acre, the last city of the crusaders in the Holy Land to fall to the Muslim infidels.

Two crewmen brought Thomas to the deck of the ship as summoned by Katherine. He needed the help given by their rough hands which grasped his upper arms to keep him upright. Not only was he weak from lack of proper food, but the brig had been so cramped that his legs were no longer accustomed to bearing his weight. And his ankles were shackled by chains of iron.

The crewman left him beside Katherine and waited watchfully nearby.

She remained silent. It would serve neither of them if she appeared anything but the vengeful noblewoman.

Thomas stared past her at the half-ruined towers, still magnificent and rising from the land at the edge of the Mediterranean Sea.

St. Jean d'Acre was a town on a peninsula surrounded entirely by sea. Once while still in Christian hands, it had been protected by a massive wall that ran across the peninsula, so that the only approach for attack was by water.

The air around him was steamy with a heat he had never felt before. The sun seemed much larger than in England, and its glare was an attack of fury. The buildings that shimmered before his eyes as the galley grew closer were formed in unfamiliar curves.

At that moment, despite the heat, Thomas felt a chill replace his anticipation.

This land is so foreign, I am doomed before I begin. Muslims have fought Christians here for centuries, and I step onto their land, not even able to . . .

Thomas took a deep breath as that new thought almost staggered him.

I have been so intent on reaching the Holy Land, I have overlooked the single most obvious barrier to my success here. I do not speak the language!

He wanted badly to discuss this with Katherine, but as he shuffled sideways to whisper his concern, the ship's captain approached.

He was a great bear of a man with swarthy skin and a hooked nose. Curiously, he wore a purple turban.

"Milady," he said respectfully, "we all wish you Godspeed in the search for your relatives. Many were lost to fine families during the Crusades, and perhaps you will find one or two still alive among the infidels."

He paused, searching for a delicate way to impart advice. "This is a strange land with strange customs. Men take insult if a woman shows her face. To be sure, you will have no difficulty finding a buyer for your wool. Yet you must wear this during all times in public, including the times you negotiate with merchants."

The captain held out a black veil.

Katherine slipped it over her head. It stopped short of the clasp at her neck which held her cloak together.

"You have my gratitude," Katherine told the captain. "Would that all might have the grace and kindness which you have extended me."

He bowed slightly, then frowned at Thomas. "Shall we whip him once to ensure meekness ashore?"

Katherine removed the veil, held it in her left hand, and touched her chin with the tip of her right forefinger as she studied Thomas. A mischievous glint escaped her eyes.

"No," she said finally. "I think the shackles should suffice."

Thomas, unshackled now that they were clear of the galley, could hardly believe his ears.

He stood with Katherine in the crowded *fonduk,* a large open-square warehouse on the eastern waterfront. It had belonged to the Venetians before d'Acre fell to the Muslims. Now, as the best trading area in a town where major trading routes met the sea, it was occupied by hundreds of sharp-eyed Arab merchants.

He stood amazed for one simple reason. The clamoring babble which surrounded him made sense.

"Don't trust his olive oil," one shout reached him clearly. "That merchant is a crooked as a snake's path!"

"Here for the finest salt!" another voice shouted.

"Silk from the overland journeys!"

"Camels for hire!"

Fragments of excited conversation filtered through his mind.

I understand each word!

And Katherine stood in front of him, her face hidden by her veil, bartering over the price of wool with an eager merchant.

In their language! Impossible!

He stood and watched the chaos around him with an open mouth. The harbor area of Lisbon now seemed like a sleepy town in comparison to this.

Camels, donkeys, and gesturing men in long, white robes and turbans in all directions. Strange animals with long, slender tails—could these be the monkeys of which he had read? Finely woven carpets, baskets as tall as men, beggars . . .

Katherine tugged on his arm.

"I have finished," she said in English. Satisfaction filled her words. "As predicted, I have doubled my investment."

"*Our* investment," Thomas felt the need to immediately correct her, although more pressing things engaged him.

He leaned forward.

"Their words!" he said. "I understand."

"As well you should," Katherine replied. "It is—"

A beggar darted up to her and chattered excitedly.

"Lady, lady, from where did you get such a fine clasp?"

Katherine reached for her neck and touched it in response.

"I—"

"Very fine! Very fine!" the beggar interrupted. "I can find someone to give you an excellent price for it!"

"I am flattered, of course, yet—"

"Double what you had expected!" the beggar insisted. Then he stopped and looked at her coyly. "Or is it a family heirloom?"

Katherine nodded firmly from behind her veil. "It will never be sold."

Unexpectedly, the beggar darted away without another word.

"Strange," Thomas said. "About the language . . ."

"Of course," Katherine reassured him. "But first, we must purchase you clothing which lets you blend among these people. And a sword."

She giggled. "And once again, you are in dire need of time in a public bathhouse."

Twenty-two years had passed since the last banner of any of the German, English, and French crusader knights had flown above the stone walls of St. Jean d'Acre, twenty-two years since shadows of those banners had danced upon the waters of the Mediterranean.

The town then had been a riot of colors. Merchants from eleven European countries had competed for sales from their great *fonduks,* all supplied from ships arriving from the sea and from camel caravans led by sharp-eyed Arab traders arriving by the Damascus road.

Yet after nearly two hundred years as the main port to the Holy Land, St. Jean d'Acre, the last of the crusader strongholds, had finally fallen to Muslim infidels. Jerusalem had fallen long before, then Nazareth — the city of Christ's boyhood, then the fortresses along the Sea of Galilee, and one by one, all of the mighty castles of the crusader knights who had battled and held the land for generations.

St. Jean d'Acre was now a mere shell of the trading town it had been. To be sure, merchants still haggled, for occasional ships still arrived. But the walls of the city and the high turrets of its remaining buildings — which seemed such a glorious illusion of strength from a distance away on the water — were, on close inspection, war-ravaged and doomed to crumble to dust.

Few now were those in the town with fair skin and blue eyes, the sure signs of Northern European heritage. And none were those who dared display the colors of any knighthood among the Muslim infidels who so thoroughly dominated the entire land that Jesus Christ Himself had walked during His brief and significant life on earth. It seemed prudent to be dressed in a way to conceal the fair skin and light eyes.

"I no longer feel half dead," Thomas grinned beneath his turban. "A rest tonight in a bed that does not shift with the waves, some food, and I will be ready to conquer the world."

Katherine smiled back.

They gazed at each other in silence for several seconds, forming an island of privacy in the hectic motion of the market around them outside the bath house.

Don't let those eyes fool you. Remember, you will only remain with her until you discover the truths you need. There is nothing more to this situation.

To cover the flush he felt beneath her gaze, Thomas bantered and gestured at his robe and turban and sword at his side. "Do I not appear the perfect infidel? Especially after you tell me how it is I understand their language."

"Perfect," Katherine agreed lightly. "We—"

She frowned.

"Thomas, to your left. Is it not the same beggar who approached me for this clasp?"

Thomas turned his head quickly enough to see the beggar grasping the sleeve of two large men and pointing in his direction.

"The same," Thomas confirmed.

All eyes locked across the space between them. The beggar and his companions, each armed with scimitars—those great curving swords—and Thomas and Katherine staring back at them in return.

"Do you find a startling resemblance between those two men and a pair of wolves?" Thomas asked softly, without removing his eyes from them.

"Hungry wolves," Katherine said. "I like this not. We should return to the inn and see your puppy instead."

They backed away quickly. And soon discovered they were prey for the two large men.

In a half run, Katherine and Thomas darted around market stalls and through crowds of people.

"This way!" Katherine cried.

"No . . ." But Thomas did not protest in time. Katherine had already started down a narrow alley.

Why have they chosen us? Thomas wondered as he ran. *Because we are foreign? Surely it cannot be because of the Druids. We have only just arrived.*

Thomas nearly stumbled on the uneven stone of the streets as he stopped and turned to run after her. His sword slapped against his side.

I pray I will not use this weapon, he thought. *These men are larger and stronger.*

The two men gained ground. They were familiar with the twists of the alley. Thomas and Katherine were not.

Each second brought the men closer. Thomas and Katherine were now in a full run, slipping beneath archways and around blind corners.

"Again! This way!" Katherine panted. "We are nearly there!"

"No . . ." Thomas moaned. He did not know the town at all, but knew with certainty her path led them away from both the waterfront and the inn.

Without warning, Katherine stopped and pounded on a door hidden in a recess in the alley.

"That is not the inn!" Thomas warned.

"Behind you!" Katherine said. She banged the door with her fist, while staring in horror at the approaching swordsmen.

Thomas did the only thing he could. He drew his sword.

Katherine pounded the door.

"You cannot avoid the assassins' pledge," the first man snarled, as he lifted his scimitar.

Thomas managed to parry the first blow, then step aside as the other swung.

I have only seconds to live, he realized. *In cramped quarters, against those great swords, I might as well be dead.*

"Katherine," he said quickly. "Run while you might."

In answer, he felt her presence plucked from his side.

The door has opened.

Another whistling blow. Thomas met it with his own

steel, and the echoing clank was almost as painful as the jar of contact that shivered up his arm.

Thomas brandished his sword and prepared for a counterattack.

If I'm to die, they will pay the price.

Both men hesitated and stepped back.

"Cowards!" Thomas cried, in the full heat of battle.

"No," came a strangely familiar voice, from the very spot where Katherine had stood only moments earlier. "They are simply prudent."

Both men stepped back farther.

"Yes," the voice continued, now directed at the two. "This crossbow truly reaches farther and faster than the sword. Go back to the men who hired you. Tell them the blood they wish to spill is now under protection."

The swordsmen nodded and quickly spun around, then hurried to the nearest corner of the alley.

Thomas, still panting, turned to look at his rescuer.

"Well, puppy," he was greeted. "Must we always meet in such troubled circumstances?"

Thomas only stared in return.

Sir William. The knight who helped me conquer Magnus. The knight who disappeared three seasons ago on his own private quest.

Thomas finally found his voice. "You describe harmless gnats like those two as trouble? Truly, you must be growing old."

Now, as when the knight had bid farewell long ago in Magnus, Thomas fought a lump in his throat.

Then, an early morning breeze had gently flapped the knight's colors against the stallion beneath him. Behind them both had been the walls of Magnus. Ahead of them had been the winding trail that had taken the knight to a destination he could not reveal.

This destination.

St. Jean d'Acre, on the edge of the Holy Land.

The sorrow Thomas felt in remembering their farewell mixed like a sweet wine with the sorrow of a remembrance of Magnus. He blinked back emotion.

Sir William smiled, switched the crossbow to his left hand, and extended his right hand in a clasp of greeting.

The knight had changed little. Still darkly tanned, hair still cropped short, now with a trace of gray at the edges. Blue eyes still as deep as they were careful to hide his thoughts. And always, that ragged scar down his right cheek.

A sudden thought struck Thomas.

"You are one of us." Although it was a guess, Thomas spoke it as a statement. "A Merlin."

Sir William nodded. "And one unable to decide whether to be gladdened or sorrowful at your arrival in this fallen town of the last crusaders."

Thomas raised an eyebrow.

"This is perhaps not the circumstance I envisioned for a joyful reunion," Sir William said, as he beckoned them in and placed an iron bar across the inside of the door. "Yet when one prays for a miracle, one does not ask the Lord to make it a convenient miracle."

Katherine smiled as she unfurled the veil which covered her face. Thomas merely gazed about the room with undisguised wonder and awe.

"I have been here before," Thomas said, "many times, in strange and troubled dreams."

"Find comfort that you have reason for this familiarity. You spent a part of your childhood in this house," Sir William said softly. "Would that I had time now to explain."

The knight's face did not reflect his urgency, despite the too recent echoes of that iron bar slammed quickly into place.

Thomas shook away his trance and half laughed. "Explain? In this town less than half a day from stepping off ship—" furrows across his forehead deepened as he shot a dark glance at his companion "—and out of the chains which had held me there because of Katherine. A half day, yet already I've been forced to flee assassins, only to have you appear as rescuer—you, a person I never expected to see again. Then you tell me that I spent part of my childhood here, in a land thousands of miles away from England."

Thomas stopped for breath. "Only a sane man would demand explanation of these mysteries."

He then shrugged and smiled to rob his sarcasm of insult. "However, no person could remain a sane man under these circumstances. So do not trouble yourself with tiresome explanations. Even if we had the time."

Katherine shook her hair loose as the veil finally fell away. The light of the lamps burnished her blond hair, so that it appeared almost bronze. Her suddenly revealed beauty drew a gasp from Sir William.

"Katherine," he marveled. "I remember you as a winsome child, but this . . . this . . ." He stopped and sighed as if love struck. "Were circumstances different and I but the age of Thomas, I would throw myself at your feet and pledge the treasure of all the earth."

Katherine wore a long cape of purple silk, held in place at the neck by an oval clasp of silver which showed an engraved sword. Her neck and wrists glittered with exquisite jewelry.

She laughed. "Death pursues us, but you men think only of desire."

She laughed again. "And to pledge the earth's treasure is farthest from the mind of your friend, Thomas. He much prefers threats, such as casting me from ships at sea."

The knight widened his eyes in mock horror, but any reply was interrupted by shouts from outside. Then, moments later, a crash into the wood of the door, as if a heavy shoulder had been applied.

Two more crashes. The iron bar held secure.

Shouts again.

"By the sounds, perhaps a dozen men," the knight said.

Another crash shook the door in its frame.

"Your crossbow will be useless at short quarters," Thomas said, nodding at the weapon the knight had laid on a nearby table. "Have we a place to our advantage in a sword fight?"

The knight shook his head. "Against infidel assassins, no place gives advantage."

"I will not die quietly," Thomas vowed.

"Who speaks of death?" the knight countered.

Sir William yanked an unlit lamp from a nearby shelf. He pulled the wick loose from the base and emptied the oil in a semicircle on the wooden furnishings of the room.

He then grabbed one of the three remaining lit lamps and shattered it on the ground.

Flames licked at the spilled oil, then burst into a small wall of fire.

The knight nodded grimly as black smoke began to fill the room.

"Let them fight this instead."

Chapter Forty-Seven

Had Thomas been able to step away from himself to observe his own reaction to the unexpected fire, he would have been slightly amused, not at his lack of panic, but at how well his childhood training served him during times of battle. For even as the flames around them began to roar, assumptions and conclusions raced through his mind.

The knight has no intention of suicide. Therefore, he must have an escape planned. The knight wasted no time to gather valuables before setting this fire. Therefore, he must have placed his valuables elsewhere.

Yet the meaning of those two conclusions are staggering. The knight has been ready to flee this house in an instant. He has anticipated this very moment!

How? Why?

The answers, Thomas vowed, would come later. Now, as shouting outside rose in response to the smoke which poured through the window openings carved in the limestone walls of the house, was the time to follow the knight.

Sir William made no noise. He only gestured for Katherine and Thomas to follow. He led them through a narrow archway into another chamber of the house.

This chamber leads to two others. I know this without doubt. There will be arched windows in one. A statue of Mother Mary in the other. And, during the morning, sunlight will stream across the statue as it did so many times when I sat on the floor and reached for lazy flies and listened to . . .

Thomas felt his heart skip a beat. Even in the haste of escape, the memories returned. This was no dream . . . no visit during sleep so that he woke with unexplained tears nearly dry across his face.

I sat in this very house! My childhood nurse spent time with me in these very rooms! Yet, how could I have forgotten?

Sir William led them to the room which indeed contained the statue of Mother Mary, then stooped suddenly and began to pry at the edge of one of the flat stones on the floor. Behind them, the heat of the fire as it spread into another chamber.

No words yet spoken . . . The stone moved aside . . . Below it, a large iron ring was recessed into wood.

Sir William flipped the ring upward with both hands.

He grunted, a sound barely heard above the fire. He pulled again and an entire section of the floor lifted.

"Take a lamp," he instructed Thomas. "Descend and wait."

Thomas moved quickly across the room, grabbed the lamp base and held it steady as he rejoined Sir William and Katherine. He looked into the darkness of the hole in the floor.

"Go quickly," the knight said. "There are steps. Katherine and I will follow."

Briefly, Thomas wondered if this was a trap. He did not yet trust Katherine fully. And by association, neither should he fully trust the knight.

He considered whether to hand the lamp to Katherine, to send her down first instead.

"Quickly," the knight urged. "I hear them breaking through the door!"

Thomas dropped down. Almost immediately, Katherine followed. With light in hand, it was not difficult now to see the downward path of the crooked steps.

Darkness closed over them as the trapdoor above lowered. The wick's flame flickered at the sudden rush of air, but Thomas protected it quickly with his upper body and the flame stayed alive.

He felt a hand on his shoulders. A soft touch.

"Thomas," Katherine's voice whispered.

His eyes adjusted to the dimness, and he held the lamp high as he descended.

"Thomas," Katherine repeated.

He shook his concentration away from the tunnel which grew in his vision ahead and below.

"Yes," he whispered back. *Where does the tunnel lead?*

"Sir William," Katherine said. "He is not with us."

Thomas set the lamp down, placed one hand on the hilt of his sword, and turned to move back past Katherine.

"No," she pleaded. "We cannot return."

"And let him die alone?" Thomas asked.

Katherine placed her hands on his shoulders as he attempted to push up the steps. "Or die together? Sir William chose to remain behind. Our deaths up there will only make his sacrifice useless."

Thomas was that one step lower, and it brought his face directly to the level of hers. For an insane moment, Thomas forgot the fire, the mysteries, and the fight above. Katherine's scent filled him as surely as the softness of her hair against his face reminded him of the touch of her arms on his shoulders.

Her eyes widened in the faltering light of the lamp, as if she too was suddenly aware that time and circumstance had fallen away.

Thomas felt her hands behind his neck begin to clasp as the pressure of her downward push on his shoulders eased and instead became an embrace. He swayed slightly, closed his eyes, and responded by moving close enough to feel the warmth of her breath on his lips. His hand left the hilt of his sword and, as if he had no control, moved to the back of her head to pull her even closer.

Insanity! She may be one of the Druids!

He opened his eyes. Her eyes were closed in trust. Such beauty. It brought him an ache of joy and sorrow to think of an eternity of her love.

Insanity! A friend above gives his life that we may flee!

She sensed his hesitation and opened her eyes. It broke the spell.

"Milady," Thomas began to apologize.

"Thomas," she said in the same moment.

They both stopped in midsentence.

Awkwardly, Thomas stepped back and down from her.

"Surely this tunnel leads to escape," he said quickly. Anything to break away from the spell of her presence. "Sir William would not have planned it otherwise. And the fire above will lead the town to panic. We must hurry to keep our advantage."

"And then?"

Thomas did not reply. He had no answer, and for that reason wanted only to concentrate on ducking through the low tunnel as he guarded the wick of his lamp from the water which dripped from the cool stone.

When they stopped to rest ten minutes later, Thomas was ready with his questions.

"Tell me," he said, determined to ignore the effect of her presence so close, "of matters of my childhood."

"How is it I should know?" she asked, almost aloof, as if she too sought to keep a distance from his effect on her.

"You . . . you are a Merlin." He had almost blurted that she *claimed* to be a Merlin. "As is the knight," Thomas finished. "Surely you and he have secrets in common."

"We are indeed Merlins," Katherine said. "Yet the fall of Magnus forced the few survivors into isolation. Sir William roamed the world while I remained in disguise among the Druids of Magnus. How much can I know of his part in our battle?"

Even now she holds back truth, Thomas thought with a trace of bitterness. *And I long to trust her and hold her and . . .*

He forced himself to concentrate on his questions.

"When the assassins pursued us from the marketplace," he said, "you led us not to the inn, but directly to the house where Sir William waited. Is that not proof of shared knowledge?"

His words echoed softly in the stone tunnel and many heartbeats passed before she replied.

"Yes, indeed," she finally began. "When Magnus fell to the Druids, Sir William, your parents, and a handful of others barely escaped with their lives. England was no longer safe. So they fled here to the Holy Land, hoping . . . hoping to find help in fighting the Druids from the valiant crusaders."

Is her hesitation a shiver of cold? Or a lie? Thomas chose to remain silent, to wait for more.

"You and I," Katherine said, "were raised here, in the house that so troubled your dreams. Your father dared not return to England. Druid spies were everywhere, and to be recognized there would give them too much warning that not all the Merlins had died. When the time was right, you and I—who would never be recognized—were smuggled back to England. I to serve in disguise as a spy in Magnus. You to receive training in that obscure abbey from Sarah, one of the most dedicated Merlins of her generation. Our hope was that you might remain unknown to the Druids, and close enough to reconquer Magnus with the knowledge given to you. It was a small hope, and with Sarah's death, even smaller."

Thomas closed his eyes at the name of his childhood nurse. She had tutored him relentlessly in games of mathematics and logic. She had corrected him with endless patience as he learned to read and write in the major languages of the world. And in all those hours and days and years of instruction, she had favored him with the love deeper than any . . .

"It cannot be," Thomas whispered.

"Thomas?" Katherine had caught the pain in his voice.

He faltered as he spoke. "I arrived at the abbey as a child. I was old enough so that now I can remember—dimly— those first days there. You tell me that the first years of my life were spent here. That I understand and believe, for is not my understanding of the tongue of this foreign country enough proof?"

He paused as another memory struck him . . . the memory of the first moment he saw Katherine's face in the moonlight when he and his army marched northward to battle the Scots. Nothing in his life had prepared him for that moment. He had learned—from betrayal by the beautiful, dark-haired Isabelle—not to trust appearance as an indication of a person's heart. Yet in the shadows of the moonlight he had felt as if he had been long pledged to the woman with the mysterious smile in front of him. Katherine . . . known since childhood.

And later, on the ramparts of the castle, when he had first stolen from her a kiss, the same certainty. What a bond they must have forged as small children, laughing and playing here in St. Jean d'Acre, unaware of the roles they must later play in a battle against the very Druids who had slain so many of their parents' friends.

Was not the bond itself—and the foreign language of the marketplace which seemed so natural—solid proof of the time of his childhood here? Yet how had those childhood memories been taken from him?

Thomas pushed those thoughts aside and pursued the one thought which had first caused his voice to falter.

"As a boy, I believed that I was an orphan, that Sarah was raising me in the monastery on the strength of money left to the church by my father, who had been a wealthy mason. You tell me, instead, that I was raised in secret as a Merlin to be part of a centuries-old battle against the unseen Druids, and that both my parents were part of that battle."

Thomas shook his head. "I can scarcely take all of this in." His voice grew shakier. "My parents were alive then, not fallen to the plague. Could it be that Sarah, the nurse who guided and taught and loved me as truly as might a mother . . . could it be she was my mother?"

Katherine's silence in the darkness of the tunnel was answer enough.

Thomas did not wipe away his tears of renewed grief. To have lost a mother twice . . .

Katherine closed her eyes and shared quietly in his pain.

There was no chance for more conversation. For above the steady dripping of water against stone came the faraway echo of approaching footsteps.

Immediately, Katherine reached between them to pinch the wick of the lamp. Thomas grasped her wrist and held it steady.

"This light will betray our presence," she protested.

Thomas thought of another time, beneath the castle of Magnus, when blind stumbling through secret passageways had nearly cost him his life, so he did not release her wrist.

"How shall we light the lamp again?" he asked. "For without light, we might never leave this tunnel." He then smiled. "And did not your training as a Merlin teach you the words of a wise general now long dead?" He paused. "All warfare is deception."

Her answer was a silent stare. Almost as if to deny their moment of unexpected closeness earlier, she was too proud to smile in return, too proud to attempt to free her wrist from his grip, and too proud to admit unfamiliarity with the quote.

The footsteps grew louder. Yet Katherine was more of a distraction for Thomas than the possible danger. It took effort not to reach upward with his free hand to softly touch the curves of her face as she looked at him with a steadiness that seemed to pierce his heart.

So he took a deep breath and forced himself to concentrate on the conversation. "Deception is what we will practice now."

Thomas released Katherine's wrist, lifted the lamp, and carried it forty steps back in the direction from which they started.

He set the lamp down and rejoined Katherine in the darkness.

"Now," he said, "when our visitor approaches, he will expect us there, ahead at the light, instead of here in the shadows."

First, Katherine and Thomas saw an approaching glow, then the light of the visitor's lamp, yet still too far away to let them identify the holder of that lamp. The visitor's footsteps slowed, however, and stopped almost as soon as the light had appeared.

This stranger sees our light, Thomas thought, *and hesitates.*

In the next moment, that faraway light disappeared.

The visitor chooses to approach now in darkness. From

caution born of fear, or caution born of evil intent?

No longer could Thomas or Katherine hear footsteps.

This visitor must pass close enough to touch us. But how soon?

Thomas nearly yelped at a sudden touch against his hand. His heart slowed quickly, though, as soon as he realized Katherine had slipped her hand into his.

They waited, side by side. Then, Thomas felt, rather than heard, the nearness of a stranger, as if the only hint of another person was air pushed ahead in the stillness of the tunnel.

Does this stranger walk with dagger or sword poised? Will I leap ahead into a sudden death?

Thomas did not answer his own silent question, for he had been taught that hesitation was the greatest enemy in the moment of action in any battle. He had also been taught the advantage of the terror of noise.

Thomas bellowed a rage that filled the tunnel as he charged into the stranger. His shoulder rammed a solid bulk. Hands were upon him instantly and Thomas punched back. Twice he hit only air, but three times his knuckles jarred against bone and Thomas continued to roar anger as he lashed out again and again at the unseen stranger.

They tumbled and rolled.

The stranger was heavier, but Thomas was faster and more desperate.

Their fight soon became silent, for Thomas had no energy to continue the roar of attack. Heavy breathing filled his face. Hands once managed to wrap around his neck, but Thomas lashed out with his knee to strike hard flesh and the hands released with a grunt of pain, only to seek him again from the darkness.

Thomas felt a face and tried to dig his fingers into the eye sockets—anything to gain the advantage in a fight that meant life or death.

In response, a sudden blow pounded his cheekbone and he fell back with flashes of light filling his eyes.

Then dimly, he heard it.

"Stop," Katherine was yelling. "Both of you stop!"

And Thomas realized the light in his eyes was from the lamp that Katherine had brought closer.

"Stop!" Katherine repeated from where she stood above them both.

Thomas felt his opponent relax and roll away from him, so he too relaxed and struggled to his feet.

The voice which greeted him was all too familiar.

"Should demons ever assume earthly form," Sir William said, attempting a chuckle of humor that became a cough of pain, "that form would closely resemble Thomas of Magnus."

Thomas groaned and began to feel his body for broken bones. "And should humans ever assume the forms of ghosts," he said, as he probed his mouth for shattered teeth, "they would do well to imitate Sir William. For considerate humans would announce their presence to friends."

Sir William staggered slightly as he tried to straighten. "I saw the lamp, but no one near. I could only assume the worst, and wonder how best to approach the enemies who had captured you."

Katherine moved forward and examined Sir William's face for cuts. "We thought you dead," she said softly.

"My own face fares poorly," Thomas hinted.

She ignored him.

"What happened?" Katherine asked Sir William. "In the house? In the fire?"

"I'll tend to my own bruises," Thomas announced, but still Katherine ignored him.

Sir William took the lamp from Katherine's hand, returned to his own lamp, and relit it. In the circle of renewed light, he sat and leaned against the tunnel wall with a moan.

"Join me," he said. "In the little time before the caravan leaves, I have much to explain, and here in the tunnel is much safer than above."

Katherine stepped forward and Thomas limped closer. It hurt him to sit. But it also hurt to stand.

"The events in the house?" Sir William began. "I wanted to lead them away from the house and the tunnel, but I also feared if I explained my intentions to fight and flee by another door, neither of you would agree to accept the safety of this tunnel. So I fought briefly, escaped the house, led the assassins on a merry chase, then entered this tunnel by the hidden exit we shall reach soon."

He turned to Thomas. "As you might guess, this escape has been ready for years. The Merlins have been in possession of the house for generations—almost since the beginning of the Crusades—and have often used the tunnel for the arrival and departure of visitors who should not be seen in the town."

"But why here in St. Jean d'Acre?" Thomas asked. It was difficult not to continue probing his ribs for bruises, but he did not want to give Sir William the satisfaction. "We are across the world from Magnus. What significance has this town to the Merlins? Or to the Druids?"

Sir William nodded. "The town itself has significance only because it is the traditional entry for those bound to the Holy Land by ship."

He let that statement hang in the silence until Thomas spoke.

"You say then that it is the Holy Land which draws Druids as well as Merlins?"

Sir William nodded. "And their spies, as do ours, watch the ships as passengers enter the town. It is the symbol on Katherine's clasp so prominent on her cloak, I believe, which led them to discover you so soon."

Yes. Had not that begger in the market inquired of its value? And had not Katherine firmly said it was a family heirloom? The distinct sword engraved in the clasp, then, what is its meaning?

Thomas was given no time to ponder, for the knight continued to speak.

"Both sides seek a great secret lost here in the Holy Land centuries ago," Sir William said. "The search has stretched over generations. The side which first discovers that secret will have the power to destroy the other."

What strangeness this is, Thomas wondered. *I am here beneath the streets of a town in the land where Christ walked, with remembered knowledge of a lost childhood,*

*in quiet conversation with a knight who once saved my
life and helped me win a kingdom, and—if Katherine's
story during our sea voyage is to be believed—I have been
destined to continue a centuries-old battle against a secret
circle of evil.*

Thomas laughed softly.

Sir William glanced at him, puzzlement clear even in the
flickering light of the lamps.

"You find humor in this?"

Thomas stood and spoke as he ran his fingers along the
rough stone of the tunnel walls.

"It is only because I feel the coldness of this stone that I
can believe this is not a dream of madness," Thomas said.
"Laughter? How else might one face the storms of life?"

"Well spoken," Sir William said. "And this is indeed a
storm. I have not yet heard what troubles have led you here
to the Holy Land. Katherine, I am sure, will tell me the sad
news later, during the long hours of travel that face us."

Thomas raised an eyebrow. "Katherine? Not I?" Instinctively, he dropped his hand to his sword. "Do you imply
that I will not be there?"

Sir William groaned and raised a hand as if fending off
attack. "Must you be so untrusting? Did I not with you
secure Magnus from the Druids?"

"Trust is the one thing I wish I could possess," Thomas
said softly. "While much has been explained, too little
knowledge has yet been given me."

He stared directly at Sir William and Katherine, considering the reasons for his mistrust. "That day at the gallows
long ago," Thomas challenged. "Why was the old man
there, the same old man who so mysteriously appeared later with Katherine as they followed me throughout England?
And you too, Sir William. Why were you there at the gallows
with the old man? I cannot believe in coincidence."

The knight answered, "We were there because of the
songs Sarah had taught you. Think back, Thomas. Had she
not always told you about a knight who would appear from
the land of the sun?"

Thomas nodded. He remembered that. He remembered

her instructions. He remembered too the chant Sarah had taught him, the chant he had heard later from the people of Magnus, that the one to reconquer Magnus would arrive as *if delivered on the wings of an angel.* Thomas remembered how Sarah had again and again told him to wait for the one knight he would need to free Magnus.

And he remembered her love. *Sarah was my mother, and not once were we able to share that knowledge.* Thomas spun away from Sir William and Katherine and bowed his head as spasms of grief shook him.

Katherine rose quickly and placed a comforting arm around Thomas.

"No," he said, not harshly, as he straightened. "This is not a time for grief. This is a time for answers."

Katherine stepped back, then slowly sat and rejoined the knight in the lamplight.

Thomas drew a deep breath. *Later, alone, I will spend time among memories and say farewell properly to the woman who gave so much of her life to me.*

Thomas exhaled. His voice remained steady as he spoke again. "You expected me, then, to appear at the gallows that day?"

"Yes," Sir William said. "How else might we get you to come forth without exposing ourselves to unseen and unknown Druids?"

"Yet, had I not appeared," Thomas countered, "you would have swung from the rope."

Sir William shook his head in gentle disagreement. "The old man was there. Had you not appeared, he would have ensured my life, and we would have begun our search for you."

"Ensured your life?" Thomas asked.

Sir William now nodded. "After all, he had arranged the time of execution to match that of the darkness of the sun."

Thomas gaped. "The old man had such power?"

Katherine's unnatural stillness suddenly drew his attention, and Thomas stopped before uttering his next words.

Sir William also turned his attention to Katherine.

"Hawkwood is dead," Katherine said quietly.

"Dead?" The word was uttered in disbelief. "But you did not speak of—"

"Dead," Katherine repeated. "Magnus is in the hands of the Druids. They rapidly expand their power among the people of Northern England, and the old man is dead."

The knight stood quickly. Urgency now filled his voice.

"Thomas, our continued survival is of utmost importance. All the more reason, then, that we separate now and travel apart. The assassins will be searching for three. And you, or Katherine and I must reach our destination."

Sir William turned to Katherine. "He shall go by caravan, you and I on foot. Tell me all during our journey. I must not delay in giving instructions to Thomas."

"Katherine," Thomas said. "That puppy. We cannot leave it to die at the inn."

"It shall be taken care of," Sir William said quickly, wanting the discussion to end. Then he took his lamp and began to lead them forward. Some thirty steps later—where he had first darkened his own lamp to approach with such caution—Sir William stooped to retrieve a package.

He gave it to Thomas.

"This must remain sealed. Guard it with every fiber of body and soul," Sir William said. "Too much of our battle against the Druids depends on its safe arrival—with you—in Jerusalem. After we visit Nazareth."

"Nazareth," Thomas repeated.

"Yes. For your father awaits you there."

Thomas woke to great shrieking groans. Startled and confused, he sat straight up, unconscious of the blanket dropping away from his upper body.

The light around him was dim and diffused to a hazy pale, and it took great effort for him to distinguish the tent walls surrounding him.

The great shrieking groans grew louder. Then he heard giggles behind him. He clutched the blanket and swung around to see two veiled servant girls, one carrying a pitcher, the other a basin. Their giggles continued.

Thomas mustered as much dignity as possible.

"The madness outside?" He stumbled through those words in their Arabic language, so strange yet so familiar. "Is it not early in the day for torture and executions?"

More giggles.

Before Thomas could inquire further, the tent flaps swirled open and a large figure entered, dark against the sunlight which streamed in behind his back.

"Be gone!" the figure roared. "Leave this man in peace!"

The girls merely giggled again, and only when the large man advanced with an upward threatening hand did they hitch up their skirts and run past him, still giggling.

It was the Arab, Muzzamar. Thomas had seen him briefly the night before, and then only in the light of a small torch, as he and Sir William bartered with great animation.

Although Muzzamar was fat, he moved with a softness that suggested athletic grace. His eyes, almost lost within that broad face, were sharp; his gray goatee, well trimmed. The deep lines around his mouth showed years of laughter, yet no man reached his age and position without an ability to dispatch the most vicious enemy, and Thomas warned himself to be on his guard.

Muzzamar groaned as he lowered himself to sit on a stool near Thomas. "This generation has little respect for their elders. In my youth, I would have been whipped for hesitation to obey any command."

The large man continued a steady stream of complaints, but used the noise of his own words as a screen, while his sharp eyes studied Thomas. During the previous night, their meeting had been hurried, and most of the attention had been on the knight who carried the purse of gold and negotiated a price of safe passage for this young stranger.

The large man saw quiet strength in Thomas, a calmness that seemed more than the steady gray eyes which watched him in return. Not for the first time, Muzzamar wondered what game these invaders played so fearlessly, here in a land that had been lost to them a generation ago.

The shrieks and groans outside renewed in pitch. Muzzamar noticed Thomas lift an eyebrow in question.

"Camels," Muzzamar explained. "Evil beasts. Smelly, stubborn, and evil. Put upon this earth only to try men's souls. They will protest their load this soundly every morning until we reach Damascus."

"Forgive my question, please," Thomas said softly. "Am I not to travel to Nazareth?"

Unconsciously, as if to reassure himself, Thomas pressed his leg against the sealed package beside him beneath the blanket.

"Of course, of course," the man said. "From here, we travel to the Valley of Jezreel. After several days passage through the valley, near Mount Tabor a road leads north to Nazareth. Some of my men will take you there as this caravan continues east to Damascus. Did not your friend explain?"

"Sir William had little time to explain," Thomas said. "He cautioned me to avoid soldiers who might inspect this caravan. He —"

"Good advice, indeed," Muzzamar said quickly, "something I cannot repeat enough. We travel in this land only by a pass of safe conduct granted by the Mamelukes. That safe conduct does not include passage for men from across the Great Sea. Should you be discovered, I cannot vouch for your life."

Muzzamar gestured behind Thomas. "Those worthless servant girls left you clothes of the desert. The head veil will protect your face from sun and wind, of course, but also from curious Mameluke soldiers. You will travel among the slaves; but even so, be advised to wear the veil at all times."

Muzzamar paused, then said, "I should not worry overmuch about the soldiers, however. This caravan carries much wealth. On these roads, we face a much greater danger from bandits."

Thomas hardly noticed the passing of hours.

It had been a new experience, to be sure, his first moments atop the great two-humped beast. The camel had been on its knees until expert hands guided Thomas into the small saddle between those humps. Then the camel awkwardly pushed itself up on its splayed legs until he sat high above the ground. Infrequently, the camel had turned its massive head and snorted foul breath as it attempted to regard its new rider. But the slave trader traveling alongside Thomas had whipped the animal's neck each time, and now it contented itself with maintaining the pace of the caravan.

For the first few miles, Thomas had marveled at the serene smoothness of this method of travel. Except for the pressure of the small saddle which he knew would leave him sore by the end of the day, he had the impression he was floating far above the ground. And to think that these great beasts could go days without water!

Thomas idly wondered if it would be practical to take camels back to England, and that led to renewed memories of Magnus. As time slipped by without his notice, those memories then led to his usual doubts and questions.

In the last few days at sea before reaching the Holy Land, Katherine had answered much, if her answers were to be trusted. The knight had also helped.

Even now, contemplating it for the thousandth time,

Thomas felt an odd mixture of thrill and relief at his new-found knowledge. *I am a Merlin, engaged in battle against a secret circle of Druids.* That explained much of his child-hood, much of the mystery behind Magnus, much about the precious books of knowledge, and about the destiny given him by Sarah, his mother.

Each time that phrase, *Sarah, his mother,* entered his mind, Thomas forced it away with vigor. He would grieve, yes, but in privacy, not among the men of this caravan that snaked slowly forward beneath the hot sun.

His new knowledge explained much of what had hap-pened at the gallows, so long ago, as he first embarked upon his quest to reconquer Magnus.

Yet new questions arose. Who had the old man been, with the power among ruling men to arrange a hanging on the day and hour that an eclipse would occur? What was this new quest in the strange Holy Land? The package he must so carefully guard?

Thomas felt dark suspicion too. Both the knight and Katherine had said that the Merlins were unable to reveal themselves to Thomas because of an uncertainty of his true allegiance. Their suspicion was simple but well-founded. Had the Druids, in the years following Sarah's death, found Thomas and converted him? Sir William, Katherine, and the old man could not know, and thus could not give him the answers he needed.

This matter of their trust was important. Both the knight and Katherine had hinted that through Thomas the Druids might find the one single secret they needed to end the centuries-old battle. *What is the secret they believe I hold? And what terrible end to the battle?*

His suspicions darkened more. *Having revealed so much, why not tell me all? Unless Katherine and Sir William do not yet trust me completely. And if I am not yet trusted completely, why reveal anything at all?*

In his confusion, Thomas groaned loudly enough to draw attention from the rider nearby. So Thomas quickly patted his belly, as if the groan had resulted from a poorly digested breakfast.

Then, he returned to his thoughts. *If I am not yet trust-ed, why reveal anything?* Sir William had had months in Magnus, ample time to draw him aside in privacy. Katherine too had had many opportunities to do the same. *Why give me answers now in St. Jean d'Acre, and not then?*

Thomas groaned again and ignored any glances. Were the answers in the package entrusted to him? Not for the first time did he consider unsealing it.

No. Thomas repeated the arguments he had given him-self. *Were Sir William and Katherine foes, they would have given me nothing that might benefit me. If they are friends, then unsealing the package would cost me their allegiance.*

Thomas closed his eyes briefly. Should he in return trust them? Enough strange events had occurred so he might full well believe *they* were Druids.

His only choice was to play this game to its end. The bait promised him was nothing less than the father he had long believed dead.

The caravan moved south along the flat road of the coastal plains. Far ahead, high, rounded hills, blue with distant haze, shimmered against the backdrop of an almost white sky.

The heat seemed an attacker. Each time Thomas wiped his face and exposed his skin to the scorching air, he breathed gratitude at the layers of fine cloth which trapped the cooler air close to his body. Long before the sun passed its highest point, one of the leather bags of water tied to his saddle was half empty.

Much more difficult than the heat was the evil of watch-ing the slaves stumble alongside the camels. A dozen of them wore layers of white for the desert heat, their heads covered against the blazing white sun. Muzzamar knew dead slaves were of little value in Damascus.

They were marked by the single rope which attached one to the other. This rope was looped around each neck, so that when one fell, he risked dragging the others down. When one slowed, he risked strangulation.

Thomas noted that they had no skins of water and vowed to ease their thirst as soon as he could.

Muzzamar, at the front of the caravan, finally raised his

sword to call a halt when the lead camels reached a stand of trees which hugged a wide well.

Thomas did not dismount until he had loosened two of his water skins from the saddle.

He nearly fell when his feet first touched the packed, sandy road. Sitting motionless for so long had cramped his legs, and it took effort to straighten them.

Thomas ignored the scowl of the slave master—for the heavy water skins were obvious in his hands—and moved to the first of the slaves. He had been warned by both Sir William and Muzzamar not to draw attention to himself, but he knew the men on foot must be in agony.

"Take this," Thomas said as he held out the water skin, "then pass it along."

The slave lifted his head. Dark eyes, glazed with exhaustion, now opened wide with surprise. The slave hesitated, briefly, then snatched the leather bag from Thomas and gulped water.

Thomas waited, then realized the slave had no intention of ending his drink, so he gently grabbed the slave's wrists and pulled the skin away.

Thomas carried the water to the next slave. While that slave drank, Thomas tried to ignore the obvious rope burns around his neck.

Then to the next and the next, until he reached the last slave held by the rope.

Unlike the other slaves, this one did not open his hands gladly to receive the water skin.

"Take this." Thomas urged the water skin on the man.

"You risk your life," the slave answered, head still down.

Thomas stepped back in surprise. *The man had spoken English.*

"Among these nomads, it is considered a weakness to show mercy," the slave continued. "And we will be fed and watered at nightfall, for they have no wish to kill us as—"

"English," Thomas blurted in that language. "You speak English!"

The slave redirected his stare from the ground to Thomas, and the eyes which rose were not the deep brown of these darker people, but a blue so piercing it almost startled Thomas.

"I speak English because I am English," the man said in a low voice. "Find it not so amazing. Many of us are doomed in this strange land, those long forgotten from a forsaken crusade. I had avoided capture for ten years. Ahead . . ."

The man shrugged. His face showed no expression. It was the face of a man who was equal to Thomas in height. How old, Thomas could only guess; but as the wind tugged against the cloth which protected the man's head, Thomas saw edges of gray at the temples of his dark hair. The wrinkles around the his mouth and eyes had not yet deepened enough to show shadow. His nose was crooked in several places, as if it had been broken more than once. His teeth were straight and without gaps; he had not eaten poorly while avoiding capture.

"Ahead," the man finished, "lies what tomorrow brings."

Thomas again pushed the water skin toward the slave. This time the water was accepted, with another shrug. The slave drank slowly, then returned the water.

"You are too young to have come with the last crusaders," the man said. "Yet your command of their tongue tells me you are not a new arrival to this land. And you are not among the slaves."

Thomas recognized it as a statement, not a question, and simply nodded in reply.

"Your story must be one of interest," the man finished Again, said in neutral tones. Again, Thomas nodded.

"Do not attempt to help me escape," the man said calmly.

Said thus, an unexpected statement with the same lack of passion as all the man's other words, the advice had the impact of a physical blow. For indeed, Thomas was contemplating that same subject.

Before Thomas could protest, the man fixed him with those uncanny eyes and unhurriedly spoke more.

"We are fellow countrymen. And, methinks, men of the same breed, for cowards and ne'er-do-wells would not stray across a world to enter the Holy Land." The man raised his voice slightly. "Yet do not offer your help. Even should you succeed, with me you would become a hunted outlaw."

A deep laugh greeted that remark.

"Well spoken, Lord Baldwin!" The words came from behind them in Arabic, for Muzzamar had approached quietly. "Words spoken for my benefit?"

Muzzamar clapped Thomas on the back. "Lord Baldwin saw me, of course. But it is still advice worth heeding. You are a stranger among us, and I suspect you know little of our history."

Muzzamar took Thomas by his elbow. "Come with me. We have a little time before our journey resumes."

Muzzamar spoke as he guided Thomas back to the trees. "You know, by now, of the Mamelukes. Two centuries ago as slaves to the Egyptians, they overthrew their masters. Later they overthrew the foreigners who built fortresses and castles all across this land."

The trader pointed east. "In those hills stood the great crusader castles. The greatest, known as Saphet, commanded the very road we travel. The Mamelukes had laid seige, and they promised safe passage to the knights upon their surrender. Yet when the gates of the castle were opened, every knight was beheaded on the spot."

Muzzamar examined Thomas for his reaction.

"So you see," Muzzamar's smile was nearly a caress of cruelty, and Thomas understood with a chill how different these people were, "we cannot afford to anger the Mamelukes. To our enemies, we are equally ruthless. And neither we nor the Mamelukes show the softness of the English."

Muzzamar tapped the water skin Thomas still held.

"We do not provide comfort to our enemies, and we show no mercy to those who betray us." Muzzamar's smile did not change as the implied threat continued. "Perhaps you feel duty-bound to help another. Take the advice offered by Lord Baldwin. Journey along your own path. I have guaranteed your safety because I have accepted gold. And I am no common bandit. I will deliver you as promised."

Muzzamar's voice then flattened with deadliness. "But should you become an enemy, you will have the choice of death or slavery. And death would be more pleasant."

Chapter Forty-Nine

On the eve of the third day of travel, Muzzamar visited Thomas in his tent.

"My young friend," Muzzamar beamed, "tonight we shall feast."

"Even more?" Thomas said. He finished drying his face. It had felt wonderful to dip in the basin supplied by servant girls and wash away the day's dust and sweat. "Surely you cannot exceed the goat's milk curds and dried figs which have sustained us thus far."

Muzzamar frowned, then laughed with understanding. "A jest!"

With a smile, Thomas nodded. A jest indeed. For the previous few days of travel had been at a forced pace. Tents had not been raised at nightfall, nor cooking fires lit. Sleep had been short, and in open air. The entire caravan had always been ready to move.

"Truly," Muzzamar said, "our people do not always eat in such a manner. And tonight, you shall taste our finest."

"No danger of bandits tonight?" Thomas asked. "Nor of Mameluke soldiers?"

"We are well into the Valley of Jezreel," Muzzammar said, as if this explained all.

"My apologies for ignorance," Thomas said. "You have been greatly occupied, and there was none other to inform me of matters of the journey."

"Of course, of course," Muzzamar said. "My own apologies for neglect of an honored guest. Yet we were in bandit-infested country, and my first duty was survival of the caravan."

"The hills on each side promised danger?" Thomas asked.

"Yes. The passage into this valley is well guarded by those hills. It favors large groups of bandits. Naturally, we are able to protect ourselves, but only at great cost, and to tarry in those hills provides the bandits unneccesary temptation. But now . . ."

Muzzamar swept his arms wide. "Now we are in the open valley. And a caravan of traders on its way to St. Jean d'Acre has joined us in its passing. There is safety away from the hills, and safety in numbers, Thomas. We shall rest here and feast. You will be welcome at the feast, for it is hardly likely that Mameluke soldiers will appear at night to inspect the caravan."

"How long will we rest?" Thomas asked. For thoughts of Nazareth and Sir William and Katherine and his father filled his every waking moment.

"The road to your destination is only a day's travel," Muzzamar said, "well within sight of Mount Tabor. From there, two of my men will guide you north into the hills to Nazareth."

Muzzamar caught the darkness of uncertainty that crossed Thomas' face.

"Come, come, Thomas. Have no fears. We have successfully passed through the dangerous country. As a small group, you and my guides will easily avoid Mameluke soldiers on the road to Nazareth. Your arrival there is a certainty."

Thomas forced a smile. For his fears had not been of arrival, but what might occur after.

Thomas groaned as he laid his head to rest. The sealed package he had sworn to guard for Sir William was wrapped in a blanket and served as his pillow. But how could he possibly sleep?

Muzzamar's promise of a feast had been only a hint of the events of the evening. There had been tambourine dancing by veiled girls, rich meats and sweets, and servants pouring wine and delivering food. The feasters from both caravans needed only sit and eat. Thomas himself had gorged, urged on by a servant who tended to him.

His stomach, overful with unaccustomed delicacies, rumbled threats of rebellion. Even as he finally drifted into sleep, Thomas tossed fitfully. His dreams gave him little rest.

He stood upon a high hill, shrouded in gray mist. The mist swirled, then cleared, and rays of sunshine broke through from behind him, sunshine that lit an entire city across the deep valley, so that the beams of light danced golden and silver on the curved towers rising tall above whitened square houses that spread in all directions along the plateau of the mountain.

From the city walls came a dark figure, small with distance. The figure slowly moved closer until Thomas could see it was a large man.

The peace Thomas felt to behold this city of dreams began to disappear, and in its place arrived a trembling panic which grew stronger as the figure approached, stronger as Thomas struggled to identify the man's face.

But the face was gray with mist, and Thomas moaned with a fear he could not explain.

"Thomas, my son," the figure called. Now the man was close enough so that Thomas could see the wrinkles of the dark cloth folded around the figure. But still, the face was featureless and gray.

"Thomas, my son," the stranger called again. "Are you a Merlin?"

Thomas tried to reply, "Father," but he could not speak, his fear was so great. There was something so threatening about this stranger who claimed to be his father that Thomas tried to reach for the sword at his side, but his hands were powerless. He stood mute and frozen.

"Thomas! Are you a Merlin?"

The figure transformed into a dragon. Yet before Thomas could scream, the dragon became Sir William, swirling out of sudden mists with a sword upraised.

Thomas tried to lift his arm against the blow, and as the sword came down, there was a roar, for the sword had struck, not downward against Thomas, but behind him at a lion that now snarled defiance against death as blood ran from its severed throat.

As Thomas turned back to thank Sir William, he caught the scent of perfume. The knight was not there. Instead, it was Katherine, her hair a halo of brightness from the sun. She reached for Thomas and he sobbed with relief.

Her arms pulled him close and she kissed him and a flare of ecstasy filled him, yet something was wrong. Her kiss was one of death, for now he could not breathe, and she would not pull away.

He struggled, trying to push her away, but his arms were still trapped at his side, and she only pressed harder.

Breathe, find breath, for he must live . . .

Thomas opened his eyes in panic. For a single heartbeat, he relaxed. It was only a dream.

Yet he still could not breathe. And above him, a giant of a man blocked the flickering light of the tent lamp.

In the next heartbeat of awareness, he realized a heavy, open hand pressed down upon his mouth and nostrils.

"Silence or death," a voice whispered.

To fulfill that promise, the figure placed the tip of a knife against Thomas' throat.

"Silence or death," the voice repeated. "Nod if you choose life."

Thomas nodded. The slightness of that movement proved the sharpness of the knife and the seriousness of the intruder—Thomas felt the knife's tip break the skin.

The hand over his nose and mouth was removed.

Thomas drew breath, but slowly, for he did not want the intruder to consider a gasp to be unnecessary noise.

Several more heartbeats passed before the figure eased backward and the pressure of the knife left Thomas' throat.

"We leave camp," the voice said. "You will not return. If we are caught, we both die."

Thomas nodded again. He dressed hurriedly, careful to place around his neck the long strap which held his pouch of gold beneath the clothing. When he was ready, Thomas reached for the sealed package that had served as his pillow, for even the threat of death did not take its importance from his mind.

"Do not forget your sword," the voice said. "For you shall travel alone and without friends."

Thomas took the sword, grateful that this stranger would not see it as a threat. And why fight now? For if the stranger had meant harm, Thomas would already be dead in his sleep.

The stranger turned and Thomas followed. They moved between the tents. Something seemed unnatural, and it did not take long for Thomas to understand. The camp did not stir with the slight movements of guards at night, the occasional scurrying of servant girls, the restless muttering of slaves in their tortured sleep. Only the grunts and stampings of the camels showed any life.

The stranger led Thomas away from the edge of the caravan. To their left was the camp of the other caravan, the traders headed for St. Jean d'Acre. This camp too was unnaturally still.

As the stranger continued his steady pace away from the camps, Thomas held his questions. When this large man in front of him indicated the silence could be broken, then Thomas would speak.

The sky above was ebony black, studded with brilliant diamonds of starlight. The moon was high and full, and cast enough pale light for Thomas to see the outlines of the far hills.

Finally, the figure stopped and turned.

"My name does not matter," the stranger said. "I was among the slaves. Yet we were not slaves. Rather bandits, biding our time."

"Band—"

The stranger held up his hand. "I have little time until my absence is discovered. What I can explain is this. It is well known that Muzzamar's caravan has many riches and is too well guarded for attack. Instead of raiding, we chose to pose as slaves until Muzzamar believed himself safe. The cook was bribed before we departed St. Jean d'Acre, before we let ourselves be put into bondage. And this night? As planned long before, all of the food of the feast was drugged. It was great fortune that brought us the other caravan to be plundered as well."

The stranger smiled as a look of comprehension crossed Thomas' face. Time and again his plate had been filled before he could rise to join Muzzamar and the others with their feasting. And each time his plate had been filled by a large slave.

"Yes," the figure said, as if reading Thomas' thoughts. "I ensured that you were kept from the food that all others ate. They sleep now. It was a simple matter for the cook to release us from our bonds and supply us with their very own weapons. It is an easy way for us to plunder, much simpler than open attack from the hills."

"Those weapons shall be used against them?" Thomas asked. "Many in camp are innocent women and children."

"Only the men shall die. This is a harsh land."

Thomas said nothing. He pondered the merits of attempting to warn Muzzamar. Yes, he had seen men die, but always in battle, not as helpless sheep.

"Your silence says much," the slave said. "Yet there is nothing you can do to prevent this. The men are heavily drugged, and your return will only ensure your death, and mine for assisting you now."

Thomas realized this was so. For a moment, wildness tempted him. Useless as his death might be, to die in attempting to warn others might prove to be a lesser evil than a haunting guilt later. But ahead were Katherine and Sir William and his father, and the fight of the Merlins.

"My own life has been spared." Thomas said in a flat tone as he tried to force his emotions of conflict aside.

"You gave us water," the slave answered Thomas. "And I have decided to repay you in kind. I wish I could give you a camel, but while your absence will be undiscovered in the confusion to come, the loss of a camel is too easily noticed. Our own leader is without mercy, and cannot know you have been spared."

Thomas absorbed this information. Others would die, and he was helpless against it. The stranger in front of him had risked his own life to save Thomas. The gift could not be discarded. He must leave.

"Truly," Thomas said, "there is no way I can repay you."

"I have heard of the man who walked this land, the man you blue-eyes claim was the Son of God. Did He not say we are all brothers? And did you not prove it with your kindness?"

The stranger extended his hand in a clasp of friendship. "Brother, may your God protect you. Shalom. Go in peace."

The stranger untied a full water skin from his belt, handed it to Thomas, and took a step away. "You must reach the hills by daybreak. It will cost us both our lives for you to be found."

Thomas reached for the stranger's arm at a sudden memory of a brave and noble face.

"The slave from my own land, Lord Baldwin?" Thomas asked. "Will he too be slain?"

The stranger snorted in irony. "During this journey, we have discovered the hell of slavery ourselves. All slaves in both caravans shall be spared and released."

Then a pause before the stranger spoke more soberly. "Whether they survive this land is another matter."

Thomas entered Nazareth at dawn. Behind him, three days of cautious travel, of slow movement along the roads at night, sleep in shadows of safety during the day. Behind him, the long and rolling hills of Galilee.

Among these hills were forests of cedar and pine, olive orchards and vineyards, fields with wheat and oats and barley. It had almost been a joy to contemplate the land as he rested hidden during the day.

Thomas was not thirsty. His water skin was still half full from a well fifteen miles earlier; and travel during the night had spared him the searing daytime heat which sucked so much moisture.

He was hungry, for he had not dared to stop at any inns or allow himself to be seen during the day. Time and again Thomas had shifted his focus from his tightened belly to think of Nazareth. There he would reach Sir William and Katherine. There he would be in relative safety.

What if Sir William and Katherine had not survived their journey? Thomas dared not think of that for how, then, would he find his father?

No, he must trust that the knight would arrive with Katherine. But he would not be foolish as he waited. They might arrive in a day or a week, time enough for Thomas to be noticed by Mameluke soldiers or other assassins. Because of that, he would satisfy his hunger, then find a place in Nazareth to wait quietly as he surveyed arriving travelers.

A rooster's triumphant crow broke the silence of his thoughts. The dawn's light was still soft, and the town ahead lay motionless in the growing shadows.

Thomas chose a large boulder to use as support and leaned back to survey the buildings ahead. The town seemed small and quiet and ordinary, hardly a place to be remembered by generations. Yet there was a timelessness about it, and Thomas let himself contemplate the burden of history that had given Nazareth and the rest of the Holy Land such significance.

It was in these moments that Thomas was most at peace, when he believed he could feel the presence of the God of his fathers and forefathers, the God who had shown the very same presence to dwellers in this Holy Land, since the beginning of recorded time.

In these moments, Thomas lost himself in a quietness, as if he could hear the voices of this land reaching to him across the centuries. Here Moses had climbed the hills to look across the Jordan River and fill his eyes with the awesome beauty of this promised land before his death. Here a great king named David had defeated invincible armies and had sung psalms of praise and love. And here, in the very town Thomas now surveyed, a boy had played in the dust of the streets; later as the Messiah, He had allowed Himself to die so cruelly on pieces of rough wood tied together in the shape of a cross.

Even as the sun warmed his back, Thomas shivered. There was strength to be received during this contemplation, he knew, and he closed his eyes in a prayer of thanks for his safety and a plea for continued help.

That prayer led him to another vision, a scene far away in a land he hoped to see again. There, a woman had started every morning with her head bowed in prayer and a young boy at her side.

Thomas blinked back a tear. As that young boy, he had barely understood her daily silence. In this moment as he remembered, his hunger faded and and he knew that now, after his journey and before Katherine and Sir William might arrive in Nazareth, now he could afford the luxury and demand of grief. Some instinct, the instinct that compels all peoples to formalize the departure of life in the ceremonies of death, told him he must perform his own ceremony for the woman who had given him so much in that faraway monastery so many years ago.

Thomas tightened his jaw to keep his face firm, and stepped away from the boulder to seek a path into the hills above Nazareth.

Thomas sat on the edge of a rock near the top of the highest hill overlooking Nazareth. A breeze flowing to cool him brought the bleating sounds of sheep grazing on a neighboring hill. But for that, the hills were silent.

Thomas closed his eyes and again remembered Sarah.

How difficult to raise a boy, to love him as a son, yet not once—even when facing death—let the boy know the teacher was also mother.

And the son, Thomas thought dispassionately, as if it were someone else who had been raised without knowing the woman had been his mother, *she must have borne the pain daily of knowing her son believed he was an orphan.*

At that thought, Thomas bit his lower lip. Memories returned. Memories of the questions he had asked about his parents, his anger at God for letting them die.

And month after month, Sarah had patiently taught him in the ways of Merlins, unable then to reveal to him his duty.

Duty that required her to sacrifice her identity as mother, duty that had let her die so far from her husband, let her die without telling me of her love for me.

Thomas bowed his head and prayed, grateful that his faith allowed him to see beyond life on earth, and to realize that the pattern of the universe was so great beyond comprehension that all he could do is trust and live as well as possible. *In the way that my mother trusted and lived.*

Thomas sat there for two hours, holding the sadness without trying to deny it. His tears and his prayers were all that he could give to the memory of Sarah.

At last he stood. Ahead, he could give more to the same duty that had called her. For that, he would have to hide openly in Nazareth. He had already chosen the method for that.

He would bribe an innkeeper to give him a room and keep it secret. During the day, he would pose as a beggar at the town gates.

After two days of begging, Thomas saw Katherine and Sir William arrive at the city gates at midmorning. With them traveled the two Muslim assassins who had vowed to kill Thomas in St. Jean d'Acre.

Chapter Fifty

His first reaction was the stillness of shock and disbelief. And the stillness of a rabbit frozen by the sudden appearance of a fox.

Do not betray your presence, Thomas told himself. *Behave as would all crippled beggars at the town gates.*

The beggars on each side of him tapped the sides of their clay bowls, so Thomas did the same with his. Yet, even though his body responded, his mind was numb.

This cannot be. Heat has caused my eyes to deceive me.

He stole another glance.

On foot, Sir William led a mule on which sat Katherine, veiled from Muslim eyes.

Beside Sir William walked two large men whose faces were engraved in Thomas' mind. Only days earlier, these men had pursued Thomas and Katherine through the street markets of St. Jean d'Acre. Only days earlier, they had forced Sir William to barricade the house and set it ablaze. And now?

Now, they walked at ease with Sir William and Katherine. There was nothing to indicate strain or tension, nothing to indicate that Sir William and Katherine were captives.

Thomas raised his head again and noticed that Sir William's sword was still against his side. *No, if they were captives, Sir William would not be armed.*

The beggars around him moaned for pity in respectful voices. Thomas did the same.

It warmed him little that Katherine insisted upon throwing tiny copper coins into each bowl. *This is the woman who now betrays me.*

Thomas ducked his head as they passed by, and silently nodded thanks for the coin thrown in his bowl. Did he imagine the scent of her perfume as dust stirred by the mule's feet settled again?

He wanted to rise, to roar in anger at the evil of their deceit. He wanted to rush Sir William, to seize his sword and attack the knight and his assassin friends. But he did not.

There was trembling in his legs and dizziness in his head, at such unexpected and colossal betrayal.

Lies. So much of what they told me must be lies.

How could I have been fool enough to believe my father is still alive? How could I have been fool enough to believe the tales of Merlin and a destiny to fulfill? And how could I have been fool enough to believe her eyes, her promises of love, and the soft touch of her lips against mine?

Thomas could not rise because weakness of despair overwhelmed him. As the murmurs of their conversation faded, he still could not raise his head to watch.

He did not bother to wipe the tears which fell shiny onto the tiny copper coin in the bowl at his feet.

It was another hour before he found the energy to grasp the cane at his side.

What to do next? Where to go?

A castle he had once conquered in the land of his birth no longer belonged to him. He was friendless in a strange land, involved in a battle he did not understand, a battle he had not chosen or invited.

Yesterday, there had been hope. Hope of finding his father. Hope of returning triumphant to Magnus. Hope of a trust in Katherine that might lead to—he barely dared think it in his bitterness—a love that would fill him with joy.

Today?

Today he must continue his disguise and walk away from these town gates leaning on his cane as if crippled, lest the ones he once thought friends discover he was in Nazareth.

Today, he had nothing. No hope, no dreams. He hobbled several more steps. He did not know or care what he should do next.

For a moment, anger flared and he almost hurled the clay bowl from his other hand. Only instinct kept him from drawing attention to himself in such a manner; so he stopped in front of a lone beggar who was nearer the town gate.

"Take this," Thomas mumbled. He leaned on his cane and offered the bowl to the seated beggar.

The beggar looked up with disbelief. "It contains copper!"

"Indeed," Thomas said. *Copper from the hands of a woman whose beauty will haunt me each time I close my eyes. Would that it be so easy to give away the memories as the coin and bowl.*

The beggar's hands shook as he accepted the bowl. "This means another cake of pressed barley for my daughter," he said with gratitude. "There are days when that seems a feast."

Thomas looked more closely at the beggar. He had a slight face and seemed in good health.

"Why are you not nearer the gate?" Thomas asked. "Where more travelers pass by?"

"It takes much of the morning for me to make my way here," the beggar replied. "Others, who arrive early, take the prominent positions."

The beggar noticed the puzzled look which crossed Thomas' face and pointed downward to the shawl over his lap.

"I drag myself here on a blanket. My feet are useless," the beggar explained. "Caught once in a grinding millstone several years after my wife died in childbirth, I cannot work, and . . ."

A smile of delight crossed the beggar's face. ". . . and I must feed my daughter. She will grow soon to be as beautiful as my wife, and then a marriage will secure her future."

The beggar continued to smile. "You see? In our lives we all have precious gifts. Perhaps, my friend, you do not have a child to love, but you are able to walk with the help of a cane, while I cannot. And when you are not rich, even a small copper coin can deliver joy . . . my joy in receiving, and your joy in giving."

"Yes," Thomas said. Despite the blackness upon him, he managed a snort of self-mocking laughter. "And to imagine. There are those in this world with strong bodies, full bellies, and pouches of gold who let themselves despair."

Thomas arrived safely at the inn and retreated to the silence of his small room. He placed his few belongings on a stool, then sat cross-legged on the floor with his back against the wall.

First, he tore open the package. A parchment, promising reward for its return. On the other pages, meaningless scrawls of Latin. A priceless package? What jest was this?

Thoughts tugged at him.

Why had Katherine brought the light near while he fought a supposedly unknown assailant? She should have stayed beside him, ready to help in the fight. Now it made sense. She knew it was Sir William and wanted the fight to end before either was hurt.

But why practice such deception?

Thomas answered his own question immediately. What better way for a Druid to convince him of friendship than find a common enemy to fight—the supposed assassins. Then, give him the mysterious package with cryptic words to further the illusion of trust.

In sudden rage and pain at the renewed thought of betrayal, Thomas slammed the floor with his open palm. The impact sobered him quickly, and he turned his back on the luxury of anger.

Regard this as warfare. There are two choices. Attack or retreat. Either action requires surprise. Yet it cannot be certain that the bribe to the innkeeper will ensure that my presence here remains secret. Therefore, action must be taken soon or surprise will be lost.

Attack? Decide what is risked. Decide what is gained if attack is successful.

Risk? One person against four. Three of the four were skilled in the arts of death. The other, Katherine, he would hesitate to put to the sword. If she wished him dead, that hesitation would prove deadly.

Conclusion? Risk is great.

What gained? If defeated and captured, could Katherine and Sir William be forced to divulge secrets? Hardly, and there would be no reason to trust their answers. If killed, they could not pursue him, but their deaths—at risk to himself—would give him little else. The other usual gain of warfare, ransom, was not helpful either.

Retreat? Decide the difficulty. Decide what is gained.

How difficult? His presence was still unknown. Retreat, then, would be simple. In these vast tracts of land, it would be impossible to find him.

What gained? His life, if indeed, they wanted him dead. But why not kill him in St. Jean d'Acre? Or why not aboard the ship? Katherine had had much opportunity then. No, they wanted more than his life. If he knew what it was they sought, then this battle would be easier to fight.

What gained? Time. Retreat gained him time to seek answers.

Thomas did not shift, so intense were his thoughts. A small lizard crept from a crack in the wall to within inches of his feet, unaware that the large object above it was alive. Thomas remained oblivious to his quiet guest.

And what is it they seek from me? Exiled in a strange land, where would he find answers to questions he barely understood?

There were only two places to begin. St. Jean d'Acre, where he had been raised as a child. He knew that to be true, for those few moments in the burned dwelling had flooded him with memories. Whatever else Katherine and Sir William had told him that might be false, he could not deny a childhood spent in St. Jean d'Acre. Not with those memories, not when he knew the language of this land. In St. Jean d'Acre, he would find someone who knew something. The tiniest scrap of new knowledge would lead him to another. And another.

It would be safer now in St. Jean d'Acre. After all, Katherine and Sir William would be in Nazareth, still waiting for him. With answers, Thomas could return, and play their game by his rules.

Or, instead of returning to Nazareth after St. Jean d'Acre, he could go next to Jerusalem. So much pointed to it. The Holy City. Perhaps he would find answers there.

Thomas smiled to the silence of the room. He still had his life. He still had his health. His freedom. And enough in gold to sustain the search.

Thomas rose quickly, a movement that scuttled the lizard to another dark crack in the wall.

"My little friend," Thomas said, "I pray that my own retreat serves me as well as yours did you."

It was a prayer much needed. For two days later, as Thomas traveled a road that narrowed between large rocks on each side, bandits attacked.

His first warning had been a slight scuffle of leather against stone. As Thomas looked over his shoulder, he saw two men dropping from the top of a boulder, only thirty paces behind.

There was no mistaking their intent. Swords raised, scarred and dirty faces quiet with deadliness, they advanced toward him.

Thomas glanced ahead to determine his chances of escape. There, four more bandits stepped onto the road. Walls of rock blocked him on both sides.

More terrifying than upraised swords was their silence and slow, patient movement. These men had no need to bluff or bluster; their purpose was profit from the victim's death, not satisfaction from toying with his fear. They would not waste energy through haste; their victim could not escape.

A part of Thomas' mind noted this objectively, just as it noted that he was their intended victim, a thought that brought him a surge of adrenaline.

Another part of his mind noted the terrain and evaluated his chances. The road wound downward from the hills of Galilee. The Valley of Jezreel was barely an hour ahead, but that fact helped little now. The huge boulders on each side of the road were too smooth to climb.

The bandits closed the circle on Thomas step by certain step.

Thomas drew his sword. One against six. His death was certain. Yet surrender, was impossible. His sword would taste blood before he died.

Thomas did not waste his breath with threats. He too had the silence of deadly intent. He began to back against a boulder for the slight protection it offered, then saw a break in the rocks beyond the four men advancing on one side.

"Use more than your sword." Thomas could hear the long ago words of Sir William as he had once coached him in the art of fighting. *"Terrain, a man's character, and surprise—all are added weapons."*

Even in this situation, the thought of Sir William and betrayal brought bitterness to the back of his throat. It brought anger too, anger which Thomas could direct at these bandits. He dropped to his knees and without taking his eyes from the four men on his left, he felt about for stones. He found two and stood.

Still, silence from the bandits. The two on his right were close enough that he could hear their breath quicken as they prepared to attack.

They expect me to attempt a break through the weakest part of their wall—the group of two, probably the stronger fighters.

So Thomas did the opposite.

He lunged at the four men on his left, and at the same time threw both stones at head level. The bandits flinched and ducked, only for an instant, and the stones clattered on the boulder behind them.

But as they ducked, Thomas swung his sword in a vicious arc and plunged directly ahead. The suddenness of his attack, the distraction of the stones, and the swiftness of his sword bought Thomas only a heartbeat of confusion. But, it was enough to get him through their ranks.

Yet, his intention was not to flee. What easier target than an open back? No, Thomas focused on the split rock ahead among the large boulders.

Was the split large enough? Yes! Thomas reached it only a step before the bandits.

He turned and faced them. Rock now protected him on

three sides. The fourth side, open to the bandits, was wide enough to give him room to swing his sword, narrow enough to limit their attack.

The largest bandit spoke to the shadow which covered Thomas.

"Fool," he spat. "You think this saves you?"

Thomas did not reply.

"You succeed only in irritating us."

Thomas still said nothing, only kept his sword ready.

"Throw us your valuables, and we will leave."

For a moment, Thomas was tempted. Then he realized they would probably retreat out of sight and wait for him to reappear in the open. And even if he did survive, without his gold, life in this strange land would be next to impossible.

So Thomas only stared at the bandit. The stalemate continued for thirty seconds.

"Search the nearby hills," the leader of the bandits then called to his men without turning his head. "Find wood and dried brush."

Two of the men scrambled away from the road.

"You see," the bandit resumed his conversation with Thomas, "I have no intention of risking even one man in direct combat. Few travelers pass here; we have much time, and a fire will easily move you from your shelter."

The man's eyes narrowed. "I will promise you this. The longer you delay us, the longer it will take for you to die."

The bandit smiled faint amusement and began to whistle tunelessly.

Thomas wondered if it might be best to bolt from his shelter. With two bandits searching for wood, his odds were now one against four.

The tuneless whistle continued. Thomas noted the layers of scars across the bandit's forearms. *He has survived many fights.*

Thomas noted the relaxed but ready stance of the other three bandits.

Neither are they strangers to battle. I will be sliced to shreds. But better to die fighting than as a helpless captive.

Thomas did not have a chance to consider further, for a short buzz interrupted the tuneless whistle. And almost in the same moment, there was a light thud.

The bandit looked down at his right shoulder in disbelief. The head of a crossbow arrow, gleaming red with blood, protuded an inch from his flesh.

Another buzz. Another thud. One of the bandits fell to the ground, clutching the shaft of an arrow already deep in his thigh.

The leader half turned. The next arrow pierced his hand and he dropped his sword, his mouth open in a soundless scream of agony.

The two other bandits were already running.

"Thomas!" a voice called. "You are safe to join me!"

English! And the unseen attacker knows my name.

Thomas stepped into the sunlight.

Above him, a dark silhouette rose at the top of a boulder.

Thomas ignored the two men moaning on the ground in front of him and took another step closer to the man with the crossbow. The sun behind him was bright, however, and much as Thomas squinted, he could not see the man's features.

Then the man dropped to the ground. "During attack, always keep the sun at your back," he instructed. "It gives you much light and blinds your opponents."

The man grinned and kicked aside one of the fallen bandits to step forward and extend his right hand to Thomas in a weaponless clasp of friendship.

The voice and face belonged to the captured crusader Thomas had last seen struggling in the bonds of slavery alongside a caravan of camels.

"I hope you will consider this a debt paid," Lord Baldwin said. "The water you once offered a poor slave in return for your life."

Katherine wished that she had been born deaf, for then she could not have heard the words which now pierced her heart.

"Thomas has failed our test." The muscles around Sir William's eyes tightened as he spoke. "We must conclude he is not a Merlin."

The test. So long ago, it seemed, she and Thomas had reached St. Jean d'Acre. And while he was in the public baths cleaning away the stench from weeks in the brig of the ship, the beggar, a spy for Sir William, had taken her to the house she remembered from her youth. There, to her surprise and delight, Sir William had greeted her, and they had hurriedly devised a way to test whether Thomas was truly a Merlin. Two others of the cause, posing as assassins, would pretend an attempt on their lives as soon as she rejoined Thomas. Then they would escape the fire by using the tunnel while Thomas believed assassins lurked nearby. In this manner, Sir William and Katherine could hurry Thomas into accepting the need for separate travel. They could also give him something of pretended tremendous value. If he appeared in Nazareth with the parcel still sealed, he could be trusted. If he did not appear . . .

"Can we not wait one more day?" Katherine asked. "Perhaps Thomas has been delayed."

And, she added to herself, *to wait means hope that Thomas can be trusted and believed.*

Sir William resumed his pacing of the inn courtyard and did not reply immediately, as if he were indeed considering her request. The sun had long since passed the highest point of the day. As the air cooled, so had Nazareth quieted and settled. The calls and babble of the town market beyond the inn was now the silence of an early evening breeze which rustled the leaves of the courtyard fig trees.

"No," Sir William finally said. "We have waited two weeks. Each day, I too have told myself that he has been delayed. But that is only wishful thinking. We must force ourselves to accept the bitter truth. Thomas has deceived and betrayed us."

Katherine heard a tiny voice speak. "Mayhaps . . . mayhaps he is dead." She was startled to realize the tiny voice was hers.

How she was torn. For if Thomas were dead, there was the consolation that he had not betrayed them, and she could always love his memory. If he were alive, she would have to learn to hate him, even though she would always harbor the slightest hope that somehow he might be part of their cause, and that her love for him could against all odds be realized.

"He is not dead," Sir William said. "No matter how much I might wish to use that for an explanation. You remember the package and how we prepared ourselves for that terrible event, do you not?"

"Yes," Katherine sighed. A great reward had been promised to the finder of the parchment inside the package entrusted to Thomas. If Thomas were killed by accident or murder, and the package opened—for what passerby or murderer would not be curious of a sealed package—there would be found the message directing the finder to appear in Nazareth with the book to receive a great reward. Yes, should Thomas have been killed, or found dead along a road, someone would have appeared, or at the very least, sent a messenger to inquire about the reward.

"Must we make this decision?" Katherine continued in the same sad voice.

Sir William stopped his pacing, moved toward her, and placed his hands upon her shoulders.

"Katherine, even a blind man could see how deeply you feel for Thomas. I have delayed my decision until now simply because of that."

A single tear trickled down her cheek.

"He has not returned with the package. It means he opened it, either because he is one of them, or because he will not be one of us. He is a fool," Sir William said softly. "A fool to choose evil, and a greater fool to walk from your love. But that is his decision, and now we must make ours."

Katherine bowed her head and patted Sir William's hand where it rested upon her shoulder. Then she turned away and, head still bowed, began to walk across the courtyard to her room in the inn.

The quietness and acceptance of her grief and pain was much more powerful than if she had protested in anger, and Sir William felt the urge to justify his decision.

He called to her back.

"Tell me again," he said, "of the trouble in England."

She paused.

He took three strides and guided her to a bench in the corner of the courtyard. Deep purple had spread across the sky as the sun dropped behind the far hills; already the brightest stars could be seen. Doves chuckled and cooed as they settled on the roofs of nearby buildings. For a moment, Katherine said nothing, as the peace of the evening fell upon them.

"England," she said, almost in a whisper. "Tell you again of England?"

Sir William nodded.

"The Druids—once hidden among the people, have conquered Magnus by openly posing as priests," she replied. "They claim power through the legend of the Holy Grail and by demonstrating miracles which are false. Now, in a large circle outward from Magnus, in one town after the other, they slowly gain converts to their cause."

Sir William nodded again, then said abruptly, "Have you ever questioned *our* cause?"

The change of subject and change in his tone startled Katherine, and for a moment, she was at a loss for words.

"You have never once questioned the sacrifices you have made to be one of us, a Merlin?" Sir William persisted. "Not during the years hidden in bandages, forced to endure the pain of an outcast freak, simply that you might report to Hawkwood the activities of Magnus? Not when other young women your age were dreaming of love and children? Not once did you question your role among us?"

"I . . . I . . ."

"And now," Sir William pushed, "as I make the decision to turn our backs on the one you *do* love, are you at peace to be a Merlin?"

Katherine drew a breath and faced him squarely with the dignity of royalty.

"I question," she said. And waited.

"That is good," Sir William said, "for a faith tested is a faith strengthened. And a faith unable to stand questions is a weak faith indeed. Now, I wish to answer your doubts."

He stared at the brightening stars as he searched for what he must say. "For your sake, I am glad mere words cannot describe the evil I have seen, the ways that Druids have killed men, how terrible their destruction of many of the best of us, when they first conquered Magnus and forced us to flee England.

"Druid ceremonies involve the ritual murder of the innocent. They believe the death of that soul transfers life and fortune to the one they choose. This death? They place the innocent into a wicker basket and lower the basket into fire."

Sir William clenched his jaw at unwanted memories. He stood, paced, and sat again before he could continue.

"As you know, King Arthur's Merlin was once a Druid. His knowledge of science and potions gave him seemingly magical powers among ordinary people. Then Merlin turned his back on the Druids and founded Magnus all those centuries ago, an island castle in a remote corner of England. There he taught others the Druid skills that were used against them, dark skills, so dark that through hypnosis, for example, we can change a man's mind, much as Thomas was caused to bury his childhood memories so very deep. But these skills can also be used for good, and the new Merlins used them throughout the country to combat the Druids in hidden warfare. That generation taught another generation to do the same, and that generation another, so that down through the centuries, the Druids could never reach their ultimate goal. Magnus served us—"

"I know this," Katherine said. "The story is told each Merlin as we come of age."

Sir William smiled. "It is important enough to repeat. And I want you to think of it as you force your heart away from Thomas."

The knight paused to remember his place in the story, then began again as if he had not been interrupted. "Magnus served us well. For hundreds of years, the Druids did not know of our existence, and time and again, from secret positions in society, we Merlins defeated them. Even after the Druids finally discovered our purpose, they could not locate Magnus, and when they finally knew of the castle of Magnus, it took generations for them to conquer it, barely years before your birth. Their surprise attack and ruthless slaughter twenty years ago all but destroyed the Merlins. Only a few of us survived."

Sir William closed his eyes again, fighting unwelcome memories. When he spoke again, his voice was strained.

"You must understand, Katherine. Generations of us have sacrificed all to fight the Druids, a terrible battle hidden from the people. Now that Magnus has finally fallen, now that there are so few Merlins, the Druids boldly and openly begin to control the people. They now seek to complete the terrible act that Merlin fought to prevent through the founding of Magnus nearly eight hundred years ago."

"That act?" Katherine asked. "Hawkwood always said I must not be burdened with the knowledge."

Sir William searched her eyes and made his decision. "That act? You shall be told, although few of the Merlins are. And you shall be told as we travel to the Holy City, Jerusalem."

"What of Thomas?" Katherine asked.

"He holds the key to the battle," Sir William said. "And we were almost fools enough to tell him where lies the final door to be opened by that key. Only this test—"

He slapped his thigh in frustration and anger. "What of Thomas? Tomorrow, when we travel, you will hear of the

Druid evil. And then, like me, you will be able to bear the pain of the fate of Thomas."

Katherine pressed her hands to her face as the knight finished his anguished words.

"There are still knights of the Crusade hidden in this land. They will be told. Thomas must be executed on sight. By sword or arrow, he must die."

They traveled on donkeys in a staggered line. Umar, one of the men who had posed as an assassin in St. Jean d'Acre, ranged the dusty road several hundred yards ahead of Katherine and Sir William. The other, Hadad, kept pace an equal distance behind. Both were alert for any signs of ambush and would cry warning at the first indication of a bandit attack.

It was not until they had departed from the high hills—so treacherous with hiding spots—and reached the road to Damascus in the Valley of Jezreel, that Sir William felt relaxed enough to drop his constant search of the land around him and finally begin conversation.

"Soon enough," he said, "we reach the valley of the River Jordan. There, we will turn south and follow the river to Jericho where another road will take us high into the mountains of Jerusalem."

"You know a great deal of this land," Katherine replied. A breeze swept through the valley, so that travel was almost comfortable. Were it not for the hard saddle and the uneven gait of the donkey, Katherine might have enjoyed the journey, for in all directions the distant hills carved a hazy horizon against the pale blue sky. But even with physical comfort, her mind and heart grieved for Thomas, and that clouded any joy she felt in the freedom of the wide expanse of the valley.

"I know little," Sir William contradicted her with a smile. "What I know comes from conversation from the two who guard and journey with us. For generations, their families have served the crusaders."

Katherine was not sure she wanted to discuss the matter which filled her with so much distress. Now that Sir William deemed conversation more appropriate than constant vigilance against bandit attacks, she wished to keep him from the subject of Thomas for as long as possible.

"Tell me," she asked, "how is it that knights of the Crusades still live in this land?"

Above them, a hawk circled and screamed. Sir William glanced upward, and the tanned skin around his eyes crinkled as he squinted against the sun. He studied the hawk briefly, then grunted, "It does not scream from alarm, but to frighten small animals into movement so that they become visible."

Then his shoulders relaxed and he faced her again. His blue eyes were serious as he studied her.

"For two hundred years," he began in response to her question, "the crusaders fought and struggled to keep this land. Enough years that entire generations were born here. Indeed, many were the noblemen who had the opportunity to return to the homelands of their fathers, yet refused. The castles established here, after all, were their true homes.

"Then the Mamelukes finally swept the land, destroying the castles and all the power of the crusaders. For many who survived, it was impossible to return to Europe. For others, unthinkable. They began to wander the Holy Land, for as nomads, they could avoid the Mameluke soldiers easily, much as we do so now by traveling in a small group and in the native dress of the people who live here."

The hawk screamed again, and Sir William paused to watch in admiration as it dove in a magnificent rush. The hawk disappeared briefly in tall grass, struggled and flapped its massive wings, then rose again, screaming in frustration that its talons were empty.

"These knights are not Merlins?" Katherine asked.

"No," Sir William said. He understood the question. "Would that there were now many of us to continue the fight. But we have no Magnus here in the Holy Land, no place to impart to them the secrets and knowledge we use to combat the Druids."

He smiled again. "However, the knights recognize fellowship, and here among enemies they have learned to assist each other where possible. You might be surprised at how quickly news can travel from outpost to outpost, through messengers trusted by these knights. I myself have many friends among them. Not Merlins, but good and capable men."

The conversation stopped and the silence between them weighed heavy. For each knew the other's thoughts. *Good and capable men now seeking Thomas for the purpose of his death.*

The donkeys swayed and plodded their sure steps for several more minutes before Katherine dared speak aloud her next question.

"Yesterday," she whispered, "you told me I would understand why Thomas must die."

And to herself she continued, *As if that is consolation for the pain I bear.*

Behind them, the hawk screamed again, now a faint cry.

"I am certain you know much of the politics of men," Sir William said. "For Hawkwood would have trained you as thoroughly as any Merlin in the old schools of Magnus."

Katherine nodded. What was there in politics that the man she loved would so coldly betray her? What was there in politics that demanded the man she loved be sentenced to death?

"There is also the politics of religion," Sir William said. "Something I wish were not so."

"Religion is a matter of God, is it not?" Katherine asked.

"I am not sure how Merlin himself might have explained it," Sir William said, "but these are my private thoughts."

Despite herself, and the dull pain of loss of hope in Thomas that made her ache every moment, Katherine felt intrigued.

"I prefer to think of faith as separate from religion," Sir William explained. "Faith is God-made, the joy and peace He gives us with our belief in His eternal presence and in His promises to us. Thus, faith is the private communication between God and each of us."

Katherine nodded. For had she not spent many hours in prayer? Had she not consoled herself countless times with such faith in her God?

"Religion," the knight said, "religion is man-made. It is the necessary structure here on earth for men to learn and teach this personal faith. The church, then, though imparting the truths of God, is made and maintained by men. Church buildings are man-made, as is the structure of the religion. We have a pope who oversees bishops, who in turn oversee priests, who in turn oversee the common man."

Katherine nodded again.

"In this man-made structure of religion, there are many men of true faith. Thus, God ensures that faith is passed from generation to generation. Yet, because religion is of this earth and of men, it is flawed. Some men use the structure of religion for their own purposes and claim faith merely for the power it gives them within the structure. You have seen, I am sure, bishops fat and well clothed, while the poor starve naked before them."

"Yes," Katherine said. "This troublesome fact leads many to doubt the truth in religion."

"Truth in *religion?* Is there truth in the stone walls of a church? No. The truth is in the contents of *faith.* One must look beyond the stone walls of the church to see it, just as one must look past the structure of religion." Sir William paused as he seached for words. "The greedy bishops are imperfect, but this does not mean the message they bring is equally imperfect. The structure in which God passes along faith is far from perfect, yet this does not mean the truth delivered by the structure is imperfect. The faith itself—the ultimate truth of God and His Son—is pure."

"I find pain in a philosophical discussion, while my heart grieves over the death sentence of Thomas."

"Yet that is my point," the knight said softly. "Because of religion, Thomas and the Druids are deadly dangerous. Can you not see what might happen in England?"

Katherine said nothing, but her knuckles were white with tension as she waited.

"Through the sham of false miracles, how long until the priests of the Holy Grail have convinced town after town to abandon one religion for another? How long until the priests of the Roman church are powerless?"

The knight closed his eyes as he spoke. "The king of England receives his power because the people believe he rules by the authority of the Roman church and by the authority of God. What then, when the people no longer believe in that authority? What then happens to the nobility, men appointed by the king to rule the entire nation?"

By his tone, these questions were not meant for reply, so Katherine said nothing.

"It is not enough horror that the Druids plan to take from the people their faith; they also plan to take total power through devastation of the land."

"How?" Katherine asked.

"How? Through a method that Merlin could not abide, a method that turned him against the Druids who raised him."

"How?" Katherine repeated.

"Do you remember the earl of York? How generations of his family followed the orders of any secret messenger who showed the ring of the Druid symbol?"

Katherine nodded. She had been told the story by the earl himself, from his place of imprisonment, a dungeon in the town he had once ruled.

"Do you remember what happened to the one ancestor who did not obey a messenger's commands?"

Katherine frowned in thought, then said, "The earl spoke of a curse which killed his great-great-great-grandfather."

"Yes. Worms consumed that ruler's body, though he was still alive. It took seven days for him to die, seven days of screaming agony."

Sir William clenched his teeth. "The Druids have a simple method to cause such death. A potion to cause deep sleep. Then a small portion of honey placed in a man's ears, and small maggots dropped within."

Katherine nearly retched. For the ears led to the inside of a man's head. How deeply would those maggots burrow? As they grew and spilled forth later, it would appear as if worms consumed the man.

"Yes," Sir William gritted in response to her reaction. "Evil horror."

He took a deep breath. "Katherine, imagine this. The masses of people begin to believe the priests of the Holy Grail. And at the slightest sign of rebellion, the firstborn of every family dies such a death. Mayhaps even before rebellion, the firstborn of the rulers die in such a way. No one would resist. England would be theirs."

He clenched his fists. "Our Merlin education gives us the history of mankind. Five hundred dark years have passed, darkness when knowledge was scarce and all people held in chains by ignorance. Only now has the light begun to appear. Advances in medicine and science are upon us, and through the written word, are shared from man to man, country to country. Mankind now begins to advance!"

Sir William stopped to draw another breath. His voice was urgent. "Katherine, there may come the day when fair laws protect every man, when abundance of food and medicine lets average people live to be forty, yes, even fifty years of age! When it will be common to read, so that all receive the pleasure you and I do from books! When ignorance is overcome and leaders of society must respond to the will of the people! This may someday arrive, even if it takes generations after you and I have left this earth. A day when such abundance and ease of living causes nations to exist in peace."

Katherine found herself holding her breath to listen to Sir William's passion.

He stopped suddenly, then dropped his voice. "If the Druids conquer and begin to rule, they will bar the people from knowledge, for their own power is derived from the ignorance of the people. They will end this slow progress that has been made by the learned men of our country. And the ages of darkness—" he faltered. "The ages of darkness will be upon mankind for centuries more."

After five days, the small group of travelers reached the town gates of Jericho. The gatekeeper gave them only a passing glance—Katherine had veiled her face as was the custom for all women in public, knowing too that it served another purpose, to hide her striking blond hair.

Once through the town gates, she noted that the streets were extremely narrow and ran crookedly in all directions. She mentioned her observation to Sir William.

"Defense," he said. "Should invaders ever break through the gates, they face the confusion of the twisting streets. And not only that; streets this narrow force armies to advance in a column only four or five men wide. Thus, four or five defenders can halt the entire army, for those behind the leading ranks of the army are unable to fight. And—" Sir William gestured upward at the sun-bleached square buildings "—while the army is slowed on the ground, defenders on top cast down rocks or boiling oil."

Katherine nodded, and then, as custom dictated, she followed meekly behind Sir William and the other two men as they searched for an inn.

At dusk, with a lighted candle in his hand, Sir William moved to the opening in the stone that served as a window.

The fading afternoon sun cast a small shaft of light into the cramped room, light almost completely blocked as the knight stood in front of the window.

The walls were gray with accumulated filth. The room was bare except for a pile of straw in one corner. Beside the straw were a pitcher with water and a bowl with figs and bread.

Earlier, Katherine had dropped her blanket on the straw, then had jumped as two rats scurried out beneath her feet to dart to the wall and scramble their way up to the window before disappearing. That surprise had not deterred her in the slightest, so eager was she to sleep on something softer than cold, hard ground.

"This inn is known to many of the forsaken knights as a safe haven," Sir William explained from the window. "Even so, I prefer not to have you sleep alone. The four of us shall share this room."

"That sets my mind at ease," she answered. She turned her head to determine Sir William's actions by the window. "For one night, it is no discomfort to be guarded in such a manner."

Sir William stepped back. Three lighted candles were now standing in the window.

"It may be more than one night," he said. "For now we wait until this signal is answered."

The knock on the door came during the second night.

It was a soft knock, yet enough to pull Katherine from deep sleep. She sat up quickly, and when Sir William opened the door, her eyes were clear and she was alert.

The three candles which burned on the the windowsill cast unsteady light across the room.

The man who slipped inside the door wore the long flowing clothing of a desert nomad. As the door shut, he pulled the wraps from his headband and rubbed his hair lightly, as if relieved to be free of its restrictions.

Katherine watched him with mild curiosity. In the flickering light, his features were blurred, but she could still distinguish a flash of white teeth as he smiled greeting to Sir William.

The two men were of same height and build. The man's hair was dark, unlike the complexion of his skin, and his first words confirmed Katherine's immediate guess. He was not a native to this land, for he spoke in slow and measured English.

"I had despaired you might never arrive," the man said.

"It was with great relief that I saw your signal in the window."

He glanced around the room and nodded at the two other men, Umar and Hadad. His eyes stopped on Katherine.

"Do my eyes mock me?" he said. "Or is this truly a vision of beauty?"

Katherine nodded in return. She did not know this man and did not want to encourage him. But the voice was deep and smooth, and she admitted to herself that few women would resent words of charm from a man who carried himself so nobly.

"Your eyes do not mock you," Sir William said. He stepped between the man and Katherine to make introduction.

Katherine took the cue and rose.

As the man stepped closer, she saw that his hair was tinged with gray at the temples. A handsome man, indeed, she thought. Another part of her mind noted sadly that handsome as he was, her mind could not release a vision of Thomas.

"This, sir, is Katherine. She is one of us."

So the man is a Merlin.

He took Katherine's hand, bowed, and lightly touched his lips against the back of her hand.

"I am honored," he said.

Katherine raised her eyebrows in question, and Sir William answered immediately.

"This, milady, is a man with vast knowledge of the Holy Land. As one of England's greatest knights, he has proven to be a great thorn in the side of the Mameluke soldiers who have attempted his capture for years."

"I am equally honored," Katherine said. "It is a pleasure to make your aquaintance, Sir . . . Sir . . . ."

Sir William quickly spoke again. "Lord Baldwin, Katherine. None other than Lord Hubert Baldwin."

"May we speak freely?" Lord Baldwin asked.

Sir William glanced at Umar and Hadad and spoke rapid words in their native language. They nodded in reply.

Then Sir William spoke to Lord Baldwin. "They will not resent it if you speak in English, a tongue they do not understand."

"And the lady Katherine?"

"She has proven herself repeatedly, Lord Baldwin. Now, with so few of us in these desperate times, she must be counted among our Merlin leaders."

High praise indeed. Katherine hoped her flush was not visible in the candlelight.

Lord Baldwin smiled broadly at Katherine. His teeth gleamed like a wolf's. Katherine tried to dismiss the thought, but failed. *A wolf, fascinating but deadly. What secrets might such a man carry?*

His words interrupted her thoughts.

"I have heard the news, of course," Lord Baldwin said. "The one known as Thomas must be killed. And it should not be difficult to find him. Not when he is a stranger among the people of this land."

Katherine flinched, but forced her face to remain as stone.

"But I know little else," Lord Baldwin said. "Why must he be killed? Did he not reconquer Magnus? Was not his father the—"

"Yes, yes," Sir William said quickly, as if he wanted to spare Katherine the pain of more thoughts of Thomas' betrayal. "Katherine, perhaps you might describe all that has happened since I departed from Magnus."

Katherine took a deep breath. "The situation in England is thus . . ."

She repeated what she had told Sir William earlier.

Lord Baldwin's frown deepened at each new piece of information.

"What can we do first?" he asked, when Katherine finished.

Sir William grinned. "Listen to the man," he said. "He says 'first.' He believes something can be done!"

Then Sir William sobered. "I too have news from England." He faced Katherine. "I withheld it from you because I believed it unfair to give you false hope. I did not know if Lord Baldwin would reach us. But now that the one knight we need is here . . ."

"Spare the flattery," Lord Baldwin growled. "Tell us what you have."

"A letter," Sir William said. He hesitated. "From Hawkwood himself. Given to a trusted messenger who delivered it to me in St. Jean d'Acre after months of journey from France."

Sir William looked to Lord Baldwin. "It arrived barely a week before Katherine did. I had no time to send you word and inform you of its contents."

Lord Baldwin dismissed the apology with a wave. "I am here now," he said. "That is what matters."

Katherine barely heard as she again forced her face to be stone. *The letter, then, was sent before Hawkwood's death.* She remembered well her entire winter in France, how she had spent hour after hour in the library of the royal palace, wondering where the old man might be during his six-month absence.

Sir William answered her thoughts. "In the letter, Hawkwood explains that he spent months traveling from monastery to monastery."

Searching for what?

Again, Sir William answered her thoughts. He reached for his travel pouch and withdrew a strange, pale material, folded flat into a small square.

Puzzlement at the material was as clear on Lord Baldwin's face as on Katherine's.

"It is called paper," Sir William explained. "Lighter and more pliable than parchment. The messenger informed me that all of Europe is now learning of its use from the Spaniards."

He handed it to Katherine. Gently, hesitantly, she unfolded it. *So much lighter than parchment,* she marveled. *And it does not crack when folded.*

Almost immediately, however, her thoughts turned to Hawkwood. For there, even in the low light, she saw his clear, strong handwriting.

"Read it aloud," Sir William urged.

She did so, in low, almost hushed tones.

From Paris this 3rd day of March, In the Year of Our Lord 1313 —

Word has reached me that matters in Magnus are worsening. Our enemies have openly begun their final campaign. In less than two years from now, I fear, they will have gained enough power among the people to succeed.

We are yet unable to trust Thomas. Our friend Gervaise is still in Magnus and watches carefully, but from him I have received no word that Thomas is one of us. And without trust in Thomas, we cannot be sure we will regain Magnus. Without Magnus, our efforts in England will be doomed.

Katherine closed her eyes briefly. Bitter sadness took her breath away. From Paris . . . Hawkwood had written this before leaving with her for England. He had been alive then. Gervaise too. Thomas had yet to betray them both. It had been a time of hope. Now . . .

"Katherine?" It was Sir William's voice, gentle and worried.

She smiled a tight smile and turned back to the letter, reading with a steadiness she did not feel.

Yet, even if England is lost to us, my friend, do not despair. It was no coincidence that we chose to flee to St. Jean d'Acre when Magnus first fell. While it has been commonly believed among us that the reason for retreat to the Holy Land was because of the crusading knights who might be of service, there is another, more compelling reason, one known only to the leaders of each generation of Merlins. A reason which forced me these last months to travel to the ancient libraries of Europe, and a reason I must pass on to you in this letter; because, should I die, the secret must not die with me. If there comes a time when I trust Thomas, he, as you are now, will be directed to the Holy Land.

Again, Katherine stopped. This time, however, she blurted her thoughts. "Hawkwood *did* direct Thomas here after the letter was written! How could he have trusted—"

Sir William placed a finger to his lips, a mild way to silence her. "Still, Hawkwood was not certain, for he did not give Thomas what remains for you to read."

Katherine accepted the reproval and bowed her head to the letter.

Our founder, Merlin, knew only little of what lies hidden in the Holy Land, for the legend of it began more than three hundred years before his birth, a time when Roman generals ruled Britain.

Even then, hundreds of years before Merlin's birth, the Druids had long been hidden among the people, suppressed by the Roman conquerers of ancient Britain. Yet, as we know too well, the Druids retained considerable power and influence through total secrecy.

There was a story passed from Druid generation to generation about the Roman general Julius Severus, who ruled Britain some hundred years after the death of Christ. This general discovered the Druid circle, but did not expose it. To let Rome know of the Druids would also let Rome know of their wealth and almost magical powers. Instead, Severus plundered the Druids in one fell swoop, taking a great fortune in gold, and the book of their most valued secrets of potions and deception.

Many of the details were lost through the centuries, but what Merlin knew was that Severus was summoned from Britain to quell a revolt, a Jewish revolt in the land of Christ. Severus could not trust his treasure to be left behind, so he arranged to take it with him.

That is all the Druids knew, for they were not sailors, and had no way of following the Roman general and his troops across half a world. That was all that Merlin knew, all that he could pass to the one he chose to lead the next generation of his followers.

Yet the Merlin leaders of each new generation were not idle. They anticipated the day that Magnus might fall, and each generation was given the task of adding to our scant knowledge of the stolen Druid wealth and secrets. When the Holy Land opened to the crusaders, we sent Merlins here to search. I have copied as much as is known in a book which must be matched with this letter.

Katherine stared at Sir William. She remembered how the jailer in Lisbon had returned to Thomas his cloak, his sword, and . . . and a book. "This book . . . Thomas carried a book. Remember how I told you that Hawkwood spent time with Thomas away from the campfire, that he remained in disguise as an old man and gave him instructions? Could he have given him the book then?"

"I had wondered," Sir William said. "Yet without this letter, the book is meaningless, only bait to draw Thomas here."

Katherine nodded. She began to read faster, anxious to know the contents of the letter.

My friend, I too have been given the task to add to that knowledge. There has been little to glean, even among the best libraries of our civilization, for history has too often been lost through the age of darkness, lost or converted to legend. What I know now, however, may be enough after all these hundreds of years of mystery.

In the land of the Franks, I stumbled across a parchment which held the words of the Roman historian Cassius Dio, who wrote a brief notice of Julius Severus and his war against the Jews. The Romans destroyed nearly a thousand Jewish villages, and a half million were slain. The Jewish rebels were finally defeated in their last refuge — caves in the Judean desert, north of the Dead Sea.

Severus, Cassius Dio writes, was recalled to Rome almost immediately after his victory in the Holy Land. It would seem unlikely he would take his treasure with him, for discovery of it by Roman officials would mean his death. Shortly after arriving in Rome, he died of sudden illness, taking his secret to the grave.

Yet there remains a peculiar fact noted by Cassius Dio. During one skirmish against the Jews near these caves, General Julius Severus lost twenty men in battle against a handful of unarmed rebels. These twenty men, Severus reported, died as a portion of the cave collapsed upon them, and their bodies could not be recovered.

Is it not more likely that these would be the twenty men who transported the treasure? For wealth that great would take such assistance. Is it not likely that the surest way for Julius Severus to guard his secret would be to kill those twenty in the cave where the treasure was buried? I believe so, and upon this now rest our hopes. Look to your friends in Jerusalem for guidance on the location of these caves.

Should Magnus be lost to us, and should you be able to recover what was so precious to the Druids, their wealth and ancient secrets may be used against them upon your return to England.

I pray this letter finds you in good health, and that the Lord God will be with us as we fight His enemies.

Katherine's fingers were trembling as she finished the letter. She looked up to a thoughtful expression on Sir William's face, and one of eagerness on Lord Baldwin's.

"I have heard rumors of the caves of refuge!" Lord Baldwin said quickly. "But I have always discounted them as myth, for stories were told of entire families living for months inside the earth. Yet this letter!"

Sir William pursed his lips. "You will assist us in the search?"

"To my death," Lord Baldwin said. He fumbled with a wineskin which hung from his belt. "And let us drink to this new hope!"

Sir William found the crude goblets supplied with the room.

Lord Baldwin insisted that Umar and Hadad join them in the toast.

The wine tasted bittersweet to Katherine. But she had only a short time to give it thought, for immediately she became drowsy.

Odd, she thought, *I was not tired, not with such important news.*

Struggle as she might, her lips would not do her bidding, and she could not voice those thoughts to Sir William.

Instead, she sat heavily, then collapsed into a stupor of wild dreams, among them that she had opened her eyes to kiss Thomas. She knew them to be wild dreams, however, for when she woke in the morning, she was bound and tied with rough hemp rope.

"Fools!"

Katherine struggled to sit so that she could turn to identify the speaker. It took her several seconds. Even as her mind was on the words, she was conscious of the terrible taste in her mouth, the thickness of her tongue, and the pounding of blood in her head that hurt as badly as the rope tight around her hands and feet.

"Ah, she wakes." The same voice continued. Cruel and taunting.

Katherine swung sideways to prop her back against the wall.

The other men, Sir William, Umar, and Hadad, were as securely bound as she. And sitting on the stool before the door was a man she recognized immediately.

Waleran. The spy who had shared a dungeon with Thomas so long ago, when Katherine had been a visitor disguised in bandages and Thomas an orphan determined to win a kingdom.

"Did you sleep like a princess?" Waleran asked. His black eyes gleamed with smugness.

Katherine felt dirty under his leering gaze. He was a nightmare, with that half-balding forehead and hair which fell scraggly and greasy onto sloped shoulders, with ears lumpy and thick, so large they almost flapped.

She refused to satisfy him with a reaction to his biting words. She merely settled against the wall and waited.

"You can release her. She is not one of us," Sir William said thickly. "But merely the daughter of a knight. One whom I have pledged safe passage across this land."

Waleran laughed. A short, harsh, mocking sound.

"Do you play me for as big a fool as you? She has spent time with Thomas; that I know from my spies."

Sir William swallowed hard, trying to work moisture into his mouth. "Thomas, as did I, served as escort. She knows nothing of his hidden reasons for remaining with her on the voyage to this land."

Another snort of laughter. "Fool. I was there in York when she entered the prison to speak to the earl. She has been involved since the beginning."

Waleran watched Katherine's face. "It was like stealing from a blind beggar," he said, "arranging to let Thomas escape York with the girl."

In spite of her determination to remain silent, a greater need brought words to Katherine's mouth; for in the passing of a heartbeat she had gained hope that Thomas was not a Druid, and she could not quench her love. "You arranged for Thomas to escape?"

"Are we so clumsy that he could march into a castle and steal from us in broad daylight? The entire matter was pre-arranged. From my cell beside the earl's, I heard every word. While you spoke to the earl, I made certain that all knew Thomas would shortly arrive at the castle."

Waleran smiled. It made Katherine think of flies crawling across the face of a corpse.

"Had I known, of course," Waleran said, "that you were with Hawkwood, I would have had you arrested right there in the prison. It would have saved all the effort of finding a way to ensure that Thomas would lead us to you."

Katherine's mind flew back to that afternoon in England, and much suddenly became clear. Thomas had been the bait to bring Hawkwood into the open. Waleran had only needed to let Thomas think he had triumphed, then follow. Thomas had not led the Druid soldiers to Hawkwood; but Hawkwood had followed Thomas, so the result was the same . . . capture the next morning, and Hawkwood's death.

She spoke her thoughts, now dreading the answer.

"Thomas is not a Druid?"

"Hardly. Were it so, I would not have taken such pains to trace his every step across the world."

Her heart rose in joy, then fell in defeat. For Sir William had passed a death sentence on Thomas. Now, unless they escaped, word could not be sent to end the sentence. And every hour in captivity was another hour closer to his death. He would die without knowing that she loved him.

"Waleran has explained," Sir William said to Katherine. "Although if your head pounds like mine, you hardly need to hear the name of the one who did betray us."

The wine. Lord Baldwin.

"Betrayal!" Waleran threw his head back and laughed. "This is a touching tale of woe. Thomas was waiting for you in Nazareth. Disguised as a beggar. He saw you with your two friends and assumed you had betrayed him."

Not only would Thomas die unaware of her love, but he would die believing she had betrayed him. Pain slammed her like a physical blow.

"How do you know of this?" Katherine demanded.

"Ahh," Waleran said, his voice now like oil. "Concern? A concern of love? This knowledge may prove to be of use."

He steepled his fingers beneath his chin and stared at Katherine. "My dear, it is simple. Lord Baldwin was not far from St. Jean d'Acre as Sir William believed, but nearby. Word of your arrival was immediate, and once he had followed you to the house and witnessed your carefully acted assassination attempt, it was an easy matter for him to anticipate the use of the tunnel; for as a Merlin, he too knew of it. Lord Baldwin then followed you to the caravan. He needed only to bribe the caravan leader to let him travel as a slave. From this position, he stayed with Thomas, and later managed to earn Thomas' trust."

Katherine looked to Sir William. The knight closed his

eyes and nodded. "You remember the hints we gave Thomas of a great secret? Lord Baldwin deduced from Thomas that our final destination was Jerusalem. As one of the forsaken crusaders, Lord Baldwin, of course, knew of the safe house in Jericho. He convinced Thomas to journey with him to Jericho, then to Jerusalem. Here in Jericho, Lord Baldwin suggested a rest, and hoped we might arrive soon. When he saw our signal, he prepared the wine, on the advice of this man."

Waleran responded to the pointed finger of Sir William with a bow. "Through Lord Baldwin and his messengers, I was informed of every single step Thomas took. Child's play, to anticipate your arrival here and arrange for the drugged wine. And what an unexpected and superb catch, that Lord Baldwin might also take possession of the letter you so stupidly revealed last night."

"And now?" Katherine asked. The letter was not on her mind. "Where is Thomas now?"

Waleran shook his head in mock disgust. "Such fools. Can you not see the obvious?"

Katherine kept her gaze steady.

"Lord Baldwin has returned to Thomas," came the reply. "He has stolen a pendant from Sir William and will use that as proof that he is Thomas' father."

Waleran smiled a smile that brought a shudder to Katherine.

"You see, my child, because of your blunder last night, we now know of the Salt Sea caves. Lord Baldwin will lead Thomas there as further proof that he is not a Druid. With that trust established, they will return to England, and Thomas will finally give us what we seek there. With our treasure restored, and with the final key to our plan, our victory will be complete."

Waleran's grimace of victory appeared to be a death mask across his face and skull.

"Once triumph is assured, three things will happen, my child. You and the knight will die, for there will no longer be reason to hold you as hostage."

Two more heartbeats passed before Waleran spoke again.

"Thomas too shall die. And England will be ours."

Chapter Fifty-Three

"Did a slave girl strike your fancy?" Lord Baldwin asked Thomas. "I feared you might never return from the market."

Thomas shook his head. *A slave girl? When the vision of Katherine fills my heart in dreams by day or night?*

Despite his thoughts, Thomas returned Lord Baldwin's smile. There was no need to burden another man with his own grief.

"Not a slave girl. Merely sweets to sustain us on our journey." Thomas held up a small square wrapped in cloth. "Combs of honey. For if we depart Jericho today, I would not refuse small comforts along our journey."

Thomas grinned wryly at the small room around them. "Not that this is the height of princely luxury."

Lord Baldwin nodded agreement and lifted his travel bag.

"Our donkeys await at the stable," he told Thomas. "And our journey is long."

They had traveled barely five miles before they reached the portion of the road that climbs the hills toward Jerusalem. Dust already caked Thomas, for there had been little rain to settle the soil of the road.

Without warning, the donkey beneath Thomas stumbled. Thomas pitched sideways but twisted to bring his feet below him quickly enough to stand.

Lord Baldwin chuckled approval.

"Well, done . . . son."

Thomas stopped dusting himself with frozen abruptness.

"Yes," Lord Baldwin answered the stare of amazement. "Son."

Thomas straightened.

"You . . . you are my father?"

"Just as you are a Merlin." Lord Baldwin dug beneath the layers of clothes that protected him from the heat. "This is the pendant that I have waited for years to bestow upon you."

His words were so unexpected that Thomas ignored the donkey as it sagged back to sit upon its hind legs. He reached for the offered pendant.

He studied it carefully, aware that Lord Baldwin's eyes were intent upon him. The delicate carvings in the pendant showed a sword stuck in a stone, with the silhouette of the castle of Magnus in the background.

"You . . . you are my father?" Though the words were repeated, his tone was not startled disbelief, but questioning hope.

"It was not chance that I was able to rescue you from those bandits outside of Nazareth," Lord Baldwin said. "Nor chance that I was part of the caravan which accompanied you away from St. Jean d'Acre."

Lord Baldwin shook his head. "It was a cause worth my while, to be with you; yet I pray I need never be a slave again."

"You followed me?" Thomas said.

Lord Baldwin nodded. "I dared not reveal myself. Not in St. Jean. Not in Nazareth. Not with that treacherous Sir William nearby. It would have been a fight to the death, and too much is at stake for me to risk such an end. Not when I couldn't tru—."

Thomas tilted his head in quizzical amusement. "Not when you couldn't trust me?" Thomas paused. "Why now? Why choose this time to tell me?"

"Because—" Lord Baldwin had no choice but to stop, as the donkey groaned in pain.

Thomas scanned the road behind him, as if measuring the distance back to Jericho.

"Is this usual for such a beast?" Thomas asked, then mused. "At least we are within sight of the town. It is not too late to turn back and find another donkey, should this one prove to be seriously ill."

"I confess this matter *is* puzzling." Lord Baldwin frowned as the donkey groaned again. "Never in this land have I seen a donkey behave so."

"Shall we wait?" Thomas suggested. "Perhaps the beast has indigestion. If we rest in the shade, it may recover."

Lord Baldwin nodded; Thomas hobbled both donkeys and reached for a pouch which hung from the donkey's saddle before climbing the rocks which led away from the road. After the climb, he stopped in the shade of a large boulder and waited for Lord Baldwin to sit beside him.

It gave them a view of the entire valley. Far away, Thomas saw, or perhaps imagined he saw, the green ribbon of trees that lined the River Jordan.

"*Father*," Thomas said, trying the strange word. "*Father*. It is strange. I do not know how to feel."

An ironic smile from Lord Baldwin. "Merlins are taught so much, but this is something even the best teacher could not anticipate."

Thomas stared at him. "You know of Merlins. You call Sir William and Katherine by name, although I had only told you that two friends betrayed me. Because you know of them, I cannot doubt you are my father."

"We will have much to share, my son." Lord Baldwin slapped Thomas on the back and smiled his handsome wolfish smile. "Much to share."

Thomas opened his travel pouch and unwrapped a comb of honey which he offered to Lord Baldwin. The older man bit into the sweetness with an eagerness that prevented him from speaking for several more minutes.

Finally, his mouth was empty of the honey.

"At first, I did not know if you were, like Sir William and Katherine, a Druid," Lord Baldwin began, after clearing his throat. "After all, how easy to pretend anger at the two friends of whom you made mention, cleverly concealing their names as if you did not know I was a Merlin. Anything to gain my confidence. But we have passed Jericho, and now I know you deserve my trust."

"Jericho?"

"My logic is thus. Sir William is a Druid. Were you a

Merlin, it would not be to his advantage to tell you of the crusader safe house there known to the knights of this land, nor to your advantage to tell you that *I* am a Merlin. Were you a Druid, he would have told you of the existence of the safe house — and instructed you to meet him there to discuss more plans to continue the deception you and he would have plotted against me. When you first told me that you might seek Jerusalem after a journey to St. Jean d'Acre, I wondered if you really meant to meet Sir William in Jericho, the one town where all travelers to Jerusalem rest."

Lord Baldwin licked the honey from his lips. "In Jericho, you did not seek the safe house, so I can happily conclude you are not an ally of Sir William. You truly are a Merlin. I can welcome you as my son. I shall earn your trust by sharing with you the great wealth of a long-lost secret. Then, we can return to England, and with what you know, defeat the Druids there."

Silence, as they both pondered those words. Not even the groaning of the donkey reached them at their secluded resting place.

"The honey is sweet, is it not?" Thomas finally said softly.

"You are generous not to take some yourself. And you have my thanks for the sweetness I enjoyed."

"Yes, very sweet. As sweet as the lies you may have told," Thomas continued in the same soft tones. He held up his hand to forestall Lord Baldwin. "I am not the fool you take me to be."

Lord Baldwin winced, but not from Thomas' words. He clutched his stomach, and his wince became a moan.

"If the honey does not settle well," Thomas said, "it is merely because of the time I spent at the market this morning in search of the poison it contains, the same poison that pains my donkey below."

Less than an hour later, Thomas was walking through the streets of Jericho. The anger on his face was not visible, nor the jutting of his jaw, for his face was hidden in the shadows of the cloth that protected his head from the sun. Yet his determination was obvious, and many were those on the crowded streets who gave way before his marching strides.

Thomas did not hesitate as he approached his destination, a small inn tucked among the poorer dwellings of the city.

He brushed aside the protests of an old man at the door of the inn, and as he climbed the stone stairs that led to the second floor of the square building, he placed his hand on the hilt of the sword.

When he reached the door, he did not knock. Instead, he pushed hard with his shoulder and popped the door inward. As he entered the swinging door, he pulled the sword loose and slashed air.

There was no one to challenge him. All four occupants of the room were lying on mats, bound, gagged, powerless to react to his sudden appearance.

Thomas turned so that he could face the half-open door. He kept his sword ready in his right hand, and with his left hand pulled the bands of cloth from his head to reveal his face.

Only then did one of the occupants react with a widening of her eyes.

"Yes, Katherine," Thomas said. There was no warmth in his voice. "Thomas. Perhaps you remember me?"

Her eyes remained wide.

Thomas glanced at the others. "Sir William," he said, with the same lack of warmth. "You prefer assassins as companions? Or do you miss my company?"

The knight only blinked. The other two men, Umar and Hadad, shook their heads.

"You have my sympathy," Thomas said to them, with no sympathy at all. "For you two shall remain here."

With that, Thomas stepped forward and, with a small knife, cut the gag from Sir William's mouth.

"One may return," Sir William warned him. "The one who guards us."

"Then he shall taste steel," Thomas said. "A fight will serve as a useful outlet for my anger. You and she and all the others have mocked me with deception for too long. Now I intend to find the truth."

Sir William merely repeated his warning. "Watch your back," he said.

Thomas ignored Umar and Hadad as he moved to cut Katherine's gag.

"Thomas . . ." she began, only to stop at the cold rage in his eyes.

"I will free you both," Thomas said, "under one condition."

He loosed a leather water bag from his belt. "The condition that you drink from this."

"Water?" Katherine asked.

"Perhaps," Thomas said. "Why ask with such suspicion? If I meant you harm, I would slit your throats instead of burdening myself with your presence as we travel."

Sir William spit remnant threads of the gag from his mouth. "Drink it, Katherine. If he insists upon such childish games, we must play. And quickly. For if our jailer returns—"

"I will drink," Katherine said calmly.

Thomas squatted to offer her the mouth of the water bag. He held her head to steady it as he poured.

This soft hair. Those deep-blue eyes. And the lips which drink.

He frowned at his weakness for those thoughts. Katherine took his frown for renewed anger.

"It is not what you think," she said.

"That remains to be discovered," Thomas said. He moved to Sir William to let him drink.

Then Thomas stood. He drank heavily from the water bag, then tied the mouth shut and hung it again from his belt.

"At the very least," observed Sir William, "let the other two men drink."

Thomas wiped his lips and shook his head.

"They mean you no harm," Sir William insisted.

Thomas shook his head again, then leaned over with the knife to begin sawing at the rope which held Katherine's ankles together.

"It will not be a favor to let them drink," Thomas said. He grunted in effort as the hemp of the rope snapped apart. "For the water we shared contains a slow-acting poison."

Past Jericho, somewhere high in the hills—Thomas did not know how far from Jerusalem—they stopped at dusk. Because the hills were so steep, there were few villages. Had Thomas even wanted to risk another night in an inn, it would not have been possible. Their choices were to travel during the night or set camp; and travel at night through these dark hills would be suicide.

Thomas began to build a fire as the others unburdened the donkeys and unrolled blankets. When they finished, they stood near the fire and watched Thomas in sullen silence.

"You see, perhaps, that I brought much food," Thomas said cheerfully. "And that our donkeys carry bundles of kindling. You may expect, then, many more nights like this."

No reply. Nor did he expect one. For all three had moved during the day in complete silence.

Thomas stood, placed his hands on his hips, and regarded them where they stood. They stared back. Lord Baldwin on one side, still pale with illness. Katherine and Sir William on the other, almost pressed together in mutual distrust of their other traveling companions.

"Come, let us eat," Thomas said in the same cheerful tones. "Then we shall talk of many things."

"Eat?" Lord Baldwin grunted. "Not your food. For what potion will you surprise me with next?"

"Come, come," Thomas said. "No trust?"

Thomas grinned at Katherine and Sir William. If it bothered him that they did not smile back in return, he did not show it.

"And you two," Thomas said, grin still wide, "you'll not trust my food either?"

They merely stared at him.

Thomas rubbed his hands together briskly, as a man might do content to be with favored guests. "Well, then," Thomas said, "let me propose this. You three cook. And I'll eat my share of the food. That way you can be assured I'll not poison you again."

Silence.

So Thomas continued, "Besides, as I'll gladly explain after our meal, the poison already within you is sufficient for your death "

The flames had died to the red glow of embers, low enough so that Thomas could see beyond the fire to the shadows cast among the boulders by the moonlight, low enough so that the piercing white of the stars reached his eyes as he sat cross-legged at the edge of the fire.

"Hear ye, hear ye, all those gathered here today," Thomas said in a low, mocking voice.

"Spare us the games," Lord Baldwin said.

Thomas raised his eyebrows, not caring that the effect would be lost in the darkness. "Such a foul disposition. Does your stomach ail you already?"

"We shared the same food," Lord Baldwin said. "Ask questions of your own stomach."

"Tsk, tsk," Thomas countered. "Must I remind you that it is not tonight's meal which should concern you, but rather the honey you ate earlier?"

Thomas grinned to remember the shock on Lord Baldwin's face as he had unbound him in the presence of Sir William and Katherine. The man had been as helpless as a baby sheep during his convulsions after the poisoned honey, and had been easy to bind and leave in the shade of the rocks until Thomas' return with the other two.

"If it is not these actions for which I will despise you," Katherine said to break a silence that had lasted since leaving Jericho, "then it will be for the taunting manner in which you treat us."

"Your feelings concern me little," Thomas said, now deadly serious. "And if you prefer rage to mockery, you shall have your wish. You and Sir William travel with assassins who tried to take my life. Lord Baldwin tells me he is my father and accuses you of being Druids, yet keeps from me his aquaintance of the two of you. Whom shall I trust? And why should your deceptions *not* fill me with anger?"

Thomas continued to speak, his voice now quiet and cold. "Merlins and Druids. Druids and Merlins. For too long now, I have been subjected to the whims of either side. For too long now, I have been uncertain of the identity of the people who so mysteriously appear and disappear in my life. That changed, however, in Jericho, and for that I owe much thanks to Lord Baldwin."

Lord Baldwin croaked from his side of the fire.

"Surprise? Or twinges of convulsions?"

The croak became a groan.

Thomas stood quickly, moved to the donkey and returned with a wineskin.

"Drink," he ordered Lord Baldwin. "Three large gulps. No more. No less."

The knight hesitated.

"Don't be a fool," Thomas said. "If I wished you dead, I would have killed you earlier."

Lord Baldwin did as directed. Thomas took back the wineskin.

"Good," Thomas said. "Your stomach shall settle shortly."

Thomas patted the wineskin. "I expect Sir William and Katherine will be in need of this as well."

"You are vile," Katherine said tonelessly.

"The pot calls the kettle black," Thomas replied, with equal lack of heat. "And I have a story to tell."

Thomas settled again at the fire, and then gestured at Lord Baldwin. "This man had spent every night of our travels in sound sleep. Until Jericho. Then, while he assumed I slept, he crept out. I followed. Much to my surprise, he reached an inn at the center of the town. I dared not remain too close, and it wasn't until he left your room that I was able to slip over myself and peer through the keyhole. Much to my surprise, I discovered he had visited a certain knight and woman who had once held my trust."

Thomas paused. "There was something unnatural in the manner of which those in the room were asleep. As if they had fallen suddenly. So I entered the room and discovered further that they had been cast into a spell of sleep, I assumed by potion, a potion easily concocted with Merlin—or Druid—knowledge."

Katherine sat straighter, a sudden movement that caught Thomas' eye.

He smiled inside. *Perhaps she does remember the long kiss I could not resist as I gazed at the perfect curves of her face in the candlelight. Perhaps I didn't imagine her eyes opening for a startled moment during that kiss.*

Thomas did not let that memory interrupt his story. "I could only conclude one thing. Whichever side each claimed—and you have both claimed to be Merlins—one was Druid. For why else would Lord Baldwin do such a thing unless he opposed you? My question, then, became simple. Who is Druid? Who is Merlin?"

Katherine groaned and clutched her stomach.

Thomas stood and offered her the wineskin. "Three gulps," he repeated. "No more. No less."

She accepted the wineskin quickly. Thomas waited until she finished, then took the wineskin.

Before he sat, he offered the skin to Sir William. The offer was declined, and Thomas sat to resume the one-sided conversation.

"Who is Merlin?" he repeated. "A simple question which presented me a difficult problem. For lies are too simple, and I have been deceived again and again."

He tapped his chin, as if thinking through the problem for the first time. "It took many hours; but, armed with the knowledge of my own training, I found a solution."

"Poison," Sir William said. His voice was strained.

Thomas brought him the wineskin as confirmation, and waited while Sir William drank.

"Yes," Thomas said, when the knight finished. "Poison. There are many known to the Merlins and Druids. Some brutally fast. Some slow. And, as you know, there are many potions to counter these posions."

Thomas smiled. "This one poison has proven to be the perfect answer. The convulsions strike once or twice a day and will worsen as death approaches. Unless the countering potion is taken."

Thomas stopped and drank from the wineskin. "As Katherine and Sir William know, I too shared that same poison. For two reasons. You need not suspect the countering potion if I drink it. And you will realize how important this countering potion is to your survival. For if we all need it, we will all stay together. One side—" Thomas pointed at Lord Baldwin, then shifted his finger to point at Sir William and Katherine "—must guard me from the other. For if I die, so do all of you."

"How so?" Katherine challenged. "With you dead, we can merely share the potion."

"And when it runs out?" Thomas asked. "How will you replace it? For the dozens of combinations of poison, there are dozens of countering potions. You will not live long enough to seek the ingredients."

Thomas held the wineskin high. "No, you will all guard me against the others. And you will all stay with me, for I shall continue to supply you with life."

Lord Baldwin snorted. "Thomas, my son, to what purpose must we remain with these two traitors?"

Thomas' face softened. "Would that I could believe you were my father."

Yet his heart urged him in the opposite direction. *If he is my father and a Merlin, then Katherine is a Druid. Can I bear that pain much longer?*

Thomas took a moment to gather new thoughts. "From Lord Baldwin's pouch I have taken the letter from Hawkwood," he said. "It speaks of a great treasure. Together, we shall find it. In so doing, we ensure that the true Merlins possess it."

"The letter," Lord Baldwin croaked. "Is it not proof that I am Merlin?"

"It has not your name in it, nor William's nor Katherine's. That you possess it says nothing."

"Then how will you know which of us is Merlin?" Katherine asked softly. "For I will tell you now that Lord Baldwin is the traitor, but you have no reason to believe."

"Believe me," Thomas promised, "I shall know. And when I withhold the antidote, the final convulsions of death from the poison shall be punishment enough for the traitor."

They approached Jerusalem shortly after dawn. For two hours they had moved along the road in the pale light that preceded sunrise.

When the sun rose high enough to cast long shadows in front of them, Thomas began to feel an inexplicable mixture of joy and dread. For these mountains and hills were as strangely familiar as the house of his boyhood in St. Jean d'Acre.

As the clouds began to break in the growing heat of the sun, Thomas found himself living the dream which had haunted him night after night, since it had first appeared during his sleep on the plains of Jezreel.

As in his dream, the hills were shrouded in gray mist.

The donkeys plodded ahead, but Thomas was scarcely aware, so riveted was he upon the view. And he wondered if indeed he were asleep and this a dream. *"The mist swirled, then cleared and rays of sunshine broke through from behind, sunshine that lit an entire city across the valley, so that the beams of light danced golden and silver on the curved towers tall above whitened square houses that spread in all directions along the plateau of the mountain."*

He rubbed his eyes and when he opened them, the city walls were still there, the beams of light dancing golden and silver on the curved towers tall above whitened houses that spread in all directions along the plateau of the mountain.

Thomas half expected, as in his dreams, that from the walls might come a dark figure, small with distance. It was early in the day, however, and no other travelers shared the road that wound down into the valley ahead of them and then up the other side to the city fortress that was Jerusalem.

Thomas felt a peace to behold the Holy City, an almost mystical wave of joy and love that sometimes filled him during prayers, a peace in the presence of One so great He had created the world.

With this peace came the fear of the dream. All Thomas need do, even in the brightness of the early morning sun, was close his eyes to see the figure and its gray face, and with that vision to feel again the trembling panic.

"Thomas, my son," he heard the figure call in his mind. Almost against his will he closed his eyes and trusted the donkey to take him forward. The wrinkles of the dark cloth folded around the figure. But still, the face was featureless and gray.

"Thomas, my son," the stranger called again. *"Are you a Merlin?"*

Thomas jerked his eyes open, straining to whisper the word "Father," and was sudddenly grateful that he was in the lead, that neither Lord Baldwin nor the others could see his discomfort.

Thomas tried to forget the end of the dream, because the donkeys were already beginning to descend into the valley at Jerusalem's feet. But the ending of his dream was there, and he could not lose it.

The figure who claimed to be his father was transformed into a dragon; yet, before Thomas could scream, the dragon became Sir William, swirling out of sudden mists with a sword upraised.

Thomas grabbed the tender skin on the inside of his arm and pinched as hard as he could. Anything to distract his thoughts.

Behind him rode Lord Baldwin and Sir William and Katherine. Ahead, the Holy City. And, if he was wrong in his desperate plan, his death.

The donkeys plodded forward.

"It has been no easy task," Thomas said, "to find scholars with knowledge of a Jewish rebellion which occurred a thousand years ago. Not when I am forced to slink from street to street with my face hidden lest my light skin give away my identity among the Mamelukes."

As Thomas shifted the weight of a small sack from one hand to the other, he did not tell his listeners of the wonder he felt to walk the same narrow streets that thirteen hundred years earlier held a procession of people who followed and ridiculed a lone Man before His death upon a cross on the hill of Calvary. Thomas did not tell his listeners of the noises and smells and sights of this fascinating city that made it a pleasure to roam in his search.

His listeners were in no mood to appreciate any descriptions, something reinforced by Lord Baldwin's next words.

"Two days in this cramped hovel, as we wait for you to return with food. Two days of wondering whether Mameluke soldiers will burst through the doors. Two days of watching the traitors opposite me, to ensure that all of us live. I have little patience for *your* difficulties. Especially because I ache to help you, to prove to you I should be trusted."

Sir William sighed with weariness. "Lord Baldwin, it is no different for us."

Thomas surveyed the room. All three did look exhausted. Dark rings under Katherine's eyes showed the strain on her. *Yet they do not diminish the beauty that shines from within.*

Thomas closed his eyes against the thought. *I cannot believe in her,* he told himself. *I cannot let my own heart betray me.*

"How long must this game continue?" Katherine asked. "It is to the point that I almost wish death would take me away from the nightly convulsions brought upon me by the poison."

Thomas shifted the sack again to the other hand.

"Did you not hear me?" Thomas asked. "I said it *has been* no easy task. Now it is completed. I have secured a map and," he held up his sack, "provisions from the market, which will let us begin the last part of our journey.

"Please begin to prepare. In a short time, I shall be ready, and I wish to leave without delay."

He did not wait for their reply, but went through the curtain which served as a door to the other room There he moved to the rough, wooden table where he removed the provisions from the sack. There were several dried roots, a handful of seeds, a vial of dark liquid, and a small clay bottle containing a fine, white powder.

Was there a movement at the doorway? Thomas glanced up quickly, but saw nothing. He began to shred the roots with a small knife, then froze at a startled scream cut short in the other room.

Before he could move, the curtain parted, and Sir William stepped through.

"You have no permission to enter," Thomas thundered.

Sir William stepped aside as Katherine half stumbled through the curtain.

"Nor you—"

Thomas stopped as he noticed the reason for Katherine's clumsy movement. A knife was held against her throat. And Lord Baldwin was pushing her forward.

"Do you wish her dead?" Lord Baldwin asked softly from behind her. His wolfish smile, which had been hidden for so many days, glinted again in triumph.

"No," Thomas said without hesitation.

"Then set your parchment map to the caves on the table."

Thomas reached into his clothing and pulled out a small roll of parchment. He placed it on the table beside the roots.

"You had impressed me," Lord Baldwin said in a conversational tone. His voice hardened immediately. "William, if you make another movement, this knife slashes her throat."

Sir William froze.

"Excellent," said Lord Baldwin. "Now stand beside Thomas. That way I can see you both."

Sir William joined Thomas at the table.

Lord Baldwin kept his left arm wrapped around Katherine. His right hand, which held the knife sharp against her throat, was steady.

He resumed his conversation.

"Yes, Thomas, you had impressed me greatly . . . until your stupidity now." Lord Baldwin studied for several minutes the various items on the table. When he was satisfied he had identified each, he nodded. "What else would you bring back from the market but more of the necessities of a countering potion? Especially if we are about to embark on our journey again."

Thomas bowed his head. "Please forgive me, Sir William. I had not expected this. It would have only taken a moment to prepare this, but now . . ."

Lord Baldwin laughed. "But now I will know the ingredients. I have no reason to remain among you."

Lord Baldwin tightened his grasp on Katherine and nicked her throat. Two drops of blood trickled downward.

"Finish your task, Thomas," Lord Baldwin snarled. "Do not delay."

Within minutes, Thomas completed mixing the ingredients.

"Pour it back into the wineskin."

Thomas did so.

"Excellent." Lord Baldwin thought for several seconds. "My choice would be that you die by the sword. My sword. But once I release Katherine, I cannot be sure of the results of battle. Not against two."

He thought for several more seconds. "Thomas, take the leather strips with which you bound me on the road from Jericho and tie William's hands behind his back."

The task lasted several minutes.

"Now, Thomas," Lord Baldwin said, "take the remaining leather strips, place them in your hands behind your back, and walk backward until you reach Katherine. She will bind your hands. At the slightest movement of threat from you, her throat will be cut."

The new task took slightly longer, for Katherine could not move quickly with the knife exerting pressure against her neck. When she had finished, Lord Baldwin reached forward and slid Thomas' sword from his sheath.

"Again, excellent," Lord Baldwin said. He pushed Thomas forward with a rude kick. "Securely bound, I can kill you at my leisure."

"No," Katherine said.

"No?" Lord Baldwin asked. He released Katherine and stepped back, sword at the ready. "You make demands on me?"

"An offer," Katherine replied. "Their lives for my assistance."

Lord Baldwin snorted. "Your assistance? You are Merlin. I am Druid."

"As you travel," Katherine said, "it will be valuable to have a companion. I hardly dare kill you, not when you have the countering potion."

Lord Baldwin examined her and smiled. "A traveling companion . . . I like it." He stopped stroking his chin. "And if I refuse your offer and kill them, but take you anyway?"

"I will fight you to my death," Katherine promised.

Lord Baldwin began to stroke his chin again.

"I will accept," he said. "But only because it gives me greater pleasure to think of these two facing a slower death from poison. For who is there to release them once you and I depart?"

"Well, my friend," Sir William said in the silence that followed the departure of Lord Baldwin and Katherine, "death is not a pleasant prospect at any time. Yet I shall seek consolation in knowing you and I share the same fight."

Thomas sighed. "The actions of Lord Baldwin prove that we do share the same fight. I am baffled, however. The assassins of St. Jean d'Acre. They traveled with you to Nazareth."

"Please forgive me," Sir William said. He explained to Thomas the reasons for their actions.

Then Sir William asked in casual tones, "How long before we die?"

Thomas smiled at the knight. "Ask that question of God. Only He knows the time of a man's passing."

Sir William did not return the smile. "A poor jest, Thomas. God did not make me drink poison."

"Nor did I," Thomas replied. "And it is difficult to resist the temptation to threaten you with death to learn my father's name."

"Merely *threaten* me with death? But the poison we drank! The nightly convulsions!"

"You may recall the predicament I faced in Jericho. Were you and Katherine Merlins? Or was it Lord Baldwin? One side claimed to be my father, yet met with you in secret. The other side—you—had threatened me with assassins, yet had also been pursued in England by Druids. I knew I had to find a way for the Druid to be revealed."

"Yes, yes," Sir William said between grunts, as he too tested his bonds.

"I devised a test," Thomas said, "knowing that any Druid would gladly abandon a Merlin to die. As you can see, my logic has proven to be correct. For Lord Baldwin took the first opportunity given him. It was not stupidity, as he so quickly assumed, that led me to announce I had returned from the market. Rather, it was bait. Bait, I might add, upon which he pounced."

Sir William shook his head. "He could easily have killed us."

"I was desperate," Thomas replied. "And had he raised the sword, I would have announced that he still needed us alive."

"My head spins, Thomas. What could he need from us? He has Hawkwood's letter and book. He has the parchment maps to the cave. He has the countering potion."

Thomas smiled. "There was no poison. Each evening meal you ingested a small amount of the juice squeezed from an insane root. Only enough to upset the stomach for ten minutes. The convulsions would have stopped whether or not you received the countering potion, which, of course, was no countering potion, but merely sweetened wine and water."

"You ate the same food we did," Sir William argued. "And *we* prepared it."

Thomas winked at the knight. "Who was it who delivered the plates for each meal? Plates—except mine—smeared with tiny drops of poison."

The knight laughed. "Well done!" Then Sir William caught his breath. "But you said we held something of importance that would have stayed Lord Baldwin's sword from our throats."

"The map to the caves," Thomas said. "Knowing I wanted the Druid to take my bait, do you think I would also give him the map?"

Another laugh from Sir William. "The parchment he took is useless?"

Thomas nodded. He waited until Sir William finished laughing. "There is more," Thomas said.

Sir William echoed, "More?"

"Yes. I expect we will be free in minutes."

"Impossible. I have given thought to our release and know it will be difficult. Glad as I am we won't die from poison, it will take hours while I use my teeth on the knots of your bonds."

"That too had been the method I thought we must use. But since Katherine departed with Lord Baldwin, our task will be much less difficult."

"Less?" Sir William strained against his bonds. "I am forced to disagree. Once we free ourselves, we must begin immediate pursuit to rescue Katherine."

Thomas began to whistle the tune of a childhood rhyme. "What is it?" Sir William demanded. "What other knowledge have you kept from me?"

Thomas continued to whistle.

"Thomas!"

"My father's identity?"

"I have sworn the secret."

Thomas resumed whistling.

"If my hands were free . . ." Sir William threatened.

"If they were free . . ." a new voice came through the doorway.

"Katherine!" Sir William blurted.

She stepped through the curtain of the doorway. She smiled at Sir William, but only for a moment, for her gaze turned almost immediately to Thomas. He stared back, hardly daring to let his face show the joy that consumed him.

Without breaking her gaze, she stepped forward and leaned over, as if to cut the bonds on Thomas' wrists with the small knife in her hand.

But she did not use the knife. Instead, she kissed him. Lightly at first as she stood leaning over him. Then she fell to her knees, dropped the knife, and held his face in both hands and kissed him again, longer this time.

How long?

Thomas did not know, for his eyes were closed and his mind was filled with her touch and scent and the feeling of her hands on his face.

Discreet coughing finally reached his ears.

Sir William coughed louder.

Katherine released Thomas, but only drew her face back several inches.

"Thank you, Thomas," she whispered. She kissed him lightly again on the tip of his nose. "Thank you, my love."

Thomas could only grin like a dancing fool. When he found his voice, he asked, "Where did Lord Baldwin fall?"

"Thomas!" Sir William's voice was a begging groan. "What has transpired?"

Katherine picked up the knife and, still on her knees, began to saw at the bonds around Thomas' wrist.

"I can explain," she said. "Lord Baldwin drank the countering potion as we began to find our donkeys. Before he could offer it to me, he fell backward, holding his stomach in agony."

"Yes, Sir William," Thomas finished for her. "My final weapon. From the market I brought back not the ingredients for a countering potion, but a vile poison."

"Your test, then, could hardly have worked more perfectly."

Before Thomas could modestly agree, Katherine interrupted. "Not so," she said to the knight, "for when Lord Baldwin fell to the poison, he rolled in such agony that he drew the attention of many passersby."

Thomas and Sir William frowned.

"Among those passersby were Mameluke soldiers," Katherine said. "They now search the city for us."

It did not seem real, the stillness of the morning air and the pastel contrasts of ancient stone buildings against olive green and brown mountains, all framed by pale blue sky. It did not seem real, the background of babble on the streets beneath the gentle warmth of the sun. And it did not seem real, to be slowly and calmly walking among the people on the streets while soldiers hunted this quarter of Jerusalem from house to house, soldiers determined to capture and crucify them.

Thomas wondered if the pounding of his heart might give him and the others away.

Crucifixion.

Could any death be more horrible? A wooden pole would first be placed into the ground, and a crosspiece fixed near the top to form a cross. Then, if they were fortunate, their arms would be roped to the crosspiece, not nailed. Should the Mameluke soldiers in pursuit choose to be merciful, the three would die quickly of suffocation, because the weight of their bodies would shut off their air passages. But should it be deemed that their agony be prolonged, the soldiers would nail their arms and feet into the wood, thus providing support for the body and making suffocation impossible. Death would occur much more slowly, from shock or dehydration or exhaustion.

Shouts of soldiers broke above the babble of the streets as they swept from house to house. *How far behind are the soldiers? And how far ahead are the gates?*

Thomas dared not lift his head to check their progress. His gray-blue eyes and fair skin would be too obvious to any

onlookers, for it had been over a hundred years since crusader knights had held the Holy City. Now, the infidel Muslim conquerors ruled, and Thomas needed to keep his face
hidden by the cloth which was draped over his head and
neck as protection against the sun.

The other two, Katherine and Sir William, walked in wide
separation and far in front. To remain in a group of three
would instantly give their presence away to any sharp-eyed
soldier.

More shouts and angry arguments, as more houses were
searched.

For a moment, Thomas let his mind wander as he again
imagined how a rabbit might feel, crouched and barely hidden among the grass with a hawk circling overhead. Any
sudden movement would draw the hawk's attention, just as
surely as anything but a pretended calm would draw the
soldiers. Yet Thomas could understand why a rabbit might
bolt under the strain of waiting beneath a hawk, even
knowing that to bolt meant certain death. It took great
effort to force himself to walk slowly, when every nerve
shrieked at him to run.

The stakes were enormous.

A terrible death through crucifixion mattered little in
comparison to the scrolled map Katherine held in her travel
pouch. He and the knight were to fight to the death, should
they be discovered. And she was to escape while they
fought. For without the scroll, a much greater battle, thousands of miles away, would be lost with cold certainty.

So much depends on escape from this city. . . .

Thomas bit his tongue to keep those thoughts away. He
could not let fear paralyze him. Instead, he directed his
mind to the events which had led to this day, any thoughts
at all, except of the soldiers in pursuit.

How long since I was exiled from England? Already half a
year. The great sweeping valleys of Magnus, a lush green
with the scattered purple patches of heather, and shrouded
with mist in the winter, were an aching memory.

He had survived a cutthroat ship's crew, and a bandit-
infested trek through the Holy Land. He had survived be-

trayals and lies; and now finally, just as he had established that he could trust the two with him, the soldiers were in pursuit. Thomas shook his head.

Walk slowly and think not of the soldiers.

So he thought of Katherine . . . of the moment she had first lifted her face to his in silvery moonlight, and how his heart had caught as if they had been long pledged for the moment, and how later, in the Holy Land the mystery of that yearning had been explained. He thought of their first fleeting kiss, one of anger and frustration at desires neither could understand or trust. He thought of how candlelight touched her blond hair, the curves of her face in the shadows of that candlelight, her half-hinted smile of inner joy and the beauty of depth of character, the slow and measured way she would gaze deeply into his eyes. If he were to lose her now, after all they had been through . . .

Walk slowly and think not of the soldiers.

Activity on the narrow twisting streets still seemed normal, a small piece of good fortune for Thomas. Obviously the people of Jerusalem were accustomed to the sight of running soldiers, for despite the shouts that carried from street to street, the bartering and selling at market booths continued.

Thomas felt a tug on the edge of his cape.

"Alms for the poor?"

He looked down into raisin-black eyes. A boy, maybe six years old.

The boy's eyes widened as he noticed Thomas' coloring. His mouth opened as he drew breath to speak his surprise.

"Alms you will have, my friend," Thomas said quickly to forestall any exclamation. "But you must grasp my hand!"

The command intrigued the boy enough that he did so and remained silent.

"Your name?" Thomas asked, his head still low as he looked at the beggar.

"Addon. I am seven."

A memory stabbed at Thomas, that of someone barely older than this boy. Tiny John, a pickpocket rascal as mischievous and cheerful as a sparrow, who might have already perished in England.

Thomas blocked the memory and concentrated on walking slowly, holding the boy's hand as naturally as if they were brothers. For if the boy bolted now and spread the word of a pale-skinned stranger...

"Addon, as you observed, I am a traveler, now confused and lost in this great city of yours. It will be worth a piece of gold if you guide me to the nearest city gates."

The boy grinned. "Essenes Gate! For a piece of gold."

Essenes Gate. As Thomas well knew, it was guarded by only one tower. Less than five minutes away. However, if a piece of gold and a feeling of self-importance kept this child silent until they had left the city walls...

"After the gates, where shall I take you?" the boy was asking.

"That shall suffice." Thomas smiled. This young guide wished to earn even more. "For then I depart."

Addon frowned. "Did you not know that is impossible?"

"Impossible?"

A quick nod from the young beggar. "The Mameluke soldiers have shut all the city gates. They guard them now."

"Addon, this is indeed your blessed day," Thomas said as slowly and calmly as possible. He could not afford to alarm the boy or raise his suspicions. "For you shall earn enough gold to feed you for a month."

Addon grinned happiness, his teeth a crescent of white against dark skin.

"There is a man ahead of me," Thomas continued in low tones. "See him yonder?"

Thomas pointed at Sir William until Addon nodded.

"Approach him and tell him the same news you gave me. Tell him I shall wait here for his return."

Addon scampered ahead.

Thomas waited in the shadow of a doorway and watched Sir William's head bend as he listened to Addon, then watched with relief as the knight turned back. To any other but Thomas, it would have been impossible to notice that the knight spoke to a veiled woman as he passed her upon his return, for he did not pause and his lips barely moved. Yet, moments after the knight passed her, Katherine stopped where she was, then began to shuffle, to wait near a stand where a vendor shouted the sale of melons.

"Thomas," the knight said softly when he reached the doorway, "news of the gates does not bode well for us."

Thomas drew deeper in the shadows. "The Mamelukes must know not only of our presence, but of the scroll and the Cave of Letters. Why else go to such measures to find us?"

Sir William's lips tightened in anger. "A sword across the throat of the man who betrayed us!"

"Think of *our* throats," Thomas retorted. "The city is sealed. Yet we cannot keep our faces hidden forever. It will be too difficult to remain unnoticed inside."

Sir William closed his eyes in thought. Moments later, he smiled. "Have you a thirst for spring water?"

"Water? We fight for our lives and—"

"Thomas, tell me of Jerusalem's history."

"There are soldiers all around! This is no place for—"

"Come, come," Sir William chided with a grin. "Surely as a Merlin you would have a glimmer of this knowledge."

Thomas snorted. "The city is as ancient as man. Its history would take hours to recite."

"Tell me, then," the knight said with a grin, "of King David."

Despite the danger he felt pressing upon them, Thomas grinned in return. How many peaceful hours of his childhood he had spent in the same tests and discussions.

"King David?" Thomas squinted his eyes shut in thought. "King David. He chose this as his capital because it sat squarely between Israel in the north and Judah in the south. Yet until David, the city had never been conquered, for it held a spring and no siege could bring it down."

"Yes," Sir William said. "The spring. Gihon Spring."

Gihon Spring. Then Thomas knew. He grinned. "We shall leave Jerusalem the same way it was conquered."

Thomas turned to Addon and spoke. "You must guide us to the inner city."

He did not finish his thoughts. . . . The inner city . . . close to the palace and soldiers' quarters.

The imposing structure of the palace was in the background, and directly ahead was the circular area where three main streets joined. At the center of that large circle, the well. Thomas surveyed the bulwark of bricked stone that surrounded the well and groaned. He could not share his dismay with anyone, because the knight and Katherine had traveled separately the entire journey back into the center of Jerusalem.

"You wish a different well?" Addon asked, in response to the low groan. "Yet there is none more ancient—"

"No," Thomas said, "a better guide we could not have found."

That was truth. For Addon had led them through a maze of narrow and obscure alleyways which made detection by searching soldiers almost impossible. Ironic then, that the first soldiers they had seen were surrounding the well.

Thomas bit back another groan.

A dozen soldiers, all within a stone's throw. More ironic, none were there as guards. Instead, they stood or sat in relaxed enjoyment of the sun and gossip. Around the well were the reasons for the soldiers' presence—the women gathered to draw water.

Their idle conversation reached Thomas. He gnawed his inner lip as he lost himself in thought.

Gihon Spring. Long ago, the shepherd boy named David, who earned a reputation as military genius and united all of Israel, had sent his soldiers up this well shaft to invade and conquer Jerusalem. Was the shaft still clear after these thousands of years?

There was only one means of discovering the answer. They must descend. But the soldiers stood between them and a desperate attempt at escape. Only a distraction could—

Shouts and the braying of donkeys interrupted his thoughts.

Thomas looked to his right in disbelief. Two donkeys plunged frantically through the small market on a nearby sidestreet. They careened through stands of fruits and beneath the awnings which provided shade. One donkey plunged back out again, draped in the blankets from a shop.

Angry shouts rose in response and men chased the donkeys in useless efforts. The soldiers turned to the confusion, at first amused, then concerned. They dashed to chase the donkeys.

"The well, my friend," came a voice from the other side of Thomas. "How long until the soldiers return?"

Thomas turned his head to look into Sir William's grin. Katherine was already halfway across the street to the well.

"How—"

"Misfortune, of course. Who could guess that a rag tied to a donkey's tail might brush against a lamp's flame?"

"Who indeed?" Thomas grinned in return.

The hubbub from the street grew. The smash of glass and roars of rage rose above the clamor.

"Addon," Thomas said. "Two gold pieces for your trouble."

Thomas began to search for words to dismiss the young boy but had no chance to speak. Addon was already backing away, his fingers firmly clasped over the gold.

"The market," Addon blurted. "In this confusion, I can fill my pockets!"

Thomas decided it was not the moment to point out that there was no honor in theft. He sprinted to join Katherine and Sir William at the edge of the well.

Thomas squeezed his eyes shut and concentrated on small mercies. With the deep unknown below, he at least worried less about the soldiers.

A heavy rope was attached to a pole at the side of the well. The rope hung at the side of the well and disappeared into the black hole; thousands of years of friction of rope against stone had worn the edges of the well smooth. The well itself was wide—toe to outstretched fingertips, Thomas could not have reached across.

"If the well does not lead to safety?" Thomas asked.

"What choice?" Sir William countered. "Gates sealed, city walls guarded, and, in all probability, a reward offered for our heads. We cannot hide among these people."

Katherine said nothing. She hastily tore the veil from her face and put it in a compartment of her cloak. She smiled once at Thomas, then without hesitation took the rope in her hands and lowered herself over the edge.

"What choice? Her action is answer enough," Thomas said. He too wrapped his fingers around the rough hemp of the rope and rolled over the edge. Sir William waited until Thomas had disappeared into the darkness, then followed.

Despite their conversation, less than a minute had passed from the time of reaching the well to when all three were clinging to the rope and lowering themselves hand over hand. No commands or soldiers' shouts reached them—no one had seen them escape.

Thomas breathed a prayer of gratitude. They were now safe from detection. He prayed they would survive the descent, and that the shaft did indeed lead outside the city walls.

For the first ten feet of the descent, they found themselves pushing away from the sides of the well. Then, without warning, the walls seemed to fall away, and it wasn't until Thomas had lowered himself another ten feet that he understood. Looking upward against the light of the sky as backdrop, he saw that the well shaft actually widened as it deepened.

The sight gave him a prickle of hope. Would not a city as ancient as this slowly build over the well through the centuries? Did this widening of the shaft not mean that perhaps there would be room to stand around the pool at its bottom?

It gave him enough hope to ignore the burning in the muscles of his lower arms.

"Thomas!"

"Yes, Sir William," he grunted. It took great effort to breathe normally, let alone speak.

"At the side of this wall. Rungs!"

Thomas grinned relief. The knight had spoken truly. A ladder of horizontal iron bars was imbedded into the stone walls of the shaft. At one time, this well had been meant for more than rope and bucket.

The rope began to swing.

"Katherine!" Thomas yelped. "This is no time for play!"

"If we . . . reach the . . . rungs," she said, "no person above . . . who seeks to . . . draw water . . . will pull against . . . our weight."

It felt dangerous, to be swaying at this dizzying speed an unknown distance from the bottom, but Thomas knew Katherine's logic was correct.

They began to sway in unison.

Moments later, Sir William managed to grasp a rung. He steadied the rope for Thomas and Katherine. Then Sir William yanked hard to test the iron bar. It did not move.

"Dare we hope this fortune holds?" he asked. He did not wait for a reply, but released the rope.

Katherine had reached a lower rung. She too relinquished the rope and began to climb downward.

With Sir William's feet about to step onto Thomas' head, there was no choice. Thomas took the rung in front of him and began to feel below for another that would hold the weight of his feet.

It took less than five minutes to reach the ground, which was a small beach circling the pool of water. And after that, through a cool and dank passageway so low they had to walk bent forward like waddling geese, it took another five minutes to reach a pile of rubble which blocked further movement. Yet from the first moment inside the passage that led away from the wide pool at the bottom of the well shaft, Thomas knew it was the most joyful walk he had ever taken. Step by cramped step, he felt like singing because of the distant white light that grew brighter as they approached. Sunlight, sunlight, and the sound of birds.

They stopped at the rubble that blocked them.

Thomas fell forward and kissed the rocks, which brought forth laughter from Katherine. Sir William caught his enthusiasm and clenched his fist in a victory salute.

"The gamble reaped great profit!" Thomas said when he stood again. "I'll not mind shredding my hands to clear these rocks, for outside are the hills and mountains."

Thomas went to the top of the pile of rubble and threw some rocks backward. The opening increased slightly.

"No, it's—"

"Not another—"

Sir William and Katherine stopped themselves, for they had begun to berate Thomas in the same breath.

The result was the same. Thomas stopped.

Sir William bowed gravely. "After you, milady," he said.

Katherine smiled. Thomas knew he would never tire of watching that gentle smile.

"I was about to say," Katherine began, "No, it's time I received an explanation."

"Explanation?" Thomas asked.

She nodded. "We were about to leave the city until Sir William turned back and whispered for me to follow. Then he lit the tails of those donkeys and told me to descend the well. I thought you had both taken leave of your senses."

"Yet you descended," Thomas marveled.

She turned grave eyes upon him. "What is trust untried? Sir William I have always trusted. And only now, in Jerusalem, have I pledged trust to you. With trust, there is acceptance. So I obeyed."

She spread her hands. "But now . . ."

"Gihon Spring," Thomas explained. "Sir William reminded me of another battle fought in Jerusalem. King David himself, those hundreds upon hundreds of years ago, won this city by sending men up the shaft of the Gihon Spring."

"You did not know for certain the passage still remained?" Katherine said.

"No, but we had little choice. And we were led to the most ancient well in Jerusalem."

Katherine nodded slow agreement, then reached upward for Thomas to help her to the top of the pile of rubble.

"Not another stone, please," Sir William said. "That is what *I* had been about to say."

"We cannot remain here," Thomas said.

"Of course not. Yet why should we expose ourselves in the light of day to flee in the heat? Tonight, while the city sleeps, we will depart. By morning, we will be far enough away to purchase horses, perhaps in Bethlehem."

Sir William turned his hands so that his palms were face up. "Feel this air. Cool and comfortable. We can rest here in safety and sleep until nightfall." He flashed a grin from a dirt-smudged face. "The treasure we seek has lain undiscovered for centuries. One day more matters little, does it not?"

Chapter Fifty-Six

By midnight, they had cleared away enough rubble to escape. Behind them, the eastern city walls. Outlined against the moonlight were the silhouettes of sentry soldiers atop those walls. Although the soldiers were barely in crossbow range, Thomas and Katherine and Sir William stayed low and crept from tree to tree as they moved directly away from the city. The moonlight was casting shadows, and detection of their presence was too much of a possibility.

Thomas hardly dared whisper until long after they had straightened and begun to walk in long, rapid strides.

"Water?" he croaked.

"None," Sir William replied. "And I share your thirst. It seems that we moved a mountain!"

They were now among a grove of olive trees, widely spaced in the dry soil. The leaves glittered silver in the moonlight, and the hills beyond were solid black against the sky and stars and scattered ghostly clouds.

"Thirst . . ." Katherine said. "I would give a king's ransom to dive into a pool. Does the scroll I carry have locations of springs nearby?"

Thomas pictured in his mind the maps he had pored over with scholars in Jerusalem. "We must turn south," he finally said, "cross the plains, and then travel to the hills of Bethlehem. That will be our nearest water. It is a journey that will last until dawn."

"Horses too we shall seek there," Sir William said. "Until now, we have ridden donkeys. While it would be prudent to continue to appear as common travelers, we must cast caution aside. Speed is of the utmost importance."

"Yet horses tire more easily," Katherine countered. "Speed matters little if it cannot be sustained under pursuit."

A slight breeze swirled, so that the shadows of the trees swayed and bounced patterns of dancers across the hard-packed ground.

"Gold is one thing we do have," Thomas mused. "Could we not purchase three or four horses each, so that when one becomes tired of the weight of its rider, we saddle a fresh one?"

Sir William clapped Thomas on his right shoulder. "Superb, my friend. We could be on a ship for England within the month."

And then? Thomas smiled at the knight in return, but already was lost in thoughts. What might happen in England? There were only the three of them.

But no . . . There is a fourth.

Sir William had yet to tell him of his father. They had hours of travel ahead, travel in the isolation of night. Thomas would be glad to fill those hours with conversation. And with questions.

They slipped among the shadows, using the receding outline of the city of Jerusalem high upon its hill to gain their bearings as they moved south. Thomas waited several minutes, then spoke again.

"Sir William, yesterday, you informed me of a self-evident truth. Lord Baldwin is not my father."

"Lord Baldwin." Sir William spat. "He hid among the Merlins for years, claiming to be one of us. Were it not for your test, we might never have known."

Katherine slipped beside Thomas as they walked. Without speaking, she took his hand and intertwined her fingers among his. The simplicity of her gesture, a quiet gift of love as they descended as fugitives through the hillside fields, touched him so deeply that his throat tightened. He did not trust himself to speak.

Sir William continued. "Thomas, you have solved one mystery. Lord Baldwin—the traitor among us—and Waleran were responsible for the fall of Magnus before your birth, the fall that sent all of us into exile here in the Holy Land."

Thomas nodded. Katherine squeezed his hand, a slight pressure of her awareness of how she affected him.

"But my father . . ." Thomas finally found his voice. "Who is my father, if not Lord Baldwin?"

"What was that!" Sir William said sharply.

"Who is my—"

"No. I thought I heard movement."

They froze. Thomas and Sir William placed their right hands upon the hilts of their swords, instantly ready to fight. Yet only shadows sifted and teased their eyes, only the sigh of the breeze greeted them.

Sir William relaxed and began to walk forward again.

This time, Thomas sought Katherine's hand.

"Who is your father?" Sir William asked. "Tell me first what you know of your childhood and the Merlins, then I shall reveal what of the rest he has permitted me."

"I am a Merlin," Thomas said. Quiet satisfaction filled his voice to call himself such. "I was raised as an orphan in an obscure monastery, near the kingdom of Magnus, which once belonged to us. The nurse who trained me, Sarah, I now know was my mother. She taught me the ways of Merlins, the use of logic and knowledge to fight our battles against the Druids."

"Yes," Katherine whispered. "You *are* a Merlin. For so long we could not trust you. Sarah's death . . ."

"My *mother's* death," Thomas said firmly. "I was not able to know her as such during her life. Please let me have that now."

Katherine lifted his hand and brushed her lips against the back of his fingers in apology.

As Thomas continued, he noted that the knight did not cease in his vigil of the shadows which surrounded them. Their conversation continued as they walked.

"My mother died before I was old enough to be told of Merlins and Druids and their age-old battle," Thomas said. "I set out to conquer Magnus with the knowledge I had been given, unaware of the hidden Druid masters of that castle and kingdom. And, for the last year, I have felt as a pawn between both the Druids and Merlins in their unseen battle."

Sir William stopped. He spun so quickly that his sword banged his leg.

"Thomas, we had no choice."

"I know," Thomas replied, almost weary. "You could not know whether the Druids had discovered me in the monastery and converted me."

"There is more," Katherine said. "More and terrible things. Sir William informed me of what the Druids truly intend, as they expand their power across England."

Sir William began to walk again. Thomas and Katherine followed. "It is a horror that sorrows me to repeat," Sir William said, now moving briskly as if to attempting to dispel anger. His dark shadow seemed to flow across the rocky ground in front of them.

"Thomas, you know full well that the Druids have begun to conquer in the most insidious way possible, by posing as priests of the Holy Grail, by proclaiming false miracles to sway the people."

"Yes," Thomas said. Few memories were closer than of his flight in exile because of the Druid priests.

The knight paused, then said, "Through the sham of false miracles, how long until the priests of the Holy Grail have convinced town after town to abandon one religion for another? How long until the priests of the Roman church are powerless?"

Thomas replied, "If that happens, the entire structure of the country is threatened! The king of England receives his power only because the people believe he rules by the authority of the Roman church and by the authority of God! If the people no longer believe in that authority, all the noblemen and the king will face rebellion!"

"To be replaced by the chosen of the Druid priests," Katherine finished for him. "But there is more at stake."

Now Sir William was clenching his fists, and he walked so quickly that Thomas and Katherine were pressed to stay in stride.

Thomas felt wonder, to see this war-hardened warrior so transformed.

"If the Druids conquer and begin to rule," Sir William

said, "they will bar the people from knowledge, for their own power is derived from ignorance. They will end this slow progress that has been made by the learned men of our country. And times of darkness..." he faltered... "times of darkness will be upon mankind for centuries more."

"This is the cause we fight," Thomas said, filled with joy at understanding the battle, and filled with dread at the enormity of the stakes.

"Yes," Sir William said. "Merlin himself founded Magnus in the age of King Arthur for this cause. An unseen battle has raged between Merlins and Druids for eight centuries, and you hold the final secrets to the battle."

"I?"

"Together, when we return to England, this secret can be unlocked, just as surely as we shall find the treasure shown on the scroll which Katherine carries. With both, we will have the chance to overcome their evil."

"Along with my father?"

Before Sir William could reply, shadows detached themselves from beneath the trees to glide and surround them.

The shadows became men, men with drawn curved swords that gleamed in the moonlight.

"Only fools travel at night," came the hoarse whisper. "Fools who pay for their mistakes with blood."

The knight reacted without hesitation. He withdrew his sword and lashed outward in a single movement so quickly that two men dropped to clutch their arms with shrieks of agony before any other bandit moved in the darkness.

Then, three men swarmed the knight, swords flashing downward in the moonlight.

Sir William danced tight circles. He struck outward with a fury of steel against steel which sent sparks in all directions and, incredibly, managed to press attack against the three.

Thomas, mesmerized by the skill of the knight's swordplay, nearly paid for that fascination with his life. Had the moon been behind a cloud, he would not have caught the glint of movement at his side. But the silver of the moon saved him, and the shine of steel gave him barely enough warning to dodge backward as a great curved sword slashed downward.

The point of that sword ripped through his sleeve, and Thomas spun around, knowing the bandit would strike again.

A vicious horizontal swing. Thomas sucked in his stomach, bending forward to pull his lower body away from the arc of the sword. Again, the swish of fabric as his cloak parted to razored steel.

Another vicious swing. This one less close, for Thomas had adjusted to the rough terrain and moved with the nimbleness of desperation.

Another attacker joined.

Thomas ducked, then sprinted to a tree. He struggled to free his own sword but was hampered by his ripped cloak.

Both attackers stayed in pursuit. Thomas edged around the tree, using it to protect his back as he fought to clear his sword.

Where is Katherine? How many bandits? Is Sir William still alive? Thomas' thoughts scrambled as he did. *We must survive! Duck this sword!*

Thomas felt the pluck of air as the sword whooshed over his head . . . A thud as the sword bit into the olive tree.

The bandit grunted at the impact and yanked at his sword to pull it free. Thomas took the advantage and, while the bandit had both arms extended to grip the sword, he kicked upward with all his strength. His foot buried itself in the softness of the bandit's stomach and sent him retching.

No time to relax!

Another woosh as the second bandit swung across. The sword bounced off the tree.

And still, the clank of sword against swords echoed through the night air. *Sir William is alive. Where is Katherine?*

Thomas stepped away from another slash and fought to clear his own sword.

The distraction was a deadly mistake, for Thomas stumbled.

He recovered with a quick half step, but the off-balance

movement threw his right foot into the arch of a root which curled above the hard ground. He frantically tried to pull free, and a bolt of tearing pain from his ankle forced him to grunt. *Jammed!*

Another frantic pull, despite the pain.

Nothing.

And the curved sword was now raised high. A snarling wolf grin from the bandit as he savored the certain death he was about to inflict upon Thomas.

"Halt!"

Katherine's voice, clear and strong, carried through the trees.

"Halt! Listen to my words!"

The sword above faltered but did not descend. Farther away, the clank of swords ended.

Thomas flicked his eyes away from the upraised sword and glanced at the bandit's face. It mirrored surprise.

A woman's voice has shocked them all into curiosity.

As if proving his guess right, the bandits craned their heads in all directions, trying to locate her voice.

"Here, in the tree," Katherine called. A shifting cloud broke away from the moon, and suddenly her silhouette was easy to see against the light. She stood balanced on a thick branch, far from the ground.

Thomas grinned. Katherine had found safety during the distraction of Sir William's instant attack.

His grin died at her next words.

"I promise you far greater treasure than the mere coins we carry! I carry a scroll which leads to great wealth," Katherine called again. Her voice remained easy to hear above the quickening breeze. To confirm her words, she waved the narrow tube of the rolled parchment.

With the attention so focused on Katherine, Thomas considered making a move for his sword, then decided against it. Katherine had managed to bring a temporary truce. He would trust she had reason to reveal the scroll. Besides, he noted more shadows moving among the trees. There were now at least a dozen, with more joining every minute. Any fight would most surely be lost.

"We are not fools," the bandit who had first spoken replied, as he edged to the tree. "Why should we believe that the scroll leads to treasure?"

"Because we will remain your prisoners until we will lead you to this treasure," Katherine said evenly. "Otherwise, our lives will be payment enough for a lie."

"Yes, I understand," the bandit said. He moved again.

"No!" Katherine said sharply.

"No?" The voice faked hurt surprise.

"No. You will not be able to reach me soon enough to get the scroll," Katherine said. She began to tear the scroll into shreds, an action easy to see in the moonlight. Pieces of the scroll fluttered away with the breeze.

"We carry the knowledge of this treasure in our heads. Now you must let us live."

Long moments of silence followed.

"This is acceptable," the bandit said. "You have made a bargain."

The bandit raised his voice. "Men! Hold your swords!"

Thomas let out a breath that he hadn't realized he'd been holding.

"Yet listen to my words, woman," the bandit finished with silky menace. "Should you not lead us to the treasure, you shall all discover how it feels to die, when your skin is peeled slowly from your bodies."

Chapter Fifty-Seven

"You *do* remember all those marks upon the scroll, don't you?" Katherine whispered to Thomas. "We *shall* find that treasure, shall we not?"

"Or die?" Thomas asked with a wry grin. "Last night, I wanted to dance for joy that you had found a way to save our lives. This morning . . ."

He shrugged to indicate the busy camp around them. Growing sunlight showed evidence of at least twenty men. That shrug brought a wince to his face. Hours earlier, the bandits had savagely bound his hands behind his back with strips of wet leather. Now dry, the leather bit even deeper into his skin.

Katherine interpreted his wince as doubt.

"I had no choice," she said quietly. "Your knowledge was our only hope."

"*Is* our only hope," Thomas corrected her. "And at the very least, you have gained us time—time we did not have last night as the swords clashed."

Thomas did not add that he wondered how much value there was in gained time. Chances of escape seemed impossible. Katherine too was bound, as was Sir William, who sat well guarded on a flat rock on the opposite side of the makeshift camp, which was hidden in a small, dusty fold of the hill. The bandits watched them constantly. Indeed, an hour had passed since the gray of dawn and as all prepared to march, this was the first moment Katherine had been able to speak privately with Thomas.

Thomas observed the bandits carefully, gauging their alertness. All of them were lean and wary, and they moved with fast, certain efficiency as they performed their tasks. *Men who hunted*, Thomas thought. *And who have been hunted. They will not be easy to deceive.*

Their own guard was now returning with a bowl of water. Like most of the others, he had a ragged black beard. A short sword was attached to one side of his belt. A scimitar, that heavy, curved weapon of destruction, was on the other side.

Water slopped over the edge of the bowl as the guard approached. Thomas licked his cracked lips as he watched the water soak into the ground.

The guard stopped in front of the them. Thomas shook his head at the offered bowl.

"The woman first," Thomas said.

The guard stared, then blinked, then grudgingly smiled. "The woman first," he repeated. "She is protected not only by Rashim, but also by one with his hands bound."

Katherine leaned forward to drink from the offered bowl. Since her hands were tied behind her back, she had to rely on the guard to tip the bowl.

Protected by Rashim. The words echoed through Thomas' mind. The leader of the bandits had seen Katherine at dawn's first light and had smiled with evil.

"She is not to be harmed in any way," Rashim had said, his face dark as he stood against the light of the sun. He had stroked his beard and smiled coldly. "Not an angel with this beauty."

There had been no threat in his words, but Thomas shivered every time he remembered the threat in his tone.

And now Rashim paced long, unhurried strides toward them, wearing the long white cloth of a nomad accustomed to endless hours in the heat. The top of his head was covered, and a black band across his forehead held the veils away from his face. His eyes flashed glittering black above a giant hooked nose. The lines around his mouth were etched deep, lines which had long since turned downward from constant snarls.

"This day has already burned long ," Rashim said without preamble. "I have readied my men for travel. At this moment, finally, I will listen to you bargain for your lives."

"Last night—" Katherine began to protest.

"Last night only saved you until morning. Convince me first that the treasure exists; then we depart. If not," Rashim shrugged, "the vultures will feast upon your bones."

He stared at Thomas, trying to cow him with a harsh, unblinking gaze.

Thomas gazed back, forcing his own eyes to hide all thoughts.

"Tell me the story," Rashim commanded.

Thomas began, in a low and calm voice, to explain. "The story begins sixteen hundred years ago—"

"Impossible!" Rashim exploded.

"Sixteen hundred years ago," Thomas continued as if he not been interrupted, "in the land from whence we come, Britain. Before the Romans conquered, Druids ruled the land. They knew secrets of science and astronomy and kept that power through secrecy."

Rashim's eyes narrowed in concentration.

Thomas did not change the levelness of his voice. "When the Romans occupied Britain, the Druid leaders formed a hidden circle within society, a circle with great wealth. Later, a Roman general discovered this Druid circle. The general, Julius Severus, who held command in Britain one hundred years after the death of Christ, did not expose what he knew of the Druids and their accumulated gold. To let Rome know of the Druids would also let Rome know of their wealth and almost magical powers. Instead, Severus plundered the Druids in one fell swoop, taking a great fortune in gold."

Thomas did not add the rest of what he knew, that Julius Severus also managed to find and keep the book of the most valued Druid secrets of potions and deception. A book to stagger the imagination with the power it might yield its owner.

"You have my interest," Rashim admitted. "But the story is centuries old, and in a land halfway across the world." Rashim took a dagger from his belt and with its tip, and as a casual threat, began to pick dirt from beneath his fingernails. "How did such a treasure—as you claim—come to be hidden here?"

"You searched us," Thomas replied. "In my possession you found a small, tightly bound book of parchment."

Rashim nodded, almost impatient for proof of a great treasure.

"That book contains the notes of many who searched through the centuries for clues to the treasure. It is meant to assist any who would hold the scroll which Katherine destroyed last night. Without the scrolled map, this book is useless."

"A book in your possession because . . ."

"That story is long and tedious." Thomas affected a sigh of weariness, hoping Rashim would not press him. It was not the time to reveal the Merlins' age-old battle against Druids. It was not the time to reveal that the small book had contained directions to the monastery in Jerusalem where Thomas had sought for scholars who would help him continue his search.

"Then make me believe that the gold did reach this land," Rashim demanded. The dagger was now clenched in his fist. "Force me to believe that it might still be hidden."

"The Roman general was summoned from Britain to quell a revolt of the Jews, here in the Holy Land. Severus could not trust his treasure to be left behind, so he arranged to take it with him. Once here, he and his Roman soldiers destroyed nearly a thousand Jewish villages, and a half million people were slain. The Jewish rebels were finally defeated in their last refuge—caves in the Judean desert near the Dead Sea."

Rashim's eyes flashed greed. "The Caves of Refuge! We all know of those," he said. "But I have always discounted them as myth, for stories were told of entire families living for months inside the earth."

"Severus was recalled to Rome almost immediately after his victory in the Holy Land," Thomas replied, with an unfriendly nod of agreement. "The treasure he had taken with him from Britain he could not take to Rome, for discovery of it by Roman officials would mean his death. And shortly after arriving in Rome, he died of sudden illness, leaving his secret in the grave."

"Why the caves?" Rashim persisted. "In this entire land, why are you certain the treasure lies in the caves?"

Thomas closed his eyes and recited what he recalled from the letter of a man now dead. "During one skirmish against the Jews near these caves, General Julius Severus lost twenty men in battle, against a handful of unarmed rebels. These twenty men, Severus reported, died as a portion of the cave collapsed upon them, and their bodies could not be recovered. Is it not more likely that these would be the twenty men who transported the treasure? Is it not likely that the surest way for Julius Severus to guard his secret would be to kill those twenty, in the cave where the treasure was buried?"

"Ahah," Rashim purred.

Thomas nodded.

Before Rashim could speak next, a bandit, almost exhausted, ran into camp and called for him.

Rashim hurried away and spent several minutes with his head bent low, listening to the man. Several times Rashim glanced back at Thomas and Katherine. Then he returned.

For a moment, he did not speak, only stared downward at Thomas.

Without warning, Rashim lashed out with his open hand and slapped Thomas across the side of his face.

"You have deceived us!"

Thomas tasted warm, wet salt. Blood from a split lip. He refused to lick it away from the corner of his mouth as it began to dribble into tiny spots onto the rocks at his feet.

Another wild lash.

Thomas stared back. He concentrated on the pain, knowing that to think of anything else would weaken his resolve not to show response.

"You have deceived us!" Rashim repeated again. He raised his hand again, but Thomas did not flinch.

Rashim dropped his hand without striking. Had he decided Thomas could not be intimidated? He studied Thomas. In return, Thomas studied him.

There were long moments of silence, broken only by the buzzing of nearby flies. An idle part of Thomas' mind noted the flies were swarming the blood at his feet.

"You told us of treasure," Rashim thundered. "But you did not tell us of soldiers!"

"Neither did we tell you of the ocean. Or of mountains. Or of birds. Or of anything else that exists in this world. What significance is there in soldiers?" It took effort for Thomas not to mumble.

Rashim half closed his eyes, as if exerting great control over his rage. He opened them again. "One is not followed by the ocean. Nor by mountains. And the birds which follow you may soon not have far to go. For they shall be vultures circling your dead body."

Rashim pointed past Thomas. "I have been told that soldiers have followed your tracks away from Jerusalem. That they are nearly within sight of these hills. Barely an hour away."

"We did not know," Thomas said. "And it does not change the matter of the wealth promised last night. Moreover, if I am dead or my friends harmed, the treasure will not be yours."

Men scurried in all directions as they loaded donkeys.

"Indeed, indeed." Rashim's smile caressed Thomas with cruelty. "Fortunately for you, the soldiers' pursuit readily confirms there is truth in your story."

Rashim lashed out one final time, hitting Thomas with such force that it loosened several of his teeth.

"Take care we don't leave you behind to be crucified," Rashim said.

"His death means you forfeit the treasure," Katherine said quietly. "He is the only one of us who studied the scroll."

Rashim laughed. "Perhaps there is different treasure to be had."

He laughed again. "Your hand in marriage," Rashim said, as he bowed to Katherine, "might well be worth the forfeit, even if an angel like you might spend our first months together mourning Thomas' early death."

On the morning of the third day of slow travel toward the Dead Sea, Thomas almost wished Rashim had removed his skin in small strips as he had threatened.

They had left the rugged hills near Jerusalem and traveled through valleys of fields and olive trees for only a short distance more. Then abruptly, they came to great and desolate ravines carved through steep ridges of sandstone and limestone.

It was difficult for Thomas to stumble ahead with his hands bound behind his back. The pressing heat squeezed sweat from every pore, sweat that immediately turned to tiny balls of mud from the choking dust. Despite the irritation inside his mouth, he refused to ask for water, and it was rarely given.

The path took them through twists and turns and difficult climbs and descents as they followed the course of the ravines. The bandits were hampered by their lack of knowledge of this forbidding terrain, and they could not race forward and risk trapping themselves in a ravine with no exit. Instead, scouts were sent ahead in various directions to report back the safest routes. They moved so slowly that it took the two full days to cover a mere twenty-five miles; on each of the two nights—because of pursuit by the Mameluke soldiers—the bandits had set up camp without daring to seek the comfort of fires.

Thus far, the bandits had made no efforts to cover their tracks. To do so properly would have taken too much time, a luxury they did not have with over one hundred soliders advancing steadily behind them, but also at a slow pace because of their numbers and the heat which worsened each step closer to the bottom of the massive rift which held the Dead Sea, some thirteen hundred feet below sea level.

Now, early in the morning of the third day, the heat was already oppressive and progress was still slow. The bandits hugged the base of cliffs so tall on each side of the narrow valley that Thomas had to crane his head backward to see where the rugged edges met the sky. Ahead, where the valley broke to open horizon, was their destination, the Dead Sea.

Thomas wished he could speak with Katherine. Or with Sir William. But Rashim kept them separated to prevent them from planning escape.

Thomas despaired. Hands bound, stripped of everything but his clothes, without water, and exhausted from heat and pain, his chances seemed hopeless. He knew the same applied to Sir William. While Katherine's hands had been unbound—Rashim treated her more gently—she too had nothing that would help them in a fight or in escape.

And they could not leave without the priceless books which had been taken from the Druids so many centuries earlier. Even if escape were possible now, they could not turn back.

Thomas reviewed what must lie ahead.

In Jerusalem, near the ruins of the temple which had been destroyed by the Romans twelve hundred years earlier, Thomas had visited a monastery which survived from the days of the Crusades. The scholars there, allowed to live by the grace of the Mamelukes, were shy and elderly, with flowing white beards that touched their chests. They had not been surprised to see Thomas, or the small book with its directions to their monastery. When Thomas had asked of the Cave of Letters and the Dead Sea, two of the scholars had stood immediately and retrieved ancient scrolls from nearby chambers. They had retraced the markings onto a smaller scroll, and then accepted quietly the gold offered by Thomas.

"When you reach the Dead Sea, go south," the scholars had told him as they ran old, thin fingers across the scroll. *"It is a land so bleak you will discover no towns on the edge of the shores. You will easily find the ruins of Engedi, for there are no other ruins, and this one is marked clearly by the dozens of collapsed stone buildings. The Dead Sea will be on your left, and deep ravines on your right. Do not enter the ravine that leads from the hills into Engedi, but travel farther. Do not enter the next ravine, nor the next. The fourth ravine will lead you to the caves of Bar Kokhba, where he and the last Jewish rebels died. Why is it you want to know, young one? How is it that you even*

have the knowledge to ask of a rebel as obscure as Bar Kokhba?"

As he walked each painful step across the scorching earth, and despite his despair, Thomas smiled to remember the unforceful curiosity which had shone from the luminous eyes of the Jerusalem scholars as they posed those final questions. Grateful that the Mamelukes found their work both harmless and useful, the scholars had no concern for politics, no concern for wealth.

"From an old one such as yourself," Thomas had answered. *"One who would have loved to spend endless hours poring through these scrolls with you."*

They had smiled mysteriously in return and nodded as Thomas left them in the quiet chambers of study.

"What cause have you to smile?" demanded Rashim.

Thomas had not noticed the attention of the bandit leader.

"I think merely of the treasure which will buy our lives," Thomas replied after a moment, for he had been so engrossed in recollection that it was not easy to dispel the feeling that he was still in the dark, cool chambers of the Jerusalem monastery. "You will fulfill your end of the bargain, will you not? You will release us after we have led you to the wealth?"

"You have my word of honor," Rashim said.

They both knew the words were lies.

At that moment, anger surged inside Thomas with the suddenness of fire exploding from dry brush. This man with the taunting smile of evil meant to take from him his life, and, far worse, take Katherine.

The anger so completely replaced his despair that Thomas forgot his helplessness, forgot that he had no weapons, no means of using any Merlin scientific secrets. Somehow Rashim would be defeated.

Long after Rashim walked away, the anger burned within Thomas, then became cold determination. He would save his life and return to England with Katherine and the knight.

A shout rose at the first sight of the water of the Dead Sea.

Thomas gritted his teeth. The Dead Sea. It meant he had until nightfall to find a way to live.

"I have heard much of this sea," Rashim said, gesturing past the wide beach. "Were not the soldiers in pursuit, I would send one of my men to test its waters."

Thomas concentrated on his balance. It was difficult to slog through the sand along its shore. Without freely swinging hands, the task was doubly hard.

"Yes," Rashim was saying, "I am told the water is so salty that men float in it like pieces of wood."

Just one more step, Thomas told himself, *one more step. And then another. We have traveled beyond Engedi. The next valley is the one which holds the Cave of Letters. Just one more step.*

Rashim grabbed Thomas by the arm as he stumbled.

"My friend," he said with a wide, false smile, "we cannot have you die."

Rashim whistled for a bandit somewhere behind them.

Thomas was too exhausted to lift his head.

The bandit ran close, and Rashim impatiently called for water.

Within moments, Thomas was drinking deeply. He did not mind the musky leather-skin taste of water hot from hours in the sun.

Rashim pulled the water bag away.

"Are we near our destination?" Rashim asked.

Thomas closed his eyes.

Rashim slapped him gently.

Thomas opened his eyes. He was able to briefly focus again.

Beyond Rashim was the beach that led to the flat, waveless water of the Dead Sea. Its waters appeared ghostly white from the glare of the sun. Wavering in the heat, yet somehow appearing close enough to touch, were the high hills on the opposite side of the sea, hardly more than ten miles away.

"Are we near our destination?" Rashim repeated. "Already we can see the dust of the soldiers behind us. Their pace quickens now that they too have reached the shore."

Thomas nodded in a delirium of confusion. All he wanted to do was lie in shade, close his eyes, and, if it were his time, finally die. His mouth had swollen and cracked from the blows dealt by Rashim earlier. His feet were blistered and his arms numb. Because his hands were bound so tightly, each jolting step seemed to pull his arms from his sockets.

"Where?" Rashim was saying. "Where from here?"

Thomas tried to mumble something.

It was not clear enough for Rashim's liking.

"Bring the girl," Rashim commanded the bandit who had brought water.

When Thomas opened his eyes again to sway where he stood, Katherine was there, in front of him.

It felt like a dream, as if all he had to do was push aside the curtains of white haze between them and he could reach out and touch her. But his arms wouldn't move.

A sharp crack brought him back instantly

Rashim's hand had flashed to strike Katherine flat across her face. A red welt appeared, showing clearly the outlines of Rashim's fingers and hand.

Rage took Thomas again, brought to him final reserves of strength. He set his feet wider, and the swaying stopped.

"Where from here?" Rashim asked again, and raised his hand to strike Katherine once more.

Rage crystallized the thoughts which tumbled through Thomas' mind. One thought took hold and grew with his rage. A thought of hope.

"Send most of your men ahead," Thomas said firmly. "They must continue along the shoreline."

"Now you give commands?" Rashim asked.

"The soldiers," Thomas said. *This small chance may be all we will be given. I must convince him.*

"Soldiers?"

"Surely if all of us turn away from the sea into the valley of the caves, the soldiers will follow. And the valley has no exit. We will all be trapped."

Rashim squinted as he considered the advice.

"We send most ahead to draw the soldiers," Rashim finally agreed. "And cover our own tracks as we go into the valley."

"Yes," Thomas said. "But Katherine and the knight must go with us."

Thomas held his breath. *What little chance we have can occur only if the bandits are divided. If Katherine or the knight continue on with the others . . ."*

Rashim shrugged.

Thomas then felt his stomach shrink with momentary fear to the hardness and size of a walnut. *He agrees easily because he cares little what happens to us when the treasure is found.*

"As you say, the girl and the knight travel with us," Rashim said with a mock bow. "After all, I am a man who bargains fairly."

Thomas took a deep breath and looked around. Hands bound, he had no other way to point except with a jerk of his head in the direction of the rocky ravine just ahead. In his mind, the directions echoed clearly. *"The fourth ravine will lead you to the caves of Bar Kokhba, where the last Jewish rebels died. There are five caves high on the sandstone walls. Bar Kokhba took his last stand in the fifth cave, the one farthest west from the Dead Sea."*

Thomas prayed it would not be the cave where he and the knight would join those rebels in the slumber of death.

One hour later, he and the knight and Katherine, along with Rashim and five of the largest bandits, stood at the top of a path, near the dark circle of a cave's entrance.

"My good friend," Rashim said. "I am pleased to discover you did not deceive us about the caves. Perhaps now it is time for you to die."

Rashim nodded once. The largest of the bandits drew a scimitar high above Thomas' head and waited for another nod.

Thomas set his jaw straight and stared straight ahead.

I have done everything I can, Thomas thought. *If this is how it must end, it is the Lord's will. I will not beg or show fear.*

The sword hung against the sky.

Thomas became vividly aware of small details—the spider which darted across a nearby boulder, the intricate shadows of the spiked leaves of brush surrounding the cave's entrance, the scream of the hawk overhead.

In that timeless heartbeat, Thomas was overwhelmed by awe. And joy. *The smallest of things reflect eternity,* he thought, suddenly unaware of the sword. *What a marvel, that a creature as insignificant as a spider may be constructed so perfectly that it moves with such grace on legs lighter than thread. What an incredible mystery, the forces which direct this bush to grow, to shoot forth branches and leaves. What a wonder, the hawk which learns to conquer even the wind.*

The passage of time became meaningless. The peace within him expanded and rushed outward, as if Thomas himself were related to the spider, the bush, the hawk.

My God, he thought, *You are Master of all of this. How can I fear death?*

"No!" a voice reached Thomas. "Do not kill him yet."

Thomas blinked.

The pain of his swollen mouth returned. The throbbing of his blistered feet, the ache of his arms. No longer did it seem he could hear the spider's steps across the boulder, no longer did it seem he rode the wind on the shoulder of a hawk.

"Do not kill him *yet?*" Rashim said. "Yet?"

Katherine nodded.

"My decision is to be with you, Rashim. Alive," she replied. "Let Thomas die as he retrieves the treasure."

Rashim stroked his chin.

"You intrigue me. Tell me more."

"Have the sword lowered," Katherine said.

Rashim nodded at the bandit, and the sword dropped from the sky.

"What if this is not the right cave?" Katherine asked. "Do we have time to search all the others? Will the soldiers remain in pursuit of your men indefinitely?"

Rashim pursed his lips together, still not fully convinced.

"And there remains this cave," she said. "If you and I are to share the treasure, I wish to see *you* unharmed. Send Thomas ahead. Let him be inflicted by vipers. Let him stumble into bottomless pits. Let him risk his life for us. If I am to be wedded to you, I wish to live in luxury."

Thomas stared at the ground. He told himself that she again was bargaining for time, forestalling as long as possible the moment of their deaths, hoping against all hopes that something might happen to set them free.

But enough truth rang from her voice for him to feel the gnawing of doubt, and he realized he would rather have died then, than discover betrayal by her inside the cave.

Rashim thought for only a few seconds.

"Find brush for torches," he directed his men. "We shall let the knight and his friend direct our way."

He grabbed Katherine by the arm and pinched her cruelly. "This one remains with me as we follow. Should she—or they—falter, I will slice her throat."

Thomas and Sir William stood side by side, ten paces ahead of Rashim and Katherine and the five other bandits.

"The strength of your arm?" Sir William whispered.

"I can barely hold this torch," Thomas replied. His fingers were still numb, even though the bonds had been cut fifteen minutes earlier.

"Begin!" shouted Rashim. His voice now reflected nervousness. This was a man accustomed to ruling other men, not searching for the tomb of dead Roman soldiers.

Rashim's command still echoed as Thomas and Sir William moved ahead. The cave roof was beyond the reach of the flames of the torch, and the light that licked into all corners cast yellow fingers and gray shadows which made it difficult to judge the depths of the passage.

"Tell me when your strength has returned," Sir William whispered as they shuffled ahead.

Only a part of Thomas's mind heard. Another part was repeating Katherine's words. *"Vipers and bottomless pits."* What was ahead of them?

Thomas focused on the ground immediately in front. The light was not strong enough to illuminate much beyond them, and to search the far shadows played too many tricks with his imagination.

"Tell me when your strength has returned," Sir William whispered again.

"We cannot attack," Thomas countered with equal softness. "He holds a knife to Katherine's throat, and we have no weapons."

"Where we find treasure, we will find the remains of soldiers," Sir William said. "Where we find those soldiers, we will find their weapons."

Yes! The knight was correct. It increased their odds, no matter how slim! Thomas grinned into the darkness ahead and immediately regretted it. His lips cracked again and he tasted his own blood.

His mind now raced. *We have succeeded in dividing this small army of bandits. Our hands are now free. We may have weapons soon. But how to get Katherine away from the knife at her throat?*

Another thought. *Will the sight of the treasure prove to be enough of a distraction? Will that give the knight the final edge he needs?*

The cave tunnel widened suddenly into a hall. Light gleamed from metal at the far corner of their vision.

"How much farther?" demanded Rashim. Thomas could hear Rashim's quickened breathing. *This fear will be to our advantage as well.*

"I cannot say," Thomas called back. "But look here. Signs of those who lived in this cave!"

The gleam of light off bronze became a wide bowl and intricately designed pitchers.

"Keep your distance from each other," Rashim warned.

Thomas and Sir William moved ahead.

Behind them, they heard the clang of metal against metal as one of the bandits prodded the vessels with a sword.

The hall narrowed again, became one passage and then almost immediately divided into two.

"Which side?" the knight asked.

"Does it matter?" Thomas said. "This entire cave must be explored."

Thomas dared not voice his single biggest fear . . . that the treasure was already plundered. Obscure and remote as this cave was, what if another had solved the riddle?

Thomas sucked in a breath. Intent on watching the ground for snakes, he noticed something the knight had missed.

A footprint.

Then he relaxed. In this still air, a footprint would be preserved for centuries.

The tunnel widened again, and looking back at the torches of the bandits, Thomas could see that the other passage, the one they had chosen to ignore, had rejoined them.

They moved into another hall and discovered a basket of skulls, a tangled fishing net, and a large basin scooped into a wall.

"Water reservoir," Sir William whispered. "Dozens of people may have lived in this cave!"

"Move quickly!" Rashim called.

Thomas hoped Rashim's knife would not tremble against Katherine's throat with the nervousness now so obvious in his voice.

Farther on, they found a bundle of letters, the edges of the parchment so well preserved that Thomas relaxed. This parchment had withstood the centuries; a footprint would do the same.

The hall ended abruptly. Thomas and the knight carefully searched for another passage but found none.

"We return," Thomas announced to the bandits who still followed ten paces behind. "There is one other passage to explore. One where this hall began."

The bandits gave them ample room to move by. *Despite the threat of a knife at Katherine's throat,* Thomas realized, *despite the weapons they hold, they still fear the knight's fighting ability.*

The realization gave him even more hope.

Now we must find the treasure. And the Druid book.

Twenty steps down the other passage, they did.

Thomas and Sir William held their torches out over the pit. The light did not extend low enough to show the bottom or the other side.

"What is it?" Rashim asked from behind them. "Why do you stop? What do you see?"

"Only darkness," the knight replied. "The darkness of a great pit."

Thomas lifted his light to survey the nearby cave floor. At the edge of the light, he saw a ladder made of rope. He retrieved it and lifted it part way so that Rashim could see it too.

"The treasure lies below," Thomas said with a confidence he did not feel. *Why else would a ladder have been left nearby?*

"Hurry then," Rashim said. "Bring me a sample."

Thomas knew he must continue to act the role of one helpless with the fear of death. It was an easy role to play.

"But you will only kill me once the treasure has been proven."

"Better than a slow death," Rashim said. From behind the torch, his fierce face was filled with shadows.

Thomas bowed his head, as if he had been beaten. Then he noticed a small line of dark powder that followed around the edge of the pit.

He dropped the ladder, fell to his knees to retrieve it, and managed to smear some of the powder on his fingers.

Strange, he thought as he turned his back and touched the powder lightly with his tongue. *This bitterness has a familiar taste. And why a line that surrounds the pit as far as I can see?*

He had no time to ponder further. Two of the bandits were at his side, holding their hands out to grasp the rope ladder. They lowered it over the side. Another bandit prodded Thomas with the point of his sword.

With pretended reluctance, Thomas began to climb downward. The bandits were so large, and held the rope so steady, that the ladder hardly moved at all with his full weight on it.

Thomas took one final look upward to mark Sir William's position. *If I find swords below, I cannot falter upon my return. I must toss him one without hesitation.*

Sir William's strong face regarded him without changing expression. Then a slow wink, and Thomas felt strengthened.

Thomas lowered himself slowly, one hand holding the side of the rope ladder, another the torch.

How far down?

He counted twenty-five steps, then touched bottom.

"What do you see?" Rashim called down.

Thomas realized that from Rashim's position, there would only be the glare of the torchlight. No one on the edge above would be able to see below the torch to what Thomas now beheld.

There were piles of large leather bags stacked along one of the smooth vertical walls of the pit. The bags bulged as if filled with stones.

Gold?

Thomas moved sideways, still carrying the torch high so that the glare of the light prevented the observers above from seeing below.

He kicked at one of the bags. The leather, dried from centuries of cool air, broke open. Chunks of gold trinkets and scattered jewels fell on the floor.

"What is it?" Rashim called again.

Thomas did not reply. He cared little for the treasure, glad only it could be used as a distraction.

I need to find swords.

Thomas moved again and nearly stumbled over a skeleton lying in a curled position, as if the soldier had fallen asleep, never to wake again.

The torchlight flickered over another skeleton. Then another. All in the same positions.

Horror hit Thomas with the realization of how these soldiers had died. Someone above had taken their ladder away.

It made too much sense. They would have carried the treasure down, then been abandoned so that the secret of the treasure's location would die with them.

"What have you found?" Rashim was saying, breaking into Thomas' spell of horror.

"The price of greed," Thomas said in a choked voice.

He pushed beyond the terrible sight. There, stacked neatly against the wall, were swords.

Thomas took two and tucked them into the belt beneath his cloak. He hurried back to the leather bags and took a handful of jewels.

Then he dropped the torch and stamped the flame into extinction.

To rise out of the darkness will give an advantage.

"What goes there?" Frustration was evident in Rashim's voice.

"Treasure!" Thomas tried to inject excitement into his voice. It was difficult. He could only hate the impulse that had driven men to let others die in this way. And for only the coldness of gold.

"Treasure!" Thomas repeated. "I cannot carry both the torch and gold."

With that, he began to climb with the awkward one-handed grip he had used to descend, but instead of a torch, he held the only hope there was for survival—jewels and gold. As Thomas neared the top, he tried to block fear from his mind. *There is so little time and but a single chance to save ourselves. One misstep and Katherine will die.*

He stepped onto firm ground.

"Yes?" Rashim demanded.

Thomas threw the gold and jewels on the floor of the cave.

Sparkles of light flashed.

Bandits whose lives were built on greed would have been inhuman if they could have resisted the impulse to look downward at the glittering of wealth.

In that heartbeat, Thomas threw open his cloak, tossed a sword to Sir William, and without pausing, charged his left shoulder into Rashim's stomach. As his legs drove forward, Thomas was reaching into his cloak with his right hand for the second sword.

Rashim fell backward. His knife clattered against the ground.

"Run, Katherine!" Thomas shouted, then whirled, sword in front, to help Sir William.

And at that moment, the world seemed to come to an end.

A great light exploded in Thomas' eyes.

He staggered and reeled as a wave of heat roared past him. If he screamed, he could not hear it among the screams of panic from the bandits.

Then, as the echoes of thunder died, and as his eyes began to adjust to the new darkness, he saw them in the light of the fallen torches. Phantoms. Twice the size of a man. Floating downward toward him.

The bandits fell face down on the ground in terror.

Dazed, Thomas barely realized that he still carried his sword.

Sir William, whose back was to the phantoms, reacted quickly to the sudden surrender of the bandits. He kicked their swords into the pit and stood above them, ready to strike any who might try to rise.

And still the phantoms descended in the dying light.

Rashim began to babble in terror, drool smearing the side of his face.

"Will . . . Will . . . William," Thomas finally managed to say.

Although he had remained standing, the explosion and the appearance of the ghostly specters had taken away his voice.

Sir William turned his head as the first phantom drifted into him. He laughed and swung his sword into it.

Thomas blinked. The weapon slashed through white cloth.

A voice reached them from the darkness. "Forgive me," the voice said. "I could think of no other way to prepare for your arrival."

Thomas thought of the footprint, the line of dark powder along the edge of the pit. That bitter taste! Charcoal, sulfur and potassium nitrate. Explosive powder.

He found himself grinning. Only a Merlin would have knowledge of this secret from the far east land of Cathay.

And the phantoms. Cloth supported by a framework of branches. Thomas himself had once been fooled by the same trick at a campfire in England. By an old man who had traveled with Katherine.

A protest of disbelief arose, then died unspoken in his throat. *The old man is dead,* Thomas wanted to utter. *The old man died the next morning by the campfire.*

But then a figure emerged from the darkness. A familiar stooped and hooded figure which had haunted so many of Thomas' dreams, the old man who had once seemed to know Thomas' every step.

Could Thomas believe what he saw? That Hawkwood was not dead?

The answer came from Katherine. She ran past the prone bandits and threw her arms around the old man.

"My child," he soothed. "If only I could have sent word."

"Hawkwood! You are here," Katherine said over and over again. "You are here and alive."

When their embrace finally ended, the old man stepped past Katherine to face Sir William and Thomas.

"It appears you had little need of assistance," he said. "I

could have waited in St. Jean d'Acre for your return. The leisure would have served my bones much better than travel through this harsh land."

Sir William grinned. "Hardly. We had not yet won this sword fight. And an entire army pursues us. I had begun to wonder when you might appear."

"You knew?" Katherine cried. "You knew Hawkwood was alive and did not tell me?"

"In a way, I did, for what promise did you overhear me make to Thomas?" Sir William said. "But against the Druids, it pays well to keep some secrets close. What if you had made mention of Hawkwood in Lord Baldwin's presence?"

Katherine nodded.

"The army," Sir William said. "We dare not tarry."

Hawkwood dismissed that danger with a wave of his hand. "Bah. An army in pursuit of us will be like a horse chasing a gnat."

He then pointed at Thomas. "Sir William, the young man has proven himself, as I predicted."

Thomas bowed his head in respect. Inwardly, he was not calm. Thoughts raced through his mind. Memories. Possibilities. Hawkwood had known their destination, this cave. He had been in the Holy Land the entire time. He knew with sudden certainty that the old man was . . .

Thomas barely dared raise his head to ask. When he did, he found himself looking at a man now not stooped, but standing with the solid strength of a man barely older than Sir William. Thomas found himself staring through the flickering light at a gentle smile in a face that was eerily familiar.

Thomas did not have a chance to ask his question. For the man answered it as his smile widened with joy.

"Hello, my son," Hawkwood said to Thomas. "It has been a long wait."

Chapter Fifty-Nine

London
July 1314

Katherine gathered her hair into a thick ponytail between her fingers. When she released the hair, she took satisfaction in feeling its weight fall upon her shoulders. *Barely a year ago,* she thought, *I borrowed shears to cut this ragged and short. Never again ... one cannot pose as a lady while looking like a boy.*

Then, almost unconsciously, she smoothed her dress with quick pats and tugs.

"Have no fear, milady," Thomas said. "You are a sight to ravage the hearts of men and to send jealousy quivering through the ladies of the court."

"Thomas," she scolded, for he had guessed correctly at her nervousness. "Must you peer at my innermost thoughts?"

"All these months of travel together ..." He shrugged. "Not once have I seen you so concerned about your appearance."

Katherine softened. Indeed, all these months of travel together. Moments of extreme danger as they avoided Mameluke soldiers in the Holy Land, fought wayside bandits, survived the most vicious storms at sea. Hours of conversation during the quieter times—beside evening campfires or on a ship's deck shifting to the waves beneath starlight. How could they not know each other? Yet they had avoided talk of the one thing nearest their hearts—love for the other—because, she could only guess, they each feared what might come to pass in England should the Druids be victors. And now, they were about to take the first step into the final battle—which if won might finally free them to dream of something more than the companionship of fellow soldiers. Now, they were about to take the first step into the final battle, and all she had as a weapon was her appearance.

"Thomas," she said, "look about you. Is this not reason enough to have concern about how others will perceive us?"

To please her, Thomas made a exaggerated pretense of scanning the Tower, the walls, and courtyard. She knew full well it had already been done; his eyes always took in every detail as he walked.

Behind them were London's narrow, twisted streets of cobblestone, the hundreds of merchants' shops, the beggars, pickpockets, musicians, storytellers, scoundrels, homeless urchins, and countless others who made the city vibrate with life and noise and stink and joy and sorrow.

Ahead, across the moat that separated the royal residence from them, were a half-dozen buildings of smooth stone block. The huge gate was open so that the interior was visible from where they stood. Some buildings were connected by hallways, some centered alone and away from the high-circling walls, and all larger than most castles in the countryside. The forbidding wall, circled by a moat all round, encompassed an area the size of a small village, which in fact, it was.

The royal residences. A part of London yet separate, these majestic buildings sat on the north bank of the Thames River. Barely a month before, Katherine and the knight and Thomas and Hawkwood had finally arrived at the nearby London docks on the same river. As their ship had slowly moved upstream against the Thames, they had all stood on the deck, drinking in the sounds and sights of London. From that vantage point, they had seen the top half of the most imposing building within the walls, the Tower. Even then, within the safety of the ship, Katherine had shivered at the sight.

The Tower.

This building, high and mighty with cramped windows cut into the stone, held the political prisoners of the King of England, Edward the Second, who himself lived in luxury less than a hundred yards away in his permanent residence. It was said that King Edward often enjoyed a stroll past the Tower after a meal, that it helped his digestion to hear the cries of agony and pleas for mercy from his enemies within.

Yet, it was not simply this awesome display of wealth and power that caused Katherine to wonder how she might appear to others. All of the people within sight were dressed in colorful silk finery. The women, with long flowing gowns and tight bodices, were assisted by maids who made sure that their skirts did not drag on the ground. Some of the more venturesome ladies wore tall, pointed hats to follow the latest in fashion.

The men also took great pains to avoid the warm, practical dress of poor peasants. As if to prove their distance from lesser creatures who wore comfortable loose breeches, as did Thomas now, the nobles wore tights. Their tunics were short and brightly colored.

The men and women strolled through the grounds, accompanied by their expensive greyhounds. It was a spectacle which gave Katherine little comfort. She shuddered at the prospect of dealing with the intrigue of the high court. But it had to be done, for it might take them days to accomplish what they so desperately needed.

They wanted an audience with King Edward himself.

"Must this servant accompany you *every* day?" sniffed the slim courtier, as he pointed at Thomas. "Your beauty and dress show royal blood, of course, but your choice of a manservant . . ."

The courtier let his voice trail away with a sniff, then continued. "Each day for the last ten mornings, I've had to suffer this peasant's . . ." the courtier searched for words capable of conveying restrained outrage ". . . this peasant's unspeakable coarseness in dress and attitude. *What* on earth will Duke Whittingham think of me when I present such a peasant along with a lady like you? After all, a chamberlain does not receive just anybody, and the Duke of Whittingham is no exception."

Katherine saw Thomas trying to maintain the sullen look

of a dull peasant. She knew him well enough to catch the twinkle in his eye, and to understand what he thought of the courtier's yellow tights and effeminate manners and voice.

She was glad, however, that Thomas maintained the long-suffering expression of a servant accustomed to abuse, and she smiled sweetly at the courtier. "This servant is my best defense as I travel through dangerous streets."

"Really?" The courtier arched a critical eyebrow.

"Yes," Katherine replied. "Already, he has killed three men with his bare hands."

The courtier jumped back slightly in alarm. Thomas growled and the courtier scurried farther away.

Thomas growled again and Katherine bit back a giggle.

The courtier nearly fell over himself as he tried to back down the corridor, too terrified to turn his eyes from Thomas. The courtier reached a corner and disappeared.

A moment later, only his head appeared, and he gasped out one last sentence. "The chamberlain will see you when the bells strike the next hour!" With that, he pulled his head from sight. The pattering of his feet retreating down the hallway drew a smile from Thomas.

"That is not a man," Thomas said. "It is a mouse. What kind of king have we who surrounds himself with the like?"

"Shush," Katherine said. "Sir William warned us the royal court would have its share of groveling flatterers and shameless bribe-takers."

"This one is both," Thomas spat. "For all the gold you have given him, I cannot believe it has taken ten days just to see the king's administrator. What price to finally reach the king himself?"

"It matters little," Katherine said, as she sat straighter on the wooden bench. "Not many receive an audience with the chamberlain, let alone King Edward. We cannot—"

She stopped abruptly as two ladies and a nobleman approached. The nobleman bowed to Katherine, while the two ladies pointedly ignored her behind their waving fans.

"Word of your beauty has reached many," Thomas observed, as they passed. "The ladies here are less than friendly."

Katherine felt herself begin to blush at his devilish grin, but she could not deny his observation. More than once during their hours of waiting in this remote castle hallway, noblemen had stopped with flimsy excuses for their sudden presence, only to be dragged away by attending ladies.

Now that they were alone again, Katherine said, "Thomas, we will only have one chance to present the reasons for an audience with the king. We cannot fail now."

"Have you not the book?"

"Of course. You bear the burden of its weight every day as we bring it here."

"Then fear none," Thomas said. "It is proof enough for the king to take action against the Druids. And no longer will we fight alone."

"Yet—"

"Yet it is enough. You will tell the chamberlain how we found the book and what it contains. The Druids will no longer move in secrecy, and without that secrecy—their greatest weapon—we will prove victorious."

Katherine knew Thomas spoke true. She had rehearsed again and again their urgent story for King Edward. No mention would be made of Merlins, only of the Druids. She would tell him that—

The church bells rang, a sound that echoed clearly in the silence of the hallway. Almost instantly, the courtier appeared at the corner. He moved no closer, only beckoned from that safe position.

Katherine followed, with Thomas close behind.

Let my words impress, she prayed silently. *Let them strike truer than any arrows.*

The courtier led them through a maze of corridors, then stopped at an arched doorway. Two guards stood in the recess of the doorway and solemnly stepped aside at the impatient snapping of the courtier's fingers.

"Go inside," the courtier said, as he pushed open the large double doors. "And expect no more than ten minutes of audience."

Katherine swept past him, smiling with quiet amusement to see how he kept ample distance between himself and

Thomas. The doors shut behind them.

It was a large enough chamber to contain its own fire-place, now filled with white ashes of a fire long past. A portrait of Edward the Second hung on the wall above the fireplace. Tapestries of deer hunts lined the other walls, and, on the far side of the room, an upright divider hid the rear portion. One large chair with leather armrests and a footstool dominated the center of the room.

No one awaited them.

"Strange," Thomas said to Katherine. "I assumed the Duke of Whittingham would be here. With all this royal riffraff rushing to and fro at such a frightful pace, it seems that he would be anxious to hear us and send us off again."

"Not when he hears my words," Katherine vowed. "It—"

She was interrupted by the opening of the doors.

A large, stoop-shouldered man in a purple cloak entered the chamber. He bowed once, then stood near the chair and placed one foot upon the footstool.

"You have begged audience," he said. And waited.

"For good reason," Katherine said. She drew a deep breath. "My servant carries a book which has lain undisturbed in the Holy Land since the time of Roman soldiers. This book contains proof of a secret circle of sorcerers and their plot which now threatens England and the good King Edward."

The large man leaned forward, so that his elbow rested on the knee elevated by his stance upon the footstool.

"My dear child," the large man said. "If you meant to intrigue me with such a bold opening statement, you have succeeded. Not that you need such a strategy to hold a man's attention, with a countenance as lovely as yours."

Katherine half bowed in a curtsy to accept the compliment, and hoped Thomas would do no more than clench his fists.

"My lord," she said quickly, "my words are truth."

"Indeed," the man said with a voice of honey. "Continue."

Katherine began her explanation much as Thomas had done in convincing Rashim that a treasure did exist. She told of the time before the Romans conquered, when Druids ruled the land. She told of the Druid secrets of science and astronomy, and of the Roman general who plundered their great wealth only to be summoned to the Holy Land, and of how the wealth lay hidden in the Cave of Letters for so many centuries. She explained how bandits had taken them, and how Mameluke soldiers had followed them along the shore of the Dead Sea.

The large man held up a hand glittering with rings.

Katherine stopped.

"How did you come into possession of this remarkable knowledge?" he asked. "And how is it you have just now returned with your story? We lost the Holy Lands to the infidels a generation ago."

"My father was a crusader knight," Katherine said. "forsaken in the Holy Land when the infidels defeated our armies. I was raised there, hidden among the peoples."

She gestured toward her fine apparel and jewelry. "I do not have royal blood, as your courtier might have assumed. Rather, the treasure that my father found provided me with passage here, and with the clothes I needed to gain entrance into royal society."

The large man closed his eyes in thought. Without opening them, he said, "You and he found this treasure in a cave. You were held hostage by bandits and pursued by Mameluke soldiers. How did you escape with the treasure?"

"The bandits were overcome with greed," she said. "My father and this servant were able to overcome them. We left the bandits in the pit in the cave for the soldiers to find."

The large man opened his eyes in sudden surprise. "For the soldiers to find?"

"Yes." Katherine explained how the soldiers had been tricked into following the main party of bandits. "As we left the cave and trekked through the ravine back to the Dead Sea, we dropped pieces of gold and jewelry, so that there was a trail of treasure leading back to the cave. When we reached the shore of the Dead Sea, we turned north. Instead of pursuing us along the shoreline, the soldiers followed the treasure back to the cave, where they were rewarded by the bulk of the treasure and by bandits held helpless beside that treasure at the bottom of the pit."

"Splendid!" the large man clapped his hands. "Absolutely splendid!"

His craggy face then became a frown of puzzlement. "Did you not feel dismay to leave such wealth behind?"

"Not when keeping it all would mean our lives," Katherine said. "Besides, what we could carry ourselves was enough. And . . ."

Katherine paused. This was the most important moment.

"And there was the book. The Druid book. It contains—"

"—nothing but the fanciful spinning of a fairytale!" came a booming voice from behind the divider.

The large man dropped his foot from the footstool and straightened to ramrod attention.

"Duke Whittingham," the large man whispered. "I did not know . . ."

"Think nothing of it," the duke said, as he stepped from behind the divider. "You had your instructions, to pretend to listen to these impostors. You could not know that I too wanted to listen. But I have heard enough."

Katherine barely registered his words, for the shock of recognition hit her like a sword blow.

"Waleran!" The uttering of his name was a low hiss, but it did not come from her lips, but like a curse from Thomas, as he too reeled with shock.

"You are dismissed," the Duke of Whittingham said to the large man.

"Yes, milord." He bowed quickly, then almost ran from the chamber. The doors slammed shut behind him.

Waleran. Not even now, dressed in royal robes, did he have a single redeeming feature to lessen his evil appearance.

"You would do well not to call me Waleran," he said. "Duke Whittingham is my title. And let me assure you, I have ways to punish those who do not address me properly."

Katherine opened her mouth once, then shut it. Her thoughts were in such disarray that she was unable to talk.

"That is better," Waleran said with a cruel leer, misinterpreting her silence as obedience. "You might have been able to escape me in the Holy Land, but you shall not be so fortunate again."

"You are such fools," Waleran laughed. His teeth were unevenly spaced and black with rot. "So easy to deceive."

"How . . . how can the king's chamberlain . . ." Katherine stopped, still nearly faint from surprise.

"How can the king's chamberlain be a Druid? Or how can the king's chamberlain accomplish so much as a Druid?"

Katherine nodded. Waleran here was not what they had expected during the long months of voyage and planning.

"Should it not be obvious? It is I who oversee all the Druid actions. And who is better placed to oversee a kingdom than the right-hand man of the king himself? And why should you show such surprise? You know the Druids have penetrated all levels of society. Surely it would seem logical that a Druid attain the position of chamberlain, especially when all the previous chamberlains were Druids. The unquestioned authority of this position gives great freedom and—" Waleran snapped his mouth shut and dropped his hand to his sword.

"Young man," he said to Thomas with a voice promising death. "Sit. Yes, immediately. On the cold floor. From there, you shall have difficulty continuing your slow movement toward me."

Thomas hesitated.

"Do you think it was an accident that you were searched? I know you do not have a weapon, and mine—" Waleran unsheathed his sword "—is coated with poison." He paused. "Now, sit! Or watch Katherine die."

Thomas lowered himself onto the stone floor with great reluctance.

"Much better." Waleran cackled, then broke into a wheeze. When he recovered his breath, he moved to the large chair in the center of the room and placed his sword beside him on the armrest. "I shall satisfy your curiosity. In turn, you shall satisfy mine."

More likely, you shall gloat, Katherine thought.

"As you well know," Waleran said, "it was I who posed as a fellow prisoner in the dungeon of Magnus during the time that Thomas and Sir William spent in captivity. I overheard nothing about that which we seek."

Katherine grinned inside. *Thomas kept his vow well. What still lies hidden in the monastery of his childhood might . . .*

"I overheard nothing about that which we seek," Waleran repeated, "and then a freak whose face was burned helped them escape."

Again, Katherine found reason for hidden satisfaction. *He does not know it was I behind those bandages.*

"It was hardly worth my efforts for what little I gained in that prison." Waleran squirmed as if remembering the dank darkness and the flea-infested straw and the scurrying of rats. "However, my time in York paid dividends, as you know."

Katherine bowed her head. *Waleran was in a neighboring cell as Thomas spoke to the captured duke of York. What he heard was enough to . . .*

Waleran cackled again. "Yes. Thomas here thought he was so brave and noble, capturing Isabelle and holding her as hostage. Little did he know we had deliberately allowed that, so that he would lead us to—"

"You saw the old man dead," Thomas interrupted with bitterness. "Was that not enough?"

Katherine kept her head bowed, this time so that Waleran would not see the gleam of triumph in her eyes. Yes, Thomas had led Waleran's soldiers to her and the old man. But Hawkwood, in the confusion of the attack, had pretended death by swallowing one of the prepared pills he always carried among the herbs and potions hidden beneath his cloak, this one made from the dried and crushed bark of rhododendrons, which caused unconsciousness, coldness of the skin, and a vastly reduced heart rate. Yes, it had been a gamble, for any of the soldiers might have run him through with a sword, but a necessary gamble. Once the Druids were convinced that he was dead . . .

"Dead, and not a moment too soon," Waleran laughed. "His death made it easy to outmaneuver you two. Following you both to the Holy Land was child's play. And such simple minds." Waleran choked on his laughter, then recovered. "Should it not be obvious that if the Merlins had men in the Holy Land, that Druids would also have their spies?"

"Lord Hubert Baldwin," Thomas spat.

"None other," Waleran said. "One of your most trusted men and one of our greater allies. Without his help, Magnus might never have fallen as it first did."

Katherine felt frozen to the ground. *So many died then. A generation of Merlins wiped out. And now the Druids will be able to move openly against an entire country.*

She lifted her head.

"You gave Lord Baldwin his instructions in Jericho?"

"Of course, milady," came the mocking reply. "He is a man of strong arm, but limited intelligence. And I did not want to soil my own hands with such matters."

"You mean you did not want to risk your life," Thomas said. "Baldwin now rots in a Jerusalem dungeon."

"He was a fool to allow himself to be taken in Jerusalem." Waleran shrugged. "No matter. I needed to return immediately to England—as a chamberlain I have freedom but not unlimited freedom—and the situation seemed to be in hand, especially since the Mameluke officials are not adverse to bribes."

Then Waleran grinned, an ugly, evil grin of stinking breath and smug triumph. "You have reported the rest. What he failed to do, you accomplished for us. What we lost so many centuries ago, you recovered and, against all odds, you returned to England."

He stood and rubbed his hands briskly. "I shall take the book now," he said.

With reluctance, Katherine nodded at Thomas.

"Not so, my dear," Waleran said. *"You* take the book

from him and slowly hand it to me. He is young enough and strong enough to attempt an attack."

Waleran placed his hand on the sword hilt as he directed his words at Katherine. "And if *you* attempt anything, I shall run you through."

Thomas removed the book from its wrappings. Katherine took it with both hands and extended it to Waleran.

He merely smiled.

"You think I will reach for it and drop my guard? Not so. Place it on the armrest and step away."

Katherine did as instructed. When she had retreated to her previous position, Waleran opened the book and glanced inside.

"Ahh, splendid," he said. "I see already many of the secrets we lost over the centuries."

He ran a soiled finger down one of the pages. "Here. A mixture of common garden herbs to induce madness . . . there, a prediction of star movement, knowledge to impress superstitious peasants."

Waleran paused. "But you already know these weapons. The eclipse during the hanging of the knight . . . that was masterful." He mused farther. "Of course, the old man is dead and I need not worry."

He slammed his fist down on the book, snapping Katherine's head upward in attention.

"Tell me," his voice was no longer contemplative, but ugly and threatening. "What did you hope to accomplish with this book?"

Katherine bit her tongue.

"Tell me!" Waleran roared. "Silence gains you nothing!"

He leapt to his feet and placed the tip of his sword against Katherine's throat.

"I need only pierce the skin," Waleran said, in a voice unexpectedly silky, "and she dies. So tell me."

"At the back," Thomas said hurriedly, "at the back of the book is the Druid outline for means of taking a country. Key towns to hold. Key people to bribe. Although it is dated by the passage of centuries, it shows intent. Proof of a Druid masterplan, to be delivered to King Edward. That, and news of what it happening in northern towns now, was to be enough for him to consider a Druid threat in this day and age. With his help, we hoped to stop you."

"Children, children," Waleran said with insincere sympathy, as he stepped away from Katherine and sat once again in his chair. "What delusions you carry. King Edward himself is a pliable fool who relies heavily on my advice. And he is so distracted now with the war against Scotland that I am allowed to dictate our domestic affairs."

Waleran laughed. "Do you think it is an accident that a hopeless battle against Scotland preoccupies him? Hardly. Once again, my advice that he should continue the war. As I said, a useful distraction that weakens the entire country."

Waleran then sighed and stared into the distance. When he spoke again, it was with the voice of a parent lecturing a child.

"Thomas," he said, "you have my thanks for securing this valuable book. But we need more from you. Give what we have always wanted from you, what you were entrusted to guard since birth."

Thomas sat silent.

"You have a simple choice," Waleran said. "Join us and gain the wealth and power of the land's most powerful earl. Or remain silent and see Katherine die."

"No!" Katherine uttered. "My life is nothing compared to what he seeks. Thomas, I die gladly."

"Thomas?" Waleran purred.

Still Thomas said nothing.

"A difficult choice?" Waleran asked. "Perhaps time in the torture chambers will loosen your tongue."

Waleran did not wait for a response.

Instead, he raised his voice. "Guards!"

The door opened instantly.

Waleran stood and pointed to Thomas and Katherine.

"Take them to the Tower."

Katherine wept freely. Though she was not alone in the Tower cell, her cries went unheard. The other occupant of the cell was Thomas, who was unconscious. Moments before, two guards had dragged him in, his head sagging like a broken puppet. They had shackled his wrists to the wall.

Now, the chains kept him from falling forward completely. His hands, attached to the chains, were behind his back, and Katherine hardly dared guess how much it tore his muscles to have his entire weight straining so awkwardly against his chest and arms.

She reached for his face. She didn't need the clank of chains which followed her every movement to remind her that it was near impossible. Her wrists were shackled as well, and her fingers stopped inches short of Thomas' face.

"My love," she cried, "awaken."

He did not.

Tears streamed down her cheeks. Five days running, the guards had taken him away during midmorning. Five days running, they had returned him less than an hour later. Each time he had been placed unconscious in those chains. Each time it had taken him longer to return to consciousness.

She longed to touch his face. In sudden rage, Katherine yanked her chains, uncaring of the stabbing pain of the cruel metal of the shackles biting into the softness of her wrist. But her fingers fell tantalizing inches short.

"Thomas," she whispered again. "Please. Please wake up."

In the quiet, a rat rustled in the straw at her feet. She cared little. Rats were as common as the fleas, and her attention was on Thomas' pale face, motionless in the sunlight that fell through a high, narrow window.

Thomas stirred. Groaned. Blinked. And slowly found his feet.

"Katherine," he croaked. Joy filled his voice. "You are still here."

She turned her head so that he would not see the tears. *How can he think of me first when they inflict so much pain on him?*

"I am still here," she said, her voice muffled by the hair which clung to her wet cheeks.

"Thank our Lord," he said. "It is my worst nightmare that I will return and find you gone. I . . . I . . . could not bear this prison alone."

"Nor I," she said simply.

As they looked at each other, Thomas brought his hand up and they reached for one another, but the chains brought them short.

"I dreamed you called me 'my love,' " Thomas said.

"I did," Katherine replied. She waited long moments, as if debating whether to speak. "It is a subject we have avoided," she said. "My love for you. Yours, I pray, for me. My own fear was this—to declare love for you, yet be helpless against the Druids."

"We are not helpless," Thomas vowed. "For I have not revealed to the torturers the secrets of my childhood monastery. Not even its location."

"To save your life—"

"No. Sir William hinted that my knowledge could turn the final battle. To reveal it now means my life is worthless."

"Yet—"

"No, Katherine. There is no 'yet.' " He grinned. It was a flash of white from a pain-exhausted face. Blood trickled from one corner of his mouth. "We shall watch for escape."

Thomas raised his voice in anger. "I say it again . . . we shall watch for escape. Then we shall return to the monastery, and I will solve the final puzzle, find what it is the Druids so urgently seek! With that, they shall be defeated."

The effort of rage cost him his last reserve of energy. He sagged again against the chains. "Then we shall talk of our love," he finished softly. "Then we shall talk of our love."

Katherine wept again, this time unable to hide her tears.

Thomas gritted his teeth and clenched his fists. Anger once more gave him strength to stand upright.

"Katherine," he began. "do not despair. You will see a chance for escape. Or I will." His voice rose again. "All we need do is reach the monastery."

A key turned in the lock.

A huge surly guard—the one who shoved food at them daily—kicked open the door. From behind him, a blare of royal trumpets.

"Make way for the king!" came a shout. A courtier dashed inside the prison cell.

Then, without further fanfare, King Edward the Second, the reigning monarch of all of England, stepped through the doorway.

He was a tall, powerfully built man with fair skin and reddish-blond hair. He carried the royal sceptre, so brilliantly studded with jewels of all colors that his purple robes and white-furred collar seemed poor in comparison.

He stood still and stared at them, his face empty of all emotion.

Katherine felt a shiver go through her. *This man need only lift a finger, and we are free. Or dead. At his command, armies of thousands march upon towns and villages.*

"This is the traitor with the tongue of stone," King Edward observed.

"Your majesty, I—" Thomas began to say.

The courtier stepped forward and slapped Thomas across the face.

"One does not address his majesty unless asked a direct question."

"I am not—"

Another slap. This one rocked Thomas back against the wall.

Katherine's eyes filled with tears again.

"I am not a traitor!" Thomas roared.

The courtier prepared to strike Thomas again.

"Enough," King Edward said.

The courtier stepped away. King Edward moved forward to examine Thomas.

"I am told our best men cannot break your spirit."

Thomas raised his head tall and met the king's eyes. "Innocence gives strength, milord."

"Indeed," King Edward said noncommittally. He turned to examine Katherine.

"And you," he said to her, "are as beautiful as the rumors."

Then he walked away from them both and filled the doorway again.

"I have heard many declarations of innocence," King Edward said, "from men as brave as you. From men who have endured the very chains you wear. Indeed, I often think it takes greater bravery to be a traitor than to serve the king. For traitors know the terrible price they will pay."

Katherine's eyes were on Thomas. He opened his mouth.

"No." With the full weight of royal authority, King Edward's command halted any words.

"There is nothing you can say to convince me," King Edward continued. "The Duke of Whittingham has told me enough, and if I cannot trust him..." King Edward shrugged as he made his jest. "If I cannot trust him, my kingdom is worthless."

Such irony. Katherine wanted to shriek. But she, like Thomas, knew it would sound like the ravings of lunatics, any talk of Druids and Merlins and kingdomwide conspiracies. Without the book, they had no hope of presenting their case. In chains, against the word of the king's chamberlain, they had even less hope.

King Edward fixed Thomas and Katherine with a stare.

"Why am I here, you might well ask, when I refuse to hear your case?" King Edward paused. "Not for curiosity."

His voice became quiet with menace.

"My son has been kidnapped," he said. "I have many enemies, all linked to the Tower prisoners, and I am here to tell each prisoner the same, so that word may spread and my son be returned. My royal proclamation is this. My son, Prince Edward, is returned safe within a week, or all prisoners within the Tower shall be beheaded."

They were fed twice each day. In the morning, their guard brought a bowl of thin, fly-specked porridge. In the early evening, it was bread—quite often drilled with holes burrowed by beetles—and a bowl of beans boiled to mush.

The guard was so large he had to squeeze sideways to get into the cell. That action usually forced him to spill a major portion from the bowls he carried. Worse, their guard enjoyed too much beer throughout the afternoon, and this led to more unsteadiness.

There was nothing unexpected about his arrival for the

evening meal. He would jangle his keys for several minutes and fumble with the lock, then kick the door open and grunt his way into the cell.

That he always drank too much beer was evident by the foul breath which overwhelmed the usual stench of the cramped prison cell. His eyes were bleary and his nose a brilliant red. Because he was so large, most of his movements meant collision with Katherine or Thomas.

Three nights closer to the eve of their execution, Katherine and Thomas received their usual warning of his arrival.

The door clanged open and the guard struggled through. This time, however, he strained harder than normal to wheeze air into his lungs. His eyes were unfocused and his entire face the red usually restricted only to his nose.

He bent to place one bowl at Thomas' feet, and barely managed to keep his balance. He then turned to Katherine. He smiled uncertainly and his breath made her choke. His large, stubbled face loomed closer, his double chins wobbled.

I'm glad my stomach is so pinched that any food will do, for this sight would dull the keenest hunger.

Her thoughts turned to sudden alarm. For the ugly face did not stop its approach.

This is not an attempted kiss!

It was not. The big man sagged forward and fell into Katherine. His bearlike arms engulfed her.

"Thomas!" she tried to shout, but the guard's weight suffocated any words which might have left her lungs.

The stench of his unwashed clothing gagged her, the rubbery feel of his flesh nauseated her, and still he pressed against her into the wall.

She tried to beat her arms against his chest, but she was pinned too securely. Yet his weight was passive, as if he were not attacking, but had . . . *collapsed?*

He rolled downward and fell in a heap at her feet.

Katherine found herself staring at the ring of keys on his belt. She hardly believed this might be. Slowly, she reached down and tugged on the keys. The guard did not respond.

It took Katherine less than a minute to find the key which unshackled her wrists.

Chapter Sixty-One

"Home!" Thomas shouted. "I . . . am . . . home!"

His words echoed through the valley below where he and Katherine stood among the shadows of large rocks.

From their vantage point, towering trees blurred the walls of the abbey hall. It was, as Katherine knew, the monastery where Thomas had been raised, believing the entire time he was an orphan.

"Home!" he shouted again. Birds scattered from a nearby bush.

"Thomas!" She tried to sound angry, but could not. His joy was too contagious. After all, they had survived a hurried trek through most of England to reach these moors so close to Magnus.

"There is none to hear me," Thomas said. "The monks have long since left." He grinned. "You'll remember the cause of that."

She did. It had been the start of his path to conquering Magnus, the beginning of all that had led to this moment above the valley.

"Come on," he whispered, as if conspiring. "Let me show you the way."

Thomas moved quickly from the exposed summit into the trees. He gave ample proof that he knew every path; he would approach a seemingly solid stand of brush, then slip sideways into an invisible opening among the jagged branches and later reappear farther down the hill.

"Hurry," he called.

The man is skipping like a boy.

Katherine smiled at his enthusiasm. No matter what their troubles, this was a time to set them aside and enjoy the sunshine, the feel of grass against their ankles, and the song of the babble of the tiny river which ran past the abbey.

Their first destination was not the abbey itself. Instead, Thomas moved directly to the river and stood at its bank. The moss of the rocks beneath the water waved in the current like tails of tiny fish.

"You know about the cave, do you not?" Thomas asked her.

Katherine nodded. "Hawkwood and I once waited for you here. It was an agony, not to be sure whether you were Druid or Merlin, not to be able to simply join you instead of follow you."

"We are together now." But he said it in such a dismissing way that Katherine knew Thomas did not want to discuss the reason for that mistrust; so she too lost herself in thought.

If his mother had not died while training him here to be a Merlin, she would have been able to impart so many more secrets as he came of age. Instead, with her unexpected death, Thomas had to struggle so long in the belief that he was alone, and unaware of his destiny as a Merlin. And we, in our isolation, feared that the Druids had found him in this obscure abbey, and had managed to turn him against us.

When Katherine looked at Thomas again, she saw his eyes were closed, his head bowed.

Minutes later, he lifted his head again. "She was a remarkable woman," Thomas finally said. "There is so much that I owe her."

Then to dispel the somber mood, he smiled. "Never would I have dreamed that I would regard this abbey with fondness."

He pointed past the abbey. "The pond there? Many was the time I could not be found by those wretched monks. Little did they know I was beneath the water, that I excelled at breathing through a reed."

He pointed at the massive gray walls of the abbey itself. "My bedchamber was there, that tiny window. I slept on a straw mattress placed atop a great wooden trunk. At nights, I escaped down those walls."

He laughed at the surprise on her face. "No, I was not a fly. There are enough cracks between the stones for a determined boy to find room for fingers and toes."

She laughed with him. And marveled at how his gray eyes seemed almost blue beneath the clear skies.

What a dream. That he and I could one day be together and never be on guard. If only our last desperate actions will—

"We have stood here long enough?" Thomas asked. "Given our followers enough notice?"

She nodded.

Thomas turned and led her to the cave.

Several bends upstream from the abbey hall, comfortably shaded by large oaks, was a jumble of rocks and boulders, some as large as a peasant's hut. Among them, a freak of nature had created a dry, cool cave, its narrow entrance concealed by jutting slabs of granite and bushes rising from softer ground below.

The knight will be waiting for us, Katherine assured herself, as they walked among the boulders. *Surely not everything we planned has gone astray.*

"Count to one thousand," Thomas suddenly said. They were still at the side of the river. Immediately to their left was the entrance, so well concealed it was difficult to see, even from ten feet away.

"Count to one thousand? Here? Now?"

Thomas laughed at the confusion that crossed her face.

"No. Those were the rules I was taught by Sarah. 'Count to one thousand. Watch carefully. Then slowly, cautiously, enter. Let no person ever discover this place.' "

Katherine nodded.

"It was a game, I thought then. Sarah taught me patience, how to wait here and listen to the sounds of the surrounding forest until I was part of it."

Thomas closed his eyes and smiled in recollection. "Inside, so cool, so safe. We spent hours in there. She taught me to read, to understand mathematics, to apply logic."

Katherine smiled in her own recollections. *The ways of a Merlin. What joy to be lost in the wonder of learning. He, here in a cave in a tiny valley in the moors of northern England. I, in a sun-baked town on the edge of the Holy Land. Both of us with a path destined to bring us to this cave. Will all of it end today or—*

"Has a trampling army arrived?" The voice came from a large figure stepping into sight from the cave's entrance.

"Sir William!" The relief in Katherine's voice surprised her. She had been depending so heavily on his being here.

"A trampling army?" Thomas snorted. "Are you so old and weak that you need an army to rescue you?"

"Hardly," Sir William said, as he accepted Thomas' offer of an extended hand. "Rather, by the sound of your progress, I expected all of England to be outside. You make enough noise to wake the dead."

Then the knight rolled his eyebrows. "Of course, waking the dead is the least of my concerns. But if you wake the babe-in-arms inside, then all wrath will fall upon us, for his majesty is prone to tantrums of temper most unseemly for one of royalty."

"The child?" Katherine asked. "He is here? Safe? With his nurse?"

Sir William nodded.

"Follow me inside," the knight said. "I will introduce you to the heir of all England, the future Edward the Third."

It was not a natural cave. Instead, it resulted from the haphazard piling of huge slabs of granite over the large boulders that lined the river. The cave was barely deeper than the interior of a peasant's hut, and was lit by a shaft of sunlight that fell between the cracks of the two of the largest slabs forming its roof. In the far corner, an oily torch burned, its smoke carried immediately upward in a draft that escaped between smaller cracks in the ceiling.

Centuries of growing moss and lichen had eroded most of the rock and made the walls seem softer than harsh granite.

Katherine did not have to stoop as she stepped through

the entrance; once inside, she discovered there was room to stretch upward, should she so choose.

She did not.

She could have moved to the left side of the cave, to an open chest that was as high as her knees and as wide as a cart.

She did not.

Instead, she looked at the other occupants of the cave.

In the corner, on a rough stool, sat a nurse, shawled in a coarse garment. In her arms, wrapped in the finest linen, was a young child.

Prince Edward. Eyes closed in sleep. A wisp of dark hair matted to his forehead. Tiny fingers clenched.

"Did his majesty travel well?" Thomas was asking.

Katherine didn't hear Sir William's reply. She was struggling with unfamiliar emotions.

She had been brought up a lonely child. The years in disguise behind bandages had ensured she did not meet other children. Never had she been allowed to hold a baby, or even come close to one.

So now, she was mesmerized by the child. His vulnerability fascinated her. That same vulnerability also made her yearn to hold and protect him.

She did not see the boy as a future king but as someone who needed love. So, it seemed, did the nurse, who leaned over the child and soothed him with low murmuring.

". . . the travel presented little difficulty." Katherine realized Sir William was replying to Thomas. "But after our arrival here! I've never known one so small could squall so loudly."

Thomas began to smirk but quickly arranged his face to a more sober expression as he noticed the glare on Katherine's face.

"Exiled here in a cold, dark cave with an uncaring knight," Katherine said. "I'd squall too." She turned to the nurse. "May I help? Does he need anything?"

The nurse shook her head without lifting her face to look at Katherine.

"May I . . . may I . . ." Katherine had become shy.

"Hold him?" the nurse asked.

"Yes."

The nurse nodded.

Katherine did not notice the amused glance between Thomas and Sir William. None of them noticed a visitor step into the cave, his shoes silent on the soft dirt.

Katherine was halfway to the child when the new voice stopped her.

"Oh, my," the voice taunted. "A touching reunion."

Katherine whirled.

Waleran. It is Waleran. As ugly as a nightmare, and leering the evil smile of rotted teeth he had last flashed as guards had taken Katherine and Thomas from his chamber to the Tower.

"Tsk, tsk," Waleran said, as Sir William reached for his sword. "This is no place for rudeness. As you can see, I do not carry a weapon."

Sir William ignored the comment and withdrew his sword.

Waleran released an exaggerated sigh. "Dealing with barbarians is so . . . so . . . fruitless."

He pursed his lips and shook his head. "William, William," he chastised. "Do you think I would be fool enough to enter this den of lions like a helpless lamb?"

Waleran replied to his own question, a man who enjoyed the sound of his own voice.

"Hardly, William," Waleran said. "Outside this cave is an army of twenty. All I need do is raise my voice, and all of you will be dead."

"Twenty men," William said. "That matters little if I slit your throat now."

Waleran snorted. "And what will become of your friends? Once I am dead, so are they. Thomas . . . Katherine . . . this child—"

For a moment, the arrogant coolness of Waleran's face slipped. "That is Prince Edward! The entire kingdom is in an uproar. And you have him here!"

Surprise became a sly smile.

"I beg pardon. *We* have him here. Perhaps you've saved me a great deal of trouble."

Before Waleran could say more, Sir William sheathed his sword.

"You will live," Sir William said, as the sword hissed back into place. "But it would be more pleasant to share this cave with a half-rotted pig."

Waleran blustered until he managed to contort his face into a sneer. He pointed at Thomas, then at Katherine. "In the very least, a half-rotted pig has more cunning than these two combined."

"Oh?" Sir William asked, with the casualness of a man holding back rage only through supreme effort.

"They believed it was an act of God that their guard suffered a seizure in the midst of their cell, that it was a miracle to escape the Tower through the use of the guard's keys."

Waleran laughed until he coughed. "A miracle? Certainly. A miracle the guard didn't die after the potion I placed in his beer. My biggest fear was that he would collapse before he reached their cell."

"You let us escape deliberately so that you could follow us here," Katherine said quietly. "Just as you once let Thomas escape York to see where that led him."

"Yes, my dear," Waleran said in a patronizing voice. "You catch onto these things so *very* quickly. And would it surprise you that every word you said in the Tower cell reached the ears of a listener?"

Katherine blushed.

"Oh, yes," Waleran said. "Every word. Such a shame. The love you two professed for each other will never flower."

He waved that away as insignificant. "Thomas repeatedly made the mistake of telling you that all he needed was to return to the monastery of his childhood. That here would be revealed the final secrets which might overcome us."

"You overheard our conversations and let us escape, just to track us here?" Thomas sounded as if he was in shock.

"Of course," Waleran said. "Nothing less than routine for the genius mind of someone who is the right-hand adviser to the king."

The nurse stirred to comfort the baby who had begun to whimper at the harshness of Waleran's voice. Her movement was slight, however; she appeared too frightened to look up at Waleran.

"This baby, Prince Edward," Waleran asked. "Why was he taken?"

"Desperation," Sir William said, after a long exhalation of breath. "There are so few of us Merlins. Messengers brought me word that Thomas and Katherine had been imprisoned. The plan to show the king the Druid book failed. I hoped King Edward would believe Druids had kidnapped his baby. It would get him to look closely at how the towns in the northern part of his kingdom have fallen to Druids posing as priests of the Holy Grail. With King Edward's help, we would stop you before you gained power."

Waleran chuckled. "What a surprise then, that *I* was there as the king's chamberlain. As you well know, King Edward will never hear of that proof. You are the last of the Merlins, and soon you will be gone."

Katherine shuddered.

"Already, we hold dozens of towns here in the north. Having King Edward's son now as hostage only makes our task easier. And within a year, Druids *will* reign supreme."

Sir William sighed. He began to pace the small cave, running his fingers through his hair in distraction. Finally, he moved to a stool near the nurse, bowed his head in defeat, and spoke. "We have truly failed. King Edward will receive no proof of your existence. You have his son as hostage. And now, you know the location of this abbey."

Waleran rubbed his hands together.

"Yes," he said. "we have finally found the childhood abbey which hid Thomas for all those years. Even if you don't tell us what we need, it will be found."

"I suspect so," Sir William said sadly, head still bowed.

"Do not suspect. Consider it truth," Waleran said. "There are twenty outside now, and more to arrive."

"More?" Katherine asked.

"I have sent messengers to all parts of England. The highest members of our circle will gather here. My original intention was to gather our best minds to find what you had hidden here. Furthermore, it seems it will give us a chance to direct the final stages of battle. England will be ours. This baby will be the heir to nothing."

Thomas finally spoke. His voice was tinged with bitterness. "Druid leaders will all meet in secrecy here?"

Waleran laughed. "You *do* see the irony. This obscure abbey was sufficient to hide you for years, even from the all-seeing eyes of the Druid web. How much better, then, for us to gather in the same remoteness?"

"All is lost," Sir William said. "The Druids have conquered the Merlins."

Katherine moved to him and placed a comforting hand upon his shoulder.

Waleran watched with a smile as hideous as the open mouth of a dying snake. "Please," Waleran said to Thomas through that smile, "save us both time and effort and tell me of what we seek."

Katherine took an involuntary look at the open chest at the side of the cave. She quickly looked away again, but not soon enough.

"Ho!" Waleran said. "Something I should not see?"

He strode to the torch, pulled it from its base, and walked to the chest.

"A single book?" Disappointment registered in his voice. "We have been searching for ten years for the great treasure that Lord Baldwin heard was rumored to appear among the Merlins, and all I find is a single book?"

"It is nothing," Thomas said quickly. "What you seek lies at the bottom of the pond."

"Play no games with me," Waleran warned Thomas. "Your whimpering voice tells me perhaps this book *is* valuable."

"I would rather die than tell you."

"Tell him all, Thomas," Sir William said. "Mayhaps we can leave with our lives."

"Yes," Waleran said in oily tones. "Tell all."

Thomas blinked once, twice, as if trying to decide.

"Spare yourselves further agony," Waleran said, "and tell me of this book." His voice rose in volume with such impatience that the boy woke and began to cry.

"Shut that whelp's mouth!" he ordered the nurse.

"No," the nurse whispered calmly.

"No? No?" Waleran's face began to purple with sudden rage. "You dare defy me? A common peasant dare defies the Duke of Whittingham? Master of the Druids? The right-hand man of King Edward? You defy me?"

The nurse lifted her head and pushed the shawl away from her face.

"I defy *you?*" she asked, as she stared Waleran directly in the face. "Ask instead if *you* dare defy *me.*"

Waleran staggered backward.

"Queen Isabella!"

"Indeed," she said. "The one person in England King Edward trusts more than you, his beloved Duke of Whittingham. And I have heard enough for you to hang."

She smiled.

"And enough for the Druids to be wiped from the face of the earth."

Chapter Sixty-Two

"Impossible," Waleran said. The slate gray of his face showed, however, that he believed it all too possible. "How . . . how . . ."

Queen Isabella stood and gracefully moved to Katherine, while Waleran's jaw worked against empty air. Katherine accepted the offered baby with awe, and hugged him warm against her chest.

The Queen of England and . . . and the future king in my arms. Surely I dream.

". . . how is it I am here—the last place on earth a traitor like you would expect?" Queen Isabella drew to her full height and pulled the shawl away from her face. Her words were brittle and unforgiving.

The peasant's shawl still wrapped her, but her posture became unmistakably royal—her back straight, her shoulders squared, and her chin held high with dignity. The pale, smooth skin of her face contrasted with her dark, thick hair and full red lips. An aura seemed to grow around her as she once again became the woman accustomed to the power that ruled an entire land.

She fixed her terrible gaze on Waleran and advanced. "I am here because of a mysterious stranger who appeared in the royal bedchambers shortly before dawn barely a fortnight ago."

Waleran shook his head as he retreated until his back touched the cave wall. "No. Only one man would be capable of such a thing, and he is dead."

"His ghost, then, appeared," Queen Isabella said without smiling. "And at first, I believed it to be a ghost. How else could a mere man slip through the royal residence and avoid the guards."

"But—"

"My first impulse was to scream. Yet something about the man's calmness . . ." Queen Isabella smiled in recollection. "This man informed me that my son Edward had been taken. King Edward was at the country estate, and I was alone, except for the guards roaming the castle, but I did not panic. There was a gentleness about this man."

Waleran began to shake, a dog waiting to be beaten.

"He invited me to see for myself if the baby was gone, that he would be waiting for my return to the royal chambers. He was not afraid, this man, for he said that if he had lied, I could call the guards. He told me if Edward truly had been taken, however, it would be in my best interest to hear the story. The baby was gone from the nursery, and I returned without calling alarm. And I listened."

Baby Edward began to cry. Katherine rocked him, but to no avail.

"That mysterious stranger informed me of a plot against the throne," Queen Isabella said. "A Druid plot. Understandably, I found the thought ridiculous. Druids were a myth, a superstition, I told him."

Katherine concentrated on the boy in her arms, but he sensed her strangeness and cried for his mother.

Queen Isabella turned away from Waleran and held out her arms for the child.

"Sir William," she said over her shoulder, "my son needs me. If you would care to finish."

"With pleasure, milady."

Katherine noticed Sir William had again drawn his sword. So engrossed had she been in the baby, she could not say when it had happened.

"Waleran, or . . ." Sir William paused as he lifted the sword, "would you prefer the Duke of Whittingham, short-lived as I pray that title may be?"

Waleran sank until he was sitting, back against the wall.

"We knew that someone, in the royal court was a Druid," Sir William said. "Thomas and Katherine were sent merely to force that Druid—you—into action. We knew that it would be of utmost importance to prevent the slightest hint of Druids from reaching the king's ears."

Waleran groaned. "You fully expected Katherine and Thomas to be thrown into the Tower."

Sir William nodded.

Katherine smiled a tight smile of relief. There had been little joy and much fear in her heart as they waited for a royal audience, knowing that execution might be the result, instead of a mere prison sentence. But they also gambled on more, something else that Katherine now could have related just as easily as did the knight.

"Waleran," Sir William said, "not once, but twice did you rely on knowledge gained from conversations overheard in prison. In Magnus while you yourself sat with Thomas and me, and in York, next to the earl himself. Once too, you used the trick of letting a foe escape, simply to follow. We thought it likely the same ploy would be used again."

"You knew I was the king's chamberlain?"

Sir William shook his head. "Thomas' father suspected. He had been traveling England for years as an old man."

"No!" Again a flash of fear. "I tell you, he is dead."

A tall man walked into the cave from where he had been waiting in the shadows of the entrance.

"If I am dead," he replied to Waleran, "then let me be your most persistent nightmare."

Waleran moaned. "I thought you dead when we conquered Magnus. Later, I knew you traveled in disguise, but I thought I'd finally beaten you outside York, when Thomas led my soldiers to your campsite."

"I am most definitely alive." Hawkwood bowed to Queen Isabella. "Your majesty . . ."

She smiled in return.

And how can she help but smile, Katherine thought. *For this man is as handsome as his son, Thomas, with the same hint of mystery and confidence, the same air of gentleness and compassion.*

"Lord Hawkwood," the queen said, "I am pleased to discover my trust in you was not misplaced."

"It was a near thing, was it not? For a moment, you nearly impaled me."

Waleran now had his arms huddled around his knees. "Im . . . impaled?" he managed to stutter.

The baby was quiet now, and Queen Isabella turned her attention again to Waleran. Katherine caught the instant transition from the warmth directed to Lord Hawkwood to the hatred and cold reserved for Waleran.

"Lord Hawkwood offered to place his life in my hands. In my royal chambers that dawn, he opened my palm, set the handle of a short dagger upon my skin, closed my fingers over the dagger, and brought my hand up so that the dagger touched his throat. He told me if I chose to disbelieve him, I could end his life right there. But if I believed, I was to arrange for a trip into the countryside, as if distraught over the kidnapping, and, unknown to King Edward, attend my own son here, while we waited."

"For me," Waleran blurted. "You expected me to arrive."

Katherine cleared her throat. "Yes. Thomas shouted at the entrance to this valley. We feared you might not have managed to follow. Then we waited at the river by the abbey, once again giving you time. Finally, we talked loudly in front of the entrance to this very cave. All to lure you inside."

Waleran lifted his head. An animal-like gleam, almost insanity, suddenly filled his eyes.

"My army outside! I may die here, but you cannot escape."

"You no longer have an army outside." By the softness of Thomas' words, Katherine knew he felt pity for the completeness of the destruction of their enemy.

"We expected you, did we not?" Thomas asked. "Many more than twenty of the finest men of Magnus were hidden in these woods. Your army has long since fallen to ambush."

They gathered—the five of them and baby Edward—in the abbey hall that evening.

Queen Isabella was given the chair closest to the fire. She and the baby were wrapped in blankets; for although it was

July, the evening chill in this northern valley had a bite, especially in an abbey hall with a cold stone floor and no heavy tapestries to slow any drafts.

Sir William was pacing the room slowly, a man of coiled energy still restless after the day's events, even with Waleran and his army safely captured.

Lord Hawkwood crouched on his knees, poking an iron into the fire to rearrange the burning wood.

Katherine and Thomas sat next to each other, opposite Queen Isabella.

They had all gathered here at the request of Queen Isabella, who had spent the bulk of the afternoon chatting with the men of Magnus, much to their delight.

Now, however, Queen Isabella wasted little time in idle conversation.

"What will draw the remaining Druid leaders to this valley?" The question was asked softly, yet Katherine sensed the steel behind it.

"Your majesty?" Lord Hawkwood expressed puzzlement, without shifting from his position near the fire.

"I have agreed to give as many men as you deem necessary to capture all the Druids who arrive in the next weeks, but I wish to know what they seek."

Sir William stopped his pacing and stood behind Thomas.

"It *is* the book, in that cave, I believe," Queen Isabella continued. "And you all seek to avoid the subject. I find it both amusing and strange that so much has been revealed about the Druids and so little about yourselves, the Merlins."

She smiled, but it did not rob the strength of her implied command to tell her all.

Lord Hawkwood prodded the fire again and did not flinch as sparks shot from a falling log. He took his time to add several more logs, then rose and faced Queen Isabella.

"You see the last of the Merlins here in this room," he said without self-pity, "so there is little to say about us."

Katherine held her breath. *Will Queen Isabella press the issue?*

Lord Hawkwood continued smoothly. "However, as you have guessed, it is the book which is of utmost importance."

"You have a habit of intriguing me," Queen Isabella said. "Please, go on."

Sir William stood. "I have brought the book from the trunk in the cave. Perhaps now is the time to deliver it to her majesty."

When Lord Hawkwood nodded, Sir William left the room, and Lord Hawkwood closed his eyes to think as he spoke. "It begins with an explorer named Marco Polo. . . ."

"Yes." Queen Isabella nodded. "The name is familiar. He dictated a book—*Description of the World*, I believe—while in prison."

"It is remarkable that you know that," Lord Hawkwood said, eyes now open. "His book is gaining popularity only now."

"Not remarkable at all. Coincidence. The man who transcribed the dictation, a romance writer named Rusticello of Pisa, spent time under the patronage of King Edward, my father-in-law. Royal courts all over Europe have copies of this book."

Lord Hawkwood grinned. "Then, milady, you shall readily understand what follows. As you know, Marco Polo explored Cathay, the unknown lands of the Far East. His patron was the great Kublai Khan, ruler of the Mongols. Polo received a golden passport from Khan, and for twenty years traveled safely through that land, recording everything he saw."

Queen Isabella nodded impatiently. "He beheld wonders, to be sure. I am told the people there have yellow skin and slanted eyes, and are extremely intelligent."

She waited while Sir William rejoined them, a large, leather-bound sheaf of parchments in his hand.

"But what," she asked, "has Marco Polo to do with *your* book here, a book to draw Druids like flies to honey."

"Consider this, your majesty. What if Polo recorded other books, not merely fanciful tales of the exotic, but books with the most advanced science of this world, books with secrets so powerful that kingdoms might rise and fall upon them?"

"I find that difficult to believe."

Lord Hawkwood turned to Thomas. "Please bring some of the exploding powder."

Thomas left silently and returned several minutes later with a small leather bag. Lord Hawkwood reached in and removed a pinched portion of dark powder.

"Potassium, your majesty," he explained. "Sulfur and charcoal. Ingredients easily obtained."

Lord Hawkwood poured a tiny trail of the powder onto the floor, near the fireplace. He twisted a twig loose from a nearby log, held the twig in the fire until it was lit, then touched that small flame to the line of powder.

Even though Katherine knew what to expect, she still marveled at the small, flaring explosion of light and sound.

Lord Hawkwood turned back to Queen Isabella. His face was blackened with smudge.

Queen Isabella did not laugh. Her eyes were still wide with wonder.

"Yes," Lord Hawkwood said, "exploding powder. The people of Cathay invented it centuries ago, yet we in Europe have no knowledge of it. Marco Polo deliberately omitted it from his descriptions of that land, and for good reason. Imagine the possibilities. If such power would be harnessed by men of evil . . ."

"It saved our lives," Thomas said.

Queen Isabella shifted her eyes to him.

"In the Holy Land," Thomas said, "Father had lined a pit with it. When it flared in the darkness, all the bandits panicked. We succeeded in our attack."

Queen Isabella nodded. "I think I understand. This book of yours, if it contains many more such secrets, would be as valuable as a kingdom."

Then she asked sharply. "How is it that you have it?"

"The Roman church confiscated it for fear of what it might accomplish and destroy," Lord Hawkwood answered. "In my own travels after the fall of Magnus, I heard rumors of it, and . . ."

Lord Hawkwood appealed to the Queen. "I would prefer not to say how it was obtained, only that I had it sent here, to this abbey, where Thomas was to be raised, away from the eyes of Druids. He would need what he learned from the book to regain Magnus."

"I will not press you for that secret," Queen Isabella said. "There is enough pain in your eyes, and you are a man of honor."

Lord Hawkwood nodded thanks.

"And the book is now mine?" Queen Isabella asked.

"If you wish," Lord Hawkwood replied.

"Why would I not wish?"

"If it falls into the wrong hands . . ." Lord Hawkwood struggled for words. "Knowledge of such a book will drive many men to desperate measures to obtain it. As it did the Druids. And in the wrong hands, a civilization may be shattered."

Lord Hawkwood began to pace, much as Sir William had done earlier. "Examine the politics of our day. The balances of power from country to country are so delicately held. Your husband may choose to take the secrets of this book and fight more than just the Scots. Other kings may begin wars to obtain the knowledge. After all, men have fought before for much less reason . . . even this exploding powder can kill men by the dozens, while ordinary warfare is much more humane."

He pointed at the baby sleeping in Queen Isabella's arms. "Too many die to leave the fatherless behind. Perhaps we can delay the advance of knowledge which might be used by evil men."

Queen Isabella stared at Lord Hawkwood and said nothing. The fire crackled and popped several times in the silence.

"You have done so much for us," she said. "King Edward, of course, will end the Druid uprising. In secrecy, of course. It would do little good for the people to be stirred by these matters."

She hugged her baby. "You have ensured that my son will inherit a kingdom, that revolt will not tear this land apart. And now, you offer this book—not copied, I presume, by any hands."

"You presume correctly," Lord Hawkwood said.

Queen Isabella looked from one to the other, gazing first

at Katherine, then Thomas, then Sir William and, finally, Lord Hawkwood.

"Because of this secrecy, history will not record what you have accomplished, and that fills me with sadness. You are worthy of much more."

She nodded at the book. "And we will engage in this final act of secrecy."

Several more heartbeats.

"Thomas," Queen Isabella then said softly, "cast the book into the fire."

Chapter Sixty-Three

"Contrary to what you might think," Lord Hawkwood smiled at Thomas, "we are not ready to depart this abbey for Magnus."

Thomas innocently raised an eyebrow. "Oh? Queen Isabella was satisfied that no more Druid leaders would arrive. Surely there remains nothing for us here."

Father gazed at son.

They stood along the river in front of the abbey hall. Midmorning sun warmed their backs. They shared the feeling of peace in a valley quiet of wind, quiet except for the distance lowing of cattle and occasional bleat of sheep.

Much had been accomplished. Day after day in the last two weeks, solitary travelers had arrived in the valley. Without fail, when captured, each had pleaded innocent to the charges of Druid conspiracy; but Waleran, as part of a desperate bargain to save his own life, had identified each as a Druid.

The full horror of the Druid secret circle had been exposed in those two weeks. Again and again, Queen Isabella had murmured shock and surprise to face each new arriving Druid. Many she knew from their positions of power—magistrates, sheriffs, priests, knights, and even earls and dukes.

Now, all were stripped of their wealth and imprisoned. In one swoop, most of the Druids across the land had been taken.

Beyond that, Queen Isabella pledged to begin action against remaining Druids who falsely posed as priests in the northern towns. Not only would the spread of their power be contained, but the base they had established in the last few years would be eliminated.

"Thomas," Lord Hawkwood said in a mock stern voice, "were you raised a Merlin?"

Thomas grinned and nodded. He enjoyed knowing he could not, even in jest, fool the man in front of him.

Strange, he thought, *to one day suddenly be forced to consider a stranger as flesh-and-blood father. Especially a man accustomed to shrouding himself in mystery.*

Yet the bond had formed. And Thomas felt himself flushing at the implied compliment.

"Yes, I was raised a Merlin," Thomas replied.

"Tell me then, instead of pretending ignorance in hopes of hearing me prattle, why is it that we are not ready to depart."

Thomas looked beyond his father's shoulder at the high walls of the abbey and at the tiny window that he had so often used for escape in the days he believed he was an orphan.

"We are not yet ready to depart, because there remains something for us here. Something we could not seek until Queen Isabella departed, for she should not know of it."

"Umm." Lord Hawkwood was noncommittal.

Thomas grinned again in pleasure. Like before, in his childhood. Exercises of the mind. Tests of logic.

"Sarah would have enjoyed this." The words came from his mouth even as they reached his thoughts. He stopped, suddenly awkward. Always, deep inside, there was the ache that she was gone.

"I grieve too," Lord Hawkwood said in the lengthening silence. "Perhaps that is the highest tribute . . . to never be forgotten."

For several minutes, they stood without speaking, in the companionable comfort of friends.

A tiny roe deer moved from the nearby trees, hesitant at first, then confident that it was alone. Thomas clapped, and the deer scrambled sideways and almost fell. The effect was so comical that each snorted with laughter.

"Life," Lord Hawkwood said. "The past should not prevent us from looking ahead and drinking fully from life, from enjoying each moment as it arrives."

Thomas let out a deep breath. "Yes."

"And one looks forward to drinking deeply this cup with Katherine?"

Thomas coughed. "Our reason for delaying departure?" he said quickly. "You were testing my observations."

Lord Hawkwood did not pursue the subject of Katherine, and instead nodded.

"There had to be more reason for the Druids to arrive here than a single book," Thomas said. "For many of these men, it involved the risk of travel and the need to explain a lengthy absence. No, there must be more."

"An interesting theory," Lord Hawkwood said. "What might you guess?"

"Before I answer," Thomas challenged, "I have my own question for you."

Lord Hawkwood waited.

"What," Thomas began, "is the single most powerful weapon available to men?"

"Not swords."

Thomas nodded.

"Not arrows. Not catapults."

Thomas nodded again.

"Not any physical means of destruction. For with the invention of each new weapon, there will be a countering defense."

"So . . ." Thomas bantered.

"So, as you full well know, my son, our greatest power is knowledge. In warfare. In business. In the affairs of our own lives. In the defense of our faith. Without knowledge, we are nothing."

Thomas pointed at the tiny window high on the abbey wall. "Were we to wager today my odds of answering your question, I would have an unfair advantage. For last night, as I puzzled yet again what might draw so many Druids to this valley, I returned to the bedchamber of my childhood."

Lord Hawkwood straightened with sudden interest. "You have not discovered—"

Thomas grinned mischief. "Ho, ho! The student knows something the teacher does not. Surely you speak the truth that knowledge is power!"

"Thomas, tell me!"

Thomas bent to scoop pebbles into his hand. One by one, he began to toss them into the river.

"Thomas . . ." Lord Hawkwood warned.

"In the Holy Land," Thomas said, "Sir William informed me that I held the final secret to the battle. Yet," Thomas pointed his forefinger skyward for emphasis, "I had no inkling of what he might mean."

Thomas tossed two more pebbles into the water before continuing. "Sir William had returned from exile in the Holy Land to spend time in Magnus with me," he said. "Had the final secret been there, he would have claimed it then. Moreover, had this mysterious object of great value been there, the Druids, who held Magnus for a generation, would have claimed it. Instead, since my departure from this abbey, both sides—Druid and Merlin—have been intent on learning the secret from me, a secret I did not know I possessed. I can only conclude that whatever it is has lain here at the abbey."

Lord Hawkwood nodded.

"Indeed," Thomas continued, "if you yourself do not know where it is located, I must conclude that it had been sent to Sarah, along with the book she chose to hide in the cave."

Again, Lord Hawkwood nodded.

"Whatever this secret is," Thomas concluded, "Sarah hid it before her death. Whatever this secret is, the Druids were willing—no, desperate—to each undertake a journey from their separate parts of England."

Thomas smiled. "Returning here to the abbey brought back to me some of my first memories of Sarah. I remember that she would sit beside my bed and help me with my prayers, or sing quiet songs of knights performing valiant deeds. And every night, her final words as I fell to sleep never differed."

His focus shifted from the edge of the valley hills to his father's face.

"Sarah would say, 'Thomas, my love, sleep upon the winds of light.' Each night she would simply smile when I asked what that meant."

Lord Hawkwood began to smile too.

"Yes," Thomas said. "Your words to me at the gallows, as a mysterious man hidden beneath cloak and hood, were almost the same."

"Bring the winds of light," Lord Hawkwood's voice was almost a whisper, "into this age of darkness."

"Knowledge," Thomas said. "The knowledge accumulated by generations of Merlins."

"Yes, Thomas," Lord Hawkwood said. "Merlin himself founded Magnus as a place to conduct our hidden warfare against the Druids. Yet he destined us for more. To search the world for what men knew. And to save that knowledge from the darkness of the destruction of barbarians."

Lord Hawkwood's voice became sad. "Time and again throughout history, gentle scholars have suffered loss to men of swords. Great libraries have been burned and looted, the records of civilizations and their accomplishments and advances wiped from the face of the earth. Few today know of the wondrous pyramids of the ancient Egyptians, of the mathematics and astronomy of the ancient Greeks, of the healing medicines of, yes, the Druids, and of the aqueducts and roads of the Romans."

In a flash, Thomas understood. "Merlins of each generation traveled the world and returned with written record of what they had discovered."

"When Magnus fell," Lord Hawkwood said, "it was more important than our lives to save the books which contained this knowledge. That is why so many of us died. Your mother and I, Sir William, and a few others escaped with the books of these centuries of knowledge, while the rest gave their lives. Why did each Druid willingly undertake a journey here when given the message by Waleran? Each assumed, rightly, there would be spoils easily divided. Books beyond value. One, two, perhaps more books for each. Books which can be duplicated only through years of transcribing. "

"Father," Thomas said quickly, because now, seeing the worry on his father's face, he found no joy in prolonging his news, "the books you sent to this abbey are safe."

"Yes?"

"Sleep upon the winds of light," Thomas said. "What better place to hide something than in the open? My mattress was placed upon a great trunk, placed so that its edges hid the lid of the trunk. A passerby, or even a searcher, of course, would think it only a convenient pedestal to keep a sleeping child away from nighttime rats. But on that trunk, I truly did sleep upon the winds of light."

Epilogue

As Thomas knelt, he thrilled to the touch of the sword atop his shoulder.

It was a private and quiet ceremony in the uppermost chambers of the castle of Magnus, with Sir William, Lord Hawkwood and, of course, Katherine, who held the sword.

"This is our own form of knighthood," she said softly. "An unseen badge of honor."

"It is enough," Thomas replied, as he rose. "Worth more than the knighthood granted by Queen Isabella, more than this kingdom officially given us by her royal charter."

Thomas felt a sorrow, however, for just as the continued existence of the Merlins had been kept from Queen Isabella, so too must he keep this part of his life hidden from those who waited below in the great hall to begin a feast of homecoming for him.

Tiny John, now bigger than the rascal sprout Thomas remembered from before his exile. Robert of Uleran, the valiant sheriff of Magnus who had survived his imprisonment and resisted all promises of the Druid priests. The earl of York, joyful to have his earldom returned. Gervaise, a man of simple faith who had often comforted Thomas and provided him escape from Magnus at the price of a terrible beating by the Druid high priests. And, a magnificent dog, the puppy Thomas had taken across half a world, then brought back again from St. Jean d'Acre.

"Our task is not complete," Lord Hawkwood interrupted Thomas' thoughts. "For I cannot believe that the Druid circle will not somehow, sometime, begin to rebuild."

He smiled. "But I believe that we as Merlins will now be

able to continue our task, searching and keeping the treasures of knowledge, and passing that task to future generations."

His voice grew fuller as he spoke with passion. "There will be a day," he said, "when a renaissance, a rebirth of the sharing of ideas, will take all of us forward into the dawning of a better age. Until then, let us ensure that Magnus stands quiet, unknown, and on guard against the age of darkness."

Sir William began to laugh.

"Well spoken, Lord Hawkwood," Sir William finally said, through a broad smile. "But first we need future generations. And *I* will not see our task complete until you and I become grandfathers."

Katherine giggled.

Thomas felt his jaw gape open. *To be sure,* he thought in confusion, *Katherine and I have pledged marriage, but we have not yet spoken of children.*

Then another thought struck him.

"What is this of which you speak?" he blurted out to Sir William. "If—"

"When," Katherine corrected.

"When," Thomas said, "our marriage results in . . . in . . . little ones, it strikes me that Lord Hawkwood alone will become a grandfather. Who is it that *you,* Sir William, expect to arrive with a babe in swaddling clothes to provide you a grandchild?"

Lord Hawkwood began to laugh in great gales. Sir William joined him, then Katherine.

Thomas fought bewilderment.

Finally, he roared to be heard above the laughter.

"What is it?"

Sir William found his voice.

"Thomas," he said, "you showed such insight into untangling the past, we all assumed you already knew."

"Knew what?" Thomas snapped. Mirth had reddened all their faces, and he did not enjoy being the source of their amusement.

Sir William moved closer and embraced him, then stood back.

"Thomas," he said, "Katherine is my daughter. Born, as you were, during exile in the Holy Land."

"But . . . but . . ." Thomas sputtered.

"Yes," Sir William said. "It will be I who gives her hand away in marriage, as you two begin to reign over Magnus. And, Thomas?"

"Yes?"

"I could not think of another man I would welcome more as my son than Thomas, lord and earl of Magnus."

Historical Notes

For 2,000 years, far north and east of London, the ancient English towns of Pickering, Thirsk, and Helmsley, and their castles have guarded a line on the lowland plains between the larger centers of Scarborough and York.

In the beginning, Scarborough, with its high, North Sea cliffs, was a Roman signal post. From there, sentries could easily see approaching barbarian ships, and were able to relay messages from Pickering to Helmsley to Thirsk, the entire fifty miles inland to the boundary outpost of York, where other troops waited, always ready, for any inland invasions.

When their empire fell, the Romans in England succumbed to the Anglo-Saxons, great, savage brutes in tribal units who conquered as warriors and over the generations became farmers. The Anglo-Saxons in turn suffered defeat by raiding Vikings, who in turn lost to the Norman knights with their thundering war-horses.

Through those hundreds and hundreds of years, that line from Scarborough to York never diminished in importance.

Some of England's greatest and richest abbeys accumulated their wealth on the lowland plains along that line. Rievaulx Abbey, just outside Helmsley, housed 250 monks and owned vast estates of land which held over 13,000 sheep.

But directly north lay the moors. No towns or abbeys tamed the moors, which reached east to the craggy cliffs of the cold, gray North Sea.

Each treeless and windswept moor plunged into deep, dividing valleys of lush greenness that only made the heather-covered heights appear more harsh. The ancients called these North York moors "Blackamoor."

Thus, in the medieval age of chivalry, 250 years after the Norman knights had toppled the English throne, this remoteness and isolation protected Blackamoor's earldom of Magnus from the prying eyes of King Edward II and the rest of his royal court in London.

As a kingdom within a kingdom, Magnus was small in comparison to the holdings of England's greater earls. This smallness was its protection. Hard to reach and easy to defend, British and Scottish kings chose to overlook it; in practical terms, it had as much independence as a separate country.

Magnus still had size, however. Its castle commanded and protected a large village and many vast moors. Each valley between the moors averaged a full day's travel by foot. Atop the moors, great flocks of sheep grazed on the the tender, green shoots of heather. The valley interiors supported cattle and cultivated plots of land farmed by peasants nearly made slaves by the yearly tribute exacted from their crops. In short, with sheep and wool and cattle and land, Magnus was an earldom well worth ruling.

In the period in which the this book is set, children were considered adults much earlier than now. By church law, for example, a bride had to be at least twelve, a bridegroom fourteen. It is not so unusual, then, to think of Thomas of Magnus becoming accepted as a leader at an early age. Moreover, other "men" also became leaders at remarkably young ages during those times. King Richard II, for example, was only fourteen years old when he rode out to face the leaders of the Peasant's Revolt in 1381.

Chapter One

Although there is no specific mention of an *eclipse* at this time in historical records, it does not necessarily mean that the eclipse did not occur. Scientific observations were almost nonexistent, and a partial eclipse could well have briefly darkened that part of England without an official recording.

Chapter Five

Gunpowder had been used by the Chinese since the tenth century A.D., but it was not until the year 1313 that any European "discovered" its explosive power; credit for its invention is commonly given to a German Friar named Berthold Schwarz. Is it possible, however, that knowledge of its ingredients may have been known to other Europeans shortly before that time?

Chapter Six

Wades Causeway is a preserved stretch of Roman road which may still be traveled today in the Wheeldale Moor of the Yorkshire area of England. It was built almost 2,000 years ago by the first Roman soldiers to reach Yorkshire in the year A.D. 70, and probably reached all the way to the coast. One of the reasons for the great success of the Roman soldiers as they conquered all of England was their roads, which let them move their armies with great efficiency.

The number of fighting *knights* in England by the year 1300 has been estimated to be only 500 to 1,000. Other landowners were called knights because they owed military service to the barons and kings above them; but they were country gentlemen, not members of a military elite.

A *barbican* was an outwork of stone built to protect the gatehouse or entrance into the castle grounds. Sometimes it was a wall of stone leading up to the gatehouse; later, as barbicans became more elaborate with their own turrets and drawbridges, they actually became outer gatehouses.

Although some scholars disagree, it is commonly held that Sun Tzu, a Chinese general and military genius who lived hundreds of years before Christ was born, compiled a book of his military theories and philosophies. This book has survived relatively unchanged for over 2,000 years. It is probable that he is the *"greatest general of a faraway land"* to which Thomas refers in his thoughts. Today, readers may find Sun Tzu's military advice in a book titled *The Art of War,* a book which General Norman Schwarzkopf made mandatory reading for troops during the Gulf War of 1991.

Chapter Eleven
Marco Polo is the Italian explorer who reached Cathay (now known as China) in the year 1275. He served the Mongolian ruler Kublai Khan for many years, and returned to Venice in the year 1295. During his travels, Marco Polo noted the Chinese custom of sending a huge man-carrying kite into the air before a ship set sail on a long voyage.

Chapter Fifteen
Even by the year 1312, *York* was already an ancient and major center in northwestern England. Located roughly eighteen miles south of Helmsley—the site of the gallows of chapter 1, York was an outpost for Roman soldiers 1,250 years before the times in which Thomas of Magnus lived. Any single man given jurisdiction over this city and surrounding area would have had considerable power.

The *Scots* posed a serious threat to the English King Edward II, who reigned from 1307 to 1327. Robert Bruce, crowned King of Scotland in 1306, nearly lost Scotland in his first battles against the English because of the leadership of Edward II's father, King Edward I. When Edward I died in July 1307, Robert Bruce was able to oppose the weaker Edward II, and began a series of successful battles. In the years 1312 to 1314, Bruce defeated a series of English strongholds, and the restoration of English power in Scotland became an impossibility. In 1318, the Scots finally captured the castle of Berwick on the English border and from there were easily able to raid as far south as the Yorkshire area.

Chapter Seventeen
It may be of interest to note that in 1297, Edward I's royal army in Flanders consisted of 7,810 foot soldiers and 895 cavalry, of which only 140 were knights.

At that time, the knight carried shield, lance, and sword into battle. His basic armor was a suit of chain mail, reinforced with steel plates at the knees and shoulders. During the 1300s, plating gradually began to replace chain mail as protection, until eventually, in the 1400s, knights were slow and heavy with complete body plating and shields were no longer needed.

While the concept of *reinforced bows* was definitely unusual to English archers during Thomas' time, other cultures, as far back as the ancient Egyptians, had experimented with bronze or bone plating to add strength to wood.

Chapter Nineteen
The isle of the *Celts* is known today as Ireland.

The earliest known records of *Druids* come from the third century B.C. According to the Roman general Julius Caesar (who is the principle source of today's information on Druids), this group of men studied ancient verse, natural philosophy, astronomy, and the lore of the gods. The principal doctrine of the Druids was that souls were immortal and passed at death from one person to another.

Druids offered human victims for those who were in danger of death in battle or who were gravely ill. They sacrificed these victims by burning them in huge wickerwork images.

The Druids were suppressed in ancient Britain by the Roman conquerers in the first century A.D. If, indeed, the cult survived, it must have had to remain as secret as it was during Thomas' time.

Today, followers of the Druid cult may still be found in England worshiping the ancient ruins of Stonehenge at certain times of the year.

Chapter Twenty
The battle tactic which Thomas used to conquer a larger force was not new. Readers today may find in *The Art of War* the same tactic used more than 2,000 years ago by the Chinese military genius Sun Tzu.

Chapter Twenty-Four
For hundreds of years before Thomas' time, it had been commonly accepted that God would judge the criminally accused through *trial by ordeal* or *trial by battle*. In trial by ordeal, the defendant was made to undergo a severe

physical test, such as burning or drowning. In trial by battle, the defendant faced his accuser in combat, usually with blunt weapons; the loser would be judged guilty and would often be hanged as a result.

In the year 1215, trial by ordeal was officially banished by the church. It would not be strange, however, for the people of Magnus to accept a self-imposed trial by ordeal or its deemed judgment, especially the one dramatically proposed by Thomas. Superstition was never very far from the people, and trial by ordeals always promised great entertainment.

Chapter Twenty-Five

Caltrops were four-pronged spikes, much like the modern-day "jacks" (except much sharper) of a game sometimes played by children with a ball.

The British Museum in London does have caltrops on exhibit, remnants of the ones used by Roman soldiers to break up cavalry charges.

Yew trees are found throughout the Northern Hemisphere. All but the red fruit of the plant is poisonous to humans. The poison contained is *taxine.* Symptoms of poisoning include nausea, giddiness, and weakness, followed by convulsions, shock, coma, and death.

Poison ingested in smoke from the yew tree, especially concentrated in the narrow upward tunnel leading into the belfry, may well have caused the "supernatural" daytime appearance and death of the bats, especially since low concentrations could harm the smaller mammals.

There is, however, another possibility, one which has interesting implications perhaps unknown to Thomas. The *oleander,* or *Jericho Rose,* a shrub which normally favors hot, southern climates, also releases a poisonous smoke when burned.

Chapter Twenty-Six

During medieval times, two main meals were served in the castle keep. Dinner was at 10 or 11 A.M., and supper was at

5 P.M. Forks had not been invented yet. Plates were not common; instead, thick slabs of bread called "trenchers" generally held the day's food.

Chapter Twenty-Eight

In the early part of King Henry II's reign, a certain clergyman in Bedford slew a knight. Despite overwhelming evidence, he was found innocent in the bishop's court, and had the gall to then insult a royal judge sent to investigate the matter.

Chapter Twenty-Nine

It is difficult for historians to agree on the historical King Arthur. Most scholars now regard Arthur's reality as probable; it is commonly held that he was born around 480.

Some argue that the castle of Camelot existed at Cadbury in southern England, while others choose nearby Glastonbury. Historians do agree, however, that the legends about King Arthur (known as the Arthurian Romances) were finally put to paper by various poets in the twelfth and thirteenth centuries, some seven centuries after the Round Table.

Most of what the old woman relates about the *Holy Grail* is part of the legend which historians today know circulated from the twelfth century on, as part of the Arthurian Romances.

As the old woman tells Thomas, the Holy Grail is thought to be the cup used by Christ in The Last Supper. Yet it must be emphasized that the Holy Grail is legend, not biblical truth. There is no single, clearly defined image of the Grail, or evidence it ever existed. In fact, even its outward shape is debated. Is it a cup? A shallow dish? A stone? A jewel? Despite, or because of, the lack of historical truth surrounding the Holy Grail, its legend held much sway over the ignorant peasants of Thomas' time, much to the dissatisfaction of the church.

A discerning reader might express amazement that in an age of wide illiteracy, an old beggar woman might know so much about the Holy Grail.

This is not surprising, however. The legend of the Holy

Grail was a well-established oral myth, and stories were commonly passed from generation to generation.

Indeed, the woman's surprise at Thomas' pretended lack of knowledge is more appropriate; but Thomas, of course, wanted to discover how much influence the false priests might have among his people.

In other versions of the legend, Joseph of Arimathaea does not go any farther than Europe, and the cup instead is passed on to a man named Bron, who becomes known as the Rich Fisher. It was told that he received this name because he had fed many from the Grail with a single fish. Bron and his company then settled at Avaron, whom many identify with Avalon/Glastonbury.

Chapter Thirty

Constructed of stone, Norman churches were often built upon the ruins of the earlier and wooden Anglo-Saxon churches. Early churches generally consisted of the *nave* where people stood for the services, and a small *chancel* at the east end of the church for the altar and priest. As time passed, towers, aisles, priests' rooms, and chapels were often added. Thus, the quieter eastern end of the church building of Magnus held the original altar.

Chapter Thirty-Three

Katherine was correct to express surprise at the existence of books so far from the libraries of kings or of rich monasteries. Books could only be duplicated through laborious hand-copying. They were so rare and valuable that some historians estimated that before Gutenberg invented the press in the early 1400s, the number of books in all of Europe only numbered in the thousands—fewer than the number found today in a single standard elementary school!

Chapter Thirty-Four

Even today, the religious miracle of unclotting blood is hailed each year in Naples, Italy, as it has been for more than 600 years. Believers there say a sealed sample of the clotted blood of Saint Januarius (martyred in the year 305) has turned into liquid each year since 1389, and the event now draws thousands, as well as a television audience numbering in the millions.

Scientists, however, claim this jamlike gel may simply consist of a mixture of chalk and hydrated iron choride lightly sprinkled with salt, a substance they say could have easily been produced by medieval alchemists.

As for the weeping statue, it is probable that the effects of condensation brought on by quick changes from heat to cold were little understood by the illiterate masses of peasants.

Chapter Thirty-Five

Modern day *York* in the the North York moors is a substantial city; but its inner core is still marked by the thick walls of ancient York, walls which still bear some of the chambers mentioned in this chapter.

Beheading traitors and leaving their heads for all to see was common and, unfortunately, one of the more merciful ways of dealing with rebels.

Chapter Thirty-Nine

Because of widespread poverty and because of the severity of prescribed punishments for theft, outlaws were common during these times. Many faced death for crimes no more terrible than poaching the king's deer. As a result, those who escaped often banded together and lived on the edge of desperation.

While historians cannot establish whether an actual historical character forms a basis for the many tales collected about him, it is not unbelievable that the outlaw Robert who rescued Katherine was indeed the legendary *Robin Hood.*

Several possible facts point to this. By the nineteenth century, some historians fixed Robin as one Robert Hood who joined Thomas, earl of Lancaster, in his 1322 uprising against Edward II. This fits with the first datable reference to Robin/Robert Hood, a *Yorkshire* place name. The Stone of Robin Hood is cited in a document of 1322.

The thirty-eight ballads about Robin Hood place him either in the forests of Sherwood, in Nottinghamshire, or in the Yorkshire forests of Barndale.

As with many heroes of legend, Robin Hood has been placed in various time periods in different ballads; some historians identify Robin Hood with the twelfth century King Richard I.

However, if the outlaw Robert Hood, so gallant to Katherine, is indeed the Robin Hood of legend, it is not improbable that in the late spring of 1313 he would reign over his band of men in the Yorkshire forests near York, some nine years before some historians place him farther away in Yorkshire's Barndale forests.

Chapter Forty

As the Vikings lost control of the North Seas late in the eleventh century, sea trade grew safer, and merchants began to need roomier vessels to carry larger shipments. By the year 1200, northern shipbuilders had developed the *cog,* which was the standard merchant and war vessel for the next 200 years. One of the most dramatic improvements of the cog was the *rudder,* a new kind of steering apparatus attached to the rear of the boat, and much stronger and more efficient for directing the boat than oars.

As Thomas notes, it was common for the merchant ships to belong to foreign exporters of wool, such as the French, Belgians, or Italians.

Chapter Forty-four

Merlin, legend tells us, was first an adviser to the King Uther Pendragon, King Arthur's father, and then an adviser to King Arthur himself. Merlin was known as the prophet of the Holy Grail—perhaps not a coincidence in light of the Druid attempts to use the Holy Grail to gain power. Finally, Merlin was legendary as a court magician or enchanter, something not unlikely for a man with the knowledge of science available to the Druids. Through his advice to King Uther Pendragon, Merlin was responsible for the formation of the Knights of the Round Table.

Is it a remarkable coincidence that Alcuin from York is found in the history books as the educated adviser summoned by Charles the Great, or Charlemagne, the famous ruler of the Franks (Germany) in the late 700s? Alcuin helped teach all the monks and priests in Charles the Great's empire learn to read and write. He also introduced a new style of handwriting known as *Carolingian Minuscule,* which used small letters and was quicker and easier than writing in capitals.

Chapter Forty-Six
The Crusades were a series of religious wars from the First Crusade in 1095 to the Eighth Crusade in 1270. These wars were organized by European powers to recover from the Muslim infidels the Christian holy places in Palestine, especially the holy city, Jerusalem. Many of the crusaders believed that if they died in battle, their souls would be taken straight to heaven.

Gradually, towards the end of the 1200s, the Muslims reconquered all the cities which had been taken from them. St. Jean d'Acre, the common destination for all ships bearing Crusaders, was the last to fall to the Muslims and remained in Christian hands until the year 1291.

Chapter Forty-Eight
A warrior race of Muslim Egypt, the *Mamelukes,* were originally non-Arab slaves to Egyptian rulers. They overthrew their rulers in the middle of the 1200s. Not only did they prove to be too powerful for the crusaders, but they were the only people to ever defeat a Mongol invasion—in the year 1260.

Chapter Fifty-One
Sir William's fear of a small group of men taking control to bring evil upon an entire country is not unfounded, especially in light of the horrible events of recent history. Adolf Hitler, for example, as a single leader atop a pyramid of power, delivered and preached a message of racial hatred that managed to manipulate thousands of ordinary people

into assisting in the murder of millions of innocent Jews.

Probably because of his excellent Merlin education, Sir William is acutely accurate in his observation of the *Dark Ages,* the term commonly given to the years 500–1000 A.D. These were centuries of decline across Europe, mostly attributed to the fall of the Roman Empire, which left a vacuum of power that encouraged civil wars and stifled classical culture. This lack of education among the common people and the suspicion between countries prevented the sharing of ideas, especially in the arts, science, navigation, and medicine. Interestingly enough, what culture there was remained preserved in remnants by monks of Ireland, Italy, France, and Britain. Not until the *Renaissance* (1350–1650) did modern civilization begin to flourish, as men across Europe began again to strive to learn and share ideas.

Chapter Fifty-Two
Papermaking was invented in China in 100 B.C., another Chinese invention that remained unknown to the Europeans for hundreds of years. The Arabs learned how to make paper by questioning Chinese prisoners of war in 768. From there, it spread throughout the Arab Empire, which at that time included Spain. From Spain, papermaking finally spread to the rest of Europe.

Historical record confirms Hawkwood's research and shows that the *Second Jewish Revolt* took place in 132 A.D. and lasted for three and one-half years. *Cassius Dio,* a Roman historian as noted in the letter, wrote a brief notice of the war which has survived to this day. In this notice, Dio relates that toward the end of the rebellion, Roman legionnaires were unable to engage the Jews in open battle because of the rough terrain, and instead were forced to hunt them down in small groups in the caves where they hid, and starve them out. Cassius Dio describes the final results this way: "Fifty of their [the Jews'] most important outposts and 985 of their most famous villages were razed to the ground; 580,000 men were slain in the various raids and battles, and the number of those who perished by famine, disease, and fire was past finding out. Thus nearly the whole of Judea was made desolate." In the nearby slave markets, there was such a surplus of Jews to be sold as slaves that the price of Jews dropped lower than that of horses.

As also noted in the letter, the Roman general *Julius Severus* was summoned from Britain to end the rebellion. Despite the fact that the timing of Druid disappearance and the stolen treasure is so close as to be possibly regarded as more than coincidental, no historical notes regarding a Druid treasure have been found. A number of the mentioned Dead Sea caves, however, were discovered in 1951–52 and 1960–61.

Chapter Fifty-Four

Insane root was widely known from Egypt to India. It is also know as "fetid nightshade," "poison tobacco," "stinking nightshade," or "black henbane." This plant contains the poisons hyoscyamine and atropine. Its seed and juice are deadly poison; even in small portions, it can cause death in fifteen minutes. Among the many symptoms are uncontrollable convulsions. It is probable that Thomas used extremely small doses of the poison to produce the results immediately after meals. It would have given two advantages: it was difficult to taste, and the slight tremor of convulsions needed no countering potion to end naturally minutes later.

Chapter Fifty-Five

Thomas feared *crucifixion* with good reason. His thoughts on the method of this horrible death are historically accurate. Readers of the Gospels will also know that there was a custom of breaking of the legs of the victims to hasten death of anyone who survived a day on the cross.

Jerusalem's history stretches back for more than 3,500 years. Its fortified walls were destroyed by invaders more than once; the last occasion by order of the Roman emperor Titus in A.D. 70, because of the first Jewish rebellion against the Roman Empire. After the fall of the Roman Empire, Jerusalem passed into the rule of the religiously tolerant

Muslims, fell again to the knights of the First Crusade in 1099, and was then taken back by the Mamelukes who rebuilt the walls and restored much of the city.

Readers of the Old Testament often forget how historically accurate is its accounting of Jewish history, as proven where modern-day archeology has succeeded in discovering the sites of such events. King David's assault via *Gihon Spring* is reported in the Old Testament (2 Samuel 5:6-10). While it is reasonable to assume that any occupants of Jerusalem since then would guard against another such assault, it should not be surprising that defenders might forget the spring could also serve as an exit.

Thomas shows an excellent sense of logic as he notes the well's walls become narrower at the top. As ancient cities aged throughout the centuries, garbage and rubble contributed to the slow building-up of the ground. Some excavations today reach thirty to forty feet deep, to reveal life of the past at certain layers of time.

Chapter Fifty-Eight
It is not unreasonable to assume that *The Cave of Letters* would lie undiscovered for the centuries from the time of the Roman general Julius Severus until it was rediscovered by Thomas and the bandits. No mention of the treasure is found in historical documents, but Mameluke soldiers would have had great incentive to keep the discovery of such great wealth to themselves. That the caves could be so well hidden and unknown is demonstrated by the fact that modern archeologists did not discover these sites until five more centuries had passed, in the years 1951–52 and 1960–61. Among the artifacts found in these caves were a basket of skulls, keys, metal vessels, parchment of palms, and fishnet. At least sixty skeletons were found.

Chapter Fifty-Nine
Readers may find it interesting that the courtier's promised "ten minutes of audience" was in those times a relatively new term. With the arrival of mechanical clocks at the end of the 1200s and the beginning of the 1300s, mankind, for

the first time had found a way to impose regularity upon time; until then, an "hour" could be measured only as a portion of daylight, which of course varied from season to season. By finally establishing an "equal hour," man gained control over the daily measure of time, and a "minute" first became a divided portion of that hour.

Chapter Sixty

England's battles against Scotland were begun by King Edward I in 1296. King Edward II did continue those battles, but to little avail. Shortly before Thomas and Katherine appeared in London for a royal audience, Edward II had lost a disastrous battle against the Scots at Bannockburn. The politics of that time would have put great pressure on Edward II for this loss; it is no wonder that he might have had little grasp on domestic affairs. Scotland, unlike Ireland or Wales, never did succumb to the English. A truce was declared in 1323.

The poison contained in all parts of the *rhododendron,* an evergreen shrub common in Britain, is carbohydrate andromedotoxin. While normally it takes over an hour for its poison to work, it is not unlikely that other herbs were added to compound its effect. Both Druids and the historical Merlin were famed for their knowledge of the poisons and medicines of plants and herbs; unfortunately, little of what they actually knew has survived.

Chapter Sixty-One

Queen Isabella, the daughter of France's Philip IV, married King Edward II in 1308 and gave birth to Edward III on November 13, 1312. Isabella later joined forces with Roger de Mortimer, the first earl of March, and they forced Edward II's abdication of the throne in 1327 to give power to Edward III. Ironically, Edward III later rebelled against Mortimer's power and had him executed.

There is no historical mention of Edward III's brief kidnapping. However, especially given the ultimatum by Edward II to put pressure on his political enemies, it might be possible that King Edward did not want to alarm the people of England during a time of instability made worse by his recent losses to Scotland. Supposing that such an event took place, Edward would have hoped to gain his son back without public knowledge of either the kidnapping or return.

Marco Polo, who left for Cathay (China) in the year 1271 with his father and uncle, was reputed to have a photographic memory. Because of that, the intensely curious and open-minded emperor Kublai Khan appointed Polo as an envoy, diplomat, and observer of an empire that covered half the known world.

For twenty years, protected by the Khan's "golden passport," Polo explored the culture, politics, and science of one of history's most dazzling yet secluded empires.

Long given up for dead, he was barely recognized when he returned to Venice with a fortune in jewels sewn into his clothing. Later, as a rich merchant, he was taken hostage in a sea war between Italian cities. From prison, he dictated a book of his recollections. This book inspired Columbus to sail for the new world nearly two centuries later.

To those who scoffed at his tall tales, Marco Polo insisted, even on his deathbed, that he ". . . never told the half of what he saw."

Yet what if he had told the other half? His first book led Columbus to discover a New World. Historians might find it curious that gunpowder—in use by the Chinese for four centuries before Polo's arrival there—is not mentioned in the published book. Yet, gunpowder was "invented" in Germany shortly after Polo returned from China. Does this suggest that some of Polo's knowledge was not made public, but rather was described in other books, missing or stolen, of his voyages?

Other Adult Fiction by Sigmund Brouwer

The Ghost Rider Series

Morning Star

Samuel Keaton wasn't looking for trouble when he rode into Laramie. Like so many other cowpunchers on payday, having a good time was uppermost in his trail-weary mind. But a few short hours later he was back in the saddle again—this time at a full gallop and trailing blood and a posse.

Moon Basket

The fall of 1874 was a bad time to start wearing a badge in Laramie. Try as he might, it seems to Samuel Keaton that, like his pay, too many things just don't add up. An unsolved bank robbery and a double murder only add to the frustration of knowing that many of the townspeople don't trust him.

Sun Dance

Coming in June '95.

Thunder Voice

Coming in October '95.